Hand-Rearing Birds

# Hand-Rearing Birds

Second Edition

*Edited by*

*Rebecca S. Duerr*
*International Bird Rescue*
*San Francisco and Los Angeles, CA, USA*

*Laurie J. Gage*
*Zoo and Wildlife Veterinary Consultant*
*Napa, CA, USA*

WILEY Blackwell

This edition first published 2020


*Edition History*
John Wiley & Sons (1e, 2007)



*Registered Office*
John Wiley & Sons, Inc., 111 River Street, Hoboken, NJ 07030, USA

*Editorial Office*
111 River Street, Hoboken, NJ 07030, USA

For details of our global editorial offices, customer services, and more information about Wiley products visit us at www.wiley.com.

Wiley also publishes its books in a variety of electronic formats and by print-on-demand. Some content that appears in standard print versions of this book may not be available in other formats.



*Library of Congress Cataloging-in-Publication Data*

Names: Duerr, Rebecca S., editor. | Gage, Laurie J., editor.
Title: Hand-rearing birds / edited by Rebecca S. Duerr, Laurie J. Gage.
Description: Second edition. | Hoboken : Wiley-Blackwell, 2020. | Includes bibliographical references and index.
Identifiers: LCCN 2019039396 (print) | LCCN 2019039397 (ebook) | ISBN 9781119167754 (hardback) |
ISBN 9781119167778 (adobe pdf) | ISBN 9781119167785 (epub)
Subjects: LCSH: Cage birds. | Captive wild birds.
Classification: LCC SF461 .G33 2020 (print) | LCC SF461 (ebook) | DDC 636.6/8–dc23
LC record available at https://lccn.loc.gov/2019039396
LC ebook record available at https://lccn.loc.gov/2019039397

Cover Design: Wiley
Cover Images: Bird's egg Dale A Smith, Four small birds Veronica Bowers, Native Songbird Care & Conservation, Different birds image Photo credit – International Bird Rescue, Sleeping birds Photo credit – Guthrum Purdin

Set in 9.5/12.5pt STIXTwoText by SPi Global, Pondicherry, India

MWEP454043140426

# Contents

## Notes on Contributors

**Yaritza Acosta** graduated from Lees-McRae College in 2012 with a Bachelor's Degree in Biology and a minor in wildlife rehabilitation. While studying there she was introduced to the Blue Ridge Wildlife Institute, where she learned most of her wildlife rehabilitation skills. After graduation, she relocated to Miami, FL and started volunteering at Pelican Harbor Seabird Station. She was brought on as staff four months later and has held a variety of positions since then. In April of 2013 she became a full-time staff member and is currently the Rehabilitation Manager for Pelican Harbor Seabird Station.

**Tracy Anderson** was the Program Coordinator for Save Our Shearwaters 2011–2019. She completed a BS in Biology and Geography at the University of Victoria and has worked in wildlife rehabilitation for over 20 years, in 3 countries: Canada, United States, and Belize. Previous positions included work at Mountainaire Avian Rescue in Courtenay, BC and British Columbia SPCA's WildARC in Victoria, BC. Tracy obtained seabird and waterbird-specific training at International Bird Rescue in California and then spent a year in Belize working with Central American species, such as parrots and toucans. She has also worked with endangered Eastern Loggerhead Shrikes. Tracy has been involved with banding passerines (songbirds) and owls and has served on the boards of several natural history and wildlife-related organizations.

**Nancy Barbachano** has been a wild bird rehabilitator for over 20 years. She volunteers with Gold Country Wildlife Rescue and Wildlife Care Association in California. She has served as Secretary for the Board of Directors of the California Council for Wildlife Rehabilitators. Nancy specializes in woodpeckers, hummingbirds, and songbirds. She has worked with the Cornell Lab of Ornithology since 2007 to determine whether or not Acorn Woodpecker babies can be released back into the wild into an existing colony. She also teaches various rehabilitation classes about bird rehabilitation locally, statewide, and nationwide.

**Michelle Bellizzi** has served in a variety of critical roles over the span of her 20-year career at International Bird Rescue. She served as the Manager of the San Francisco Bay-Delta Wildlife Center between 2003 and 2015 where she oversaw the care of approximately 3000 patients per year. While managing the rehabilitation program, she supervised the hand-rearing, re-nesting, and fostering of shorebirds, gulls, cormorants, alcids, ducklings, herons, and egrets. She has also responded to more than 30 oil spills around the globe, from Alaska to Argentina. Between her rehabilitation and response work, she has had the opportunity to work with a wide variety of species, ranging from pelagic seabirds, penguins, and terrestrial birds, as well as oiled beaver, muskrats, snakes, turtles, and a variety of amphibians.

**Veronica Bowers** has been working exclusively with passerines since 1999. She is director and founder of Native Songbird Care and Conservation (NSCC), located in Sebastopol, California. NSCC is a state and federally permitted wildlife rehabilitation facility and cares for approximately 1000 songbirds each year. Veronica teaches songbird rehabilitation workshops and species-specific classes to rehabilitators throughout North America. During the winter, she can be found in Central and South America birding and studying migratory songbirds in the field. Her favorite bird is the Cliff Swallow, but all other insectivorous and migratory passerines run a very close second.

**Andrew Bowkett** started his career studying enrichment and visitor effects in primates as a student at Paignton Zoo in Devon, England. He subsequently switched focus to field-based conservation and research projects overseas, including working hands-on with endangered birds in Mauritius and a PhD on Tanzanian duikers. He currently coordinates conservation projects in sub-Saharan Africa and southeast Asia, and supervises zoo-based research on birds, reptiles, and amphibians back at Paignton Zoo. Andrew holds honorary teaching and research positions at the Universities of Plymouth and Exeter, is a member of the IUCN SSC Antelope Specialist Group, and chairs the Field Conservation Committee of the British and Irish Association of Zoos and Aquariums.

**Nikki Buxton** is a founder-Director of Belize Bird Rescue (BBR). The facility was created in 2004, and BBR has been working with the Belize Forest Department since then to reduce or eliminate the illegal trade in wild-caught parrots. BBR has developed an innovative rehabilitation program for former-captive and hand-reared wild parrots with documented results addressing inappropriate diet, husbandry-related conditions, and adverse behaviors through careful flock-building, enclosure management, and nutrition. Parrots soft-released following rehabilitation at BBR are documented thriving and breeding in the wild. BBR also hand-rears endangered Yellow-headed Amazon chicks, releasing over 100 back into the wild since the program began in 2014.

**Laurie Conrad** began her career in aviculture and rehabilitation in 1989 at SeaWorld in San Diego. Her hand-rearing experience includes small mammals and numerous exotic bird species. Laurie represented SeaWorld in the collaborative Light-footed Clapper Rail recovery conservation program from 2001 to 2018. She served on several Association of Zoos and Aquarium Taxon Advisory Group steering committees, presented at numerous conferences, and coordinated two North American Species Survival Programs. Laurie co-organized the Third International Flamingo Symposium in 2014 and acted as the IUCN Flamingo Specialist Group Ex situ Coordinator for North America. Laurie also worked at the San Diego Zoo Global Avian Propagation Center, where she specialized in hand-rearing and incubation.

**Kateri J. Davis** lives with her husband in Oregon, USA, and together they run the Davis Lund Aviaries where they specialize in raising and breeding a large variety of softbilled birds. Kateri has been involved with birds her entire life and has been working with softbills since the early 1990s. She currently has about 130 birds of 25 different species in her aviaries and ships offspring to zoos and other private aviculturists around the USA. She is the author of the Birdhouse Publication books *Turacos in Aviculture* and *Mousebirds in Aviculture*, and has written many softbill articles for publication in magazines and journals.

**Rebecca S. Duerr** is the clinical veterinarian and research director at International Bird Rescue's two wildlife clinics in California. After earning a BS in marine biology from San Francisco State University, she completed DVM, MPVM, and PhD degrees at UC Davis, with graduate work on the care of oiled Common Murres and on the nutritional energetics and physiology of Common Murres and Western Grebes. She serves on the Board of Directors of the National Wildlife Rehabilitators Association and is a frequent speaker at avian and wildlife conferences. She enjoys sharing her enthusiasm for how incredibly cool and strange birds are with the world, and particularly loves repairing birds that have been injured by the unfortunate actions of humans.

**Maureen Eiger** is the Director and founder of Help Wild Birds, Roanoke, Virginia's only nonprofit wildlife rehabilitation organization that exclusively rehabilitates all species of migratory birds. She holds state and federal wildlife rehabilitation permits, and has been rehabilitating birds for over 10 years. She is a contributing writer to the *North American Bluebird Society Journal,* the Roanoke *Star Newspaper,* various Audubon and bird club newsletters, and the blog 10000 Birds. Maureen teaches classes about birds at state wildlife conferences, bird clubs, colleges, Master Naturalists, and other organizations. Maureen is an avid birder; she was Vice President of the Roanoke Valley Bird Club and a Virginia Bluebird Society Board Member. One can say her life is very "birdy."

**Nancy Eilertsen** has been a wildlife rehabilitator since 1988. She is the founder and director of East Valley Wildlife based in Phoenix, Arizona, and is state and federally licensed. She is a coauthor of *A Flying Chance* passerine rehabilitation manual.

**Elizabeth Penn (Penny) Elliston** earned a MSc at Johns Hopkins School of Hygiene and Public Health, now the Bloomberg School, and has worked with epidemiological teams in India and Africa. One of the founders of Wildlife Rescue of New Mexico, she has been working with hummingbirds and other avian species since 1980. She has authored and coauthored a number of papers on hummingbird growth, care, and behavior.

**Meryl Faulkner** was a full-time home care volunteer with Project Wildlife, a rehabilitation group in San Diego County, for more than 20 years, and is currently retired. She raised and rehabilitated various avian species, and also skunks, but specialized in sea and shorebirds. She captive-reared and rehabilitated California Least Terns and Western Snowy Plovers (sometimes hatched from salvaged eggs) for local, state, and federal agencies.

**Mark Finke** has worked in the area of comparative animal nutrition for more than 30 years and has published more than 30 peer-reviewed articles on nutrition in insects, birds, mammals, and reptiles. He has a PhD from the University of Wisconsin with a dual major in nutritional sciences and entomology. He runs a consulting business specializing in pet food formulation and product development. Mark supports several rehabilitation groups by helping them develop diets for specific species and situations.

**Lisa (Elisa) Fosco** is a wildlife biologist and a licensed veterinary technician. She has been involved in wildlife rehabilitation for over 30 years and was an instructor for the International Wildlife Rehabilitation Council for 14 years. Lisa has published several papers on owls and has also participated in several radiotelemetry studies documenting the dispersal and survivability of captive-reared owls. She has managed large scale wildlife centers in both the US and Canada.

**Elaine Friedman** a former Federal Food and Drug Administration pharmaceutical chemist, has been a wildlife rehabilitator and educator since 1986. Working and volunteering at numerous wildlife rehabilitation and education centers in the Bay Area, Elaine's original focus was on multiple species, but later shifted to focus on corvids. In 1999, Elaine founded Corvid Connection, a wildlife education nonprofit organization. Through writing, speaking at wildlife rehabilitation symposiums, and mentoring and advising educators and rehabilitators, her focus now is on transferring years of experience and knowledge to benefit all corvid species, rehabilitators, and educators, and to help the general public learn to live peacefully with the wildlife they encounter.

**Laurie J. Gage** was the Director of Veterinary Services for Six Flags Marine World in Vallejo, California, for 23 years, the Director of Veterinary Services for The Marine Mammal Center in Sausalito, California, and was a clinical veterinarian at the Coyote Point Museum and the Los Angeles Zoo, where she worked with a large variety of mammals and birds. She served as the Big Cat and Marine Mammal Specialist for the United States Department of Agriculture for more than 15 years. She edited Hand-Rearing Wild and Domestic Mammals (Blackwell Publishers 2002) and the first edition of this book, plus co-authored the Wild Orphans section of several editions of the Merck Veterinary Manual.

**Marjorie Cahak Gibson** is Founder and Executive Director of Raptor Education Group, Inc. (REGI), a wildlife rehabilitation, education, and research facility, located in Antigo, Wisconsin (www.raptoreducationgroup.org). A former president of International Wildlife Rehabilitation Council (IWRC), she teaches wildlife rehabilitation classes internationally and maintains an active schedule consulting with wildlife professionals worldwide about avian species. Marge has been active with avian field research and wildlife rehabilitation for over 40 years and has cared for thousands of avian patients from Bald Eagles and Trumpeter Swans to warblers and hummingbirds.

**Dana A. Glei** has been a rehabilitation volunteer at the Bird Rescue Center (BRC, Santa Rosa, CA) since 2012. She took a special interest in towhees after completing her first baby bird season and discovering the challenge they pose for rehabilitators. In collaboration with others, she researched and helped implement strategies for improving the care and rehabilitation of young towhees that cannot be reunited with their parents. She has presented talks and workshops on towhee care at wildlife rehabilitation centers and symposia to help train new "towhee whisperers." In her day job, she holds a PhD in sociology and works as a demographer studying health and mortality among the human population.

**Michele Goodman** received her veterinary medical degree from the University of Pennsylvania School of Veterinary Medicine, and completed an MHS degree at Quinnipiac University in biomedical health sciences. During school, she worked as a research assistant and animal health consultant at the Livingston Ripley Waterfowl Conservancy. She lectures on waterfowl rehabilitation and medicine, parasitology, and avian health in aviculture around the country and internationally. Michele is currently participating in several research initiatives on sea ducks and pochards. She is an instructor for the Wildlife Medicine Course at the University of Pennsylvania School of Veterinary Medicine. Michele has served as President of the National Wildlife Rehabilitators Association and is the Director of Veterinary Services at the Elmwood Park Zoo.

**Aimee Greenebaum** is the Curator of Aviculture at the Monterey Bay Aquarium. She received a Bachelor of Science in wildlife biology from Kansas State University. She has been working with birds for about 20 years and has been with the Monterey Bay Aquarium's Husbandry Department for 15 years. She manages the aquarium's avian exhibits, including the shorebirds, Common Murres, puffins, African Penguins, Red-footed Booby, and Laysan Albatross, as well as the aquarium's Snowy Plover rehabilitation program.

**Jo Gregson** is the Curator of Birds at the Paignton Zoo Environmental Park in Dover, England. She is the Vice chair of the Ratite and Charadriiformes Taxon Advisory Groups and also sits on EAZA hornbill and stork committees. Presently she is involved in the Socorro Dove *Zenaida graysoni* and Pink Pigeon *Nesoenas mayeri* reintroduction projects. Jo has spent seven years managing a team of aviculturists working toward the translocation of the Cirl Bunting *Emberiza cirlus* to the UK county/region of Cornwall. She is currently working closely with VIETNATURE adding her skills and expertise to the Edwards's Pheasant reintroduction project. Jo believes that well-practiced aviculture can lead to conservation success.

**Sophie Hebert Saulnier** earned a DVM from the University of Montreal, and has been in practice at the Montreal Avian and Exotic Animal Hospital since 2010. She taught animal health technology and gives regular presentations to the general public and to veterinary students in Quebec. She spent a year in Belize working with Belize Bird Rescue, a multi-species wild bird rescue center specializing in the rehabilitation for release of wild-caught (poached) parrots. She has also worked with various psittacine conservation projects throughout the Americas.

**Linda Henry** has been a supervisor at SeaWorld San Diego's Penguin Encounter since 1983. Henry was a lead team member in five penguin propagation projects involving the incubation and hand-rearing of seven species of penguins from eggs collected in the Antarctic. These projects helped to establish penguin hand-rearing and incubation guidelines and contributed to the knowledge of penguin growth rates. Linda co-authored chapters in *Reproduction for the Penguin Husbandry Manual* (1994, 2005) and the *Penguin Care Manual* (2014). Henry is currently the SSP® Program Coordinator for King Penguins and Candidate Program Leader for Emperor Penguins. Henry is an advisor on lighting to the Penguin Taxon Advisory Group.

**Linda Hufford** is an avian wildlife rehabilitator permitted in the state of Texas and through the U.S. Fish and Wildlife Service since 1995.

**Susie Kasielke** started her career as an Animal Keeper at the Los Angeles Zoo in 1977 and earned a BS degree in Avian Sciences at the University of California, Davis. She was Curator of Birds at the LA Zoo from 2001 to 2016. She is currently the Avian Biologist for the Toledo Zoo and Aquarium. Through her involvement in the California Condor Recovery Program, she worked with the staff at LA Zoo and partner facilities to develop and refine propagation, incubation, and rearing methods for California Condors and many other species. She teaches workshops on avian egg incubation for zoo and avicultural groups around the world. She has also taught aviculture at Pierce College and is a guest lecturer at Moorpark College, UCLA, and UC Davis.

**Ashton Kluttz** is the Executive Director of the Bird Rescue Center (BRC, Santa Rosa, CA), and holds a BA degree in Environmental Studies from Washington College (Chestertown, MD) and certification as a Registered Veterinary Technician. She began her career as a wildlife rehabilitator at The Marine Mammal Center, where she served as a marine mammal stranding intern. From 2009 to 2013 she worked at the Bird Rescue Center as a Shift Supervisor, and advanced to

Rehabilitation Hospital Manager and Director of Avian Care from 2013 to 2019. Through consultation with other facilities and under her direction, BRC dramatically improved their success with difficult species such as towhees and House Finches. In 2019, she became Executive Director.

**Liz Koutsos** earned a BS in Animal Science from the University of Maryland, and MS and PhD degrees in Nutrition from University of California, Davis. Her research focused on interactions between nutrition and immunity in a variety of avian species. After serving as faculty at California Polytechnic State University, San Luis Obispo, Liz joined Mazuri Exotic Animal Nutrition in 2006, as the lead nutritionist and then as Director. In 2016, she became an independent consultant, focusing on the nutrition of aquatic animals, elephants, insects, dogs, and cats. In 2017, Liz began working with EnviroFlight, the first U.S. commercial producer of dried black soldier fly larvae, meal, and oil, and assumed the role of President in 2018. She is an Adjunct Professor at North Carolina State University, and a Smithsonian Research Associate.

**Romy Klusener** has been working at the Southern African Foundation for the Conservation of Coastal Birds (SANCCOB) in Cape Town, South Africa since 2012 and is experienced in seabird rehabilitation as well as the incubation, hatching, and hand rearing of seabirds to be released back into the wild. These include African Penguins, Cape Cormorants, Bank Cormorants, Hartlaub's Gulls, Kelp Gulls, African Black Oystercatchers, and Northern Rockhopper Penguins. She has also worked as a seabird rehabilitator and cared for a variety of seabirds.

**Nicole LaGreco** graduated from Arcadia University with a degree in Animal Behavior. Her interest in hand-rearing birds began as a keeper at Zoo Atlanta, when she had the opportunity to rear several species. She was able to further her passion by joining the San Diego Zoo's Avian Propagation Center team in 2006, and worked her way up to her current position, Animal Care Manager. She has been involved in several conservation projects including head-starting the critically endangered Mangrove Finch. The Avian Propagation Center has a long history of successfully hand-rearing hornbills and members of the order Coraciiformes.

**Jennifer Linander** earned dual BS degrees in Environmental/Marine Biology and Zoology with a minor in Wildlife Biology from Humboldt State University. She has spent more than 10 years volunteering and working in wildlife rehabilitation caring for myriad species of birds and mammals, ranging from songbirds to pelicans and squirrels to bears. Most notably she spent over four years working at International Bird Rescue's San Francisco Bay Delta Center, where she earned the position of Senior Rehabilitation Technician, caring for and raising injured and orphaned aquatic birds.

**Isabel Luevano** has been a wildlife rehabilitator for nine years working exclusively with aquatic avian species. She holds a BS in Marine Biology from Sonoma State University and is the Wildlife Center Manager for International Bird Rescue's San Francisco Bay Delta Center, where 2000–4000 wild aquatic birds of all ages undergo rehabilitation annually. She has presented on the care and raising of young aquatic avian species as well as created multiple protocols for raising the less common species of aquatic bird chicks International Bird Rescue receives.

**Jessika Madison-Kennedy** has been working with birds for 15 years and has been a wildlife rehabilitator for 12 of those years. Jessika managed the avian nursery at the Wildlife Rehabilitation Center of Minnesota from 2010 to 2017 and currently acts as their Avian Outreach manager, collaborating with local vet tech programs and creating opportunities for students to learn how to work with injured and orphaned wild birds. Jessika is also a resource advisor for the Avian Rearing Resource in the UK, an organization that creates, gathers, and shares hand-rearing techniques for captive populations in zoos and conservation programs around the world. Her focus is on difficult to raise insectivorous species, shorebirds, and hummingbirds.

**Jesse Menne** completed her Bachelor of Science in Ecology and Evolution at University of California, Santa Cruz. Wanting to pursue a career with wildlife, she took an internship with the Wildlife Rehabilitation Center of Minnesota in 2013. While completing her Veterinary Technology degree, Jesse managed the Waterfowl Nursery for three seasons. Jesse is currently the Waterfowl Nursery Liaison, as well as a Certified Veterinary Technician for the Wildlife Rehabilitation Center of Minnesota. She has raised over 3000 ducklings and developed standardized protocols for the many species the center treats.

**Jayne Neville** operates Mount Vernon Songbird Sanctuary (formerly The Recovery Wing) in Southington, CT, a nonprofit organization focusing on the conservation of songbirds through education, rehabilitation, and preservation of their habitat, and has been rehabilitating songbirds since 1997. Semi-retired, she focuses her expertise on insectivores, hummingbirds, woodpeckers, Killdeer, chimney swifts, and swallows. Jayne taught The Basics of Songbird Rehabilitation for many years for the State of Connecticut Department of Environmental Protection exam and all-day training seminar for new rehabilitators. Jayne also teaches wildlife rehabilitators in and out of the country at wildlife rehabilitation conferences. She is past President and Vice President of Connecticut Wildlife Rehabilitators Association.

**David A. Oehler** has been committed to animal care and conservation since 1985. In 1993, he began in-situ programs with Alcids in Alaska while simultaneously rearing hundreds of puffin, guillemot and auklet chicks for ex-situ programs. In 2001, he began to study penguin colonies on Isla Noir, Chile, which lead to his founding of Feather Link, a local NGO. As Curator of Ornithology at the Wildlife Conservation Society, Bronx Zoo, he participated in programs involving the rehabilitation of African Gray Parrots, Little Penguin health assessments, and additional conservation programs. David serves on the board of the Asa Wright Nature Centre in Trinidad and conducted Oilbird monitoring/tracking programs along with ongoing bat acoustic studies. He currently is with the Nashville Zoo at Grassmere in the position of Vice-President.

**Libby Osnes Erie** started working in wildlife rehabilitation in 1993. She has worked extensively with terrestrial and marine wildlife in the California central coast region. She was a participant in the California Department of Fish and Game Oiled Wildlife Care Network from 1995 to 2004 and a California Council for Wildlife Rehabilitators board member from 2000 to 2006. She also has worked as a wildlife rehabilitator in Colorado and Washington. She is a volunteer with the Washington State Animal Response Team (WASART) and the Washington State Department of Ecology oil spill response network. Libby is a California registered veterinary technician and a Washington licensed veterinary technician. She has an MS in Marine Science, specializing in marine mammals and birds.

**Jean Pichler** is an educator with over 35 years of high school teaching experience. She is a volunteer moderator for the Institute for Wildlife Studies Bald Eagle Restoration Program live-streaming nest cameras on the Channel Islands (CA) and moderated the Humboldt Bay (CA) Eagle Cam. Jean is a co-founder of the nonprofit Biodiversity Education and Research Foundation, providing education opportunities for citizen scientists to learn about Bald Eagles and the environments in which they live.

**Nora Pihkala** raised and bred exhibition chickens in the 4-H youth program in Southern California. She obtained both her BS in Avian Sciences and a DVM from the University of California, Davis. Following veterinary school, she practiced companion animal medicine, including backyard poultry. Currently, her professional interests lie in public health practice. Her favorite chicken breeds remain Silver Spangled Hamburgs and bantam Barred Plymouth Rocks.

**Megan Shaw Prelinger** is a former wildlife rehabilitator specializing in aquatic birds and oil spill response, working with International Bird Rescue from 2000 to 2010. Living in San Francisco, CA, she leads birding walks for San Francisco Nature Education, teaches a course on diving birds for Golden Gate Audubon Society, and has presented widely on aquatic bird rehabilitation. She is also an independent scholar and cofounder of the Prelinger Library, a private research library in San Francisco.

**Guthrum Purdin** earned a BS in Marine Biology from San Francisco State University and his DVM from the University of California. While making a living as a jeweler and then a movie propmaker in Hollywood, he began working with wildlife as a volunteer at The Marine Mammal Center in Sausalito, CA where he was active for 18 years. He went on to work professionally with birds and land mammals before deciding to pursue a career in veterinary medicine. In the past 30 years, he has worked with and provided medical care for a myriad of animal species, both wild and domestic, and has served as the primary veterinarian for several of California's large wildlife hospitals. He has a particular fondness for passerines and California sea lions.

**Yuko Sato** is a 2012 graduate of Purdue University's veterinary medicine program. She joined Iowa State University in August 2015 after completing a poultry residency and serves as the university's Poultry Extension Veterinarian and Diagnostic Pathologist. She has been a diplomate of the American College of Poultry Veterinarians since 2015. Sato works broadly with commercial and backyard poultry producers within and outside the state of Iowa.

**Renée Schott** has been involved in wildlife rehabilitation since 2003, working in various centers across the country, before starting at the Wildlife Rehabilitation Center of Minnesota in 2010. Renée teaches courses at the University of Minnesota School of Veterinary Medicine, does relief work at The Univ. MN Raptor Center, is a Course Instructor for the International Wildlife Rehabilitation Council, and lectures on wildlife rehabilitation and medicine all over the country. Renée's professional interests include wildlife rehabilitation welfare and clinical medicine, and advancing the profession.

**Louise Shimmel** has been a state and federally permitted wildlife rehabilitator since 1985, working for five years with all species, and then specializing in raptors. In 1990, she founded Cascades Raptor Center, a nature center and wildlife hospital in Eugene, Oregon, to focus on environmental education, as well as rehabilitation. The Raptor Center now sees over 30 000 visitors each year. She served for seven years on the board, including two years as president, of the International Wildlife Rehabilitation Council, was an IWRC Skills Seminar instructor for five years, has reviewed articles for the IWRC Journal of Wildlife Rehabilitation since 1989, authored an article in Seminars in Avian and Exotic Pet Medicine, contributed a number of articles to the IWRC Journal, and presented at numerous conferences.

**Dale A. Smith** is Professor Emeritus, University of Guelph, following a career in the Department of Pathobiology at the Ontario Veterinary College, Ontario, Canada. She educated generations of veterinary students in the clinical medicine of avian and exotic pet species, zoo animals, and wildlife; and graduate students in the pathology of these same species. She has lectured and published extensively, and has been involved in international development programs throughout her career. An alumnus of the joint Toronto Zoo/University of Guelph graduate program in Zoo Animal Medicine and Pathology, she spent several years teaching veterinary students in Zimbabwe before returning to Guelph. Her interest in ratites began in Africa and has survived the "boom and bust" industry cycle in North America.

**Kappy Sprenger** began working in wildlife rehabilitation in Los Gatos, California in 1985, caring for both mammals and birds. In 2002, she moved to Maine where she has continued as a rehabilitator, accepting all avian species but specializing in the fish-eating birds (particularly loons) and all precocial species.

**Nicky Stander** graduated from University of Plymouth in the UK with a BSc (Hons) in Animal Science (Behaviour and Welfare). Since 2010 she has held the position of Seabird Rehabilitation Manager the Southern African Foundation for the Conservation of Coastal Birds (SANCCOB) in Cape Town, South Africa and has played an instrumental role in the implementation of the Robben Island Seabird Ranger project.

**Carol Stanley** has been an aviculturist for over 20 years. During that time, she has kept and raised a variety of avian species, including many psittacine species, as well as cranes, kookaburras, and Chilean Flamingos. As a Model Aviculture Program (www.modelaviculture.org) certificate holder, she has provided birds to AZA institutions. As past board member and current president of the Avicultural Society of America, (ASA), Carol has contributed to organizing ASA's Annual Education Conference for over 13 years, which are hosted by AZA institutions such as the San Diego Zoo. Carol is art director and editor of the Avicultural Society of America Avicultural e-Bulletin, which features avian education for ASA members (www.asabirds.org). She is an avid avian photographer, author, and speaker.

**Marie Travers** earned a BA in Psychology from University of Massachusetts, Boston, and has been working with wildlife since 2001. She has since worked as Wildlife Rehabilitation Manager at Lindsay Wildlife Museum and as Assistant Manager at International Bird Rescue, establishing herself as an aquatic bird specialist and oil spill responder, a role she continues today. She has been employed as an oiled wildlife specialist/rehabilitation manager with Focus Wildlife since 2013, and has done contract work at several other wildlife rehabilitation facilities. Marie is co-founder of Bird Ally X and serves on the board of the Wild Neighbors Database Project (creators of the Wildlife Rehabilitation Medical Database). She co-authored the book *An Introduction to Aquatic Bird Rehabilitation.*

**Linda M. Tuttle-Adams** is a lifelong naturalist, avid birder, photographer, writer, and artist. Since 2008, she has held staff and volunteer positions for Wildlife Rehabilitation and Release in Grass Valley, CA, and has rehabilitated many bird species. Linda received a BS in Biology from the University of California at Santa Cruz, and spent six years as a curatorial assistant with the California Academy of Sciences in the Ornithology & Mammalogy Department. She has participated in two atlas projects for breeding birds of Napa/Sonoma Counties and Nevada County, with her illustrations depicted in both atlases. Her passion is baby bird identification, and she is currently working on a book on the subject, for which she is painting over 400 depictions of nestling and fledgling baby birds.

**Diane Winn** is the Executive Director of Avian Haven, a wild bird rehabilitation practice of approximately 2500 admissions per year, based in Freedom, Maine (Marc Payne is Avian

Haven's co-founder). She has published several peer-reviewed articles, and given numerous conference presentations, on various aspects of wild bird rehabilitation, including nestling diets and emaciation protocols.

**Patricia Witman** was the Avian Care Manager for the Zoological Society of San Diego at the San Diego Zoo's Avian Propagation Center for 17 years. Her responsibilities included creating protocols for any of the avian species from which eggs or chicks were removed from the parents for hand-rearing. Pat first became involved with hand-rearing hornbills in 1987. This department has continued to have a very high success rate with other related species, including the Micronesian Kingfisher.

**Martin Vince** has been keeping and breeding toucans both in private and professional aviculture since the 1970s. Vince worked for 20 years in AZA accredited zoos, including terms as population manager for the Toco Toucan as well as significant leadership roles in numerous other avian conservation programs. Now a software engineer, Vince remains close to professional and private aviculture, still taking pleasure in sharing and writing about birds.

# Preface

The second edition of this book was originally planned to be a simple update to the chapters from the first edition, with a few more chapters added for species not covered last time. After years of discussions with the previous authors of the first edition and colleagues at wildlife rehabilitation centers, zoos, and universities, as well as veterinarians and bird enthusiasts, we opted to create a more thorough revision and expansion. The original plan seemed like a reasonably straightforward thing that should only take a year or so to complete ... but then Dr. Duerr would have flashes of inspiration, and another chapter or two were added, until there were 50.

The second edition is organized much like the first but includes 12 more chapters covering species or groups of species not covered in the first edition, and also includes color photographs this time, which helps illustrate many concepts pertinent to birds. Our chapter authors are experts, and are passionate about the species for which they have carefully documented their successes in the hand-rearing process. They have shared their tips and knowledge in this edition and we hope this book will be helpful for anyone faced with raising most species of birds.

We would have loved to have chapters covering the more rare or endangered species of birds but we have limited the chapters to those birds most frequently in need of hand-rearing at wildlife centers, zoos, and private bird facilities. That being said, many endangered birds being hand-reared will have useful information available on near-relatives within these chapters.

We reiterate that hand-rearing birds is often more art than science and hope the information we share in this book will help others who are new to this discipline, or who wish to find new methods to consider. There are many different ways to successfully hand-rear a given species, and our authors have kindly agreed to share theirs. The reader shouldn't hesitate to read chapters on species other than the species of their immediate concern, as many authors have tips and tricks for food presentation, housing, and other useful ideas that may be the perfect thing for a different circumstance. We also hope bird enthusiasts everywhere enjoy reading the chapters within for pleasure and curiosity's sake too. Birds are endlessly fascinating, and the ways our authors have managed the quirks of each species make for entertaining reading. Enjoy.

*Rebecca S. Duerr DVM MPVM PhD*
*Laurie J. Gage DVM Dipl. ACZM*

## Acknowledgments

Endless thanks to our authors for being game to revise chapters, start new chapters from scratch, dig through their photo collections for that perfect shot to accompany their own chapters and each other's, plus patiently put up with the several years it took to bring it all together. Thanks also to the nonauthor photographers who were so kind to share their stunning photographs that add so much to this book. This project has been a labor of love for the editors and many of the authors as well. With that being said, we have a lot of people to thank.

Laurie would like to thank the veterinary and bird staff from Marine World Africa USA (now Six Flags Discovery Kingdom) for sharing their skills and knowledge of hand-rearing many different species of birds and mammals and igniting my passion for sharing practical tips and information with others. Thanks to my friend, the amazing Dr. Becky Duerr for her endless work and enthusiasm for this project, as she had far more chapters to edit than I did, and yet she still had the time to fix little details in my chapters, such as those pesky weight graphs. Always a force of nature, this book would not have been possible without Becky's perseverance.

Becky would like to thank Jeri O'Donnell for editorial assistance and her perfectionist's sharp eye. Many thanks to International Bird Rescue's current and former staff for not only being awesome rehabilitators willing to do yet more work by writing, collaborating, and editing chapters, but also for tolerating (and managing) their perpetually overextended and distracted veterinarian. Special thanks to IBR current and former staff for taking such compelling images of our patients: Cheryl Reynolds, Jennifer Linander, Isabel Luevano, Julie Skoglund, Michelle Bellizzi, Kylie Clatterbuck, Miranda Starr, Marie Travers, and the late Jay Holcomb. Thanks to the most fabulous PhD advisor I could have ever hoped for, Dr. Kirk Klasing, who vastly expanded the way I think about birds and their challenges, and is always willing to talk about the often-odd quirks of their immunology, nutrition, and physiology. Thanks to the 1990s staff of Wildlife Rescue Inc. in Palo Alto, CA for getting me a good start with birds and making me aware Dr. Klasing existed; you never know how your words and actions will shape the lives of the people you work with. Thanks to my friend and partner in this undertaking Dr. Laurie Gage, without whom this book would never have happened, who not only wrote me a reference letter to get into vet school long ago, but put up with all the delays in getting this second edition finished. And of course, a thousand thank yous to my husband of 30+ years who got me interested in birds in the first place, Dr. Guthrum Purdin, for not only putting up with my chronic writing and editing but also for contributing as an author and chapter reviewer.

*Rebecca S. Duerr DVM MPVM PhD*
*Laurie J. Gage DVM Dipl. ACZM*

# 1

# Baby Bird Basics

*Rebecca S. Duerr*

## Introduction

Many circumstances occur where people hand-rear birds. A small number of easily-raised species are propagated to become human foods. Other species are kept as companion birds, or in zoologic collections as part of conservation programs, or when a health problem occurs with parents or chicks. Several hundred thousand injured and orphaned wild birds are presented for care annually in the United States alone (Borgia 2004), with an unknown number of wild birds hand-reared for release back into the wild throughout the world. In some of these circumstances, a strong human–animal bond is crucial, while in others, special techniques may be needed to avoid development of this bond to allow the young bird to grow up wild, both physically and psychologically.

There are over 9600 recognized species of birds in the world, taxonomically divided into 32 orders, although as more genetic information is acquired, this number continues to evolve. This diversity garners broad differences between species during hand-rearing, many of which will be discussed in the chapters of this book. Throughout the hand-rearing process for any species of chick there are certain commonalities of care that will be discussed in this chapter. Chapter 2 provides information to narrow down the species of an unknown chick, and Chapter 3 provides extensive details around incubation and hatching of eggs, including advice on assisting a chick with a difficult hatch. Subsequent chapters cover the finer details, quirks, and needs of specific species or groups of species. Most avian orders have at least a few representatives covered in this book, and a major goal is to provide at least general guidance for any species of bird by discussing the needs of commonly hand-reared examples of close relatives.

## Human Safety and Biosecurity

Some species of young wild birds may be dangerous to novice handlers. Heron relatives may forcefully stab with their bill, even through the air holes in a pet carrier; young raptors have very strong talons with which to pierce whatever human body part they can grab; juvenile pelicans may strike at faces with their very powerful bills. Wild chicks, or any chick that is frightened, may attempt to protect itself with whatever weaponry it has, due to the reasonable expectation that any creature that is not its parent is likely planning on making the chick lunch. Protective goggles and thick leather gloves may be needed with some species.

*Hand-Rearing Birds*, Second Edition. Edited by Rebecca S. Duerr and Laurie J. Gage.

Viral, bacterial, fungal, and parasitic diseases are common in wild birds, and may be problems in captive collections as well. Caregivers with health concerns should discuss the risks of activities involving handling of chicks with their physician. Good hygienic practices are always warranted when handling animals of any kind, especially wild animals. Personal protective equipment such as a face mask, gloves, dedicated clothing, and foot baths may be useful to both reduce caregiver exposure to zoonotic diseases and to reduce exposure of chicks to human flora and pathogens. Although many parasitic diseases of wild birds require intermediate hosts and as such are not commonly transmitted within care centers (e.g. helminths), some are zoonotic (e.g. *Giardia lambla*) or transmissible between birds (e.g. *Trichomonas* spp.). Bacterial pathogens may become problematic in kitchen or other areas (e.g. *Salmonella* spp.). Viral diseases are of particularly high concern when raising poultry (see Chapter 7), and fungal organisms may become a risk in some environments or when feces is allowed to accumulate in housing.

Disposable gloves are useful, and frequent handwashing is imperative. Routine cleaning and disinfection of caging, food dishes, and feeding implements helps control risks to everyone involved, both birds and their caregivers. Nursery protocols should be thoughtfully planned to avoid pathogen transmission between groups of chicks, while also allowing for appropriate socialization as dictated by each chick's intended adult lifestyle. An avian veterinarian can be extremely helpful in planning nursery protocols that protect both human and animal health.

## Criteria for Intervention

Chicks found in the mouth of a dog or cat, alone in an inappropriate location such as the middle of a parking lot or prone on a baking hot sidewalk, or that are cold, injured, covered with parasites or ants, entangled in a foreign material, or otherwise in obvious trouble, are indeed in need of rescue. Alert, active, fully-feathered, mobile chicks that are found without evidence of trauma or distress in the environment in which their parents nested, whether that is a backyard or natural area, should be left alone. If the parents are providing care and the chick is uninjured, the risk of "cats in the neighborhood" is not sufficient reason to bring a found chick into captivity. This risk is faced by most wild birds in the world, and it is always preferable for a wild animal of any species to be raised by its parents. This enables the youngster to best learn the finer details of species-specific social and survival skills it will need to navigate its wild environment.

### Precocial vs Altricial

There are two principle types of chick development, although this is an oversimplification of the diverse strategies birds have evolved for raising their young. *Precocial* chicks are those that hatch with their eyes open and are mobile and able to leave the nest shortly after hatching, following after the parent who provides protection, warmth, and guidance regarding what to eat. These chicks are sometimes found alone, apparently parentless. Once precocial chicks hatch, the family group usually leaves the nest area. Consequently, it may be very difficult to reunite separated chicks with their parents, although some species will foster extra chicks if an appropriate family group with chicks the same age can be located. Precocial chicks in obviously bad locations, such as running in the street, should be immediately rescued or shepherded out of traffic to rejoin their family. Mallards will sometimes nest in urban fountain planters or near swimming pools, and when chicks hatch, they leap into the water, cannot get out, and eventually drown. Often all that is needed is to place a ramp that allows chicks to exit the water.

*Altricial* chicks hatch blind, naked, helpless, and completely dependent on the parents for every aspect of care. The family is dependent on the nest site remaining safely hidden from predators until the chicks grow up, which is generally a short few weeks. If a chick is found, check it for injuries; look for blood, asymmetrical limbs, parasites, and other problems. If these are found, the chick will need captive care. Fallen, uninjured chicks may be replaced in the nest if its location is known. Always check to make sure that the chicks in the nest are of the same species as the chick being replaced, although some chicks may be days older or younger. If the whole nest structure has fallen and the chicks appear uninjured, the nest can be replaced by placing it in a larger wicker basket (or other container with drainage holes) that is attached to the tree as close as possible to its former location. Choose the location such that the nest is high enough to be safe from predators and not in direct sunlight. Nests that have been replaced should be monitored from a distance to ensure that the parents return to feed the chicks. If it is near dark and the parents have little daylight in which to find the new nest, bring the chicks inside and provide warmth overnight before re-nesting them in the morning. Unfeathered altricial chicks too young to be outside the nest that are unable to be reunited with parents will need hand-rearing. It is a myth that humans having handled a chick will cause a parent bird to reject it or abandon its nest. Persistent disturbance, however, can cause nest abandonment.

Altricial chicks normally have periods of time when they are fully feathered and old enough to begin exploring their environment, but are not yet able to fly away from danger. These older chicks are still cared for by the parents, but no longer require moment-to-moment attention. Chicks of this age group are at high risk for capture by domestic pet predators or kidnapping by well-intentioned people. If chicks of this description are in an area, keep dogs and cats inside for the few days it will take the birds to become fully flighted. Monitor such chicks from a distance to watch for parental attention. The parents will usually visit the chick frequently for feedings. These chicks quickly finish growing flight feathers and soon will be able to follow the parent in flight while learning to be proficient at foraging and other skills.

Parents of certain species may "dive bomb" humans or pets in an effort to save their young from perceived or real predation. The best thing to do in this circumstance is to allow the birds privacy to finish raising their young, which should be over within a few weeks. It may be seen as a hardship to vacate one's backyard for a short period of time, but bear in mind that one's backyard may be the only habitat the birds have. They cannot move and finish raising their chicks elsewhere. It also may be against federal, state, provincial, or other laws to remove migratory bird nests or chicks, as many species have legal protections.

If a person observing from a distance has not seen a parent visit a suspected orphaned chick within an hour or more of continuous observation, the chick may be in need of care. If the parents are known to have been killed or injured, the chicks should be rescued, because they will starve without parental support.

The Humane Society of the United States has a webpage with links to each state's listings of permitted rehabilitation groups at https://www.humanesociety.org/resources/how-find-wildlife-rehabilitator. The International Wildlife Rehabilitation Council (IWRC) maintains a website that provides answers to frequently asked questions about orphaned chicks and other wildlife issues at https://theiwrc.org/resources/emergency, and includes contact information for organizations both outside and inside North America.

## Legal Considerations

The chapters in this book make the assumption that any reader applying the knowledge contained herein to protected species possesses the appropriate permits. See local, state, provincial, or federal wildlife permit offices, and regional wildlife rehabilitation associations for information regarding rules. For example, in the United States, both the general public and veterinarians are prohibited from keeping migratory birds without valid permits from both the U.S. Fish and Wildlife Service and applicable state authorities, which may have additional rules regarding possession of birds. The vast majority of wild orphans found are protected by this ruling. In the U.S., as Good Samaritans helping a wild bird in need of care, the public is required to transfer the bird to a permitted wildlife rehabilitator immediately. Wild birds requiring medical treatment may only be kept by veterinarians who do not possess rehabilitation permits for 24 hours after the bird's condition has been stabilized, after which time it must be transferred to a permitted wildlife rehabilitator (50 CFR 21.12: Code of Federal Regulations 2018). If a veterinarian is unable to locate a permitted migratory bird rehabilitator, the Regional Migratory Bird Permit Office must be contacted for assistance, see https://www.fws.gov/birds/policies-and-regulations/permits/regional-permit-contacts.php. Many states maintain lists of currently permitted rehabilitators within websites of state Fish and Game, Parks and Wildlife, or Division of Natural Resources Departments. For example, Texas Parks and Wildlife lists all permitted Texas rehabilitators by county at https://tpwd.texas.gov/huntwild/wild/rehab/list and a California list is available at www.wildlife.ca.gov/Conservation/Laboratories/Wildlife-Investigations/Rehab/Facilities.

There are several nonnative species found throughout the United States that are commonly encountered as orphans, such as Rock Pigeons (*Columba livia*), Eurasian Collared-Doves (*Streptopelia decaocto*), European Starlings (*Sturnus vulgaris*), and House Sparrows (*Passer domesticus*). Their care and possession is not regulated in some states, but may be illegal in others. European Starlings and Rock Pigeons make excellent pet birds and starlings can even learn to speak words. However, identification must be verified because native wild chicks may appear quite similar. Release of nonnative species into the wild is discouraged by most wildlife biologists and natural resource managers, and may be illegal in some areas because many nonnative species have deleterious effects on native bird populations. In other parts of the world, these species may be protected in their native ranges and possession may require permits from regulatory agencies.

## Record Keeping

Most wildlife regulatory agencies have minimum standards for record keeping that require tracking individual wild animals undergoing rehabilitation, and permanent captives may also require permits for possession. Check with regulating agencies for further information. At a minimum, the following information should be kept for the sake of the individual: species, age, location and date found, reason for hand-rearing, medical problems, final disposition, release location, and release date. Detailed information on the location where the chick was found will serve as a guide for suitable habitat for release and in some circumstances may place the bird back with relatives that may still recognize it. For permanently captive birds being hand-reared, information regarding parentage also may be pertinent; for example, to avoid inbreeding, especially when hand-rearing endangered species.

A detailed medical record should be kept on each individual, with results of the initial examination recorded, and any updated information added as it happens. This should include daily body weights, progress of treatments, and pertinent notes on behavior. For examples of a paper version of a record, see Appendix 1. Many caregivers are moving to using cloud-based electronic databases such as the Wildlife Rehabilitation Medical Database (WRMD, www.wrmd.org), which has the added benefit of allowing caregivers at multiple locations to access an animal's record. It is helpful when large numbers of diverse species are being raised en masse, with different volunteer caregivers, to have a "Feeding Instructions" sheet on each housing unit that tells the next caregiver when to feed, what to feed, how much to feed, and any tips for food delivery. Electronic printouts from animal care databases, white boards, chalk boards, reusable color cage flags, and other types of communication regarding chick needs are used at various facilities to indicate species, feeding frequency, medications, and other pertinent information. These sorts of communications can also serve to flag individuals with specific health concerns. Data collected from good record keeping can be used to assess successes and failures, and can be used to advance animal care protocols.

## Initial Care and Stabilization

### Housing and Thermal Support

The main rule of initial baby bird care is warmth, rehydration, and feeding, in that order. Warm chicks before giving fluids, and then hydrate them until they start passing droppings, only then is it safe to commence feedings. Feeding a cold or dehydrated baby bird before it is warm and hydrated may kill it, even if it is begging. Most chicks found in need of care will be cold, significantly dehydrated, and very stressed. Provide a visual barrier against people and other animals. Do not place birds next to barking dogs, staring cats, noisy children, or other disturbances.

Because avian body temperatures are much higher than that of humans, chicks should always feel warm to the touch. If the chicks are cool or cold, provide supplemental heat. A wet wash cloth inside a sealed plastic bag or hot water bottle warmed in a microwave oven can provide a rapid ad hoc source of heat. These sources of warmth tend to cool rapidly, so must be rewarmed frequently. Take care that steam from a heated, moist surface will not reach the chick and scald it. Chemical handwarmer packs or microwavable pet warmers are also an option. Always have cloth or tissues between chicks and any heat source to prevent excessive heating, and check the chick frequently. Chicks may also arrive hyperthermic, in which case additional heat is contraindicated until the chick has cooled to a more normal temperature.

Both altricial and precocial chicks should be placed in a climate-controlled incubator if available, or other high-temperature, moderate-humidity enclosure. See Figures 1.1 and 1.2; also see specific chapters for examples of appropriate nests and housing for chicks. Heat lamps may be used but are less desirable for nonmobile chicks since it is easy for chicks to overheat and become dehydrated under these if they cannot move away. Typically, the smaller the body size and less feathered the chick, the higher the temperature required, with moderate humidity to help prevent dehydration. Older chicks of any body size require less thermal support once stabilized, although chicks that arrive malnourished may benefit from thermal support longer. Start with a very warm 90–100 °F (32–38 °C) 40–50% humidity environment to normalize the bird's body temperature. Chicks 5–10 g or less may require even higher environmental temperatures (100–104 °F, 38–40 °C). Larger-bodied chicks, such as waterbirds, do well in well-padded pet carriers with one half placed on a heating pad set on "low." Beware leaving large birds in incubators or brooders very long, as

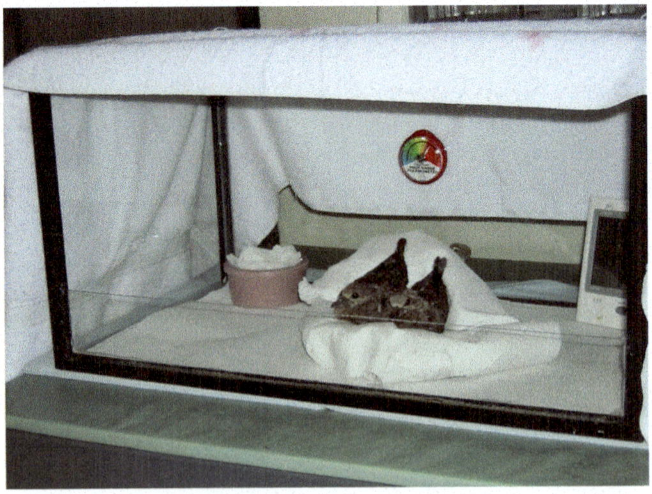

Figure 1.1 Modified glass aquarium incubator, turned sideways to hold heat better. Front opening has Plexiglas "baby gate" high enough to prevent escapes, attached with aquarium cement; dish of soaked paper toweling to add humidity, thermometer, two hot pads underneath with two more on top if needed. Cloth flap folds down over opening between feedings.

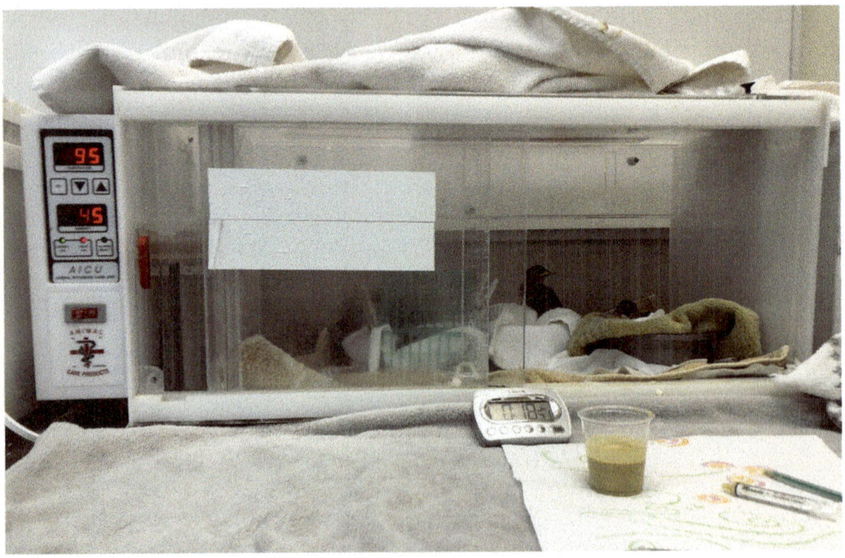


Figure 1.2 Animal Intensive Care Unit from Lyon Technologies, Inc. provides an excellent controlled environment for chicks requiring high temperatures and humidity.

they can go from hypothermia to hyperthermia surprisingly quickly. Also be aware that chicks able to stand may also be proficient at running and jumping. Do not handle the chick more than necessary. Be judicious in application of heat to chicks with head injuries, because high temperatures may exacerbate brain swelling.

If the bird is not able to stand – whether due to age, weakness, or injury – it should be placed in a soft support structure such as a rolled cloth "donut" or tissue-lined nest (see Figure 1.3) appropriate for its body size. Do not allow a chick to lie on its side or in other abnormal positions or on flat

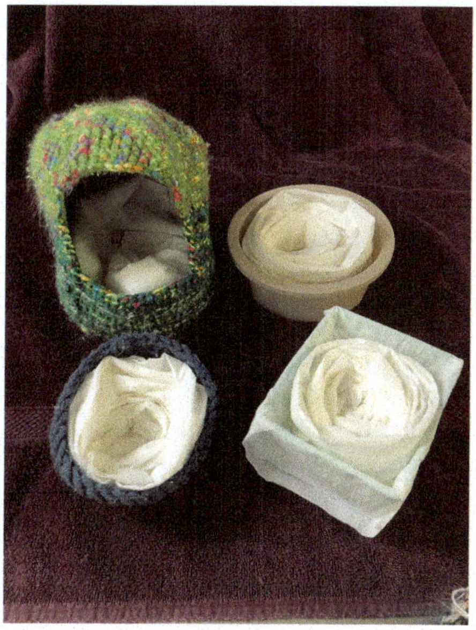

Figure 1.3 Nest substitute examples, clockwise from upper left: Knit nest with tall roof to simulate a nest cavity, ceramic dish nest, berry basket nest, knit nest, all have rolled tissue bedding inserts to provide substrate for toes to grip. *Source:* photo courtesy of Guthrum Purdin.

surfaces. Chicks should be placed in an appropriately sized nest to support their body with the head slightly elevated and the legs folded beneath the body. Weak precocial chicks can also benefit from the comfort of a nest support until stronger. Altricial hatchling or nestling age chicks in poorly-shaped nests may seem restless and continually try to get out of the nest. Re-evaluate the nest replacement if this occurs. Some chicks may be more content with a soft tissue or light piece of cloth draped over the top of the nest to simulate parental brooding. Cavity nesting species may be more comfortable in dim lighting.

Precocial chicks are very stressed by being alone and may be comforted by the addition of a clean undyed feather duster and small mirror to simulate companionship. However, avoid allowing the chick to spend all its time gazing into the mirror, rather than eating and drinking. Remove the mirror if it is preventing normal activities. Be sure the mirror and other cage furnishings are secured to prevent hazards to chicks. Some waterbird chicks, such as grebes and loons, are physiologically unable to stand due to the anatomy of their legs; these species need to be placed on ample soft bedding to prevent pressure sores on their legs or keels.

Monitor chicks frequently for signs of discomfort. Normal avian body temperature is approximately 104–108 °F (40–42 °C), but this varies by species and the stress of handling and restraint. It is not practical to measure the temperature of small-bodied birds, but each chick should always feel warm to a warmed human hand; cloacal temperature can be measured in larger chicks but care must be taken to not cause injury with the thermometer. Cold chicks are often lethargic and poorly responsive. Nest-bound chicks that are too hot may hang their heads over the edge of nests, lay with their necks stretched out, hold their wings away from their body, or keep their mouths open although not gaping or begging. Hot chicks that are able to stand and ambulate will attempt to move away from the heat source or may pant or gular flutter. Overheated birds are likely to become lethargic and dehydrated if the overheating is allowed to persist, and may cease producing droppings. Dehydrated chicks may feel hot or too firm to the touch; a normally hydrated chick's body feels fleshy and soft. Dehydrated chicks may have wrinkled skin over the abdomen, reduced skin elasticity, sunken eyes, slow eyelid responsiveness, stringy saliva, and dry mucous membranes.

## Correcting Dehydration

Human infant electrolyte solutions (unflavored) are excellent for oral rehydration of baby birds, as is lactated Ringer's solution or 2.5% dextrose in 0.45% sodium chloride. Do not use rehydration solution recipes for humans that contain sucrose, as many species of birds lack the ability to digest disaccharides such as table sugar or fructose. Glucose and dextrose are appropriate for all species, but not all newly-acquired chicks are likely to be hypoglycemic because faunivorous birds typically maintain their blood glucose through obligate gluconeogenesis rather than from dietary sources of sugars.

When the bird is warm and calm, it may be hydrated orally and/or subcutaneously (SQ). Gaping (begging) altricial chicks should be orally hydrated until they produce droppings. Give a few drops of warm oral fluids every 15–20 minutes with a small syringe (Figure 1.4) or eye dropper, and allow the bird to swallow completely before giving more. Once comfortable with the amount the chick is able to swallow, the amount may be raised to 2.5–5% of body weight (25–50 ml/kg). Oral fluids may be administered to larger chicks by gavage tube (Figure 1.4). Initial amounts should again be small and frequent, 1–2.5% body weight (10–25 ml/kg) with gradual increases in volume to 5% body weight (50 ml/kg), until the bird is strong and alert. If the chick was fed inappropriate foods by the rescuer, continue oral hydration until the inappropriate foods have passed through the gastrointestinal tract.

Anatomic differences can drive the best method of rehydrating chicks. In species with a crop (e.g. pigeons, doves, parrots, vultures, some passerines, hummingbirds, flamingos, hawks), tubing into the crop, which sits outside the ribcage on the neck portion of the esophagus, is often very effective; however, many bird species lack a crop (e.g. owls, herons, grebes, loons, pelicans, cormorants, some passerines, others), in which case gavage tubings must be given deeper, with the end of tube targeted at the expansible thoracic esophagus in some, or even deeper into the proventriculus in others. Older chicks of species with long necks may require especially long gavage tubes to avoid depositing fluids mid-esophagus where regurgitation becomes more of a risk. Subcutaneous fluids may be preferable in some species to avoid risks of regurgitation.

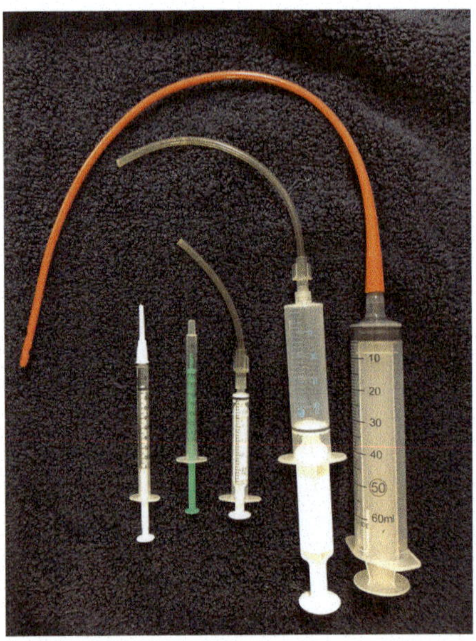

Figure 1.4 Feeding implements left to right: 1 ml O-ring syringe with plastic cannula tip; 1 ml syringe; 3 ml O-ring syringe with short cut section of IV extension set tubing (note cut end has been burned to round sharp edges); 20 ml syringe with cut section of IV extension set tubing (note cut end has been burned to round sharp edges); 60 ml syringe with red rubber feeding tube. *Source:* photo courtesy of Guthrum Purdin.

Use the smallest gauge needle possible when giving subcutaneous fluids; a 25–30 gauge works well for small chicks, 23–25 for larger-bodied chicks. Tiny altricial hatchlings less than 5 g may bruise regardless of how small a needle is used; hence, hydrate these chicks orally whenever possible. Intravenous fluids may be feasible in larger chicks, the medial metatarsal vein is the best option in many species. In this author's opinion, intraosseous fluids are not advisable in wild chicks due to risks of damage to long bone growth plates and joints by caregivers inexperienced with using this method in young birds.

Precocial chicks, such as ducklings, may drink and eat on their own once they are warm and feel safe. Provide water in shallow dishes with rocks or other space-occupying masses to prevent the birds falling into the water and drowning or becoming cold and wet. Small precocial chicks such as quail or killdeer are often extremely stressed when brought into captivity, and may arrive in care well below hatch weight after a period of extreme stress. Debilitated precocial chicks may require hand hydration one drop at a time with a wet cotton swab or small syringe moved along the bill until a swallowing motion is observed (see Chapter 24). These chicks may be hypoglycemic and benefit from administration of glucose.

If a chick is depressed or not swallowing well, oral rehydration must be done very carefully because there is a substantial risk of aspiration of fluids into the respiratory system. It may be better in this circumstance to wait for the animal to absorb SQ fluids, rather than giving oral fluids too quickly. If SQ fluids are not an option, give tiny amounts of oral fluids deep into the mouth and ensure that the bird swallows everything before giving more.

Start altricial birds on a hand-feeding diet after they begin passing droppings (see specific chapters for diet information). If an altricial chick does not begin passing droppings within 1 hour of giving rehydration fluids, begin feeding a hand-feeding diet, but keep the diet dilute and the meal size small until droppings are seen. See Chapter 2 for assistance identifying the chick, and then proceed to the most appropriate chapter for further instructions and information on what to feed.

## Baby Birds are Not Baby Mammals with Feathers

***Day/Night Schedules:*** Most commonly encountered species are primarily diurnal (day-active) animals, and unlike mammalian neonates, require 8–10 hours of uninterrupted sleep. Most birds do not feed their young at night. Chicks will develop several problems if kept awake to feed all night, including crop or gut motility problems, and will show increased susceptibility to infection due to reduced immune competence. It is not advisable to keep the bird awake all night to be fed because the chick may die of exhaustion if not allowed to rest. Even sickly or injured chicks benefit from a solid night's sleep and generally will awaken stronger than when put to bed. Fretting over the chick all night is in no one's best interest, especially the chick's. Once the sun goes down or the lights are off, chicks settle in to go to sleep. Altricial chicks often stop passing droppings and appear to spend the night metabolically recovering from the stress of the day. First thing when the lights go up, chicks awaken, begin actively begging for breakfast, and pass an overnight dropping after the first meal. This strong day/night schedule means that chicks will remain active and expecting more food until the lights go off; hence it is beneficial in nurseries to start turning the lights down as the day's feedings wind down in the evening, and then shut the lights off when feedings stop so that chicks do not waste energy fruitlessly begging. End of day cleaning activities should happen as quietly and dimly lit as possible.

***Nighttime Admissions:*** If a bird is brought into care at night, any life-threatening conditions should be treated and rehydration therapy initiated, and then the bird should be allowed to remain warm, dark, and quiet until transferred to an experienced caretaker in the morning. However, if the bird is extremely young or debilitated, a feeding or two once it is warm and rehydrated may be beneficial before bedding it down for the night. Freshly hatched chicks have the benefit of a yolk sac that may continue to provide nutrition for 12–24 hours after hatching.

## Physical Examination

Each chick should receive a complete physical examination once it is warm, and exams should be repeated regularly during care in order to spot problems before they become serious. Exams should be performed in a habitual, systematic manner to avoid missing subtle problems possibly missed if distracted by glaringly obvious abnormalities. With practice, a complete physical should only take a few minutes.

### Visual Exam

A visual exam should include the container in which the chick arrived. Any droppings, blood, parasites, or food should be noted. Assess the chick's general posture and attitude: Is it alert or depressed, standing or prone, showing normal movements or convulsing, open-mouth breathing or regurgitating? Is the head drooping or held tilted or straight? Are the wings symmetrical? Does it have an obvious fracture? Is the chick abnormally unsteady when walking or trying to perch if it is old enough to do so? Is it dragging any limbs? Limping? Are there visible areas of swelling? Are there signs of bleeding or disturbed areas of feathering? Are there any unusual odors? What is the species and age? Is the chick covered with food? If so, what kind?

### Hands-on Exam

Restrain chicks carefully for a full physical examination. Be as gentle as possible and do not allow the chick to become chilled again. The exam can occur in numerous short periods spread out over several hours if necessary. If the chick shows any open-mouth breathing during handling, stop and allow the chick to rest and become calm before further handling. If a major injury is found immediately, stop active bleeding and then complete the rest of the physical examination, evaluating the major injury last. Prognosis for recovery from a single severe injury may be good; multiple serious problems hold a much graver prognosis.

***Skin Tone:*** If the chick is unfeathered, what is the color of its skin and flesh? Although skin color varies, most altricial chicks should be pinkish. Although some species may have black, green, or yellowish skin, white and gray are not often normal colors for the flesh of young birds. With a modicum of experience one can spot a bird that is pale due to anemia or poor perfusion. Ectoparasites are a common cause of anemia.

***Eyes:*** Is the chick old enough to expect the eyes to be open? If so, are they open? Any chick fully feathered or old enough to stand should have its eyes open. Are they caked with food? Wild chicks that have been fed by the general public often have food in their eyes that requires irrigation with ophthalmic saline solution. Are the eyes symmetrical? Is the bird tending to hold one eye closed? Check pupil size and response to light, although this may be difficult to interpret in young birds. Birds have voluntary control over iris muscles; hence, a lack of pupillary light response does not mean the bird has a vision problem. Are the pupils dilated or constricted? Look for lacerations and scratches, hemorrhage, conjunctivitis, discharge, or swelling of the eyelids. Are there any cloudy or opaque areas to the lens or cornea? Is there blood visible inside the eye? Is the third eyelid functioning? Is its movement normal or slow? Is the iris normally positioned within the globe? If warranted, use fluorescein stain to examine for corneal ulcers and examine the retina with an ophthalmoscope.

***Nares and Bill:*** Check the nares and bill for discharge, patency, symmetry, dried food, masses, or parasites. Fly eggs or freshly hatched maggots are easily overlooked, but are frequently found in the nares. Soft swellings may indicate parasites such as bot fly larvae which will need removal. Beak fractures and dislocations are sometimes seen. Examine the beak for cracks, bruises, and proper occlusion. In all wild species in North America, with the exception of crossbills, the top and bottom beak tips should be well aligned.

***Mouth:*** Check the color of the oral mucous membranes. Bird species vary widely in normal oral mucous membrane color from yellow to purple to pink to black, and some species have unusual markings inside the mouth. The conjunctiva or skin tone may be a better gauge of perfusion than the mouth in some species. Look for parasites or blood within the mouth. The presence and state of gape flanges at the corners of the mouth will help determine how old the bird is, because these regress as the bill matures. These flanges are sometimes torn in injured chicks. Stringy saliva suggests significant dehydration. Look for plaques, swelling, discharge, and abscesses in the mouth. Some species, such as roadrunners and cuckoos, have normal markings within the mouth that must not be mistaken for lesions. *Trichomonas gallinae* affects many species and may result in malodorous whitish plaques and masses within the mouth, throat, or crop. Similar lesions can be seen with vitamin deficiencies or viral, yeast, and bacterial infections. Perform a wet mount of a throat swab to differentiate potential pathogens if suspicious lesions are present.

***Ears:*** Are there any signs of parasites, blood, or infection in the ears? Are there any lacerations, discharge, or swelling? Young chicks with head injuries may show a protuberant everted ear canal.

***Scalp and Skull:*** Is there evidence of swelling, bruising, or lacerations on the head? Gently palpate the skull for indentations, scabbed areas, or crepitus. The skulls of chicks are not fully calcified and normally feel soft. If a chick appears to have a wound such as what might be a skull puncture, clean the wound carefully and use the chick's neurologic status as a guide for prognosis. Scalp lacerations exposing the skull should be closed or dressed as any other wound. Old, dry, skull-exposing lacerations often heal well when dressed to keep moist and clean.

***Crop:*** Palpate the crop for contents if the species has a crop. Is it empty or full? Does it feel like normal food or is it mushy or hard? Is it leaking contents from a laceration? Crop lacerations are quite common in young doves and pigeons or birds caught by predators. Impactions are common for chilled, dehydrated birds with food in the crop due to lack of gut motility. In some cases, when the material is either unlikely to pass or is decomposing, it may need to be removed once the chick is warm and well-hydrated. Crop infections may be a primary problem in an unthrifty chick. Yeast infections are common and may show as a gassy crop. Microscope examination of a direct smear from a crop swab is often informative.

***Abdomen:*** Gently palpate the abdomen. It should feel soft. Many altricial hatchlings have abdominal organs that are easily visualized through the skin. Markedly dehydrated chicks may have firm or hard-feeling abdominal organs and wrinkled skin over the abdomen, both of which may resolve with fluid therapy. Chicks that have fallen onto hard surfaces may have blood visible inside their abdomen or even herniated viscera. Hatchlings with intraabdominal bleeding do not do well. However, older chicks may recover, depending on the severity. Hernias can be surgically repaired. Use the chick's attitude as a guide for prognosis. Precocial chicks sometimes present with an umbilical hernia or infection, or an unabsorbed yolk sac that has not been normally resorbed. Check the vent for lesions, diarrhea, patency, crusted droppings, and normal sphincter tone. Gently wash the vent with warm water if necessary, without soaking or chilling the chick.

***Nutritional Status and Body Wounds:*** Assess body condition by palpating the muscle mass of the breast and over the hips. Look and feel for areas of scabbing, bruising, and feather loss or damage. In most passerines, one can blow air to part the feathers, allowing a view of the skin between the feather tracts. This works well to spot punctures, lacerations, bruising, and subcutaneous emphysema (air under the skin). In the author's experience, emaciated or malnourished chicks with major injuries do not do well, but well-fleshed chicks may recover fully from surprisingly severe injuries.

***Skeleton:*** Inspect the limbs and joints. Gently palpate, flex, and extend all limbs and each joint separately. Note the presence of pain, heat, swelling, deformities, and asymmetries, limitation of motion, bone firmness vs rubberiness, crepitus, dislocation, or fractures. Midshaft tibiotarsus fractures are quite common, with many times more leg fractures than wing fractures seen in chicks. Check for lacerations, other lesions, and missing nails and toes. Lacerations are especially common around the knees and thighs of small birds, especially if caught by cats. Evaluate muscle tone of the tail as limpness may indicate a spinal injury. Palpate the vertebral column and hips for injuries or deformities. Spinal deformities are sometimes seen in certain species. Examine each toe and ensure it is normally formed and pointed in the right direction. Do the feet grip?

Fractured limbs must be considered life-threatening in wild chicks because they need to have fully functional limbs in order to qualify for release. With a small amount of handling or thrashing in a cage (or restraint for radiographs), a formerly fixable fracture may quickly become a limb that requires amputation, which is usually a death sentence. Hence, it is very important to keep the chick from flapping or kicking a fractured limb while finishing the rest of the exam. As soon as the bird is stable enough to tolerate the handling, the fracture should be at least temporarily immobilized. Fracture stabilization and repair is described in Stocker (2005) and in great detail by type of bird in Duerr and Purdin (2017). Permanent placement for disabled wildlife is often not available. If a wild chick is likely to be disabled to the point of not being able to function in the wild, euthanasia should be considered.

Chicks with metabolic bone disease (MBD) may show rubbery or deformed long bones on physical examination and perhaps one or more folding fractures. Mild cases may present with subtle fractures or angular deformities of the proximal tarsometatarsus or other long bones. If able to be corrected into a normal shape, these fractures may heal well with light stabilizing external splints while the chick's dietary deficiencies are corrected (see individual chapters). Once placed on a balanced diet, many birds will quickly calcify their long bones if the diet is corrected to a calcium to phosphorus ratio of at least 2 : 1 (mg to mg); insufficient calcium is the usual reason for MBD in wild chicks (Klasing 1999). If there are marked or uncorrectable skeletal deformities, euthanasia should be considered.

***Feathers:*** Evaluate feather condition. Malnourished chicks often exhibit poor feather condition with ragged or broken feathers, adhered feather sheaths, and stress marks (aka stress bars, fault bars). Abnormally whitish feathers are sometimes seen in malnourished crows, jays, House Sparrows, and others. Missing or broken feathers may also provide evidence of predator attack. Ectoparasites such as mites and feather lice are common.

***Droppings:*** Normal droppings vary widely by species, but in most small-bodied altricial chicks, feces are enclosed in a mucus envelope. When these species have diarrhea, encapsulation is lost and the droppings are wet, messy, sometimes malodorous, and often soil the chick. If the bird is emaciated, droppings look or smell odd, or the bird has diarrhea, a feces examination and a mouth/crop swab should be performed to look for parasites or budding yeast (e.g. *Candida* spp.). Fecal examination may need to wait until the bird passes significant feces. Routine fecal examination of all wild birds admitted for care is prudent, and fecal exams later in care can catch parasitism problems not identified at admission – bear in mind that parasites also take time to grow up and start passing eggs to be found in fecal matter. Bacterial infection is another common cause of diarrhea in chicks. Gram stains of feces may be informative.

## Common Medical Problems

In addition to the previously discussed hypothermia and dehydration, common medical problems encountered in chicks presented for care include one or more of the following: lacerations from attack by cats or other predators; fractures and soft-tissue trauma due to falling from nest or cat attack; emaciation secondary to either parasite load, parental separation, or poor care by finder (including eye or skin infections from being covered in food); malnutrition with poor feather condition with or without accompanying MBD; malnutrition or maldigestion due to diet quality or quantity, heavy parasite loads, crop infections due to yeast or bacteria, and other problems, including contagious diseases.

### Wounds

Chicks should be warm and well-hydrated before wound care occurs and it is preferable to give the bird a break for rest, warmth, and food between bouts of treatment if wounds are extensive or the chick is very stressed. Do not allow a chick to become cold while wound care occurs. Pain medications are merited prior to treatment; depending on age, species, and available resources, anesthesia may or may not increase the chick's probability of a good outcome. Wear disposable exam gloves when possible to avoid contaminating a wound with human bacteria.

Chicks with wounds should be placed on a course of broad-spectrum antibiotics, such as amoxicillin with clavulanic acid, at 125 mg/kg orally twice daily (Hawkins et al. 2018) until the wound heals. Be sure antibiotics are not discontinued until the wound has completely healed; merely being covered with a scab does not count as "healed" as scabs often cover serious problems. Some wildlife veterinarians continue antibiotics for several days after external wounds have healed to reduce the likelihood of complications, especially in cases of body cavity punctures.

Wounds should be cleaned, debrided, and closed primarily whenever possible, both to speed healing and to reduce development of stress bars on growing feathers. Rapid healing is especially important in wild chicks that must have perfect plumage at release. The longer the bird must stay in captivity, the more likely it is to develop additional physical or behavioral problems.

The nature of the injury may be obscured by dried blood, debris, or disarrayed feathers. For tiny chicks (or older eyes doing the examining), magnification and good lighting is helpful. Begin with gross removal of debris from the wound with sterile or disinfected forceps, hemostats, or other appropriate tools. Cotton swabs and gauze also can be helpful. The younger and smaller the chick, the more delicate the skin; be very careful to not tear it. Pluck toward the wound whenever possible to avoid ripping the wound larger, or hold flat-tipped forceps on the skin at the base of each feather with your other hand to reduce tension. Follow the wound margin to fully identify the extent of the lesion. Do not remove flight or tail feathers if at all possible, especially when in blood as it is preferable to allow soft tissues to heal with a feather in the follicle. If partially-grown blood feathers are broken and bleeding, they may need removal. Species vary in how plucking is tolerated, how difficult particular feathers are to remove, and how follicles respond. Never cut or shave feathers. Be very conservative in removing feathers from swimming species; use tape to hold feathers back during wound closure instead.

Once gross debris has been manually removed, follow by irrigating the area with warm sterile 0.9% NaCl or other sterile physiologic fluid with or without dilute chlorhexidine, betadine, or other disinfectants. Irrigation is contraindicated in wounds that include an opening into the bird's air sac system. If uncertain whether irrigating a wound will risk drowning the bird, cleanse the area repeatedly with sterile gauze or swabs moistened with sterile irrigation fluids.

During wound cleaning it may become apparent that an important structure is involved in the wound. Prognosis and outcomes are highly dependent on what structures are involved. There are some tendons that can be lost without a perceptible effect on function, but losing a large bundle of tendons that completely control, for example, flexing or extending the hock joint, is not compatible with being a releasable wild bird. Quality of life must be assessed for captive birds with similar loss of function. The outcome of these cases is usually dependent on what function has been lost, but it is often worth attempting treatment to see what functionality is retained, especially in a young bird already metabolically busy creating new tissue during rapid growth. A wound that seems very large and concerning on a 70g gosling may seem minor one week later when the chick weighs >500g.

The author's preference is to close all open wounds via sutures or glue, especially in crowded wild-bird nursery situations. The more dressing changes a chick needs in a busy nursery, the less likely it is to actually happen in a timely manner. All abnormal-looking tissue should be removed from the wound if it is to be closed. For skin lacerations that do not have much tension, surgical tissue glues may provide adequate closure. Sutures are preferred for wounds with tension or located in high-mobility locations, such as adjacent to the knee, where glue will not hold. Semipermeable self-adhesive dressings such as hydrocolloid blister bandages or Tegaderm® (3M) cut to size may be used for wounds that are unable to be sutured or glued. There are many wound care products that are appropriate for use in young birds; however, merely dabbing some cream onto a wound does not foster optimal wound healing. Silver sulfadiazine cream is often used to treat exposed wounds if secondary intention healing is necessary, because it has both antifungal and antibacterial properties and it is water-soluble. Avoid the use of petroleum-based products such as ointments due to their inevitable undesirable contamination of feathers.

One advantage birds have over mammals is that bone exposure in wounds is usually much less concerning, and with appropriate care these areas heal very well. See Duerr (2016) for repair of degloving injuries to the neck and scalp, and Duerr (2018) for information regarding repair of keratin damage exposing pelican mandible, which is also applicable to bone exposure in any species near the feathered skin–bill keratin border.

### Subcutaneous Emphysema

Subcutaneous emphysema (air under the skin) is a common result of a cat attack or severe impact, in which one or more air sacs have been ruptured and leak air into subcutaneous spaces. This often resolves without treatment, but it may be helpful to remove the pressure if it is interfering with mobility or if it is causing the bird to become depressed. If necessary, puncture the bubble with a sterile needle, avoiding any visible skin blood vessels. Many cases will reinflate quickly and may require repeat punctures several times over the course of a few days. This problem may manifest 24–48 hours after presentation.

### Fractures

Fracture repair instructions, including splints and wraps and surgical repairs appropriate for most species of chicks, are available in Duerr and Purdin (2017). Dry brown bone at an open fracture generally is an indicator that the area is unlikely to heal with full return to function. Open joints are always of serious concern and healing that results in a fully functional joint is uncommon.

Wild birds may become depressed if encumbered by heavy or confining splints, and wraps may damage growing feathers. Hence, minimally restrictive wraps and lightweight splints are recommended. Only use tapes that can be removed without pulling out feathers and do not leave a sticky residue behind. Whenever possible, allow the chick to use their legs as normally as possible during healing; weight-bearing speeds bone healing. It is often contraindicated to immobilize a joint that is actively growing; creative solutions that allow the chick to grow normally while healing a skeletal injury are often needed. This includes sometimes doing nothing and not immobilizing the fracture at all, with the chick treated with cage (e.g. nest) rest.

If a fracture must be immobilized, consider:

- Baby bird bone often lacks enough density to hold fixators and pins.
- The bone may be twice as long in a week or so; growth may either engulf an intramedullary pin and render it irretrievable or the fracture may no longer be supported by the pin.
- The joints are also developing; maintaining range of motion in joints is imperative for the bird to have normal mechanical properties of the joint when it has finished growing.
- If the chick is headed for wild release, flight feathers must be able to continue growing unimpeded by any wraps or splints or pins.
- Chicks that need to be able to fly when adults must absolutely have fractures reduced prior to fixation to avoid loss of long bone length.
- Cross pins in an external fixator may hold a long bone at a certain length while it is trying to grow – this can either result in a bone that bends to conform to the fixator length, or in a bone that grows past the fixator while it pushes past the pins in slow motion. There are, however, circumstances when pins are appropriate in growing birds, see Duerr and Purdin (2017).

## Parasitism

For details regarding the most common and many uncommon parasites of wild birds, see Atkinson et al. (2008). With certain exceptions (e.g. Capillarids) (Yabsley 2008), helminth (i.e. multicellular, worm-like) parasites typically have a life cycle that involves one or more intermediate hosts, thus concerns for transmission from bird to bird during care are minimal in the absence of intermediates. Others, such as protozoan parasites, may be able to directly infect birds sharing housing or cause reinfection after treatment if housing is contaminated, although some require vectors to transfer infected blood such as ticks (e.g. *Babesia* spp.) or mosquitos (e.g. avian malaria), which to some extent can be controlled in captive environments. Individual chapters in this book discuss parasitic infestations relevant to the species covered. See Hawkins et al. (2018) for a thorough review of antiparasitics used in birds.

In general, the social needs of wild chicks during development outweigh the need to keep birds infested with parasites alone until deemed clear of parasites. With few exceptions, at least one conspecific companion should be paired with an infested chick; most single chicks should never be kept alone for more than a short period.

From a longer-term view, it is a likely benefit to wild chicks to have been exposed to the normal parasites of their species – a subclinical infestation of normal parasites is ideal. However, many chicks received for care are debilitated in many ways, recovering from starvation or injuries or both. Consequently, reducing a chick's parasite burden while it recovers and finishes growing up is reasonable. Once the bird is released it will be re-exposed to its usual parasites and will hopefully be able to manage them when in better health. The goal is not to completely eliminate parasites but to keep them in check during recovery.

***Ectoparasites:*** Mites, ticks, lice, flies, fleas, and leeches can cause severe debilitation due to anemia in chicks and spread many blood-borne diseases. Mites and lice are often treated with ivermectin at 0.2–0.4 mg/kg once orally (Hawkins et al. 2018); however, ivermectin takes many hours to have an effect, which seems an eternity while chicks (and caregivers) are crawling with mites. Many rehabilitators and wildlife veterinarians lightly dust the bird with Sevin Dust (GardenTech) in severe cases, which works very quickly. The National Pesticide Information Center has a factsheet on this class of chemicals available online http://npic.orst.edu/factsheets/carbarylgen.html#products. However, due to concerns about hazards to handlers and birds from skin and respiratory exposure, many have moved away from using carbaryl-based products in favor of permethrin or piperonyl butoxide/pyrethrin-based products, such as Ultra Care Bird Mite and Lice Spray (8 in 1 Pet Products). Gloves and good ventilation are recommended when applying chemical pesticides – each bird may only be sprayed once but the caregiver may be exposed a thousand times a year. Cover the bird's eyes when spraying with any chemical. See each chemical's Safety Data Sheet (SDS) before handling. Bathing the chick is another option to reduce mite numbers if the bird is strong enough to tolerate the stress; do not allow the chick to become chilled during the washing or drying process. Feather lice can cause substantial damage to plumage, and affected birds should also be sprayed with mite/lice spray. Look for oval tiny nits at the base of feathers. Nitenpyram (Capstar, Novartis) tablets can be dissolved in water and used as a flush to kill maggots in wounds. Ticks often drop off when they have finished having a blood meal, and may be affected by ivermectin. Flat flies (Hippoboscidae) are common on young pigeons, owls, and others in North America. These fast-moving dorsoventrally flattened flies may cause excitement or horrified reactions in caregivers when a fly suddenly pops out of a bird's plumage and flies at or onto the caregiver. They are resistant to fly swatters and are typically killed by an aggravated thumbnail after a madcap chase around the clinic. Waterfowl may have leeches residing within the sinuses.

***Endoparasites:*** Internal parasites should be diagnosed by direct wet mount and fecal examination, and treated accordingly. However, not all endoparasites can be diagnosed by fecal examination. Either the parasites are not being shed at the time of examination, or they are not shed in feces. Some helminths can be diagnosed from mouth swabs, such as oral capillaria in ducks or respiratory flukes in pelicans. Although gastrointestinal parasites are common, the GI tract is not the only bodily system affected by parasites. Soft swellings anywhere on the body not explainable and treatable as injuries may be due to parasites. Ocular flukes may cause havoc to the eyelids and nictitans. Multiple diagnostics may be necessary.

## Acknowledgments

Many thanks to Julie Skoglund and Guthrum Purdin for reviewing this chapter. Thanks also to the multitude of wildlife rehabilitators and veterinarians who have allowed me to pick their brains over the past 30 years, and to the thousands of birds that have taught me about their needs.

## Sources for Products Mentioned

Animal Intensive Care Unit: Lyon Technologies, Inc., 1690 Brandywine Avenue, Chula Vista, CA. 91 911, https://lyonvet.com.
Capstar (Nitenpyram): Novartis Animal Health, (800) 637-0281.
Sevin Dust: GardenTech, PO Box 24830, Lexington, KY 40524-4830, (800) 969-7200.
Tegaderm: 3M Corporate Headquarters, 3M Center, St. Paul, MN 55144-1000, (888) 364-3577.
Ultracare Mite and Lice Bird Spray: 8 in 1 Pet Products, Hauppauge, NY, (800) 645-5154.

## References

Atkinson, C.T., Thomas, N.J., and Hunter, D.B. (eds.) (2008). *Parasitic Diseases of Wild Birds*, 595 pp. Ames, IA: Wiley Blackwell.

Borgia, L. (2004). NWRA membership survey 2003: results and comparisons. *Wildlife Rehabilitation Bulletin* 22 (1): 37–42.

Code of Federal Regulations (2018). Title 50: Wildlife and Fisheries, Part 21 – Migratory Bird Permits, Subpart B – General Requirements and Exceptions, §21.12 General exceptions to permit requirements. U.S. Government Printing Office.

Duerr, R.S. (2016). Surgical repair of keel lesions and lacerations in aquatic birds. Proceedings of the Association of Avian Veterinarians Annual Conference at ExoticsCon, Portland, OR, pp. 83–88.

Duerr, R.S. (2018). Successful surgical management of pouch and bill injuries in pelicans. Proceedings of the Association of Avian Veterinarians Annual Conference at ExoticsCon, Atlanta, GA, pp. 363–367.

Duerr, R.S. and Purdin, G.J. (eds.) (2017). *Topics in Wildlife Medicine, Vol. 4: Orthopedics*, 206 pp. St. Cloud, MN: National Wildlife Rehabilitators Association.

Hawkins, M.G., Barron, H.W., Speer, B.L. et al. (2018). Birds. In: *Exotic Animal Formulary*, 4e (eds. J.W. Carpenter and C.J. Marion), 167–375. St. Louis, MO: Elsevier.

Klasing, K. (1999). *Comparative Avian Nutrition*, 350 pp. Cambridge, MA: CAB International.

Stocker, L. (2005). *Practical Wildlife Care*, 335 pp. Oxford, UK: Blackwell Publishing Ltd.

Yabsley, M.A. (2008). Capillarid nematodes. In: *Parasitic Diseases of Wild Birds* (eds. C.T. Atkinson, N.J. Thomas and D.B. Hunter), 463–497. Ames, IA: Wiley-Blackwell.

# 2

# Identification and Aging

*Linda M. Tuttle-Adams*

## Introduction

Identifying the species and assessing the age of chicks, especially those that arrive mostly naked or with a few downy feathers, can seem daunting (Figure 2.1). However, there are many reasons to make the effort as soon as possible, because species and age play an essential role in such decisions as reuniting versus fostering, diet, housing, and psychological development needs. This chapter describes the primary characteristics that help identify a chick's species (or at least place it in a family group) and help assess its age.

Although many of the basic needs of baby birds are similar, each species has unique requirements based on its physiological and psychological makeup. For example, except for some baby finches that need regurgitated seeds, nearly all passerine nestlings are fed arthropods (mainly insects). Misidentification can result in a baby bird being fed the wrong diet, which may have consequences for its health.

The difficulty with chick identification begins with a lack of readily available and comprehensive guides like those covering adults. Creating a guide to cover just the 900+ North American breeding species would be an insurmountable task, as it would need to include all the stages of development and subspecies variations. Additionally, there are many gaps in the knowledge about some species because of their secrecy in breeding behavior and inaccessibility of nests (Rodewald 2015). Relying on photos alone to identify a chick comes with its own set of issues, such as color interpretation and, of course, the inability of photos to convey behaviors and vocalizations. Moreover, photos often lack such information as size, weight, and location. One needs to know what key features to look for before searching through references, so it's essential to study the bird itself and recognize key features in order to reduce errors and arrive at a correct identification.

Social development is a very important aspect to address when captive-rearing birds. A necessary form of learning where a chick learns to recognize others of its own species is called imprinting. Imprinting occurs during a time in a young bird's life called the "sensitive period," beginning with the onset of focused vision (Bateson 1966, 1979; Welty and Baptista 1988). In precocial birds that hatch with their eyes open, imprinting on a parent (called filial imprinting) is immediate. In altricial birds, filial imprinting occurs around the second week of life, or later depending on species, when the eyes are fully open. After this initial period, birds may go through a period called sexual imprinting, when they learn mate preferences. During the

*Hand-Rearing Birds*, Second Edition. Edited by Rebecca S. Duerr and Laurie J. Gage.

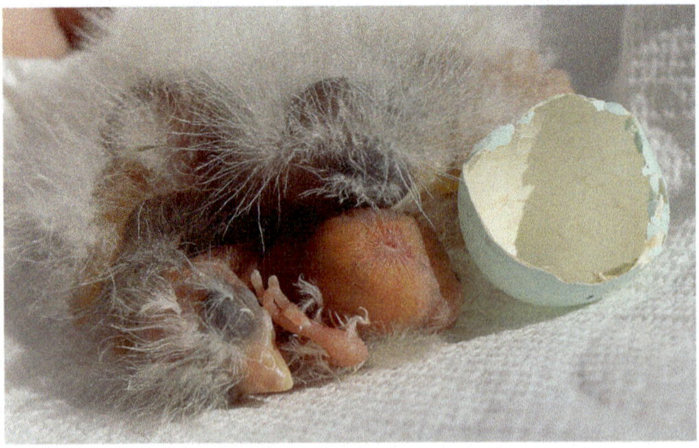

Figure 2.1 Just-hatched House Finch (1.5 g) with blue egg. Note grayish-brown down and beak shape already conical/finch-like. Gape color is pink. Gape flanges will swell and become more yellowish.

imprinting phase birds may also learn what foods they need to find, where their birthplace is, information about migratory paths, and in many species, songs and other species-specific communications. Incorrect imprinting occurs when a young animal imprints on something other than its own species, in which case it may not be accepted by its own kind and thus will be incapable of reproducing in the wild. Species known to be susceptible to incorrect imprinting are gallinaceous birds (turkey and quail), waterfowl (ducks, geese, swans), coots, raptors (especially some owls), some columbids (pigeons and doves), woodpeckers, roadrunners, corvids, Pygmy Nuthatch, icterids (blackbirds and orioles), and other small songbirds (Immelmann 1972; ten Cate and Vos 1999). For these species, it is critical that the first object they see is (in descending order of importance) a conspecific adult, a conspecific juvenile, or a combination of a taxidermy mount, a conspecific nest buddy, a mirror, and a photo of an adult. Traditional views of imprinting are that it is not reversible, but more current studies have shown that imprinting may be more flexible or forgiving than once believed (Hoffman and DePaulo 1977; Bolhuis et al. 1990). Until more is known, caregivers should take precautions and not make casual assumptions about the learning capabilities of chicks, especially those not well-studied. Many ways to prevent imprinting issues are mentioned in this book. The first step is to make a correct identification as early as possible.

Since identification is a process of comparison and elimination, it is essential to have a thorough knowledge of the most common species that live and reproduce in your area. That way, when an unusual bird arrives, it can be compared to eliminate common species and species that do not live in the area. Diligent questioning of the finder is helpful for gleaning clues about the chick's species, such as type of nest and whether parents were seen. However, caregivers need to discern whether a finder's information is based on opinion or perception rather than on knowledge and understanding. For example, a chick found on the ground below a colony of mud nests may not be a Cliff Swallow, since other species such as House Sparrows occasionally take over such nests.

The anatomic features of the chick from head to toe often can be used to identify a chick to the level of species, but it takes skill and a keen eye. This chapter will present several tables in which physical characteristics can be used to differentiate among taxonomic groups.

## The Key Characteristics

### Altricial Versus Precocial

There are two main divisions into which baby birds are divided, *altricial* and *precocial,* although there are numerous gradations between these extremes. Altricial chicks are blind, more-or-less naked, and helpless at hatching. Parents care for altricial chicks in the nest until they are old enough to venture into the outside world, usually at several weeks of age. Altricial chicks include all songbirds, raptors, herons, and many others. Precocial chicks have their eyes open, a full coat of warm downy feathers, and the ability to leave the nest as soon as they have dried off after hatching. Parents of precocial chicks typically provide warmth at night and protection from predators, and – although chicks are able to eat on their own – the parent shows them what to eat, how and where to find it, and what to avoid. Precocial chicks include most waterbirds, such as ducklings and shorebirds, plus chickens, quail, pheasants, and other Galliformes.

### Bill Shape

The beak or bill of a bird is one of its most distinguishing external features. Even without feathers, a bird can be placed in a particular family based on its beak. Passerine hatchlings have shorter beaks than passerine adults, but within a few days the contour of the beak begins to reveal the family, whether a flycatcher, a finch, or a thrush. The size of a flycatcher's beak may vary by species, but all are wide and flattened. Most have bristles at the base and slightly hooked tips. Finches and sparrows have short, stout, conical beaks, with a decurved culmen, and the commissure is abruptly angulated. Thrushes and mimids have large beaks and a big gape relative to head size (see Figure 45.3). Their beaks are variable in length (short to medium), straight, and slender, with the culmen decurved toward the tip. Beaks of precocial chicks are miniature versions of the adult beaks because these chicks are more developed at hatch.

### Mouth Color

In passerine birds, mouth color is a reliable feature for identifying family group, with some exceptions. The oral cavity of the mouth is lined with soft membranes, variously colored according to species, and consistent within most family groups. Some colors are more intense than others, some have spots or markings on the tongue or roof of the mouth, and some have colors in the UV range. The surrounding parts of the passerine mouth lining the edge of the bill, egg tooth, and gape flanges (swollen corners) are predominately white, yellow, or cream-colored (Clark 1969). If it has been determined that the chick is a passerine, the interior mouth color will considerably narrow the field, with choices in the yellow to orange range (Table 2.4) or pink to red range (Table 2.5). It should be noted that although many insectivores have colors in the yellow range and many omnivores and granivores have colors in the red range, there are several exceptions within the trophic categories (Ficken 1965). There are also some variations to keep in mind. Intensity of mouth color changes as the chick develops and may even change throughout the day. Color and intensity may be much reduced in unhealthy or cold chicks. Prominence of gape flanges varies by species, is reported to be more conspicuous in hole-nesting species (Kilner and Davies 1997), and regresses as young birds become self-feeding.

## Skin Color

For some species, true skin color in chicks can be difficult to assess because the skin is transparent, letting underlying tissues affect the color's appearance. As a result, skin color is not always a reliable identification feature. Most altricial nestlings hatch with a pinkish appearance that darkens even within the day. However, a few species appear to have yellowish-orange skin (as in some thrushes) or reddish skin (as in some blackbirds). Within columbids, the Mourning Dove hatches with blackish-gray skin while the Rock Pigeon has pink skin. Hatchling cuckoos and roadrunners have black skin.

## Feet

Table 2.1 presents foot topography, which is very helpful in determining species identity. A bird's feet, considered by most biologists to be the portion of the legs that includes the tarsometatarsus (or tarsus) and toes, are covered variously with feathers or scales or are smooth (booted) without scales or plates. The pattern of skin or scales and presence of feathers on the feet, as well as shape of the tarsus, can place a bird in a particular family. We do not provide a comprehensive listing of the various definitions and descriptions of these coverings; some, however, are presented in the tables.

Table 2.1 Types of foot topography.

| Type | | Description | Typical Birds |
|---|---|---|---|
| Anisodactyl | | Three toes pointed forward, one toe (hallux) pointed back. | Most common arrangement. Herons, egrets, quail, turkey, pheasant, nighthawks, ibis, storks, guineafowl, pigeons and doves, vultures, spoonbill, falcons, and all passerines. |
| | | Sharp, decurved talons. | Accipitridae family of raptors. |
| Zygodactyl | | Two toes pointed forward, two toes pointed back. 4th toe permanently reversed. | Woodpeckers (except three-toed and black-backed), cuckoos, roadrunners, most parrots. |
| | | 4th toe reversible. Same as above, toes can rotate to look like x or + shape. | Owls, Osprey, turacos. |
| Pamprodactyl | | Hallux can rotate forward so all four toes point forward. | Swifts (some species hold toes anisodactyly). |
| Syndactyl | | Third and fourth toes fused together for most of their length. | All Coraciiformes (kingfishers) and hornbills. |
| Webbed | Palmate | Forward three toes fully webbed with small hallux placed high on metatarsus. | Waterfowl, loons, flamingo, gulls, terns. |
| | Semipalmate | Partial web between front toes. Hallux absent or reduced. | Plovers (such as killdeer) and other shorebirds, ibis, herons. |
| | Lobate | Lobes of skin around toes, not attached to each other. | Grebes, phalaropes, some diving ducks. |
| | Semilobate | Separate lobes on each joint of toes. | Coots |
| | Totipalmate | Webbing connecting all four toes (hallux pulled medially). | Pelicans and cormorants, boobies, tropic birds, frigatebirds, anhinga. |

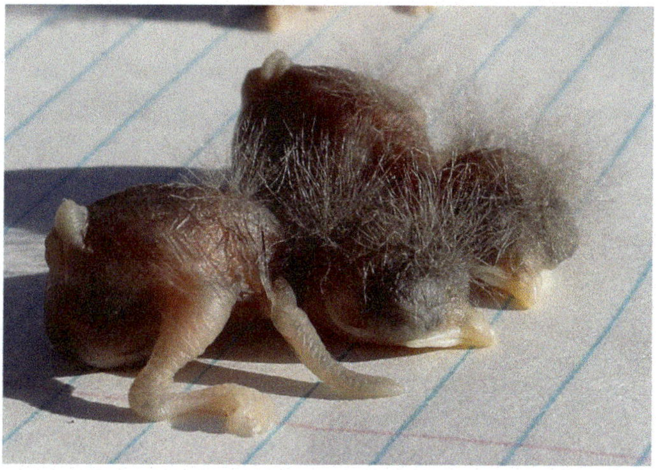

**Figure 2.2** House Wren hatchlings (~1 g). Note tufts of dark gray down only on dorsal tracts, thickest on crown. They can use their wings to propel themselves, and the rear end is characteristically pointed upwards.

## Plumage

Natal down – its presence or absence and, if present, its color, pattern of distribution, and abundance of neossoptiles (first feathers) – can help identify a species (see Figure 2.2). The natal down of precocial species is abundant and covers the entire chick. Precocial chicks of Galliformes have a particular species-specific pattern when viewed dorsally. Woodpeckers, kingfishers, swifts, hummingbirds, some vireos, some wrens, House Sparrows, and Cedar Waxwings hatch completely naked, do not develop true down, and develop their juvenile plumage as their first feathers. Corvids hatch naked or with barely visible down that thickens by day two or so. Some birds, such as kites and falcons, grow two successive coats of down before they molt into their juvenile plumage.

Plumage patterns and markings on the head or tail can sometimes aid identification. Many sparrows have white outer tail feathers (rectrices). Some species are strongly counter-shaded, such as the Black Phoebe, which is dark dorsally with white underparts. Most thrush chicks are spotted. Orange patches on the top of the rump could indicate a Cliff Swallow; rufous undertail coverts could indicate a Gray Catbird. Most young birds resemble the adult female for purposes of protection, but a few species, such as bluebirds, will show the adult color and can be sexed at 12 days. The posterior margin of the tail is another key in that it assumes various shapes: square in Accipiters, rounded in ravens, pointed in pheasants and Mourning Doves, and forked in terns and Barn Swallows.

## Size and Weight

Another aid to identification is to compare the weight and size of a young bird to the weights and sizes of species of similar measurements *at the same age*. Also, check to ensure the chick does not weigh more than the adult of the species being considered. In general, a fledgling altricial chick should weigh less than or about the same as an adult female, except in the case of species (e.g. swallows) that weigh more than the adult when they fledge. One way to tell American Robin and Northern Mockingbird nestlings (often mistaken for each other) apart is to note that at all stages of life, the robin will always be larger and weigh more than the mockingbird.

### Developmental Clues

If hatching is not witnessed, a chick's age can be estimated without taking measurements other than weight, via known developmental stages of the family group. Measurements of wing chord, tarsus, gape, and culmen are reliable variables *if* there are standards available for the species for comparison. Table 2.2 demonstrates age by feather development and typical behavior in most passerines. Eyes of altricial young *begin* to open at a predictable age, thus helping to reinforce age estimates; however, illness or injury may complicate evaluation. Eye color is helpful in aging species in which iris color changes as the bird matures, such as Spotted Towhees, Brewer's Blackbirds, and many hawks.

## Putting It All Together

Consider a sample identification process. A baby bird arrives, found on the ground, no parents or nest observed. Is the chick precocial or altricial? If fully covered in down, it's precocial, so note the down pattern on the dorsal view and check the type of foot (webbed, partially webbed, chicken-like). If naked or mostly naked with some down on the dorsal view, it's altricial. Note the foot arrangement. If zygodactyl, check for key features of woodpeckers; if they are not found locally, consider other zygodactyl type birds. All passerine birds are altricial with an anisodactyl toe arrangement. Is it passerine or nonpasserine? What is the weight and size? Then note the beak shape and length (relative to head). What is the color of the mouth interior and gape flanges and are they thin or thick? If the skin is pinkish, the baby could be one of several species. If its skin is yellowish-orange, consider robin or bluebird; if reddish, look at blackbird species. At this point, the identification should be narrowed down to a family or two. Describe the natal color and abundance of the down or, if the bird has some juvenile feathers, note the colors. Consult the tables on all clues found, and compare the chick's weight with that of the adult of the species being considered. Regardless of an early guess at an identification, go through all the steps for confirmation. Also, always consider geography and typical species encountered in the area while remembering that nature can throw a curve ball.

The next tables present key nestling characteristics and developmental (age) markers for a selection of species from most taxonomic orders. Table 2.3 covers nonpasserine species organized by type of development and foot topography. Tables 2.4 and 2.5, organized by interior mouth color, cover a selection of passerine chicks of common or widely distributed North American breeding species. Closely-related species in other parts of the world with broad distribution may be present as examples in the tables; close taxonomic relatives also often have similar captive requirements. Data in the tables were extracted from the Birds of North America (BNA), an online reference of the life histories of over 760 breeding birds in the U.S. and Canada (Rodewald 2015), numerous scientific publications, data collected personally from bird carcasses (frozen and prepared), personal observations of wild and captive songbirds, and conversations with many songbird rehabilitators across the U.S. and Canada. Tables 2.4 and 2.5 are a sampling from a comprehensive collection of key characters of 200+ passerine species, which will be included in a soon-to-be-published guide by the author on *How to Identify Baby Birds*.

Although learning to identify and age young birds takes practice, research, and patience, it can be very rewarding. As the lives of birds become better understood, the standards of care for birds in captivity improve. Caregivers – whether they specialize in a species, a family group, or birds with similar lifestyles – are able to save time and costs and to provide housing enrichment and social atmosphere that better simulates the birds' natural lives. Early, definitive identification of baby birds that must be hand-raised by humans greatly enhances their ability to survive and thrive in nature once released.

Table 2.2 Stages of life and development of passerine birds.

| Stage of Life | Days | Description |
|---|---|---|
| Hatchling Stage | 0 (hatch day) | Skin is thin and transparent. Down may be sparse or thick in one area or all over, or there may be no down at all. Eyes are closed and bulbous. Unable to thermoregulate; must be brooded by parent. Weak. |
| | 1 | Pinfeathers may be becoming visible (pigmented) beneath skin in dorsal tracts. Begs for food. |
| | 2 | Most feather tracts, especially primaries, show through skin. First food calls. |
| | 3 | Beak darkens and begins to take shape. Gape flanges thicken and become brighter. Mouth interior color intensifies. Egg tooth may have disappeared. Feather tracts continue to darken as pins grow. Down may thicken. Eyes are partly open (slits). Most can raise head and gape. May use wings as props. |
| Nestling Stage | 4–5 | Beginning of rapid growth stage and increase in weight. Pinfeathers develop along tracts. Ventral feather tracts are visible, but belly and chest area up to neck are bare. Primaries pierce through skin. Eyes still opening. Begins to use legs. Evacuates at edge or over nest rim. Voice is stronger. |
| | 5–6 | Some temperature control. Beginnings of motor coordination. |
| | 7–8 | Eyes are fully open (may be longer for cavity-nesting species). Rapid growth of motor coordination. Well covered with feathers. Primaries unsheathing. Down feathers, if present, are still attached to feather tips. Flutters when begging. Makes new calls for location and feeding. Freezes, cowers, crouches, and may snap bill when alarmed. Responds to alarm call of parent. |
| | 9–10 | Fully feathered; wing and tail feathers still growing. Temperature control nearly established; siblings keep each other warm. Juvenile plumage covers entire skin surface. Preens, scratches head, moves about, exercises wings, stays awake for longer periods, responds to parent's alarm calls, is alert to sights and sounds outside nest, may peck at objects on or near nest rim. Fear response very strong, if nest discovered or disturbed, may jump before it would normally fledge. |
| | 12–13 | May still have a few downy feathers protruding from head. Pecks at objects outside of nest. May be antagonistic toward siblings. Can perch, walk, and hop. May perch on edge of nest or may venture out onto a branch and flutter wings. |
| | 14–15 | Leaves nest. Exceptions: cavity-nesters and long-winged species take about 20 days. Longer for some cavity nesting species. To 44 days for large corvids. |
| Fledgling Stage | 9–22 | 70–80% of adult weight (or more depending on species). Breast feathers have grown in to cover ventral body. Tail is about half grown. Wings are not as long as those of adult. Can perch, walk, hop, or run well, but flight capability varies. In general, some species do not fly well at first; not capable of sustained flight for a few weeks. Cavity nesters fly better right out of nest than open-cup nesters. At first, fledgling remains mostly immobile and silent except for food calls and stays apart from nest mates. Sleeps in adult position with head under wing. Begins wiping beak, pecking at objects, and picking up food off the ground or catching insects in the air (swallows, flycatchers), working at grass heads (finches), or scratching at ground (sparrows). Pursues parent(s) for food, begging in horizontal rather than vertical position. Bathes, suns, and preens. |

Table 2.3 Key characteristics of representative NON-PASSERINE species, arranged taxonomically.

| Species | Feet (Tarsus/toes) | Weight (g) | Development and Integument | Beak / Mouth | Vocalizations | Other |
|---|---|---|---|---|---|---|
| **DUCKS, GEESE, SWANS (Anatidae):** Anisodactyl toe arrangement and palmate. Precocial young. | | | | | | |
| **Canada Goose** (*Branta canadensis*)<br>Refs: 1, 4, 7 (bna.cangoo.02) | Dark gray to black. | Hatch: 68–103<br>Adult: 2640–4858 Weight/size varies by subspecies. | Down: thick, yellow to greenish yellow with olive pattern colors and dark round cap on crown. Plumage becomes "dirty" olive-gray with distinctive cheek patch. | Just hatched: pale blue-gray to blackish gray, rounded at the tip. Egg tooth light and prominent. | Locator and recognition calls: single *peeps* or warbling *trills*, can become loud and intense when distressed. | Iris: blue-gray at hatch, then dark brown. |
| **Wood Duck** (*Aix sponsa*)<br>Refs: 1, 4, 7 (bna.169) | Brownish yellow and boldly patterned with black webbing. | Hatch: 19–28<br>Adult: F: 635, M: 681 | Down: thick, light yellow base color, darker on back with a few yellow patches (shoulders and rump), buffy yellow under and on face. Crown brown with defined dark stripe from eye to back of head, no eye stripe between eye and bill. Yellow lighter than mallard. | Just hatched: gray brown upper mandible; lower dull yellowish pink. Nail reddish brown, pale pink toward tip. Pale yellow egg teeth with lower bilobed. | A few days before hatch, give "click" calls. When alarmed, give high-pitched *peep*. Will *hiss* at predators or make shriek sound to alert others. | Iris: brown or grayish brown, Leave nest after last egg hatches. Jump to ground from nest cavity in tree. |
| **Mallard** (*Anas platyrhynchos*)<br>Refs: 1, 4, 7 (bna.658) | Orange with some gray-brown patterning. | Hatch: 31.8<br>Adult: F: 1095, M: 1246 | Down: fully covered, thick, yellow base color. Head: brown forehead, ear spot, and eye stripe that runs from base of bill through eye to back of head. Brown patches on back and wings. Hybrids or domestics may have odd coloring. | Just hatched: pink-beige with black spotting and black tip. Egg tooth. | Quiet pips or *pipi* (contentment), loud *peep* (distress). Air-alarm call (after 1 week): shrill *pii*. | Iris brown. Leave nest 13–16 hrs after hatching, tended by hen only, |

| | | | | | | |
|---|---|---|---|---|---|---|
| **Common Merganser** (*Mergus merganser*)<br><br>Refs: 1, 4, 7 (bna.442) | Olive-brown. | Hatch: 46.2<br><br>Adult: F: 1232, M: 1709 | Down: fully-covered, head dark brown to black, white eye stripe, white cheeks, rufous patch on neck, tawny brown patch over eye with dark streaks from bill to below eye, white ventral surface, flanks and dorsum dark brown, white patches on rump and wings. | Just hatched: slender, gray, relatively shorter than adult, not duck-like. Sharply serrated in adults. | Unknown. | Iris grayish brown. May remain in nest a day or so after hatching. May rest on back of hen. |
| **QUAIL, NEW WORLD (Odontophoridae)**: Anisodactyl toe arrangement. Precocial young. | | | | | | |
| **California Quail** (*Callipepla californica*)<br><br>Refs: 1, 7 (bna.473) | Dark gray.<br>Short hallux. | Hatch: 5–7<br><br>Adult: F: 162, M: 186 | Down: fully covered, buffy white background, rusty on dorsal and buff white below. Two dorsal stripes down back, one under each wing. Back of head has large dark brown patch with buff border. Dark spot at ear openings. Down pattern similar to Gambel's Q. but yellower. | Very short and gray (similar to chicken chick). | Just hatched emit "trill" call, then peeping or *pseu-pseu* call when distressed. Become highly stressed when alone or cold and may peep quietly with eyes closed. | Iris lighter brown than adult. Leaves nest right after hatch with parent. |
| **PHEASANT, TURKEY, AND RELATIVES (Phasianidae):** Anisodactyl toe arrangement. Precocial young. | | | | | | |
| **Ring-necked Pheasant** (*Phasianus colchicus*)<br><br>Refs: 1, 7 (bna.572) | Pink-white, become browner with age. Short hallux. | Hatch: 18.5<br><br>Adult: F: 953, M: 1317 | Down: fully covered, color varies. Light parts pale tawny to yellow buff, dark (or rufous) stripes on flanks and dorsum. Black spots over ears, black patches on wings. Sides of crown and brow cinnamon. | Short and chicken-like, pink horn-colored with black at base of upper beak. Egg tooth not retained very long. | 3 types of calls. Contentment: *Ter-rit* or *ter-wit*; caution: *Terreep* or *turreep*; flock call *tee-erp* or *pre-erp* (repeated). | Iris dark brown. Leaves nest with hen soon after hatch. |

(*Continued*)

Table 2.3 (Continued)

| Species | Feet (Tarsus/toes) | Weight (g) | Development and Integument | Beak / Mouth | Vocalizations | Other |
|---|---|---|---|---|---|---|
| **Wild Turkey** (*Meleagris gallopavo*)<br><br>Refs: 1, 7 (bna.22) | Buffy yellow at hatch turning vinaceous pink. | Hatch: 47<br><br>Adult: F: 3200, M: 6100 | Down: fully covered, cinnamon to tawny forehead and on back, breast and sides lighter. Sides of head pinkish buff to yellow. Chin, upper throat, and breast near white. Dark brown blotches on crown, nape, and upper body. Wings: primaries (1–7) project from sheaths at hatch. | Chicken-like but heavier, lower pale pinkish, upper darker pink. | Newly hatched chicks give a soft "purr" sound. Chicks give 3 types of peeping calls and a *putt* call when threatened. Poults give whistling (locator) call at 7 wk. when separated from brood. | Iris: sepia. Leave nest soon after hatching. |
| **GREBES (Podicipedidae):** Anisodactyl toe arrangement and lobate; legs situated far back on body, walking awkward. Semi-precocial young. | | | | | | |
| **Pied-billed Grebe** (*Podilymbus podiceps*)<br><br>Refs: 1, 7 (bna.410) | Grayish black. Asymmetrical lobes. | Hatch: 13.3–16.2<br><br>Adult: F: 358, M: 474 | Down: two downy stages. 1st: short, thin, back and sides black with 4 white stripes. Crown has 2 v-shaped stripes. Head and neck with black marks extending to white chest. Spot on crown and bar on nape cinnamon-rufous. | Bill: high, laterally compressed, tip has slight hook and decurved; pink with black in middle and white egg tooth on upper and lower mandible. Gape pink to reddish. | First few weeks, soft *seep-seep* calls associated with adult bringing food. Also, a *ee-ee-ee-ee-ii-ii-iah* call. When distressed a single, frequent *peep* note is given. | Iris black until end of first week, then changes to dark brown. Eye-ring rufous. Can swim shortly after hatching. Fed by both parents. Ride on parents' backs when small. |
| **Western Grebe** (*Aechmophorus occcidentalis*)<br><br>Refs: 1, 7 (bna.26a) | Slaty, near black with greenish lobes. | Within 1 day of hatch: 21.7, 34.4, 36.0.<br><br>Adult: F: 1199, M: 1429 | Down: dense, velvety, dark gray above, white below. Crown is bare and straw-yellow, turns scarlet when begging or when apart from parents. Clark's down: light gray. | Bill: black. White egg tooth on upper tip corresponds with white spot on lower. | Not known to make calls before leaving nest. | Iris black, then pale gray. White eye ring and lores. Rides on back of parent. |

| | | | | | | |
|---|---|---|---|---|---|---|
| **PIGEONS AND DOVES (Columbidae)**: Anisodactyl toe arrangement. Altricial young. | | | | | | |
| **Rock Pigeon** (*Columba livia*)<br>Ref: 7 (bna.13) | Pink to slate. Nails grayish black.<br>Note: Band-tailed Pigeon squabs have yellow feet. | Hatch: 15.2<br>Adult: F: 340, M: 369 | Skin: pink. Down: long, silky, light to bright yellow on head and body, may have reddish tint. | Leathery with smooth texture. Pinkish to dark gray, light at tip. | During feeding, make "squeaky" *peeps* become louder and more persistent as chick develops. | Eyes open: 4–5 d. Iris: medium or grayish brown. |
| **Mourning Dove** (*Zenaida macroura*)<br>Refs: 1, 7 (bna.117) | Olive gray turning geranium pink. | Hatch: 5–6<br>Adult: F: 115, M: 123 | Skin: blackish gray (olive) or yellowish. Down: off-white or cream. 2–3 d: primaries and tail feathers developing. 8–9 d: crown feathers appear. | Dark gray, leathery and smooth, lumpy around nares. Sharp egg teeth upper and lower beak tip. Gape: gray in squabs. | Weak *peeps* at first become louder with growth. | Eyes partly open: d 4–5, fully open 6–7 d. |
| **CUCKOOS AND ROADRUNNERS (Cuculidae)**: Zygodactyl toe arrangement. Altricial young. | | | | | | |
| **Black-billed Cuckoo** (*Coccyzus erythropthalmus*)<br>Refs: 1, 7 (bna.587) | Slate gray. Very strong. | Hatch: 7.4<br>Adult: 50.9 | Very alert and active. Skin: shiny black. Down: gray, "hair-like" on dorsal surface and thighs.<br>d 6: looks like "porcupine" as long contour feathers emerge. d 7: appears fully feathered.<br>Note: hatchling Yellow-billed Cuckoo has white down. | Slate gray.<br>Mouth: lining red or pink, with "complex pattern of large, creamy-white papillae," on palate and tongue. | Sounds like buzzing insect while begging. At 6–7 d when disturbed, makes grating "bark" call. | Eyes: lids and eye-ring yellow, partly open<br>2 d, fully open 4 d. Leave nest: ~6–7 d, unable to fly until 21–24 d. |
| **Greater Roadrunner** (*Geococcyx californianus*)<br>Refs: 1, 7 (bna.244) | Black. | Hatch: 14<br>Adult: 376 | Altricial, but very alert and active. Skin: black, has oily appearance. Down: white. | Black (pink at commissure) and triangular, narrower by fledgling. Black tongue tip. Mouth: lining red with 4 white markings and white hard palate. Rictus red. | Young chick makes rasping, buzzing, and hissing sounds with mouth open. Juveniles make calls similar to adult female "whine." May have critical period during which they learn calls. | Gapes when touched. Leave nest: 11 d. Fly: 17–18 d. |

(*Continued*)

Table 2.3 (Continued)

| Species | Feet (Tarsus/toes) | Weight (g) | Development and Integument | Beak / Mouth | Vocalizations | Other |
|---|---|---|---|---|---|---|
| **NIGHTHAWK, POORWILLS, AND NIGHTJARS (Caprimulgidae)**: Anisodactyl toe arrangement. Semiprecocial young. | | | | | | |
| **Common Nighthawk** (*Chordeiles minor*) Refs: 1, 7 (bna.213) | Small weak legs. Brown turning black, then plumbeous (d 17), metal gray d 20. | Hatch: 5.8–6.1 Adult: 79.3 | Down: soft, dark gray, paler underside. d 5: pins emerge on wings. d 13: appears fully feathered, primaries partially unsheathed. Very dark gray malar stripes. | Bill: tiny, pale mouse gray, turns darker 3–10 d, purplish gray at 17 d. Very wild gape. | Unknown. | Hatch with eyes open. Leave nest: 18 d (can walk around), 23–23 d, short flights. |
| **Common Poorwill** (*Phalaenoptilus nuttallii*) Refs: 1, 7 (bna.32) | Light grayish-brown. Small relative to body size. | Hatch: no information. Adult: 47.7 | Down: sparse, buff, darker dorsally. | Small and black with tubular nostrils. Gape very large. | Young raised in captivity did not make sounds until 25 d of age. | Hatch with eyes open. Fed regurgitated insects by adults. d 2: can move short distances. Leave nest: 20–23 d. |
| **SWIFTS (Apodidae)**: Pamprodactyl toe arrangement. Altricial young. | | | | | | |
| **Chimney Swift** (*Chaetura pelagica*) Refs: 1, 7 (bna.646) | Tarsus very short, toes strong with gray claws, can cling vertically as hatchling. Hallux rotates forward. | Hatch: 1.0–1.5 Adult: 23.6 | Skin: pink. Down: none. d 4: pins visible under skin in tracts, pierce through skin d 5–6. Wings unsheathed 10–12 and contour feathers ~ d 12–14. Has small wing claw near alula, helps cling on vertical surface. | Small, weak, light gray. Mouth: drab interior, no gape flanges. | Hatchling begging sounds: weak, squeaking sounds, at 3 d *cheh, cheh, cheh*; 5 d louder *chuh, chuh, chuh*. At 5 wk. make "chipper call" of adult. Disturbance calls of young a rasping *raah, raah, raah*. | Eyes open: d 14–16. Leave nest: 28–30 d, fly well. |
| **HUMMINGBIRDS (Trochilidae)**: Anisodactyl toe arrangement. Altricial young. | | | | | | |
| **Anna's Hummingbird** (*Calypte anna*) Refs: 1, 7 (bna.226) | Tarsus is short; toes are very tiny. | Hatch: <1 Adult: 4.3 | Skin: black. Down: "smoky fuzz" in 2 lines of tracts running along the spine. 7 d: numerous pinfeathers. 13–14 d: head is feathered, flutters wings. 18–19 d: extends tongue. | Short and squat. Mouth interior yellow. | Sharp *Tzip* call is most frequent at any age. Begging sound is a high, short *seet* call. | Eyes open: 5 d. Begging call: high thin *seet*. Leave nest: 23–24 d. Dependent on female parent 1–2 wk. |

| | | | | | | |
|---|---|---|---|---|---|---|
| **RAILS (Rallidae)**: Anisodactyl toe arrangement; some (e.g. coots) are semilobate, others not. Precocial young. | | | | | | |
| **Virginia Rail** (*Rallus limicola*)<br><br>Refs: 1, 7, 9 (bna.173) | Fuscous (or dusky brown), adult size 3–4 wk. | Hatch: 5–5.8<br><br>Adult: 84.1 | Down: glossy black, bare on crown. Wings have claws. Able to walk almost immediately, swim same day as hatch. | Bill: pale pink, dark band around center, widens as chick grows. | Young chicks *pee-eep*, then calls (1–2 syllables) become more intense when separated from family members. | Fed by parents 1st 3–7 d or up to 21 d. Leave nest: 3–4 d post-hatch, may return for a few days. |
| **American Coot** (*Fulica americana*)<br><br>Refs: 1, 7 (bna.697a) | Very large, greenish-gray or blackish-gray, and lobed on each toe joint. | Hatch: 19–22<br><br>Adult: F: 560, M: 724 | Down: thick, black. Tips of down "stiff, curly, and hair-like," long and orange on dorsum and wings, short and yellow on ventrum. Ruff of "wirelike" down encircles neck. Crown is scarlet with little down. Skin above eyes blue. By 15 d, colored body plumes are gone. Full adult plumage 50–60 d. | Bill: orange-red to blood-red at base, with black tip and white egg tooth. By 15 d bill bright orange-red. | 4 call types of captive raised chicks: twitter, *wit-ou*, squawk, and *yeow*. | Quickly mobile but fed by adults at first. Somewhat self-feeding by 8 d, seldom fed after 28 d. Joint (pollex) on wing that bears the alula has 1 mm claw. Fly at 75 d. |
| **CRANES (Gruidae)**: Anisodactyl toe arrangement. Precocial young. | | | | | | |
| **Sandhill Crane** (*Antigone canadensis*)<br><br>Refs: 1, 7 (bna.31) | Long legs, yellowish or pinkish. Short hallux higher than plane of other toes. | Hatch: 114.2<br><br>Adult: 2982–5797 (subspecies vary) | Down: thick, fully covered (including crown), rusty brown color, grayish-white underparts. Dark mark in front of eye. Dark brown on upper back (diamond-shaped) and on rump. | Narrow, beige-pink, darkening toward tip. | 3 calls: pipping, (trills and peeps), contact (high-pitched yelp), and stress (slurred notes that are loud and rapid). | Eyes: dark umber or gray.<br>A few hours after hatch able to sit on hocks and stand (weakly). Leaves nest and begins feeding next day. |

(*Continued*)

Table 2.3 (Continued)

| Species | Feet (Tarsus/toes) | Weight (g) | Development and Integument | Beak / Mouth | Vocalizations | Other |
|---|---|---|---|---|---|---|
| **STILTS AND AVOCETS (Recurvirostridae):** Anisodactyl toe arrangement and semipalmate, lack hallux. Precocial young. | | | | | | |
| **American Avocet** (*Recurvirostra americana*)<br><br>Refs: 1, 7 (bna.275) | Long, olive tinge in juvenile. Hallux is clawed and very small. Webs are more developed between 3rd and 4th digits. | Hatch: 19<br><br>Adult: F: 302, M: 307 | Down: fully covered. Dorsal view is drab with cinnamon tones, crown and back mottled jet-black. Cream to white underparts. Gray nape. Dark lines beginning at shoulders meet into single line at mid-back, becomes spotty toward tail. Thin black line through eye, solid or broken or indistinct. | Short, jet-black, nearly straight in nestling. | Make a *chip-chip-chip* call when stressed or captured. | Leave nest 1–24 hr. after last chick hatches. Able to follow parents by walking or swimming, stronger by 2nd day. Fly: 27 d. |
| **PLOVERS (Charadriidae)**: Anisodactyl toe arrangement and semipalmate. Precocial young. | | | | | | |
| **Killdeer** (*Charadrius vociferus*)<br><br>Refs: 1, 7, 9 (bna.517) | Partial webbing (for swimming); lacks hallux. Tarsus pink-buff. Nails black. | Hatch: 9.6–10.1<br><br>Adult: F: 101, M: 92.1 | Down: completely covered, mottled buff, brown, black on back. White on forehead, chin, throat, belly, and neck ring. Black stripe runs back from the eye. Wreathlike black stripe around crown. Broader black band collars neck. Black mid-dorsal stripe (normally broken). | Glossy black, short, blunt wedge. Mouth interior: pink or grayish-pink. | High-pitched piping calls when distressed such as when separated from parents. | Eye ring: bare, yellowish- gray; changes to red by juvenile. Iris dark. Able to leave nest soon after hatching. Become motionless if approached. Fly: 20–31 d. |
| **SANDPIPERS AND RELATIVES (Scolopacidae)**: Anisodactyl toe arrangement and semipalmate. Precocial young. | | | | | | |
| **Marbled Godwit** (*Limosa fedora*)<br><br>Refs: 1, 7 (bna.492) | Long, blue-gray tarsus with small hallux. | Hatch: 37<br><br>Adult: F: 391, M: 326 | Down: fully covered. Dorsal view is pale buff-brown dappled darker with dark crown, spotted on temporal region. Underparts are pinkish buff. Wings: buff brown. Diamond mark on lower back. | Egg teeth on upper and lower disappear at 1–2 d. | Unknown. | Able to walk and peck at food at hatch. Fly: 26–30 d. |

| | | | | | | |
|---|---|---|---|---|---|---|
| **MURRES, AUKLETS, AND RELATIVES (Alcidae):** Anisodactyl toe arrangement and palmate, lack hallux. Semi-precocial young. | | | | | | |
| **Tufted Puffin** (*Fratercula cirrhata*)<br><br>Refs: 1, 7 (bna.708) | Dark gray, pinkish gray web between toes and back of tarsus. | Hatch: 61–70<br><br>Adult: F: 744, M:806 | Down: fully covered. Light and dark morphs. Most sooty black upper, sooty gray below, few with white belly. Orbital ring black. | Bill: triangular shape, blackish, cere undeveloped. | Begging: continuous *peep, peep, peep*. | Eyes open at hatch, black. Both parents care for young. Fledge before capable of flight ~38 d. |
| **Common Murre** (*Uria aalge*)<br><br>Ref: 7 (bna.666) | Toes very large relative to body, dark gray. Able to stand day after hatch. | Hatch: 75.8<br><br>Adult: 991 | Down: fully covered, medium gray, pale below; replaced with contour feathers at 6 d. d 14: dark gray mask, contrasting white throat and cheeks. | Just hatched: conical wedge shape, tapers to point, blue-gray. Mouth pale pink beige to purplish. | Chicks emit short peep calls 1st wk. increasing in length and frequency by 2nd wk. | Nest in colonies on cliff ledges along cold coastlines of Northern Hemisphere. Leave nest before flighted: 23–24 d. Iris: dark. |
| **GULLS, TERNS, AND RELATIVES (Laridae):** Anisodactyl toe arrangement and palmate. Semi-precocial young. | | | | | | |
| **Herring Gull** (*Larus argentatus*)<br><br>Refs: 1, 7, 9 (bna. hergul.03) | Pink at first; turn buffy brown with pinkish-gray webbing between toes. | Hatch: 60–75<br><br>Adult: F: 1023, M:1147 | Down: completely covers, thick and long, pale gray background with dark blotches on dorsal surfaces and thighs. Spots on head and throat fine, gray-black. Underparts are paler. | Just hatched: wedge shaped, black or horn-colored. Tip 1/3 pink buff with pinkish base. Pinkish egg tooth lasts 2–3 days. | Begging call: soft *peeps* at first, becomes a more high-pitched intense *peep*. "Shrill waver" call when being chased or caught. | Eyes: open at hatch, iris is dark. Leaves nest shortly after hatch. |
| **Common Tern** (*Sterna hirundo*)<br><br>Ref: 7 (bna. comter.03) | Pink at first, turning more orange by 14 d. | Hatch: 15<br><br>Adult: 120 | Down: thick, completely covered. Cinnamon brown to gray brown on back, wings, and sides. Dorsum lined with indistinct black spots or streaks. Throat, sides of neck and lores brown-black. White underparts. | Beak: pink with black tip. Lower may turn orangish by 14 d. | Peep softly when begging (pecking bill of parent), becomes squeaky *cheeping* 3–6 d, and > 6 d, a *kri-kri-kri-kri-kri*. When distressed or alone, emit a *zeee*. | Eyes: open at hatch with dark brown iris. Able to stand and walk. |

(*Continued*)

Table 2.3 (Continued)

| Species | Feet (Tarsus/toes) | Weight (g) | Development and Integument | Beak / Mouth | Vocalizations | Other |
|---|---|---|---|---|---|---|
| **LOONS (Gaviidae):** Anisodactyl toe arrangement and palmate; legs situated far back on body, walking awkward. Semi-precocial young. | | | | | | |
| **Common Loon** (*Gavia immer*)<br>Refs: 1, 7 (bna.313) | Grayish black. | Hatch: 71.4–108.5<br>Adult: F: 4657, M: 5974 | Down: thick, blackish-brown, slightly lighter on undersides, belly white. Second down (at 3 wk) paler than 1st. | Grayish black, darker near base. | Contact and begging call: *peep-peep-peep*. Also, "yelp" and "wail" by 2nd wk. | Iris: reddish-brown. Fly at 12–13 wk. |
| **ALBATROSS, SHEARWATERS, AND RELATIVES (Procellaridae):** Anisodactyl toe arrangement, and palmate, no hallux. Altricial young. | | | | | | |
| **Manx Shearwater** (*Puffinus puffinus*)<br>Refs: 1, 7 (bna.257) | Tops and webbing between toes pinkish, underside of toes dark gray. | Hatch: 32–50<br>Adult: F: 439, M: 468 | Down: two stages.<br>1st fluffy, long, soft, grayish brown above, paler below.<br>2nd down (6–12 d) darker and coarser.<br>Primaries unsheathe at 4 wk. | Grayish black, lower mandible paler. | Begging: soft *cheep* or piping calls. May squeak or "chortle" when excited. | Nest in burrow on cliff or outcropping, in colony on islands. Leave nest 62–70 d (after parents abandon at ~60 d). |
| **CORMORANTS (Phalacrocoracidae)**: Totipalmate. Altricial young. | | | | | | |
| **Double-crested Cormorant** (*Phalocrocorax auritus*)<br>Refs: 1, 7 (bna.441) | Dark brown, turn dull black. | Hatch: 27.6–34.7<br>Adult: F: 1831, M: 2089 | Skin: shiny brown body, mostly pink on head and neck. Down: hatch mostly naked, by 6–7 d short down appears; by 14 d a thick, black "wooly" coat covers nestling. d 16–19: throat pouch is yellowish. | Beak: culmen 9 mm (avg). Egg tooth remains until d 4–7. Mouth is pink in nestling and juvenile. | Chicks *chirp* when begging or stressed (too hot), also *hiss* when threatened. | Hatchling: barely able to lift head. Eyes open by 3–4 d. Leave nest: 3–4 wk. before flight. Fly at 6–7 wk. |
| **PELICANS (Pelecanidae:** Totipalmate. Altricial young. | | | | | | |
| **Brown Pelican** (*Pelecanus occidentalis*)<br>Ref: 7 (bna.609) | Cream white in nestlings >24 d old. | Hatch: 54.9–87.0<br>Adult: F: 3174, M: 3702<br>Calif subsp. larger | Skin: pink at hatch, purplish-pink d 2–4, more purple by d 5–6. Down: naked except distal portion of wing; white down on rump d 10–12; fully covered by d 21–25. Juv. plumage complete by d 70. | Greenish gray in nestlings; wedge-shaped at first and "short," compared to adult, achieving full adult length after fledging. Slight hook at tip. | When begging chicks make a "shrill, rasping *squawk*." | Hatchling: unable to lift head, eyes are open but nictitating membrane not yet functioning. |

| | | | | | | |
|---|---|---|---|---|---|---|
| **HERONS, EGRETS, BITTERNS (Ardeidae)**: Anisodacytyl toe arrangement. Altricial or semi-altricial young. | | | | | | |
| **Snowy Egret** (*Egretta thula*)<br><br>Ref: 7 (bna.489) | Tarsus darker than toes, vary yellow to gray-black. Toes yellow-green by 34 d. Long legs. | Hatch: 20<br><br>Adult: 371 | Skin: grayish, tinted greenish in areas. Down: white, fully covered except wings, long on crown. Juv plumage mostly covers bird by 2–3 wk. | Long, pointed, varies yellow to gray-black, all black by 7 d (some become yellowish w/darker tip). Mouth interior pale pink. | Begging for food is a buzzing sound of 2–3 syllables. | Eyes: dark blue around eyes, turns gray by 7 d. Iris: pale gray, becomes lighter, then very pale by 34 d. Able to climb out of nest onto branches by 8–12 d. Leave colony ~ 6–7 wk. |
| **Black-crowned Night-Heron** (*Nycticorax nycticorax*)<br><br>Refs: 1, 7 (bna.74) | Long relative to body, dull buff/brown at hatch turning yellowish to gray-green by 30 d, yellow by 2 yrs. Toes drab on top, yellowish on bottom. Pink-ivory nails. | Hatch: 24.2<br><br>Adult: 810 | Skin: pink shades. Down: varies gray to rufous-brown on dorsum, neck, head; lighter gray on ventral. White filamentous down on crown (resembles a crest) and femoral tract. Natal down remains for weeks.<br>Acquires adult plumage in second year. | Light drab upper, grayish tip. Becomes yellowish 5–10 d then black with yellowish sides 50 d. Eventually long and pointed.<br>Mouth interior pinkish. | Food begging: *pip, pip, pip* or *Yip, yip, yip*. Older nestlings make *Yak, yak, yak* or *Chuck, chuck-a-chuck, chuck, chuck*. | Iris: grayish or greenish at first.<br>Both parents care for young. Fully feathered at 4 wk. Fly: 6 wk. |
| **IBIS AND SPOONBILL (Threskiornithinidae):** Anisodactyl toe arrangement. Semi-altricial young. | | | | | | |
| **White-faced Ibis** (*Plegadis chihi*)<br><br>Refs: 1, 7 (bna.130) | Pink. | Hatch: 30.7<br><br>Adult: F: 546, M:697 | Skin: pink, crown reddish pink (may change to light orange 3 wk). Down: brownish black, darker above, back of crown with white patches. | Short, straight, pinkish, black tip, base and middle band. Begins to decurve d 12. | Begging: trilling *cheeeeeeu* at high-pitch while bobbing head. | Eyes: partly open at hatch, fully open d 2. Adults feed young by regurgitation for 6–7 wk. Leave nest: 10–12 d, unable to fly. Fly: 28 d. Leave colony 6–7 wk. |

(*Continued*)

Table 2.3 (Continued)

| Species | Feet (Tarsus/toes) | Weight (g) | Development and Integument | Beak / Mouth | Vocalizations | Other |
|---|---|---|---|---|---|---|
| **VULTURES (Cathartidae):** Anisodactyl toe arrangement. Altricial young. | | | | | | |
| **Turkey Vulture** (*Cathartes aura*)<br><br>Ref: 7 (bna.339) | Gray at first (washed with feces), then pinkish. | Hatch: 60<br><br>Adult: 2006 | Down: long, white and fluffy, shorter on head. Face, throat, and crop areas black and bare. Down thickens and turns "dingy white" by 25 d. Traces of down left at 60 d. Head turns red by first spring. | Beak: dark, short, hooked, with large nares that are perforate. | Lacks syrinx but able to make sounds. Hatchling hisses weakly at first, then variations of hissing sounds when disturbed. | Eyes: may be open at hatch, iris gray. Leave nest: approximately 60 d after hatching with short flights at first, extended flight at 70–80 d. |
| **HAWKS, EAGLES, KITES (Accipitridae):** Anisodactyl toe arrangement, raptorial feet. Altricial or semi-altricial young. | | | | | | |
| **White-tailed Kite** (*Elanus leucurus*)<br><br>Refs: 1, 7 (bna.178) | Yellow. | Hatch: 17.4<br><br>Adult: 346 | Down: 1st coat is vinaceous buff on upper, buffy white on chin and sides, lighter on lower back sides. 2nd down (d 7), gray or bluish-gray and longer. Fully feathered 40 d. Juvenile plumage retained at least 4 months. | Black, hooked. Gape: red. | Unknown. When threatened gape and raise wings but make no sound. | Iris: brown (red in adult).<br>Leave nest: 1st flight ~ 4–5 wk. post-hatch. |
| **Golden Eagle** (*Aquila chrysaetos*)<br><br>Refs: 1, 7 (bna.684) | Pale pink colored at hatch, then yellow. Feathered to toes. | Hatch: 100<br><br>Adult: F: 4627, M: 3900 | Down: 1st down short, white or with pale gray. 2nd (d 6) long, thicker, white down. | Black, hooked, raptorial, with prominent egg tooth. Cere: yellowish white in nestling. | Hatchling: chirp. Nestling calls usually for food begging: chirps, cheeps, chitters. 15 d: *tsik*. 25 d: *seeir*, then loud pssa or *tsycuk tsycuk*. | Eyes: partly open at hatch but cannot see well. Feed selves 40 d (food brought by parents). Fly: 63–70 d. |

| | | | | | | |
|---|---|---|---|---|---|---|
| **Red-tailed Hawk** (*Buteo jamaicensis*) Refs: 1, 7 (bna.52) | Unfeathered, yellow, become more yellow in juvenile. | Hatch: 58 Adult: F: 1224, M: 1028 | Down: 1st down short, buff-white or grayish-white, no down on femur. White occipital spot may be visible. 2nd down: shorter, thicker, white. d 9: 7th primary emerges, down pale gray. d 29–30: head 90% downy, occipital spot still evident. | Black, hooked. Gape: cream to buff. | Young chicks emit soft *pipsee* calls. Older young make loud, rapid *klee-uk* calls. | Iris: dark, light yellow in juv. Leave nest: d 42–46, sustained flight 6 wk. |
| **OWLS (Tytonidae)**: Zygodactyl toe arrangement, raptorial feet. Altricial young. | | | | | | |
| **Barn Owl** (*Tyto alba*) Refs: 1, 7 (bna.1) | Long, with grayish white down on tarsus to toes (naked on back of tarsus). | Hatch: 12–21 Adult: F: 357-566, M: 306-474 Weights vary by subspecies | Skin: pink areas. 1st down: sparse, short, and grayish white on dorsal surfaces, lacking on belly and sides of neck. 2nd down (12 d): long, dense, white to pale gray or buff. | Hooked, raptorial, ivory color. | Young owlets twitter when fighting with siblings or seeking attention. Food call is raspy *scheuh*. Also hissing and other sounds. | Iris: pale blue at first. Leave nest: 50–55 d, fly at 60 d, independent by d 76–86. Young in brood vary greatly in size. |
| **OWLS, TYPICAL (Strigidae):** Zygodactyl toe arrangement, raptorial feet. Altricial young. | | | | | | |
| **Great Horned Owl** (*Bubo virginianus*) Refs: 1, 7 (bna.372) | Pink. | Hatch: ~35 Adult: F: 1142–1768, M: 914–1318 Weights vary by subspecies | Skin: pink. 1st down: pure white on dorsal surfaces. 2nd down: long, soft, grayish buff or yellowish-white or grayish-white, mottled on back. Ear tufts: fully grown 26 wk. | Hooked, raptorial, slate gray color | Rasping chirp, then whimper becoming louder and more intense with growth. Juvenile males do not hoot until late fall/ early winter, females more in spring. | Eyes: open 9–11 d, iris becomes yellow by 30 d. Branch at 6 wk., first (short) flights 7 wk., more sustained 9–10 wk. Long dependency. |
| **KINGFISHERS (Alcedinidae):** Syndactyl toe arrangement. Altricial young. | | | | | | |
| **Belted Kingfisher** (*Megaceryle alcyon*) Refs: 7, 9 (bna.84) | Tarsus very short, 2nd and 3rd toes fused together, short hallux (pointed back), "heal pads." | Hatch: 9–13 Adult: 148 | Skin: bright pink. Down: none. d 6: pins emerge in humeral tract. d 13: dorsal surface covered in feathers. d 16–18 appear fully feathered. | Blackish, heavy, longer than head, lower mandible longer than upper. Mouth: lining pink, no gape flanges. | Rattle call at 5–7 d. | Nest: burrow in bank near water. Nestling diet: fish and arthropods. Leave burrow: 27–29 d, can fly. |

(*Continued*)

Table 2.3 (Continued)

| Species | Feet (Tarsus/toes) | Weight (g) | Development and Integument | Beak / Mouth | Vocalizations | Other |
|---|---|---|---|---|---|---|
| **WOODPECKERS (Picidae):** Zygodactyl toe arrangement. Altricial young, no down. | | | | | | |
| **Downy Woodpecker** (*Dryobates pubescens*)<br><br>Refs: 7, 9 (bna.613) | Pink. Large "heel" pads. | Hatch: 1.55–1.77<br><br>Adult: 27.7 | Skin: pink, translucent. Down: none. | Beak: pink-white, upper shorter than lower. Tip of tongue white and shiny. | Contentment call: low-intensity *pip*.<br>Begging call: rasping. | Eyes: partly open d 4, fully open d 8. Gape flanges: light pink, disappear d 11–12. Leave nest: 20–25 d, fly well. |
| **Red-Cockaded Woodpecker** (*Dryobates borealis*)<br><br>Refs: 1, 7 (bna.85) | Pale pink-white. Large "heel" pads. | Hatch: 3.3<br><br>Adult: F: 47.4, M: 48.6 | Skin: bright pink. Down: none. d 4–5: pins visible. d 7–8 red colored spot on forehead of males. | Beak: upper pink-white and shorter than lower. Gape flanges: white and prominent, curve upwards. | Begging: rasping squeak.<br>Contentment: low-intensity peeping. | Eyes: open ~ d 10, iris brown with buff-yellow ring. Leave nest: 26–29 d, partly dependent on adults 2–5 more months. |
| **Northern Flicker** (*Colaptes auratus*)<br><br>Refs: 1, 7 (bna.norfli.02.1) | Pink. | Hatch: 5.5<br><br>Adult: 142 | Skin: pink or brownish-orange becomes reddish, then blackish. Down: none. | Beak: pink. Gape flanges: white. | Buzzing call until fully feathered. Before fledgling emit *peah* call. | Leave nest: 25–28 d. |

| | | | | | | |
|---|---|---|---|---|---|---|
| **FALCONS (Falconidae):** Anisodactyl toe arrangement and raptorial. Altricial or semi-altricial young. | | | | | | |
| **American Kestrel** (*Falco sparverius*)<br><br>Refs: 1, 7 (bna.602), 9 | Yellowish tinge, turn pale yellow; talons whitish pink. d 21: whitish pink, talons nearly black. | Hatch: 8–12<br><br>Adult: F: 103–132, M: 90.8–113 | Skin: pinkish. Down: 1st down white, sparsely covering, belly bare. 2nd down: thick, yellowish-white. Juv plumage covers body by d 14 and sex is distinguishable. Fully feathered d 21, remnants of down on crown and upper wing coverts. | Bill and cere: white-pink; not yet hooked, falcon "tooth" evident. Becomes dark gray at tip d 21. | Begging: *peep* at first, increasing to a shrill *cheep*. 2 wk. *whine, chitter*, and *klee*. | Eyes: partly open d 1–2 post-hatch, fully open d 7. Iris: bluish-black.<br>Sounds: *peep* then "*klee*" d 3.<br>d 21: skin around eye bluish-green and bare. Leave nest: 28–31 d. |
| **PARROTS AND ALLIES (Psittacidae):** Zygodactyl toe arrangement. Altricial young. | | | | | | |
| **Monk Parakeet** (*Myopsitta monachus*)<br><br>Ref: 7 (bna. monpar.03) | Gray. | Hatch: 4.07–5.45<br><br>Adult: F: 112, M: 114 | Down: sparsely covered with yellowish down. d 18: primaries begin to emerge.<br>d 28: body feathers half developed. | Large, hooked, yellowish-brown bill, notched on upper mandible. Feathered cere. | Noisy, raucous. Food-begging: complex, many notes. | Leave nest: 40 d (wild), 50 d (captive). |
| **Red-crowned Parrot** (*Amazona viridigenalis*)<br><br>Ref: 7 (bna.292) | Gray. | Hatch: 11.5–13.5<br><br>Adult: 316 | Down: sparsely covered with whitish down. In captive raised birds: feathers first appear 35 d, fully feathered 8 wk. | Large and hooked. Bill and cere cream yellow. | Imitate adults but at higher pitch. Begging calls: rackety. | Leave nest: 53 d. |

Table 2.4 Guide to identification of representative hatchling and nestling songbirds: YELLOW TO ORANGE MOUTHS. All have anisodactyl feet.

**Abbreviations: d: day, H: hatchling 1–3 days, N: nestling, Fl: fledgling, Juv: juvenile, F: female, M: male.**

| Species | Mouth color | Gape flanges | Integument | Legs/feet | Approx. Weight (g) | | Other Features and References |
|---|---|---|---|---|---|---|---|
| | | | | | **H to Fl** | **Adult Mean (SD)** | |
| **Western Kingbird** (*Tyrannus verticalis*) | Yellow-orange | Bright yellow, swollen | Down: white.<br>Skin: reddish to pinkish.<br>Fl: tail has whiter outer edges, darkish "mask" beak to eyes. | Copper to smoke gray | d 0: 2–3<br>d 7: 16–17<br>Fl: 36 | 39.6 (2.8) | Nest: open cup. Leave nest: 13–19 d, independent by 2–3 wks.<br>Refs: 1, 7 (bna.227) |
| **Willow Flycatcher** (*Empidonax traillii*) | Yellow-orange | Pale yellow then brighter yellow | Down: gray.<br>Skin: Pinkish.<br>Beak: buffy orange to pink<br>d 9: buffy wing bar evident. | | d 0: 1.4–2.2<br>d 4: 7.2<br>Fl: 12.5 | F: 13.7 (1.5)<br>M: 13.1 (1.4) | Nest: open cup in fork of slender branch. Leave nest: 12–15 d, earlier if disturbed. Eyes partly open: d 6.<br>Sounds: H faint *weep-weep*, Fl *peep*.<br>Refs: 1, 7 (bna.533) |
| **Say's Phoebe** (*Sayornis saya*) | Reddish-orange | Yellow and thin | Down: Sparse, light gray.<br>Juv: upperparts browner than adult, 2 distinct cinnamon buff wing bars. | | d 0: 2 (est.) | 20.9 (2.5) | Nest: open cup (resting on ledge or pocket, or nest of other species). Leave nest: 13–21 d.<br>Ref: 7 (bna.374) |
| **Loggerhead Shrike** (*Lanius ludovicianus*) | Yellow-orange palate, scarlet throat, orange tongue | Yellow-orange | Down: sparse, white on back, tan in wings.<br>Skin: gray but appears pinkish-orange.<br>Beak: orange yellow. | Pink-orange, nails, hooked | d 0: 2.8–3.5<br>d 8: 21<br>Fl: 48 | 50.5 (3.0) | Eats small vertebrates, carrion, insects. Nest: open cup. Leave nest: 17–21 d, dependent until 3–4 wks post-fledge.<br>Refs: 1, 7 (bna.231) |

| | | | | | | | |
|---|---|---|---|---|---|---|---|
| **Red-eyed Vireo** (*Vireo olivaceus*) | Yellow to bright orange | White to light beige | Down: sparse, gray or brownish gray on dorsal areas.<br>Skin: pinkish-orange, turns gray. | Pinkish buff, turn lead gray | d 0: 1.5–1.8<br>d 6: 12.5 | 16.8 (1.0) | Nest: open cup. Leave nest: 10–12 d.<br>Eyes partly open 6 d.<br>Refs: 1, 7 (bna.527), 8, 9 |
| **Horned Lark** (*Eremophila alpestris*) | Bright orange-yellow | Thin, yellow | Down: very long, pale creamy buff-yellow on head and back Skin: brown.<br>3 small dark spots on tongue. | Pinkish- colored, then light neutral gray | d 0: 2.4<br>Fl: 22.3 | 32.2 | Nest: shallow cup on ground. Leave nest: 9–12 d, independent 21–30 d post–fledge. Eyes open: 4 d.<br>Refs: 1, 2, 7 (bna.195), 8, 9 |
| **Purple Martin** (*Progne subis*) | Lemon-yellow | Light yellow, prominent | Down: none.<br>Skin: reddish pink. | Short legs. | d 0: 3–3.5<br>d 6: 20–24<br>Fl: 47–52 | F: 54.1 (4.8)<br>M: 53.5 (3.8) | Nest: in cavity. Leave nest: 28–31. Eyes partly open: 6 d, fully open 9–10 d.<br>Refs: 1, 7 (bna.287) |
| **Cliff Swallow** (*Petrocheli-don pyrrhonota*) | Yellow-orange | Creamy white, somewhat prominent<br>at first | Down: light gray on head and dorsum.<br>Skin: Light pink or bright reddish pink.<br>Buffy orange feather patch on dorsal rump shows early. | Short pink legs, small chubby feet. | d 0: 1.5–2.2<br>d 10: 22.1 | 21.6 (2.0) | Nest: in colonies of mud nests under over-hangs. Leave nest: 21–24 d, parental care 3–5 d post-fledge. Highly social. Sounds: barking type *chirp*.<br>Refs: 1, 7 (bna.cliswa.03), 8, 9 |
| **Black-capped Chickadee** (*Poecile atricapillus*) | Bright yellow | White | Down: pale mouse gray on dorsum.<br>Skin: pinkish-orange. | Legs pinkish gray. | d 0: ~1<br>d 15: 11 | 10.8 (0.8) | Nest: in cavity. Leave nest: 16 d, stay with parents 3–4 wks. Sounds: hatchling makes faint calls.<br>Refs: 1, 7 (bna.39), 9 |
| **Bushtit** (*Psaltriparus minimus*) | Orange-red to orange-yellow | Cream or pale yellow | Down: none at hatch.<br>Skin: pink.<br>First feathers appear crest-like on crown. | Long, delicate legs, light pink feet. | d 0: <1–2<br>d 3+: 3.5–4 | 5.3 (0.4) | Nest: cryptic pendulum (sock like). Leave nest: 14–15 d (or 18–20 d). Sounds: 3–syllable “locator” call. Eyes open: 7–8 d. Females have blue eyes.<br>Ref: 7 (bna.598) |

(*Continued*)

Table 2.4 (Continued)

**Abbreviations: d: day, H: hatchling 1–3 days, N: nestling, Fl: fledgling, Juv: juvenile, F: female, M: male.**

| Species | Mouth color | Gape flanges | Integument | Legs/feet | Approx. Weight (g) | | Other Features and References |
|---|---|---|---|---|---|---|---|
| **White-breasted Nuthatch** (*Sitta carolinensis*) | Bright yellow | Creamy-yellow | Down: gray, with 2 rows of horizontal tufts on head; gray tufts going down back.<br>Skin: pink. | Long legs, big feet.<br>Fl: pinkish buff. | Fl: 18 | 21 | Nest: in cavity. Leave nest: 23–24 d (14–16 d, or 19–26) d. Eyes open: d 13.<br>Refs: 1, 7 (bna.54), 8, 9 |
| **Brown Creeper** (*Certhia Americana*) | Yellow | White, become yellow | Down: long, grayish-black down on superciliary and occipital regions in 3 rows/6 feathers each.<br>Skin: pink.<br>Tail short w/ stiff feathers. | Short legs, long toes and nails. Pinkish buff. | | 8.1 (0.5) | Nest: behind bark or in cavity. Leave nest: 13–16 d. Eyes open: 8 d.<br>Sounds: older nestlings *ts–tssi*.<br>Fledglings prefer to cling to vertical surfaces.<br>Refs: 1, 7 (bna.669) |
| **House Wren** (*Troglodytes aedon*) | Yellow or orange-yellow | Cream to pale yellow, somewhat prominent | Down: long tufts of mouse gray or drab brown, concentrated on crown, occipital, and dorsum.<br>Skin: dark gray or pinkish. | Pale pink, then dark gray. | d 0: 1–1.7<br>d 6: 8<br>d 9–10: 10 | F: 11.1 (0.8)<br>M: 10.8 (0.6) | Nest: in cavity. Leave nest: 15–17 d, (or 13–18 d) may leave early (after 10 d) if disturbed. Sounds: distinctive begging chatter.<br>Refs: 1, 7 (bna.380), 8 |
| **Bewick's Wren** (*Thryothorus bewickii*) | Yellow with orange tinge | Light yellow, becomes dark yellow with orange tinge | Down: long, grayish-brown.<br>Skin: pinkish.<br>2 dark spots on tongue.<br>Superciliary line shows by d 11. | Pinkish, turn light horn. | d 0: 1.4<br>d 11–13: 10 | 9.9 (0.8) | Nest: in cavity. Leave nest: 14–17 d (or sooner if disturbed), fly well at 21 d, remain w/parents another 2 wks. Eyes open: 5–6 d. Sounds: Chirping at 8 d.<br>Ref: 7 (bna.315), 8 |

| | | | | | | | |
|---|---|---|---|---|---|---|---|
| **Blue-gray Gnatcatcher** (*Polioptila caerulea*) | Bright yellow | Pale yellow | Down, skin: no info. Outer rectrices white.<br>Tongue: 2 dark spots. | Light gray | d 0: < 1<br>d 9: 6.2 | 5.8 (0.3) | Nest: cup with high walls. Leave nest: 10–12 (or 10–15).<br>Refs: 1, 7 (bna.23), 8, 9 |
| **American Dipper** (*Cinclus mexicanus*) | Orange-yellow, darker interior | White | Down: pale gray, sparse, on head and dorsum.<br>Skin: orange on flanks and abdomen, pink on dorsal. | | d 3: 10<br>d 16: 55 | F: 54.6 (4.8)<br>M: 61 (2.2) | Diet: aquatic invertebrates and small fish.<br>Nest: ball-like "hut" of moss often behind waterfall or on midstream rock. Leave nest: 18–25 d.<br>Ref: 7 (bna.22), 8 |
| **Wrentit** (*Chamaea fasciata*) | Deep orange | Yellow | Down: none.<br>Skin: Light pink.<br>First contour feathers gray-brown. Eye area dark. | Straw colored legs, darken by d 5. | d 0: 1.5–1.6<br>d 10: 11.4 | F: 14.2 (1.1)<br>M:15.3 (1.1) | Nest: cup. Leave nest: 15–16 d, cannot fly. Remain in family flocks 30 d post–fledge. Sedentary, must be returned to natal territory. Calls: *wheat*. Iris: yellow, turns pale 15 d.<br>Refs: 1, 7 (bna. wrenti.02.1), 8 |
| **Eastern Bluebird** (*Sialia sialis*) | Ocher yellow | Cream to yellow, color and prominence varies | Down: dingy gray or dark drab.<br>Skin: Pink.<br>Fl: browner than adult, dusky spots and streaks. | Pinkish-colored, then black. | d 0: 1.7–3.1<br>d 6: 20<br>d 10: 25 | 27.5 (3.3) | Nest: in cavity, open cup rare.<br>Leave nest: 17–18 or 19 d, remain in family groups 3 more wks. Eyes open: 5–6 d.<br>Refs: 5, 6, 7 (bna.381), 8 |
| **Hermit Thrush** (*Catharus guttatus*) | Orange-yellow | Yellow | Down: few tufts of dark gray on head, alar, and lower ½ dorsal.<br>Skin pinkish. | Dull pink. | d 0: 4.1<br>d 9: 25<br>d 12: 24.8 | 30.1 (3.1) | Nest: cup. Leave nest: 10–15 d (12 avg), earlier (d 10) if disturbed. Eyes partly open: 3 d, fully open 4–5 d.<br>Ref: 7 (bna.261) |

(*Continued*)

Table 2.4 (Continued)

**Abbreviations: d: day, H: hatchling 1–3 days, N: nestling, Fl: fledgling, Juv: juvenile, F: female, M: male.**

| Species | Mouth color | Gape flanges | Integument | Legs/feet | Approx. Weight (g) | | Other Features and References |
|---|---|---|---|---|---|---|---|
| **American Robin** (*Turdus migratorius*) | Yellow to yellow-orange | White exterior, pale yellow inside corners | Down: whitish on head, back, wings, turns creamy then gray.<br>Skin: yellowish.<br>1st feathers rust-tipped, speckled dorsal and ventral, chin and throat white. | Long legs, toes more delicate than starling. | d 0: 4.1–6.7 (5.5 avg)<br>Fl: 48–50 | 78.5 (7.4) | Nest: cup-shaped, grass with mud.<br>Leave nest: 14–16 d (possibly earlier), independent by 4 wks post-fledge, stay in natal area up to 4 months. Eyes partly open: d 5. Hatchling sounds: staccato *trill*.<br>Ref: 7 (bna.462) |
| **Gray Catbird** (*Dumetella carolinensis*) | Yellow to yellow-orange | Creamy white | Down: dark brown or gray to blackish.<br>Skin: blackish-gray.<br>Black at bill tip and base of tongue. | | d 0: 3<br>d 4: 12.8<br>Fl: 28.5 | 35.3 (2.5) | Nest: open cup, low. Leave nest: 8–12 d (or 10.5–15 d), fed by adults up to 12 d post fledge.<br>Refs: 1, 7 (bna.167), 9 |
| **Brown Thrasher** (*Toxostoma rufum*) | Creamy yellow, orange in throat | Whitish, thin | Down: grayish-white on dorsal surface.<br>Skin: pinkish.<br>Juv: buff wing bars and spotting. | Deep vinaceous then brown. | d 0: 4.8<br>d 9: 45.5<br>Fl: 41.5–52 | 68 | Nest: cup, low, dense shrubs (with thorns). Leave nest: 11–12 d (range 9–13), run well. Eyes: H dusky brown,<br>Fl olive gray, (adult orange yellow).<br>Refs: 7, 9 (bna.557) |

| | | | | | | | |
|---|---|---|---|---|---|---|---|
| **Northern Mockingbird** (*Mimus polyglottos*) | Yellow | Off white or creamy yellow | Down: plentiful dark gray or sepia-brown, gray and white first feathers.<br>Skin: light pink w/yellow tint. | Long legs. White nails turn dark. | d 0: 2.7–4.5<br>d 6: 26<br>d 16: 40 | 48.5 | Nest: open cup. Leave nest: 10–15 d (avg 12), fly well 8 d post-fledge. Eyes: iris dark gray to gray-green in juvenile.<br>Sounds: H and N make single high-pitched *peep*.<br>Ref: 7 (bna.7) |
| **European Starling** (*Sturnus vulgaris*) | Bright yellow or orange | Lemon yellow, thick, **very** prominent larger lower mandible | Down: very long, thick, light brown and grayish-white on head, dorsum and humerus.<br>Skin: pink.<br>Juv: gray-brown plumage, blackish bill, turns yellow in first winter. | Long legs. | d 0: 5.5–7<br>d 17–18: 78<br>Fl: 71 | F: 84.4 (4.2)<br>M: 87.6 (4.8) | Nest: in cavity. Leave nest: 18–21 d<br>Eyes partly open 6 d, fully open 8 d.<br>Sounds: H single squeaky note, later raucous. Beaks of juv and non-breeding birds are dark, turning bright yellow during breeding.<br>Ref: 7 (bna.48) |

North American family groups with yellow-orange mouth interiors: Tyrant flycatchers, shrikes, vireos, larks, swallows, chickadees, titmice, verdins, Bushtits, nuthatches, creepers, wrens, gnatcatchers, gnatwrens, dippers, sylviid warblers (Wrentit), thrushes, mockingbirds, thrashers, and starlings.

Table 2.5 Guide to identification of representative hatchling and nestling songbirds: PINK TO RED MOUTHS. All have anisodactyl feet.

**Abbreviations: d: day, H: hatchling 1–3 days, N: nestling, Fl: fledgling, Juv: juvenile, F: female, M: male.**

| Species | Mouth color | Gape flanges | Integument | Tarsus/Toes | Approx. Weight (g) | | Other Features and References |
|---|---|---|---|---|---|---|---|
| | | | | | **H to Fl** | **Adult Mean (SD)** | |
| **Blue Jay** (*Cyanocitta cristata*) | Pink | White, thin | Down: none.<br>Skin: pink, darker by d 2. Tongue lavender gray. | Lavender gray | d 0: 5.5<br>d 12: 58<br>d 21: 72 | 88 (5.8) | Nest: open cup. Leave nest: 17–21 d. Eyes partly open: d 5, fully open d 11.<br>Ref: 7 (bna.459), 9 |
| **Black-billed Magpie** (*Pica hudsonia*) | Deep pink to red | Pale pink to white | Down: none.<br>Skin: pink, turns grayish and yellowish. | | d 0: 6.3 (est.)<br>d 9–15: 63–129<br>Fl: 180.5 | F: 66 (14.3)<br>M: 89 (10.3) | Nest: domed, mud cup and anchor. Leave nest: 24–30 d, stay with parents for 6–8 wks. Eyes open: 7 d.<br>Ref: 7 (bna.389) |
| **American Crow** (*Corvus brachy-rhynchos*) | Med pink to red | White or pinkish and small | Down: none to sparse.<br>Skin: pink then turns black by d 5–10. | Pinkish at hatch, then grayish black, long and heavy. | d 0: 15.6 (avg)<br>d 15–18: 210–255<br>Fl: 390 (avg)<br>Weights vary by region | F: 474<br>M: 538 | Nest: bulky cup. Leave nest: 28–35 d, fed up to 4 mos. Post–fledge. Eyes partly open: 5–6 d, fully open 10–13 d. Blue eyes begin to turn gray at about 60 d. Sounds: Weak at first, 4 d variety of *churrs, cheeaps, wa-eeks, yumyumyum* when fed.<br>Ref: 7 (bna.647), 9 |
| **Golden-crowned Kinglet** (*Regulus satrapa*) | Orange-red | Pale yellow | Down: Few tufts of gray down on head and above eyes. Skin: pinkish skin. | Large relative to body size | d 0: < 1<br>d 1: 1.5–2 | F: 4.5 (7.8)<br>M: 4.9 (7.7) | Nest: pendulum. Leave nest: 14–19 d, independent 15–17 d. Eyes partly open: 5 d, fully open 11 d. Sounds: *tsip*.<br>Ref: 7 (bna.301) |

| | | | | | | | |
|---|---|---|---|---|---|---|---|
| **Cedar Waxwing** (*Bombycilla cedrorum*) | Deep pink to bright red | Creamy-yellow, thin | Down: none.<br>Skin: pink, darkens d 1.<br>d 3: yellow waxy tips on tail. Black "mask" feathers last to unsheathe. | Weak until d 9.<br>Juv: legs brown | d 0: 2.8–3.3<br>d 7: 18.4–19.5<br>d 14: 26<br>Fl: 25–30 | F: 32.6(2.3)<br>M: 30.6 (2.2) | Nest: open cup in fork. Leave nest: 14–18 d. Eyes begin to open 6–7 d, open 8 d. Sounds: 5th d: faint *buzzing* or *chirping*. Begging call: long excited trill using several *chip* syllables. Opalescent markings inside mouth at corners.<br>Ref: 7 (bna.309), 8, 9 |
| **Phaino pepla** (*Phainopepla nitens*) | Pinkish-beige | Yellow | Down: white, long tufts on head and wings, center of crown is bare.<br>Skin: grayish or purplish-black. | Short and chunky, pinkish to gray. | | 22.1 | Nest: open cup. Leave nest: 19–20 d. Refs: 1, 7 (bna.415) |
| **House Sparrow** (*Passer domesticus*) | Pinkish, pinkish-yellow, or red | Varies white, then lemon<br>yellow, prominent | Down: none.<br>Skin: pink to red. Light gray feather tracts appear 6–10 hours after hatch, then darken. | Short and chunky, pinkish to gray. | d 0: 2–3<br>d 6: 14<br>d 14: 27.5 | F: 28.4 (1.4<br>M: 28.6 (1.4) | Nest: cavity preferred, in crevice or on ledge. Leave nest: 14–16 d, fed by parents 2 wks post-fledge. Eyes partly open 3–4 d; fully open 5 d. Sounds: melodic, single *chirp*.<br>Ref: 7 (bna.12), 9 |
| **American Pipit** (*Anthus rubescens*) | Reddish-orange | Very pale yellow | Down: fairly thick, long, brownish-gray, shorter and lighter underparts.<br>Skin: pinkish. | | d 0: 1.6–2.4 | F: 20 (0.8)<br>M: 21.1 (1.4) | Nest: open cup on ground. Leave nest: 13–16 (avg. 14) d. Eyes open: 4–5 d.<br>Refs: 1, 7 (bna.95) |
| **House Finch** (*Haemorhous mexicanus*) | Pink, then dark pink to bright orange- red | Pale yellow at hatch, then yellower (cream at corners) | Down: abundant, white or grayish brown on all dorsal areas. Rows of whitish down on head (2 rows on crown and a small row above each eye). Skin: pinkish yellow. | Short, stocky legs and feet. | d 0: 1.5–1.8<br>d 5: 6.4–7.7<br>d 16: 18.8 | 21.4 (1.3) | Nest: open cup. Leave nest: variable, avg. 16 d, or earlier (d10) if disturbed. Eyes partly open 3–5 d, fully open 7 d, self-feeding ~ 3wks after fledging. Sounds: none at hatch, later a high-pitched *peeping*.<br>Ref: 7 (bna.46) |

(*Continued*)

Table 2.5 (Continued)

**Abbreviations: d: day, H: hatchling 1–3 days, N: nestling, Fl: fledgling, Juv: juvenile, F: female, M: male.**

| Species | Mouth color | Gape flanges | Integument | Tarsus/Toes | Approx. Weight (g) | | Other Features and References |
|---|---|---|---|---|---|---|---|
| **American Goldfinch** (*Spinus tristis*) | Pinkish red or "geranium" pink | Pale, creamy yellow | Down: few wisps of pale grayish on head, legs, wings and abdomen Horseshoe shape on head from frontal to occipital and back to frontal.<br>Skin: reddish.<br>Peach wing bars once feathered. | Short, pink at first. Then turns dark grayish brown. | d 0: 1.5<br>d 6: 7<br>d 13: 12 | F: 12.5 (0.7)<br>M: 13.1 (0.9) | Nest: cup. Leave nest: 11–17 d (earlier if disturbed), dependent on parents 3 wks post–fledge. Eyes partly open 3 d, fully open by 7 d. Sounds: faint, high-pitched begging calls, become louder by d 8.<br>Ref: 7 (bna.amegfi.02.1), 9 |
| **Eastern Towhee** (*Pipilo erythro-phthalmus*) | Red, fades to pink | Bright yellow, fades to pale yellow | Down: grayish in sparse tufts.<br>Skin: pinkish-beige. | Long legs with big feet, by d 8 tarsus as long as adult. | d 0: 3<br>Fl: 24.7 | F: 38.8 (2.3)<br>M: 41.3 (2.4) | Nest: cup on or above ground. Leave nest: 10–11 d (earlier if disturbed), fed by parents 3–4 wks after fledging. Eyes begin to open 4 d, fully open 5–6 d. Juv eye: reddish brown.<br>Refs: 1, 7 (bna.262) |
| **Song Sparrow** (*Melospiza melodia*) | Red (ruby) | White to yellow | Down: Sparse black or sepia-brown on back, thighs, wings.<br>Skin: yellow to bright orange. Bottom of toes dull to bright yellow. | Short, pink to yellow orange, then grayish-brown. | d 0: 1.5<br>d 5: 11<br>d 15: 19 | F: 19.5 (1.3)<br>M: 20.5 (1.1) | Nest: cup. Leave nest: 9–12 (possibly up to 16) d. Eyes partly open: 4 d, fully open 6–7 d. Sounds: quiet *chirp*, very first basic songs appear 13–15 d.<br>Refs: 1, 3, 7 (bna.704), 9 |
| **Dark-eyed Junco** (*Junco hyemalis*) | Deep pink to red | Bright yellow.<br>Relatively thick, not prominent | Down: dark gray dorsally, dense and above each eye, about 5–7 mm long.<br>Skin: reddish with orange tint.<br>White outer rectrices when feathered. | Pink gray legs and tan nails. | d 0: 2.2<br>d 6: 14<br>d 11: 17.3 | F: 17.9 (1.0)<br>M:<br>19.3 (1.0) | Nest: cup. Leave nest: 9–13 d (earlier if disturbed). Eyes begin to open: 2 d, fully open 6 d.<br>Ref: 7 (bna.716) |

| | | | | | | | |
|---|---|---|---|---|---|---|---|
| **Eastern Meadow lark**<br>(*Sturnella magna*) | Pinkish | Bright yellow | Down: pearl gray<br>Skin: pinkish-orange or orange-red. | Pinkish buff. | d 0: 5<br>Fl: ~ 59 | F: 76<br>M: 102 (11.2) | Nest: cup. Leave nest: 10–12 d, run well, short flights. Eyes open 4 d. (Western Meadowlark is similar).<br>Refs: 1, 7 (bna.160) |
| **Baltimore Oriole**<br>(*Icterus galbula*) | Reddish | White or yellow, thin | Down: long, whitish on head and back. N: olive gray on back, orange-yellow below. Skin: pink. | Gray or bluish gray. | d 0: 2–2.5 | F: 31.8 (1.6)<br>M: 33.9 (2.0) | Nest: pendulous, usually near tip of tree branch. Leave nest: 11–14 d. Sounds: chattering.<br>Ref: 7 (bna.384), 9 |
| **Red-winged Blackbird**<br>(*Agelaius phoeniceus*) | Red | White, thin | Down: scant buffy or grayish along main tracts.<br>Skin: orange to pinkish-red N: bald around eye, cheek and throat. | Long legs, white nails at first, turn dark. | d 0: 3.8<br>d 7: 26<br>Fl: ~ 36 | F:39.5 (2.3)<br>M: 65.3 (3.6) | Nest: cup, woven reeds. Leave nest:<br>11–14 d, climb out of nest and move around in reeds before can fly. Eyes open 6 d.<br>Ref: 7 (bna.184), 9 |
| **Brown-headed Cowbird**<br>(*Molothrus ater*) | Deep pink to cherry red | Varies from white to yellow, thin | Down: olive-gray.<br>Skin: pinkish skin.<br>Bald face. | Long legs, big feet, black tipped nails. | d 0: 1.8–3.1<br>d 7: 20<br>d 12: 32 | F: 38.1 (2.5)<br>M: 48.7 (2.6) | Nest: do not build own nest, obligate brood parasite. Leave nest: 8–13 d (avg:10–11). Eyes open 2 d. Sound: continuous, high-pitched, vibrating.<br>Ref: 7 (bna.47), 9. |
| **Common Grackle**<br>(*Quiscalus quiscula*) | Bright pink | Whitish at corners only | Down: thick medium gray brown.<br>Skin: pink and apricot.<br>Bare apricot/ yellowish face. | Long tarsus, long toes, nails white to tan. | d 0: 5.6–6.7<br>d 10: 45<br>d 17: 75 | F: 92.2 (7.3)<br>M: 120 (7.1) | Nest: cup shape, usually in conifer. Leave nest: 10–17 d. Eyes partly open 2 d, fully open 7 d.<br>Ref: 7 (bna.271) |
| **Common Yellowthroat**<br>(*Geothlypis trichas*) | Deep red or red–orange | Bright yellow | Down: dark gray on head, back, wings.<br>Skin: light orange.<br>Buffy wing bars once feathered. | Pinkish beige, lemon yellow nails. | H: 1.74–2<br>Fl: 10.3 | F: 9.2 (0.6)<br>M: 9.7 (0.6) | Nest: cup on or near ground. Leave nest: 9–10 d. Eyes open 4–5 d.<br>Refs: 1, 7 (bna.448), 9. |

*(Continued)*

Table 2.5 (Continued)

**Abbreviations: d: day, H: hatchling 1–3 days, N: nestling, Fl: fledgling, Juv: juvenile, F: female, M: male.**

| Species | Mouth color | Gape flanges | Integument | Tarsus/Toes | Approx. Weight (g) | | Other Features and References |
|---|---|---|---|---|---|---|---|
| **Yellow Warbler** (*Setophaga petechia*) | Reddish orange | Bright yellow | Down: scant light smoke gray (or cream) on head, back, wings, thighs.<br>Skin: reddish. | Pinkish buff. | d 0: 1.5<br>d 7: 9 | F: 9.2 (0.5)<br>M: 9.6 (0.5) | Nest: cup. Leave nest: 9–12 d (as early as 8–9 d). Eyes open 3–5 d.<br>Refs: 1, 6, 7 (bna.454), 9 |
| **Northern Cardinal** (*Cardinalis cardinalis*) | Deep pink or red-orange | Whitish, thin. N: creamy and thicker | Down: sparse, long, medium gray on back.<br>Skin: Pinkish-apricot, black as adult. | | d 0: 3.5<br>d 7: 23<br>Fl: 27.1 | F: 41.8 (2.9)<br>M: 43.5 (1.9) | Nest: bowl shape in fork. Leave nest: as early as 9 d. Sounds: begging call loud by d 5.<br>Refs: 1, 7 (bna.440) |
| **Black-headed Grosbeak** (*Piranga melano-cephalus*) | Reddish apricot | Yellow or ivory white | Down: sparse, grayish-white in occipital areas and along main tracts.<br>Skin: apricot-orange, paler by d 1–4.<br>Lemon-yellow underwing coverts show early. | Apricot orange; pinkish beige by d 5. | d 0: 3<br>d 3: 6<br>d 4: 10 | F: 46.1 (3.3)<br>M: 48.2 (4.8) | Nest: cup. Leave nest: 10–14 d. Eyes open 8 d. Sounds: faint high-pitched *peeps*, then continuous *whee–you*, builds to loud begging when parent arrives.<br>Refs: 1, 7 (bna.143) |

North American family groups with pink-red mouth interiors: corvids, kinglets, waxwings, silky-flycatchers (Phainopepla), Old World sparrows (House or English Sparrow), pipits, wagtails, finches, longspurs, New World sparrows, Yellow-breasted Chats, icterids (including meadowlarks and orioles), wood warblers, cardinals (including tanagers, grosbeaks, some buntings, and Dickcissel).

## Acknowledgements

Many thanks to Guthrum Purdin DVM for the original version of this chapter, which offered an excellent guide to follow. My husband, Kyle, with a shared passion for photography and gift for spotting birds, has assisted me with nesting bird field studies over many years. I also want to thank the many wildlife rehabilitators who shared their photos of birds in care as well as preserving those that did not survive so that I could study them.

## References

Superscript indicates reference used as source for tables

[1]Baicich, P.J. and Harrison, C.J.O. (2005). *Nests, Eggs, and Nestlings of North American Birds*, 2e, 347 pp. Princeton, NJ: Princeton University Press.

Bateson, P.P.G. (1966). The characteristics and context of imprinting. *Biological Review* 41: 177–220.

Bateson, P.P.G. (1979). How do sensitive periods arise and what are they for? *Animal Behaviour* 27: 470–486.

Bolhuis, J.J., de Vos, G.J., and Kruijt, J.P. (1990). Filial imprinting and associative learning. *Quarterly Journal of Experimental Psychology* 42B (3): 313–329.

ten Cate, C. and Vos, D.R. (1999). Sexual imprinting and evolutionary processes in birds: a reassessment. *Advances in the Study of Behavior* 28: 1–31.

Clark, G.A. (1969). Oral flanges of juvenile birds. *The Wilson Journal of Ornithology* 81 (3): 270–279.

[2]Dunning, J.B.(ed. M. Ghadrdan), 117 pp (2018). *Body Masses of North American Birds*. Eugene, OR: The International Wildlife Rehabilitation Council.

Ficken, M. (1965). Mouth color of nestling passerines and its use in taxonomy. *The Wilson Journal of Ornithology* 77 (1): 71–75.

Hoffman, H.S. and DePaulo, P. (1977). Behavioral control by an imprinting stimulus. *American Scientist* 65: 58–66.

Immelmann, K. (1972). Sexual and other long-term aspects of imprinting in birds and other species. *Advances in the Study of Behavior* 4: 147–174.

[3]Jongsomjit, D., Jones, S.L., Gardali, T., et al. (2007). A Guide to Nestling Development and Aging in Altricial Passerines. *U.S. Department of Interior, Fish and Wildlife Service, Biological Technical Publication, FWS/BTP-R6008-2007,* Washington, D.C.

Kilner, R. and Davies, N.B. (1997). Nestling mouth colour: ecological correlates of a begging signal. *Animal Behaviour* 56 (3): 705–712.

[4]Nelson, C.H. (1993). *The Downy Waterfowl of North America*, 302 pp. Deerfield, IL: Downy Station Press.

[5]Pyle, P. (1997). *Identification Guide to North American Birds, Parts I and II*. Bolinas, CA: Slate Creek Press.

[6]Ridgway, R. (1902). The Birds of North and Middle America, Pt. 2. *Bulletin of the United States National Museum No. 50*.

[7]Rodewald, P. (ed.). (2015). The Birds of North America: https://birdsna.org. Cornell Laboratory of Ornithology, Ithaca, NY. (Individual species papers are indicated by BNA number under each species in Tables 2.3 and 2.4.)

Welty, J.C. and Baptista, L. (1988). *The Life of Birds*, 4e, 581 pp. Orlando, FL: Harcourt Brace Jovanovich Publishers.

[8]Wetherbee, D.K. (1957). Natal plumages and downy pteryloses of passerine birds of North America. *Bulletin of the American Museum of Natural History* 113 (5): 339–436.

[9]Wetherbee, D.K. and Wetherbee, N.S. (1961). Artificial incubation of eggs of various bird species and some attributes of neonates. *Bird-Banding* XXXII: 141–159.

# 3

# Incubation

*Susie Kasielke*

## Introduction

Artificial incubation of bird eggs, like everything we do to care for animals, requires both art and science. A large body of scientific work on avian embryonic development has been done to optimize production in the commercial poultry industry. Fortunately for those working with nondomestic birds, the process of development and hatching of avian embryos is highly conserved across all species, so most of the knowledge derived from domestic species can be directly applied to other taxa. Variation among species is seen in incubation periods (terms), temperature and humidity requirements, and, to some extent, the hatching process. This is where the art, our collective avicultural expertise, refines science-based techniques to achieve optimal hatchability.

Artificial incubation may be used as a tool to increase production in rare and endangered species, as many birds will lay replacement eggs if the first clutch of eggs is removed. In this case, timing of removal of eggs may be carefully planned. Most often, however, artificially incubated eggs have been rescued due to parental abandonment or other emergency situations. In some cases, a combination of natural and artificial incubation may give the best results. Certain species, such as raptors, have better hatchability if eggs are naturally incubated – either by actual or foster parents – for one quarter to one third of the incubation term, before placing under artificial incubation. With a new or contentious pair of birds who may squabble over incubation duties with freshly-laid eggs, replacing them with artificial or "dummy" eggs during most of the term will protect valuable eggs from breakage. Once parents have settled in and proven themselves with dummy eggs, the real eggs may be carefully returned to them, usually at internal pip, to allow parental hatching and rearing.

In order to manage the process of artificial incubation, and to some extent natural incubation, it is important to first have a thorough understanding of the structure of the egg, the functions of its components, the development of the embryo and its extraembryonic membranes, and the hatching process. This chapter will provide a cursory review of these. The reader is strongly encouraged to take advantage of more detailed references on the subject (Romanoff and Romanoff 1949, 1960; Hamburger and Hamilton 1951; Anderson-Brown 2002) and to practice incubation techniques with chicken eggs or other domestic species.

When the egg is laid, the embryo, known as the blastoderm at this stage, is positioned over the least dense area of yolk and so rises to the uppermost position regardless of the orientation of the egg during early development. The yolk is surrounded by layers of albumen, including the chalazae,

*Hand-Rearing Birds*, Second Edition. Edited by Rebecca S. Duerr and Laurie J. Gage.

which keep the yolk suspended in the egg and prevent the embryo from sticking to the shell. In addition to serving as a source of water and protein for the embryo, the albumen contains antimicrobial proteins that are barriers to infection. Surrounding the albumen are two nonliving membranes: the inner and outer shell membranes. The air cell forms between these two membranes, at the blunt end of the egg in most species, initially as the egg contents cool and contract after laying and during incubation through evaporation of water through the pores of the shell. The shell provides not only physical protection but the primary source of calcium and other minerals for the developing embryo. The shell is covered by the cuticle layer which ranges from glossy to chalky to barely visible in various species. This coating helps regulate water loss and, along with the shell and shell membranes, provides a mechanical barrier to infection. The embryo begins to develop before the egg is laid and does so initially in a flat plane, with the four extraembryonic membranes extending outward from the body wall.

The **yolk sac** is the first of these living membranes to develop. It is a highly vascular structure, initially forming a roughly circular pattern of vessels as it begins to envelope the yolk. Before other membranes have formed and because, along with the embryo, it is in contact with the inner surface of the shell membranes at the uppermost point of the egg, it serves as the first respiratory organ for the embryo, providing a limited amount of gas exchange. As it grows, it becomes thicker and develops folds lined with villi to increase surface area for the uptake of nutrients, much like the mature intestinal wall. The yolk is the primary nutrient source for the embryo, and for the chick even after hatch for a few days, and contains maternal antibodies, providing some passive immunity to the embryo, which has no active immune function.

The **amnion** is the next membrane to develop, also extending outward from the body wall. This nearly transparent membrane is minimally vascular. It grows up and over the embryo, eventually closing and filling with fluid that will cushion the embryo during development. The amnion also contains fine muscle fibers that contract rhythmically to prevent the embryo from sticking to it until embryonic muscles are developed enough to perform this function.

The **chorion** is formed by the extension of the amnion folding back on itself from the seam where it sealed over the embryo. It extends out to line the entire inner shell membrane, fusing with it and with the allantois, which is the last membrane to form.

The **allantois** is highly vascular. It emerges balloon-like from the hind gut of the embryo, continuing to expand and coming in contact with the chorion, with which it fuses, forming the **chorio-allantoic membrane** (CAM) or **chorioallantois.** The fluid that expands and is contained by the allantois is urinary waste, with uric acid crystals held in suspension until shortly before hatching when the concentration causes them to precipitate out of suspension into strands of opaque, white urates. The chorioallantois is the primary respiratory organ for the embryo throughout most of incubation, allowing transpiration of oxygen, carbon dioxide, and water vapor from its dense vascular network across the shell. It also forms the albumen sac, which ruptures its contents into the amniotic fluid just after the middle of incubation, allowing the embryo to consume the albumen protein that facilitates its final growth stage. Lastly, the chorioallantois transports calcium and trace minerals, etched from the shell, to the developing embryo.

## Hatchery Facilities and Equipment

Before the first egg arrives, the hatchery must be well organized and equipped. While few facilities have the resources to build and equip an ideal hatchery, most of the following principles can be achieved in any facility with some creativity and attention to detail.

Because eggs and chicks are vulnerable to infection and disturbance, the hatchery should be treated as a quarantine facility with access restricted to only essential personnel. The design should allow the primary functional areas to be separated and a one-way traffic flow, from cleanest to dirtiest, should be maintained. The incubation room, with only intact eggs, has the least contamination. Before they are externally pipped, eggs should be moved to the hatching room as the shell waste and feather dander of hatched chicks can provide substrates for microbial growth. Once hatched and rested, chicks should be moved to the chick-rearing room where food, feces, and more feather dander create the greatest source of contamination. Tools and equipment should also follow this one-way path, being thoroughly disinfected before returning to previous areas.

Construct rooms with materials that allow all surfaces to be washable, including floors, walls, and ceilings. Only equipment and supplies in current use should be kept in the room and eliminate all clutter. Historic paper records and reference materials are invariably dusty and should be stored elsewhere. Rooms should have adequate ventilation with frequent air changes and, ideally, a separate system for each functional area. The environment should be kept at 65–70 °F (18–21 °C) and must be as dry as possible to minimize microbial growth and optimize incubator function.

In developing the hatchery design, consideration should also be given to every aspect of its function. An efficient design facilitates easy servicing of incubators, routine weighing and candling of eggs, frequent cleaning, and maintaining and moving equipment.

Although the skill of the person operating an incubator is far more important than the machine itself, investment in high-quality equipment invariably pays off. There is no one incubator that is best and in fact all have potential quirks. The number and type acquired will depend on each facility's species, number of eggs, and budget. Discussion of options with those in established hatcheries is helpful in making these decisions. For many operations, a good strategy is to have at least three incubators, all set at the same temperature but at different humidities so that eggs can be moved among them as needed rather than making risky adjustments during incubation.

Most incubators currently available for avicultural incubation are table-top models, making it possible to have several in a relatively small room. Nearly all employ a forced-air system in which air is circulated by a fan, creating a relatively uniform temperature throughout the cabinet. Popular brands available in the United States include: Grumbach (Grumbach USA LLC), Georgia Quail Farm (GQF Manufacturing), Brinsea (Brinsea Products), Rcom (Rcom Company). A. B. Newlife incubators (A.B. Incubators) can be ordered only from the United Kingdom, but have been used in some U.S. facilities with good results. Brinsea has been marketing a "contact" incubator which is intended to more closely simulate natural incubation. The air above a flexible plastic membrane is heated by a forced-air system. This membrane is then in contact with the tops of the eggs in the tray underneath, creating a temperature gradient from the top to bottom through each egg, which is somewhat similar to a still-air system. Inexpensive incubators made primarily for classroom use with chicken eggs are usually not reliable enough for avicultural incubation. The Humidaire Incubator Company is now out of business but their popular table-top Models 20 and 21 – as well as their older free-standing Model 50, Ostrich, and Gooser incubators – may be worth purchasing used, although replacement parts may be difficult to find. The Petersime Company has also discontinued making their excellent free-standing incubator Models 1 and 4. Sunny Creek Farms in Minnesota acquires and sells used incubators, incubator parts, and operating manuals.

Nearly all current models have electronic temperature controls that are accurate and dependable. Older incubators may employ mercury contact thermometers or ether wafers to control temperature. Contact thermometers are also accurate but have a fatal flaw in that when they fail, the heating element stays on rather than shutting off and eggs are rapidly overheated. Ether wafers were once the most common incubator thermostats and are still used as a back-up temperature control system in some incubators. They are slightly less accurate than electronic controllers. They deteriorate over time and should be replaced annually.

Humidity may be provided by an automatic humidifier with either an evaporative pad or fine mist, or by simple evaporation from open water reservoirs. Automatic humidifiers are usually accurate and effective but are difficult to clean and disinfect, particularly during use. Unless mounted into the machine, most open reservoirs are easily changed out for cleaning. If not, using simple water pans in lieu of the humidifier built into the machine may be easier. Humidity is controlled by increasing or decreasing the surface area of water, usually by adding or removing pans. To ensure consistent humidity, pans should be straight-sided, made of nonreactive material such as stainless steel or plastic, and kept full at all times. With multiples of the same sized pans, both changing humidity and changing pans is easily done. All humidity systems should use distilled water or reverse-osmosis treated water only to prevent mineral buildup and microbial growth.

Turning mechanisms fall into three types: trays that are rotated, rollers on which eggs rest, and grids (or bars) that either push eggs along a substrate or hold them over a moving substrate. Rotating trays are usually safe as eggs do not actually move but many do not rotate through an adequate radius of 90°. Used properly, rollers provide sufficient turning radius for most eggs, although small eggs receive more turning and large eggs receive less. If rollers are improperly spaced, eggs may "ride" the rollers and receive little or no turning. Eggs with a more conical shape tend to "walk" toward one end of the rollers. Placing eggs point-to-point will minimize this. Grids or bars that push eggs have a greater chance of breaking eggs, but this potential varies greatly among machine designs.

Incubators may also be used as hatchers, but these functions should be done in separate machines to prevent contamination of incubating eggs and to accommodate changes in temperature and humidity during the hatching process. Machines designed specifically for hatching are also available. In addition to the models listed above, Brinsea, Rcom, and A. B. Newlife make hatchers. Spare parts, especially thermostats and fan motors, for both incubators and hatchers should be kept on hand to quickly repair mechanical problems during incubation.

It is important to invest in high-quality thermometers. Better mercury, mercury substitute, digital, and bi-metal-dial thermometers with a range bracketing that of incubation and readable increments of 0.1 °C or F should be used. All should be calibrated annually. Use of mercury has been prohibited in many areas due to safety risks but a proprietary blue "spirit" liquid is now used as a substitute in certified and other high-quality thermometers. A laboratory-grade ASTM-certified mercury or mercury substitute thermometer, Model 18F or 18C (VWR Scientific, Fisher Scientific, or Cole-Parmer), is useful for this but is not typically used directly in incubators as they are expensive and fragile. Digital thermometers and thermometer/hygrometers, certified as "traceable" from scientific supply vendors, have the advantage of being able to stay on continuously, allowing accurate readings without opening the incubator door. Similar-looking models are available from some incubator vendors but have not performed as well and do not stay on continuously. Inexpensive digital room thermometers and alcohol or red "spirit" thermometers are not accurate enough for egg incubation.

Humidity in egg incubators has historically been measured using wet-bulb thermometers, otherwise known as sling psychrometers, but these devices are being replaced by digital hygrometers in most applications. One end of a cotton wick is placed over the bulb of a secondary thermometer and the other end in a small water reservoir, usually a glass tube. Often only the reading of this wet bulb is used to record humidity, but true relative humidity is actually calculated from the differential between the dry and wet-bulb temperatures. The same wet-bulb temperature will indicate different humidities at different dry temperatures. If the wick is not rinsed daily and changed at frequent intervals, increasingly inaccurate readings will result and it may become a source of contamination in the incubator. Dial hygrometers give direct relative humidity readings but must be calibrated for the humidity range in which they are used. Digital hygrometers are the most accurate and reliable, but it is important to buy a high-quality model and to calibrate them at least annually.

Precise scales are essential for effective egg weight-loss management. Digital scales are more affordable than in the past. Scales should be laboratory quality, if possible. The range of egg sizes seen in the hatchery will determine the capacity and weighing increments needed for effective egg weight-loss management. For eggs weighing less than 30 g at lay, the scale should weigh in increments of and have an accuracy of 0.01 g. For eggs greater than 30 g but less than 500 g, increments and accuracy of at least 0.1 g are needed. If the only eggs incubated are from large ratites and weigh over 500 g, whole gram increments and accuracy are sufficient.

In most hatcheries, it is important to have an egg candler with the greatest light intensity available. The original Lyon High-Intensity Zoo Model Candler (Lyon Electric), which used a halogen bulb, is still in use in many facilities. Lyon later replaced this with an LED model. An old-fashioned slide projector, adapted to focus the beam and prevent light leaks, works nearly as well as the original halogen candler. The technology for tactical LED flashlights (Fenix, Surefire, and others) has advanced, and models providing 1000 lumens or more can be an excellent option for candling, with a home-made cone-shaped aperture. For facilities incubating only small, white eggs, such as parrots, less powerful candlers are fine. LED flashlights available in hardware stores work well for this and those with a flexible neck are ideal for checking small eggs in the nestbox. Prototype models of infrared and ultraviolet light candlers have been used for imaging with eggs that are difficult to candle with white light, but are not commercially available.

A room dehumidifier is necessary in humid climates and with species whose eggs have difficulty losing sufficient weight such as condors and ostrich. An emergency back-up generator is indispensable, even if it produces only enough power to run one machine. A portable incubator/brooder can be quite useful, especially if eggs must be transported long distances between facilities or from the field, or in freezing weather. A small portable brooder (Avey Incubators) may be used on an airplane (contact the airline well in advance for security assistance) and can be run on 110 V household current, a car cigarette lighter outlet, or portable batteries.

## Hatchery Sanitation

A rigorous sanitation protocol will minimize egg and chick mortality due to infection. Access to the hatchery should be restricted to essential personnel and only the equipment and supplies in immediate use should be stored in the rooms.

Before the onset of the breeding season each year, the hatchery and all its equipment should be thoroughly cleaned and disinfected. A strong disinfectant such as Rescue (formerly Accel; Virox Technologies) or Virkon-S (Virkon), is recommended. The interiors of incubators and hatchers are now most often disinfected with such a product between uses but great care must be taken to rinse and air all parts and ensure that sensitive electronics are not damaged, as the solution is somewhat corrosive. In the past, formaldehyde fumigation was the preferred method, but due to serious human health hazards this is now strictly regulated or prohibited by state laws. All machines should have any needed annual maintenance done, and then be run to test and stabilize them before eggs are likely to arrive.

Once the hatchery is operational, routine cleaning of the rooms should be done at least weekly. This should include wiping down all working surfaces and places where dust might accumulate, washing the floor, and cleaning water reservoirs in the incubators. Hydrogen peroxide-based, chlorhexidine and quaternary ammonium disinfectants are good choices for this. Chlorine bleach is inexpensive but creates noxious fumes and is corrosive to equipment. Water pans and wet bulb wicks should be replaced with freshly sterilized (autoclaved) or disinfected pans and wicks. Water reservoirs that cannot be removed for cleaning should be drained and flushed periodically during the season. A disinfectant footbath placed outside the door reduces contaminants that may be tracked into the rooms. Trash receptacles may be kept outside to minimize the potential for contamination in the room.

Staff working in the hatchery should organize daily work to minimize the potential for contaminants to enter the hatchery. Most of the hatchery work should be done before cleaning messy enclosures and similar chores. Some facilities choose to use protective clothing, such as lab coats or coveralls, over work clothes in the hatchery, but this may also serve as a reservoir of contaminants in the rooms. Wash hands thoroughly with soap and water (not only hand sanitizer) before servicing incubators and observe aseptic techniques. When handling eggs, the use of exam gloves in addition to handwashing may be desirable.

## Egg Handling and Storage

Many factors affect hatchability even before the egg is laid. These include genetics, nutrition, and exposure to toxins, as well as physiological factors such as age and disease, and behavioral influences such as stress or physical trauma that can affect egg formation. Much research has been done on all of these and many other publications are available for reference (Landauer 1967; Romanoff and Romanoff 1972; Kuehler 1983).

Additional factors influence hatchability once the egg is laid but before incubation starts. Infection of the incubating egg is one of the main causes of reduced hatchability. Microbial contamination of the shell can come from feces, nest material, or human hands. Physical trauma, such as cracking or breaking of eggs, is an obvious cause of egg mortality, but any jarring, shaking, or vibration can disrupt the loosely-adhered cells of the blastoderm, much like a sand painting, and cause abnormal twinning, duplications, or complete failure of the embryo. Allowing an egg to roll or turn over and over in the same direction can cause the chalazae to wind up like rubber bands and break, causing the embryo to stick to the inner shell membrane.

Environmental conditions prior to incubation affect hatchability. At a temperature of 70 °F (21 °C) or higher, embryonic development will initiate but different tissues will form at abnormal rates often resulting in embryonic mortality. Eggs will also lose too much weight through water evaporation if held at ambient humidity.

Many taxa, such as waterfowl, do not begin incubating until the clutch of eggs is complete. Eggs of these species tolerate short periods of storage better than those of single-egg clutches, such as flamingos, or multiple-egg clutches of species that begin incubation with the first egg, such as parrots. When incubating a lot of eggs of certain precocial species, such as ostrich or pheasant, it is desirable to synchronize hatching by storing eggs and then setting a group at once. Such eggs may be stored up to seven days without significant decrease in hatchability. Ideal parameters for egg storage are 55–60 °F (13–15 °C) and 70–80% relative humidity. Refrigerators designed for wine storage can be set to the appropriate temperature and humidity can be provided the same ways as in an incubator. Ventilation is not crucial, but it is important to prevent condensation moisture from getting on the eggs. Eggs can be stored in cardboard egg flats or clean sand and should be rotated through at least a 90° angle once daily. Stored eggs should be allowed to warm gradually, usually overnight, to room temperature before being set in the incubator.

## Initial Care of Eggs

Eggs that have been partially incubated prior to transfer to the hatchery must be placed in the incubator as soon as possible, especially if they have already become chilled. More time may be taken with unincubated eggs. In either case, eggs should be handled with exam gloves or paper towels and should be transported to the hatchery carefully to avoid rough handling or jarring. Many types of transport containers have been used, from cardboard boxes to buckets to small ice chests, which are filled or lined with cushioning materials such as clean paper or cloth toweling, waterfowl down, or small seed such as millet. Hot water bottles or chemical warming packs may be used if transport time or outdoor temperature puts eggs at risk of prolonged cooling. Ensure these do not come in direct contact with the eggs and that the eggs are maintained below incubation temperature, as even slight overheating would damage developing embryos. For longer trips, portable electronic incubators or brooders made for chicks (Avey Incubators) are useful, with the option of using wall outlets, car cigarette lighter jacks, or rechargeable batteries for power. Containers should be hand-held during transport if possible, to reduce the risk of shaking and jarring.

Once at the hatchery, carefully examine the egg both directly and with the candler. Cracks and flaws may not be obvious until the egg is candled. These should be carefully marked with a blunt pencil during candling to ensure that potential openings for infectious agents will be completely sealed. An identification number can also be written on the shell in pencil. A fine black marker may be necessary for heavily pigmented eggs. Embryonic and membrane development, if initiated, should be described along with any anomalies in or on the egg.

Soiled eggs should have loose, dry material such as down, nest substrate, or feces gently brushed off with a dry paper towel, gauze sponge, or swab, depending on the size of the egg. Large deposits of dried fecal material can be mostly removed by carefully sanding with a clean, fine sanding block, emery board, or dry scrub pad, taking great care not to disrupt the cuticle or shell. This will leave a visible stain or thin coating which should be left undisturbed.

Eggs should never be spot-cleaned with liquid. Even using an antiseptic or disinfectant solution fluid on the shell can facilitate the movement of infectious microbes through the pores of the shell and into the egg. In commercial production of domestic species, unincubated eggs may be dipped in a disinfectant solution to reduce contamination. This is done with products designed specifically for this purpose and using strict protocols of concentration, temperature, agitation, and immersion time. The temperature of the solution must be sufficiently higher than the egg contents but not so high as to kill the embryo. If the solution is too cool, the egg contents will shrink, drawing surface contaminants rapidly into the egg. Dipping is generally contraindicated for nondomestic bird eggs, especially with more delicate or thin-shelled eggs. Eggs that have, or may have, received any incubation should not be dipped. Fumigation with formaldehyde gas has been used to disinfect eggs but is more strictly regulated and no longer used now as the fumes are highly toxic to humans. Formaldehyde gas has been shown to cause lethal embryonic defects in the eggs of nondomestic species. Other methods of disinfecting eggs, such as exposure to ultraviolet light, have not been shown to be effective. The best way to prevent soiling of eggs and resulting infections is to ensure a clean nest environment whenever possible.

Cracked, flawed, punctured, or dented eggs are often hatchable if carefully repaired. If not repaired, they are vulnerable to infection and excessive weight loss. Even if there is a slight leakage of albumen or blood, repairs can usually be made. Eggs leaking yolk material, however, are not repairable. Various materials have been used to repair eggs, with some more suitable than others. Tape and wound dressing products do not make an adequate seal over an opening in an egg. Similarly, surgical tissue glue or other cyanoacrylate glues are too fluid and do not fill in fine cracks or punctures. In a laboratory setting, where a large number of eggs are undergoing invasive procedures, high melting point paraffin is typically used but is less practical in a small hatchery. Clear nail polish is quick-drying and has been used successfully, especially with small eggs, but it contains volatile solvents that have the potential to be toxic to the embryo. White glue (polyvinyl acetate – PVA) – such as Elmer's Glue All® or Wilhold – although slow-drying, is an excellent, nontoxic material for repair that also provides some structural support and is waterproof when dry. School glue is not appropriate as it is made to be washed out of clothing and may rehydrate in the humid incubator.

White glue should be applied with a sterile swab and using aseptic technique, thoroughly sealing the entire crack or puncture but only covering the affected area so as not to interfere with chorioallantoic respiration. For large dents or cracks which compromise the structural integrity of the egg, thin, sturdy paper toweling (or gift wrap tissue for tiny eggs) may be used to create a papier mâché patch. The patch should be torn (not cut) just larger than the area to be supported and carefully pressed onto a layer of glue, eliminating air bubbles, and sealed over with another layer of glue. Because white glue will become more fluid at incubation temperature and may run down the side of the egg, the egg should be placed in a paper-towel lined dish on the bottom of the incubator or on a leveled tray until the glue is thoroughly dried. If necessary, slight hand-turning can substitute for machine turning during this time. It is better to take this precaution, even with a small repair, than to come back later to find an egg glued to the tray.

Eggs compromised by cracks or excessive soil that are too valuable to discard should be incubated in a separate machine from sound eggs, if possible, or, if this is not an option, at least in a separate tray.

## Incubation Parameters

Natural incubation conditions create a temperature gradient from the top to the bottom of the egg, humidity varies within the nest microclimate and turning occurs with varying timing and radius. Artificial incubation does not strictly mimic the natural process, but rather should strive to achieve the same outcome. Eggs should hatch in the same time period, or incubation term, for the species as is seen under parental incubation. The chicks should be able to hatch without assistance and be vigorous after hatching. And as with any scientific effort, these results should be consistently repeatable.

### Temperature

Incubating machines may be either still-air or forced-air. While still-air incubators, those with a radiant heat sources that circulate air by convection rather than fans, create a temperature gradient, the temperature is difficult to control, ventilation is poor, and capacity is limited due to the necessity of setting eggs in a single layer. Temperature in a still-air incubator is usually, but not always, measured at the top of the egg. When using parameters developed by others, it is important to verify how and where temperatures are taken. Nearly all incubators in current use have a forced-air design, with air circulated by a fan that creates a uniform temperature throughout the cabinet. Only forced-air incubation parameters will be discussed here.

Domestic poultry species are normally incubated at 99.5 °F (37.5 °C) and this temperature works well for many nondomestic species. Particularly large eggs with longer incubation terms typically require lower temperatures. For example: 96.5 °F (35.8 °C) is typically used for Antarctic Penguins; 98.0 °F (36.7 °C) for condors and other large vultures; 98.5 °F (36.9 °C) for ostrich and large raptors; and 99.0–99.2 °F (37.2–37.3 °C) for psittacines. The smallest eggs, such as small passerines, and others with shorter incubation terms may hatch best at temperatures of 100.0–100.5 °F (37.8–38.1 °C).

If the temperature is a little too high, embryonic development will be slightly accelerated but at different rates in different tissues. If chicks hatch, they are likely to be reduced in size, have rough umbilical seals, and be thin and noisy. During hot weather, power failures affecting air conditioning may cause overheating in incubators despite the power loss to the machines. Embryos usually tolerate temporary drops in temperature but not increases in temperature once incubation starts. An increase of even 1.0 °F (0.5 °C) is often fatal in a few hours or less. If eggs must be moved in an emergency, such as a machine or power failure, they should always be moved to a machine with the same or lower temperature. They may be returned to the original temperature once normal power is resumed.

If the temperature is too low, embryonic development will be retarded, again with different rates in different tissues if this is extreme or prolonged. It is not usually lethal unless to an excessive degree or duration, but chicks are often large, sluggish, and sticky with incomplete yolk sac retraction or partially open umbilical seals. Power failures causing cooling for more than a few hours will prolong development. Although embryos may survive the initial insult, detrimental effects are usually not seen until the hatching process is initiated and some late mortality may occur.

During the hatching process for commercial poultry, the incubation temperature is dropped by 0.5–1.0 °F (0.3–0.5 °C) which has been shown to improve hatchability. This seems to work well for nondomestic species as well, although it has not been scientifically tested.

### Humidity

Avian eggs lose weight during incubation, usually 15% ±3%, by water evaporation through the pores of the eggshell. Because this is a physical process, not a metabolic process, it is not influenced by the stage of embryonic development and follows a linear pattern throughout incubation. Under artificial incubation conditions, this weight loss is managed by controlling the humidity in the incubator.

Domestic poultry are normally incubated at 45–55% relative humidity, at least to start. This is a good starting point for most nondomestic species. Eggs of species such as ostrich that are from exceptionally dry climates, however, are incubated without supplemental water in the incubator and may require a room dehumidifier. Similarly, eggs from wet-climate species will require higher humidity from the start.

Eggs should be weighed as soon after laying as possible and weight loss tracked throughout incubation to ensure successful hatching. If the humidity is too high, weight loss will be insufficient and embryos are likely to be edematous and/or malpositioned or have residual albumen/fluids (potentially resulting in drowning). Chicks that do hatch may have unretracted yolk sacs and/or open umbilical seals and will be lethargic. Humidity that is too low will result in excessive egg weight loss. This causes poor bone mineralization due to impaired calcium transport and weak, dehydrated (red) chicks with rough/bloody umbilical seals. Ambient humidity is naturally low at high altitudes and even parent-incubated eggs may lose too much weight. In this situation, good strategy is to remove eggs for artificial incubation at an appropriate humidity and give the parents dummy eggs, returning their own eggs just before hatching.

For artificially hatched eggs, the humidity in the hatcher should be increased as soon as eggs are externally pipped in order to limit the drying of shell membranes, which can restrict the embryos' movement. The amount of humidity needed varies by species, but those eggs with longer pip-to-hatch intervals are at greatest risk of having dry membranes.

### Turning

Eggs must be turned at regular, frequent intervals during incubation to facilitate normal membrane development and nutrient uptake and to prevent the embryo from sticking to the inside of the shell. Chickens turn their eggs every 35 minutes on average, while most incubators with automatic turning mechanisms turn eggs hourly. Some machines can be set to turn at longer or shorter intervals, but hourly turning is generally sufficient for nondomestic species. While commercial poultry eggs are set with their air cells uppermost and rotated around the short axis in order to maximize the number of eggs that will fit in the incubator, nondomestic species are not adapted to hatch well in this position. They should be set on their sides and rotated around the long axis. Eggs must be turned in opposite directions each time to prevent rupture of the chalazae and should turn through a radius of at least 90°. Supplemental hand-turning, usually two to three times daily through ~180° in opposite directions, may improve hatchability, particularly in large eggs. In machines that do not turn through at least 90°, additional hand-turning is essential to ensure completion of the chorioallantoic membrane (CAM). When automatic turning is not available and eggs are hand-turned, they must be turned a minimum of five times daily, preferably more, but always an odd number of times to prevent eggs from being in the same position overnight every night.

### Ventilation

Because embryos are respiring throughout incubation, they are sensitive to abnormal levels of oxygen and carbon dioxide in the incubator. In most avicultural settings, only a few eggs are incubated at a time so ambient outdoor oxygen and carbon dioxide concentrations are naturally maintained in the incubator as long as the hatchery is adequately ventilated. The exception to this is at high altitude where the oxygen concentration in the air is lower. In that case, testing and supplementing oxygen levels in the incubator can increase hatchability. Commercial incubation facilities, however, must always work to ensure adequate ventilation, especially late in incubation when eggs are generating high levels of carbon dioxide. During a power failure with incubators containing large numbers of eggs, opening the incubator for ventilation within an hour becomes more important than keeping it closed to conserve heat.

## Candling

Candling is the primary method for monitoring embryonic development. Excellent photos of candled eggs, healthy and not, at all stages of development are available on the internet (Ernst et al. 2004a) and in published materials (Jordan 1989; Delaney et al. 1999). Many eggs have pigmented shells that make candling difficult or even of little value later in incubation. It is important to have a room that can be completely darkened and to use a candler with the strongest light available. The brighter the candler, the hotter the light, so great caution must be used to avoid damaging eggs. Eggs should not be held against the light for more than a few seconds at a time and their surface should be felt to ensure they do not overheat. Even strong LED lights generate heat when used for longer periods.

Before eggs are placed in the incubator, they should be candled to evaluate shell quality, check for cracks and flaws, note yolk quality and mobility, and determine air cell formation and position. During incubation, development of the embryo and its extraembryonic membranes should be monitored to the extent possible, based on visibility. The progression of the air cell can be tracked by tracing its margin on the shell with a blunt pencil at regular intervals, usually every 3–7 days.

The first observable evidence of development is often the shadow of the blastoderm, appearing as a faint crescent along one edge of the yolk, although this is not visible in all fertile eggs. The yolk will also begin to increase in size and appear more fluid as water from the albumen moves into the yolk material. By 15–20% of the incubation term (3 days of 21 for the chicken) the embryo and yolk sac vessels should be clearly visible in even the smallest eggs. Practiced eyes will be able to discern this even in the most heavily pigmented eggs, although candling will quickly become impossible as vessels line the shell in such eggs. Note that while it is possible to confirm fertility by candling once the embryo has reached the stage of blood development, it is not possible to confirm infertility by candling alone. In eggs that remain "clear" on candling, fertility can only be determined by breaking them open and carefully examining the contents.

It is useful to record landmarks of development, such as heartbeat, eye pigment, membrane progression, and embryonic movement, and other detailed comments on candling observations, including sketches. Review of past records can help determine whether eggs are progressing normally, but only if notes are descriptive and detailed.

Initially, the yolk sac will appear clearly as a roughly circular red "spider" shape with the embryo in the center. As this membrane surrounds the yolk and becomes more complex, it will appear less distinct, an effect that is soon compounded by the vessels of the CAM as they line the inside of the shell. This "streaky" stage is often incorrectly interpreted to be the breakdown of vessels. Eggs at this stage have even been removed from incubation by those who were convinced they were dead or dying. The vasculature of the CAM eventually becomes more distinct and heavier. It should completely line the inside of the shell soon after the middle of incubation, usually forming a visible "seam" along the back side of the egg. Insufficient turning radius and setting eggs with the air cells uppermost will prevent the CAM from completing. This is easily checked by candling the egg from the small end.

The first indication that the hatching process has begun is the apparent sudden enlargement of the air cell, termed "draw down." This is caused by the slight separation of the inner and outer shell membranes rather than a true increase in air cell size. The inner shell membrane that has been taut above the embryo during incubation is now loosely draped like a blanket, allowing the embryo more flexibility of movement. Prior to internal pip, the shadow of the embryo's beak may be seen pushing against the membrane. The hatching contractions will appear irregular and jerky. Once the embryo has internally pipped, or pierced into the air cell, regular, rhythmic respiration is observed. After external pip, candling can verify whether the outer shell membrane has been pierced, ensuring the embryo's access to outside air. As the hatching process progresses, candling at the small end and sides can be used to monitor the regression and shutdown of the CAM vessels, at least in light-shelled eggs. This is especially useful in deciding if and when hatching assistance can be safely initiated.

## Egg Weight-Loss Management

Eggs must lose the appropriate amount of weight during incubation in order to hatch successfully. Generally, this is about 15% of the initial egg weight at laying, or fresh weight, for most species. Because this is not a metabolic function but occurs by the physical process of water evaporation through the pores of the eggshell, it is linear and can be manipulated by increasing or decreasing the humidity during incubation. Carefully monitoring and controlling egg weight loss is key to hatching success.

Eggs should be weighed as soon after laying as possible. Using a starting weight taken after eggs have started incubation will result in inaccurate weight loss calculations that may affect hatchability. If a true fresh weight taken within 24 hours of laying cannot be obtained, it can be approximated by the following formula:

$$\frac{CW}{1-\left[\frac{CD}{TD}(0.15)\right]} = FW_{\text{est}}$$

Where $CW$ = current weight, $CD$ = days incubated from setting to current, $TD$ = total days of incubation expected (incubation term), and $FW_{\text{est}}$ = estimated fresh weight. This equation assumes that the egg has had a weight loss trend of 15% under the incubating parents, as represented by the term "0.15" in the equation. This number can be adjusted as indicated by individual circumstances.

Another, more accurate method of estimating egg fresh weight is to use a species-specific constant, $K_w$ (Hoyt 1979; Burnham 1983). This relies on the shape of eggs, more specifically the relationship between egg dimensions and volume, that is unique to each species and can only be determined based on data from large number of eggs:

$$K_w = \frac{FW}{LB^2}$$

Where $K_w$ = observed weight coefficient, $FW$ = fresh weight, $L$ = length of egg (mm), and $B$ = breadth of egg (mm). Coefficients for intensively managed species, including Peregrine Falcons (Burnham 1983), California Condors (Kasielke personal communication), and Attwater's Prairie Chickens (Bailey personal communication) have been determined from existing data. Estimated fresh weights for future eggs with known length and breadth can then be calculated as follows:

$$K_W LB^2 = FW_{\text{est}}$$

Once the fresh weight is known or estimated, the expected weight loss can be calculated and the actual weight loss tracked graphically. This can be done using computer software designed especially for hatchery management, such as Tracks Software Egg Log, a generic spreadsheet application, or simply graph paper and pencil. Egg weight is plotted on the $y$-axis, with a scale range from fresh weight to fresh weight less 20% (approximately). Days of incubation are plotted on the $x$-axis, with the set date as day 0 and continuing a few days beyond the expected incubation term. If the expected weight loss is 15%, lines that bracket this, usually 13% and 17%, should be plotted on the graph (Figure 3.1). Then, as actual egg weights are plotted, it will be easy to see whether the weight loss is staying within the expected range and whether the slope of the line projects the appropriate trend.

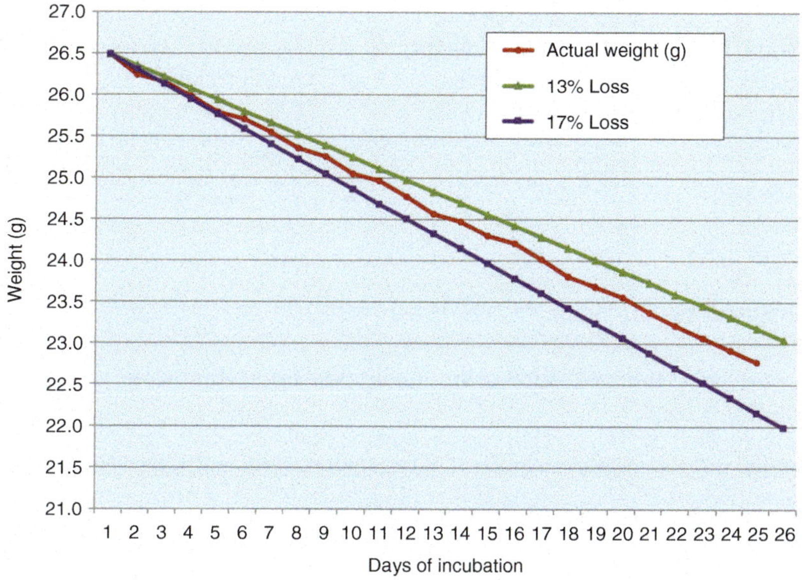


| Days | Actual weight (g) | 13% Loss | 17% Loss |
|---|---|---|---|
| 0 | 26.49 | 26.49 | 26.49 |
| 1 | 26.24 | 26.35 | 26.31 |
| 2 | 26.16 | 26.21 | 26.13 |
| 3 | 25.98 | 26.08 | 25.95 |
| 4 | 25.79 | 25.94 | 25.77 |
| 5 | 25.71 | 25.80 | 25.59 |
| 6 | 25.55 | 25.66 | 25.41 |
| 7 | 25.36 | 25.53 | 25.23 |
| 8 | 25.26 | 25.39 | 25.05 |
| 9 | 25.05 | 25.25 | 24.87 |
| 10 | 24.97 | 25.11 | 24.69 |
| 11 | 24.78 | 24.97 | 24.51 |
| 12 | 24.57 | 24.84 | 24.33 |
| 13 | 24.48 | 24.70 | 24.15 |
| 14 | 24.30 | 24.56 | 23.97 |
| 15 | 24.21 | 24.42 | 23.79 |
| 16 | 24.02 | 24.29 | 23.61 |
| 17 | 23.81 | 24.15 | 23.43 |
| 18 | 23.69 | 24.01 | 23.25 |
| 19 | 23.56 | 23.87 | 23.07 |
| 20 | 23.38 | 23.74 | 22.89 |
| 21 | 23.22 | 23.60 | 22.71 |
| 22 | 23.07 | 23.46 | 22.53 |
| 23 | 22.92 | 23.32 | 22.35 |
| 24 | 22.78 | 23.18 | 22.17 |
| 25 | | 23.05 | 21.99 |

**Figure 3.1** Egg weight loss – Saint Vincent Amazon, *Amazona guildingii,* egg 2017 (*Source:* data courtesy of Houston Zoo). Because frequent, small adjustments to humidity were initiated early in incubation, the weight loss trend was kept on track which resulted in a successful self-hatch.

If the date the egg was laid or incubation started is unknown and cannot be estimated, it is more difficult to manage weight loss. Such eggs should be set with parameters used successfully for the same or similar species and the progression of the air cell closely tracked. Understanding when the size of the air cell is appropriate for the stage of development can help determine whether the egg weight loss trend is normal. If there are records for eggs of very similar size, the expected daily weight loss for the current egg(s) can be estimated.

Ideally, eggs should be weighed daily and at the same time each day. This is particularly important during the early part of incubation as it becomes increasingly difficult to change an established weight loss trend later in incubation. When incubating very large numbers of eggs, weight loss can be recorded and managed for the average of all eggs or for a representative subset.

## Record Keeping

Consistent, detailed record keeping is essential to successful hatching of eggs, analyses of results, and ongoing refinement of techniques of artificial incubation. The following basic data should be collected on each egg and/or clutch:

- species;
- individual egg identification number;
- dam's and sire's identification, age, and reproductive history;
- history of individual egg or clutch;
- lay date;
- set date (the date either natural or artificial incubation commenced);
- expected term;

- expected egg weight loss;
- fresh weight (egg weight on lay date, actual or estimated);
- incubator and hatcher (identify individual machines);
- temperature and humidity settings prescribed.

Each time the egg is handled for weighing, candling, or moving to a different machine, the following data should be recorded:

- day of incubation (lay date = day 0);
- date and time;
- actual temperature and humidity;
- current egg weight;
- candling observations, changes to the incubation environment, and other comments;
- initials of the person recording data.

These data may be recorded directly into a spreadsheet or egg management software program for egg management during incubation, including monitoring of egg weight loss, and later analysis of overall hatchery results.

In addition to egg incubation records, data on individual incubators and hatchers should be recorded. Subtle problems with individual machines may only become obvious through poor hatchability. Records will help identify specific problems, such as excessive temperature fluctuation or failed turning mechanisms, and indicate needed repairs or other solutions. The following information should be recorded on each machine:

- make, model, serial number, and local identification;
- date, time, temperature, humidity, and egg tray position at least twice daily and whenever the machine is opened;
- type of event, including routine monitoring, servicing the machine (adding water, cleaning reservoirs, etc.), adjustments to parameters, weighing, candling, or movement of eggs, and seasonal cleaning or repair;
- initials of the person recording data.

Similarly, monitoring room temperature and humidity on an ongoing basis will aid in management of the hatchery.

## The Hatching Process

As the time of hatching nears, the embryo approaches its maximum size, occupying nearly all the space within the egg except for the air cell. The gas exchange capacity of the chorioallantois becomes insufficient, causing the onset of hypoxia (low $O_2$ in blood) and hypercapnia (high $CO_2$ in blood). The embryo consumes the remaining fluids while positioning for hatching. The spine is aligned with long axis of egg, with the dorsal side corresponding to "highest" edge of air cell, and the head is between the thighs in the small end of the egg. The head gradually moves up alongside the body to under the right wing, positioning the egg tooth under the air cell (inner shell membrane) (Figure 3.2). The hatching muscle along the back of the neck engorges with lymph to enhance leverage. At this stage, the entire head may be edematous despite normal egg weight loss, but pulmonary respiration will normally dissipate this edema. Correct positioning is correlated with adequate egg weight loss, incubation position (on side versus air cell up), and adequate ventilation (excess $CO_2$ often causes upside down embryos).

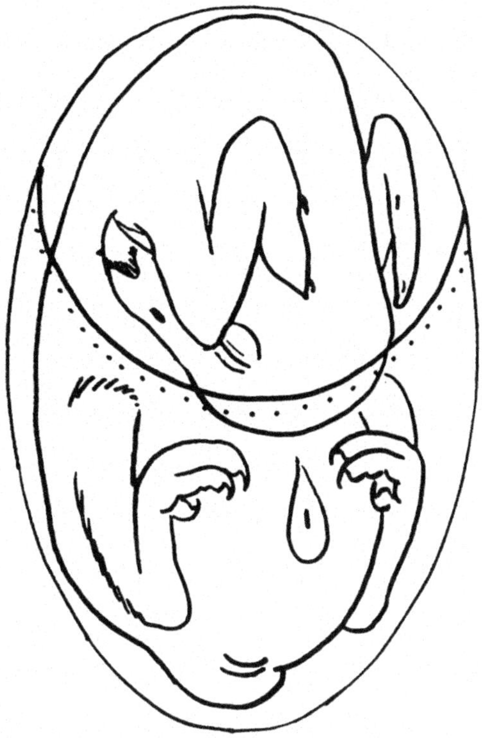

Figure 3.2 California Condor embryo in correct hatching position with head under right wing. *Source:* drawing credit: Mike Clark, courtesy of the Los Angeles Zoo.

The first indication that the hatching process has begun is air cell "draw down" seen on candling as the inner and outer shell membranes begin to separate. This occurs at about 85% of the incubation term. The inner membrane is then draped over embryo rather than being held taut and the air cell margin appears irregular. Internal pip occurs as contraction of the hatching muscle causes the egg tooth to pierce the inner membrane. Pulmonary respiration is then initiated. This may be audible, including vocalization in response to stimulation by the parent or surrogate. The contractions subside as gas exchange improves and the embryo rests. With exposure to air and the rubbing movements of the embryo, the chorioallantoic vasculature begins to recede, initially around the air cell, and finally at the umbilical seal just prior to hatch. External pip occurs as hatching contractions resume in response to decreasing $O_2$ and increasing $CO_2$ and the egg tooth pierces the shell. The contractions again subside as gas exchange improves and the embryo rests.

The yolk sac is gradually drawn into the abdomen, facilitated by embryonic movement. By hatching, the yolk sac is fully internalized behind a tight umbilical seal. The remaining yolk continues to be a food and water source for the chick for up to three days as it transitions to feeding or being fed. It also continues to provide maternal antibodies while the chick's immune system gains competence.

The pip site is broken up as hatching contractions resume in response to decreasing $O_2$ and increasing $CO_2$. The embryo rests only briefly at this stage. Rotation occurs with sustained hatching contractions combined with the embryo pushing with its legs. The embryo rotates in counterclockwise direction (viewed from air cell end), from one half to more than a full circumference of egg. Hatching occurs as the embryo pushes the cap off and frees itself from the shell (Figure 3.3). The chick then rests and dries off. Residual chorioallantoic vessels protrude from the seal but normally dry quickly. The chick may remain on its side for some time, even continuing to push as if

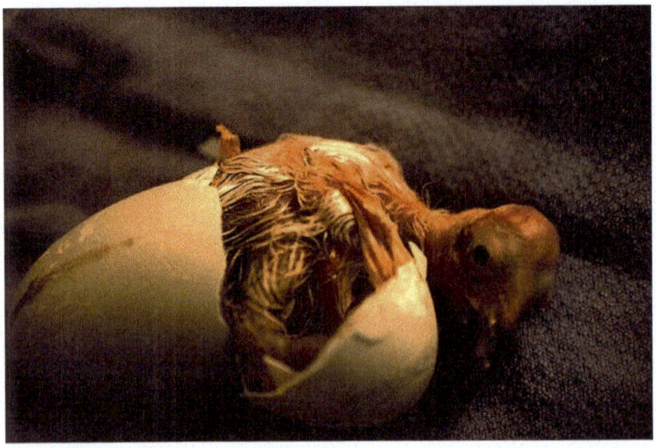

Figure 3.3 California Condor chick hatching. *Source:* photo credit: Mike Wallace, courtesy of Los Angeles Zoo.

still hatching. Healthy, artificially hatched chicks are usually ready to move from the hatcher to the brooder when they can maintain sternal posture, will give a feeding response, and usually will have defecated. They should be weighed and have their umbilical seals swabbed with a tamed iodine solution such as Betadine.

## Hatching Assistance

Even under ideal conditions, a proportion of embryos will fail to hatch, often due to malpositioning. Because of this, the imperfect nature of artificial incubation, and the likelihood that eggs are in the hatchery because they were already compromised, it is sometimes appropriate to assist the hatching process (Kasielke 2010). There is no simple formula for all species, or even individual species, to determine when this is necessary. Careful observation of many healthy eggs, particularly during the hatching process, will make it more obvious when something is going wrong.

Failure of the embryo to make expected progress during the hatching process warrants more frequent observation and possibly assistance. When malpositioning is suspected, eggs can be radiographed, ideally using a digital system, or with film and/or screens that give very fine detail. A piece of thin surgical wire can be loosely taped along the surface of the egg as a marker to correspond with a pencil line drawn on the shell. In order to determine which structures are in front of others, four views will be useful: presumed V–D (ventral-to-dorsal, with the lowest edge of the air cell uppermost), then rotated 45° counterclockwise (viewed from air cell end) around the long axis three times so that the last view is presumed to be right lateral/dorsal oblique. Interpreting the images takes considerable time and patience as the bones are poorly calcified and overlay one another.

If the embryo has internally pipped but failed to make progress within the expected time, providing an air hole may be helpful at this stage. A small hole, ~2 mm, can be drilled at the apex of the air cell, well away from the embryo, using a small rotary tool (Dremel Micro #8050) with a clean diamond-coated or other abrasive bit. A 16- or 18-gage hypodermic needed may also be used as a drill, but extreme caution must be used to avoid slipping and injuring the embryo. Some embryos require no further assistance and go on to hatch on their own, making us wonder if the assistance was necessary in the first place.

If the embryo has failed to internally pip and is either losing strength or becoming frantic, it may be necessary to manually provide an internal pip. A larger hole can be made in the shell nearer the tip of the beak and a hole made through the membranes over the beak and nares, using blunt dissection technique to minimize bleeding. The level of blood flow to the CAM and location of large vessels can be checked by moistening a sterile swab with sterile water (or normal saline or lactated Ringer's solution) and gently pressing or rubbing the area. If necessary, repeating this process will eventually reduce the refill rate of the vessels, making it safer to break the membranes.

Once this is done, it is most often necessary to fully assist the embryo from the shell when it is ready. Both the retraction of the yolk sac and the shutdown of the chorioallantoic vessels take time. Ensure both these have occurred before the shell is completely removed. Candling all areas of the egg is helpful in monitoring vessels. It is difficult and sometimes impossible to see whether the yolk sac is exposed, but removing too much shell will allow the embryo to push out prematurely. In the meantime, the hole in the shell should be covered with cellophane tape or a dressing material such as Tegaderm that is perforated or loose around the edges to allow air exchange while retaining moisture. Membranes usually become too dry during a lengthy assisted hatch and can even shrink, compressing the embryo. Application of sterile water or isotonic solutions seems to aggravate this drying, but oil-based artificial tears or ophthalmic ointment, used sparingly, will ensure membranes remain pliable. Ensure the tip of the beak and the nares remain clear.

There also is a risk of infection at this stage, because both the membranes and the yolk sac are exposed to the air and microbes in the environment. Using sterile, or at least aseptic, technique will minimize the risk. Because California Condors have a protracted hatching period – an average of 72 hours from external pip to hatch in self-hatching eggs – at the Los Angeles Zoo, it is routine to treat them prophylactically with antibiotics when the egg must be opened for assistance. An antibiotic least likely to cause kidney damage, such as Rocephin (Roche Pharmaceuticals), is dripped onto the inner surface of the CAM.

Malpositioned embryos with the beak not near the air cell are more difficult to assist. Radiographs can determine the position of the beak and an air hole made directly over the beak. This is certain to result in some bleeding but usually not enough to be life threatening. Because it has not pipped into the air cell, the embryo will not have that additional space to allow movement and yolk sac retraction. An additional small hole should be drilled at the apex of the air cell and the egg positioned such that the weight of the embryo will gradually push out the air at that end, gaining more room to move. This is also a good technique for embryos that externally pip on their own away from the air cell. These may even hatch without further assistance, although they warrant frequent checks.

Most chicks, even those requiring hatching assistance, will have fully retracted their yolk sacs and tightly closed their umbilical seals. A few, however, may have partially or fully unretracted yolk sacs. If there is a small amount exposed and the seal is slightly open, it may be possible to ease the yolk sac into the body cavity and suture the seal closed. If the seal has tightened around a small knob of yolk, the chick can be kept especially clean until the material dries and eventually sloughs off. If there is a large part or all of the yolk exposed, it is usually surgically amputated. Great care must be taken when tying it off as there is normally a loop of intestine external to the body cavity until the yolk sac is retracted. Chicks that have had their yolk sacs amputated will require supportive care, including feeding frequent small amounts as early as possible, as well as a course of antibiotics.

## Egg Necropsy and Analysis of Hatching Failures

Thorough analysis of hatching failures is crucial to future hatching success. This chapter will provide a simple outline for this process. The reader is strongly encouraged to review more detailed references on the subject (Kuehler 1983; Langenberg 1989; Joyner and Abbott 1991; Ernst et al. 2004b).

The two most useful statistics are fertility and hatchability, and they are expressed as percentages. Fertility is the ratio of the number of fertile eggs to the total number of eggs received. For commercial poultry, this is usually 90% or more. Similar fertility should be seen in aviculture as well with mature, healthy, compatible birds. Hatchability is the ratio of the number of hatched eggs to the number of fertile eggs set (not the total number of eggs – infertile eggs are incapable of hatching). This is typically 87–93% in commercial poultry hatcheries but tends to be a bit lower in aviculture, even under good conditions, for a variety of reasons.

This expected or normal mortality falls into specific developmental periods. One third, or about 2–5% of all expected mortality occurs during the first few days of incubation and is primarily due to chromosomal anomalies when the gametes form. The remaining two thirds, about 5–9%, occur during the last few days of incubation and are usually associated with the hatching process, including malpositions. There should be little or no mortality during the middle of incubation.

Break out and examine all unhatched eggs, including those that are "clear" on candling. If all clear eggs are assumed to be infertile, efforts will likely be made to solve a fertility problem when, in fact, there may be a hatchability problem with a vastly different cause.

The first step in a thorough egg necropsy is a review of the parental history and the incubation record. The egg should be candled to locate the embryo, air cell, and any unusual characteristics. It may be desirable to take microbial culture samples from the shell surface and/or egg contents, particularly the yolk contents, but the embryo will likely have been dead for more than a day resulting in a high number of decay organisms and masking infectious ones. It is sometimes very difficult to determine whether an embryo is still viable and usually wise to risk leaving the egg under incubation a few days longer. If egg infections are suspected, the interior of the incubator may be swabbed for culture, particularly water sources.

Clear eggs and those with younger embryos are best opened in water. The shell can be cracked (much like for cooking), and the egg held submerged in a bowl of water while the shell halves are eased apart. Broken yolk is likely to obscure everything else, so it may be necessary to carefully strain and rinse the egg contents to find membrane tissue or a tiny embryo. Eggs with older embryos can be opened with forceps, beginning with a hole over the air cell and carefully noting the condition of the extraembryonic membranes and fluids, and the position of the embryo as the shell and shell membranes are removed. Even badly decomposed eggs may yield useful information. Using a standard system of characterizing embryos by developmental stage (Hamburger and Hamilton 1951), breakout results should be characterized as follows:

***"Clear" on Candling:***

- I = infertile – blastodisc centrally dense white, not "donut-shaped" as in fertile egg;
- PD = positive development – no discrete embryo but white membranous tissue on the surface of a watery yolk;
- FND = fertile, no development – rare case of development ceasing at lay due to genetic defect or thermostabilized blastoderm.

***"Blood Ring" on Candling:***

- BWE = blastoderm without embryo – membranes and blood only;
- ED = early dead embryo (see below).

***Obvious Dead Embryo on Candling:***

- ED = early dead embryo – H&H stage 1–19 (≤3 days in chick embryo);
- MD = mid-dead embryo – H&H stage 20–39 (3–14 days in chick embryo);
- LD = late dead embryo – H&H stage 40–45 (≥14 days in chick embryo).

All embryos should be examined to determine if they are normal for their developmental stage and whether that stage is consistent with the number of days of incubation. Positioning of very late dead embryos, those near hatching with little or no free fluid in the egg, should be noted as either normal or one of seven recognized malpositions:

1) head between the thighs (normal early pre-hatch position);
2) head in the small end (upside down);
3) head under left wing;
4) beak directed away from the air cell;
5) leg over head;
6) head over right wing (should hatch normally);
7) crosswise in egg (spine aligned with short axis).

These embryos may be dissected for more detailed gross and histological examination as would be done for a newly hatched chick.

Hatching failures due to obvious causes, such as insufficient egg weight loss, are easy to diagnose with individual eggs, and often easy to prevent in the future. Most causes of poor hatchability will be subtle and difficult to detect, so careful analysis of data over time will prove invaluable. For example, if there is a high incidence of mortality during mid-incubation, it may be traced back to a nutritional problem with the breeding birds or to a source of infection of the eggs. The problem may be as simple as a malfunctioning turning mechanism on a particular incubator. Diligent and detailed record keeping followed by objective data analysis is the best way to ensure optimum hatchability.

## Sources of Products Mentioned

A.B. Incubators: Unit 1, Church Farm, Chelmondiston, Ipswich, Suffolk, IP9 1HS, United Kingdom, +44(0)1473-780-050, www.abincubators.co.uk.

Avey Incubators/Precision Incubators: P. O. Box 279, Hugo, Colorado 80821, (719) 297-7010, https://www.precisionincubators.com.

Brinsea Products, Inc., 704 North Dixie Avenue, Titusville, Florida 32796, (321) 267-7009, (888) 667-7009, http://www.brinsea.com.

Cole-Parmer, 625 East Bunker Court, Vernon Hills, Illinois 60061, (800) 323-4340, (847) 549-7600, sales@coleparmer.com,www.coleparmer.com.

Dremel, 1800 West Central Road, Mount Prospect, Illinois 60056-2230, (800) 437-3635, www.dremel.com.

Fenix Lighting, Littleton, Colorado, (888)775-9996, customerservice@fenixlighting.com, https://www.fenixlighting.com.

Fisher Scientific Worldwide, One Liberty Lane, Hampton, New Hampshire 03842, (800) 766-7000, http://www.fishersci.com/us/en/home.html.

G.Q.F. Manufacturing Company, 2343 Louisville Road, Savannah, Georgia 31415-1619, (912) 236-0651, www.gqfmfg.com.

Grumbach USA LLC, 111 N Arlington Heights Rd, Arlington Heights, Illinois, 60004, (772)607-0590, sales@grumbach-usa.com, https://www.grumbach-usa.com/Default.asp.

Rcom Company, P. O. Box 780871, Wichita, Kansas, 67278-1038, (912)239-5612, info@r-com-hatcher.com, https://www.r-com-hatcher.com.

Roche Pharmaceuticals, Hoffman-La Roche, Inc., 340 Kingsland Street, Nutley, New Jersey 07110, (973) 235-5000, www.roche.com.

Sunny Creek Farms, 15378 160th Street, Red Lake Falls, Minnesota 56750, (218) 253-2291, (218) 253-2211, dshirrick@gmail.com, http://sunnycreekhatchery.com.

Tracks (Egg Log), http://trackssoftware.com.

Virkon Disinfectants, Pennsylvania, (800)441-9408, www.virkon.com.

Virox Animal Health, 2770 Coventry Road, Oakville, Ontario L6H 6R1, Canada, (800) 387-7578, www.viroxanimalhealth.com.

VWR Scientific, 1310 Goshen Parkway, West Chester, Pennsylvania 19380, (800) 932-5000, (888) 897-5463, technicalproductSupportNA@vwr.com, https://us.vwr.com/store.

## References


Anderson-Brown, A.F. (2002). *The Incubation Book*. Surrey: Hancock House Publishers.

Burnham, W. (1983). Artificial incubation of falcon eggs. *Journal of Wildlife Management* 47 (1): 158–168.

Delaney, M.E., Tell, L.A., Millam, J.R., and Preisler, D.M. (1999). Photographic candling analysis of the embryonic development of Orange-winged Amazon parrots (*Amazona amazonica*). *Journal of Avian Medicine and Surgery* 13 (2): 116–123.

Ernst, R.A., Bradley, F.A., Abbott, U.K., and Craig, R.M. (2004a). Egg Candling and Break Out Analysis. *Oakland: University of California Division of Agriculture and Natural Resources Publication 8134*. http://anrcatalog.ucanr.edu/pdf/8134.pdf.

Ernst, R.A., Bradley, F.A., Abbott, U.K., et al. (2004b). Common Incubation Problems: Causes and Remedies. *Oakland: University of California Division of Agriculture and Natural Resources Publication 8127*. https://anrcatalog.ucanr.edu/pdf/8127.pdf.

Hamburger, V. and Hamilton, H.L. (1951). A series of normal stages in the development of the chick embryo. *Journal of Morphology* 88: 49–89; Reprinted in Developmental Dynamics 195:231–272(1992); http://homepage.univie.ac.at/brian.metscher/ Hamburger51_ChickStages.pdf. https://www.swarthmore.edu/NatSci/sgilber1/DB_lab/Chick/hamburger.pdf.

Hoyt, D.F. (1979). Practical methods of estimating volume and fresh weight of bird eggs. *Auk* 96: 73–77.

Jordan, R. (1989). *Parrot Incubation Procedures*. Ontario: Silvio Mattacchione & Co.

Joyner, K.L. and Abbott, U.K. (1991). Egg necropsy techniques. Proceedings of the Association of Avian Veterinarians Annual Conference in Chicago, IL, pp. 146–152.

Kasielke, S. (2010). When good eggs go bad: hatching assistance and egg necropsy. Proceedings of the American Association of Zoo Veterinarians Annual Conference, South Padre Island, TX, pp. 126–131.

Kuehler, C. (1983). Causes of embryonic malformations and mortality. Proceedings of the American Association of Zoo Veterinarians Annual Conference, Tampa, FL, pp. 157–170.

Landauer, W. (1967). *The Hatchability of Chicken Eggs as Influenced by Environment and Heredity, Monograph I (Revised)*. Storrs, CN: University of Connecticut.
Langenberg, J. (1989). Pathological evaluation of the avian egg. Proceedings of the American Association of Zoo Veterinarians Annual Conference, Greensboro, NC, pp. 78–82.
Romanoff, A.L. and Romanoff, A.J. (1949). *The Avian Egg*. New York: Wiley.
Romanoff, A.L. and Romanoff, A.J. (1960). *The Avian Embryo*. New York: MacMillan Co.
Romanoff, A.L. and Romanoff, A.J. (1972). *Pathogenesis of the Avian Embryo*. New York: Wiley.

## Further Reading

Abbott, U.K., Brice, A.T., Cutler, B.A., and Millam, J.R. (1991). Embryonic development of cockatiel (*Nymhicus hollandicus*). *Journal of the Association of Avian Veterinarians* 5 (4): 207–209.
Gilbert, S.F. (2003). Chick Embryo Staging. Swarthmore College. http://www.swarthmore.edu/NatSci/sgilber1/DB_lab/Chick/chick_stage.html.
Hamilton, H.L. (1952). *Lillie's Development of the Chick*. New York: Holt, Reinhart & Winston.
Harvey, R. (1990). *Practical Incubation*. Surrey: Birdwood Holt Pound.
Kuehler, C.M. and Good, J. (1990). Artificial incubation of bird eggs at the Zoological Society of San Diego. *International Zoo Yearbook* 29: 118–136.
Rahn, H., Ar, A., and Paganelli, C.V. (1975). How bird eggs breathe. *Scientific American*: 46–55.
Weaver, J.D. and Cade, T.J. (1991). *Falcon Propagation*. Boise: The Peregrine Fund.

# 4

# Ratites

*Dale A. Smith*

## Natural History

Ratites are flightless birds in five orders of the infraclass Palaeognathae: ostriches, emus, cassowaries, rheas, and kiwis (Gill and Donsker 2015). The term "ratite" comes from the Latin *ratis* meaning raft and refers to the flat smooth sternum that is characteristic of these birds. Ostriches, emus, and rheas are raised commercially for meat, leather, and feathers – and in the case of the emu, oil. Cassowaries and kiwis are handled more as specimens in zoological or display collections, or – particularly for the kiwi – as part of conservation and rehabilitation projects. All species have lived for 30 years or more in captivity. The tinamous are the sixth group of birds in the Palaeognathaea, and are flighted. Some commercial raising of tinamous has been undertaken.

The ostrich (*Struthio camelus,* Order Struthioniformes, Family Struthionidae) was originally found throughout Africa and extending into the Middle East. Wild birds are currently found in greatly reduced numbers in geographically limited pockets. Four subspecies have survived: the North African Ostrich (*Struthio camelus camelus*), the Somali Ostrich (*Struthio camelus molybdophanes*), the Masai (East African) Ostrich (*Struthio camelus massaicus*), and the South African Ostrich (*Struthio camelus australis*) (Folch 1992e). In the 1800s, North African and South African Ostriches were interbred in South Africa to produce the domesticated South African or Cape Black Ostrich (*Struthio camelus domesticus*). Because of the color of the skin on the legs and necks of males during the breeding season, North and East African birds are commonly known as *Red-neck,* and Somali and South African birds as *Blue-neck*. Ostriches are the largest living birds; males commonly stand 6.5–9.8 ft. (2–3 m) in height and may weigh up to 400 lb (180 kg). Females are smaller with weights up to 330 lb (150 kg). Male birds have black and white plumage; females and juveniles are brownish gray. Ostriches have relatively large wings and two unequally sized toes pointing forward.

The emu (*Dromaius novaehollandiae,* Order Casuariiformes, Family Casuariidae) is found in a variety of open and semiarid habitats through most parts of Australia (Folch 1992b). Birds stand up to 6 ft. (1.8 m) in height and weigh up to 110 lb (50 kg); females are slightly taller and heavier than males. Both sexes have brown and black feathering. Emus have vestigial wings and three forward-facing toes.

The rhea is native to South America (Order Rheiformes, Family Rheidae) (Folch 1992d). There are two species: the Greater or Common Rhea (*Rhea americana*) and the Lesser or Darwin's Rhea (*Pterocnemia pennata*). The Common Rhea, the species raised commercially, may stand up to 5 ft.

*Hand-Rearing Birds*, Second Edition. Edited by Rebecca S. Duerr and Laurie J. Gage.

(1.5 m) in height and weigh 44–55 lb (20–25 kg); the Lesser Rhea is approximately half this size. Rheas have gray-brown plumage and are not sexually dimorphic, although males are slightly larger and darker. Rheas have moderately sized wings and three forward-facing toes.

Cassowaries (Order Struthioniformes, Family Casuariidae) are found within tropical rainforests in Australia, Papua New Guinea, and Indonesia (Folch 1992c). There are three species: the Southern or Double-wattled Cassowary (*Casuarius casuarius*), the Northern or Single-wattled Cassowary (*Casuarius unappendiculatus*), and the Dwarf Cassowary (*Casuarius bennetti*). The Southern Cassowary, the species most commonly held in captivity, measures in height 4.3–5.6 ft. (1.3–1.7 m), with weights of 64–75 lb (29–34 kg) for males, and up to 125 lb (58 kg) for females. Northern and Southern Cassowaries are similar in size; Dwarf Cassowaries are smaller. Cassowaries have glossy black hairlike feathers and brightly colored featherless facial and neck skin, with colored wattles hanging from the sides or front of the neck. Cassowary wings are vestigial and end in a claw. Cassowaries have three forward-facing toes ending in strong, and sometimes very long, nails.

Kiwis (Order Apterygiformes, Family Apterygidae) live in forested zones in New Zealand. Five species of kiwi exist: the Southern Brown (*Apteryx australis*), North Island Brown (*Apteryx mantelli*), Okarito or Rowi (*Apteryx rowi*), Little Spotted (*Apteryx owenii*), and Great Spotted (*Apteryx haastii*). These small birds, the larger females weighing up to 7.7 lb (3.5 kg), are nocturnal, spending their days in burrows (Folch 1992a; Sales 2005). Kiwis have long decurved beaks with nostrils at their tips; they rely more on scent and hearing than they do vision. Kiwis have three cranial-facing and one rear-facing toe.

Tinamous (Order Tinamiformes, Family Tinamidae) are relatively small, compact, partridge-like birds belonging to 9 genera with 47 species (Cabot 1992). Body weight ranges from 43 g for the dwarf tinamous (*Taoniscus nanus*) to 1800 g for the Solitary Tinamou (*Tinamus solitarius*). Tinamou species can be found in a variety of forest, scrub and grassland habitats from north-west Mexico through much of South America. Tinamou eggs have a highly polished, glossy surface and a wide range of colors, depending on species.

The information contained in this chapter refers primarily to the species held most commonly in captivity, the ostrich, emu, and rhea, unless otherwise noted.

## Criteria for Intervention

In captivity, natural incubation and parental raising of ratite chicks is unusual. In commercial settings, ostrich, emu, and rhea eggs are collected, artificially incubated, and most commonly raised apart from adults, although they may occasionally be fostered back to breeding pairs. Ratite chicks are precocial but would normally stay with their parents for a period of months. Chicks may be recognized as requiring intervention at the time of hatching, or might be removed from their groups of conspecifics for reasons including obvious illness (e.g. anorexia, dehydration, depression, inactivity), injury, developing limb deformities (e.g. torsional, valgus, varus), and significantly delayed growth (Figure 4.1).

Ratite chicks are normally alert, social, and inquisitive and, especially ostriches, are highly stressed by changes in management and by being isolated from their companions. Extensive picking at nonfood items may indicate stress and be a predictor for poor-doing ostrich chicks, with anorexia, gastric stasis, and death resulting (Deeming and Bubier 1999).

The days of incubation and percentage of weight loss during incubation follow normal distribution curves; hence, a spread of values within a hatch is to be expected. Specifically designed and commercially available computer programs and computerized incubation systems are also

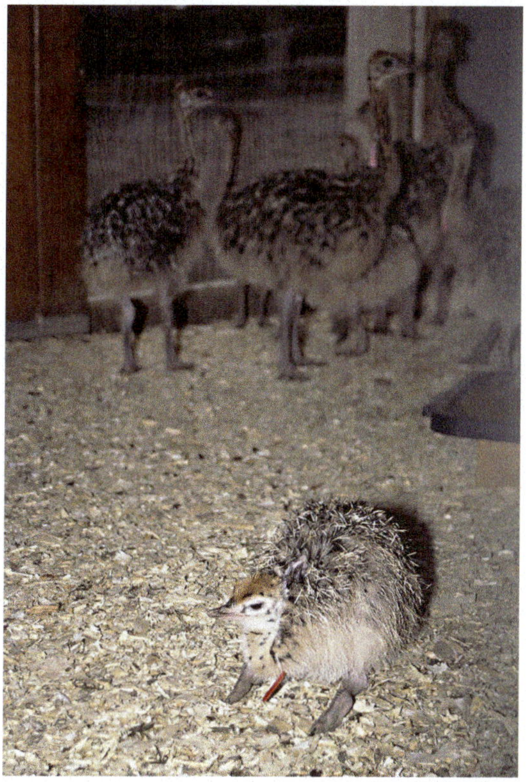

Figure 4.1 Depressed young ostrich separating from other chicks.

available. Careful record keeping and frequent assessment of incubation parameters and growth of chicks is essential to maximize production and for early identification of management errors and impending health problems.

## Record Keeping

Commercial ratite farms keep extensive records on breeding, egg laying, incubation parameters, egg weight loss during incubation, hatch times, and chick growth and development.

## Incubation of Eggs

Ratites are seasonal breeders, with egg production linked to increasing daylight in ostrich, rhea, and kiwi; decreasing daylight in emu; and availability of food sources in cassowary (Folch 1992a–e; Biggs 2013). Eggs are laid in depressions in the ground; hence, environmental cleanliness is important to reduce egg contamination and maximize hatching success. They should be collected and given a specific identity as soon as possible after lay. Eggs are often stored after collection to synchronize incubation of groups of eggs. Hatchability generally decreases with increased storage time, i.e. after 7–10 days for ostrich eggs. Ostrich eggs are stored at 50–68 °F (10–20 °C) with twice-daily turning during this period. Emu eggs are stored at temperatures of 40–60 °F (4.5–15.5 °C) and may be more tolerant of longer storage periods (Minaar 1998). Hatching rates of ratite eggs, especially ostrich, are considerably less than those for commercial poultry.

Table 4.1 Incubation parameters for ratites.

| Species | Egg Weight (g) | Temperature | Relative Humidity | Days of Incubation | Weight Loss over Incubation | Approx. Chick Weight at Hatching (g) |
|---|---|---|---|---|---|---|
| Ostrich | 1300–1700 | 36.0–36.5 °C<br>96.8–97.7 °F | 20–40% | 42 | 15% | 860–1100 |
| Emu | 550–600 | 36.1–36.4 °C<br>97.0–97.5 °F | 25–40% | 50–52 | 10–15% | 360–400 |
| Rhea | 500–800 | 36.4 °C<br>97.5 °F | 30–60% | 36–40 | 15% | 330–530 |
| Cassowary | 500–800 | 35.5–36.7 °C<br>95.9–98.1 °F | 57–64% | 47–57 | 12–15% | 330–530 |
| Kiwi | 400–450 | 35.5–36.5 °C<br>95.9–97.7 °F | 60–65% | 70–90 | | 280 |

Although recommended incubation parameters are listed in many texts and references (Jensen et al. 1992; Tulley and Shane 1996; Huchzermeyer 1998; Minaar 1998; Doneley 2006; Romagnano et al. 2012; Biggs 2013), considerable variation can result from farm and location-related factors, such as type of incubator, number of eggs being hatched, and ambient temperature and humidity. General incubation guidelines are presented in Table 4.1.

The environmental quality inside the incubator is of paramount importance to embryo development and growth. Eggs should be examined and weighed at weekly intervals to ensure that weight loss and embryo development are progressing appropriately. As in other avian species, abnormal embryo development and embryonic mortality may be associated with elevated or depressed temperature or humidity, with inadequate or inappropriate egg-turning, or with bacterial or fungal contamination. Adequate air flow through the incubator is particularly important to provide sufficient oxygen for the large embryos and to ensure that incubator temperature does not rise excessively. Specific incubators are manufactured for ostriches and emus in order to provide the appropriate frequency and mechanics of egg rotation. Ostrich eggs are set air cell up, and are rotated over a 90° arc, 45° each side of vertical. Emu and cassowary eggs are generally laid on their sides and are rotated back and forth around the long axis with a series of roller bars. Visual assessment of embryonic development (i.e. candling eggs) requires strong light sources to pass through the thick shells of ostrich and rhea eggs. An infrared candler may be used for dark-shelled emu eggs (Figure 4.2).

## Initial Care, and Stabilization

Ratite eggs are moved to a hatcher 1–4 days before the end of incubation to provide higher humidity, slip-free flooring, and reduce contamination in the incubator. Chicks may take 1–3 days from internal pipping (entry into the air cell) to external pipping (opening of the shell). It may take several hours to days for the chick to fully emerge from the egg. Ratite chicks open their shells by a combination of pushing with their legs and head. Hatching problems are almost always a result of weak chicks due to incubation difficulties, inadequate nutrient stores provided by the hen, or embryonic developmental anomalies. It is a quite common practice to assist hatch in ostrich chicks

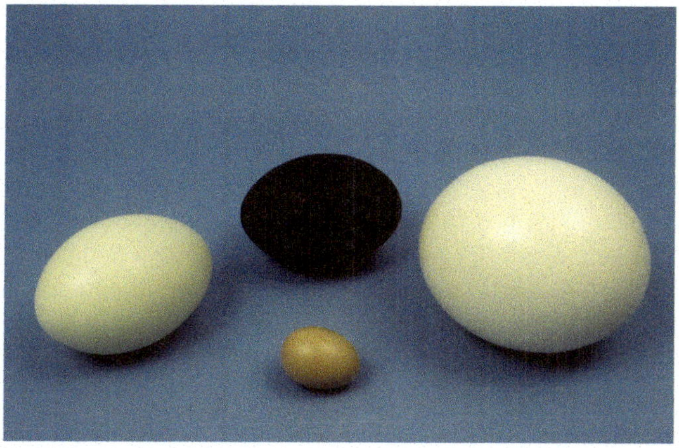

Figure 4.2 Rhea, emu, and ostrich eggs (left to right), with chicken egg in foreground for scale.

by chipping away some of the egg shell once external pipping begins; however, prematurely forcing the hatch may result in bacterial contamination of the yolk sac. After hatching, chicks are inspected to ensure that the yolk sac is completely internalized and the navel closed; if not, the navel is treated with a topical disinfectant, e.g., a povidone-iodine solution, and covered with a bandage or other temporary protection. The navel should be closed before the chick is removed from the hatcher. A visible identification tag is placed to allow accurate record keeping. Microchips are sometimes placed in the large pipping muscle at the back of the neck at this time. Splaying and leg injuries can occur as the chicks move around and attempt to stand; in some facilities tape hobbles are placed on all chicks for first few days to prevent this. Chicks are left in the hatcher for a few hours up to a few days, depending on their strength and activity.

Chicks of several days to several months of age may be sexed by direct cloacal observation. The bird is restrained on its back and the cloaca gently everted to reveal the male phallus or much smaller female clitoris. Experience is required for accuracy, and caution should be taken in guaranteeing the sex of young birds.

## Common Medical Problems and Solutions

Ratites are susceptible to a variety of infectious and noninfectious disease conditions. Evaluation of incubation and hatching records should be the first step in the clinical evaluation of poor-doing or ill ratite chicks. Problems seen within the first week of life often reflect the quality of the egg (and hence the nutrition of the hen) and incubation and egg handling procedures. Congenital abnormalities can occur. Mortality rates are generally highest for the first 3 months of life; beyond 6 to 8 months ratite juveniles are generally hardy, as are adult birds. Ostrich chicks appear to be more easily stressed and more prone to infectious diseases than the other species of ratites. Noninfectious conditions, particularly those predisposed to by management factors, are the primary causes of losses on many farms. Major outbreaks of infectious disease are less common.

Chicks should be observed at rest before restraint and handling in order to assess mental alertness and demeanor, and the respiratory, nervous, and musculoskeletal systems. Ratites are normally extremely curious. Birds should be assessed for conformation, stance, and gait because leg deformities are a significant problem. Scoliosis and other spinal deviations occur and may be the result of genetics or problems during incubation. Stunted growth and poor feathering are evidence of chronic disease or maladaptation.

Supportive care, including provision of supplementary heat and fluid and nutritional support, is critical regardless of the primary concern. Because there are no medications licensed for use in ratites in the majority of countries of the world, veterinarians must prescribe and use drugs in an "off-label" manner as governed by their veterinary associations. Medications may be administered orally via stomach tube, or birds may be manually pilled. Many will even preferentially peck at and consume tablets or capsules because of their unusual appearance. Placing medication in the food or water may be appropriate in some circumstances providing there is adequate intake. Esophagostomy tubes have been used for long-term nutritional supplementation; ratites do not have a crop in which to store food. Injections can be made subcutaneously, into the muscle masses of the legs or lumbar area, or intravenously via the medial metatarsal vein. In larger juveniles, the jugular – or in the ostrich, the brachial – vein is also used. In older birds intended for the slaughter market, intramuscular injections can result in condemnation or trimming of meat.

Young ratites are easily caught and handled. Small chicks may be supported under the body with the legs folded or left to hang. Birds may also be laid upside down in one's lap to examine the abdomen or legs. As chicks grow, their running speed increases exponentially and it is important not to cause injury by panicking the birds or by rough handling of the legs during catching. The use of corrals or chutes, or boards used for herding, can aid in isolating and capturing individual birds in need of attention. Juvenile birds may be lifted off the ground from behind, leaving their legs dangling free. After a short period of kicking, most birds relax and may be carried without a struggle. Older juvenile birds should be treated like adults, which are large and strong and may seriously injure the handler.

Common medical problems in ratite chicks include yolk sac retention and infection, nutritional deficiencies, developmental limb deformity, gastric impaction, enteritis, respiratory disease, and fading ostrich syndrome. For a more detailed description of these and other diseases of ratites the reader should consult the veterinary literature (Jensen et al. 1992; Tulley and Shane 1996; Huchzermeyer 1998; Tulley and Shane 1998; Verwoerd 2000; Jakob-Hoff 2001; Doneley 2006; Morgan 2008; Romagnano et al. 2012; Biggs 2013; Kummrow 2014).

## Yolk Sac Problems

Yolk sac retention and infection are generally identified in birds under two weeks of age, but may result in more chronic ill-thrift. Chicks with yolk sac problems are often reluctant to feed and fail to gain weight and grow at the same rate as their clutchmates. The yolk sac should be completely retracted into the body at the time of hatch, the navel closed before removal from the hatcher, and the yolk sac completely resorbed by 2–3 weeks after hatch. The kiwi is the exception to this; almost half the yolk mass is present at hatching, and may provide nutrients to the chick for up to 17 days (Prinzinger and Dietz 2002). The abdomen in chicks with persistent and infected yolk sacs is fuller than normal, and the normal intestinal tract and its contents cannot be palpated. Ultrasound examination can help confirm the diagnosis. Improper incubation and hatching parameters resulting in delayed umbilical closure, prematurely assisted hatching, and inadequate hygiene leading to umbilical infection are the common predisposing factors. If only a small portion of the sac remains external at hatch, it may sometimes be replaced in the abdomen and the navel sutured or bandaged closed. Large or abnormal portions of the sac should be removed surgically and the yolk sac stalk ligated and umbilicus closed; however, these chicks are often weak and reluctant to eat. In older chicks, surgical removal of the sac and systemic antibiotic therapy are required, along with supportive care.

### Nutritional Deficiencies

A wide range of nutritional deficiencies have been suggested to occur in ratite chicks; however, these are often based on clinical signs that might be seen in domestic poultry rather than actual knowledge of the conditions as they occur in ratites. Classic and phosphorus-deficient (particularly in rheas) rickets, vitamin E/selenium-responsive myopathy, and suspect vitamin B deficiency syndromes – including dermatitis and curled toes – have been identified in ratites. Some ostrich chick management protocols include injection with a vitamin E/selenium product shortly after hatch. Recently hatched emu chicks with twisted necks or that "tumble" and roll may respond to vitamin B supplementation.

### Leg Deformities

Long-bone deformity is probably the most widespread problem in young chicks. A number of interrelated factors are likely involved in the development of this condition. These include overfeeding (excessive calorie intake) or excess dietary protein leading to too rapid growth, nutritional deficiencies and imbalances (e.g. calcium, phosphorus, vitamin D, vitamin E, selenium, methionine, choline, manganese, zinc), damage to the leg during hatching or within the hatcher, inadequate exercise, and genetic predisposition. The extremely rapid growth rate of ratite chicks exacerbates any nutritional imbalances that may be present. The most successful methods for prevention appear to be providing large pens to encourage exercise, reducing the protein level of the chick diet to under 20% within approximately 2 weeks of hatching, and reducing the total amount fed.

Leg deviations may be rotational – that is, around the axis of the bone – or to the side. The resulting turnout of the lower leg and foot can be severe enough to completely prevent the bird from standing or walking. The tibiotarsal bone is most frequently affected, but not all cases are alike. Because of the rapid growth rates, problems may literally appear overnight and can progress rapidly. Lateral displacement of the gastrocnemius and other tendons can occur either at the same time, or secondarily. A variety of splinting and surgical procedures have been attempted, with almost uniformly poor results unless the leg is splinted correctly within a few hours of the onset of the problem.

A separate problem seen in ostrich chicks is rotation of the large toe. This problem usually responds well if corrective splints are immediately applied. Again, a variety of causes have been suggested, including genetic predisposition and riboflavin deficiency.

### Gastric Impaction and Stasis

Ratite chicks will eat and possibly impact on various foreign objects and almost any substrate: sand, gravel, straw, long grass, or plastic turf materials. Emus seem slightly less prone to this than ostriches or rheas. Ingested foreign bodies may also perforate the proventriculus or gizzard causing septic peritonitis, similar to hardware disease in cattle. Management activities that may predispose to impaction include irregular feeding routines, rapid changes in diet, lack of grit, movement of birds onto a substrate that is novel to them, and any change in routine that stresses the birds. Gastric stasis can also occur in ostrich chicks in the absence of ingested foreign material, with low or high environmental temperature and gastric infection implicated in addition to the factors listed above. Clinical signs may be acute and resemble colic as seen in other species, or they may be chronic and include listlessness, reduced appetite and fecal output, decreased size and increased dryness of fecal pellets, and stunted growth. The impacted proventriculus or ventriculus may be palpable in the abdomen, but often plain or barium contrast radiographs are necessary. If the condition is identified quickly, laxatives may assist in passage of the proventricular and ventricular contents, but in most cases surgical removal is required. The prognosis depends very much on the condition of the bird at the time of surgery; the survival rate is poor for weakened birds.

Proventricular and ventricular function may also be disrupted by localized infections by fungi, including *Candida*, *Aspergillus* spp., and avian gastric yeast (*Macrorhabdus ornithogaster*). These are often secondary to immunosuppression or another insult.

### Enteritis

Enteritis may be an important problem in chicks less than 6 months of age. Inadequate sanitation, combined with the propensity of chicks to be coprophagic, may result in outbreaks of disease. The establishment of a normal intestinal flora within the first days of life is considered important in preventing enteric infections. A variety of pathogens have been implicated, including gram-negative bacteria such as *Escherichia coli, Campylobacter jejuni, Pseudomonas* sp., *Salmonella* spp., and *Clostridium* spp.; *Brachyspira hyodysenteriae* in rhea; and paramyxo-, reo-, corona-, adeno-, and herpes viruses. Systemic infection frequently follows bacterial enteritis. Cloacal prolapse may occur secondary to diarrhea and straining and has also been associated with cryptosporidial infection in ostrich chicks. Appropriate antibacterial therapy should be provided along with fluids and supportive care. Investigation into underlying sanitation and management protocols is essential to prevent and control outbreaks of enteritis.

### Parasitic Disease

A variety of internal and external parasites have been identified in ratites. The most clinically significant of these is *Libyostrongylus douglassi,* the proventricular worm of ostriches. Clinical signs in affected chicks include anorexia, weight loss, depression, and death. Enteric coccidiosis is an important cause of illness and mortality in captive kiwi chicks, particularly those raised at high density. Regular fecal evaluation and deworming programs are essential for parasite control.

### Respiratory Disease

Upper and lower respiratory disease may be significant in chicks under 6 months of age. Clinical signs include conjunctivitis, rhinitis or sinusitis, and respiratory distress. A variety of bacterial, fungal, mycoplasmal, and viral agents have been implicated, including *Pasteurella hemolytica, Bordetella avium, Pseudomonas aeruginosa, Hemophilus* spp., and *Neisseria* sp. Ostrich-specific mycoplasmas have been identified in South Africa (Botes et al. 2005). Aspergillosis is a disease of particular concern to ratite farmers. Infection occurs by exposure to overwhelming numbers of fungal spores in situations with poor husbandry (in the brooder or later), or after reduction in a bird's immune function due to concurrent disease or other stress. Poor ventilation leading to high levels of ammonia in the barn may predispose to outbreaks of respiratory disease. Aspergillosis may be seen as explosive outbreaks in flocks of young chicks. Smoldering infections in individual older birds may become clinically apparent under stressful conditions – for example, after transport to a new farm. Birds may show minor or nonspecific clinical signs even when severely affected. Treatment is rarely effective, but a variety of systemic and aerosolized antifungal medications have been recommended.

### Fading Ostrich Syndrome

A specific cause of this syndrome, whose features include anorexia, gastric stasis, and extremely high mortality in ostrich chicks less than 6 months of age, has not been determined. A combination of management-induced stress and immunosuppression and one or more infectious agents is likely responsible. Careful attention to management, hygiene, and biosecurity appears to be the best prevention at present.

### Other Conditions

Other husbandry-related diseases include trauma, predation, exertional myopathy, hypothermia, heat stroke, intestinal accidents, and plant, heavy metal, or chemical poisoning.

## Diet and Feeding Procedures

Ratites, with the exception of kiwis, are primarily herbivores; however, their digestive systems and natural diets differ (Cillers and Angel 1999; Sales n.d.). Ostrich, emu, and rhea graze on a variety of low energy vegetation in semiarid environments. Gastrointestinal transit time is more rapid in the emu (5–6 hours) than in the ostrich (36–39 hours for immature birds) or rhea, species that rely more heavily on hindgut and cecal fermentation. Commercial feeds are formulated specifically for ostrich, emu, and rhea, and for birds of different ages and are sold by a several major feed companies (e.g. Mazuri®), as well as local feed coops. Cassowaries feed on a variety of fruits of the tropical forest, but in captivity are fed a mixture of fruit, pellets, and sometimes small amounts of animal matter (e.g. chicks, rats, meat) (Folch 1992c; Biggs 2013). Kiwis are insectivorous, feeding primarily on earthworms and a variety of soil invertebrates (Folch 1992a; Sales 2005).

Although the larger ratite chicks rely on the yolk sac for nutrients and fluid for up to a week after hatching, a pelleted or crumbled starter ration should be offered soon after hatching to encourage development of normal feeding behavior and early weight gain (Deeming and Bubier 1999). Without older birds to act as role models, newly hatched chicks may need assistance to identify food and water. White dishes with patterns on the bottom, or freshly chopped greens, or brightly colored vegetable matter floating in the water or placed on dried feed may encourage interest (Figure 4.3).

Chicks may feed more readily from the ground than from dishes or pans. For biosecurity reasons, species such as domestic chickens should not be placed with the chicks to encourage eating. It is a matter of debate whether grit is necessary for birds fed a pelleted diet; however, the following general recommendations have been made for grit size: starter (2/16 in.; 3 mm) at hatch to 3 weeks; grower (2/16 in. × 3–4/16 in.; 2 mm × 5–6 mm) at 4–7 weeks; developer (4/16 in. × 6–8/16 in.; 6 mm × 9–13 mm) at 8–16 weeks; and turkey (6/16 in. × 10/16–14/16 in.; 9 mm × 16–22 mm) after 16 weeks (Mazuri/PMI Nutrition International 2012).

There is no universal program for chick nutrition (Minaar and Minaar 1992; Minaar 1998; Sales n.d.). Most chicks are initially fed a ratite crumble or starter with at least 20% protein free choice. If specific ratite diets are not available, a pelleted feed with approximately 15–20% protein could be substituted (Sales n.d.). Dietary utilization of nutrients is poor initially as the digestive and absorptive capabilities of the gastrointestinal tract mature over the first few weeks of life. The establishment of normal GI flora is felt to occur within the first week of life. Some producers place fresh feces from healthy adult or juvenile birds in the pen with chicks in order to transfer the appropriate

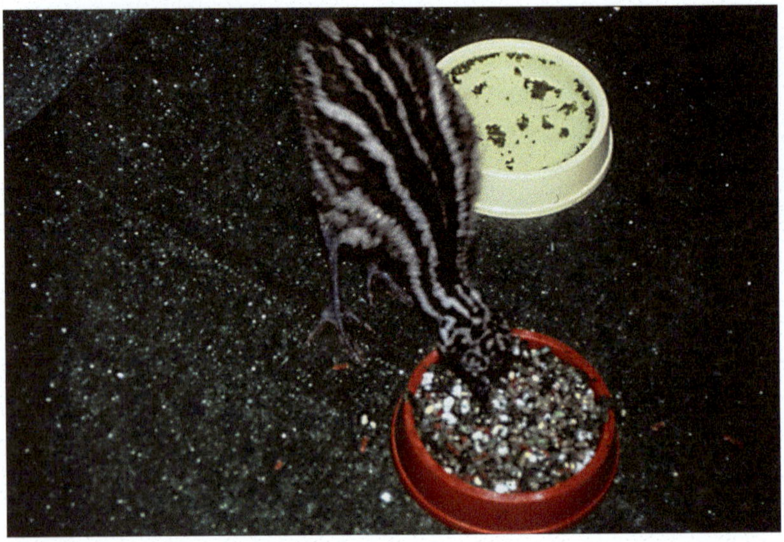

Figure 4.3 Emu chick eating from feed top-dressed with fresh greens to encourage foraging behavior.

bacterial and protozoal organisms. This practice has also led to severe disease outbreaks. Some farmers feel that probiotics assist in development of balanced flora, but this has not been substantiated scientifically. Fresh water should be provided at all times; automatic livestock waterers are useful for older birds. Birds will cease eating if water is not available.

At approximately 2–3 months of age, the protein level of the feed is progressively decreased to reach 13–15% by the time birds are 6–10 months of age (O'Malley 1996; Cilliers and Angel 1999; Mazuri/PMI Nutrition International 2012). Feeding frequency should also be decreased to limit growth rates. Chicks placed in outdoor paddocks will supplement their food intake by grazing. Maintenance and breeder rations are used for birds over a year of age, as appropriate.

## Expected Weight Gain

Commercial species of ratites grow rapidly. Ostrich chicks may increase in height by 30 cm per month and can reach 4 kg in weight by 1 month of age, 9–14 kg by 2 months, 20–30 kg by 3 months, and 40–50 kg by 4 months (Huchzermeyer 1998). Ostrich chicks develop their juvenile plumage at approximately 3 months of age, and gain adult plumage and weight by the second year of life. Emu chicks gain juvenile plumage at approximately 2 months of age; full adult plumage and full height are reached at approximately 1 year of age. Emu chicks should achieve hatch weight by day 6–7, will weigh approximately 1.5 kg at 1 month, 6 kg by 10 wks, 16 kg by 20 wks, and continue to grow steadily until reaching adult weight (O'Malley 1996).

## Housing

A number of references describe the management of young ratites (Jensen et al. 1992; Minaar and Minaar 1992; Tulley and Shane 1996; Huchzermeyer 1998; Minaar 1998; Verwoerd et al. 1999; Glatz and Miao 2008; Biggs 2013). Chicks are moved from the hatcher into a brooder pen – a confined area with supplementary heating to compensate for the young birds' poor thermoregulation – and then into larger pen or paddock areas, preferably with access to the outdoors if climate conditions permit.

Pen size is dependent on the size and number of animals in the group but should be sufficient to allow the birds to move about freely and to exercise as they grow. A rough guide for brooder pen size is 8 ft.$^2$ (2.4 m$^2$) with 2 ft. (0.6 m) sides (Jensen et al. 1992). The temperature is gradually dropped from an initial high of 90 °F (32 °C) to approximately 79 °F (26 °C). Chicks are kept in groups so they can socialize and huddle together for comfort and warmth at night. Similar-sized chicks should be kept together to prevent bullying and crowding at feeders. Ideal stocking densities have not been determined. As birds grow, they are given access to larger pens and, depending on ambient temperature, may be confined to or simply provided with heated areas at night. Localized heat may be provided by underfloor and radiant heaters.

Runs must be well drained with good footing and should be practical to clean and sanitize. All in–all out systems and leaving pens fallow after a group of chicks has been in them helps reduce pathogen load. Chicks respond poorly to changes in their environment; therefore, it is recommended to keep groups of birds together during the growing period, and whenever possible to maintain them in the same physical location until they are well established.

It is essential that even the youngest chicks be given sufficient room to allow adequate exercise. In the wild, young birds of all species follow their parent(s) for many kilometers each day. Lack of exercise is felt to be one of the main predisposing factors for the variety of leg deformities seen in growing birds. Minimum pen area is approximately 40 ft.$^2$ (3.7 m$^2$) for birds less than 2 months of age, or less than 20 lb (9 kg) in weight, and 225–250 ft.$^2$ (21–23 m$^2$) for older or heavier birds (Raines 1998). Pens should be rectangular with lengths of 100–200 ft. (30–60 m) and a minimum width of approximately 10 ft. (3 m) (Jensen et al. 1992; Minaar 1998; Raines 1998). Width and total pen size will depend on the number of chicks in the group. In colder climates, the use of large greenhouse structures is effective in providing chicks hatched in winter months – for example, emus – with exercise as well as exposure to sunlight and natural light cycles (Figure 4.4).

Older birds are kept outdoors in fenced paddocks or pens. To prevent injuries, fences should be 6 ft. (1.8 m), have a smooth and solid top rail, and be easily visible. Shade should be provided in the summer, and in temperate climates protection must be given from the coldest weather and wind. Adult ratites of commercially raised species are able to tolerate full winter temperatures if appropriate shelters are present; however, icy or slippery footing may be dangerous for the birds. Barns are rarely heated unless they also contain young birds.

It is critical that ratites are exposed early to the types of bedding used on the farm. The rate of proventricular impaction in ostrich and rhea chicks is extremely high and is often associated with changes in management that include alterations in bedding substrates. Chicks that will be put out on grass should be watched carefully for early signs of impaction if they have not had access to the outdoors as young birds.

## Preparation for Socialization or Introduction to Captive Flock

Young ratites are sociable and become easily accustomed to human contact. Caution should be taken working with birds as they gain adult sizes, particularly as they reach sexual maturity and in breeding season. Cassowaries and male ostriches can be extremely dangerous.

In general, young birds are not aggressive toward each other; however, some caution must be undertaken when chicks or juveniles are reintroduced to similarly aged conspecifics. Smaller birds

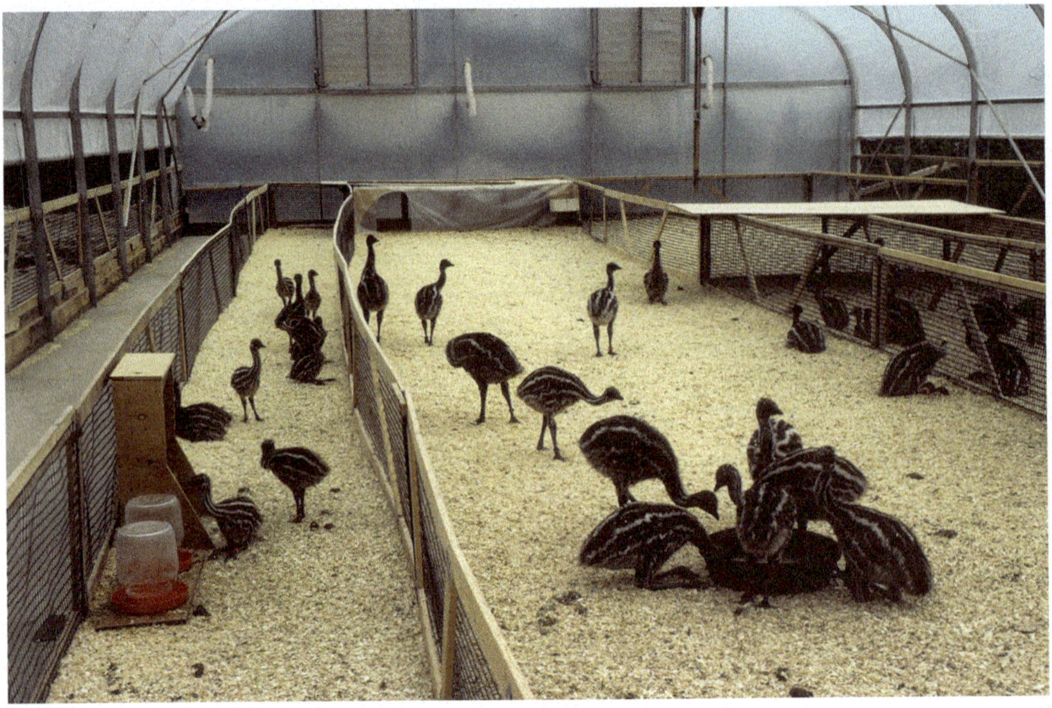

Figure 4.4 Emu chick pens in a large plastic greenhouse.

may be at a disadvantage getting to food and water sources. Rabbits and pygmy goats have been used as "company" and role models for young chicks that are raised on their own.

## Acknowledgments

I would like to thank Sharon Patterson for assistance with manuscript preparation, and Alison Downie, Dr. Graham Crawshaw, and Dr. Colin Peace for reviewing the manuscript for the first edition of this book.

## Sources for Products Mentioned

Mazuri, PMI Nutrition International, LLC, PO Box 66812, St. Louis, MO 63166, www.mazuri.com.

## References

Biggs, J.R. (ed.) (2013). Captive Management Guidelines for the Southern Cassowary *Casuarius casuarius johnsonii*, 2013 edition. Cairns Tropical Zoo. http://aszk.org.au/wp-content/uploads/2015/05/2013_FINAL_bird_hm_casso_COMPLETE.pdf.

Botes, A., Peyrot, B.M., Olivier, A.J. et al. (2005). Identification of three novel mycoplasma species from ostriches in South Africa. *Vet. Microbiol.* 111: 159–169.

Cabot, J. (1992). Order Tinamiformes. Family Tinamiformes (Tinamous). In: *Handbook of the Birds of the World*, vol. 1 (eds. J. del Hoyo, A. Elliott and J. Sargatal), 112–125. Barcelona: Lynx Edicions.

Cilliers, S.C. and Angel, C.R. (1999). Feedstuff evaluation and metabolisable energy and amino acid requirements for maintainence and growth in ostriches. In: *The Ostrich: Biology, Production, and Health* (ed. D.C. Deeming), 105–128. Wallingford, Oxon: CABI Publishing.

Deeming, D.C. and Bubier, N.E. (1999). Behaviour in natural and captive environments. In: *The Ostrich: Biology, Production, and Health* (ed. D.C. Deeming), 83–104. Wallingford, Oxon: CABI Publishing.

Doneley, B. (2006). Management of captive ratites. In: *Clinical Avian Medicine*, vol. 2 (eds. G.J. Harrison and T.L. Lightfoot), 957–989. Palm Beach, Florida: Spix Publishing.

Folch, A. (1992a). Family Apterygidae (Kiwis). In: *Handbook of the Birds of the World*, vol. 1 (eds. J. del Hoyo, A. Elliott and J. Sargatal), 104–108. Barcelona: Lynx Edicions.

Folch, A. (1992b). Family Dromaiidae (Emu). In: *Handbook of the Birds of the World*, vol. 1 (eds. J. del Hoyo, A. Elliott and J. Sargatal), 98–102. Barcelona: Lynx Edicions.

Folch, A. (1992c). Family Casuaridae (Cassowaries). In: *Handbook of the Birds of the World*, vol. 1 (eds. J. del Hoyo, A. Elliott and J. Sargatal), 90–97. Barcelona: Lynx Edicions.

Folch, A. (1992d). Family Rheidae (Rheas). In: *Handbook of the Birds of the World*, vol. 1 (eds. J. del Hoyo, A. Elliott and J. Sargatal), 84–88. Barcelona: Lynx Edicions.

Folch, A. (1992e). Family Struthionidae (Ostrich). In: *Handbook of the Birds of the World*, vol. 1 (eds. J. del Hoyo, A. Elliott and J. Sargatal), 76–82. Barcelona: Lynx Edicions.

Gill, F.B. and Donsker, D.B. (2015). IOC World Bird List (v 5.2) 2901–2903.

Glatz, P.C. and Miao, Z.H. (2008). Husbandry of ratites and potential welfare issues: a review. *Aust. J. Exp. Agric.* 48: 1257–1265. https://doi.org/10.1071/EA08136.

Huchzermeyer, F.W. (1998). *Diseases of Ostriches and Other Ratites*. Onderstepoort, South Africa: Onderstepoort Agricultural Research Council.

Jakob-Hoff, R. (2001). Establishing a health profile for the North Island brown kiwi (*Apteryx australis mantelli*). *Kokako* 8 (2): 6–9.

Jensen, J.M., Johnson, J.H., and Weiner, S.T. (1992). *Husbandry and Medical Management of Ostriches, Emus and Rheas*. College Station, Texas: Wildlife and Exotic Animal Teleconsultants.

Kummrow, M. (2014). Ratites or Struthioniformes: Struthiones, Rheae, Cassuarii, Apteryges (ostriches, rheas, emus, cassowaries, and kiwis), and Tinamiformes (tinamous). In: *Fowler's Zoo and Wild Animal Medicine*, vol. 8 (eds. R.E. Miller and M.E. Fowler), 75–82. St. Louis, MO: Elsevier Saunders.

Mazuri/PMI Nutrition International. (2012). Mazuri ratite starter. Online at http://www.mazuri.com/product_pdfs/5M32.pdf.

Minaar, M. (1998). *The Emu Farmer's Handbook*, vol. 2. Grovetown, Texas: Nyoni Publishing Company.

Minaar, P. and Minaar, M. (1992). *The Emu Farmer's Handbook*. Grovetown, Texas: Induna Company.

Morgan, K. (2008). *Kiwi First Aid and Veterinary Care*. Wellington, New Zealand: Science and Technical Publishing, Department of Conservation http://www.doc.govt.nz/documents/science-and-technical/sap245entire.pdf.

O'Malley, P.J. (1996). An estimate of the nutritional requirements of emu. In: *Improving our Understanding of Ratites in a Farming Environment*. (ed. D.C. Deeming), 92–108. Oxfordshire, UK: Ratite Conference.

Prinzinger, R. and Dietz, V. (2002). Pre- and postnatal energetics of the North Island brown kiwi (*Apteryx mantelli*). *Comp. Biochem. Physiol. A Mol. Integr. Physiol.* 131: 725–732.

Raines, A.M. (1998). Restraint and housing of ratites. In: *The Veterinary Clinics of North America – Food Animal Practice (Ratites)* (eds. T.N. Tulley and S.M. Shane), 387–399. Philadelphia, Pennsylvania: WB Saunders.

Romagnano, A., Glenn Hood, R., Snedeker, S., and Martin, S.G. (2012). Cassowary pediatrics. *Vet. Clin. North Am. Exot. Anim. Pract.* 15: 215–231.

Sales, J. (2005). The endangered kiwi: a review. *Folia Zool.* 54: 1–20.

Sales, J. (n.d.). Feeding guidelines for ratites in zoos. http://www.eznc.org. http://www.eznc.org/docs/Ratitestandard2.pdf.

Tulley, T.N. and Shane, S.M. (eds.) (1996). *Ratite Management, Medicine, and Surgery*. Malabar, Florida: Krieger Publishing.

Tulley, T.N. and Shane, S.M. (eds.) (1998). *The Veterinary Clinics of North America – Food Animal Practice (Ratites)*. Philadelphia, Pennsylvania: WB Saunders.

Verwoerd, D.J. (2000). Ostrich diseases. *Rev. Sci. Tech.* 19 (2): 638–661.

Verwoerd, D.J., Deeming, D.C., Angel, C.R., and Perelman, B. (1999). Rearing environments around the world. In: *The Ostrich: Biology, Production, and Health* (ed. D.C. Deeming), 191–216. Wallingford, Oxon: CABI Publishing.

# 5

# Ducks, Geese, and Swans

*Marjorie Cahak Gibson*

## Natural History

Ducks, geese, and swans are well known in every part of the world and have a long history of association with humans. They often are the subject of literature, music, and art of all forms, and are an intimate part of human culture (Stromberg 1986). From ancient writings, to Shakespeare's sonnets, to children's literature, references to these magnificent birds that both fly and swim hold a unique place in our lives (Price 1994). Several species of geese and ducks have been domesticated and bred as farm flocks. Some are legally hunted during certain seasons.

Order Anseriformes, family Anatidae, includes 154 species of swans, geese, true ducks, and whistling ducks. The group is commonly referred to in North America as "waterfowl" and "wildfowl" in Britain (Weller 2001). Species vary dramatically in size, posture, plumage, diet, and breeding habits. Adult body weights range from 0.5–30 lb (230 g to 14 kg).

Members of the Order Anseriformes are easily recognized as waterfowl even when newly hatched. Young are down-covered and leave the nest immediately or within a few days of hatching (Figure 5.1). Many species share similarities of structure and form, including large heads, horizontally flattened blunt beaks, long necks, heavy bodies, and webbed feet (Altman et al. 1997; Weller 2001). Smaller species fledge in 6 weeks; the larger ones do not fledge for 10–12 weeks. There is great diversity in natural history and diet, and therefore substantial variation in the way these species are cared for as patients in a captive state.

Waterfowl live in aquatic habitats that include lakes, streams, rivers, oceans, and estuaries. In recent years, several species have shown great adaptability of nesting habitat, expanding their territories into highly urban areas. This adaptability comes with mixed success. A generation ago, urban nesting ducks and geese were rare and generally regarded with fond curiosity. As urban nesting increased, public opinion gradually reflected less fondness, and more concern for sanitation and inconvenience (Erickson 2006). Accommodating territorial adults near a nest site becomes annoying and downright risky. Many species of waterfowl, including swans, have become comfortable with the manicured landscaping of corporate campuses or other urban sites. This is particularly so when landscaping includes a lake or other water elements designed to replicate nature. Rehabilitators become involved when nesting sites are placed too near humans, an adult becomes territorial, or when young have hatched within enclosed courtyards or similar areas that have no foot access to natural habitat.

*Hand-Rearing Birds*, Second Edition. Edited by Rebecca S. Duerr and Laurie J. Gage.

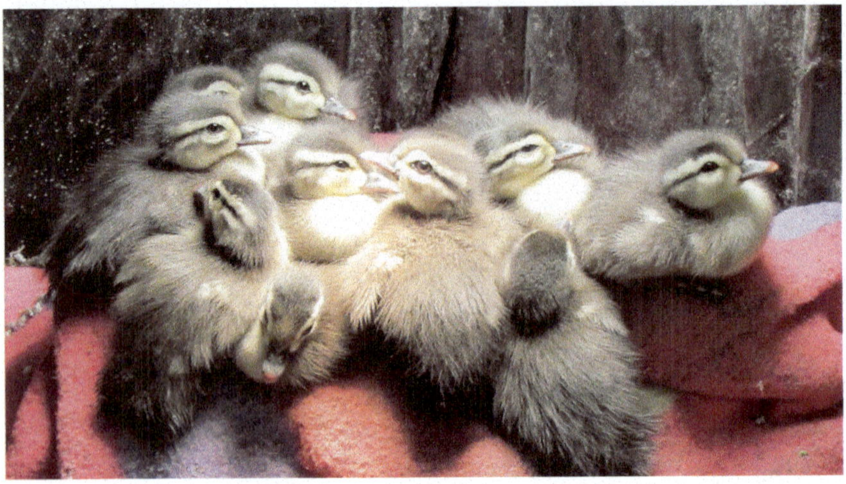

Figure 5.1 Newly admitted hypothermic Wood Duck ducklings warming under warming lamp. Large heads, flattened beaks, and webbed feet are structures common to all waterfowl chicks.

These species have strong wings, necessary to carry their heavy bodies into flight. The wings are also used effectively for defense. Swans and geese are well known for aggressive defense of their territories and protection of young. Aggression also occurs outside of breeding season in birds that are maladjusted or imprinted to humans. Swans, the largest of the Anseriformes, can be dangerous and have been known to break ribs and arms, cause concussions, and even render human rescuers unconscious with brutal wing beating. They should not be underestimated in terms of strength and tenacity. Do not attempt to rescue an adult or nearly grown swan that is swimming, as they have the advantage when in water. It is important to work as a team when rescuing large waterfowl.

Several species have declined significantly in population in recent years; others have responded to conservation habitat restoration and nest box development efforts (Erickson 2006). With endangered species, captive breeding and reintroduction continue to be utilized. The rehabilitator must be able to recognize species within the region that are of threatened or endangered status, in case one is admitted for care. Special permits are often required by state or provincial government to work with threatened and endangered species.

Waterfowl of various species are kept and captive-bred by aviculturists throughout the world (Tarsnane 1996). Because of this, a wealth of information on captive care is available online through waterfowl breeder associations, including housing and veterinary care for common species (Wobeser 1981). Excellent age and species-specific commercial diets can be obtained through most farm feed stores. The Mazuri® brand makes several commonly-used products. Due to the wide variation in species nutritional requirements, it is important to have good references in one's library to anticipate specific habitat, behavior, or diet questions.

This chapter focuses on the rehabilitation of wild Anseriformes, with emphasis on releasing the birds rather than giving lifelong captive care. Challenges exist for sensitive species that do not thrive well. Much of the literature deals with domesticated rather than wild waterfowl, so allowances have to be made. Chicks, both domestic and wild, do best with the companionship of others of their species. Networking with other wildlife rehabilitators that care for waterfowl to match single chicks with conspecifics is a good idea for best survival and success. Also see Chapter 6 for specific information on more marine-oriented species such as eiders.

### By Any Other Name

Ducks, geese, and swans are commonly known by the following terms for gender and age:

*Ducks:* The female is a hen, the male is a drake, and young are ducklings.
*Geese:* The female is a goose, the male is a gander, and young are goslings.
*Swans:* The female is a swan, the male is a cob, and young are cygnets.

## Criteria for Intervention

Reasons for young waterfowl to be admitted to rehabilitation include "kidnapping" by people, separation from parent shortly after hatch, cat or dog bite, or hypothermia with cold or inclement weather. Newly hatched waterfowl attract people. The small size and soft downy appearance of a hatchling contributes to many wild young being taken from nature into human homes. Most of these kidnapped chicks will be stressed, hypothermic, and malnourished when finally admitted to wildlife rehabilitation centers.

### Calls from the Public

For the person calling seeking advice about young waterfowl that are still in the wild, it is important to tell them to give the adult space and privacy in order to come back to a site if they have been startled and scattered due to disturbance. Suggest that the caller observe from a safe distance, out of sight of the adult birds, for at least an hour, unless the youngster is in immediate danger. Offering natural history information about the species will be helpful in determining whether the chick is an orphan. If the youngster is already captive, but still at the capture site, urge the finder to locate the family with the purpose of reuniting, if possible. If the finder and the youngster are away from the capture site, stress that the youngster must remain warm and dry. People are often not aware of the need for supplemental heat, particularly with precocial young that are downy, mobile, and appear self-sufficient. Reinforce that the young are brooded by the adults in nature and are not able to maintain body heat on their own for several weeks after hatch or until contour feathers grow in.

A complete history is important. Ask specific questions such as where was the chick found? What type of habitat? This will give information for species identification. Were adults in the area? The chick may be a species that can be reunited with the adults. What were the circumstances of the finding? There may be other injured youngsters at the site. How long has it been in captivity? Who has handled the chick? If children are involved there may be unintentional internal injuries to the patient. What is the behavior now? Is it peeping loudly, lying still, jumping, or gasping? Has it been in contact with domestic fowl during captivity? If so, isolation may be necessary due to possible exposure to common diseases of domestic waterfowl.

### Reunion with Parents

Reuniting families can be successful but must be done with care and follow-up observation. Some species are agreeable to reuniting and even adopting additional foster chicks; others will reject chicks, even kill them, usually by drowning. The general rule is if the family or area from which a youngster was taken is known, reunion can be attempted within the day. Some rehabilitators have had success with species such as the Canada Goose and Trumpeter Swans accepting foster chicks if the adult has goslings or cygnets of the same age. Other rehabilitators report unhappy experiences with the same. Wild counterparts reject human-imprinted waterfowl due to their atypical behavior.

### Transportation to Wildlife Facility

The chick should be transported as soon as possible. Instruct the transporter that the chick should kept quiet, away from dogs, cats, and small children before and during transport. A transport box no more than twice the size of the bird will lower stress and keep the youngster secure. A cardboard box with small air holes works well. A clean towel or dry grass on the bottom of the box will prevent chicks from sliding and possible splaying of their legs from poor traction. Do not transport with a water bowl. Spilled water will wet the chick and cause hypothermia. Provide supplemental heat during transport, such as a warmed rice bags, hot water bottles, or the equivalent. Pad the heat source with towels so the chick is not directly in contact with it. A stuffed animal, feather duster, or calm and gentle holding may comfort the youngster during transport.

## Initial Care and Stabilization

Newly hatched waterfowl, regardless of the species, have the following common needs: heat, water, and nutrition, given in that order. A young waterfowl patient that is hypothermic is considered critical and must be tended to immediately. It is important to bring the temperature up quickly or death will result. Before a physical exam can be done, the bird must have a normal core body temperature. Hypothermic chicks should not be given oral food or water; however, small amounts of warmed sterile isotonic subcutaneous fluid may be given if skill and equipment allow. The digestive system does not function until the core body temperature is restored. Massage the patient to stimulate response and increase circulation. To warm a chilled bird, a heating pad set on low, and covered with a towel, can be used. Nonresponsive patients should never be left on heat without constant monitoring. Heating pads and lamps can overheat debilitated patients unable to move from the heat. Death may result.

Once the chick is stabilized, offer warmed electrolyte fluid, such as human infant rehydration solutions, to the tip of the beak. In small species, this can be from the tip of a finger. A spoon or syringe will work with larger birds and allow you to dip the beak into the fluid or allow small amounts of fluid to naturally flow into the closed beak without forcing the beak open. The action of swallowing when accompanied by fluid will stimulate gastrointestinal motility. Once hydration is complete, tube-feed with a weak mixture of baby cereal and water. Use small amounts at first until the chick defecates. Size appropriate French catheters or metal feeding tubes can be used based on the body size of the chick. The tube-feeding amount should be as small as 0.1 ml for the smallest ducklings to 2 ml for a cygnet. Initial tube-feedings are meant to further stimulate peristalsis rather than filling the crop. Once stable, these species should eat and drink on their own. When the chicks are stable and mobile, they can be put into a brooder set up as described below.

Young waterfowl may nibble at food, giving the appearance of eating, without actually ingesting anything. Do not assume they are eating without observing closely. Weighing chicks and documenting weight gain is important during the first 2 weeks of life. Stimulation that mirrors wild circumstances may be needed for sensitive species to encourage them to begin eating and drinking. Mallard ducklings are calm and eat eagerly unless injured. For that reason, they can be used as models to encourage more sensitive species to eat. Canada Goose goslings can provide the same service for larger waterfowl.

### Tips on Teaching to Drink and Eat

Ducklings and other newly hatched waterfowl may not drink or eat easily on their own once separated from their parents. Observe the young bird. If it does not drink on its own, take it in hand and gently tip its beak into the water dish. After a few efforts the chick should began to drink on its own. If it does not, repeat the process until it drinks on its own. Offering electrolyte solution alternately with water is a good practice for the first week of life.

Cavity-nesting ducks have natural techniques to stimulate eating. By their natural history it is known that within the first day, these ducklings take their first step out of the nesting cavity and tumble to the ground. This tumble is sometimes from impressive heights, without apparent injury. Their first meal follows this event. The most common cavity-nesting ducks in North America are Wood Ducks, Mergansers, Buffleheads, and Common Goldeneyes. All are considered high-stress and difficult to raise in captivity. When orphaned, the "fight or flight" response takes over these sensitive species and they go into stress overload. To help them over the trauma we can simulate a new start in life. Taking a hint from their natural history, the best thing to do with a newly hatched cavity-nesting species is to literally "drop" it from several feet into the brooder. When the chick lands, life begins anew. This may seem like a crazy method, but it works for most youngsters. Be certain of the species before attempting this method of stimulation. Ground-nesting species are not made for "taking the plunge" into life.

Use fresh water as opposed to saltwater, even if the bird is an ocean or marine species such as the King Eider. The salt gland, which enables marine birds to excrete excess salt, is poorly developed in ducklings (Weller 2001). Saltwater will be fatal until chicks are nearly feathered.

### Restraint

Young waterfowl are very active and can escape even a firm grasp. A towel dropped over the top of the back of a patient and wrapped under the legs is helpful in securing the bird and preventing damage to the legs and developing wings.

Adult birds can be restrained in the same manner as chicks. Adult waterfowl use their wings as a method of defense. It is important to maintain control of the wings, keeping them firmly against the restrainer's body, as well as the legs, to prevent injury to the bird or the rehabilitator (see Figure 5.2).

### Foster Parents

Foster parents are adult ducks, geese, and swans that function as parents for orphaned chicks. They are an invaluable resource for rearing young waterfowl species once the chicks are stabilized, healthy, and eating on their own. Foster parents are usually former rehabilitation cases that are unable to be released to the wild. Most of the best foster parents are adults that have reared chicks in the wild. Imprinted birds rarely work as foster parents and have been known to kill chicks. Foster parents should be physically healthy enough to provide a good role model in terms of proper vocalizations, swimming, selecting appropriate food items, eating, and offering youngsters a normal view of the behavior of their species. In cooler climates or during inclement weather, chicks may need to be removed from the foster parents at night and taken to a heated area until they are mostly feathered.

When introducing foster parents to chicks, provide a quiet, safe, and protected area where the adult can be alone with the chicks to get to know them. Observe the new family without being

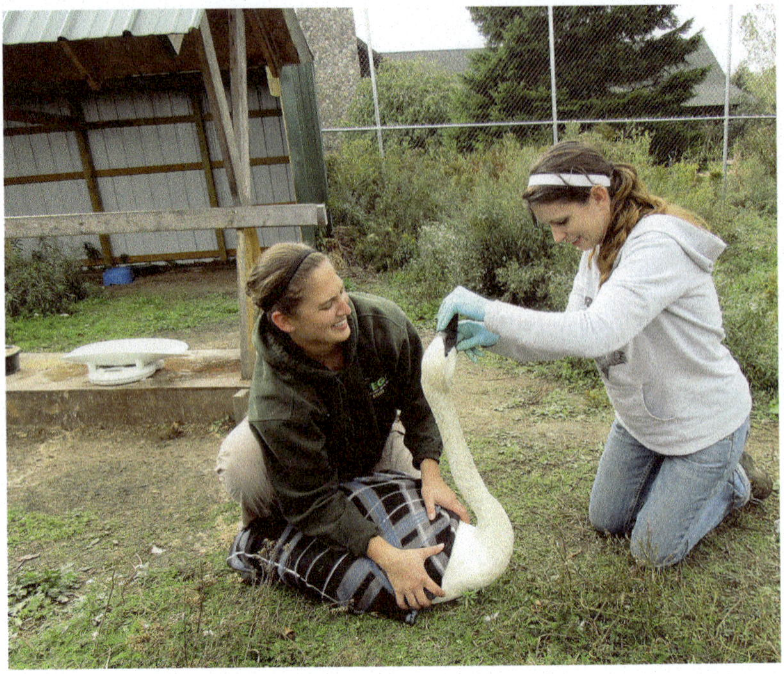

Figure 5.2 A sheet over the wings of a Trumpeter Swan works well to control the bird's wings, protecting both the handlers as well as the swan during health checks.

intrusive until both the adult and chicks are interacting well with each other. Species-specific foster parents are the best; however, mixed groups of ducklings and geese have also been successful.

## Common Medical Problems and Solutions

### Infectious Diseases

Waterfowl carry many types of parasites, not all of which are dangerous to them, as well as viruses, bacteria, and other disease-causing agents (Wobeser 1981; Ritchie 1995; Altman et al. 1997). Wild birds should be prevented from contact with domestic birds. Disease transference can occur and spread during migration (Ritchie 1995). See Chapter 7 for more in-depth information on common diseases and parasite problems in domestic Anseriformes. Many treatments are good for one species and harmful to another. It is therefore important to consult an avian veterinarian with waterfowl experience. Some states have required testing for diseases such as Newcastle disease, duck plague, avian influenza, and others. Check governmental requirements before networking with rehabilitators out of state or transferring birds to out-of-state migratory areas for release.

### Bumblefoot

Foot problems are common with wildfowl that are raised or kept in captivity. In natural habitats, waterfowl live and rear young around lakes, wetlands, and ocean estuaries. Water, muddy, or bog areas effectively massage the foot constantly as the bird walks or swims. Hard or harsh substrates are unnatural to the footpad and contribute to callusing and bumblefoot (pododermatitis), particularly in heavy-bodied waterfowl. Bumblefoot is a serious disease in large waterfowl and is fatal in many cases as it often progresses from damaged skin to infected damaged skin to infected deeper tissues, eventually causing tendonitis, joint infections, and/or osteomyelitis (bone infection and destruction). For this reason, birds should not be kept on cement floors without padding. Substrates used in housing waterfowl should allow the foot to sink into the substrate with each step (Ritchie et al. 1994). Appropriate substrate includes carpet (when housed indoors), artificial turf, pea gravel, sand, and natural soil.

Waterfowl in captivity should be examined regularly for signs of foot lesions, particularly at the central footpad and the bony prominences of the toe joints. As a preventive measure, in addition to using appropriate substrates, massage the foot with a small amount of Vermont's Original Bag Balm monthly or whenever the bird is handled. If calluses or irritated areas are visible, warm-water pulse massage and foot massage treatments with bag balm should be done twice per week to prevent bumblefoot from progressing. Prevent feathers from contacting oil or bag balm as the bird may lose its waterproofing if it becomes greasy.

### Splayed Legs

Leg splaying can result when a young bird slips on unstable substrate, stretching ligaments beyond normal range. If caught early, it can be corrected by using VetRap™ (3M) or similar material to "soft-splint" legs in a natural position (this is also sometimes called "hobbling"). The feet should be separated by normal standing/walking distance. The bird should be able to walk and maintain normal behavior with the splint on its legs. Standing and walking while splinted is important to maintain muscle tone and development. Depending on the severity of the problem, the legs should remain splinted for a few days to a week. Adjust the splint daily in a newly hatched bird to accommodate the rapid growth (Altman et al. 1997). See Goodman et al. (2017) for information regarding management of orthopedic problems in wild waterfowl.

### Mud-balling

Mud-balling occurs when material, such as mud or feces, adhere and form a ball around the foot of a young bird. If the problem becomes severe, the bird may be unable to walk or move naturally. Mud-balling sometimes occurs in nature in habitats with clay soil and in brooders during captive-rearing. Most cases that develop in brooders are due to wet feces sticking to the feet and combining with wood shavings or other substrates. Early intervention is important to prevent foot or leg deformity or death from exhaustion. See Chapter 8 for photographs and more information on mud-balling (Welty and Baptista 1988).

### Trauma

Damage to the wings, face, and beak may occur when a bird comes into contact with wire fencing or occasionally in a territorial dispute with another bird. Injuries can be very severe, causing blindness and even death of a patient. If a bird is observed pacing a fenced area in escape attempts or coming into physical contact with it, remove the bird from the pen immediately until privacy screening or a solid barrier on the perimeter fence can be installed. If bleeding or injury is evident, stop bleeding with pressure, wash the area, and apply topical water-soluble antibiotic cream to prevent secondary infection. Older chicks sometimes act as bullies, and may damage the growing flight feathers of other chicks by nipping at them; always be attentive to how groups of chicks are getting along with each other.

### Angel Wing

Waterfowl chicks should be watched carefully for development of *angel wing,* a condition thought to be nutritionally based. In this condition, the flight feathers at the wingtip flip up and out, giving the appearance that suggests its name. It is also referred to as *airplane, reversed, slipped,* or *sword wing.* There are several dietary factors that may contribute to the malady. Diets high in sulfur-producing amino acids, deficiency of vitamin E and manganese, plus high protein for some species, have been cited as factors (Ritchie et al. 1994). A diet high in carbohydrates and sugar, such as when young waterfowl are fed white bread, also contributes to the problem. The physical problem begins when the weight of the flight feathers and gravity pulls the carpal joint down and out. Angel wing can be corrected if intercepted early. Wrapping the wing to itself in a natural position for a few days may correct the problem. Wraps must not be left on longer than a few days in consideration of the young birds' rapid growth rate. Be careful to apply wraps such that they do not damage the growing blood feathers. Untreated, the wing will be permanently deformed and the bird will not be releasable.

### Lead Poisoning

Lead poisoning is a serious and unfortunately common problem in waterfowl coming into rehabilitation. In the United States alone it was estimated that 2.4 million waterfowl die yearly from lead poisoning (Ritchie et al. 1994). Birds come into contact with lead in the wild in various ways, including swallowing lead sinkers commonly used for fishing, lead shot from bullets, or ingestion of mine wastes. The possibility of lead poisoning should be considered with all swans and, to a lesser degree, geese.

Birds admitted with lead poisoning may have a variety of symptoms that include low weight, weakness, inability to walk or use legs well, wing droop, and the signature grass-green feces. Often feathers on the chest and crop area may be soiled due to vomiting. Patients with lead poisoning also will be generally lethargic, anemic, and dehydrated. Not all symptoms need to be present and will vary with the patient, species, amount of toxicity, and source of lead. Many will be unable to digest food. Vomiting is common. In these cases, fluids should be given subcutaneously. Oral tube-feeding in small amounts can be attempted, keeping in mind that aspiration may result if the bird regurgitates the oral diet. If the crop empties and the bird is defecating, a more liquid diet can be fed (see the section on Emaciation Diet for Debilitated Waterfowl later in this chapter). Offer the bird water, but do not allow it to eat grain or solid food until the digestive system is functioning normally.

Blood testing and diagnostic imaging play an important role in the diagnosis of lead poisoning, and early diagnosis and treatment is imperative. If metallic densities are observed on x-ray, gastric lavage or endoscopic removal of metal pieces (Ritchie et al. 1994) may be required. Consult an avian veterinarian in lead poisoning cases. Calcium disodium versenate or dimercaptosuccinic acid (DMSA) are often used to chelate lead from the blood stream.

Many states have banned the use of lead for waterfowl hunting, but lead shot is often used in small and large game hunting as well as fishing. Lead does not degrade in the environment. Swans, in particular, encounter lead pellets when water levels are low and they eat material from the bottom of lakes or streams. Conservation groups often have material available on nontoxic alternatives to lead sinkers and lead shot that may be helpful to create an awareness of the problem.

### Botulism

Young waterfowl may present with botulism. *Clostridium botulinum* grows in anaerobic conditions, when bodies of water become warm and have poor flow. This bacterium produces a toxin that paralyzes the neuromuscular junctions of affected animals. Birds are exposed when they eat invertebrates in the water that have the toxin in their tissues. Affected birds display varying degrees of paralysis of the neck, legs, and wings, and often have odorous diarrhea. Severe cases may have difficulty breathing. Mild to moderately affected birds have an excellent prognosis. Unlike lead poisoning, this disease may result in dozens or even hundreds of birds of mixed species presenting at once, often from a particular water source.

Because this disease is an intoxication rather than an infection, antibiotics are of no use. Provide birds with supportive care, including an initial tube-feeding of activated charcoal dissolved in water and then frequent small amounts of oral fluids to flush any remaining invertebrates from the intestines. After 24 hours of frequent tube-feedings, switch to a more nutritious tube-feeding formula, such as the emaciation diet given in this chapter. Keep birds clean and comfortable, with heads elevated above the body to reduce regurgitation and ease respiration. A laundry basket with a towel over thick bedding of shredded paper makes appropriate temporary housing for affected birds to prevent problems with pressure sores on legs. Apply eye ointment several times daily because some birds may be unable to blink. Unlike mammals, birds recover from botulism very quickly, often within 1–2 weeks. Many birds will regain the ability to hold their heads up within 2–4 days and will be able to stand and eat within a week.

## Human Imprinting

Human imprinting of newly hatched waterfowl is a serious problem and must be avoided. Imprinting is a very fast and efficient learning mechanism in the very early hours and days of a young birds' life. The effects are an irreversible behavior pattern, and these species imprint very easily on humans. Raising a single, newly hatched waterfowl chick without a foster parent, adult model, or conspecifics assures the chick will be imprinted to humans. Large-bodied imprinted waterfowl can be dangerous to humans and should be kept with care at a facility that understands the behaviors associated with imprinting. They should not be allowed to range freely. Newly hatched waterfowl can be irreparably imprinted to humans in the matter of a day in most species. Maladjusted individuals become aggressive to humans, particularly once they reach sexual maturity. It is often those individuals that are the source of urban legends of attacks on humans. People destroy what they fear. The result of one person's negative experience with an imprinted individual can cause the reputation of large waterfowl to be called into question with such voracity that many normal wild birds are destroyed in response to human fear. Human-imprinted individuals that have been reared from hatchings, once released to the wild, NEVER integrate into the wild population and become normal. They are not candidates for release to the wild and should be held in permanent captivity situations or euthanized.

## Habituation

Habituation is a social situation where individuals past the age of imprinting become accustomed to something that does not have a negative effect on them, but does not alter their sense of who or what species they are or their instinctive behavior. For instance, ducks being fed in a park are comfortable with people coming and going and may seem tame, when in fact they are only habituated to the situation. Habituation can change with circumstances and is not a permanent condition. It may, however, be enough of a behavior problem that the bird needs to stay in captivity extra long in order to socialize with its own species and become warier of humans before release.

## Diets

Diet variation is a huge issue when rearing waterfowl. One species may do very well on commercial duckling starter; the next species may need live food to survive. It cannot be stressed enough that birds coming into care at a rehabilitation facility must be correctly identified to care for them successfully (Baicich and Harrison 2005). There are a few "first" foods that waterfowl young respond to universally. These "first" foods are not meant to be the only food offered. The health of young waterfowl requires a varied diet.

### First Foods

After stabilization feedings, introduce wild-growing duckweed or watercress. It is one of the best first foods for young waterfowl. Duckweed contains tiny invertebrates important for rapid growth. Wild ducklings, goslings, and cygnets readily eat natural greens (Stromberg 1986). Duckweed can be legally collected from lakes or streams and maintained under refrigeration for a week or more. With fresh water, gently rinse as much as needed for a day's feeding until the water runs clear but most natural material remains (Figure 5.3). Wild greens have organisms that occur naturally in the wild. In the past, some sources have expressed concern about introducing potentially pathogenic organisms to young waterfowl. That concern may be valid for those birds that are domestic or remain captive; however, this author suggests rehabilitated birds will experience these upon release and it is better to do that with a natural immunity developed from hatch.

Float the greens in a shallow pan of water and place it in the brooder box (Figure 5.3). Water dishes should have a ramp to facilitate access into and out of the pan for small species. Change water and rinse greens frequently, or when soiled with feces. If there is no access to natural duckweed, finely chopped romaine lettuce can be used. Small amounts of dried or frozen blood-worms, available in pet store tropical fish departments, human baby cereal available in grocery stores, or Waterfowl Starter (Mazuri) crushed into a powder can be added to the duckweed water to increase protein and food taste experience. More advanced chicks will appreciate the addition of small minnows and insects to the duckweed water.

Many young birds refuse to eat dry food. Wetting food may increase success. However, wet mash sours easily and should be changed at least twice per day. Commercial starter pellets come in a

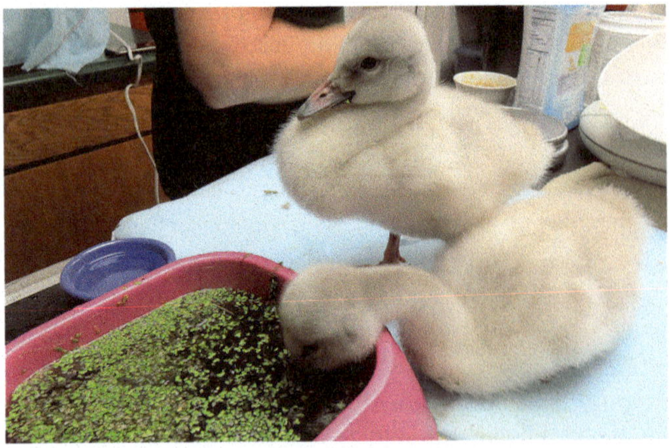

Figure 5.3 Young swan cygnets showing interest in duckweed in water bowl.

variety of sizes. They can be crushed into a powder for very young waterfowl. For reluctant eaters, the powdered starter can be sprinkled over the youngsters' backs. While preening, the chick will naturally get some of the powder into its mouth and this may stimulate the eating process. Soaked feline and canine growth pellets, such as Science Diet™ (Hill's® Pet Nutrition, Inc.), and crushed hard-boiled egg can be used as part of a successful starter diet for young waterfowl.

"Shoveling" best describes the method of eating for Anseriformes. The beak works as a strainer to take in tiny invertebrates and grasses. Dry mash can be a hazard to swallow when it forms a paste with the bird's natural saliva. Water must be near the food to allow normal food intake. Pellets are preferred to mash in most species, because they are easier to eat.

Listing foods for all Anseriformes is a nearly impossible task due to the great variety in diet. The best information available for species that are not addressed in this chapter is a field guide that includes diet information (Elphick et al. 2001). As a rule, youngsters eat insects or invertebrate protein for their first few weeks or month of life and graduate to the wide variety of foods that the references list for adults as they develop to maturity. Local, natural areas will be the guide as to what insects, invertebrates, or other listed diet items are available during nesting season and therefore used as food for waterfowl. General foods are minnows, crayfish, insects including grasshoppers, crickets, bloodworms, waxworms, and mealworms, as well as a variety of natural grains and grasses.

Shallow dishes or saucers make appropriate dishes for ducklings. Dishes with the size and depth of a cake-pan are needed for goslings and cygnets. Water founts, available in most farm equipment supply stores for domestic fowl, may be used. Include pea gravel on the bottom of water founts and dishes to prevent the youngsters from entering the water and possibly drowning. As odd as it sounds, waterfowl young do drown in shallow water. Water must be changed frequently and dishes washed to prevent bacterial growth and subsequent illness.

Aggressive behavior at the food dish suggests that more food or a different variety of food is needed. Increased urgency in peeping occurs when chicks are either imprinted, hungry, or lonely. If the feces are normal consistency and the chick is eating, it may not be eating adequately. It may be advisable to supplement tube-feedings a few times to see whether the vocalizations calm. Offer a new food variety, such a small minnows or active insects. Examine the vent of chicks that appear fluffed, lethargic, or are avoiding other chicks. Soft feces can dry and build up on down near the vent and not allow the chick to defecate. In this case, wash the area with warm water until the material is removed.

### Emaciation Diet for Debilitated Waterfowl

- 2 oz (56 g) human baby mixed grain cereal, such as Gerber's brand.
- One 2.5 oz (71 g) jar of Gerber's baby meat food (beef, chicken, turkey or veal).
- One 2.5 oz (71 g) jar of water.
- One 2.5 oz (71 g) jar of human infant electrolyte replacer, such as Pedialyte.

Whip ingredients together, adding more water if needed, until the diet will pass through an appropriately sized French red rubber feeding tube (catheter tube) or metal feeding tube. Make the diet thinner for very weak patients.

The diet should be prepared fresh for each feeding in the amount needed. Feed the amount that fills the crop and is able to be moved out of the crop in an hour. If the chick regurgitates or fluid comes up, cut back the quantity given. Continue tube-feedings until the chick is eating on its own. Offer food items when the chick is able to stand. The diet must be warmed to 85 °F (30 °C) when administered. It should not be too hot or crop burns will result. Microwave heating is not recommended due to uneven heating of the food particles. Feeding a cold diet may put a fragile patient into shock and result in death.

## Housing

Waterfowl vary greatly in size. As another general rule, chicks of the same size and age can be put together even with species variation. Mixed housing has advantages and disadvantages that must be weighed up. A singleton of any species will likely not survive. If it does, the chick may imprint on the caregiver and not be releasable to the wild. Older chicks may suffocate, injure, or not allow newly hatched young to feed. Use care if this is the only option for housing. Older chicks that have begun to eat on their own may encourage and teach younger ones how to eat and drink. Observe the birds carefully for any aggression and separate immediately if it occurs, especially if mixing age groups. Networking with other waterfowl rehabilitators is suggested and very helpful with housing multiple species or varied ages. When smooth surfaced dishes are used or slick surfaced floors, be sure to cover the bottom with pea gravel or other material to assure stable footing and prevent splayed legs from developing.

### Brooder

Brooder boxes can be made from a variety of materials. Dry brooders have no option for swimming; wet brooders do. Each has benefits and drawbacks. Experience, including what species is most common in the region and the numbers of patients expected, will be the best method of selecting which box and brooder type will work for your facility. Many waterfowl breeders use a walk-in wooden box about 6 ft. (1.8 m) high to accommodate highly active cavity-nesting duck species as well as geese and swans. Other breeders find that a rectangular plastic storage container makes a very good brooder for most young waterfowl. A large cardboard box works well as a dry brooder. The size of the container will vary according to the species and numbers of chicks.

A box 42×24×36 in. (1×0.6×0.9 m) will accommodate up to eight newly hatched ducklings. Some species of ducklings, "jumpers," or larger waterfowl require taller containers. Cardboard can be used to increase the height of the brooder box. Do not use wire, because some species of cavity-nesting ducks hatch with toenails and will use the wire as a stairway to escape. Larger waterfowl may injure their beaks on wire. Pea gravel, coarse sand, and Astroturf® pieces all make a good substrate for the bottom of the brooder. Wood shavings, straw, and newspaper may be ingested by chicks and should not be used as substrate. Wet carpet and towels can harbor fungus and must be replaced when they are wet or soiled. Fine sand may irritate the eyes of hatchlings. Hard substrate, such as cement, will cause foot problems and should not be used. For the first few days of rehabilitation, place a white muslin cloth or towel on top of the substrate to allow easy assessment of the chicks' droppings, both for color and consistency, indicating problems from not eating or digestion issues (Figure 5.4) (Rupley 1997).

A heat lamp firmly fixed to one corner of the brooder box should keep the temperature under the lamp between 95 and 99 °F (35.0–37.2 °C). In the case of rearing only a few chicks, the lamp can be as simple as a reflector-style clip-on lamp with a 40–60-W heat producing bulb. Raising or lowering the lamp can easily adjust the heat. Commercial brooders and heat lamps are available at farm supply stores if caring for larger numbers of hatchlings.

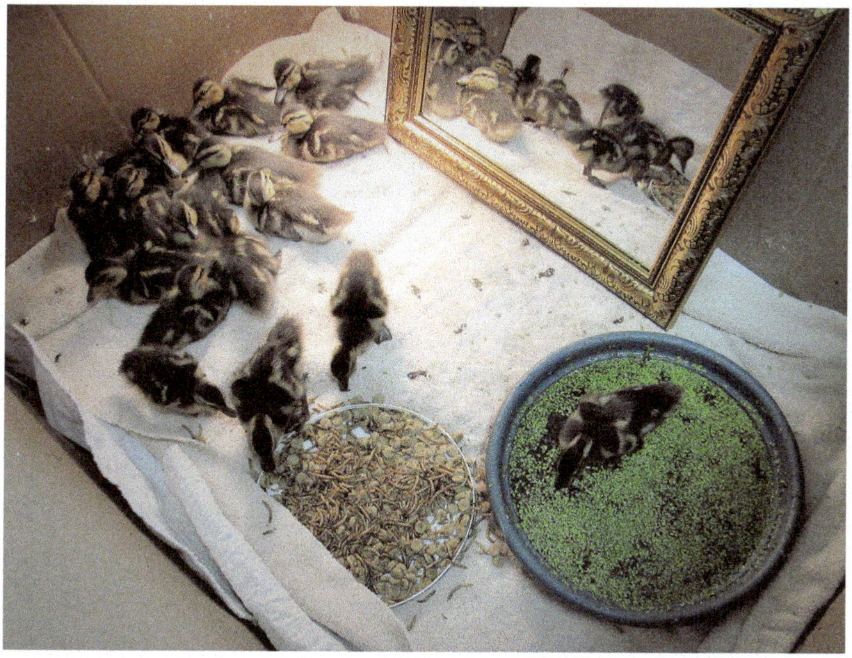

Figure 5.4 A box set up for young ducklings. A mirror is helpful, especially with small groups or a single duckling. Note duckweed in a flat pan of clean water and dried mealworms on top of saturated science diet canine growth kibble. A white muslin fabric floor cover aids in detecting digestive problems in recently admitted ducklings, while providing nonslippery footing.

Observation of behavior will be the best guide to several factors including whether the heat lamp is adequate, too cold, or too warm; whether the brooder box space is adequate, or a larger area is needed; and whether enough food is available. Chicks that huddle under the heat lamp are cold and need increased heat. Chicks that stand away from the heat lamp or have their wings hanging are overheated. Chicks should be allowed ample room to walk and exercise without being crowded (Ritchie et al. 1994; Tarsnane 1996; Altman et al. 1997).

If caring for a single youngster, a clean cotton mop head (Ritchie et al. 1994) or feather duster and a mirror in combination with a windup alarm clock that ticks may offer the chick security (Figure 5.5). If using a feather duster, check for preservatives on the feathers that may give off toxic fumes when wet.

## Access to Swimming

Young waterfowl are nidifugous (i.e. leave the nest shortly after hatching), and when with their parents can eat, swim, and dive soon after hatch (Ritchie et al. 1994). Having said that, chicks are not waterproof when hatched and depend on their parents or parent to waterproof them, preening on oil from the adult oil gland. Putting young chicks that have not had parental assistance in waterproofing into the water will be fatal, due to hypothermia or drowning. Once the chicks are stable and eating, usually several days after admission, begin to expose young birds to brief warm-water swims for a minute or two (Figure 5.6), and then put them back into the dry brooder under heat 95–99 °F (35.2–37.2 °C). If the chicks begin to shiver in the water, take them out immediately and put them in the brooder. Short periods of swimming will encourage preening, which is necessary

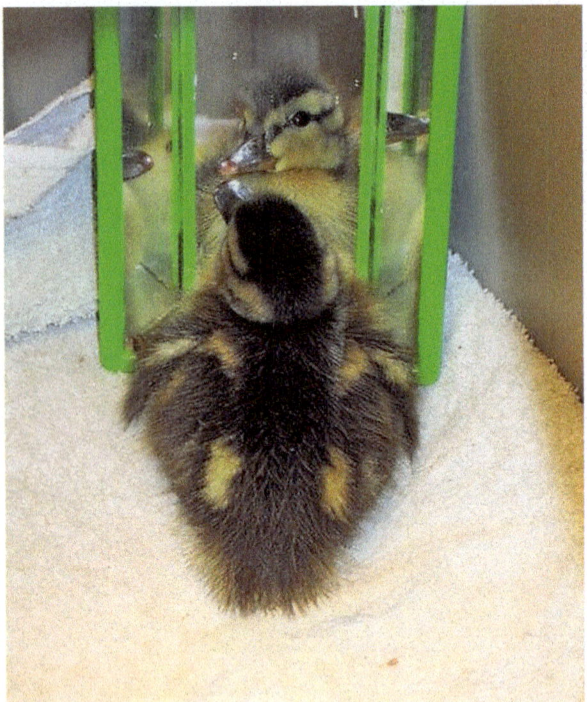

Figure 5.5 A solitary duckling with a mirror to help the chick not feel alone, which is very stressful.

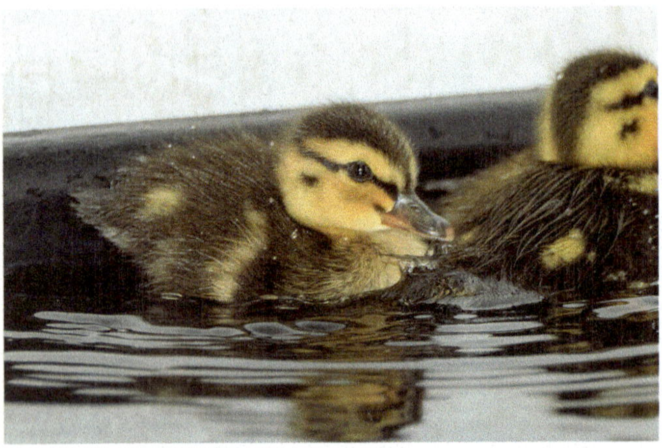

Figure 5.6 A Mallard duckling during swim time. Chicks must be able to exit the water to warm and preen. *Source:* photo courtesy of International Bird Rescue.

for the plumage to become waterproof. Chicks that have become contaminated with food or feces will have more problems becoming waterproof and will need many short swims to work out the problem areas. Dry brooders should be used initially until the young birds are eating well and are comfortable with finding the heat lamp when chilled. Supplemental heat will be required for most waterfowl young until they are feathered. However, heat lamp temperatures can be gradually lowered to 75 °F (24 °C) by age 3 weeks and maintained at that temperature, allowing the young to choose heat if they desire.

Feather development varies by species and even between broods. Young waterfowl that have undergone physiological stress from starvation, injury, or even captivity itself in very sensitive species, may have delayed development and need more time in a dry brooder. As a rule, young waterfowl should be maintained in a confined area with the option of a heat lamp until fully feathered. Due to the wide range of problems that may affect development with birds in rehabilitation, the rehabilitator will be the best judge of when it is safe to move young from an indoor brooder to an outdoor pen. Weather, including rain or other inclement conditions, will be a factor.

## Outside Pens

Intermediate pens housing juvenile birds should have both indoor and outdoor access. The inside area should be protected from the elements and have a heat lamp, food, and water available. The size of these areas depends on how many young are in care. An outdoor grassy area 20 × 20 × 6 ft. (6 × 6 × 1.8 m) will accommodate eight juvenile ducks. Overcrowding waterfowl can cause stress and disease. Pens made to raptor specifications work well because the young have access to natural sun and rain and protection from predators (Gibson 1996). A solid visual barrier 2–5 ft. (60–152 cm) high from the ground, depending on species, lowers stress and injury due to contact with fencing.

Water is a common requirement for waterfowl (Figure 5.7). All need access to some form of pond or swimming pool prior to release to the wild. Swimming will ensure that feathers are waterproofed, as well as providing needed exercise and experience. A children's swimming pool works well for a small number of birds. Use a ramp to assist chicks in and out of the water. Larger ponds should be used for larger species or large numbers of ducklings. Waterfowl are messy eaters and defecate

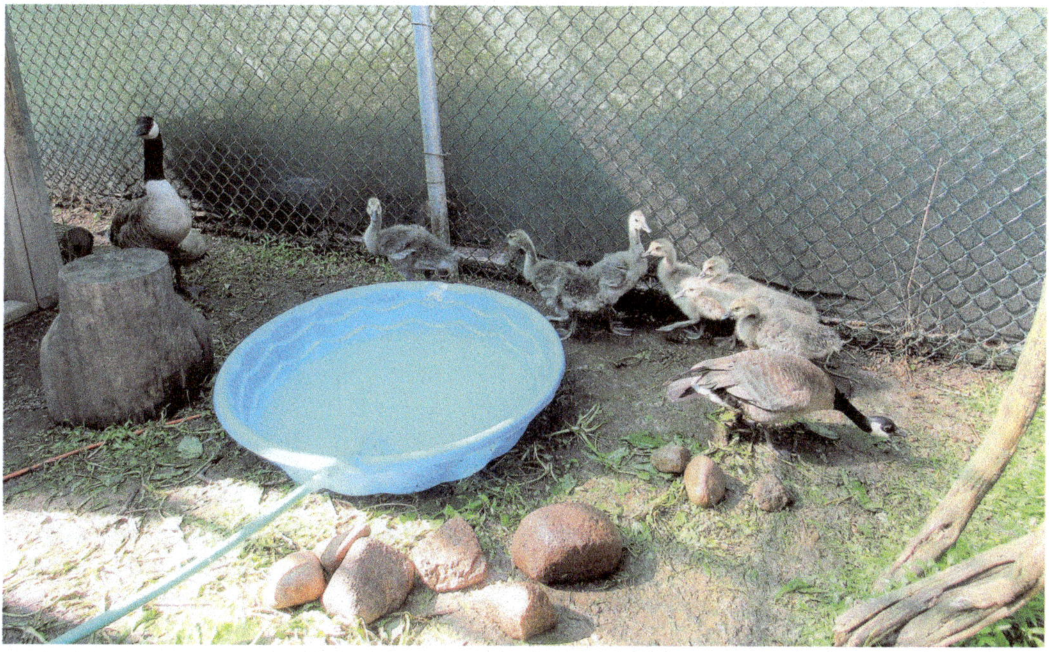

Figure 5.7 Foster parent Canada Geese rear normal well-adjusted geese without imprinting to humans. The water in outdoor enclosures must remain clean with easy access for birds to safely get in and out. Smaller species or younger chicks may need a ramp to enter this pool.

frequently. Food and feces often end up in ponds. Water must be kept clean, with pools being drained and the water changed often. A good filtration system should be installed in larger ponds.

### Keeping Predators Out

The best approach to protecting patients from predation is to take steps to exclude predators and not attract predators to the pens. Do not leave excess food out and clean up spilled grain outside the pen should it occur. Solid barrier fences will block visual attraction. Trees near or bordering enclosures may allow avian predators to perch or climbing predators to use them as a launching platform to access the enclosure; these should be eliminated. Digging animals, such as skunks, can be discouraged with buried 1 × 0.5 in. (2.5 × 1.3 cm) galvanized wire. The wire should be buried at a depth of 2 ft. (0.7 m), straight into the ground, and angled outward from the pen another 2 ft. (0.7 m). The use of galvanized moderate- to heavy-gauge wire is wise because less substantial wire will deteriorate in the ground and require costly maintenance or replacement every few years. Some rehabilitators have had success using multiple strands of electric fencing on the outside of the perimeter fencing. This technique will discourage climbing predators, such as raccoons, mink, and fishers. Several strands of electrical fencing starting inches from the ground and going to approximately 5 ft. (1.5 m) from the ground are generally adequate to discourage most predators. Check with local wildlife officials for a list of predators that frequent the area and for regulations for legal means to control them. Humane trapping using live traps or other methods may be needed for persistent predators. Local regulations affect the translocation of live-trapped predators. Under no circumstances should poison be used to control predators. The chance of poisoning nontarget species is great, including the patients being protected. The enclosure should be covered with wire on the top to prevent avian or climbing predation, as well as wild visitors that may bring parasites or other problems to pens, and premature release.

## Release

Youngsters remain with the adult until fully feathered and, in some cases, through the first winter. Fully feathered juvenile ducks, familiar with natural foods and proven to be waterproofed, can be released into prey-abundant natural habitat. Waterfowl releases are ideally done away from human activity in protected wildlife areas. Release should be done in the morning to allow young birds time to adapt, integrate with the wild population, and find cover for the night.

If the waterfowl in care must migrate from the area, keep the migration needs of each species in mind and allow time for the young to integrate into a flock. Monitor release sites for local and regional plans to assure no herbicide or pesticide programs for weed abatement have been or will be used in the waterway. Check with local officials to assure damage control waterfowl population abatement methods are not planned or underway in the release area.

Larger species may stay in family groups through the first winter. If migratory flocks can be located, most species of geese can be successfully released into the flock. If larger numbers of geese of the same species are reared together at a rehabilitation center, they form a "family group" and do well released together. Rehabilitated adults can be integrated with juvenile birds and released with the young birds. Swans can be aggressive with cygnets that are not their own. A close working relationship with state and federal wildlife agencies is important to develop a release plan for larger species that may require overwintering and a spring release for greater success.

## Exotic Species

Aviculturists, game farms, and zoos care for and breed a vast array of waterfowl species, not all of which are native to a region or even a given continent. Because many of these birds can fly, escape is always possible and does occur. Some species may adapt well and thrive, while others die from starvation or exposure in an environment to which they are not suited. Exotic species compete and often conflict with native species. If a facility admits a patient that is not native to the area, do not release it even if it was found in the wild. Finding a captive placement for the bird with a zoo or game farm is the best solution for the individual bird and for the future of native wildlife.

## Acknowledgments

In honor of E95, a Trumpeter Swan, an early member of the State of Wisconsin Trumpeter Swan Reintroduction Program and Raptor Education Group, Inc. patient. He changed our world and will always have a place in our hearts. Thanks to the State and Federal programs, aviculturists, and conservation groups that continue to contribute to habitat and species preservation, assuring a place for our magnificent waterfowl.

## Sources for Products Mentioned

Mazuri Waterfowl Starter: Mazuri, P.O. Box 66812, St. Louis, MO 63166, (800) 227-8941, www.mazuri.com.

Science Diet: Hill's Pet Nutrition, Inc., Consumer Affairs, P.O. Box 148, Topeka, KS 66601-0148, (800) 445-5777, www.hillspet.com.

Vermont's Original Bag Balm, P.O. Box 145, Lyndonville, VT 05851, (844) 424-2256, www.bagbalm.com.

## References

Altman, R.B., Clubb, S.L., Dorrestein, G.M. et al. (1997). *Avian Medicine and Surgery*, 944–959. Philadelphia, PA: W.B. Saunders Co.

Baicich, P.J. and Harrison, C.J.O. (2005). *Nest, Eggs, and Nestlings of North American Birds*, 2e, 347. Princeton, New Jersey: Princeton University Press.

Elphick, C., Dunning, J.B. Jr., and Sibley, D.A. (2001). *The Sibley Guide to Bird Life and Behavior*, 73–77. New York: Alfred A. Knopf, Inc., 190–211.

Erickson, L. (2006). *101 Ways to Help Birds*, 320. Mechanicsburg, Pennsylvania: Stackpole Books.

Gibson, M. (1996). The ABC's of housing raptors. *Journal of Wildlife Rehabilitation* 19 (3): 23–31.

Goodman, M., Schott, R., and Duerr, R. (2017). Waterfowl (ducks, geese, and swan). In: *Topics in Wildlife Medicine, Vol. 4: Orthopedics* (eds. R.S. Duerr and G.J. Purdin), 99–119. St. Cloud, MN: National Wildlife Rehabilitators Association.

Price, A.L. (1994). *Swans of the World in History, Myth and Art*, 196 pp. Tulsa, OK: Council Oak Books.

Ritchie, B.W. (1995). *Avian Viruses: Function and Control*, 525 pp. Lake Worth, FL: Wingers Publishing, Inc.

Ritchie, B.W., Harrison, G.J., and Harrison, L.R. (1994). *Avian Medicine: Principles and Application*, 1384 pp. Lake Worth, FL: Wingers Publishing Inc.

Rupley, A. (1997). *Manual of Avian Practice*, 265–291. Philadelphia: W.B. Saunders.

Stromberg, L. (1986). *Swan Breeding and Management*, 95 pp. Pine River, MN: Stromberg Publishing Company.

Tarsnane, S. (1996). *Waterfowl Care, Breeding and Conservation*, 288 pp. Blaine, WA: Hancock House Publishing Ltd.

Weller, M.L. 2001. Ducks, geese, and swans. In: *The Sibley Guide to Bird Life and Behavior*, 588 pp. C. Elphick, J.B. Dunning, and D.A. Sibley (eds.), Alfred A. Knopf, Inc., New York.

Welty, J.C. and Baptista, L. (1988). *The Life of Birds*, 4e, 581 pp. Orlando, FL: HBJ College Publishing.

Wobeser, G.A. (1981). *Diseases of Wild Waterfowl*, 2e, 324 pp. New York: Plenum Press.

## Further Reading

Anderson Brown, A.F. and Robins, G.E.S. (2002). *The New Incubation Book*, 206–213. Blaine, WA: Hancock House Publishing Ltd.

Gibson, M. (1997). Natural history: square one for wildlife rehabilitation. *Journal of Wildlife Rehabilitation* 17 (1): 3–6, 16.

Newton, I. (2007). *The Migration Ecology of Birds*, 984. Cambridge, MA: Elsevier Academic Press.

Rogers, L.J. and Kaplan, G. (2000). *Songs, Roars and Rituals, Communications in Birds, Mammals, and Other Animals*, 224 pp. Cambridge, MA: Harvard University Press.

Sibley, D.A. (2000). *The Sibley Guide to Birds*, 70–103. New York: Alfred A. Knopf, Inc.

# 6

# Sea Ducks

*Michele Goodman*

## Natural History

Sea duck species comprise the tribe "Mergini" within the family Anatidae, which includes eiders, scoters, mergansers, goldeneyes (including Bufflehead), and a few monotypic species including the Harlequin Duck, the Long-tailed Duck, and the extinct Labrador Duck. For detailed accounts on the natural history of North American waterfowl, see Baldassarre (2014), and for international species accounts, see Kear (2005). Sea ducks, as expected, spend much of their time on the water and can be poorly adapted to walking on land. Many species do not reach sexual maturity until 2 or 3 years of age. Within the group, there is considerable diversity relating to habitat selection and use as well as dietary preferences. All species are primarily carnivorous, feeding on benthic invertebrates and other aquatic animals. Mergansers are nearly exclusively piscivorous. Sea ducks are skilled divers, generally using their large feet to propel them underwater; some species (primarily eiders) use their wings to paddle underwater. As a group, many sea ducks have declining populations and are the subject of interest among conservationists (Bowman et al. 2015). Captive breeding efforts are ongoing for threatened species like Steller's Eider, Scaly-sided Merganser, and Brazilian Merganser while investigating the possibility for future reintroductions.

## Record Keeping and Duckling Identification

Private aviculturists and zoological institutions should strive to keep detailed records on the waterfowl in their care including info on parentage, egg-lay dates, egg weights and dimensions, fertility data, hatch dates, and hatch weights. Much of this information is not available to wildlife rehabilitators, but the location of stranding and details of care prior to admittance should be obtained from the person relinquishing the animal. Paper or digital records should be kept on each animal with daily progress notes. Chick weights should be recorded twice daily until the ducklings are eating sufficiently to maintain weight. The collection of frequent weights is a valuable tool for implementing a nutritional support program, discussed later. See Appendix 1 for a sample wildlife rehabilitation animal record and Chapter 1 for information regarding record keeping.

While it is often desirable to identify each bird individually, this can be challenging with rapidly growing waterfowl. Cable ties (or zip ties) are useful for individual bird identification as they are inexpensive and come in a wide array of colors. The use of different colors makes identification of

*Hand-Rearing Birds*, Second Edition. Edited by Rebecca S. Duerr and Laurie J. Gage.

an individual straightforward without having to capture it to read a band number. It is essential that any identification be checked daily as these can cause constriction injuries if they become too tight (which can happen in a very short period of time). The benefit of individual identification has to be weighed against the stress associated with handling the birds daily for band checks; this activity should be timed with other necessary interventions to minimize handling.

For older birds, Tyvek™ wristbands designed for humans can be cut to size and placed on the tarsometatarsus, and then used to facilitate individual bird identification. Like cable ties, they are inexpensive and come in a wide array of colors. Identification numbers can be written with a permanent marker on the wristband.

As an alternative to individual bird identification, birds can be maintained in natural clutches such that only siblings are housed together in a group. This method is often preferable in a wildlife rehabilitation setting when large groups of waterfowl are often managed within a short period of time. Any individual that presents separately or has specific medical issues can be individually banded and added to an established clutch of the same age.

## Criteria for Intervention

In an avicultural or zoological setting, it is common practice to remove eggs from a nest several days prior to hatch for artificial incubation. This allows the eggs to benefit from natural incubation and, following removal, often stimulates the adult birds to re-nest, which increases overall productivity. Sea ducks are far less common in captivity than other types of waterfowl and can be challenging to breed as these species generally have higher mortality rates, so there is an interest in maximizing productivity. It is up to the individual aviculturist or zoo to determine whether they want to attempt to parent-rear a second clutch, assuming that the birds will produce a second clutch; many factors influence this decision, including time of year and facility. Common Eiders (*Somateria mollissima*) are dedicated mothers and are often allowed to parent-rear offspring and raise young in a crèche.

When dealing with wild sea ducklings, intervention is often necessary as they should not be seen without a parent. There are often few opportunities for wild fostering of orphaned ducklings. Common Eider exhibit the unusual rearing strategy of crèche formation such that groups of females with ducklings aggregate. Wild fostering attempts can be successful with young Common Eider provided that the crèche is not disturbed during the attempt. State waterfowl biologists are an excellent resource to help with wild fostering of Common Eider ducklings to ensure minimal disturbance to the crèche.

## Initial Care and Stabilization

Initial care varies immensely depending on whether the duckling is captive-bred or presented as a wild orphan. Captive-bred ducklings pulled for artificial incubation hatch under low-stress conditions, are kept warm from hatch, and are offered appropriate food and water. Ducklings presented to wildlife rehabilitators are often debilitated and have been held by finders for varying lengths of time and offered a variety of often inappropriate food items.

Regardless of whether the duckling is captive-bred or presented for rehabilitation, the focus should be on providing heat and on encouraging self-feeding behavior. Ducklings not hatched under ideal conditions should be warmed in an incubator. A heat lamp or heating pad can suffice but care has to be taken to prevent hyperthermia if ducklings are too debilitated to move away from the heat source. Sea ducklings generally require lower temperatures than other groups of waterfowl.

Sea ducklings, as well as pochards and stifftails, can be challenging to rear in captivity; ducklings may be dehydrated, hypothermic, and exhausted on presentation. Despite being labeled as precocial, due to the typical debilitated state of wild chicks at presentation, supplemental nutrition and hydration is often required until the chick is able to eat sufficiently to maintain weight.

On admission, ducklings should be placed in a warm, dark, escape-proof container. Once they are warmed appropriately, they can be rehydrated orally with warm isotonic rehydration solution such as Plasma-Lyte or Normosol®-R. Unflavored pediatric electrolyte solutions can be used if the aforementioned solutions are unavailable. To administer oral rehydration fluids to neonatal sea ducklings, a #8 French rubber urethral catheter can be cut to a 1 in. (2.5 cm) length, the end can be burned or filed to remove sharp edges, and then attached to a 1 ml slip tip syringe (Figure 6.1). Depending on the type of catheter purchased, the flared base of the catheter may have to additionally be cut to fit snugly on the syringe. The shortened urethral catheter is placed past the glottis and the warmed fluids are delivered slowly. Ducklings will generally tolerate 10% of their body weight administered orally in this way every 2–4 hours.

Downy waterfowl are waterproof from shortly after hatch; they do not require brooding from adults to transfer oils (Goodman 2017). That being said, orphaned sea ducklings presented for rehabilitation are often debilitated and may have lost overall waterproofing due to inappropriate food presentation, inappropriate water presentation, or hypothermia. Once warm and rehydrated, ducklings should be placed in a hybrid or wet brooder with an overflow to keep surface water clean (see Housing section below). Food should be provided on both the dry portion of the brooder and in the swimming or wet portion of the brooder. Sea ducklings should be given supervised access to swimming water as soon as stable and rehydrated; they are unlikely to eat out of a dish and are prone to captivity-associated disorders when denied swimming water. The development and maintenance of excellent waterproofing and feather condition is an essential component of successful sea duck rearing.

Ducklings that are unable to maintain waterproofing in a hybrid brooder should be maintained in a dry brooder or plastic tub setup with a poultry fount, heating pad, and hide area with food presented on white paper towels (Figure 6.2). Ducklings should be placed in cold swimming water with floating food multiple times a day for gradually increasing periods of time as their feather condition improves. Initial swim time may be 5–10 minutes; once the chest or head feathers become wet, the ducklings should be removed and placed back in a dry brooder. This gradual introduction to swimming water stimulates preening behavior, which results in improved water resistance. Nutritional support may need to be provided during this period as sea ducklings and related species are less likely to eat on land.

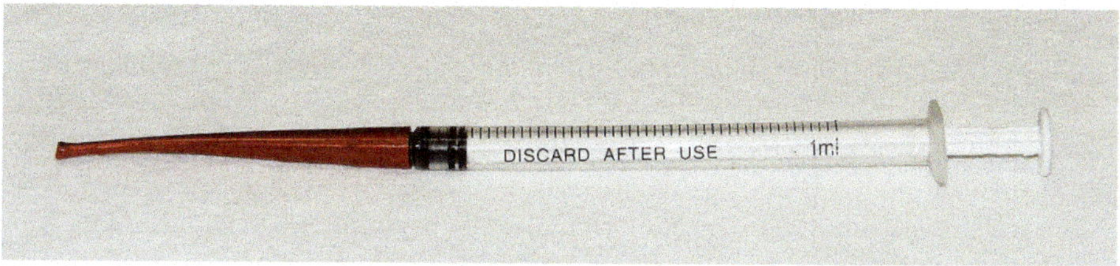


Figure 6.1 Syringe (1 ml) with cut urethral catheter and cut end burned to round sharp edges, which may be used to administer hydration fluid to small chicks.

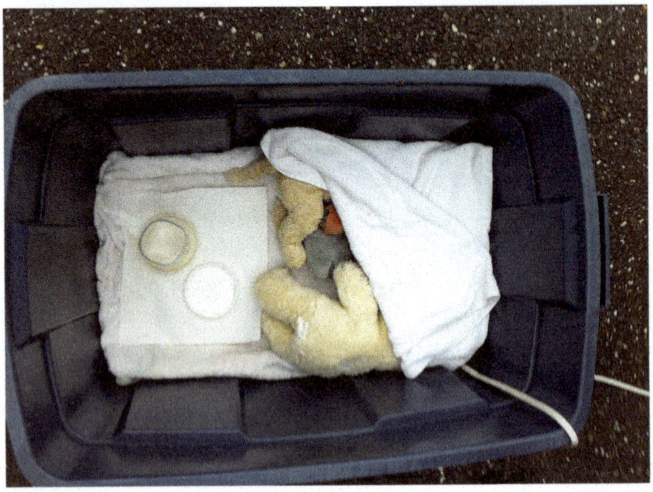

Figure 6.2 Dry brooder for critical care with poultry fount, heating pad, and hide area.

## Common Medical Problems

Developmental disorders that are seen occasionally in other waterfowl species – like angel wing, perosis, and angular limb deformities – are rarely seen in captive-reared sea ducklings. For techniques for management of orthopedic problems in wild sea ducks, see Goodman et al. (2016). There are, however, a few conditions that sea ducklings can develop in captivity, including wet feather and keel lesions. Of these conditions, wet feather is more common and refers to a duckling that loses waterproofing primarily on the breast; lack of overflowing water may play a role. Over time, the barbs and barbules responsible for the structural integrity of the feather deteriorate. Affected birds will swim low in the water and will eventually refuse to spend time in the water. Keel lesions occur primarily as a result of inappropriate husbandry, which for sea ducklings generally means overcrowding or inadequate access to swimming water such that the birds spend too much time on land bearing weight on their sternum. Birds with wet feather may be predisposed to developing keel lesions once the condition progresses to the point where they refuse to swim. Affected birds become debilitated and are more susceptible to secondary opportunistic infections, such as aspergillosis (Friend 1999). Prevention is the best approach for both of these conditions; once a bird develops either of these conditions they are unlikely to resolve even with intensive supportive care and/or a full molt.

Establishing and maintaining feather condition and waterproofing is often the greatest indicator of health; ducklings with excellent feather condition are reared uneventfully (Figure 6.3). Ducklings that struggle to maintain waterproofing may be more susceptible to infections with bacteria, viruses, fungi, and parasites. Waterfowl are susceptible to a wide variety of pathogens that are reviewed elsewhere (Backues 2015). Aviculture facilities commonly encounter *Plasmodium* spp. in certain sea duckling species such as Common Eider; this can be diagnosed by microscopic evaluation of a blood smear and is routinely treated with antimalarial medications (Miller et al. 2017). Endoparasites, while uncommon in sea ducklings, may be encountered in facilities that feed live prey that may harbor intermediate host life stages for which waterfowl are the definitive host; food items like crayfish are best avoided. Routine care for waterfowl in care should include periodic fecal examinations particularly prior to moving to a new enclosure. Positive fecal examinations

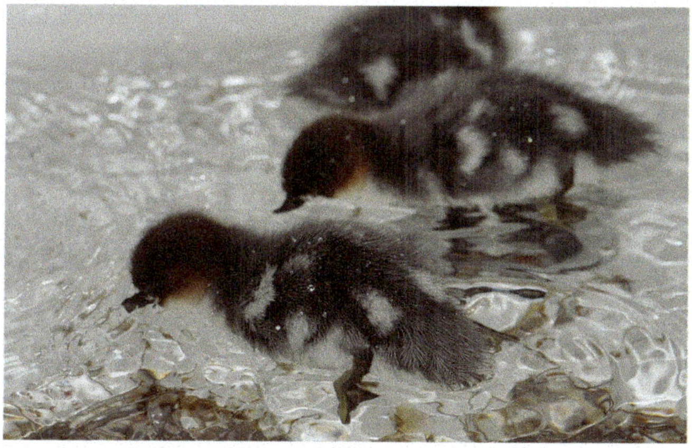

Figure 6.3 Common Merganser chicks foraging for live fish in small pool. Note downy chicks appear dry and fluffy even when swimming, which shows normal chick waterproof plumage. *Source:* photo courtesy of Ian Gereg.

should be evaluated based on the life cycle of the parasite and should be treated with the appropriate anthelminthic drug when indicated.

It is worth mentioning that many regions have hunting seasons for sea ducks; in the U.S., FDA regulations under the Animal Medicinal Drug Use Clarification Act may apply to these species and prohibit or restrict certain classes of drugs in food animals. To view the current list of prohibited or restricted drugs, visit www.farad.org. Waterfowl are considered a Minor Food Animal Species.

## Diets

There are several essential components to the diet of sea ducklings, including a staple diet and numerous natural food items that are integrated based on species specifics. The staple diet should be a commercial pellet specifically designed for wild waterfowl. Mazuri™ manufactures an extruded Waterfowl Starter pellet that floats when placed in water. Floating items promote natural foraging behavior and are ideal for a wide variety of waterfowl species. As ducklings grow, they can be transitioned onto a maintenance diet; Mazuri offers a Diving Duck extruded pellet as well as a Sea Duck Diet; these products float and are suitable for all sea duck species. Any of these staple diets can be soaked in warm water and blended to make a gavage formula suitable for debilitated or anorexic waterfowl. Nonextruded pellets do not float and tend to foul the water, which negatively impacts birds feather condition and can lead to loss of waterproofing. While the extruded products manufactured by Mazuri are less likely to contaminate the water surface, an overflow is strongly recommended to reduce negative effects on feather condition and waterproofing. Feeds manufactured for commercial poultry, pet poultry, or labeled as "all flock" products should be avoided for sea ducks and most waterfowl in general.

In addition to a high-quality staple diet, sea ducklings require a wide variety of natural food items in order to establish self-feeding behavior and grow appropriately. In the wild, sea ducklings have access to dozens of different species of aquatic invertebrates and insects. In captivity, the commercial options are limited but are nonetheless an essential component of sea duckling rearing. A certain amount of experimentation may be required when working with different groups of sea ducklings to ensure that they are eating the natural prey items offered to them. Commercially available aquatic invertebrates are available as both frozen and freeze-dried. In most cases, the frozen variety is preferred for sea ducklings as it sinks; most sea ducklings seek prey underneath the surface of the water. Freeze-dried invertebrates float on the surface of the water and may be used in addition to frozen invertebrates to stimulate self-feeding behavior. Of the commercially available aquatic invertebrates, frozen krill tends to be the most versatile prey item and is readily consumed by nearly all species of sea ducklings (smaller ducklings require that the krill be chopped). Mergansers benefit immensely from live fish and are capable of capturing live prey (if the fish are sized appropriately) from a few days old. Live fish can be obtained from a local bait shop or pet store or can be harvested (depending on local regulations) from ponds and/or streams. When feeding thawed frozen items (particularly fish), thiamine supplementation should be provided to avoid deficiencies (Miller et al. 2017). Feeder insects (primarily mealworms) should also be incorporated into a sea duckling's diet. Live insects create movement on the water surface which can trigger self-feeding behavior. Live insects should be maintained on an appropriate substrate and should be gut-loaded approximately 12–24 hours prior to feeding with a commercially available gut-loading diet to maximize nutrient composition prior to consumption (Fidgett and Gardner 2014). Transitioning ducklings onto a staple diet may be challenging for some species once acclimated to whole prey.

Certain species of sea ducklings (namely goldeneyes along with certain mergansers) along with the majority of pochards and stifftails consume a moderate amount of aquatic plant material. In captivity, either duckweed (*Lemna* spp.) or chopped greens can be offered floating on the water surface.

The provision of an appropriate staple diet along with a variety of natural food items does not necessarily indicate that the ducklings will eat sufficiently to maintain weight. Ducklings should be weighed twice daily for at least the first week in care. Ducklings that lose weight in care have a poor chance of survival without intervention. Intervention includes a combination of gavage feeding and drip feeding. These interventions are intended to provide supplemental calories while encouraging the ducklings to self-feed in an effort to minimize any weight loss while the ducklings are learning how to self-feed. Gavage feeding and drip feeding can be alternated throughout the day every 2–4 hours to maximize success. Whenever possible with critically debilitated animals, one overnight feeding should be provided to reduce weight loss overnight. Supplemental nutrition is generally provided for 7–10 days or until the ducklings are eating sufficiently on their own to maintain weight. Adjustments are made throughout this time to the volume and feeding increments to slowly increase the amount of formula being administered per feeding while increasing the time between feedings.

### Gavage-Feeding

Use the same type of syringe with an attached cut urethral catheter. Gavage-feeding small amounts of formula will help ducklings maintain weight while they transition to self-feeding. The two primary diets appropriate for gavage-feeding sea ducklings are Mazuri® Nestling Handfeeding Formula or Mazuri Waterfowl Starter. The Nestling Handfeeding Formula is a powder for reconstitution with hot water. The Waterfowl Starter should be soaked in warm water and blended to a paste consistency that can fit through the urethral catheter. Ducklings can tolerate gavage feedings equal to 10% body weight every 2–4 hours. When gavage-feeding, ensure that the cut urethral catheter is primed with formula prior to feeding to avoid air administration. With practice, the process of gavage-feeding should take no more than 15 seconds per duckling. Both of the formulas above can also be used for debilitated juvenile and adult waterfowl. Feeding equipment should be thoroughly cleaned and disinfected between uses.

### Drip-Feeding

Using a 1–3 ml syringe, a mixture of freshly thawed aquatic invertebrates (small species like plankton, bloodworms, brine shrimp, and daphnea work well) are drawn up into the syringe with a small amount of water. This water and invertebrate mixture is then dripped onto the bills of the ducklings every 2–4 hours. It takes a few drip-feedings for ducklings to acclimate to this method, but this gives them a taste for the invertebrates that they will ultimately consume in a wet brooder.

## Housing

Sea ducks and related species have strict housing requirements to maximize rearing success. Dry brooders are generally inappropriate for sea ducklings unless being used during the initial care period while waterproofing is being established (see Initial Care section). Sea ducklings require constant access to swimming water in order to thrive in captivity. Swimming water can be provided through various types of hybrid wet brooders and then ultimately in an outdoor aviary as the ducklings grow.

### Hybrid/Wet Brooder

The terms *hybrid* or *wet brooders* are used primarily in avicultural and zoo settings and refer to either an above-ground box or an in-ground structure that features both swimming water and a dry loafing area. The dry loafing area is usually located to one side of the brooder but can be created in the center of a brooder as a sort of island. Hybrid or wet brooders promote natural foraging behavior and are highly effective for the successful rearing of sea ducklings as well as many other waterfowl species, as they allow the ducklings free access to swimming water at all times to maintain excellent waterproofing.

Brooders should include a number of additional features. A hanging heat lamp should be provided over part of the loafing area that can be adjusted to the desired height based on the age of the ducklings; halogen heat lamps (QC Supply) offer the added feature of water resistance as the bulb will not explode if it gets inadvertently sprayed with water. A water line that allows a constant flow of clean water to feed the swimming area should be available, along with a drain with an overflow. An overflow is easily achieved with the use of a standpipe; the standpipe drains excess water which keeps the surface water clean. When using a standpipe, cross-bars should be added to prevent small ducklings from being able to get stuck in the pipe. When feeding small invertebrate prey items, a fine mesh can be stretched over the standpipe to allow water to drain without losing valuable food; monitor the standpipe for clogging or flooding when using mesh (Figures 6.4 and 6.5). Regardless of whether in-ground or above-ground, a brooder must provide a gentle slope or ramp to allow ducklings to get in and out of the swimming water easily. The dry area of the brooder is often covered with an easily washable, drainable substrate, such as unbacked vinyl coil matting (Cactus Mat). A combination of staple diet and natural food items should be provided in the swimming water; the staple diet should also be provided on the dry side of the brooder (either sprinkled directly onto the substrate, onto a paper towel, or offered in a shallow tip-proof dish close to the water).

Brooders may have to be cleaned two to four times daily depending on brooder size. If a brooder needs to be cleaned more than four times daily, the brooder is either too small or there are too many ducklings housed in the brooder. Maintaining a clean brooder environment for the ducklings

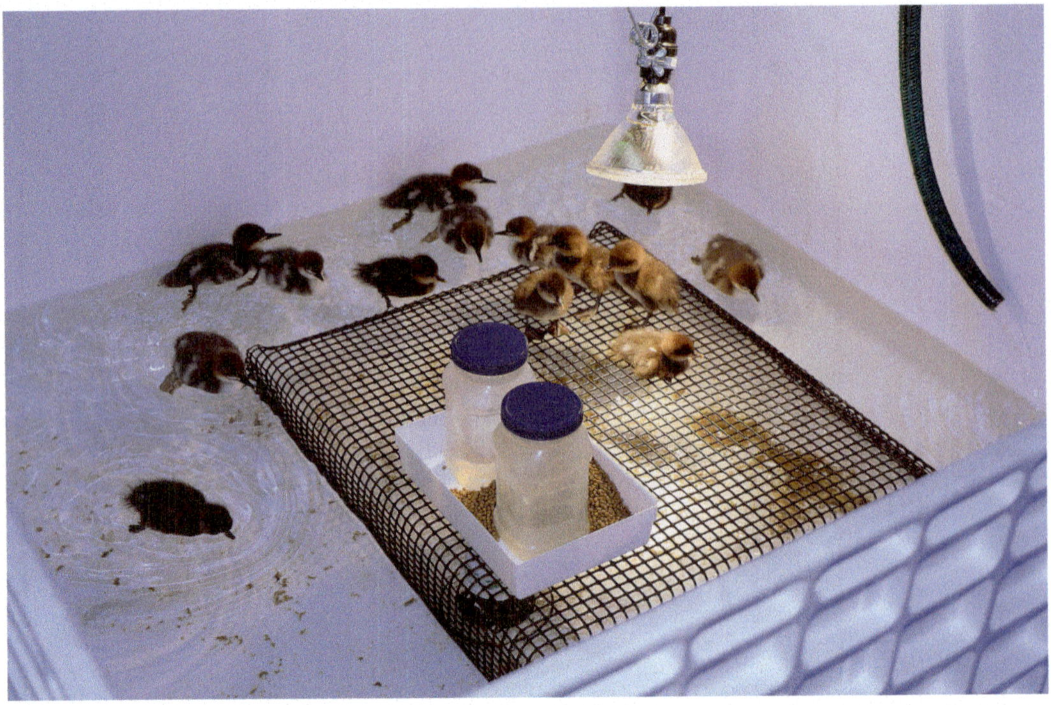

Figure 6.4 Hooded and Scaly-sided Merganser chicks in a wet brooder with access to both live and prepared food and a haul-out area with heat lamp. A hose producing a small stream and a standpipe drain provide a constant turnover of surface water. *Source:* photo courtesy of Arnold and Debbie Shouten.

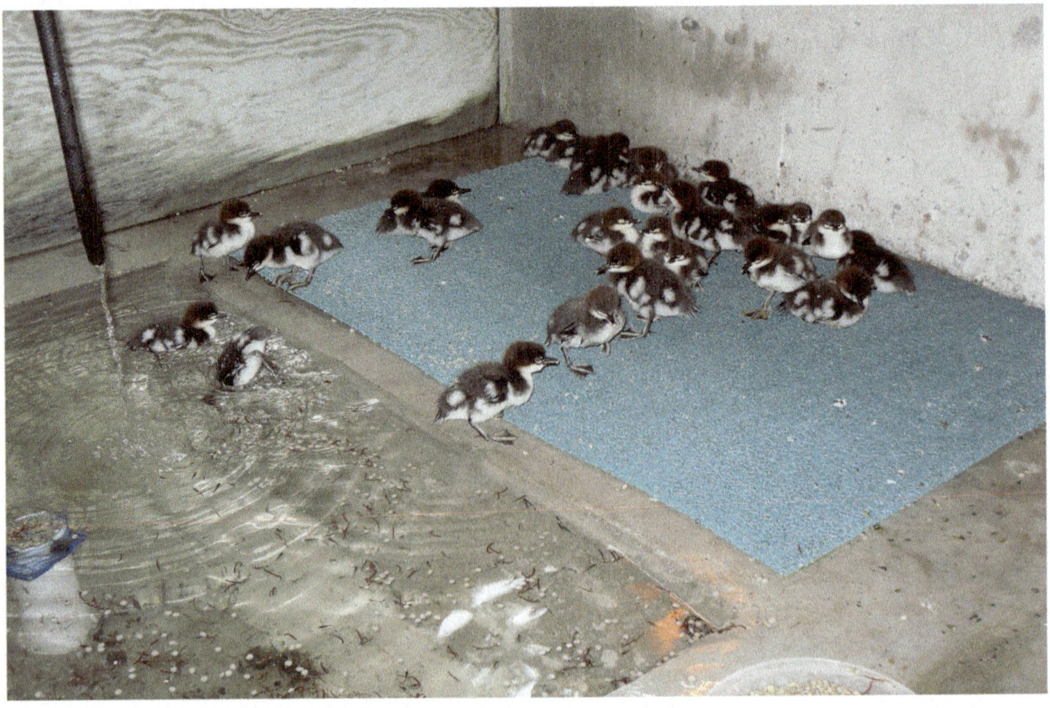

Figure 6.5 In-ground wet brooder: chicks can forage for live fish and easily exit the water to rest in a heated area with matting that helps prevent bumblefoot.

may require the provision of increased ventilation via a fan or air conditioner to prevent excess humidity. High levels of humidity may contribute to an increased incidence of wet feather and may predispose the ducklings to opportunistic infections like aspergillosis.

## Preparation for Wild Release

The size of an outdoor aviary for sea ducklings will vary depending on whether the ducks will be conditioned for release or maintained in permanent captivity. Wildlife rehabilitators are encouraged to review the Minimum Standards for Wildlife Rehabilitation (Miller 2012) for information on caging materials and sizes; keep in mind that recommended cage sizes are minimums and should be exceeded whenever possible. Regardless of the ultimate size of the outdoor enclosure, an in-ground swimming pool deep enough for swimming and diving is essential (Figure 6.6). The overall pool dimensions will vary based on species and number and age of ducklings in care. Concrete ponds with drains and overflows are often preferable to natural dirt ponds as they are easy to keep clean and there is a lower risk of intestinal parasites. As with the brooders, an overflow maintains high-quality surface water which promotes excellent waterproofing.

### Release

Transport kennels should include net-bottom cage inserts for all sea ducklings; this protects the ventrum from soiling if the bird(s) defecate during transport (Holcomb 1988). A net-bottom insert can be fashioned from PVC pipe made into a rectangle (using 90° corners) the same size as the

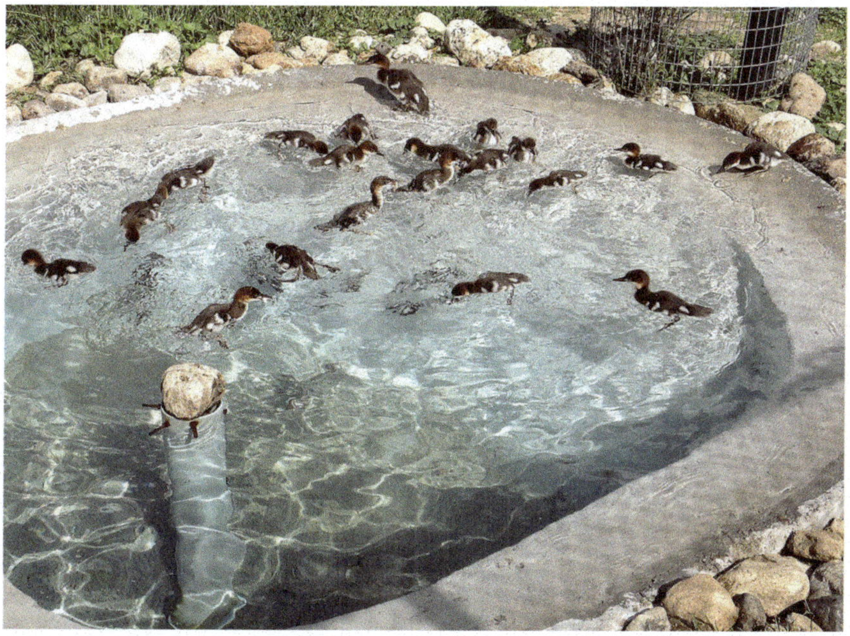

Figure 6.6 Pre-release aquatic housing with an in-ground pool and a naturalistic surround providing a diversity of substrates. Note the standpipe providing surface water drainage, while the opening is partially blocked by a rock to prevent ducklings from falling down into the pipe. *Source:* photo courtesy of Ian Gereg.

floor of the kennel. Knotless netting is then stretched tight over the PVC pipe frame and secured with rope on the underside of the frame. Natural history should dictate release timing for waterfowl in a wildlife rehabilitation setting. Waterfowl should be conditioned to be able to obtain natural food items prior to release and should have perfect feather condition and waterproofing. As a general guide, sea ducklings should have all of their contour feathers and should have at least 50% of the length of their primary and secondary feathers grown in. While it may seem advisable to wait until ducklings are fully flighted prior to release, this can present challenges if the ducklings startle out of their release kennel and fly away from the suitable release habitat. Waterfowl should be released in groups, in an area with known conspecifics, first thing in the morning in dry weather to allow a full day to acclimate to their environment.

## Acknowledgments

Many thanks to Arnold and Debbie Schouten at Dry Creek Waterfowl for sharing photos from their facility and to Ian Gereg for sharing his photos and for his assistance and support.

## Sources for Products Mentioned

Aquatic Bird Rearing Cubicle, Leucopsis Products, Ambler, PA, 19002, www.leucopsis.com.
Cactus Mat 1451 Vinyl Coil Scraper Mat Unbacked, 930 West 10th Street, Azusa, CA 91702, www.cactusmat.com.
Halogen Heat Lamp, QC Supply, PO Box 581, Schuyler, NE, 68661-0581, www.qcsupply.com.
Knotless Netting ⅜" Stock 1011, Memphis Net and Twine, 2481 Matthews Avenue, Memphis, TN, 38108, www.memphisnet.net.
Mazuri, PMI Nutrition International, LLC, PO Box 66812, St. Louis, MO 63166, www.mazuri.com.

## References

Backues, K.A. (2015). Anseriformes. In: *Fowler's Zoo and Wild Animal Medicine*, vol. 8 (eds. R.E. Miller and M.E. Fowler), 116–126. St. Louis, MO: Elsevier Saunders.

Baldassarre, G. (2014). *Ducks, Geese, and Swans of North America*. Baltimore, MD: Johns Hopkins University Press.

Bowman, T.D., Silverman, E.D., Gilliland, S.G., and Leirness, J.B. (2015). Status and trends of North American sea ducks: reinforcing the need for better monitoring. In: *Ecology and Conservation of North American Sea Ducks* (eds. J.-P.L. Savard, D.V. Derksen, D. Esler and J.M. Eadie), 1–28. Boca Raton, FL: CRC Press.

Fidgett, A.L. and Gardner, L. (2014). Advancing avian nutrition through best feeding practice. *International Zoo Yearbook* 48: 116–127.

Friend, M. (1999). Aspergillosis. In: *Field Manual of Wildlife Diseases: General Field Procedures and Diseases of Birds* (eds. M. Friend and J.C. Franson), 129–134. Madison, WI: USGS.

Goodman, M.D. (2017). Ducks, geese, and swans: An introduction to waterfowl medicine. Proceedings of the Association of Avian Veterinarians Annual Conference, Washington, DC, pp. 55–67.

Goodman, M., Schott, R., and Duerr, R. (2016). Waterfowl (ducks, geese, and swan). In: *Topics in Wildlife Medicine, Vol. 4: Orthopedics* (eds. R.S. Duerr and G.J. Purdin), 99–119. St. Cloud, MN: National Wildlife Rehabilitators Association.

Holcomb, J. (1988). For the new rehabber: net-bottom caging for waterfowl. *Wildlife Journal* 11 (1): 3–4.

Kear, J. (2005). *Ducks, Geese and Swans*. Oxford: Oxford University Press.

Miller, E.A. (2012). *Minimum Standards for Wildlife Rehabilitation*, 4e. National Wildlife Rehabilitators Association: St. Cloud, MN.

Miller, E.A., Goodman, M.D., and Cox, S. (2017). *NWRA Wildlife Formulary*. St. Cloud, MN: National Wildlife Rehabilitators Association.

# 7

# Domestic Poultry

*Nora Pihkala and Yuko Sato*

## Natural History

Several species of birds in the orders Galliformes (chickens, turkeys, quail, pheasants, partridges) and Anseriformes (ducks, geese) have been domesticated for use as food, sources of feathers, or pets. All species covered in this chapter hatch precocial chicks that are fully covered with downy feathers and are able to run and eat on their own shortly after hatching. Although parents of these species do not regurgitate food for their young, they do show their chicks what to eat and provide warmth and protection from the environment and predators.

Raising chickens, quail, and turkeys as a backyard hobby and for exhibition in poultry shows are popular pastimes. All manner of poultry are raised, from crossbreeds to purebred chickens, turkeys, ducks, geese, pheasants, and quail. Although many people choose to raise these birds in elaborate coops, poultry are hardy birds and do well under most circumstances provided that appropriate nutrition, environmental conditions, and protection from predators are provided.

Duck and goose chicks have three toes facing forward that are fully webbed for swimming, with feet that are usually orange. The rear digit is reduced but present slightly above the plane of the foot. Galliform chicks have an anisodactyl toe arrangement with three toes facing forward and one back.

Because state and federal permits are required to be able to rehabilitate wild birds, it is critical to identify the species of the chick(s). Contacting your local wildlife rehabilitation center or avian veterinarian or even searching the internet is a good option for positively identifying stray chicks. It often requires a professional eye to tell the difference between a domestic and a wild chick of similar species. As a general rule, chicks of most wild species have mottled or striped coloring, and are never bright yellow. However, domestic chicken chicks, turkey poults, ducklings, goslings, and game bird chicks can also have mottled or striped coloring, depending on the breed or variety. Wild rail chicks are often very small, fluffy, and black, and may be mistaken for chicken or quail chicks; they are best differentiated by their extremely long thin toes. Wild relatives of the species covered in this chapter are covered in Chapters 5, 6, and 8.

### Domestication of Chickens

Chickens (*Gallus gallus domesticus*) belong to the order Galliformes, family Phasianidae, and were domesticated from the Red Jungle Fowl native to Asia. Chickens were originally domesticated for cockfighting, and it was for this purpose that chickens spread throughout the world (Smith 1976).

*Hand-Rearing Birds*, Second Edition. Edited by Rebecca S. Duerr and Laurie J. Gage.

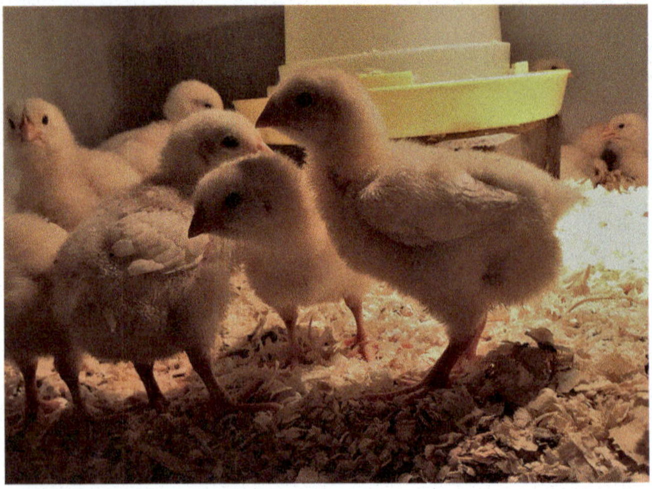

Figure 7.1 Active, alert chicks under a heat lamp in a brooder. *Source:* photo courtesy of Dan Famini.

At some point, chickens also became valued for their contributions to the table, namely in the form of eggs and meat (Figure 7.1).

Humans have bred chickens selectively for favorable traits, concentrating on livability and production, usually incorporating environmental considerations into breeding. This is apparent when studying the various classes of standardbred chickens, organized by world region by the American Poultry Association, an organization dedicated to advocating purebred poultry and their origins. The American class of chickens, for example, comprises 13 breeds of chickens, all of which characteristically have rounded bodies and thick, loose plumage to insulate against New England winters and provide a balance between egg production and meat quantity. These are currently classified as dual-purpose chickens. In contrast, the Mediterranean class of chickens encompasses seven breeds of chickens characterized by a long, lean body shape and plumage held close to the body for hot summers, frequently dark plumage, high alertness to evade predators in year-round foliage, and keenness to forage widely while producing a high number of eggs. Most of these are categorized as laying-type chickens. Commercial broiler chickens are the best example of meat-type chickens, and their sole purpose is to produce meat. See American Poultry Association (2015) for further descriptions, illustrations, and breed histories of purebred domestic poultry. It is not the intention of this chapter to address raising commercial meat and egg-producing chickens, because these birds and situations have specific management needs.

## Domestication of Other Galliformes

Because turkeys, pheasants, quail, and partridges were domesticated more recently than chickens, there are fewer domestic breeds of these game birds. Turkeys are thought to have been domesticated from North and Central America's Wild Turkey (*Meleagris galapavo*) in Mexico by the Aztecs as meat birds. They were introduced into Europe in the mid-sixteenth century (Richardson 1897). Varieties such as the Royal Palm and Narragansett were developed in Europe and North America and can still be found in hobbyists' yards and poultry shows. Today's predominant modern meat turkeys are strains of the Broad Breasted White breed, developed for quick rate of growth and lack of visible feather tracts after processing. These birds are strikingly different from wild turkeys and exhibition turkeys. If left to grow to full size, strains of modern meat turkeys can weigh upwards of

50 lb (22 kg) or more. Illustrations and descriptions of domesticated turkey breeds can be found in American Poultry Association (2015).

Pheasants were first domesticated in Asia Minor (Quarles 1916). Breeds include the Ringneck, Amherst, Reeves, Mongolian, Silver, and Golden. American breeders have crossbred pheasants to suit commercial purposes, but it is often difficult to distinguish pure breeds from cross breeds. Today they are popular birds raised for release at hunting clubs. Jumbo Ringnecks of 7 lb. (3 kg) have been developed for the tables of many fine restaurants (Hayes 1995). In the early twentieth century, Ringnecks were successfully introduced into many areas of the U.S., where wild populations continue to thrive or are replenished by regular releases.

The most commonly encountered domesticated quail breeds are Japanese and Bobwhite Quail. Japanese Quail (also known as Pharaoh Quail, *Coturnix japonica*) were domesticated in Japan in the eleventh century, initially for their singing and as pets (Hayes 1995). These birds reach sexual maturity at 6 weeks of age, and are prolific producers of small eggs, for which they are currently raised. They have also been a popular bird for scientific research because of their quick growth, hardiness, and ease of rearing. Bobwhite Quail (*Colinus virginianus*) originated in North and Central America, and there are many subspecies found throughout the continent. It is not clear when they became domesticated, but they adapt easily to different environments. With many variations in color pattern, they are raised for hunting clubs just as pheasants are. A jumbo Bobwhite of 22 oz. (620 g) has been developed for the table; wild and other nonjumbo breeds usually weigh 7–8 oz (225 g). Hayes (1995) is a good reference for more information on domesticated game bird rearing.

### Domestication of Anseriformes

The wild Mallard (*Anas platyrhynchos*) is thought to be the first duck domesticated and is the progenitor of all domesticated ducks except the Muscovy (*Cairina moschata*). Evidence suggests that Mallards were domesticated around 500 BCE in Southeast Asia or Italy. Muscovies are thought to have been domesticated in Colombia, likely over 1000 years ago (Holderread 2011). Ducks spread throughout the world after their domestication because of their versatility in producing meat, eggs, and feathers. Common breeds of ducks include Pekins, Runners, Khaki Campbells, Rouens, and Swedish. Please see American Poultry Association (2015) and Holderread (2011) for descriptions and illustrations of domestic duck breeds and their development. The latter also provides more detailed information about raising these birds.

The FAO (Food and Agriculture Organizations of the United Nations) recognizes 96 domestic goose breeds or genetic groups of geese around the world, although there are probably more. Despite limited available information, it is thought that geese were among the first animals to be domesticated about 3000 years ago in Egypt, although some research suggests that it may be earlier. Domestic geese of the world derive from two different lineages: the wild Greylag goose (*Anser anser*) from Europe and wild Swan goose (*Anser cygnoides*) from Asia. Despite its adaptability and genetic diversity, commercial goose production is only important in few countries in Asia and Europe (Buckland and Guy 2002).

## Criteria for Intervention

Individual chicks are often brought to veterinary clinics or wildlife rehabilitation centers by good Samaritans or are found wandering neighborhoods or streets after becoming lost. Chicks may be identified that are starving or do not eat or drink well, or that display other nonspecific symptoms of illness such as ruffled feathers, depressed posture and attitude, thinness, and pallor. Chicks suffering from gastrointestinal problems may present with diarrhea. Those with respiratory problems may present gasping for air, with open-mouthed breathing (be aware of concurrent causes of open-mouthed breathing, such as heat stress), and/or with *snicking* (quickly shaking head in one direction while making a sneezing or clicking sound). They may also cheep loudly if distressed; healthy and comfortable chicks chirp in soft tones. More dramatic presentations include cannibalism, external parasitism, and traumatic injury.

It is important to keep in mind when handling domestic poultry that they can be carriers of bacteria that may be harmful to humans, specifically *Campylobacter* and *Salmonella*. These bacteria naturally can occur on the feathers and skin of poultry and in their feces, and do not cause illness to the birds themselves. However, these bacteria can cause illness in humans such as vomiting, diarrhea, abdominal cramps, and fever. Recent outbreaks of salmonellosis from handling young chicks have been documented by the U.S. Centers for Disease Control and Prevention (CDC). Children, pregnant women, the elderly, and immune-compromised individuals are at greatest risk from handling *Salmonella*- and *Campylobacter*-infected poultry and surfaces that come into contact with poultry (such as feeders and waterers), although otherwise healthy adults are also susceptible. The CDC has several recommendations for reducing the chance of pathogen spread when handling poultry of any age, including washing hands with soap and water immediately after touching poultry or anything in their environment. Additional recommendations are found on the CDC's website (US CDC 2018).

## Initial Care and Stabilization

Regardless of species or whether being cared for permanently or temporarily, the first thing a new chick requires is warmth. When examining chicks, use warm hands and avoid placing them on cold surfaces. Particularly cold chicks may shiver and may cheep loudly. In this case, chicks should be warmed under a heat lamp before further evaluation is attempted unless immediate action is required (such as significant bleeding). Because these species are precocial at hatching, they are able to thermoregulate within a wider temperature range than altricial species. However, chilling chicks stresses them, and they should be handled in a warm room.

When birds of apparently different species are presented, they should immediately be separated and raised apart from each other. Young game birds should not be raised with chickens, turkeys, ducks, or geese because they are very susceptible to diseases these other species may carry, and the larger birds may peck at the game birds, causing injury.

All young poultry need a source of heat until fully feathered. The least expensive option is to arrange a screen-covered heat lamp so that the distance from floor to lamp is 1.5–2.5 ft. (0.5–0.75 m), depending on the lamp wattage. The bulb should be red rather than white to discourage cannibalism in older chicks. Incandescent bulbs or infrared bulbs rather than fluorescent, CFL, or LED bulbs should be used because they radiate sufficient heat. However, care should be taken when using heat lamps to prevent burns and fires. The floor temperature should be approximately 100 °F (37.7 °C) directly under the lamp for newly hatched chicks. A 1–2 ft. (0.3–0.6 m) high brooder ring is placed under the lamp in a circle to act as a corral to keep chicks from straying too far from the heat source. It is unwise to use a square-shaped enclosure because some species will pile in corners and suffocate. This ring can be removed after the first week. The best rule of thumb for achieving the proper temperature is to observe the distribution of the chicks at rest under the lamp. Chicks should be in an even and fanned pattern outward from the lamp. If they are piled under the lamp, the temperature is too cold; if they are pressed against the brooder ring, the temperature is too hot or there may be a draft.

Solitary chicks may benefit from the addition of a feather duster or even a mirror in their enclosure, because many chicks of these species are stressed by being alone. Frequent handling of chicks destined to become pets will assist them in becoming socialized to humans, but chicks must be allowed ample time to eat and drink throughout the day. Children should be instructed about this because many children enjoy carrying chicks around, but may inadvertently prevent them from obtaining adequate nutrition.

Many chicks need some introduction to food and water. If the flock size is large, about 25% of the flock can have "formal instruction," and those can be counted on to "teach" the rest. Instruction consists of dipping the beak into the water and feed a few times. Select the feed type once the species is known. Chick starter feed and game bird starter feed should be readily available at most feed stores and are preferred over scratch (which is not nutritionally complete). Starter feed typically comes in mash and crumble forms, both of which are suitable for feeding, though very young chicks may find mash easier to ingest. Waterers must have a small lip for the chicks to drink from; even smaller if the species has tiny chicks. Generally, preferred waterers are a bell shape that allows water from the center holder to refill the lip as needed. Never use waterers that are big enough for the chicks to fall into. Newly hatched chicks are unstable on their feet and have trouble righting themselves if flipped over. This can result in mass drowning if waterers consist of open dishes. If this is a concern, placing marbles or stones in the waterers reduces the depth of the water and the possibility of entrapment. Gradually, the waterers can be replaced with larger units to accommodate the growing birds.

Healthy or mildly dehydrated chicks may begin drinking on their own or after a few turns of beak dipping. Weak chicks may attempt to swallow but may not be able to hold up their heads. In this situation, after dipping, tip the chick backward gently, using a thumb and index finger to gently support the beak; observe them swallowing. Once they have swallowed, dip their beaks into the water again. Repeat the dipping and tipping until they no longer drink.

The goal throughout initial treatment is to stabilize birds and reduce stress as much as possible. Stress causes depression of the immune system and otherwise weakens chicks' defense against disease (Saif 2003). Stressors include chilling, nutritional deficiency (including due to decreased appetite), dehydration, excessive handling (particularly of game birds), and overcrowding.

## Physical Examination

***General:*** Is the bird thin? Feel the bird's breast and note the keel bone; the more prominent, the more underweight the bird. Does the bird appear pale? Is the bird lethargic? Is the bird hunched over or showing an otherwise abnormal posture? Are there signs of trauma (puncture wounds, broken skin)?

***Integumentary (Skin and Feathers):*** Is the skin dry and clean? Are there any cuts, scrapes, or abscesses on the body? Are there any bumps or nodules on the skin? Are feathers ruffled and held away from the body? Examine the feet and legs. Do leg and foot scales lie flat and appear smooth, or are they raised and crusted? Are the pads of the feet clean and intact, or is there thickened skin or an apparent "scab"? Examine feathers and skin near the vent and tail base very closely for signs of external parasites. Use a magnifying glass to examine the base of the feathers and along the feather shafts and barbs (Figure 7.2). If legs and toes are feathered (a breed characteristic in some chickens), examine feathers there also. Examining feather plucks under a microscope can help identify the type of parasites. Lice and mites are the most common types of ectoparasites. Poultry

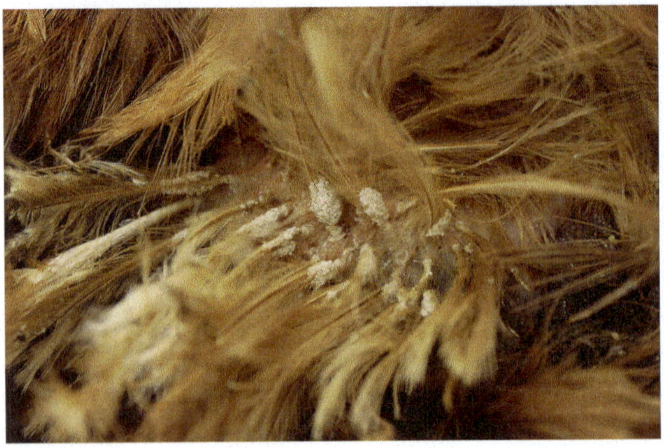

Figure 7.2 Lice eggs (nits) encrusted at the base of feathers.

have their own type of flea, the stick-tight flea, which is usually found on facial skin and on the comb. Poultry also have their own type of tick.

***Eyes, Ears, Nose, Throat:*** Hold the bird's mouth open and gently extend the head and neck so that the mouth and esophagus can be visualized. Note any lesions in the mouth, including in the choanal opening. Whitish masses may indicate a yeast or parasitic infection (possibly *Candida albicans* and *Trichomonas gallinae*, respectively) or a systemic fowl pox infection. An avian veterinarian can differentiate these conditions with additional testing. Shine a penlight or small flashlight down the trachea (or transilluminate across the trachea) and look carefully for tiny red worms known as gapeworms (*Syngamous trachea*). Care must be taken during this procedure because gapeworms reduce breathing capacity, and added stress can asphyxiate the birds. Look carefully at the eyes and note whether the eyes appear clear or cloudy. Note whether the bird appears blind in one or both eyes. Note whether they have pus or other discharge around the eyes that can indicate infection or irritation. Is nasal discharge present, and, if so, what does it look like (thick, frothy, bloody, watery, opaque)?

***Cardiovascular:*** Heart rate is difficult to assess in chicks owing to birds' normally high heart rate. Examine mucous membranes of the mouth (or just inside the vent) and describe color. Pale pink color (in light pigmented birds) may indicate anemia, poor perfusion (blood reaching tissues), or blood loss. Birds with dark or blue pigmented skin are difficult to assess.

***Respiratory:*** Is the bird having difficulty breathing? Is it rasping, gasping, or coughing?

***Gastrointestinal:*** Examine the vent area. Are there signs of diarrhea such as dried, crusted feces around the vent and adherent to surrounding feathers? Are there worms in any adherent feces? Evaluation of internal parasites is best done with a fecal examination by a local veterinary clinic.

***Neurological:*** Is the bird able to walk? Does the bird exhibit gait abnormalities, incoordination, lameness, or leg weakness? When resting, does the bird have tremors (other than shivering)? Does the bird rest on its hocks? Is the bird *stargazing* (turning its head so that it is looking toward the sky)?

When receiving many chicks, it may not be practical to perform physical exams on all birds. In this situation, observe all birds as a group before handling individual birds. Note their general appearance, behavior, and gait. Performing physical examinations on a few representative birds can provide a quick overview of what may be going on with other birds in the flock.

## Record Keeping

A detailed history should be obtained from the person presenting the chicks, if available. If the chicks were found, they should be asked where they found them, how long they have had them, whether they attempted to feed or water them (and the results), and what environmental conditions they had been exposed to (such as cold nights). If an owner is presenting you with chicks that he or she is raising, finding out about the growing environment, feed, vaccination history, history of exposure to other birds, and history of avian disease on the premises can potentially yield helpful information about underlying causes of disease or injury. Specifically, ask about housing, feeding, and environmental conditions.

***Housing:*** Are chicks raised in a brooder or loose with other birds? Of what material is the brooder made? If it is a nonporous material, do they clean and disinfect after each brood? With what disinfectants? If they use cardboard boxes to brood, do they reuse them for brooding? From what source do they get the cardboard boxes?

***Feed:*** What are they feeding? Where do they purchase it? Does the feed ever have an "off" or musty smell? If so, do they feed it? How do they store the feed? Do they feed additional feed such as table scraps or scratch feed? What type of feeder is used? Does it appear that the chicks are having difficulty eating?

***Environment:*** Are chicks brooded indoors or outdoors? If they are brooded outdoors, are they raised near or have access to other birds? If so, what species? Are chicks exposed to drafts? To direct sunlight? To rain? What type of litter is used? Is newspaper used during brooding? When is litter changed? Does litter ever get wet and caked? Is mold ever found when litter is changed?

## Common Medical Problems and Solutions

Most pet poultry, unless used for show, rarely encounter the same intensity of disease exposure that commercial poultry do. However, domestic poultry are afflicted by a plethora of contagious diseases of tremendous concern to regulatory agencies, and people who keep these species as pets or for small-scale production of eggs or meat should be aware of these issues. Nonetheless, keeping poultry can be very rewarding and many perceived "disease" conditions are actually the result of environmental or feed mismanagement or are unusual presentations of normal events (such as molting). Vaccinations, with a few exceptions, are unnecessary for backyard poultry and can be difficult to obtain in the proper dose size. Most vaccines are sold in bottles of 500–10 000 doses, and mixing errors can be devastating. In addition, medication is also frequently tailored for commercial flock sizes, and dilution errors for small flocks are common. If vaccines are given, be sure to document all dilution calculations in case of possible overdosing. Due to space constraints, a thorough discussion of most infectious diseases will not be included here. Please see Boulianne (2013) for an excellent and inexpensive resource for most avian diseases for chickens, ducks and geese, and game birds.

The following sections are not meant to be comprehensive, but include some of the more common conditions that are encountered in backyard poultry practice. Note that for any insecticides or medications listed, it is important to follow application instructions and the drug withdrawal requirements for human safety. Insecticides and medications and their residues can remain in muscle tissue or eggs, which can be harmful to humans. Following withdrawal requirements helps ensure that consumption of any meat or eggs from treated birds does not cause harm to the consumer.

### Cannibalism

Domestic Galliformes are naturally cannibalistic; game birds especially should be observed for cannibalistic behavior. Cannibalism usually does not begin in earnest under 2–3 weeks of age. If observed in young chicks, it is generally the result of insufficient feed or diarrhea (soiled vents can be attractive pecking targets). In older birds with noninfectious causes, methods of controlling pecking include reducing light intensity, reducing bird density, increasing the number of feeders, providing environmental enrichment, and conditioning of the beaks. Remove moderately to severely cannibalized birds and segregate them until their skin has healed completely. Avian skin regenerates quickly and with little to no scarring, particularly in younger birds. If an individual bird has been pecked severely but no isolation facilities are available, spraying the affected area with pruning tar (used for trees) is a good solution. The tar protects the skinless area from fluid loss, is nontoxic even when used on open wounds, and has the advantage of identifying the perpetrators by staining their beaks black. If small numbers of birds are the aggressors, these birds can be given red spectacles ("peepers") that attach to their nares or be fitted with red contact lenses, which are available at most poultry supply stores. If many of the birds are acting cannibalistic, making environmental adjustments such as reducing light intensity, checking feed, or simply putting a tinted (e.g. red) light bulb may help with the behavior.

### Bumblefoot

Bumblefoot or pododermatitis occurs when the footpad is abraded or punctured, allowing *Staphylococcus* bacteria to infect the wound. Bumblefoot is readily identified on physical exam as a well-defined, thickened "callus" (granuloma) on the footpad sometimes seen with or without a penetrating ulcer. A granuloma is a collection of hardened inflammatory cells. Granulomas may be very large and when removed result in pain and expose underlying tissue to further infection. Consult an avian veterinarian, who will definitively diagnose the condition and may prescribe a course of antibiotics. Although more commonly encountered in older, heavier birds, bumblefoot can be seen in chicks. Keeping litter clean and dry, and not allowing it to get caked up, can reduce the incidence of this condition. Use soft yet supportive litter such as rice hulls or wood shavings. Avoiding exposure to sharp objects can reduce the chance of injury to footpads and prevent *Staphylococcus* infection.

### Crop Impaction

Chicks are naturally curious and will peck at anything that interests them. When chicks ingest nonfood particles such as sand or sawdust, their crops may become filled with this nondigestible material. Birds may stop eating and the crop may appear pendulous and feel very full. In older birds, crop impaction may indicate Marek's disease (MD) (see "Viral Diseases"), which can cause paralysis of the vagus nerve and loss of gut motility.

### Infectious Diseases

When infectious diseases are suspected, an avian veterinarian should be consulted. He or she will observe the birds, perform diagnostic tests, and make specific treatment and prevention recommendations. Since January 1, 2017, a new U.S. Food and Drug Administration rule named the Veterinary Feed Directive has put tighter regulation of the use of antibiotics, meaning that drugs can only be obtained using a prescription under the supervision of licensed veterinarians (see AVMA 2018). This often requires further work-up with additional testing at a laboratory. If a veterinarian knowledgeable in poultry medicine is not available, one or more birds may be submitted to the nearest veterinary diagnostic laboratory. Birds submitted will be humanely destroyed and undergo necropsy and pathology to determine the cause of disease.

### Ectoparasites

External parasites (ectoparasites) such as mites, lice, and ticks are a concern in both commercial and small flock poultry producers. Two common mites of poultry are the Northern Fowl Mite and the Red Mite. The Northern Fowl Mite is most common around the vent, tail, and breast of the bird. They are easily observed and are a reddish-brown color. The Red Mite feeds only at night, making daytime diagnosis difficult. They can be found in cracks and seams near the bedding areas and appear as white fuzz balls or salt-and-pepper-like deposits. Red Mites will cause feather loss, irritation, and anemia. Insecticides are available for treatment of both mites. Effective insecticides, such as permethrin sprays and dusts may be used for treatment of both types of mite and are available at feed or home and garden stores. Apply the product liberally, ensuring that it reaches the skin, paying special attention to the skin around the vent and base of the tail. Consult the label on specific products used for indication, application instructions, and the withdrawal period. Other approved insecticides are listed in Townsend (2018).

There are several types of lice that live on poultry, and lice or nits can be observed at the base of the feathers. An important thing to note is that only chewing lice, not the blood-sucking kind, infest poultry. With severe infestations, growth and egg production can be affected. Again, permethrins are effective in treating lice.

Fowl ticks comprise a group of soft ticks, which parasitize many species of poultry and wild birds. Ticks are easily missed because they spend relatively little time on the bird. Heavy infestations can cause anemia or tick paralysis, and ticks can be vectors for *Borrelia anserina* (spirochetosis). Spraying of buildings with permethrins or pyrethroids (e.g. cyfluthrins) is the treatment of choice.

### Endoparasites

Large roundworms and tapeworms are the most common poultry worms and are generally the result of soil contamination and poor management. Unless infestations are heavy, clinical disease is usually not evident. Piperazine can be used for roundworms (repeat in 10–14 days) and dibutyltin dilaurate for tapeworms. Do not use these compounds in laying hens. Proper litter management will reduce parasite loads and reinfection.

Control of coccidia is one of the most common and more costly problems of commercial and backyard poultry raising. Coccidia are found primarily in the intestinal tract of most poultry, but may occur in the kidney in geese. Coccidiosis is generally observed in young birds of 1–4 months. The disease causes diarrhea that may be bloody and frequently leads to death. Coccidia thrive in moist, heavily soiled litter, and disease is often a result of excessively high bird density. Prevention can be obtained by supplying coccidiostats in the feed (amprolium is a common type of coccidiostat found in medicated poultry starter feeds) or ordering chicks that are vaccinated from the hatchery (e.g. Murray McMurray hatchery). Outbreaks of disease can be treated, usually with either a treatment dose of amprolium or sulfa drugs; however, consult with a poultry veterinarian to make sure the birds are not dying from secondary infections leading to lethal conditions such as necrotic enteritis. Sulfa drugs cannot be used in laying hens.

**Viral Diseases**

Marek"s disease (MD is a common viral disease of chickens. The primary lesions are tumors of the viscera, muscle, skin, eye, and peripheral nerves. Nerve lesions can be an early indicator of the disease resulting in a condition termed "range paralysis." Birds with visceral tumors will often have only cachexia (wasting) as a clinical sign. Tumors of the muscles and skin are frequently palpable. MD cannot be treated but can be prevented by vaccination at hatch. When acquiring backyard poultry or hatching your own, every attempt should be made to vaccinate against MD. Vaccinations are not effective if applied to birds older than 1–2 weeks of age. Clinical MD generally affects birds 6–14 weeks of age; however, it is not uncommon in older birds. If tumors are found in the viscera of deceased birds, carcasses should be submitted to a diagnostic laboratory for differential diagnosis between MD and another common viral lymphoid tumor disease, avian leukosis. Avian leukosis is found in birds older than 14 weeks and tumors are very similar to those found with MD. Avian leukosis has no treatment or vaccination.

Infectious bronchitis virus (IBV) causes a rapidly spreading respiratory disease in young chicks. Laying hens experience reduced production and egg abnormalities. Certain strains of IBV will also cause kidney disease. Chicks that are infected early in life may have temporary voice changes and/or permanent damage to the oviduct, which will prevent them from laying eggs. Although IBV is highly transmissible, most birds will recover with supportive treatment. Antibiotics can be applied to the water in order to prevent secondary infection. Vaccines are available; however, doses are too large (10 000 or more) for backyard chickens, which are usually not vaccinated unless they come in contact with other chickens (neighbors, shows).

Newcastle disease virus (ND) affects numerous species of birds and is the reason for establishment of quarantine regulations for birds entering the United States. Virulent ND is very likely fatal; outbreaks have occurred in the recent past in both commercial and backyard poultry. ND does exist in milder forms in the U.S., and is primarily characterized by respiratory disease and an egg production drop. Mortality is variable and depends upon the strain of the virus. As with IBV, vaccination is available, but is generally given only to pet poultry that are exposed to other birds.

Fowl pox virus causes nodular and scab-like lesions primarily on the unfeathered portions of the bird's skin (dry form). Occasionally, pox virus can cause lesions in the mouth and trachea causing death due to suffocation (wet form). Once the bird recovers from the disease, immunity is generally lifelong. Not all pox outbreaks are caused by fowl pox virus but can be caused by related strains such as pigeon pox, turkey pox, psittacine pox, quail pox, etc. Strains are usually species-specific but can occasionally affect other species. One strain may not cross-protect with another. Vaccination is available and should be applied to flocks on premises with a previous history of pox or with presence of pox in nearby birds. Poxvirus is transmitted through contact of infected lesions with open wounds and through insect bites (mosquitoes), although wet pox can be spread without a break in the skin.

Avian encephalomyelitis (AE) occurs in chickens, turkeys, pheasants, and quail and primarily causes tremors and paralysis in young chicks 1–3 weeks old. Nearly all commercial flocks are infected, but clinical disease is low due to protection by maternal antibodies. AE can be transmitted vertically in eggs laid 5–13 days post-infection, and it is an enteric infection under natural conditions. The spread is more rapid in floor-raised birds than in those cage-raised. There is no treatment, and vaccination of breeders (both chicken and turkey), so that maternal antibodies protect the young during early life, is critical to prevention. Because many specialty breeders, particularly those that sell stock to feed stores, do not vaccinate, AE is a fairly common viral disease in backyard birds. Vaccination should be given to hens after 8 weeks of age but by at least 4 weeks prior to onset of laying.

### Bacterial Infections

There are many different species in the bacterial genus of *Salmonella*. Generally speaking, *Salmonella pullorum* and *Salmonella gallinarum* are reportable diseases and cause the greatest problem for poultry; *Salmonella enterica* serotype Typhimurium and serotype Enteritidis are important for the public health aspect. Pullorum (*S. pullorum*) is egg-transmitted and causes a diarrheal disease in young chicks and turkey poults resulting in high mortality. Adult birds are asymptomatic carriers. Diagnosis is based on disease history and isolation of the bacteria. Prevention is achieved by purchasing birds from disease-free flocks, such as participants of the National Poultry Improvement Plan (NPIP) program. Treatment is not recommended because it can cause birds to become carriers. Fowl typhoid (*S. gallinarum*) occurs in chickens, turkeys, and many other game and wild birds. Fowl typhoid is similar in disease presentation and diagnosis to pullorum, although mature birds can show clinical signs of fowl typhoid. Prevention is again achieved by obtaining disease-free stock. Clinical signs are infrequently observed in poultry infected with *Salmonella enteritidis* and *Salmonella typhimurium*. Flocks can be monitored by regulatory blood testing and obtaining egg samples or environmental samples for culturing the organism.

Chronic respiratory disease in poultry (primarily chickens and turkeys) is generally caused by *Mycoplasma gallisepticum* infection. Pathogenicity of the organism is enhanced by co-infection with other organisms. Clinical signs of respiratory disease develop slowly in a flock and feed consumption drops. Infection of the sinuses is common in turkeys. Serology and identification of the organism can be used for diagnosis. Contact your veterinarian or local veterinary diagnostic laboratory for testing options. Prevention, as with the Salmonellas, rests with the establishment of a clean flock by eliminating the infected flock, complete sanitation, and obtaining clean stock. Live vaccination is available on a state-by-state basis. Treatment is expensive, and the disease often recurs after cessation of treatment. Other important mycoplasmas in poultry include *Mycoplasma synoviae* (infectious synovitis) and *Mycoplasma meleagridis* (venereal infection and airsacculitis).

Colibacillosis is caused by the organism *Escherichia coli* (*E. coli*) and is usually secondary to other infections such as IBV and mycoplasmosis. A wide variety of clinical signs can be observed, and the organism occurs in most species and age groups. Vigorous adherence to biosecurity and sanitation programs will effectively prevent the organism from causing disease. Many antibiotics can be used for treatment, and sensitivity to the antibiotic should be ascertained. Treatment is usually successful if the disease is in the early stages.

### Fungal Diseases

Aspergillosis (brooder pneumonia) occurs in many poultry and nonpoultry species of birds. Birds under 3 weeks of age are most commonly affected, and infection is obtained from hatchers or brooders that are contaminated with fungal spores. Morbidity is variable and mortality can be high in clinically affected birds. Culturing the fungus or demonstration of typical fungal hyphae in fresh preparations from lesions are used for diagnosis. Prevention is obtained by thoroughly cleaning hatchers, incubators, waterers, feeders, and ventilation fans and by keeping litter clean and dry. Treatment is expensive and may not be effective. Ketoconazole and nystatin have been used.

### When to Notify State Authorities

Reportable diseases are those diseases that cause severe morbidity and/or mortality, are economically harmful, or spread very rapidly. Veterinarians and rehabilitators are very important first lines of defense in identifying reportable and potentially devastating avian diseases such as virulent Newcastle disease virus (vNDV) and avian influenza. It was a veterinarian in private practice who first discovered the presence of vNDV in California in both 2002 and 2018 and reported it to the state food and agriculture department.

The World Organization for Animal Health (OIE) is an international animal health group that has over 160 member countries. The OIE has several objectives, including collecting data on animal diseases. It has created a list of reportable avian diseases: avian infectious bronchitis, avian infectious laryngotracheitis, avian mycoplasmosis (*M. gallisepticum*), avian mycoplasmosis (*M. synoviae*), duck virus hepatitis, fowl typhoid (pullorum disease), fowl cholera (*Pasteurella multocida*), psittacosis (avian chlamydiosis), infection with avian influenza viruses, infection with influenza A viruses of high pathogenicity in birds other than poultry including wild birds, infection with exotic ND virus, infectious bursal disease (Gumboro disease), and turkey rhinotracheitis (OIE 2018). Additionally, each state may have deemed additional diseases as reportable; contact the state Department of Agriculture for additional reportable diseases.

When suspecting that birds presented may have a reportable disease, contact your veterinarian and quarantine all birds until the authorities give more specific instructions. Time is an exceptionally important factor in controlling disease outbreaks, and state departments of agriculture urge anyone who suspects a reportable disease to contact them as soon as these diseases are suspected. Clinical signs of reportable (and nonreportable) diseases are often nonspecific and may include depression, lethargy, inappetance, decreased water intake, ruffled feathers, and decreased egg production. It is when a disease outbreak results in dramatic, acute morbidity and/or mortality, lasts for a prolonged period of time, and/or spreads rapidly within a flock that the authorities should be notified.

## Diet Recipes and Feeding Procedures

More is known about the nutritional needs of chickens than of any other animal, including humans. Specific dietary formulations are available for young, growing chicks; for young, growing turkeys, pheasants, and quail; and for ducks and geese. Feed may be purchased in 25–50 lb. sacks at any feed store. In suburban areas, some hardware stores or garden centers may sell feed in sacks as well as by the pound. Sacks of feed are very economical and practical when several chicks are being raised. However, when raising only one to two chicks, such large quantities of feed may grow stale before they can be consumed and are more likely to become moldy or parasitized. In this situation, purchasing 3–4 lb. of feed at a time may be more expensive, but it will help ensure that feed is palatable and safe for consumption. Storage of feed in dry, cool areas (e.g. garage) is recommended to keep feed safe from contamination.

For very young chicks, a small handful of feed should be placed on a plastic or disposable tray with sides no higher than 0.5 in. (1 cm). Disposable foam or cardboard trays are convenient and may be purchased inexpensively at craft and hobby stores. Foam trays that have been used to hold raw meat should not be used due to the risk of bacterial contamination. Egg carton tops may also be used if the sides have been cut short. Chicks are naturally curious and peck instinctively at objects around their toes. By placing chicks on top of the food they will become familiar with it. They also imitate one another; if one chick learns to eat the others will follow suit. If chicks do not seem interested in food, gently stir the feed with a finger as the chicks observe. The movement will help stimulate them to eat. Observe that all the chicks are eating and drinking before leaving them for any period of time. Usually by 1 week of age, chicks will be able to use a chick feeder. Introduce a chick feeder after the first few days. Chick feeders have the advantage of being covered to keep older chicks from scratching out feed and wasting it. As chicks grow they will learn to eat from the feeders, and the trays should be removed.

When feeding young chickens, a chick starter ration should be fed until 6 weeks of age, when they should be switched to a grower ration. Feed is available in dry mash, crumbles, and pellets. Pellets are often too large for chicks and should be avoided. Mash is very palatable but can be wasteful; chicks also tend to pick through the mash to ingest preferred grains (usually corn), potentially leading to nutritional deficiencies. Crumbles ensure nutritional adequacy and are usually small enough for even youngest chicks to easily ingest. If crumbles prove to be too large for chicks to eat easily, mash should be fed instead. If no mash is available, crumbles may be further pulverized by placing some crumbles into a resealable plastic freezer bag and grinding with a rolling pin. At 18–20 weeks of age, a laying ration should be fed to both male and female birds.

Young turkeys, pheasants, and quail have higher requirements for protein and calcium. These birds should be fed game bird starter feed until 6–8 weeks of age. Ideally, game bird conditioner or game bird developer ration should be fed thereafter until 16–20 weeks of age. A game bird layer ration may be fed thereafter. Although game bird diets are generally well-balanced nutritionally, individual species can have different nutritional needs. It is advisable to use a mineral mix in chicks' water until their species and breed can be established, and then feed accordingly. Use mineral mixes specifically formulated for birds; consult your feed store on their available products and follow instructions carefully.

An important exception to feeding game birds is the Japanese Quail. They reach sexual maturity rapidly and may begin laying eggs as soon as 6 weeks of age. They should be fed a game bird starter mash until 6 weeks of age. Game bird layer mash or crumbles should be fed thereafter.

Ducks and geese have their own feeds as well. Feed starter ration for the first 2 weeks, grower until 8 weeks of age, developer until 20 weeks of age, and a maintenance or laying ration thereafter. Waterfowl feeds are not as widely available as chicken and game bird feeds. Consult with knowledgeable feed store personnel or feed manufacturer representatives about which feeds are appropriate in the absence of waterfowl feed. A good description of feed substitutions and additions when waterfowl feed is not available can be found in Holderread (2011).

When raising young chickens with ducks and geese, an all-purpose grower feed such as Purina Mills® Flock Raiser® may be fed to all young birds up to 18–20 weeks of age. (This feed may also be feed to turkeys after 8–10 weeks until 30–32 weeks.) However, it is vital that turkeys, pheasants, and quail be fed a game bird starter until 8–10 weeks of age. It is equally important that young chickens *not* be fed game bird starter, because this feed has excessive levels of calcium and protein, which may lead to problems with maturation of the long bones. Because there are several feed millers in the U.S. and their formulations or feeding programs may vary, consult the feed dealer for recommendations on raising mixed flocks. Diets fed to diverse species may not meet the requirements of one or more of the species; hence, it is preferable to feed diets specific for the type of bird being raised.

There are other considerations when selecting and feeding poultry diets. It is highly recommended to feed a diet containing a coccidiostat such as amprolium. Coccidiosis is a protozoal disease caused by species in the genus *Eimeria,* which inhabit the small intestine of most poultry. Coccidiosis is a leading cause of fatal diarrhea in young poultry. Coccidiostats prevent *Eimeria* from undergoing its normal lifecycle in affected animals and are safe to use in even the youngest chicks. They should be used until 16 weeks of age (Mississippi State University Extension 2018). Feeding diets containing premixed coccidiostats is the easiest and safest method to reduce or eliminate coccidiosis, because only FDA-approved drugs are allowed in feeds. Follow the feed manufacturer's recommendations on drug withdrawal before consuming meat or eggs.

Antibiotics should not be used in chicks unless bacteria have been found to be the agent of disease. During the first few weeks of life, a chick's digestive tract is being colonized by many beneficial microflora. These microflora serve to aid digestion as well as to successfully compete with pathogenic bacteria such as *E. coli*. When antibiotics are given to young chicks without a specific therapeutic goal, beneficial microflora are destroyed, thus leaving the digestive tract open to colonization by pathogens. Use of antibiotics in any bird should only be done in consultation with a licensed veterinarian; for example, if a chick has been injured by a predator such as a dog or cat, see your veterinarian for treatment.

When young chickens are eating well, dietary supplements should not be given because feeds are nutritionally complete. Feed stores may offer scratch feed, but this is more of a treat for adult birds. Scratch contains little nutritive value and may contribute to obesity if fed excessively. Feeding kitchen vegetable scraps is acceptable for adult birds but should not be fed to chicks because they may potentially cause diarrhea.

When chicks are ill they may refuse to eat dry food. In this case, they may prefer a wet mash or gruel. Wet mash (gruel) is highly palatable, contributes to hydration, and is simple to make. In a large saucepan or Dutch oven, place three parts water and one part mixed grains. Grains such as rolled oats, crushed wheat, milo, and wheat bran can be purchased in bulk at many grocery and natural food stores. Heat over medium-high heat, stirring occasionally. When it starts to boil, reduce heat to low and continue to stir occasionally until most liquid is absorbed, from 10 to 30 minutes depending on the amount made. Cool completely and add one teaspoon to one tablespoon of cod liver oil (depending on amount made), stirring thoroughly. If the gruel is difficult to stir once cooled, add a little water until it is of a cooked oatmeal consistency. Because this gruel is not nutritionally balanced, it should be used only to nurse ill chicks to health until they can eat dry food on their own.

Poultry feed should be protected from the elements and from pests such as rodents and beetles. Depending on the amount obtained, feed may be stored in sturdy containers ranging from plastic breakfast cereal storage canisters to plastic or metal trash cans. Lids should be tight fitting. In warm, humid climates, mold may be a problem, particularly when it cools at night and moisture condenses within the container. To prevent mold growth, feed should preferably be stored indoors or other areas in which there is not a wide variation in temperature. Moldy feed should *never* be fed to any animals because of its potential toxicity. Mold in feed may be identified by its appearance (green, black, or rusty-colored "fuzz") or by its musty odor. This also applies to the unfortunate practice of well-meaning people feeding moldy bread to pond ducks and their chicks.

Water is the most important nutrient. Ensure that fresh, clean water is available at all times and is changed daily or whenever it is soiled with feces, litter, or feed. When water is changed, the waterer should be scrubbed out using a sponge or brush, because algae and bacteria may accumulate quickly. Chicks will begin scratching behavior at 7–10 days of age. At this time, water availability should be verified several times per day because of chicks' propensity to kick feed and litter into their water.

A few types of waterers are available. Plastic founts are readily available at feed stores and are easy to use. They usually have an opaque white reservoir and red base (red attracts chicks' attention). They are easily disassembled for filling and cleaning, and the threaded screw-on type is most secure. For a small number of chicks, a quart fount waterer is preferable to a gallon size fount as the lip is shallower and narrower, discouraging drowning. To further discourage chicks from falling into water, clean aquarium gravel or marbles may be placed so that water depth is 1/8–1/4 in. (3–6 mm).

## Expected Weight Gain

Because poultry come in many sizes, there is great variation in normal expected weight gain. A good indicator of appropriate growth and development for any poultry species is to simply feel the keel bone (sternum) and the musculature on either side. Ideally, the tip of the keel should be surrounded by full, round pectoralis muscles. A sharp keel with sunken pectoralis muscles indicates that a bird is very thin; nutritional and gastrointestinal parasitic causes should be investigated.

## Housing

Preferably, brood chicks indoors until they are 4–5 weeks old or until the weather outside is relatively warm, at least 70 °F (21 °C). Brooding inside allows close observation and protection from predators and the elements should the heat lamp fail.

When brooding chicks, the most convenient housing is a plastic Tupperware box or sturdy cardboard box with high sides of at least 24 in. (60 cm) (Figure 7.3). For chickens, turkeys, ducks, and geese, this height should prevent chicks from jumping out. For game birds, placing a piece of cut wire mesh over the box should prevent chicks from jumping out (the wire can easily be cut to accommodate the heating lamp).

Space requirements vary depending on species and age of the chicks. These requirements are particularly important to consider when raising game birds, because they are easily stressed and are prone to cannibalism when too closely confined.

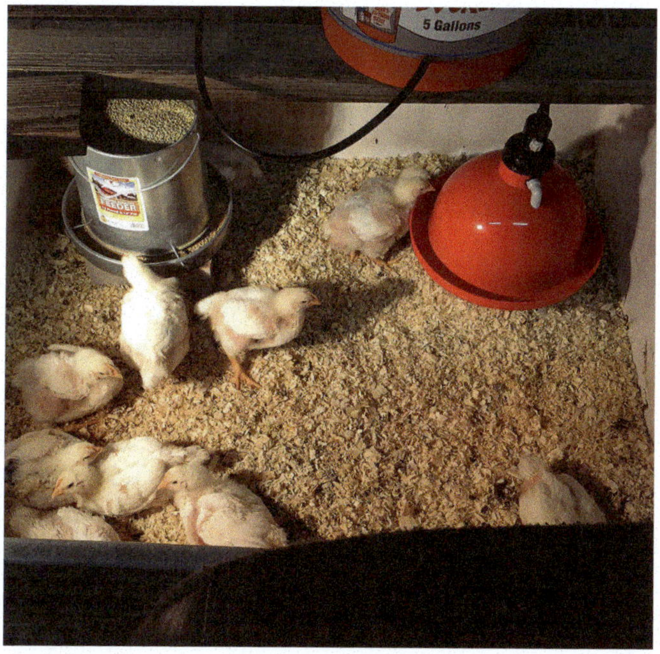


**Figure 7.3** Simple brooder setup, with heat lamp at one end, ample feed for all chicks, and a waterer with an additional water reservoir above the brooder. Some species of chicks can jump quite high, so ceilings on brooders should secure birds from escape (not shown). *Source:* photo courtesy of Dan Famini.

Appropriate litter material can include wood shavings or rice hulls. Avoid sand or sawdust because chicks may ingest these materials, causing crop impaction. Also, newspaper or other slick surfaces should never be used because young chicks' legs easily slide out underneath them. Because they are weak and their bones and joints are still very malleable, chicks may become permanently deformed if their legs are splayed out for extended periods of time. Deformed chicks may never walk or may walk abnormally, causing unnecessary joint problems throughout life.

A heat source may be set up as described above in the "Initial Care and Stabilization" section. Caution must be used because there is a fire hazard with this setup due to the intense heat production from the 24-hour light. Make sure the lamp is sturdily affixed and that the lamp edges are at least 4 in. away from any flammable materials. Other suitable brooder options can be found in chapters about the wild counterparts of these species (see Chapters 5, 6, and 8). As mentioned previously, very young chicks should be observed for behavior and comfort under heat lamps before leaving them unsupervised. Regardless of species, decreasing temperature by 5 °F (2.8 °C) each week results in comfortable chicks as the temperature drops to match the rate of feather growth.

## Biosecurity

Losses from disease can be reduced substantially by adhering to biosecurity practices. The biggest single source of disease is other birds, both from the same species and from different species. The second biggest offender is human traffic. No person or animal should be allowed to visit the flock if they have been around other birds. A general guideline for commercial poultry employees is a down-time of 48–72 hours after contacting other poultry. Practicing common sense, such as having farm-specific clothing (coveralls, boots) and not entering your flock after visiting a fair or other flocks, goes a long way. Frequent transgressors are domestic animals (dogs and cats) and rodents. These animals can mechanically transmit disease or be biological vectors. Attractants for animals need to be removed; feed must be kept in rodent-proof containers and spilled feed rapidly cleaned up. Carcasses should be removed immediately and disposed of appropriately; observe local environmental regulations. If burial is chosen, carcasses can be covered with lime in order to reduce the likelihood of being dug up by animals. Good rodenticide and insecticide programs are essential. Waterers and feeders must be cleaned and disinfected at least every 2–3 days and houses cleaned when litter becomes moist. Store feed in containers that are not sun exposed, which can cause condensation when the containers cool at night and subsequent mold growth. Use feed rapidly and store no more than a 1-week supply. Foot pans filled with sanitation products such as a dilute iodine solution can reduce the risk of carrying in organisms on boots; when the iodinated water becomes clear, it needs to be replaced. Alternatively, have farm-specific boots for taking care of your birds or use disposable booties for guests, especially in cold weather when the water pans are frozen. All equipment must be thoroughly cleaned and disinfected before use. Organic matter left on equipment can render even the best disinfectant useless. Again, different bird species should not be mixed and in best conditions, ages should not be mixed as well. In facilities with multiple ages in one site, the general rule is prioritizing young birds that are more susceptible to health challenges vs old birds (i.e. visit from young to old).

All birds leaving the premises and encountering other birds (i.e. shows) should be quarantined for 4–6 weeks in a separate area. Be sure to not give medicated feed during quarantine. Any equipment used at shows – such as cages, feeders, waterers, and egg flats – needs to be disinfected before storage or reuse. If housing birds being quarantined for any reason or that are ill, be sure to work with these birds last to avoid exposing healthy birds to potential disease organisms.

Additionally, in the U.S., many Cooperative Extension offices have pamphlets on specific poultry husbandry and best management practice topics. These pamphlets are written by poultry scientists and veterinarians and are the most accurate and up-to-date sources of information, particularly regarding region-specific diseases and husbandry matters. Materials from Cooperative Extension are usually free and scientifically sound.

## Behavioral Training for Pet Birds

Many species of poultry make excellent, personable pets. Ducks and chickens in particular are often kept as pets. In order to raise a bird so that it is well socialized to humans, be sure to handle it frequently while it is growing up, as you would any pet. Young chicks that are exposed to close human contact and activity become very accustomed to people and often seek their company. Certain breeds lend themselves better to being pets; heavier breeds such as Plymouth Rocks and Cochins are generally calmer than high-strung Mediterranean breeds such as Leghorns. See American Poultry Association (2015) for more examples of "friendlier" breeds.

## Acknowledgments

The authors would like to thank Dr. Pat Wakenell for her contributions to the first edition of this chapter, much of which remains here.

## Sources for Products Mentioned

Poultry diets: Purina Mills, St. Louis, MO, https://www.purinamills.com/products.

## References

American Poultry Association (2015). *The American Standard of Perfection*, 406 pp. Mendon, MA: American Poultry Association, Inc.

American Veterinary Medical Association. (2018). Veterinary Feed Directive (VFD) Basics. https://www.avma.org/KB/Resources/Pages/VFD123.aspx (accessed 6 March 2018).

Boulianne, M. (ed.) (2013). *Avian Disease Manual*, 7e, 300 pp. Kennett Square, PA: American Association of Avian Pathologists.

Buckland, R. and Guy, G. (eds.) (2002). *Goose Production. FAO Animal Production and Health Paper 154*. Rome, Italy: Food and Agriculture Organization of the United Nations http://www.fao.org/docrep/005/Y4359E/y4359e03.htm.

Hayes, L.B. (1995). *Upland Game Birds: Their Breeding and Care*, 350 pp. Valley Center, California, self-published.

Holderread, D. (2011). *Storey's Guide to Raising Ducks*, 336 pp. Pownal, VT: Storey Publishing.

Mississippi State University Extension. (2018). Feeds and nutrition. http://extension.msstate.edu/agriculture/livestock/poultry/feeds-and-nutrition (accessed 16 August 2018).

Office International des Epizooties (OIE)/World Organization for Animal Health (2018). *OIE-Listed Diseases, Infections and Infestations in Force in 2018*. Paris, France: OIE http://www.oie.int/animal-health-in-the-world/oie-listed-diseases-2018.

Quarles, E.A. (1916). *American Pheasant Breeding and Care.* Wilmington, DE: Hercules Powder Company.

Richardson, E. (1897). The Turkey: its natural history and origin of name. In: *Turkeys and How to Grow Them* (ed. H. Myrick), 1–4. New York: Orange Judd Company.

Saif, Y.M. (ed.) (2003). *Diseases of Poultry*, 11e, 1231 pp. Ames, IA: Iowa State Press.

Smith, H.E. (1976). *Modern Poultry Development: A History of Domestic Poultry Keeping*, 215 pp. Hampshire, England: Spur Publications Company.

Townsend, L. (2018). Insecticide control on poultry. University of Kentucky Extension publication ENT-28. University of Kentucky, Lexington, KY. http://pest.ca.uky.edu/EXT/Recs/ENT28-Poultry.pdf (accessed 6 March 2018).

U.S. Centers for Disease Control and Prevention. (2018). Keeping backyard chickens and other poultry. (accessed 8 April 2018).

## Further Reading

Smith, T.W. (2016). Feeding quail. Mississippi State University Extension publication 2383. http://extension.msstate.edu/sites/default/files/publications/publications/P2383_web.pdf.

# 8

# Wild Turkeys, Quail, Grouse, and Pheasants

*Marjorie Cahak Gibson*

## Natural History

Worldwide, there are 300 species in five families considered to be in the order Galliformes (Gill and Donsker 2019). In North America, these include grouse, pheasants, turkeys, quail, and curassows. These terrestrial birds have added much to human history and continue to play a huge role in human life through art, literature, and, notably, economics. They are considered by many to be the single most important source of protein in the world today.

These species are terrestrial, meaning living and foraging on the ground, although they do roost in trees. Although equipped with strong wings, they are not known for their flight ability due to the round, short structure of the wing. Flight is in short, powerful bursts. These birds have chicken-like feet, which are feathered in some species and are equipped with hard nails for scratching the ground to expose food. They do not swim. The main method of escaping from predators is by running or taking evasive action. If forced to defend themselves, they use their strong legs, feet, nails, and occasionally spurs to thwart attackers. The wings can be used aggressively as clubs to beat enemies, or in some cases rehabilitators or rescuers.

Most species have cryptic coloration, feathers that match their environment. Some, like ptarmigans, molt and change color seasonally. This cryptic form of camouflage allows individuals to blend into the habitat, remaining inconspicuous to people and predators.

Wild Galliformes most likely to be encountered in wildlife rehabilitation facilities include pheasants, quail, grouse, partridges, ptarmigans, prairie chickens, turkeys, peafowl, and jungle fowl. Due to widespread domestication and hybridization of several species, caregivers should make every effort to correctly identify the patient, as it may be a domestic fowl, an escaped exotic species, a native species, or even a threatened or endangered species. In some regions, populations of native species such as quail and Prairie Chickens have declined dramatically, causing the birds to be listed as threatened or endangered. Nonindigenous species have been introduced regionally in North American by sportsmen and organizations in attempts to establish new hunting opportunities. Some introduced species, such as the Ring-necked Pheasant, have become so common in regions of the U.S., that they are considered native by some. See Chapter 7 for information on hand-rearing chickens and other domestic Galliformes.

*Hand-Rearing Birds*, Second Edition. Edited by Rebecca S. Duerr and Laurie J. Gage.

Game birds hunted for sport and food are frequently raised commercially. Game birds are also known for their beauty and are kept in zoos and private aviaries as ornamental birds. The most common species for commercial game farm production are pheasant and quail. These species adapt easily and do well with a commercial game bird diet. Although many species are common and easy to raise, some in this order are among the most difficult birds to raise and maintain in captivity. Many are secretive in nature, fastidious, and difficult to study in the wild, so little is known about their life history and diet. Unfortunately, a native bird taken into wildlife rehabilitation is frequently one of the most challenging species to treat. Information on domestic fowl diseases and housing techniques may be helpful, but many aspects of rearing wild species differ, sometimes in dramatic ways.

## Identification Is a Must

Among the vast numbers of wild species within this order, many are specialists in terms of diet (Elphick et al. 2001) and disease sensitivity (Altman et al. 1997). Correct identification is therefore extremely important when a young Galliformes is admitted into care. Some field guides have descriptions of the young as well as habiat, range, nest, and eggs. One excellent resource is *A Guide to the Nests, Eggs and Nestlings of North American Birds* (Baicich and Harrison 2005).

Although obtaining a history is important with any patient, the specific habitat of grouse and other sensitive species makes the information of where the chick was found invaluable in identifying a wild patient and may directly affect the successful rehabilitation of the individual bird.

It may be determined that a patient is an exotic species. It may have escaped from a local game farm or zoo. If that is the case, the bird can simply be returned to the owner. Or, the new patient may be a domestic chicken. Some breeds of chickens when hatched are striped and resemble wild grouse, pheasant, or quail. Because of the commercial nature of many Galliformes, private ownership may be a factor. Depending on your city, state, or provincial laws, this may have legal ramifications, and attempts to find the owner should be made.

Many Galliformes are legally hunted. It is beneficial to know hunting laws and have information available regarding legal hunting seasons. Some states or provinces may discourage rehabilitation of game birds. Be sure to check permits to clarify this status before a game bird is admitted as a patient.

## Highly Precocial Chicks

Galliformes chicks are highly precocial at hatch. Nests with rare exceptions are located on the ground, because these are terrestrial birds and the young leave the nest soon after hatching. At hatch, the primaries of many species are already formed (Ritchie et al. 1994; Sibley 2000). Chicks are downy, striped, or mottled in color and blend in with their surroundings. Although able to forage soon after hatch, chicks rely on adults to locate food (Williams 1991). Most chicks feed themselves; however, some species, including turkeys, kill insects first before placing food directly into the mouth of their young (Skutch 1976). Chicks are sensitive to cold and require brooding by the adult until well-weathered. Chicks are capable of limited flight within 5–10 days. Many species have large families numbering up to 25 chicks per nest. The adult communicates with chicks before hatch and shortly after, cementing parental imprinting and voice recognition. Many species not only identify their mother's voice, but that of each sibling as an individual as well (Skutch 1976; Williams 1991; Gibson 1998). For this reason, fostering can be difficult.

### Galliformes Glossary

- *Beard:* Stiff feathers on the chest of a tom turkey but occasionally a female as well.
- *Caruncles:* Fleshy bumps on the neck of a turkey that turn red with excitement. Both males and females have caruncles.
- *Hen:* Female turkey (Figure 8.1) and other game birds.
- *Jake:* Young male wild turkeys under 1 year of age.
- *Jenny:* Young female wild turkey under 1 year of age.
- *Lek:* Area where birds gather for courtship displays to attract mates. Game birds including grouse use leks.
- *Poult:* Young wild turkey under 6 months of age.
- *Roost*: Congregation or gathering of turkeys in trees, usually for safely and nighttime protection.
- *Snood:* Fleshy bump on the face of a turkey above the beak, which inflates by becoming engorged with fluid. Both males and females have a snood.
- *Spurs*: Are used in defense. Made from keratin and situated on the leg of many Galliformes.
- *Strut*: Tom turkeys' flagrant courtship ritual to attract hens.
- *Tom*: Adult male turkey.

## Criteria for Intervention

Regulating agencies may have rules discouraging the rehabilitation of game birds or hatching eggs of disturbed nests. Check with wildlife officials in the area to clarify responses to the public.

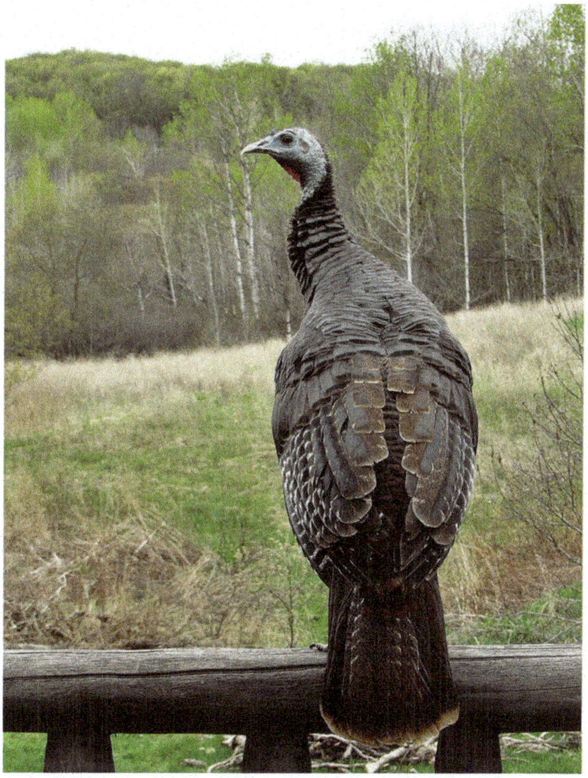

Figure 8.1 Wild turkey hens are smaller than males. They have the same features on their head and neck as males, however those features – the snood, caruncles, and dewlap – are less pronounced on hens than on males.

## Eggs

Youngsters may be kidnapped by well-intentioned people or energetic children. Ground nests are sometimes located by buildings or agricultural projects. Often, eggs from these will be collected before the finder calls a wildlife center for advice. Wildlife center personnel may be asked to come and remove eggs, so a building project can advance on time. Nest disturbance is illegal for native species. Unless otherwise stated, federal permits for rehabilitation are issued for native birds that are injured or orphaned, but not for eggs not yet hatched. Therefore, hatching eggs that are collected by the public is not covered under wildlife rehabilitation permits and not something that can be offered to the public. It is important to be well-versed in federal and state migratory bird laws before responding to such calls. Offer natural history information to the caller. The fact that the eggs hatch within 3 weeks of being laid and the young leave the nest soon thereafter can be a comfort to those waiting to begin a building project in the same area where a nest has been discovered.

## Chicks or Young Birds

Young gallinaceous chicks are admitted to wildlife centers due to the death of a parent on the road or injuries from domestic dogs or cats. Chicks hatched in cold or inclement weather may be weak and unable to keep up with a highly mobile family. The wildlife rehabilitator plays an important role keeping wild youngsters with their natural parents through dissemination of information to the public. Most Galliformes hatch between 18 and 26 days. Once hatched, they can leave the nest area within hours but need brooding from the adult to survive.

If a caller has questions about a hatchling that is not yet captive, urge the caller not to touch the chick unless it is in immediate danger. Reassure the caller that the adult is likely close by and will respond to the voice of her chick once human disturbance abates.

If the caller has the chick in captivity but is still in the area where it was found, urge the caller to release it and leave the immediate area, giving the adult bird an opportunity to reunite with the chick. Observation from a distance is suggested for a period of 1 hour.

If the chick is injured, or other reasons exist whereby reuniting with the adult is not an option, underscore the need to keep the chick warm and confined. Galliformes brood their chicks, keeping them close to their bodies. Situations that mimic brooding, such as wrapping a towel around the chick in a warmed environment, will lower stress and give the best chance for survival.

## Adults

Adult Galliformes are most frequently injured when hit by cars, shot, or caught in a barbed-wire fence (Erickson 2006). Diseases such as avian pox and lymphoproliferative disease (LPDV), a type-C retrovirus, have been known to affect wild turkeys and cases are reported to be on the increase. See Chapter 7 for more information on diseases of concern. Instruct the caller to gently remove the injured bird from the area, place it in a cardboard box with towel or leaf material on the bottom, and transport it as soon as possible to a wildlife rehabilitation facility. Wild adult Galliformes are highly stressed in captive situations. Callers should be cautioned against transporting wild Galliformes in wire caging as injuries due to caging are highly likely.

### Transportation to Wildlife Facility

Transport to a wildlife center should occur as soon as possible, preferably immediately. A transport box no more than twice the size of the bird will lower stress and keep the youngster secure. A cardboard box with air holes works well. A towel or tee-shirt on the bottom of the box will prevent chicks from sliding and possible leg splaying. Do not transport with a filled water bowl, as spilled water will wet the chick and cause hypothermia. Provide supplemental heat during transport. Heating pads, warmed rice bags, a hot water bottle, or an equivalent may be used when padded with towels, so the chick is not in direct contact with the heat source. A stuffed animal or feather duster may comfort the youngster during transport.

## Initial Care and Stabilization

Chicks of these species are often tiny at hatch, sometimes weighing 1 g or less (Figure 8.2). They are very susceptible to stress and cold. The condition of a hypothermic patient is always critical. It is vital to bring the temperature up quickly or death will result. Before a physical can be done, the bird must have a normal core body temperature. Hypothermic birds should not be given food or water orally. The digestive system does not function until the core body temperature is restored. To warm a chilled bird, a heating pad set on a low setting can be used or a heated box or incubator set at 97–99 °F (36.1–37.2 °C) (Anderson Brown and Robins 2002). Nonresponsive patients should never be left on the heat without constant monitoring because heating pads and lamps can overheat debilitated patients that are unable to move away from the heat. Death can result. Massage the patient with a warmed towel to stimulate response and increase circulation.

Physical examination of chicks should be brief to avoid stress. Much of the exam can be done by observation in the brooder. Check for an egg tooth on the patient to determine whether the patient is a hatchling. The egg tooth assists hatching and remains visible only a few days. It is important to remember that many species hatch with primary feathers, and thus may be assumed to be older. Check the vent to make sure it is clean and not pasted. Soft feces can dry and build up on down

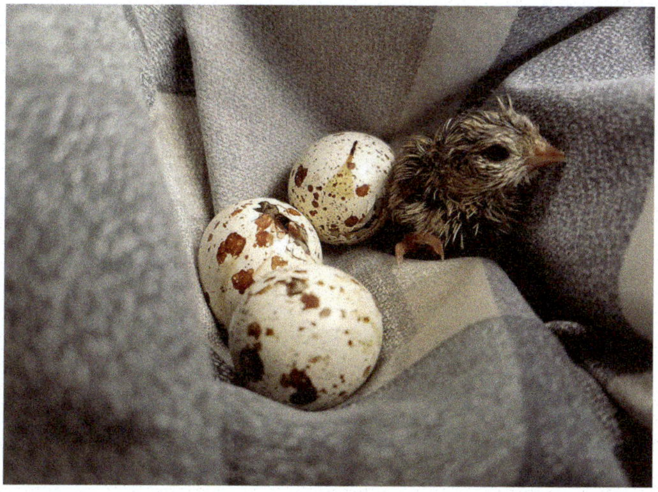

Figure 8.2 Hatching California Quail eggs – the freshly hatched chick is still wet but looks alert, other chicks are just pipping. *Source:* photo courtesy of International Bird Rescue.

near the vent and stop the chick defecating. If the vent is not clean, wash the area with warm water until all material is removed.

Offer a drop of warmed water or electrolyte fluid (Pedialyte®, 0.9% sodium chloride, or lactated Ringer's solution) off the tip of a finger after the chick has opened its eyes and has a swallowing reflex. Allow the chick to drink in this manner. Once the chick is strong enough to stand, add a light mixture of protein to the fluid and continue to offer drops from a fingertip (see the recipe in Chapter 23 in the section titled "Emaciation Diet for Crane Colts"). Because many of these species are so tiny, syringe- or pipette-feeding can overwhelm their ability to swallow and they may drown. Continue feeding the light mixture until the chick defecates. Tube-feeding should be initiated in small amounts (0.05 ml for quail). Initial tube-feedings are meant to stimulate peristalsis rather than to fill the crop.

## Common Medical Problems and Solutions

Wild Galliformes chicks, unlike their domestic counterparts, are very easily stressed birds. Those raised in captivity are more susceptible to disease and parasites: the stress of captivity likely plays a role. When raised with the parent in a natural habitat, they are more likely to die from predation than disease (Bump et al. 1947; Woodward 1993). Although not clearly understood, wild-raised chicks and adults benefit from the large variety of natural insects and foliage available, perhaps by boosting their immune systems and providing natural remedies. Some naturally ingested plants have secondary compounds and chemicals that are toxic, and yet are easily digested and tolerated by species such as grouse (Elphick et al. 2001). For this reason, using litter from a forest floor or other habitat native to the patient may improve success rates. The treatment of parasites and disease in domestic Galliformes is covered in Chapter 7.

Preventing disease is much better than treating after it occurs. Due to the small size and sensitivity to stress of Galliformes chicks, diagnosis through blood work is not practical, although older birds may have blood collected from the cutaneous ulnar vein when needed. For the same reason, treatment is frequently not successful once the process has begun. The rehabilitator's focus should therefore be on prevention and early detection.

Bacterial diseases such as salmonellosis or colibacillosis (due to *Escherichia coli* infection) may develop through a contaminated water or food source. Water should be changed several times a day for young patients, and food should not be allowed to sour or become contaminated by feces. Observe the birds' droppings and respond to changes such as diarrhea quickly. Keep the vent clean and be alert for pasting that can occur with digestive problems. A bird with a pasted vent cannot defecate adequately and may die.

A single chick of any wild Galliformes species reared alone is unlikely to survive, and most certainly will not be normally imprinted, despite the best efforts of the rehabilitator. Networking with other rehabilitators is important as Galliformes chicks imprint readily, often within a day or two, when raised in captivity without conspecifics. Imprinted or hand-reared young will rarely survive in the wild. Those that do survive often become aggressive to humans once they reach sexual maturity. Aggressive behavior can cause serious injury to humans and damages the reputation of the species with the public. The reasons for this have been discussed earlier in this chapter. The chances of survival increase dramatically when another chick of similar size is introduced. Ideally, the species should be the same, but since in the world of wildlife rehabilitation that is not always possible, a similar species may be used as a companion. The conundrum is that many wild species are sensitive to diseases carried naturally by another, which may not manifest itself as clinical disease in the second. This sensitivity continues through adulthood, and as a rule birds should never be raised in mixed flocks or crowded conditions.

In the wild, even though species may share a common habitat, they usually do not have enough close contact to allow disease transference. In many species, very little is known about disease transference and textbooks on avian medicine freely discuss this (Altman et al. 1997), though new information is continually being discovered. Check with an avian veterinarian experienced in game birds for specifics of diseases, species incompatibility, and drug sensitivities. Use antibiotics sparingly in wild Galliformes as they may suppress the birds' immune systems. Antiprotozoals may be necessary in some species, particularly turkeys, and are often included in commercial turkey diets.

Commercial feeds, which are developed specifically for certain species, may be toxic to other Galliformes. For instance, feed developed for chickens may be toxic to pheasants and partridge due to the addition of halofuginone. Commercial turkey food containing antiprotozoals can inhibit cecal flora and cause death in grouse and other sensitive species (Altman et al. 1997). For this reason, natural food is best for the wild Galliformes.

## Mud-balling

Mud-balling may occur with ground-dwelling birds, both in the wild and in captive care (Figure 8.3). The problem begins when wet conditions turn the soil sticky, allowing it to adhere to the feet of young birds (Welty 1982). Multiple layers build up around the feet until they are encased around a ball – thus the term *mud-balling*. This may cause death from exhaustion as the bird struggles to free itself, or is unable to walk, eat, or maintain other normal behaviors. In captivity, this process can occur in brooders with very young chicks, or in outdoor facilities. Wet feces mixed with any soft substrate, such as wood shavings, can also cause balling. Foot deformities can result from even minor cases if not corrected quickly. The hardened material acts as a cast, retarding growth in

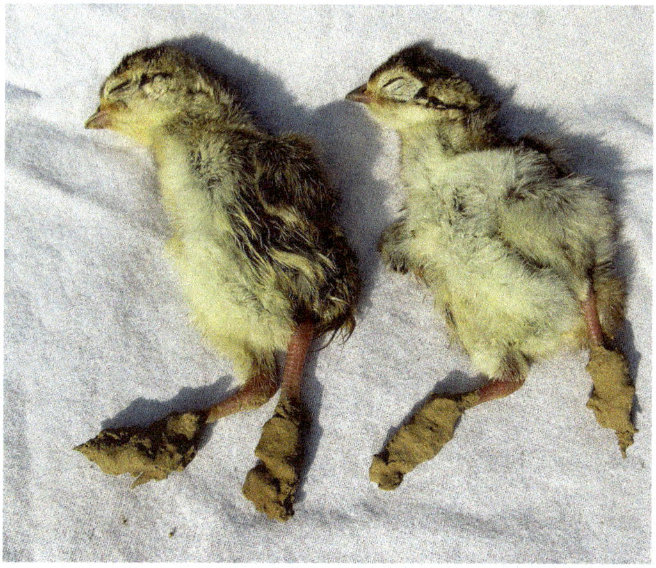

Figure 8.3 Mud-balling causes foot deformity and death in young Galliformes if not noticed early. It occurs in wet conditions allowing mud and feces to collect on the feet of a chick.

rapidly growing young. Treatment consists of soaking the feet in warm water to soften the material. Be careful pulling it off because fractures may occur, or the skin may be torn.

### Splayed Legs

Splayed legs can happen when a young bird slips on unstable substrate, stretching ligaments beyond their normal range. If caught early, it can be corrected using Vetrap (3M) or similar material to "soft-splint" the legs in a natural position. The feet should be separated by normal standing or walking distance. The bird should be able to walk and maintain normal behavior with the splint on its legs. Standing and walking while splinted is important to maintain muscle tone and development. Depending on the severity, the legs should remain splinted for a few days to a week. Adjust the splint daily on newly hatched birds to accommodate their rapid growth (Altman et al. 1997).

### Cannibalism

Cannibalism may occur in all Galliformes when kept in captivity. Many theories exist on the causes of this, from nutritional deficiencies, to overcrowding, to poor sanitation (Woodward 1993). It is likely that multiple factors play a part in the phenomenon. Providing adequate space and good food in plentiful amounts is a proper place to start for prevention of this destructive behavior. Stress from human or domestic animals should be kept to a minimum.

While in brooders, chicks will often pick at the toes or legs of others. Check the victim for bleeding or physical abnormality, such as crooked toes, that could attract attention. Feces or bedding adhered to the vent or feet may resemble bits of food and cause picking by other chicks. All areas that are open sores should be treated with antibiotic ointment. Open wounds must be healed before reintroducing birds that have been cannibalized by cagemates.

Removing an aggressive bird for even a short time seems to break the cycle of picking, and it may be enough to solve the problem. Introducing fresh greens with roots and soil still attached may also distract the birds and resolve picking.

Birds in outdoor facilities pick feathers of others or themselves when under either physiological or environmental stress. Check all factors, including making sure there is adequate high-quality food available, no predator harassment, and a stress-free environment. Domestic animals, including dogs that live on the property, can be responsible for stress. The birds see domestic pets as predators and will react as such. Release may be the best option if you are unable to locate the stressor.

## Diet

Wild Galliformes have very specific food needs. Although some can survive on prepared commercial diets, many cannot. Unfortunately, there is no hard and fast rule to indicate which will be relatively hardy patients and which are delicate beyond expectation for even the most experienced rehabilitator.

As a generalization, species that have been raised commercially, such as pheasants and quail, are hardy and have a high success rate when raised in captivity. By contrast, wild turkeys and grouse are delicate in captive care. Wild turkeys differ in many ways from domestic varieties, including the fact that they have 35% more brain capacity than domestics.

There is often wide variation in food habits for grouse species. Complicating things, these diets change with the season. Considering there are 16 grouse species in the northern hemisphere alone, it is virtually impossible to give successful diets for each within this chapter. The best approach is for the rehabilitator to become familiar with the species found in each region and their diets. This is one reason a history and location where the bird was found is more important for Galliformes than for most patients. Young patients of these sensitive species will require extra effort to successfully raise to release.

Getting youngsters to eat can be challenging. The first food of grouse chicks is ants or other tiny insects. The rapid movement of an insect attracts chicks, and they are usually stimulated to begin eating. A large-sized dog food bowl will work as a miniature habitat for a small shovel of active ants. Ants can overwhelm youngsters and bite them, so be sure to monitor them well.

Wild grasses or weeds pulled from the ground with some soil left on the root (Hayes 1992) are very interesting to chicks. Most instinctively begin scratching the roots, eating as they do. Be sure the grass is safe, nontoxic, and has not been sprayed with pesticide. The act of eating will encourage chicks to eat other food offered. Kitten or puppy pellets (Hill's Science Diet), soaked overnight in the refrigerator with an equal amount of water, should be offered in a shallow dish. Before serving, add tiny mealworms, bloodworms, waxworms, tubifex worms, or naturally occurring insects from the region. Some commercial game farm growers suggest crumbling a red dog treat and using it to top food. The red color is said to attract the attention of the chicks (Woodward 1993).

If a young patient still refuses to eat despite the above measures, try sprinkling dry baby cereal or crumbled dried insects on the chicks' backs. During the natural preening behavior, they will invariably get some food in their mouths, recognize it as food, and begin eating. If all else fails, use a drop-by-drop method with the emaciation diet described earlier in this chapter. Tube-feeding can be used but is stressful to these delicate species.

Water (Hayes 1992) should be provided in shallow nonslip saucer-like dishes lined with pea gravel or coarse sand substrate. This prevents the chick from slipping and splaying its legs. Some sand may also be eaten for grit to aid digestion. Chicks should be prevented from ingesting large amounts of sand as impacted crops can result. Commercial chick water founts are available at most farm supply stores and work well. Colorful marbles put in the drinking water prevent tiny game birds from drowning while attracting interest to the water supply (Hayes 1992; Woodward 1993; Ritchie et al. 1994). As chicks get older, water and food can be supplied in plant saucers. A good product for use with wild patients will be sturdy, be made of nonslip and nontoxic materials, and be easily cleaned.

Once the youngsters begin to eat, continue providing soaked kitten or puppy pellets topped with small mealworms, tubifex worms, bloodworms, and other insects as a staple diet during the first month of life. The saturated pellets must be changed several times per day to prevent souring. Add grasshoppers, crickets, and finally grain as the chicks grow and show interest in new foods. Wild natural greens cut into tiny bite-size pieces are a good addition to the diet. Romaine lettuce can also be used. Cutting the greens into small bits will help prevent large pieces from impacting in their crops – adults perform this service for chicks in the wild.

## Housing

### Brooders

Commercial brooders used for chicken or game farms also work well for wild chicks. If the brooder has been used in the past for domestic species, clean and sterilize it well. Many wild species are highly susceptible to diseases found in domestic chickens and turkey poults. Commercial brooders are designed to brood many chicks at a time and may not be the best choice if you have only a few to rear.

If only a few chicks are in care, a smaller setup may be more practical. A clean cardboard box, 16 × 20 × 20 in. (40 × 50 × 50 cm), or plastic storage container is a good option. A clip-on reflector heat lamp, found in the hardware section of many stores, should be firmly secured on one side of the box. A 40–60-W incandescence bulb is usually adequate to provide a temperature of 95–99 °F (35–37.2 °C). Check the temperature under the heat lamp and move the lamp either up or down to reach the correct temperature.

Single chicks rarely survive. For that reason, it may be helpful during the first few days of confinement to house the chick with a day-old bantam chick or older chicks to lower stress and encourage eating. However, be aware of the possibility of bacterial, viral, or other infectious diseases that can be transferred in these cases. It is recommended that any domestic fowl be from a closed flock or vaccinated for common diseases before they come into contact even briefly with a wild individual.

Mixed-age housing has advantages and disadvantages that must be weighed. Older chicks may suffocate, injure, or not allow newly hatched young to feed. Use care if this is the only option for housing. Older chicks that have begun to eat on their own may encourage and teach younger ones how to eat and drink. Observe the birds carefully for any aggression and separate immediately if it occurs. Networking with other rehabilitators is suggested and very helpful with housing multiple species or varied ages.

A windup alarm clock (alarm disabled), a "womb" or white noise sound product, or mirror with a clean feather duster or cotton mop head (Ritchie et al. 1994) may be helpful to provide the youngster with a substitute parent figure. If using a feather duster, make certain no chemicals or preservatives have been used. Toxic fumes may result when chemically-treated feathers become wet. Synthetic feathers may be the safest for this use. White muslin fabric placed on top of the substrate during the first week of life allows the caregiver to observe the feces and be alert to digestive problems or whether the young birds are eating. The fabric also helps prevent chicks from developing an impacted crop by ingesting large amounts of plant material or sand. Other substrates that work well for the brooder can be coarse sand, pea gravel, clean soil, or natural dry leaf litter. A firm substrate will prevent young birds' legs from slipping and splaying out. Fine sand can cause eye problems in young chicks. Wood shavings (not cedar), or natural leaf litter from the chick's natural habitat combined with pea gravel can be used as substrate as the chicks mature.

No matter what substrate is used, it must be kept clean and dry to prevent bacterial growth and disease. Some people suggest wooden boxes; although they work well, they retain moisture and are more difficult to sanitize after use (Woodward 1993).

The behavior of the chicks will be the guide as to whether the temperature is too warm or cold. Chicks that are too cold will huddle under the heat lamp and hesitate to come out to eat or drink. If they are too hot, they will droop their wings and stand away from the lamp. A heat lamp on one side of the box enables them to choose to stay close or move away from the heat if needed.

As chicks develop and become more active, they will require larger and taller brooder boxes and lower temperatures. Lower the temperature in 5 °F (2.8 °C) increments weekly, or more quickly if chicks display signs of being too hot. Many Galliformes chicks can fly within a few days to a week of hatch. For that reason, a top for the brooder box is essential to keep the chicks inside. Chicks will need to remain under a brooder for 5–6 weeks. When they are fully feathered, they may be moved to an outdoor area. A supplemental heat source and protected indoor area must remain available in cooler climates until the birds have acclimated completely.

## Outdoor Facilities

Galliformes are often prey for other animals and therefore have a strong stress reaction to the sight and sound of predators. Seeking cover and hiding is their reaction to fear. Birds do not eat or drink well when forced to "hide" from predators, even as their metabolism and need for calories increases with the added stress.

Pens made to raptor specifications work well, offering the birds access to natural sun and rain and protection from predators (Gibson 1996). A visual barrier installed at least 3 ft. high around the perimeter of the enclosure will lower stress in captive birds by providing privacy. Galliformes destined to be released to the wild do best in enclosures planted with native plants, berries, apple trees, and other nontoxic plants to provide cover. The author uses dwarf variety fruit trees to prevent damage to the netting covering of the pen. A shelter, such as a lean-to or building, should also be provided for severe weather and shade protection if needed.

The size of the enclosure will depend on the species of the bird in care. Natural soil is the best substrate for these species. The enclosure should be freshly tilled at least once per season, or before young Galliformes are introduced, to prevent infection with parasites and disease left by previous inhabitants that may be harbored in the soil. If the substrate of the enclosure is pea gravel or other material it should be sanitized. Cover the substrate with several inches of natural litter (leaves, decaying bark, and soil) from a forest floor in the region. Leaf litter is a natural habitat and will give young birds an opportunity to exercise normal foraging behaviors. Sand in one area of the pen is beneficial. Galliformes use sand or light soil as a grooming aid and as grit for digestion.

The size of the pre-release enclosure will depend on the species of bird in care. The enclosure size of 30×30×10 ft. (9×9×3 m) will accommodate 5–10 young grouse until release. Crowding increases stress and opportunities for disease. Natural logs, some hollow to provide shelter, are useful and will help birds become accustomed to "wild habitat" prior to release.

It is natural for Galliformes to live with a parent, usually the hen, until they are fully feathered – sometimes through the fall of their first year (Figure 8.4). Some adults, such as males and juveniles approaching adult status, are often not compatible. Many species are territorial and will be aggressive to others in the group. Watch for signs of this behavior and separate those individuals

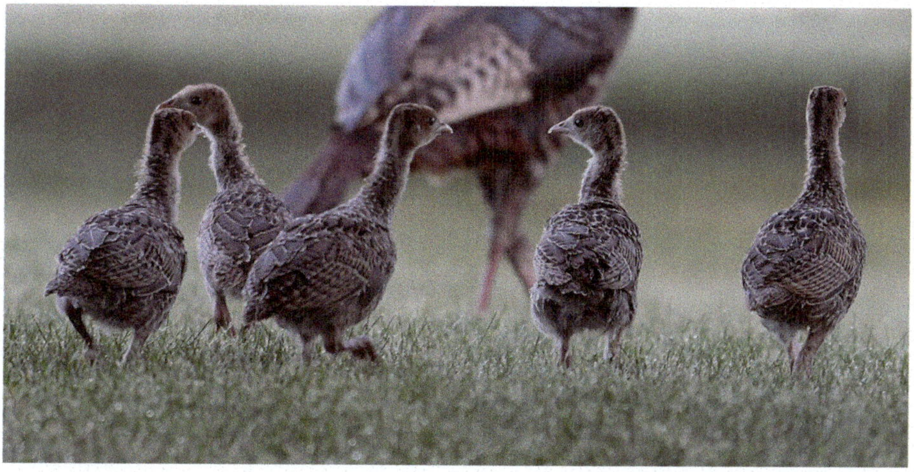

Figure 8.4 Young wild turkeys with an adult. *Source:* photo courtesy of Al Scherwinski.

that cause injury. Injured birds that are bleeding also must be removed for their safety until no fresh injury is visible.

### Predator Guards for Housing and Enclosures

The first step in protecting patients from predation is to not attract predators to the area. Grain spillage should be cleaned up and no excess food left outside the pens. Solid barrier fences block visual temptation for predators. Trees bordering enclosures may allow avian predators to perch and climbing predators to access the enclosure, so they should be carefully evaluated. Digging animals such as skunks can be discouraged with 1 × 0.5 in. (2.5 × 1.25 cm) hardware cloth buried 2 ft. (60 cm) straight into the ground and angled outward from the pen another 2 ft. (60 cm). The use of galvanized heavy gauge wire is wise because less substantial wire may deteriorate and require costly maintenance. Some rehabilitators have success using multiple strands of electric fencing on the outside of the perimeter fencing, starting inches from the ground and placed about 1 ft. (30 cm) apart to a height of approximately 5 ft. (1.5 m), which is generally adequate to discourage most predators. Check with local wildlife officials for a list of predators that frequent the area and regulations for legal means to control them. Humane trapping using live traps or other methods may be needed for persistent pests. Local regulations may affect the translocation of live-trapped predators. Under no circumstances should poison ever be used to control predators. The chance of poisoning nontarget species is great. For the most complete protection, the enclosure should be covered to prevent avian predation, premature release, or wild visitors that may bring parasites or other problems to the pens.

## Release Criteria

Everything about wild Galliformes is unique – and release is no different. Most species do not fly well, migrate, or move great distances; therefore, dispersal is not an option for these birds as it is with many avian species. It is important for them to be released into a good habitat, with natural food availability, and away from humans and domestic animals. Release should occur after the bird is fully feathered, acclimated to outdoor temperature, and experienced with natural food. Galliformes are prey for many animals in the wild. The formation of family groups offers the birds protection and for some species, such as wild turkeys, are a key method of survival. This behavior is especially true of hens; however, all young Galliformes benefit through their first winter or until they can assimilate into the local population.

Many Galliformes are hunted. Consider the hunting season dates in timing release. For best survival, release birds after the hunting season ends or a few weeks before to allow the bird to acclimate without threat. Post-release supplemental feeding is generally not needed.

## Author's Note

The rehabilitation of wild Galliformes can be challenging. Wildlife rehabilitators have contact with species that are rarely handled, particularly as chicks. Working with these delicate species gives the wildlife rehabilitator an opportunity to be a valued partner in natural history information development and disease research. It is essential to keep good records of diet, housing, and treatment regimes. Both successes and failures with every aspect of care are important and should be shared with the wildlife community. Full necropsies of mortalities should be done to document possible emerging disease processes, which may be poorly understood. Adding to the knowledge of a species is an important endeavor and one in which the rehabilitator can play an active role.

## Acknowledgments

I owe much to my parents and grandmother who filled my young life with Galliformes both wild and domestic and to Tori the Turkey (Figure 8.1), a wild turkey that has graced our life for many years and continues to teach us about the intelligence and adaptability of the wild turkey.

## Sources of Products Mentioned

Feeder insects: Arbico Organics, PO Box 8910, Tucson, AZ 85738–0910, (800) 827–2847, https://www.arbico-organics.com.

Feeder insects: Bassett's Cricket Ranch, Inc., 365 S. Mariposa, Visalia, CA 93292–9242, (800) 634–2445 or (559) 747–2728, Fax 559–747-3619, https://store.bcrcricket.com.

Feeder insects: Grubco, 7995 North Gilmore Rd., Fairfield, OH 45014, (800) 222–3563, www.grubco.com.

Feeder insects: Rainbow Mealworms, Inc., P.O. Box 4907, 126 East Spruce Street, Compton, CA 90220, (310) 635–1494, www.rainbowmealworms.net.

Hill's Science Diet: Hill's Pet Nutrition, Inc., P.O. Box 148, Topeka, KS 66601–0148, https://www.hillspet.com.

## References

Altman, R.B., Clubb, S.L., Dorrestein, G.M., and Quesenberry, K. (1997). *Avian Medicine and Surgery*, 944–959. Philadelphia: W.B. Saunders Co.

Anderson Brown, A.F. and Robins, G.E.S. (2002). *The New Incubation Book*, 206–213. Blaine, Washington: Hancock House Publishing Ltd.

Baicich, P.J. and Harrison, C.J.O. (2005). *Nest, Eggs, and Nestlings of North American Birds*, 2e, 347 pp. Princeton, New Jersey: Princeton University Press.

Bump, G., Darrow, R.W., Edminster, F.C., and Crissey, W.F. (1947). *The Ruffed Grouse: Life History, Propagation and Management*, 179–226. New York State Conservation Department.

Elphick, C., Dunning, J.B. Jr., and Sibley, D.A. (2001). *The Sibley Guide to Bird Life and Behavior*, 73–77. New York: Alfred A. Knopf, Inc., 233–245.

Erickson, L. (2006). *101 Ways to Help Birds*, 73–74, 76, 203. Mechanicsburg, Pennsylvania: Stackpole Books.

Gibson, M. (1996). The ABC's of housing raptors. *Journal of Wildlife Rehabilitation* 19 (3): 23–31.

Gibson, M. (1998). Putting baby back. *Journal of Wildlife Rehabilitation* 21 (2): 33–40.

Gill, F. and Donsker, D. (eds.). (2019). IOC World Bird List (v9.1). doi: https://doi.org/10.14344/IOC.ML.9.1.

Hayes, L.B. (1992). *The Chinese Painted Quail, Their Breeding and Care*, 161 pp. Leland Hayes' Gamebird Publications.
Ritchie, B.W., Harrison, G.J., and Harrison, L.R. (1994). *Avian Medicine: Principles and Application*, 1384 pp. Lake Worth, Florida.: Wingers Publishing Inc.
Sibley, D.A. (2000). *The Sibley Guide to Birds*, 134–149. New York: Alfred A. Knopf, Inc.
Skutch, A.F. (1976). *Parent Birds and Their Young*, 312–315. University of Texas Press.
Welty, J.C. (1982). *The Life of Birds*, 3e, 754 pp. Philadelphia: Saunders College Publishing.
Williams, L.E. Jr. (1991). *Wild Turkey Country*, 160 pp. Northword Press.
Woodward, A. (1993). *Commercial and Ornamental Game Bird Breeders Handbook*, 181–188, 272–290, 357–359. Hancock Wildlife Research Center.

## Further Reading

Atwater, S. and Schnell, J. (1989). *The Wildlife Series: The Ruffed Grouse*, 130–138. Mechanicsburg, Pennsylvania: Stackpole Books.
Delacour, J. (1978). *Pheasant Breeding and Care*, 18. T.F.H. Publications Inc., 443–448.
Gibson, M. (1997). Natural history: square one for wildlife rehabilitation. *Journal of Wildlife Rehabilitation* 17 (1): 3–6, 16.
Johnsgard, P.A. (1988). *The Quails, Partridges and Francolins of the World*, 202–205. Oxford University Press.
Johnsgard, P.A. (1999). *The Pheasants of the World: Biology and Natural History*. Smithsonian Institution.
Landers, L.J. and Mueller, B.S. (1986). *Bobwhite Quail Management: A Habitat Approach*, 39 pp. Tall Timbers Research Station and Quail Unlimited.
Martin, L.C. (1993). *The Folklore of Birds*, 69, 153. The Globe Pequot Press.
Rogers, L.J. and Kaplan, G. (2000). *Songs, Roars and Rituals, Communications in Birds, Mammals, and Other Animals*, 20, 83, 90. Cambridge, MA: Harvard University Press.
Rupley, A. (1997). *Manual of Avian Practice*, 265–291. Philadelphia: W.B. Saunders Co.

# 9

# Loons

*Renée Schott and Jesse Menne*

## Natural History

Loons occupy their own Family (Gaviidae) and Order (Gaviiformes). There are five species of extant loons: the Common Loon (*Gavia immer*), the Yellow-billed Loon (*Gavia adamsii*), the Pacific Loon (*Gavia pacifica*), the Arctic Loon (aka Black-throated Loon) (*Gavia arctica*), and the Red-throated Loon (*Gavia stellata*). All loon species are Northern hemisphere, migratory birds that breed in or near Northern freshwater bodies but overwinter in marine environments, generally south of where they breed. They are heavy-bodied diving birds with legs positioned so caudally on their body, they are largely incapable of walking on land. They prefer bodies of water that are clear (easier to see fish), have a surface area large enough for takeoff, and minimal human interference. Pacific and Arctic Loons require 30–50 m of open water for takeoff under calm conditions. Red-throated Loons need 15–40 m, depending on wind. Common Loons, and probably Yellow-billed Loons, require up to 200 m for takeoff, but can lift off in substantially shorter distances if taking off into high winds. Common Loons do relatively well in human inhabited areas (Titus and VanDruff 1981; Caron and Robinson 1994); they breed closer to human populations than any other loon species, and so are the most likely young loon to be admitted for wildlife rehabilitation. Almost all human experience raising loons has been with Common Loons (Barr 1996; Kenow et al. 2014). This chapter will be based on care of Common Loons, but likely much of the techniques and information can be extrapolated to other species of loons. Hereafter, "loon" is used to imply "Common Loon" unless otherwise noted.

Loons feed primarily on fish but will also eat insects, annelids, mollusks, amphibians, and only rarely vegetable matter. Loons rely on stones present in their ventriculus to help them digest the prey they swallow whole as they do not cast pellets.

Common Loons potentially live to more than 30 years old (Tischler 2011; Piper et al. 2017). It is estimated that ~50% of Common Loon juveniles will survive to 3 years of age (Piper et al. 2012). Loons mature at age 3 and on average obtain breeding territory around age 5. They are long-lived, slow to mature, and have low fecundity. Loons nest within 2 meters of water, on shore, or on other similar areas, like a muskrat lodge (Tischler 2011). Made by both sexes, the nest is typically formed using a collection of plant material. Nest sites are often used year-to-year. Loons are territorial; a mated pair will defend an area of water (5–50 ha) from other loons. Loons may share a lake with other loons, but they have distinct territories within the lake and nest in separate bays/areas. Loon chicks are semi-precocial, and swim after hatching, although they will ride on the parent's back to

*Hand-Rearing Birds*, Second Edition. Edited by Rebecca S. Duerr and Laurie J. Gage.

conserve heat and energy and to avoid predators. They stay in shallow water with one parent 24/7 for the first 3 days of life. After a few days the family moves to a "nursery" area of the lake and doesn't return to the nest. After the first 3 days, the chick may stay alone in the nursery area unless summoned by the parent. Loons most commonly have one or two chicks, rarely three or four (Timmermans et al. 2004), and the chicks often compete for food, leaving one smaller than the other; siblicide can occur (Tischler 2011). Juveniles first start to fly at 11–13 weeks of age and migrate between late-September and freeze-up of lakes (Barr 1996).

## Criteria for Intervention

Any chick with visible injuries should be brought to a licensed wildlife rehabilitator. In the authors' and other's experiences (Diane Winn, pers. comm.), over half of the young loons presenting to wildlife rehabilitation are ill or injured; less than half are healthy orphans. A chick should rarely be alone on the shore that is not their nest. A grounded loon chick, other than during the first 24 hours after hatching, indicates possible illness, injury, or abandonment.

Exceptions are as follows:

- Moving: Adult loons sometimes move their chicks overland from a nesting lake to a nearby lake that provides better opportunities for forage. The parents may be a bit ahead on the journey, so the finder may presume the chick is alone.
- Defecation: Occasionally, loons move onto shore and, when 2–4 m from water, they turn to face the water, defecate, and then return to water. This behavior has been observed in young loons and adult loons. The function is unknown but may act as a territory marker (Evers et al. 2010).

## Record Keeping

Loons are incredibly territorial during the breeding season (Evers et al. 2010); it is assumed this is why, in the authors' experience, parents will not foster a chick that is not their own. It is important the exact location where the finder found the chick is recorded in case it can be reunited with the parents. Detailed husbandry records should be kept including daily weight, diet offered, how much was eaten, and any observations (e.g. behavioral changes). Regular physical exams out of water should be conducted and details recorded weekly. The first indication of injury or illness is often subtle, such as changes to appetite, weight, or physical exam (Kenow et al. 2014). See Appendix A for a sample wildlife rehabilitation animal record.

## Initial Care and Stabilization

Loons are generally a high-stress species, so minimize handling and any interaction. A thorough physical exam should be conducted on admission. Pay close attention to waterproofing, keel/hock/foot injuries or pressure sores, attitude, and perform a thorough respiratory tract (lungs and all air sacs) auscultation if possible. A visibly wet chick should be assumed to be hypothermic. If the chick is hypothermic, offer warmth but monitor for hyperthermia. When a chick is able to thermoregulate and visibly dry, they should be removed from the incubator and placed in appropriate housing (see below). Once warm, the chick can be rehydrated. If the chick is drinking readily from

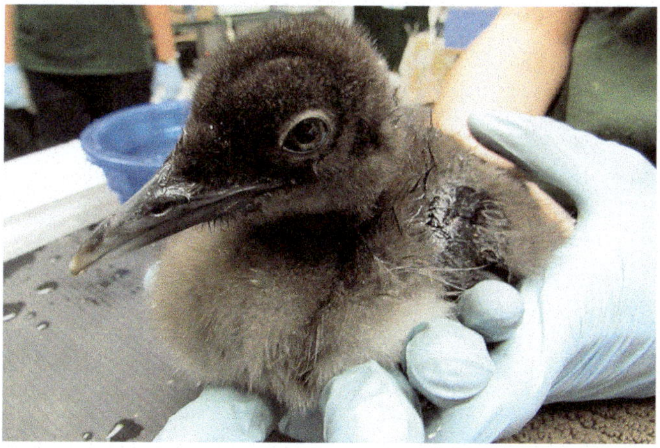

Figure 9.1 Common Loon chick with wet area on wing after hydration offered from a small tub. *Source:* photo courtesy of Marge Gibson.

a pool or dish, then reassess hydration 4–12 hours later (Figure 9.1). If they are dehydrated and not drinking, fluids can be gavaged at 30–50 ml/kg or sterile isotonic fluids given subcutaneously at 50 ml/kg. It should also be noted that those who have raised loons from hatching have not noticed signs of malimprinting (Diane Winn, Kevin Kenow, pers. comms.).

## Common Medical Problems

### Lethargy

Older, healthy, wild-caught loon chicks should become progressively more aggressive and feistier with age. They should be stabbing at your hands and eyes when handled. However, chicks hatched in captivity may be much more docile toward handlers. Any deviation from this is abnormal and a thorough physical exam should be performed. It can be difficult to catch small declines in attitude. It is recommended to weigh the chicks daily in a standardized manner (i.e. before morning feeding). Declining body weight may be the first sign of something wrong, so weighing chicks daily is paramount.

### Pressure Sores

Loons have evolved to spend almost 100% of their lives on water and thus lack any significant soft tissue padding over the plantar surface of their feet, hocks, and keels (Figure 9.2). Chicks kept off water or who are hauling themselves out too frequently will develop lesions here. They are very difficult to manage; thus, prevention is best. See "Haul-out" section below under "Housing."

### Aspergillosis

Loons are very susceptible to aspergillosis (White et al. 1976; Forrester et al. 1997; Stone and Okoniewski 2001). Typically, it is secondary to another stressor; however, that stressor may simply be captivity or growth. In Kenow et al. (2014), 47% of hand-reared chicks had evidence of

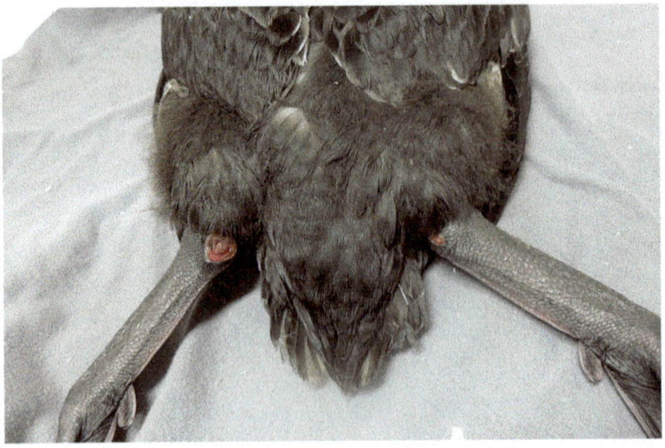

Figure 9.2 Loons are prone to development of hock lesions when housed out of water for any reason.

aspergillosis on necropsy; no prophylactic medications were administered to these chicks. The authors of this chapter give all loon chicks in captivity 10–12.5 mg/kg voriconazole orally twice daily for the duration of their rehabilitation. Sporanox or Itrafungol may be acceptable alternatives; however, the authors have not used these products. Compounded itraconazole from the chemical powder should be avoided due to lack of bioavailability in cats (Mawby et al. 2018). Other rehabilitators (Diane Winn, pers. comm.) do not give antifungal prophylactic medications to loon chicks and anecdotally have not seen an increase in aspergillosis infections. It is unclear whether the side effects of voriconazole outweigh the benefits of perceived aspergillosis prevention.

### Lead and Mercury Toxicosis

Because of their high percentage fish diet and the propensity for accidentally picking up fishing sinkers instead of stones for digestion, loons can develop methylmercury and lead toxicosis. Lead toxicosis is a very common problem for loons and has been shown to decrease overall populations (Grade et al. 2018). Lead toxicosis and fishing tackle ingestion are common in adults, but less so in chicks. Nevertheless, an initial radiograph should be taken to look for metal opacities in the body and a blood lead level evaluated for previous exposure, especially in any ill chicks without obvious injury. Mercury toxicity is less likely in a loon chick than an adult. Loons are used as environmental indicators for exposure to methylmercury in aquatic systems (Depew et al. 2012).

### Traumatic Injuries

Traumatic injuries may result from entanglement in fishing line, an altercation with a boat, attack from a nonparent adult loon, or, rarely, siblicide attempts. Injuries should be treated as other seabird species, with particular care being taken to preserve waterproofing and prevent pressure sores.

## Reuniting with Parents

Reuniting a healthy chick with its parents is ideal, and the best chance of survival for the chick. It is very difficult to "kidnap" a healthy chick and often there is underlying illness or trauma; consequently, an obligatory medical work up should be conducted prior to considering family reunification. This should include a thorough physical exam including lung/air sac auscultation, blood lead level, and an un-positioned awake radiograph to look for metal opacities. Once the chick is deemed healthy, the original lake where the chick was found must be scouted. Are both parents present? Are there any other chicks? What size are the other chicks compared to the current chick? How confident are you that this is the correct set of parents? If the answers to all these questions are known and favorable, reuniting *may* be possible. However, this does not guarantee the reunification will be successful. It is recommended to be ready for rescue should the identified adult loons turn on the chick. If a sibling is present, it may or may not be aggressive toward the chick or outcompete it for food. Additionally, if the chick was in captivity for an extended period of time, the parent loons may have already re-nested.

## Fostering

Fostering a chick to a different set of parents often doesn't work. The pair may already have chick(s) who will aggressively drive away the stray chick or the parents may recognize the chick as foreign and drive it away or kill it themselves. Rarely, fostering has appeared to work; however, long term follow-up was not possible (Marge Gibson, pers. comm.). Other methods that appear to work include separating the native chick from the parents, and placing the native chick next to the foster one, so the parents are confused about who is who and they don't see you adding another chick (Kevin Kenow, pers. comm.). Anecdotally, the younger the chick is, the more successful the fostering is likely to be. Adult loons are difficult to maintain in captivity owing to stress and husbandry standards, and therefore aren't kept as foster parents or exhibit animals. Captive adult loons undergoing rehabilitation may attack a foreign chick introduced to its enclosure.

## Captive Diet

Common Loons primarily eat a variety of fish (cisco, perch, suckers, small white fish, common and golden shiners, and trout) but are opportunistic when choices are limited. Wild loons have been known to consume crayfish, aquatic insects, amphibians, and rarely vegetable matter in addition to fish (Barr 1996). Loon chicks under 5 days old have been observed to eat various larvae and adult insects found on the surface of lakes, such as dragonflies, waterbugs, and whirligig beetles (Barr 1996). It is likely loons seen pecking at vegetation are eating invertebrates within the vegetation. However, some rehabilitators have noticed repeatedly that young loons will eagerly seek out and consume decayed and fresh vegetation as soon as they are placed in a natural enclosure; additionally, one rehabilitator has noticed a few instances in which a young loon appeared to have digestive problems that improved after being offered decayed leaves (Diane Winn, pers. comm.).

In the rehabilitation process, fish have been provided as the primary food source. The maximum size of fish offered should correspond to the size of the chick's beak/gastrointestinal tract as loons swallow their prey whole. Small to medium sized fish (10–70 g) are preferred as larger fish can be difficult to swallow. Crappie minnows (i.e. from a bait shop) work well for smaller chicks, whereas fathead minnows and small suckers are excellent for larger juveniles. Other fish species can be used but may be prohibitively expensive or hard to acquire alive. If possible, a variety of fish is ideal for nutrition and hunting practice. Different fish species have different evasion tactics, speed, and nutritional composition.

Fish are best offered live, as chicks instinctively chase and peck moving objects. But fish may need to be stunned and offered via forceps to very young chicks. Dead fish can be offered; however, this increases the chance of fish oil contamination in the water which may possibly compromise waterproofing. It may also limit the time spent learning to hunt and compromise the overall nutrition of the fish. Fish that is individually flash frozen and then thawed can be fed but care must be taken to hand-feed or place the fish on the haul-out or pool's edge, so as not to overly contaminate the water. Fish that have been fed thawed include capelin, silversides, rainbow trout, or lake smelt.

Even if using live fish, it is impossible to replicate the chick's natural diet. The authors recommend a daily multivitamin supplement that contains thiamin, such as Sea-Tabs® (Pacific Research Labs, Inc.), and others have used ThiaminE Paste (Mazuri® Exotic Animal Nutrition).

### Storage of Live Fish

Minnows are best stored in a refrigerator or an industrial cooler. Multiple air bubble stones are necessary to keep minnows alive. For a 10-gal tank, two to three bubblers are needed depending on how many minnows are housed. A simple fish tank filter works well and should be cleaned as needed. If tap water contains chlorine, a dechlorinator must be used to treat the water before live fish are added. This includes the fish tank, water dishes, and pools for the loon or the live fish will die quickly.

## Feeding Procedures

In the wild, chicks rely on parents for food exclusively for the first 8 weeks of life and start transitioning to self-feeding after that. Parents often continue to offer some fish up to and after 14 weeks of age. However, many chicks will catch and eat fish when offered hourly. A fish consumption chart can be filled out every hour to record how many fish or the mass of the fish the chick is consuming (Table 9.1). Before hand-feeding, offer small fish in a dish or shallow pool; if the chick successfully eats fish on its own, hand-feeding may be unnecessary. Reducing hand-feeding may reduce habituation and unnecessary stress.

Keep offering fish until the chick is satiated. Daily weights will help decide whether hand-feeding is needed. The number of fish offered each feeding will depend on the size of the fish, the size of the chick, the chick's stress level, and if the chick is self-feeding.

### How to Hand-feed

Hand-feedings should be done in a pool as adult loons only feed chicks while the chicks are swimming. This will also prompt them to practice shallow dives, preen, and drink. If a hatchling is not drinking water on its own, then water should be offered each feeding. This can be done by dipping a hemostat into the pool and dripping water on the chick's beak. The chick should swallow the water droplets (Barr 1996). Adults feed chicks by holding fish crosswise in their beak and present the fish within reach of chick. The chick then grabs the fish and with some movements of the beak and head manipulate the fish to swallow it head first. Mimic this behavior by presenting a small fish crosswise in forceps; if the chick does not take it, wave the fish in front of its face side to side to entice. If the chick is still reluctant, drop the fish into the pool and repeat the offering. It can take several attempts to get a chick to take the offering (Barr 1996; Kenow et al. 2014). Take a break if the chick begins to get too stressed.

Table 9.1 Fish consumption chart for loon chicks.

Please make note of **how many fish are left** in the dish and **how many new fish you add**.
Check and record numbers of remaining fish, dead fish, and fish added **hourly**
Use **dechlorinated water** only and remove dead fish

| Date: | | | | Date: | | | | Date: | | | | Date: | | | |
|---|---|---|---|---|---|---|---|---|---|---|---|---|---|---|---|
| Time | # fish left | # dead removed | # fish added | Time | # fish left | # dead removed | # fish added | Time | # fish left | # dead removed | # fish added | Time | # fish left | # dead removed | # fish added |
| | | | | | | | | | | | | | | | |
| | | | | | | | | | | | | | | | |
| | | | | | | | | | | | | | | | |
| | | | | | | | | | | | | | | | |
| | | | | | | | | | | | | | | | |
| | | | | | | | | | | | | | | | |
| | | | | | | | | | | | | | | | |
| | | | | | | | | | | | | | | | |
| | | | | | | | | | | | | | | | |
| | | | | | | | | | | | | | | | |
| | | | | | | | | | | | | | | | |
| | | | | | | | | | | | | | | | |
| | | | | | | | | | | | | | | | |

### Self-feeding

At 7–10 days old, a chick should be able to chase and catch some prey (Kenow et al. 2014). Success may be minimal, but if offered a large enough school of fish, chicks should maintain and gain weight. Once the loon chick is sufficiently eating on its own and gaining weight, they can be weaned off hand-feeding.

Using the fish consumption chart (Table 9.1), caregivers can record how many fish or the mass of the fish consumed or having died, and then replace a specific number of fish to equal a certain size school of fish. The size and number of fish offered each hour is based on the individual, not necessarily the age of the chick. For young fledglings, typically 10 fathead minnows are offered each hour. The goal is to have some fish leftover, finding a balance between the bird's consumption and not leaving the pool fishless. Increasing the number of fish is based on how much the bird eats daily; once a balance is met, fish are increased each week by 5–10 minnows. By 6 weeks of age, minnow schools are between 35 and 45 based on consumption. Larger schools may be necessary for larger pools or those in natural lake environments. It's important for the chicks to be successful; therefore, increasing the number of fish offered may be necessary. To help increase the success rate of hunt and capture, fish can be injured by clipping the side fins shorter on one side and/or clipping the tail (Michelle Kneeland, pers. comm.). This causes the fish to swim more erratically. Erratic swimming creates movements attracting the loon to pursue the fish and increasing the chance of capture. Clipping fins on a few fish each feeding is enough to help build the chick's success.

Chicks are fed live fish every hour up to release in order to maintain pristine water conditions for waterproofing in a 1.8-m square pool. Dead fish give off oils and these can compromise the chick's waterproofing. At each feeding, dead fish should be removed and replaced with new live fish. It is not uncommon for a chick to catch prey and then discard it. Either the chick is satiated, can't swallow the fish, or simply doesn't like that fish, perhaps due to spines or hard scales (Barr 1996). If the pool has a larger surface area and adequate water turnover, fish oil is less of a problem.

It is ideal that loon chicks do not associate humans with food to reduce the risk of the chick approaching people or boats after release. Therefore, ideally add fish to the pool behind a blind or through a PVC pipe. The PVC pipe can be lifted so the fish splash in the water to catch the eye of a loon chick that is not eating well (Michelle Kneeland, pers. comm.). Otherwise it can remain underwater as fish are added each feeding.

## Expected Weight Gain

Birds should be weighed daily to ensure each chick is gaining weight (Figure 9.3). Typically, loon chicks gain 100–200 g every 3 days. Once the chick's primary flight feathers are fully grown, weight begins to plateau. It is known that chicks may not eat as much when stressed (i.e. moved to different pool for cleaning) and this may affect daily weights (Kenow et al. 2014).

## Housing

For a debilitated chick, it may be prudent to start off in a wet-dry or completely dry setup. Orphaned loon chicks often have underlying illness or injuries, so it is not uncommon for death to occur within 48 hours of admission to a wildlife rehabilitation facility. Once the chick is strong/stable enough, it is important to get the chick on water as soon as possible to prevent pressure sores. Housing for loon chicks must change as they grow and become more waterproofed.

## All Ages

All chicks should be placed into a brooder box with a shallow pool once admitted (Figure 9.4). Shallow water reduces the chance of accidental drownings and allows the bird to stabilize if needed. After 24–48 hours, if the chick is healthy, bright, alert, and responsive, it can be moved to a small or large pool depending on maturity. The depth of the pool will depend on age and

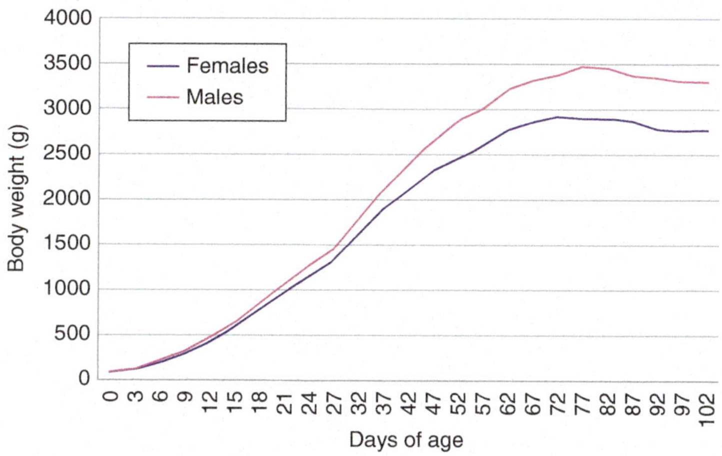


Figure 9.3 The average weight gain of 18 female and 14 male Common Loon chicks. *Source:* data courtesy of Kevin Kenow.

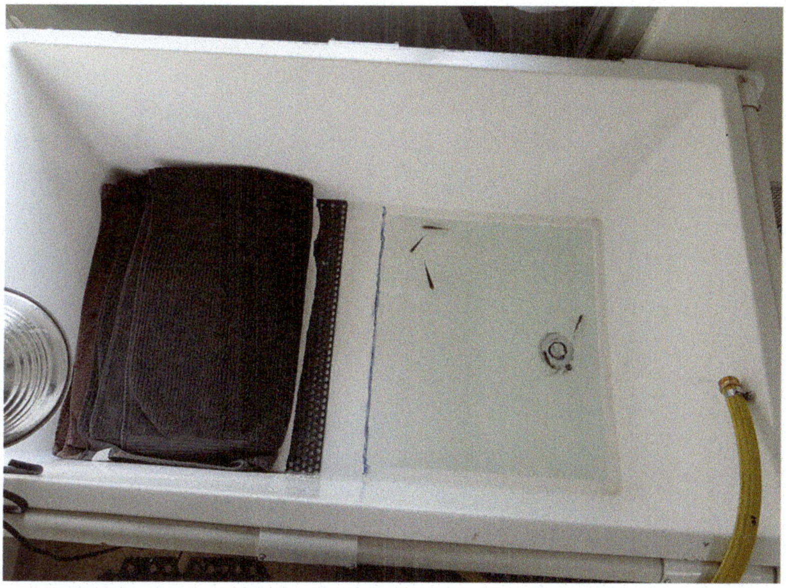

Figure 9.4 Wet brooder box with well-padded haul-out area, heat lamp, and clean water in which to offer live fish.

waterproofing. Moving chicks to larger pools is based on self-feeding success, waterproofing, and thermoregulation. Once a chick has moved to a pool, it is vital there is flowing surface water. Flowing water is necessary to maintain a loon's waterproofing. Either an overflow system or a closed filtration system is used (Jimmy Pichner, pers. comm; Kenow et al. 2014).

### Haul-outs

No matter where chicks are housed, they should have a place to haul themselves out of water. This area should be (i) large enough for all individuals to haul-out at the same time, (ii) flat, (iii) only 1–2 in. higher than the water level, (iv) soft and dry, and (v) have good drainage. An example is a frame made out of PVC tubing with soft netting stretched over it to allow drainage and flexibility. Foam (i.e. pool noodles) can be wrapped around the PVC to allow it to float and a chenile microfiber bath mat (with no backing) on the top will offer a soft surface to prevent pressure sores (Figure 9.5). Kenow et al. (2014) used a haul-out that was much firmer but otherwise satisfied all the above requirements and resulted in no pressure sores: Standard Tenderfoot flooring (Tandem Products, Minneapolis, MN).

### Wet-dry Setup

Hatchlings and debilitated young loons should be placed in a brooder box with a platform or haul-out and a shallow pool (Figure 9.4). Provide an inch of padding on the platform or a netted bottom with open air underneath; chenille-tufted bathmats without the rubber backing work well alone or on top of the netted bottom. A heat lamp on the low setting should be above the platform. The shallow pool should have an overflow system where excess water flows out of the system at the surface and a hose is left on a trickle. This maintains clean surface water and is necessary for the chick's waterproofing. If the pool is not level with the platform, a ramp must be provided. Small fish should be offered in the pool to help encourage chicks to peck at moving objects.

Once the caregiver is confident the chick is well waterproofed, the pool size can be increased. Original Rearing Cubicles (Leucopsis Products, www.leucopsis.com) are plastic brooder boxes which are excellent for gradually increasing pool size. Pipes can be added to this system at different heights, increasing the pool depth as needed. The pipes also act as exit point for the overflow system, keeping surface water clean. It is ideal to get loon chicks on water as quickly as possible, so

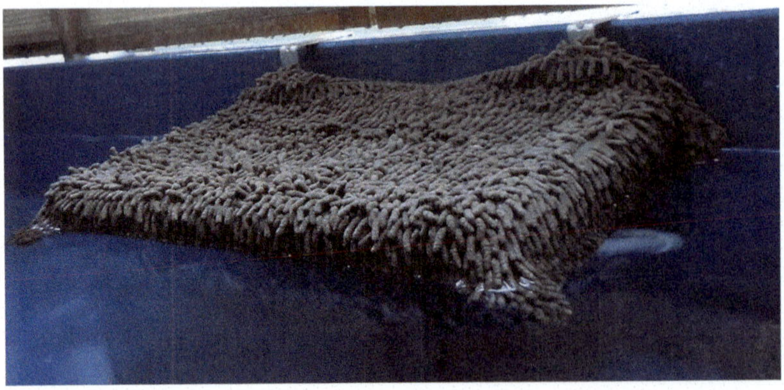

Figure 9.5 Chenille bathmat covering netting on a PVC frame which acts as a soft area for the bird to haul-out of the water without acquiring hock or toe lesions. *Source:* photo courtesy of Diane Winn/Avian Haven.

this method of gradually increasing pool depth from 6 in. (15 cm) to 14 in. (35 cm) works well. Debilitated young loons may be in the Original Rearing Cubicle until healthy, while healthier chicks may outgrow it in a few days.

## Transitioning to a Pool

A small haul-out should be provided in the pool. The chick may need to be placed on the haul-out a few times in order to learn what it is. Once the Original Rearing Cubicle is filled with water and the haul-out is provided it is important to check on the chick. Checking every 15–30 minutes may be necessary based on the age and waterproofing of the chick. Peeking through a window or curtain is ideal for observation to limit interaction. While observing, note if the chick is staying waterproofed or if it is wet, waterlogged, sinking, or appears cold. If this occurs, the chick should be moved back to a wet-dry setup with a heat lamp. If the chick is doing well, observations can be decreased to every hour and correlated with feedings. Once the chick hauls itself out, observations can stop. Some chicks may not use the haul-out and the caregiver must use their judgment on whether they think the chick can stay in the pool for the entire day. It may take a few days for birds to learn to use the haul-out. If concerned about the chick overnight, place the bird back into the wet-dry setup. After several days of the deeper water in the brooder box, it is likely the bird is ready to move to a larger pool.

## Pool

Pools should be a color that will contrast the fish given to the chick. Loons depend on good light for hunting. The authors used a white water storage tank (Vertical Storage Tank, Norwesco, St. Bonifacious, MN), and cut off the top to leave a pool of 67 in. (1.7 m) diameter and 18 in. (45.7 cm) water depth; this was then retrofitted with a closed filtration system (Figure 9.6). Larger pools are ideal, but expense and space are factors in rehabilitation. A pool large enough to encourage foraging,

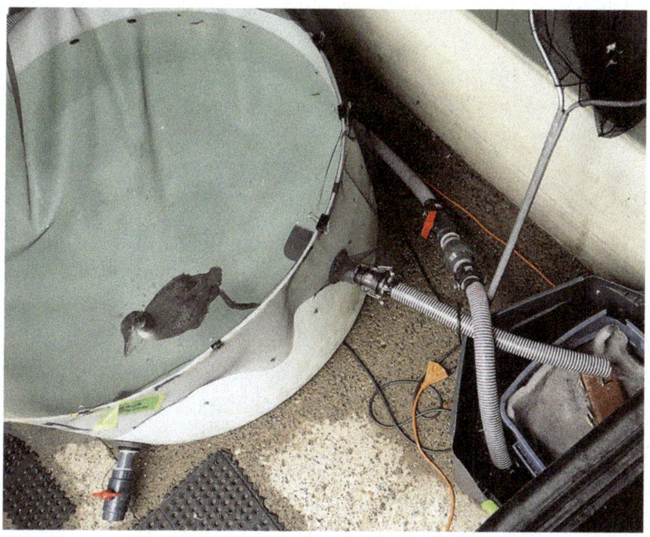

Figure 9.6 Top view of a Common Loon in a pool with a screen cover and closed filtration system that provides constant surface water skimming and replacement of water after it passes through the filter.

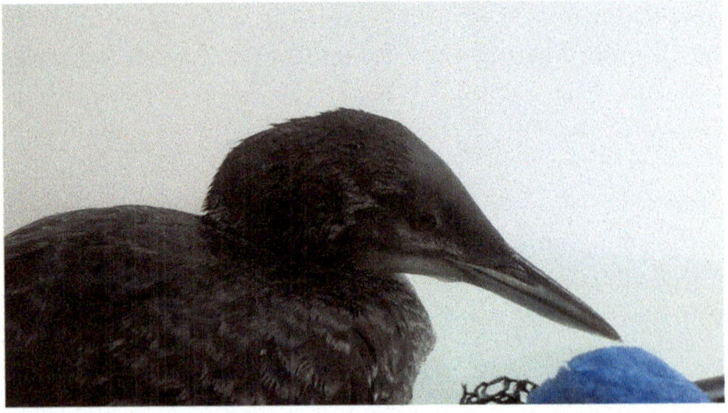

Figure 9.7 A loon chick that is not waterproof on its head, note the feathers clump together rather than remaining fluffy.

chasing, and diving should be sufficient for a loon chick. Pools need above-water walls sufficient to allow birds comfortable space above the water and a visual barrier to provide privacy, plus a netted ceiling that prevents attempted escape if birds were to attempt launching themselves over the side of the pool.

There are several types of pool systems that can be used to maintain waterproofing in diving birds. One is the overflow-trickle system. This system requires holes or thin horizontal slots in the pool wall at the desired height and a hose left on continuously at a trickle (see Figure 10.7 for image of drainage slot). The overflow out of the drain holes creates water movement at the surface, keeping the surface water clean. Dead fish, feces, and debris fall to the bottom of the pool. Trickle systems are not ideal if water conservation is a concern. Water is constantly flowing and draining out of the pool, wasting significant water each day. A filtration system can be used instead. An exit port is created at the wanted height of the pool and a flexible pipe is attached. The exiting water flows into the filter. The filter consists of a 5-gal bucket with holes drilled 1 in. from the bottom at 1.5 in. apart. The top layer of the bucket has a foam-like filter material that removes large debris (e.g. dead fish, leaves) from the system. Next is a bag of charcoal and finally 3–4 in. of bio balls. Water exits the bucket through the drilled holes and is now in the storage tote with the sump pump. The sump pump pushes water back into the pool. The piping connected to the sump pump hangs just above the water surface. This flow of water at the surface maintains a small current flow in the pool, keeping the water clean. Similarly to the trickle system, dead fish, feces, and debris fall to the bottom of the pool. In both scenarios, the bottom must be siphoned frequently to remove debris. If filtration systems malfunction, the water becomes too dirty and the chick's waterproofing may be negatively affected. Pools may need to be cleaned as frequently as every or every other day, depending on the number of chicks present. Chicks can be placed in a kennel or in a smaller pool with a trickle system during cleaning.

The chick should be observed for becoming waterlogged for the first few days (Figure 9.7). The haul-out should still be provided. In a pool, chicks use more energy chasing and catching fish, therefore increasing food demand. It is not uncommon for a slight weight drop in the first few days as the chick adjusts to the new pool, but the chick should start to gain weight again after a few days.

## Moving Outside

Ideally, chicks should be moved outside as soon as possible. Loons are at high risk for aspergillosis. Depending on indoor and outdoor air quality, being outside may either reduce or increase this risk (Burco 2010). Adequate air filtration systems may decrease the fungal spore load in the indoor air.

Once a chick can thermoregulate on their own, they no longer need a heat lamp and can move outside. Younger chicks can move outside during the day, weather permitting, and be moved in overnight. Once a chick has their white belly feathers and no access to a haul-out, they should stay outside overnight as well. Birds that are waterproof should do well in all weather conditions. It is recommended to have tarp or other shelter over part of the pool in case of severe storms. This also provides shade on sunny days. Chicks have been observed for waterlogging when left in pools during severe thunderstorms and have done well.

### Conspecific Aggression

Loon chicks in the same brood will exhibit aggressive behavior among themselves to establish a pecking order. Loons hatched in captivity exhibit this same behavior after hatching, but the behavior stops after dominance is established and all other chicks assume a submissive posture (Kenow et al. 2014). Chicks from different broods may have an increased incidence of aggressive behavior toward conspecifics, especially if the pool area is small, or the birds are older than a few weeks of age. Care should be taken in introducing loon chicks more than 2 days of age apart from one another, and consideration should be given to housing them separately if group housing fails. However, socialization is natural and is likely important for developing behaviors and skills. Up to six loon chicks have been successfully reared together from age 1 month to release in pools of 49 $m^2$ (Kenow et al. 2014). Chicks should always be approximately the same size and weight before introducing them to chick(s) from another brood.

## Preparation for Wild Release

### Waterproofing

Birds must be fully waterproofed to survive after release. An air bubble surrounding the loon as it dives under water can be observed in well-waterproofed birds. When on the surface, chicks should be completely dry and water beading observed. No areas of the body should be wet to the skin in a waterproof bird.

### Hunting Skills

It is important that the bird can successfully hunt on its own and maintain its body weight. Hand-feeding should be completely stopped and daily weights maintained or increased while the bird only self-feeds on live prey. If dead fish was used as the main diet, it should be switched to live fish only for at least 2–3 days prior to release.

### Age of Release

In the wild, loon chicks are very independent by week 12 and usually make their first flight attempt (Barr 1996). Loon chicks can be released as early as 9 weeks old if they are doing well capturing prey (Michelle Kneeland pers. comm.), but closer to 12 weeks is more consistent with natural history. If a chick becomes very restless, is pacing, and stops eating, but is otherwise doing well, it may be a sign it is ready for release (Michelle Kneeland pers. comm.); however, a chick that stops eating also may be sick (Kenow et al. 2014). Use behavior and body weight to differentiate, and radiographs may be helpful if respiratory disease is suspected. Ultimately, age at release will depend on the individual bird.

## Release

Release lakes should be known to have loon sightings, but release should not take place within an active territory occupied by adult loons. Loons prefer large lakes with adequate fish and clear water. Both these criteria are important when selecting a release spot. Release hand-reared chicks in areas with aggregations of juvenile loons whenever possible. These locations demonstrate an adequate fish source and good hunting grounds. It will also allow the chicks to observe other loons' hunting techniques. Releasing in a group setting likely increases the success of survival after release. Allowing enough time to develop hunting skills in a natural environment is important when selecting release spots where lakes freeze. It is also recommended to either release on a lake that prohibits boating or after Labor Day (in the U.S.) when there are fewer people out on lakes.

## Acknowledgments

The authors cannot thank Kevin Kenow and Jimmy Pischner enough for their advice when raising the authors' first set of young loons. Kenow's loon natural history expertise has also been invaluable when releasing young and adult loons. Special thanks to Diane Winn and Michele Kneeland for sharing their experiences raising loons. A final big thank you to Kevin Kenow and Diane Winn who thoroughly reviewed this chapter and for contributing their experiences. It takes a village ... even with loons!

## Sources of Products Mentioned

Mazuri products: Mazuri, PMI Nutrition International, LLC, PO Box 66812, St. Louis, MO 63166, www.mazuri.com.
Original Rearing Cubicles: Leucopsis Products, Wayne, PA 19087, www.leucopsis.com.
SeaTabs: Pacific Research Labs, Inc., 730 Saddlebrook Dr., Ramona, CA 92065, www.prlvitamins.com.
Vertical Storage Tank: Norwesco, Inc., 4365 Steiner Street, St. Bonifacius, MN 55375–0439, (800) 328–3420, www.norwesco.com.

## References

Barr, J.F. (1996). Aspects of Common Loon (*Gavia immer*) feeding biology on its breeding ground. *Hydrobiologia* 321: 119–144. https://doi.org/10.1007/BF00023169.

Burco, J.D. 2010. The ecology of aspergillosis in seabirds. PhD Dissertation, 149 pp, University of California Davis.

Caron, J.A. and Robinson, W.L. (1994). Responses of breeding Common Loons to human activity in upper Michigan. *Hydrobiologia* 279–280 (1): 431–438. https://doi.org/10.1007/BF00027874.

Depew, D.C., Basu, N., Burgess, N.M., et al. 2012. Derivation of screening benchmarks for dietary methylmercury exposure for the Common Loon (*Gavia immer*): rationale for use in ecological risk assessment. Environmental Toxicology and Chemistry 31(10): 2399–2407. doi: https://doi.org/10.1002/etc.1971.

Evers, D.C., Paruk, J.D., McIntyre, J.W., and Barr, J.F. (2010). Common loon (*Gavia immer*), version 2.0. In: *The Birds of North America*. (ed. A.F. Poole). Ithaca, NY, USA: Cornell Lab of Ornithology https://doi.org/10.2173/bna.313.

Forrester, D.J., Davidson, W.R., Lange, R.E., et al. 1997. Winter mortality of Common Loons in Florida coastal waters. Journal of Wildlife Diseases 33(4): 833–847. doi: https://doi.org/10.7589/0090-3558-33.4.833.

Grade, T.J., Pokras, M.A., Laflamme, E.M., and Vogel, H.S. (2018). Population-level effects of lead fishing tackle on Common Loons. *Journal of Wildlife Management* 82 (1): 155–164. https://doi.org/10.1002/jwmg.21348.

Kenow, K.P., Meier, M.S., Mccoll, L.E., et al. 2014. Hand-rearing, growth, and development of Common Loon (*Gavia immer*) chicks. *Zoo Biology* 33(4): 360–371. doi: https://doi.org/10.1002/zoo.21130.

Mawby, D.I., Whittemore, J.C., Fowler, L.E., and Papich, M.G. (2018). Comparison of absorption characteristics of oral reference and compounded itraconazole formulations in healthy cats. *Journal American Veterinary Medical Association* 252 (2): 195–200.

Piper, W.H., Grear, J.S., and Meyer, M.W. (2012). Juvenile survival in Common Loons *Gavia immer*: effects of natal lake size and pH. *Journal of Avian Biology* 43 (3): 280–288. https://doi.org/10.1111/j.1600-048X.2012.05633.x.

Piper, W.H., Brunk, K.M., Flory, J.A., and Meyer, M.W. (2017). The long shadow of senescence: age impacts survival and territory defense in loons. *Journal of Avian Biology* 48 (8): 1062–1070. https://doi.org/10.1111/jav.01393.

Stone, W.B. and Okoniewski, J.C. (2001). Necropsy findings and environmental contaminants in Common Loons from New York. *Journal of Wildlife Diseases* 37 (1): 178–184. https://doi.org/10.7589/0090-3558-37.1.178.

Timmermans, S.T.A., Eoin Craigie, G., and Jones, K.E. (2004). Common loon pairs rear four-chick broods. *The Wilson Journal of Ornithology* 116 (1): 97–101. https://doi.org/10.1676/03-071.

Tischler, K.B. (2011). Species Conservation Assessment for the Common Loon (Gavia immer) in the Upper Great Lakes. *Report prepared for USDA Forest Service, Ottowa National Forest by Common Coast Research & Conservation*, Hancock, MI. 54 pp.

Titus, J.R. and VanDruff, L.W. (1981). Response of the Common Loon to recreational pressure in the boundary waters canoe area, Northeastern Minnesota. *Wildlife Monographs* 79: 57.

White, F.H., Forrester, D.J., and Nesbitt, S.A. (1976). Salmonella and aspergillus infections in Common Loons overwintering in Florida. *Journal of the American Veterinary Medical Association* 169 (9): 936–937.

# 10

# Grebes

*Jessika Madison-Kennedy and Rebecca S. Duerr*

## Natural History

Grebes comprise 20 widely-distributed species of waterbird that can be found on each continent except Antarctica. They are the only members of the order Podicipediformes. The seven grebe species found in North America are Black-necked (or Eared), Clark's, Horned, Least, Pied-billed, Red-necked, and Western. The Western Grebe is best known for a display known as "rushing," where two birds race across the surface of the water in a graceful and coordinated courtship dance. Grebes are migratory; however, some can be considered casual migrants and will move to large inland bodies of water that remain open or will relocate to nearby coastal waters for the winter.

All grebes spend most of their time on the water, live as members of flocks, swim exclusively with their feet, and have legs situated far back on their bodies. This adaption gives them excellent swimming and diving capabilities, but makes walking on dry land challenging and unwieldy. Due to the difficulty in maneuvering out of water and the inability to take off in flight from dry land, grebes are often found grounded and are mistakenly thought to have broken legs by their finders. Besides having unique leg positioning compared to other avian species, grebes can also be easily identified by their distinctive feet, which have a laterally flattened tarsometatarsus and three large, lobed toes that fold together to reduce water resistance on the upstroke, but open to become powerful and wide swimming paddles on the downstroke (Figure 10.1). Grebes have a feather structure that allows them to adjust their buoyancy by trapping air against their body. By controlling the amount of air trapped under the feathers, they are able to move above and below water with ease. Grebes can catch small fish and invertebrates by diving or by slowly and stealthily submerging themselves under the water.

Fish are the main food for most species of grebes. Grebes also eat a wide variety of aquatic invertebrates including various insects, leeches, crayfish and other crustaceans, and snails and other mollusks. Grebes will also eat frogs, tadpoles, and other small aquatic vertebrates. Natural diets vary not only from species to species, but within the same species, based on what is available within a specific habitat. Grebes are opportunistic and the body of water in which they live will largely dictate their diet. For example, Pied-billed Grebes in general favor fish such as carp, minnows, catfish, sculpins, killifish, sticklebacks, gizzard shad, and sunfish; but those living in the fishless wetlands of Manitoba primarily survive on a diet of tiger salamanders (Muller and Storer 1999).

*Hand-Rearing Birds*, Second Edition. Edited by Rebecca S. Duerr and Laurie J. Gage.

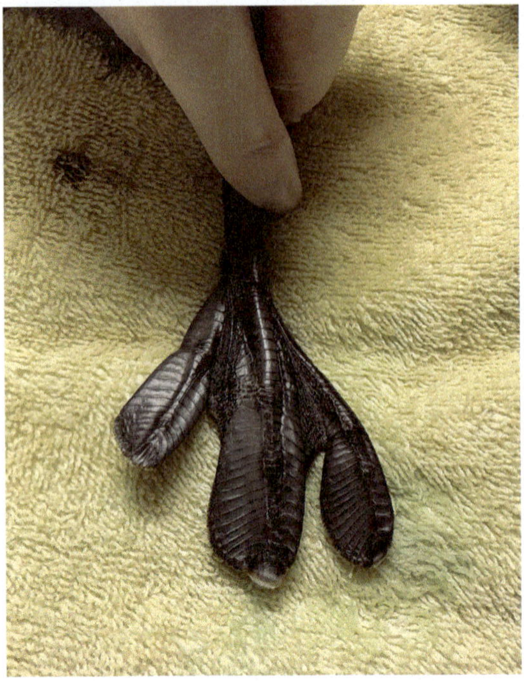

**Figure 10.1** Foot of a Pied-billed Grebe chick. Other grebe species often have reduced webbing between the digits and stiffer toes overall. *Source:* photo courtesy of Wildlife Rehabilitation Center of Minnesota.

Grebes nest where they live, and build floating nests of cattails, grasses, and other vegetation in freshwater lakes, ponds, slow moving rivers, estuaries, and marshes. They situate their nest where thick vegetation grows out of the water, and a portion of the heat necessary for incubation is thought to be provided by decomposing vegetation built into the nest (Muller and Storer 1999). There are variations from species to species, but 3–10 light-blue to white eggs are laid and incubated for approximately 21–23 days for smaller species: Black-necked, Pied-billed, Horned, and Least; and smaller numbers of eggs incubated for 25–28 days for larger species: Western, Clark's, and Red-necked. Both parents cooperate to incubate and care for the young when they hatch. Hatch weight also varies from species to species and ranges up to 30 g in Western Grebes (LaPorte et al. 2013). Grebes are highly susceptible to breeding failure due to human disturbance on lakes by water recreational vehicles, and nests may be left high and dry if the water levels of reservoirs drop during breeding (Plumas Audubon Society 2016). Western and Clark's Grebes are known to hybridize and may produce young during fall or winter in southern regions (e.g. Southern California).

The semi-precocial young are mobile, covered with dense down, and have their eyes open at hatching; however, they require parental care for food, warmth, and protection from the elements and predators. Hatchling grebes will spend most of their time during the first few weeks of life nestled on their parents' backs, with short forays into the water to drink, defecate, practice swimming, and to learn how to forage for food. Parents share the responsibility of carrying the chicks equally. When transferring duties, one parent will "dump" the chicks off their back into the water only for the other parent to come and let the chicks climb onto theirs; dumping the chick into water also stimulates the chick to defecate. The unencumbered parent will then forage for food and offer it to the young grebes (LaPorte et al. 2013). It takes 6 weeks for hatchling down to transition to juvenile plumage, with flight feathers coming in around 10 weeks of age. Grebes become independent of their parents at about 8–12 weeks of age, depending on the species. At 6 months of age, grebes reach 75% of their adult size and will find a mate and breed within 1 to 2 years of age.

Fledgling age Western and Clark's Grebes have shown parenting behavior toward hatchlings in rehabilitation, even allowing hatchlings to climb on their backs (Elliott 2007).

Grebes and their young are especially vulnerable to predation during the nesting season and will employ various tactics to evade predators when confronted with danger. If a predator approaches, nesting parents may sit tight, lunge at the predator, or attempt to flee if the chick is old enough to be able to attach itself to the parent by clamping its beak securely onto the tail. Parents who see a predator while they are away from the nest may feign injury or try to distract predators from any vulnerable young that are in danger (Muller and Storer 1999). For grebes, predation can come from the land, the sky, or the water. Known predators include gulls, large fish, birds of prey, raccoons, and mink. Eggs are also subject to predation from ravens, crows, and rats.

## Criteria for Intervention

Disruptions and accidents caused by human activity are the most common reason for chicks to come into a rehabilitation setting. Young grebes are often discovered separated from their parents due to disturbances by boats that cause the young to fall off their parent's back and become separated from them. Injuries from boat propellers or entanglements with fishing line are also known to occur. There is some anecdotal evidence of chicks being adopted by others into their colony, but more research needs to be done and, in most cases, chicks are suffering from dehydration, weakness, aspiration, or injury; thus, human intervention is warranted. Wild fostering is never a viable option for unhealthy or compromised chicks.

It is important to understand the needs of rearing a grebe to the point of release before undertaking their rehabilitation. The ability to maintain a constant supply of appropriate foods and provide adequate pools for swimming needs to be taken into consideration; transferring chicks to a facility with these capabilities is ideal. When working with these birds, careful attention must be paid to preserving waterproofing and the prevention of captivity-related secondary problems.

## Record Keeping

Detailed information should be collected from the person presenting the chicks. Find out the circumstances under which the chicks were found, if they were fed or given water, how long they have been in the person's possession, and if they were exposed to compromising environmental conditions for any length of time. It is good practice to assign patient numbers to each bird that is received and, if there are multiple birds being rehabilitated, employing temporary plastic leg bands will help keep patient identities straight.

In addition to the information collected upon presentation, the following details should be recorded for each patient: species, admission date, location found, reason for admission, admission weight, medical problems, and final resolution. Dated medical records should be maintained throughout the rehabilitation process that include findings from examinations, any treatment prescribed, amount and kind of food offered, amount and kind of food consumed, medications administered, daily body weights, general behavior, and responses to treatment. Information collected over time from multiple patients can help serve as guidelines for administering future rehabilitative care, and can help define expected ranges for growth, weight, and development. Collected data can also aid in optimizing the treatment of certain illnesses and injuries. See Appendix A for an example of a rehabilitation medical record and Chapter 1 for more information on record keeping.

## Initial Care and Stabilization

It is important to stabilize newly admitted orphans before handling them excessively and before administering any invasive care. Orphans are likely to be dehydrated, cold, exhausted, and hungry, so addressing these basic needs should be the first priority. Give the chick a quick, cursory examination to see if there are any life-threatening injuries that require immediate action, and then place the bird in a dark, quiet brooder to warm them. This quiet time will also allow the chick to recover from the inevitable stress that preceded presentation. Brooders should have a soft, padded substrate and should be set to 86 °F (30 °C) with a humidity level of 40–50%. A cardboard box or plastic container with a heating pad set to low and placed under a soft towel works well for warming grebes of any age. The heating pad should only fill half of the space, to allow the bird to move away from the direct heat source if they become overheated. After about 15–20 minutes the chick should be warmed and ready for a thorough examination. Warmed birds will be more active and alert and will start to vocalize.

After a complete examination, birds that can hold their bodies and heads upright and seem physically stable should be placed in a shallow tub of water so they will drink (Figure 10.2). The water should be warmed to 80–85 °F (26–29 °C). If the bird will not drink on its own, use a finger to gently tip the head forward, dipping the beak into the water. This maneuver should prompt the bird to drink. If a few attempts are unsuccessful, and if the bird is able to hold its head upright, fluids should be delivered using an orogastric tube. If the chick becomes waterlogged or struggles, end the first swim session immediately, towel dry the bird, and place it back on heat to dry before oral fluids are given. If the chick self-hydrates and doesn't run into trouble during the first short swim, it can proceed to routine care described in later sections. If needed, subcutaneous (SQ) fluids may be given; however, these can be difficult to administer due to the dense down, so should only be administered by a care provider who is skilled in this method of hydration. Intravenous (IV) fluids are easily given in older chicks into the medial metatarsal vein, but young chicks may be too small for this route. Lactated Ringer's solution (LRS) and Normosol-R® are isotonic fluids and work

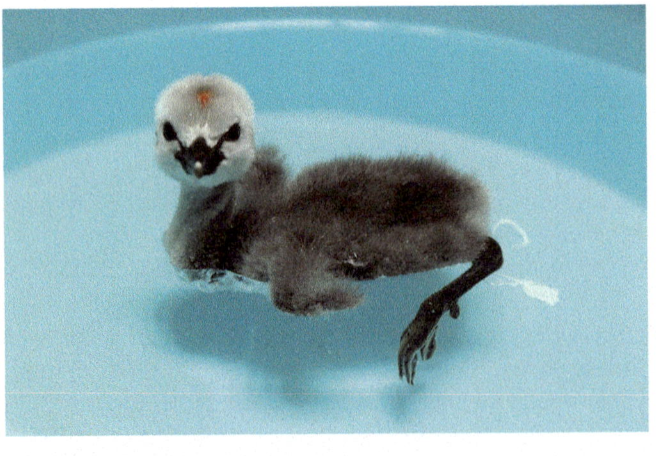

Figure 10.2 Swimming stimulates grebe chicks to defecate. This Western Grebe chick is having a quick swim in a small tub. Note the chick is floating comfortably and his downy plumage appears dry. Chicks must be kept scrupulously clean to maintain waterproof plumage. *Source:* photo courtesy of International Bird Rescue.

well for rehydration. Human infant oral rehydration fluids, such as unflavored Pedialyte®, may be given orally by orogastric tube. Fluids should always be warmed to 102.2–104 °F (39–40 °C) before administration (Perlman 2016).

Grebes in general require more fluids than would be expected by their body size to avoid clinical dehydration and may become dehydrated whenever kept out of water for any reason. Healthy birds that are only mildly dehydrated can be given one to two oral doses of fluids at 2.5% of their body weight. Once these are absorbed and the chick is active and alert, or after about an hour, they may be offered food. Moderately dehydrated birds, with tenting of the skin or dry mouth, require a few more doses of fluids at hourly intervals. The oral cavity of severely dehydrated birds is pale in color with reduced, stringy saliva. Their eyes are sunken and tented skin is slow to return to its normal position; the chick's skin may feel firmly attached to its underlying tissues (i.e. their skin feels "shrink-wrapped"). Severely dehydrated birds require a more prolonged course of rehydration, and IV fluids are recommended if the chick is large enough to access the medial metatarsal vein; 10–20 ml/kg of warmed sterile isotonic electrolytes as a slow bolus two to three times per day using a 25-gauge butterfly catheter works very well.

The digestive system cannot function when the bird is significantly dehydrated. Feeding should be initiated as soon as possible, but only after the bird's hydration level and behavior normalize. Once the bird is warmed, then hydrated, and then fed, it should begin defecating and can be considered stable and ready for continued rehabilitation.

## Common Medical Problems and Solutions

### Large Grebe GI Syndrome

Typically, grebes come into care suffering from dehydration, starvation, and hypothermia. Large grebes are especially prone to developing dysbiosis, intestinal and cloacal bloating, diarrhea, and cloacolithiasis when emaciated and severely dehydrated; hence, aggressive fluid therapy is warranted in debilitated large grebes. Hemodilution has not been observed in severely dehydrated Western or Clark's Grebes receiving up to 20 ml/kg bolus IV fluids up to three times daily in conjunction with seven times a day tubings of fluids and dilute diets at 50–70 ml/kg. Some debilitated grebes will drink when swimming, but others do not; thus, frequent access to water is not a guarantee against dehydration, and cloacoliths may form even in birds housed in water around the clock. Movement of the legs during swimming appears necessary for normal elimination in grebes, and extremely debilitated grebes often benefit from swimming in warm water.

Grebes that produce gritty droppings are at risk for development of cloacolithiasis, which can progress to necrotizing cloacitis which permanently damages the cloaca wall. The author (RD) has found treatment with aggressive fluid therapy combined with a combination of a gastric protectant (sucralfate 1 ml/kg orally q8h), an antibiotic (Trimethoprim sulfamethoxazole 100 mg/kg orally q12h), a laxative (lactulose 0.3 ml/kg orally q8h), and an anti-inflammatory (meloxicam 0.5 mg/kg orally q24h) has substantially improved survival from this problem. Clinical signs of this syndrome include lethargy, hunched posture, cold body temperature despite waterproof plumage, gritty droppings, blood in droppings, abdominal bloating, and/or prolapsed vent. Grebes with more than small amounts of blood or tan pieces of tissue (usually sloughed intestinal wall) in droppings should be humanely euthanized due to a poor prognosis.

### Aspiration Pneumonia

Aspiration pneumonia can occur if food or water is introduced into the lungs or air sacs either by inappropriate feeding techniques, or due to a weak bird becoming submerged and inhaling water before coming into rehabilitative care. Due to their watery habitats and frequent interaction with boats, a compromised chick can easily inhale water, so rehabilitators should be vigilant for symptoms of aspiration pneumonia in new grebe patients. If it is available, an oxygen-rich environment should be provided to birds with signs of respiratory distress, and antibiotics may be indicated.

### Aspergillosis

Grebes are susceptible to aspergillosis, although antifungals are not usually given to healthy chicks. Prophylactic antifungal medications may be prudent in grebes with other significant health problems, such as wounds or aspiration.

### Trauma

Fledgling grebes are sometimes presented with traumatic impact injuries. Large-bodied grebes require a long water runway to take off; hence, after a wing fracture, recovery of normal flight capabilities can be difficult or impossible to assess before release. Because grebes maneuver with their legs to find prey, normal lower extremity function is absolutely necessary for successful release. Tibiotarsus and tarsometatarsus fractures and hock joint luxations hold a poor prognosis due to anatomic surgical and medical management challenges. Toe fractures may be splinted but luxations do not heal well and may warrant amputation. See Duerr (2017) for guidance on the treatment of orthopedic injuries in grebes.

Supplemental heat should be withheld from patients with traumatic head injuries to keep possible swelling at a minimum. Nonsteroidal anti-inflammatory drugs (NSAIDS), such as meloxicam, may be given to help with pain and to reduce swelling. Head trauma patients should be contained in a dark, quiet enclosure at an ambient temperature of 70–75 °F (21–24 °C). Unsteady patients who are potentially unable to swallow and self-feed safely should be fed via orogastric tube until stable.

Grebe chicks are sometimes caught by predators such as cats or hawks, and may have wounds requiring surgery. Hawk talon punctures may cause subcutaneous emphysema (air under the skin) that may not resolve until holes into the body cavity (usually located deep to a small skin scab) are sutured. Grebe chicks caught by cats or other mammalian predators should be treated with antibiotics, such as amoxicillin with clavulanic acid (125 mg/kg orally q12h), until wounds have completely healed, and even very small wounds may impact waterproofing and benefit from closure. See Duerr (2016) for the surgical techniques necessary for the repair of lacerations in diving birds.

### Endoparasites

Grebes often carry heavy burdens of intestinal parasites such as tapeworms. Chicks entering care at older ages may need deworming, such as with praziquantel at 20 mg/kg once, with a repeat dose 10 days later. Ivermectin is used for feather lice and roundworms at 0.2–0.4 mg/kg orally once; again, this is usually only a problem in older chicks or adults.

### Avoiding Captivity-related Problems

Great care should be taken to avoid captivity-related issues that can compromise a grebe's chance for wild release. Although these issues are less common in chicks than adults, foot and hock lesions may occur when skin is abraded on hard substrates or when the skin dies due to pressure between a hard surface and a bony prominence, such as at toe joints. These lesions can become contaminated and infected, and may progress to infection of the underlying bone or joint. Prevention of these captivity-related problems is far superior to treatment. Grebes unable to remain in water during their rehabilitation due to injury or contamination may benefit from applying preventative foot wraps or keel protectors, or being kept in a soft-sided, net-bottom cage. See Goodman et al. (2016) for examples of appropriate nonaquatic housing for diving birds. That being said, grebes that are waterproof and thermoregulating should be housed in water, as prolonged dry housing inevitably causes severe problems.

Grebes, even as young chicks, maintain their waterproofing by preening their feathers to regularly organize the fine structure of each feather's barbules and barbicels to create a barrier impermeable to water. Preening also distributes oil from the uropygial gland that keeps the feathers supple and helps maintain the integrity of the feather structure. The loss of waterproofing can adversely impact every aspect of a grebe's rehabilitation. Compromised waterproofing is a common result of becoming soiled by food or feces in a captive setting that fails to meet their needs. Loss of waterproofing can also be present due to an injury sustained in the wild where there is an exposed wound and feather damage, or it can occur when feathers have been exposed to contaminants such as oil before the bird has come into care. When waterproofing is lost, diving birds not only lose the ability to control their buoyancy but also have no protection from the wet and cold, and will eventually succumb to hypothermia.

Birds suffering from a loss of waterproofing will need repeated, carefully controlled sessions in clean water to preen and restore their feather condition. During this time, rehabilitators should take care that the bird never becomes chilled, and carefully monitor improvements to feather condition. Grebes that are heavily contaminated may need to be washed or rinsed if unable to waterproof themselves within a small number of days. Debilitated patients may lack the ability or energy to preen, so their feather condition should be carefully and constantly monitored. It is critical that the water in pools used to house waterbirds is kept scrupulously clean at all times.

## Diets

Since each species of grebe has evolved adaptions for catching and eating their prey, as well as adaptations to specific hunting environments, it is important to become familiar with the natural history of any grebe species in care. There are many commonalities among grebe species. In general, similar diet and rehabilitative care may be applied to all grebes. As a rule, the size and the shape of the bill reflect the types of prey the particular species eats. These bill characteristics should be taken into consideration when choosing foods. Grebes swallow their food whole, so take care to ensure that offered foods are not too large for the bird's mouth. That being said, Pied-billed Grebe chicks have been photographed swallowing surprisingly large crayfish whole.

It can be difficult to replicate the wide variety of foods that a grebe would consume in the wild, but best efforts should be made to present the patient with foods that are as similar as possible to what they naturally would find and consume. Grebes primarily eat fish, plus insects and other invertebrates, and therefore this is the diet they need in captivity.

Grebes should be offered live feeder fish and insects such as crickets and mealworms. Various small-sized live feeder fish may be obtained from a bait or pet store and easily kept in a 30 l or larger aquarium with a filtration system. Live crickets can typically be found at most pet stores. It is always best to add as much diversity into the diet as possible to encourage food recognition and good self-feeding behaviors, as well as to provide nutritional variety. Appropriate live fish include rosy reds, minnows, fingerling carp, threadfin shad, crayfish, herring, and small smelt. Insects that may be fed include crickets, mealworms, water fleas, and water beetles. Pools and water containers should always be treated with a dechlorinating agent 20 minutes before adding live fish, if the water has chlorine in it. Live fish should be kept in water that matches the temperature of the pool to which they will be added so they do not die quickly.

Live food is ideal but not always available, and may be expensive. Thawed frozen fish can be used but this does not help teach the chick hunting skills. Dead fish should always be supplemented with 35 mg of thiamine and 100 mg of Vitamin E per kilogram of fish. The optimal calcium-to-phosphorus ratio is 2 : 1 and small-bodied fish may have poor ratios similar to mealworms. Deboned fish is very high in phosphorus and low in calcium, so extra calcium will need to be provided to make up the deficit if deboned fish is being fed. Twelve grams of calcium carbonate powder (4800 mg of elemental calcium) should be added to each kilogram of deboned fish, resulting in 0.4–0.8% of the complete diet (Perlman 2016). Deboned fish are also deficient in many other nutrients, as the organs are the primary sources of many vitamins such as A and D. If small pieces are needed to feed a particular chick, be sure to feed the viscera in addition to muscle tissue. Similarly, young chicks eat fish roe eagerly, but it is also deficient in many nutrients, especially calcium.

If tube-feeding is necessary, a slurry can be made by blending fish in a food processor until a consistency is achieved that will easily move through a syringe and orogastric tube. The addition of insects will add nutritional diversity to the diet. Prepared diets should always be fed at room temperature, refrigerated if not used immediately, and used within 24 hours. Cold food can be allowed to sit out for a short length of time to take the chill off; however, slurry should not be heated to warm it up since fish cooks at very low temperatures and heating will affect the bioavailability of the nutrients in the diet.

Grebe chicks are regularly fed soft contour feathers by their parents beginning shortly after hatching, and they continue to consume them throughout adulthood. Feathers are mainly obtained from the parents' own bodies while they preen, but occasionally they are found floating on the water and taken either by one of the parents or by the self-feeding chick. The consumed feathers form into a compacted mass that creates a plug in the gizzard. This plug slows food passage and allows more chemical digestion to occur before further passage. A second distinct mass of feathers is typically found in the pyloric pouch, which finally prevents indigestible matter from entering into the intestine. Research suggests that the purpose of eating feathers is to slow down the digestion process (Jehl 2017). The undigested material and some of the feather matter are regularly regurgitated as cast pellets, which may assist in minimizing the presence of gastric parasites (Piersma and Van Eerden 1989). Feathers have been found to comprise over 50% of the stomach content for several species of grebe, indicating that their consumption is intentional and relevant to the grebe's digestive system (Muller and Storer 1999). Since grebes seek out notable quantities of feathers to feed to their chicks, these should be made available to grebes at all stages of their care in captivity. Donor feathers should be small clean contour feathers and can be obtained from grebes that did not survive rehabilitation or older current patients. Chicks will usually eagerly eat these feathers (Figure 10.3).

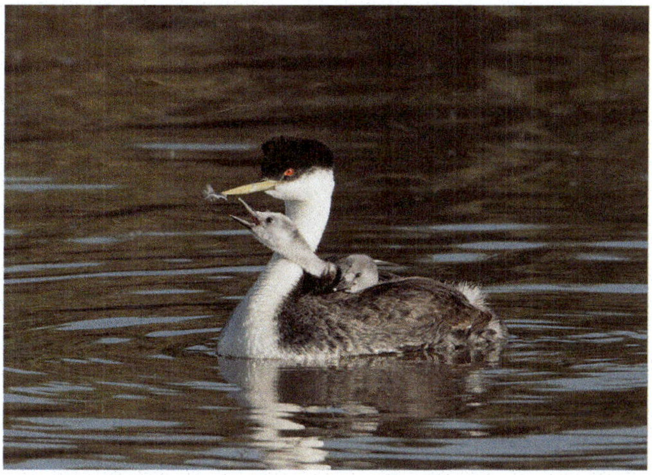

Figure 10.3 Adult Western Grebe feeding a contour feather to a chick nestled on its back. *Source:* photo courtesy of Ron Dudley.

## Feeding Procedures

Grebes hatch with their eyes open, maneuver to the edge of the nest, enter the water, and climb on their parent's back just hours after hatching. Hatchlings understand how to accept food from their parents' beaks immediately, and are fed this way for the first 2 days of life. By the third day, they are already attempting to eat from the surface of the water and are developing critical hunting and foraging motor skills. It is important to allow even very young captive grebes to demonstrate their ability to self-feed before resorting to other feeding methods. By first observing what the chick is capable of, one can gauge the level of intervention, if any, that is needed. Any grebe more than 10 days old should be capable of self-feeding unless it is compromised due to exhaustion, illness, or injury. Counting the fish or insects provided, and those remaining after the chick eats, allows quantitative tracking and recording of consumption.

Once a grebe's ability to self-feed is known, it, along with the bird's age and condition, may be used to help determine what feeding method is most suitable. Birds that are debilitated or otherwise not interested in eating can be gavaged by orogastric tube, or force-fed by placing food deep in the mouth, well behind the glottis. Willing eaters may be hand-fed with a blunt-tipped hemostat if they happen to be very young or if they do not have the stamina or strength to forage (Figure 10.4). Capable eaters should be allowed to self-feed on food placed in the water.

It is important to weigh birds daily to make sure they are consuming enough food, especially while the bird is new and their self-feeding abilities are being assessed. A good rule of thumb is to make sure they are receiving in milliliters the equivalent of 5% of their body weight in grams per feeding. Consistent weight gain should be seen daily; if a chick is losing weight rather than gaining, carefully re-evaluate the bird, as a medical problem may have been overlooked or a new problem may have developed. It is easy to miss small puncture wounds in the fluffy plumage. Scabs are sometimes revealed at wet spots.

### Hatchlings

Young chicks should be fed to satiation hourly during daylight hours and should be encouraged to self-feed before any attempts at hand-feeding are made. This is accomplished by placing them in a small tub with water that is 65–75 °F (18–24 °C) and 3–4 in. (8–10 cm) deep and contains small fish,

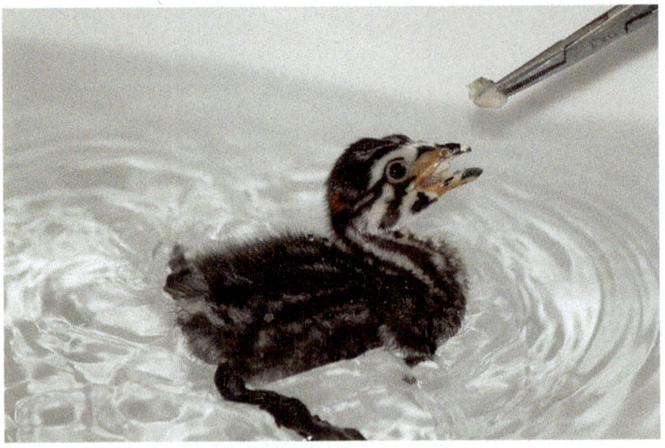

Figure 10.4 Pied-billed Grebe chick being offered small pieces of whole fish from hemostats. *Source:* photo courtesy of International Bird Rescue.

or in a dry enclosure with crickets. Be sure to step out of sight to avoid distraction and allow them to focus on the movement of the food. Food in motion is highly attractive and helps the young grebe develop its food recognition skills. Performing this exercise before more assisted meals provides the needed motivation of hunger. Small feathers should be offered alongside food or floating on the water at feeding time. After the bird has defecated and eaten its fill, allow it to climb out on your hand and return it to the dry nest container, being sure to keep all enclosures clean between visits. Even if the chick is being hand- or tube-fed, it requires hourly short swims in order to stimulate defecation. Such chicks will only need to be in the water for long enough to drink and defecate, after which they will call and demonstrate a need to be removed. If cries are heard between swim sessions, offer food via hemostats, and increase the amount of food being fed. Methods of assisted-feeding are described below.

#### Hand-feeding

Offer food to the bird's beak with a hemostat, ideally while the bird is swimming or, if necessary, while in the dry nest box. Allow for some learning time while the bird learns how to accept food this way. They may shake the food and fling it around while they master maneuvering it from beak into mouth.

#### Tube-feeding

Appropriately-sized soft rubber French urogenital catheters can be cut to the required length and work well for tube-feeding when attached to a luer tip syringe (see Figure 6.1). Any feeding tube should have a soft, rounded end to avoid injury; hence, any cut tubing must have its cut end burned or filed to remove sharp edges. Draw up the desired amount of food, plus slightly more to fill the tube, and make sure there are no air pockets in the syringe. Depress the plunger to fill the tube prior to feeding, to avoid introducing air into the stomach. Hold the tube next to the bird to gauge the length that you will need to reach the stomach at the back of the rib cage, and either mark the tube or place a finger there. Do not get any food on the bird's feathers or handle the bird with dirty hands. Gently open the beak at its tip, and insert the tube at the bill's commissure (where the upper and lower portions of the beak meet), down the right side of the bird's throat, passing over and avoiding the glottis. Extend the neck so the tube can be gently guided down the esophagus on the right side of the neck. A correctly placed tube will move easily and can be seen beneath the skin as it passes down the side of the neck. Stop once you feel any resistance or the mark at the top of the tube has reached the commissure. Keep the neck extended to avoid reflux as you deliver the contents of the feeding syringe. If the tube is not luer locked in place, it is helpful to hold the tube–syringe junction, to avoid accidental separation as you put pressure on the plunger. Carefully watch the throat, and at any sign of upwelling (reflux) of food, immediately cease feeding. In this case or when the syringe is empty, gently remove the tube. If reflux should occur, immediately release the bird and allow it to clear its oral cavity on its own.

**Force-feeding**

Carefully insert a fingernail between the upper and lower beak near the base or at the tip and then slide it to the base and open the mouth from a point near the face. Place small insects, fish, or slivers of fish in the back of the mouth using a blunt-tipped hemostat and allow the bird to swallow. If not swallowing, gently close the beak, extend the neck, and stroke the neck downward to move the food toward the stomach. Do not dirty the neck feathers with fishy fingers if doing this.

### Fledglings

At the fledgling stage, healthy grebes should be self-sufficient and becoming skilled at diving for food; they should be fully feathered with their waterproofing intact. They will spend more time in the water and should be allowed free access to a large pool with a haul-out. Fledglings should be offered as many live fish as possible, but will usually accept small, thawed frozen freshwater fish or slivers of large fish of the correct size for their mouth. Take care that slivered fish does not contaminate water or plumage with fish juices. Feathers should be continually available for ingestion until release. Food should be provided to healthy fledglings three to four times per day during regular intervals during daylight hours. Offering slightly more food than the fledgling can consume will ensure they are fed to satiety. Some species of grebes may eat their own body weight in food per day during certain stages of growth. If ravenous hunger is observed, increase the available food so that there is always more than enough to ensure the chicks are getting plenty to accommodate a growth spurt.

## Expected Weight Gain

There is no compiled information available about daily weight gain averages for grebes, only species-specific generalizations based on different geographical areas. The best approach is to make sure that weight gains are observed and to use the body condition and behavior as a guide. If a grebe is growing, active, and alert, appears generally healthy, and is offered as much food as it is able to consume, it is likely to be growing at a normal rate. Grebes will vocalize their hunger, so this too can help determine when more food should be provided. Body weights should be collected daily to ensure the bird is gaining weight continuously and to give rehabilitators data toward establishing typical and normal patterns of growth, for different grebe species. Weight gain information for small numbers of chicks in rehabilitation are shown in Figure 10.5.

## Housing

Very young, sick, or injured grebes should be housed in a brooder, or a container with a heat source that can be set to 86 °F (30 °C) with soft padding as a substrate. Feathers must be kept in pristine condition, so bedding should be changed at least twice per day to keep the feathers from becoming soiled. Grebes should be given ample opportunities to take short swims in water so they can

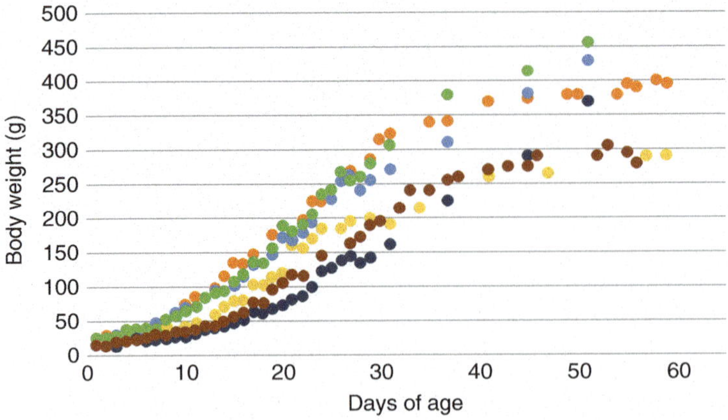


Figure 10.5 Weight gain of six Pied-billed Grebe chicks during rehabilitation. The split curves at maximum weight likely reflect the sexes of the chicks, as males are generally about 100 g heavier than females.

exercise, feed, and defecate naturally. Young grebes should not be left alone in water, however, until they are fully waterproofed. Allowing grebe chicks to swim before, during, and after feedings for as long as they are able will help them develop strength, keep their gastrointestinal tract motile, aid in keeping feathers clean, and allow them to practice their diving skills.

There are several ways to approach housing for young grebes, but all methods should take two key points into consideration: the bird must have easy access to a dry area, and the water needs to remain clean at all times to preserve feather condition and to keep pathogens at a minimum. As chicks become more adept at swimming and foraging, the depth of the water can be increased to allow for more diving and maneuverability. Self-feeding chicks can be housed either in a multi-container system of one dry nest and two tubs of water (where the water is continually changed in both, but at any given time in the container they are not using), or they can be offered a pool that has a trickle filtration system which, once set up and running, is a very efficient and reliable way to keep the water continuously clean.

As grebes grow and become self-sufficient, their housing needs will change. To keep their feet and keel protected from abrasions, grebes should only be exposed to very soft, padded surfaces until the bird is able to spend all of its time in the water. Ample access to water and pools is critical, and should be introduced as soon as possible, based on each bird's ability and health rather than by age or size. Grebes are flock birds and socialization is crucial for their development, so young chicks should be housed with similarly sized conspecifics whenever possible. Solitary birds should have a mirror placed along the water line. Some species, such as Pied-billed Grebes, can become aggressive as they mature, so older birds should not be left together unattended until you are certain they are getting along. Rehabilitators must familiarize themselves with the behavioral tendencies of any species in care when considering putting groups of birds together, as some birds can be aggressive when housed with others of their own or other species.

Swimming containers should increase in size as the grebe chick grows and needs more space to swim, forage, and dive. A dishpan or medium plastic tub works well for a 50–60 g hatchling, whereas a 200 g bird needs at least a bathtub-sized pool. Plastic storage tubs of various sizes, children's pools, and plastic stock water troughs can all make suitable swimming habitats for grebes in captivity. Whatever container is used, it should be appropriate to the bird's needs and should have several inches between the top edge and the surface of the water, so the grebe cannot propel itself

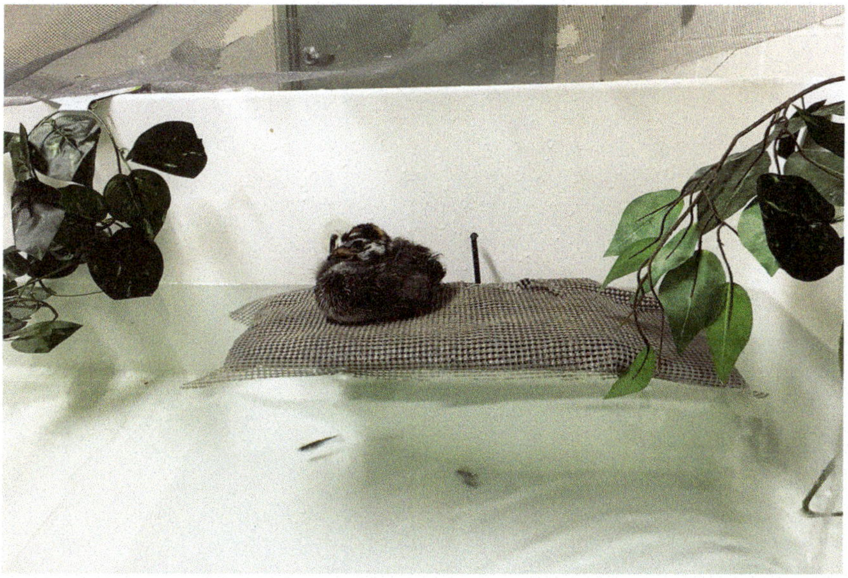

Figure 10.6 A young Pied-billed Grebe resting on a haul-out made from a wire platform that is covered in soft, porous shelf liner material and secured to the side of the pool. A heat lamp may be placed over the haul-out if needed. *Source:* photo courtesy of Wildlife Rehabilitation Center of Minnesota.

over the side. The water depth should be determined by how deep the bird can dive. It is important to provide housing based on the close observation of each bird's capabilities and consideration of its medical history. Some larger birds may require a large pool, but also may need to be moved to a safe, dry enclosure overnight if supervision is necessary.

The wet brooder shown in Figure 10.6 is set up to accommodate a healthy young Pied-billed Grebe. The haul-out is above the water line and has a nonslip soft mesh for a substrate, small live fish are available for the chick to capture; other food offerings can be placed on the haul-out island as needed to supplement once the chick is self-feeding. A heat lamp can be placed over the haul-out until it is no longer needed. Netting covers the top of the pool and a hose is set on low so a small amount of water is added while a small amount is also allowed to drain out to keep the water from becoming soiled and stagnant. Knotless netting and other substrates could also be used for the haul-out, but must always be nonabrasive to delicate grebe feet.

The recommended pool size for grebes that are completely self-feeding and independent is 6 ft. (1.8 m) diameter × 2 ft. (0.6 m) deep (Miller 2012). When upgrading to a larger pool, it is prudent to spend some time carefully observing the bird's ability to swim, forage, and generally navigate the larger space, before leaving the bird unattended.

All pools should have an accessible, dry haul-out area so the bird can rest, preen, and warm itself when needed. Haul-outs for young chicks can be made by tightly stretching knotless, nylon netting over a 1 × 1 ft. (30 × 30 cm) × 1–2 in. (2.5–5 cm) thick piece of closed cell foam, or be constructed by wrapping Select Grip Easy Liner© shelf liner tautly around a PVC frame made of four 1 ft. (30 cm) pieces of 1 in. (2.5 cm) PVC pipe and four 1 in. (2.5 cm) unthreaded 90° PVC elbow joints. Larger birds should have a haul-out that is either made from a similarly covered 2 × 2 ft. (60 × 60 cm) PVC frame, or a piece of foam that is 2 × 2 × 3 ft. (60 × 60 × 90 cm) and covered in 1 in. (2.5 cm) knotless nylon netting (Figure 10.7). Haul-out coverings can be secured with zip ties and the whole unit positioned so birds can easily climb onto them and should be attached to the pool side or anchored

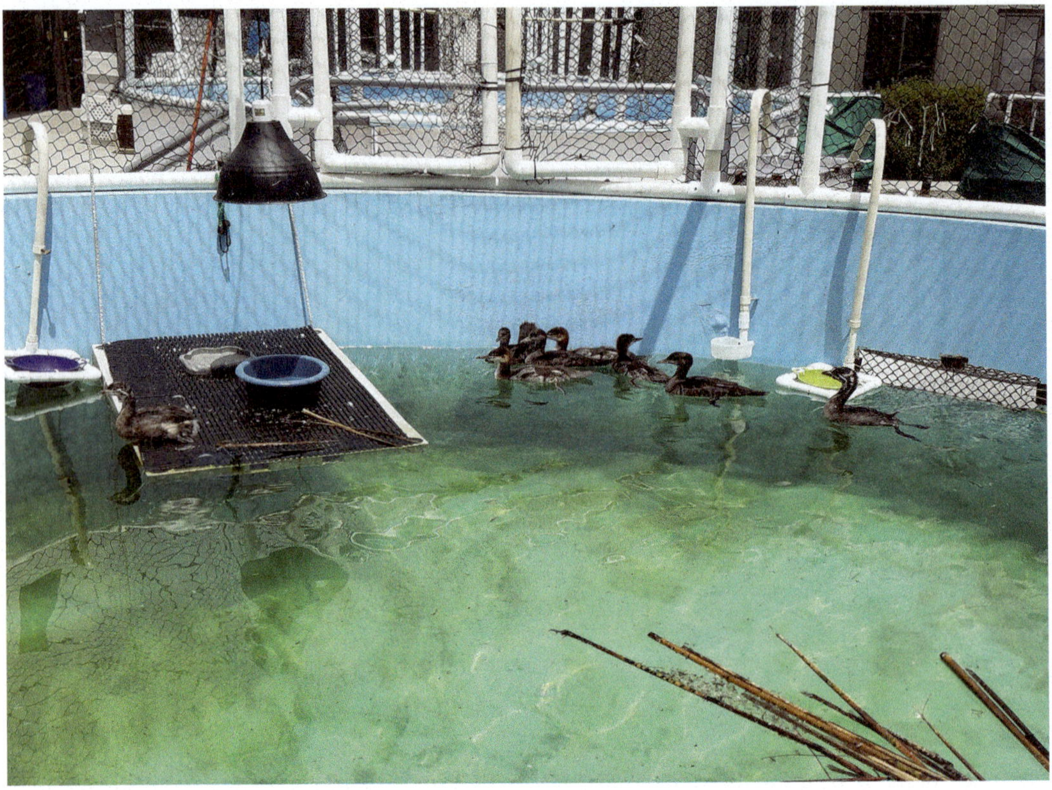

Figure 10.7 Large pool set up for fledgling Pied-billed Grebes (with similarly-sized mergansers). Note the angled haul-out with heat lamp and assortment of food dishes supplementing supplies of live fish with other foods. *Source:* photo courtesy of International Bird Rescue.

to the bottom of the pool with a rope tied to a weight such as a brick. Take care to position the cut off zip ties such that sharp areas are not accessible to the birds.

Pools should ideally be located outdoors in a quiet, protected area and water temperatures should be kept around 65–70 °F (18–21 °C). If the weather is unseasonably cool, a heat lamp should be provided for younger birds and positioned above the haul-out to help them maintain their body temperature. Most heat lamps will indicate the correct distance that they should be placed from the bird, so one should take care to set it up appropriately. The area should be protected from both aerial and ground predators and should have a visual barrier to give birds a sense of security and keep visual contact with their human caregivers to a minimum. Netting can be used over pools to provide overhead protection, but will also allow natural sunlight into the enclosure. If a bird is kept indoors, full-spectrum lighting on timers that mimic natural photoperiods should be supplied.

Birds that are waterproofed, have transitioned from hatchling down to juvenile down, and are capable of swimming for extended lengths of time should be housed full time outdoors in the largest pool that is available, at least 6 ft. (1.8 m) diameter × 2 ft. (60 cm) deep. At this point, no external heat source should be needed. Larger birds may leap out of the pool if startled so a 1 ft. (30 cm) protective barrier or surround should be in place at the top of the pool to keep them contained. Any flexible material that can withstand moisture can be used. Some examples are: waxed cardboard, flexible plastic, netting, or a fiberglass window screen secured to stakes, and linoleum. Solid materials have the advantage of providing additional privacy for the birds. Netting should be used to provide a ceiling for the pool to prevent premature release in birds able to take flight from small pools, and to provide protection from aerial predators.

A filtration system is recommended for efficiently keeping larger pools clean and is a worthwhile investment when rehabilitating waterbirds. Not only is the patient disturbed less frequently, since the entire pool does not need to be cleaned out as often, but the water is continuously kept moving so there is less risk of feather damage as just one instance of unnoticed soiled water can compromise waterproofing on a bird. Existing pools can generally be modified to accommodate the addition of a filtration system. See Chapters 6 and 9 for more tips and information about waterproofing, brooders, and pools suitable for grebes.

If no filtration system is available, a hose can be placed at one edge of the pool with the water set to a low trickle. A drainage hole should be placed at the water line on the other side of the pool so the surface water is allowed to drain off. Overflow cleaning should be done periodically for pools without filtration systems. This can be done by filling the pool to the top edge and letting the water overflow for several minutes. This will help flush out and minimize contaminants from food and feces building up in the water. Swimming pool nets and siphons should be used daily to remove larger debris that settles to the bottom.

## Preparation for Wild Release

Grebes can be considered ready for release when they are 8–12 weeks old, capable of hunting live fish, completely waterproof, free from illness or fully recovered from any injuries, and appropriately wary of humans. Flight feathers should be mostly grown in at this stage, but do not need to be fully mature prior to release. Waterproofing can be tested by removing the haul-out for 48 hours and then checking to ensure that the contour feathers are completely dry without any compromised areas that are wet to the skin anywhere on the body. Keep a close eye on any grebe that is being tested in this way and intervene if the waterproofing test shows signs of failure.

Birds should be released near the location where they were found into a suitable habitat that ideally has other grebes of the same species. Birds should only be released when mild weather is expected for at least 3 days so they have an opportunity to get their bearings and adapt to life in the wild. It is important to track migration timing if a grebe is ready to be released close to or during migration. During this time, it is important to always introduce a newly released bird into a flock so they can join any migration movements of their wild conspecifics.

## Acknowledgments

Many thanks to Sandie Elliott for her work on the first edition of this chapter, and for caring for grebes for many years. Thanks to the staff and volunteers of both Wildlife Rehabilitation Center of Minnesota and International Bird Rescue for their efforts on behalf of grebes.

## Sources for Products Mentioned

Leg Bands: National Band and Tag Company, 721 York St, Newport, KY 41072–0430, (800) 261–8247, www.nationalband.com.

Netting: Duluth Fish Nets, 4976 Arnold Road, Duluth, MN 55803 USA, (800) 372–1142, www.duluthfishnets.com.

Stock Water Troughs: Agri Supply, 409 US East Highway 70, Garner, NC 27529, (800) 345–0169, www.agrisupply.com.

Filtration System Equipment: The Pond Guy, 15425 Chets Way, Armada, MI 48005, (866) 766–3435, www.thepondguy.com.

## References

Duerr, R.S. (2016). Surgical repair of keel lesions and lacerations in aquatic birds. Proceedings of the Association of Avian Veterinarians Annual Conference at ExoticsCon, Portland, OR, pp. 83–88.

Duerr, R.S. (2017). Other diving and marine birds (grebes, loons, alcids, others). In: *Topics in Wildlife Medicine Vol. 4: Orthopedics* (eds. R.S. Duerr and G.J. Purdin), 137–144. St. Cloud, MN: National Wildlife Rehabilitators Association.

Elliott, S. (2007). Grebes. In: *Hand Rearing Birds* (eds. L. Gage and R. Duerr), 81–90. Ames, IA: Blackwell.

Goodman, M., Schott, R., and Duerr, R.S. (2016). Waterfowl (ducks, geese, and swans). In: *Topics in Wildlife Medicine Vol. 4: Orthopedics* (eds. R.S. Duerr and G.J. Purdin), 99–100. St. Cloud, MN: National Wildlife Rehabilitators Association.

Jehl, J. Jr. (2017). Feather-eating in grebes: a 500-year conundrum. *The Wilson Journal of Ornithology* 129 (3): 446–458.

LaPorte, N., Storer, R.W., and Nuechterlein, G.L. (2013). Western Grebe (*Aechmophorus occidentalis*). No. 026a. In: *The Birds of North America Online* (ed. A. Poole). Ithaca, New York: Cornell Lab of Ornithology.

Miller, E.A. (ed.) (2012). *Minimum Standards for Wildlife Rehabilitation*, 4e. St. Cloud, MN: National Wildlife Rehabilitation Association.

Muller, M.J. and Storer, R.W. (1999). Pied-billed Grebe (*Podilymbus podiceps*). No. 410. In. In: *The Birds of North America Online* (ed. A. Poole). Ithaca, New York: Cornell Lab of Ornithology.

Perlman, J. (2016). Nutrition and nutritional management. In: *Avian Medicine*, 3e (ed. J. Samour), 28–29. St. Louis, Missouri: Elsevier.

Piersma, T. and Van Eerden, M.R. (1989). Feather eating in Great Crested Grebes *Podiceps cristatus*: a unique solution to the problems of debris and gastric parasites in fish-eating birds. *Ibis* 131 (4): 477–486.

Plumas Audubon Society. (2016). Audubon's Aechmophorus Grebe Conservation Project, Comprehensive Monitoring Report: 2010–2016 Almanor, Antelope, Davis, and Eagle Lakes, Plumas and Lassen Counties, California. http://www.plumasaudubon.org/uploads/1/1/8/1/11812806/pas_grebe_monitoring_2010-2016_nov_2016.pdf (accessed 20 August 2018).

# 11

# Flamingos

*Laurie Conrad and Susie Kasielke*

## Natural History

There are six species of flamingo: Greater Flamingo (*Phoenicopterus roseus*), American Flamingo (*Phoenicopterus ruber*), Chilean Flamingo (*Phoenicopterus chilensis),* Lesser Flamingo (*Phoeniconaias minor*), Andean Flamingo (*Phoenicoparrus andinus*), and Puna Flamingo (*Phoenicoparrus jamesi*). All have similar natural history characteristics. They feed primarily on aquatic invertebrates and algae by filtration, form monogamous pairs, breed in dense colonies of thousands to over a million pairs, and are long-lived. As colonial wading birds, flamingos nest on or near water sources and rely on water for building nest mounds of mud and reducing predator activity. A single egg is laid atop a volcano-shaped mound built by the pair. Both the sire and dam incubate the egg for 27–30 days and feed the chick with crop milk, produced in the lining of the adult crop. In the wild, chicks are reared in crèches, allowing parents to leave the colony to feed while a few adults provide "day care." Chicks fledge at 65–90 days.

## Criteria for Intervention

### Wild Colonies

Rescue of chicks from wild colonies depends on the species, population concerns, likelihood of intervention causing additional chicks to become abandoned, and the governmental regulations and cultural norms in the affected habitat. Disturbance or water level fluctuations may cause nest abandonment, and abandoned flamingo eggs and chicks will not survive without intervention if not already part of a crèche. In the right conditions, eggs may hatch days after abandonment leaving chicks to die on the mound. Legislative issues combined with animal welfare and conflicting input from stakeholders may delay intervention while decisions are agreed upon, particularly with no disaster management plan. Delays in care lead inevitably to worsening condition and prognosis for rescued chicks. It is ideal for wildlife regulatory agencies to have a management plan based on possible contingencies in advance, particularly in places where a large breeding area is within an urban district or is heavily observed by a concerned public. Intervention that results in rescue of hundreds to thousands of chicks requires resources equivalent to a large oil spill, with a management structure to supply knowledgeable and timely decision-making, sufficient experienced caregivers, and appropriate housing, food supplies, and funding.

*Hand-Rearing Birds*, Second Edition. Edited by Rebecca S. Duerr and Laurie J. Gage.

While human intervention in wild flamingo colonies is rarely needed, in 2000, a jaguar ran through a flamingo colony in Ría Lagartos Biosphere Reserve, Mexico, disrupting the breeding and causing the abandonment of over 1000 American Flamingo eggs and an estimated 400 chicks. Caretakers, including professionals from SeaWorld and other Association of Zoos and Aquariums (AZA) organizations, assisted in hand-rearing chicks at Xcaret and Rio Lagartos with many ultimately released back into the Yucatan wetlands.

Environmental conditions influencing water levels and breeding conditions for Lesser Flamingos resulted in thousands of adults abandoning eggs and chicks at Kamfers Dam in Kimberley, South Africa in January, 2019. Thousands of chicks were rescued with the best of intentions but without preplanning, resources, or onsite experience to support the rescue. Ultimately, a vast array of stakeholders became involved in the care of the chicks: NGOs; wildlife rehabilitation centers and veterinary hospitals; private facilities; the Kimberley community and SPCA; zoological facilities within Africa and supporting organizations from around the world; along with different layers of South African governmental oversight. Although many chicks were in extremely poor condition at rescue, several hundred were successfully released; outcomes and post-release survival of rescued and rehabilitated chicks remains a work in progress at the time of writing. This immense collaboration to save thousands of birds increased awareness about the species and the massive resources necessary to rescue flamingo chicks. Scientists, rehabilitators, and zoo professionals continue to gather intellectual data to document the lessons learned and to improve best practices.

## Captive Breeding

Flamingos are wary of intrusion into nesting areas, but in zoological settings hands-on management is usually necessary and can be done safely with the appropriate protocols. Abandoned eggs and compromised chicks may need to be removed for care. Colony and mound management, coordination and planning reduce the interruption of the colony and improve parent-rearing opportunities, reducing the need to hand-rear birds.

Flamingos synchronize breeding as a colony, but hatching may occur over 2 to 3 months. Birds require leg banding for identification to track the sire and dam of chicks. Identifying mounds only may result in errors because of the changing colony dynamics throughout the nesting season. SeaWorld California (SWC) has routinely entered the flamingo breeding site since the early 1990s and performed maintenance and chick checks. The colony habituated to intervention over time and the birds now defend the sites and do not leave the mounds mid-season. At the end of the season when only a few pairs remain at the site, the birds may leave the breeding area to find safety within the colony.

Adult pairs may push another pair off of a mound and destroy the less dominant pair's egg or drop or abandon an egg. Intervention to retrieve eggs requires caregivers to analyze the genetic value of the egg and the activity and stage of development of remaining eggs on surrounding mounds. For example, an overdue egg may be left abandoned between mounds rather than disturb birds near a hatching egg. Pairs given an artificial egg will incubate the "dummy" egg which provides opportunities for fostering eggs. When removing the egg from the mound, label it with mound and egg numbers in pencil. Candle eggs and map out mound activity to record visual data necessary for assessments. Pairs may build mounds that are cylindrical rather than volcano-shaped. Chicks may not be able to climb back on some mounds and become damp and chilled or injured by adult flamingos. Nest area maintenance allows chicks to return to steep mounds. Add buckets of dirt to build bridges between mounds or on one side of the mound while the eggs are candled and prior to chick hatch. Adding water by misting birds or running a hose into channels between the mounds provides water for the birds to continue to mound-build throughout the season. Chicks on neighboring mounds can be removed for health checks and will be accepted back by the parents when placed back on the mound or vicinity of the parents. As long as the parents have heard the chick vocalizing, they will still accept chicks 2 weeks or more after removal from the nest site. When a Great Blue Heron threatened flamingo chicks at SWC, chicks of various ages were pulled to the hand-rearing room for over 2 weeks and then returned to the parents without issue. Empty mounds can be knocked down allowing the chicks to crèche on flat areas as chicks stop spending time on the mounds.

## Record Keeping

Best practices in husbandry and animal care require keeping accurate and thorough data. Record individual identification numbers, daily weight, percent weight gain per day, feeding frequency and volume fed per feeding, housing temperature, and water feedings for each chick. Include comments on behavior and developmental changes, environmental changes (temperature and housing), and fecal output. Also note medical issues and treatment for each chick. Recording weights on a weight comparison chart is recommended to analyze differences in chick weight gains per individual. Record observations and changes made to feeding guidelines.

## Incubation of Eggs

Incubate flamingo eggs at 99.0 °F (37.2 °C) and 45–50% relative humidity (RH). Move the egg to hatcher parameters of 98.0 °F (36.7 °C) and 55–60% RH once the egg pips externally. Cease turning at this time and set the egg in the hatcher on a nonslip surface such as rubber shelf liner. Refer to Chapter 3 for further information.

## Initial Care and Stabilization

Once the chick hatches; lower the temperature of the hatcher to 97.0 °F (36.1 °C) and reduce the humidity to 50% RH. Swab the chick's umbilicus with a sterile povidone-iodine swab. The umbilicus should be closed and clean appearing. The newly hatched chick will appear wet, but will dry with a fluffy white or gray appearance as it rests in the hatcher. The chick's legs are pink at hatch and appear swollen. They will lose the swollen appearance after a few days and the skin will appear to be "peeling" as the legs grow – this is normal. Weigh the chick and record all data. Color mark the chick's down with permanent markers or food coloring for identification. Move the chick to the brooder once it appears dry, alert, and responsive, usually 3–4 hours after hatch.

Flamingos are typically housed in open enclosures in zoological facilities, which requires the birds to be flight-restricted. This may be accomplished by pinioning, or removal of the carpal segment of one wing, at 2–6 days of age. The procedure is fairly simple but must be done by or under the supervision of a veterinarian. The small amount of blood generated may be submitted to a laboratory (Animal Genetics) for gender determination via DNA. Pinioning birds later is a major surgical procedure and typically results in a poorly healed site. Flight restriction can also be done by clipping off flight feathers but requires birds to be handled every few months, which is not well-tolerated. Most zoological facilities insert a small, subdermal microchip implant (an integrated circuit device or Radio Frequency Identification Device (RFID) transponder encased in silicate glass), typically placed in pectoral muscle, that contains a unique identification number that can be linked to information contained in an external database (AVID® Identification Systems).

## Common Medical Problems and Solutions

### Omphalitis/Open Umbilicus

Wet hatches from eggs that have not lost sufficient weight during incubation and contaminated water sources in incubators can both cause incomplete closure of the umbilicus and/or infection caused by gram negative bacteria (see Chapter 3). Antibiotics or surgery may be necessary for chicks that hatch with an open umbilicus. Consult with a veterinarian.

### Pododermatitis

"Bumblefoot" or pododermatitis is an infection on the plantar surface of the foot. Proper substrate on a soft but textured material with a flat surface combined with exercise reduces bumblefoot. Discourage chicks from standing on a hard, flat surface for prolonged period of time. Provide non-slip matting, grass, or a similar substrate and encourage frequent walking. If a chick develops cracks or ulcers on the bottom of the foot, clean and disinfect the area and use Super glue® or tissue glue to close the crack. Antibiotics may be necessary to prevent infection. Once a crack develops, the foot should be monitored closely. Flamingos will walk onto mats soaked in dilute disinfectant (Nolvasan®) if placed in front of feeders. The solution should just cover the mats to prevent flamingos from ingesting it.

### Leg Abnormalities

Inadequate diet, exercise, and/or sunlight exposure can easily result in leg problems, including slipped tendons and rotation. Flamingos raise young on cone shaped mounds for about the first week of life until the chick is large enough to begin walking around the nest site in increasingly further distances from the mound. Parents brood the chick tightly the first 24 hours and then increase the exposure to sunlight rather rapidly after the first week. Flamingo nesting sites are generally found in brackish, wetland habitats on mudflats in direct sunlight. Provide indoor-raised chicks with adequate exposure to UVB light for proper vitamin D metabolism. Vitamin D and calcium are integral nutrients for proper leg development. Standard fluorescent, incandescent, and halogen lights provide a poor substitute for sunlight (Gehrmann 1987). Provide an outdoor exercise area if weather permits (Figure 11.1).

Proper diet and exercise reduce leg issues, but if these occur many can be corrected when caught early. Kinesio Tex Gold™ tape creates tension on the flamingo leg to encourage growth in the correct direction to correct angular limb deformity issues (Collinsworth 2014). If caught early enough, the growth plates on the bird's leg have not closed, allowing the corrective changes to occur. Legs should be visually checked daily throughout the growth phase. Limping is often one of the first symptoms of growth issues which can be painful to the chick. Severe cases of angular limb deformities may require the bird to be placed in a sling during care. Flamingo chicks should be standing for short periods by day 3 and are able to climb off the mound by day 10. Hand-reared flamingos

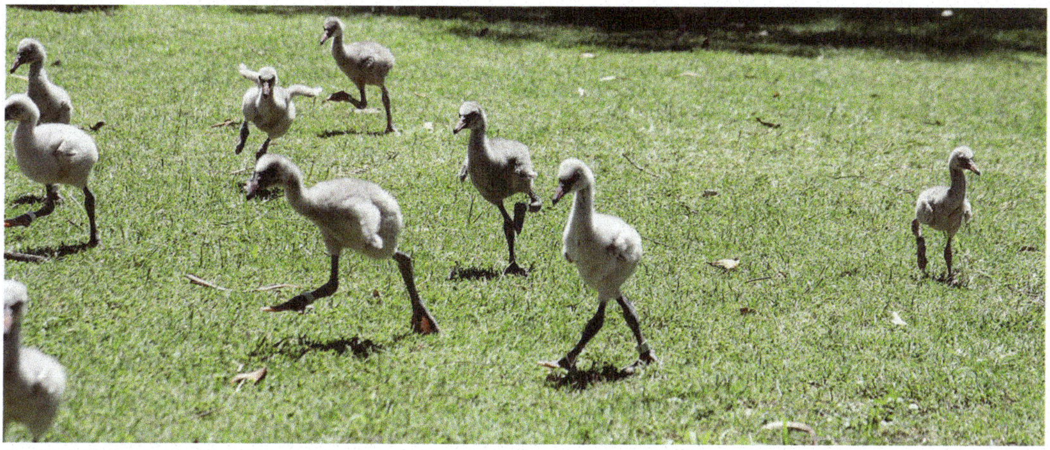

Figure 11.1 Rescued American Flamingo chicks hand-reared at Ría Legartos Biosphere Reserve, Yucatan Peninsula, Mexico.

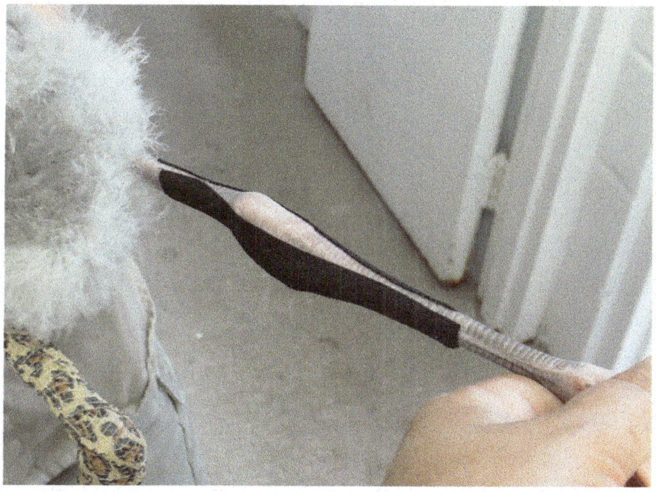

Figure 11.2 Kinesio tape applied to correct leg/joint deviation in a flamingo chick. Corrective tape is then lightly covered with soft, flexible bandaging tape. *Source:* photo credit: Shelly Collinsworth, courtesy of Fort Worth Zoo.

should be encouraged to stand and walk regularly from day 3 until housed in the adult habitat. Small or crowded enclosures may lead to leg issues (Figure 11.2).

## Feces and Pathogens for Flamingos

Assess fecal output at each feeding. Expect to see the fecal color change during the first few days. Yellow-colored feces after hatch are common as the chick is still processing its yolk. Fecal color will initially appear dark orange and may change to a dark green color (bile) as it transitions from the yolk to water to formula. Feces may look red or oily when krill in the diet is processed. Feces should be a quick "projectile squirt." If a chick is seen straining or produces thick and small droppings, replace the next scheduled feeding with oral water feedings and continue until hydration is improved (see "Hydration" in Chapter 18). Consult with your veterinarian when diarrhea, solid light brown, sweet, or sour smelling feces are noted.

### Mosquito-borne Diseases

Flamingos are susceptible to several common mosquito-borne diseases, such as avian malaria, avian pox, and West Nile virus (Shannon 2007). Juvenile flamingos at many zoos are vaccinated against West Nile virus. Caregivers raising birds released into wild habitats should seek approval and coordinate prophylactic treatments with governing agencies from the in situ country/region.

## Imprinting

Flamingos easily and willingly follow caretakers around enclosures or out of enclosures while exercising. Many zoos currently imprint and habituate flamingos as animal ambassadors and flagship species for habitat conservation and education. Birds reared in captivity will pair up and breed at 3–4 years of age. SWC's ambassador flock of 25 birds build mounds, lay eggs, and rear chicks despite participating in daily guest interactions. Incubating females stay at the nest while the remaining colony leaves the exhibit to interact with park guests. The males from breeding pairs defended the nest site and successfully reared chicks despite frequent contact with people and nest intervention. The results show that habituated flamingos will display normal breeding behaviors and reproduce once mature.

Birds reared without the additional handling and interaction required to raise ambassadors rarely truly imprint on people when reared within a "crèche" or a small group of birds, but will habituate to being hand-fed during their dependent period. Flamingos focus on feeding and bickering with conspecifics when talking and unnecessary handling is reduced. Chicks reared for release to the wild have been reared in this manner and even seemingly human-imprinted birds will integrate into the colony as they wean.

## Diet

The sire and dam both produce crop milk that is fed to the chick during the rearing period. Most zoos feed modifications of a pellet-based diet with fish, krill, and egg or, less commonly, a simpler egg-based diet when hand-feeding chicks (Shannon 2007). The diets strive to meet the nutritional needs of the growing chicks. The SWC diet in Table 11.1 is a pellet-based diet. Modifications made over a 20-year period have resulted in proven success and changes made to the recommended diet may not yield the same hand-rearing results. Leg development issues with use of the egg-based diet were reported by three facilities in 2018. It is not clear whether the issues were diet-related or due to other causes but similar issues have not been reported with the pellet-based diet. Once a preferred diet is chosen for hand-rearing, talk with others who have used the diet to inquire about hand-rearing challenges and avoid duplication of issues. Hand-rearing techniques and diets continue to evolve and professionals usually share techniques willingly.

Blend ingredients well (about 60 seconds). Strain the formula into a bottle using a fine mesh strainer and a funnel. Label the bottle with the date and time. Store refrigerated formula for up to 24 hours or freeze small portions for up to 30 days. Warm a portion of chick formula by floating a

Table 11.1 SeaWorld California (SWC) Flamingo hand-rearing diet.

| | |
|---|---|
| 1 cup (237 ml) | Mazuri Flamingo Bits |
| 1300 ml | Filtered drinking water |
| 75 g | Krill (thawed, water squeezed out) |
| 75 g | Herring (heads, tails, and fins removed) |
| 75 g | Hard-boiled egg yolk |
| 1 tsp (4.8 g) | Vionate powder |
| ½ tsp (2.4 g) | $CaCO_3$ powder |
| 250 mg | Vitamin B1 (thiamine) |
| 600 IU | Vitamin E (squeeze oil into mix from capsule before blending) |

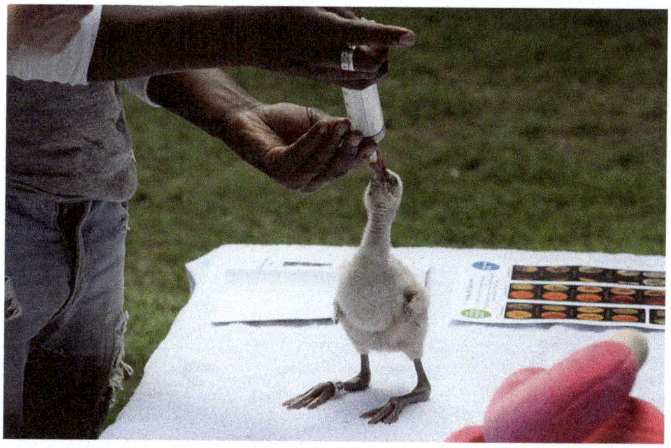

Figure 11.3 Oral feeding of flamingo chick via catheter-tipped syringe.

small container in hot tap water prior to each feeding. Do not microwave the formula. Discard the unused remainder after each feeding.

## Feeding Procedures

Stabilize the chick's temperature and ensure hydration prior to feeding. Chicks pulled for medical reasons should be stabilized and examined by a veterinarian. Two different feeding methods yield successful results. Many caregivers prefer administering hand-rearing diets with a syringe and a catheter tube, by gavage. Tubing birds with a long feeding catheter during triage situations in a recovery effort or emergency response saves time and is the faster method; however, it holds some risks. Flamingo crops are located very ventrally and their necks are very long. If tubes are not placed deep enough into the crop and food is deposited in the esophagus, birds are at risk of life-threatening regurgitation and aspiration. Feeding chicks directly into the mouth, via syringe, allows the chick to refuse feedings which acts as an indicator of inadequate chick thermoregulation or hydration (Figure 11.3). Syringe-feeding without a catheter may also lead to earlier self-feeding. Warm the diet to 98–100 °F (37–38 °C). The diet should feel warm to the touch, but not hot. The chick may refuse the hand-feeding diet if it is too cold, while formula that is too hot can burn the chick's crop. The volume of the hand-feeding diet received by each chick increases progressively with age until the chicks are 5 weeks old, and thereafter stabilizes (Burch and Gailband 2000) (Table 11.2). Chicks initially parent-reared may take several attempts before they solicit a feeding or give a feeding response. Chicks that refuse to eat may need to be tube-fed.

Provide two water feedings prior to introducing the diluted formula when chicks have been partially parent-reared. It is normal for flamingo chicks to ingest dirt from around nest sites and initial fecal output may look like "dirt" output.

Fecal output will transition from green to brown to krill-colored if feeding a krill-based hand-feeding diet. Fecal output should appear watery, but will normally change color. If the chick does not give a feeding response and brooder and diet temperatures are consistent and within set parameters, dilute the formula to a 50 : 50 formula-to-water ratio. Provide drinking water by day 5 so that the chick can begin to self-regulate.

### Day 1

The chick's gut is still processing yolk material at this stage, and overfeeding can overwhelm the gut resulting in stasis. Feed about 1 ml water prior to feeding the hand-rearing formula. Feed 50 : 50 (formula-to-water) every three hours for the first six feedings. Dribble the formula into the chick's bill via a 1 cc syringe at a 45° angle. The chick will eat while sitting down. The neck should always be outstretched during feedings and the chick will vocalize and sway its head back and forth as if it is feeding from its parents. Initially, the head may need to be supported using a thumb and forefinger held in a circle under the chick's lower mandible. Immediately check the environmental and food temperature when a chick refuses to eat. Assess hydration by looking at fecal output, eyes, and by performing a "tent" test on the nape of the bird's neck. Usually, fecal output is the most obvious indicator of hydration, and must be monitored closely. The dilution of the formula controls hydration of the chick. The SWC chick diet is very thin and appears "watery." Monitor the chick's hydration throughout the rearing process and dilute the hand-feeding diet if needed. Attempt to give water orally if the chick refuses the formula and has food remaining in its crop.

### Day 2

Weigh the chick daily before the first morning feeding and calculate percent gain or loss. Chicks may lose up to 15% of their initial weight in the first few days as they use the remaining yolk reserve. Feed the chick 75 : 25 (formula-to-water) six times per day. The volume may exceed 10% of bird's weight per feeding. Feed to a full crop and watch fecal output. Gradually increase the formula amount throughout the day. Feed 1–2 ml of water midway between each feeding. Water is quickly absorbed and does not reduce the nutrient content of the hand-rearing diet as diet dilution does. Satisfy caloric intake without sacrificing water intake. Assess fecal consistency and quantity as indicators of hydration when increasing the strength of the formula. Watch for dehydration during the transition period and anticipate the need for supplemental fluids.

### Day 3

Feed 100% formula five times per day. Feed conservatively by starting at the volume from the last feeding on day 2 and increasing the volume gradually. The chick may likely need to continue to

Table 11.2 SeaWorld California (SWC) Flamingo hand-rearing guidelines.

| Age (days) | Housing, Temperature, and Humidity | Feeding Frequency | Diet | Volume | Comments |
|---|---|---|---|---|---|
| 0 | 96–97 °F (35.6–36.1 °C) in Hatcher | 1 × day | Do not feed for 12–24 hours.<br>Give water if chick hatches in the afternoon.<br>25 : 75 formula: water<br>Warm food via hot water bath.<br>Feed with 1 cc syringe. | 1–2 cc | Chick will dry off in hatcher and use yolk sac. |
| 1 | 95 °F (35 °C)/50–60% RH in Animal Intensive Care Unit (AICU) | 6 × day | 50 : 50 formula: water<br>Feed with 1 cc syringe. Give water between feedings for at least six feedings. | 10% of a.m. body weight per feeding. | If the fecal volume is low, evaluate increasing formula volume. |
| 2 | 94 °F (34.4 °C)/50–60% RH | 6 × day | 75 : 25 formula: water.<br>Feed with 1 cc syringe.<br>Give water between feedings for at least six feedings. | 10% of a.m. body weight per feeding | Do not overheat chick.<br>Check leg development daily. Expect weight loss. |
| 3–4 | 93 °F (33.9 °C)/50–60% RH | 6 × day | Transition to 100% formula.<br>Feed with 1 cc syringe.<br>Supplement with 1–2 cc water in between feedings as needed. | 10% of a.m. body weight per feeding | Provide access to sun 30 min daily from now on.<br>Encourage standing and walking. Ensure daily exercise, increasing as tolerated, from now on. |
| 5 | 91 °F (32.8 °C)/50–60% RH | 4 × day | 100% formula<br>Feed with 3 cc syringe.<br>Supplemental water feedings as needed.<br>Introduce to self-feeding. | ≥10% a.m. body weight per feeding | Evaluate hydration in between feedings.<br>Provide shallow flat dish with 1 in. (2.5 cm) of water and bits or crushed pellet sprinkled in. Change every hour.<br>Expect a weight gain. |

(*Continued*)

Table 11.2 (Continued)

| Age (days) | Housing, Temperature, and Humidity | Feeding Frequency | Diet | Volume | Comments |
|---|---|---|---|---|---|
| 6–7 | 90 °F (32.2 °C)/50–60% RH | 4 × day | 100% formula<br>Feed with 3 cc syringe.<br>Supplemental water feedings as needed. | same | Chick should be standing and walking.<br>Chick should reach hatch weight. |
| 8–9 | 88 °F (31.1 °C)/50–60% RH | 4 × day | 100% formula<br>Increase size of feeding syringe as needed. | same | Move to outside holding during the day. |
| 10–12 | ~85 °F (29.4 °C)/ambient humidity<br>in floor “corral” with heat lamp | 4 × day | same | same | |
| 13–14 | ~82 °F (27.8 °C)/ambient humidity | 3 × day | same | same | Continue to change food tray out frequently.<br>Monitor leg growth. Watch for bowing or uneven growth. |
| 21 | | 2 × day | same | same | Continue to change food and water in trays frequently.<br>Should be able to stay outside in temps 55 °F (12.8 °C) and above. |
| 28 | | 1 × day | 100% formula<br>Feed pellet diet ad lib. | same | Continue to monitor leg development. |
| ~35 | | wean | Feed pellet diet ad lib. | | |

receive water feedings in between formula feedings. Return to 75 : 25 if the chick does not clear its crop by the next feeding, refuses food, or has thick fecal output. Hydration is more important than weight gains on day 3 and it is normal for the chick to have a weight loss on day 3. The transition to 100% formula and also the transition to self-feeding is subjective, and there is species, as well as individual, variation. Carefully assess fecal output and hydration as volume and frequency of feed decisions are made.

### Day 4–5

Reduce feedings to four times daily. Expect to see a weight gain on day 5, although the chick might not reach hatch weight until day 6. Begin encouraging self-feeding as soon as the chick can stand by offering food items in water (crushed Mazuri® Flamingo Pellet, Mazuri Flamingo Bits, and/or krill). Mazuri Flamingo Complete and Mazuri Flamingo Bits currently provide the necessary nutrients for use as a chick pellet during weaning. Other commercial flamingo diets have not yielded the same results. Change food and water trays every hour initially to encourage self-feeding and ensure freshness.

Throughout this process, be sure to weigh the chick and assess the weight gain from the previous day. If the weight gain is over 20%, feed a volume of 10% of the morning weight per feeding and do not increase the volume throughout the day. If the daily weight gain is below 5%, gradually increase the feed amounts throughout the day. When determining the initial morning amount, look at the volume fed at the last feeding, the evening before. If the chick refused formula or did not take the full amount, assess hydration and the frequency of feedings. As feeding volumes increase, the frequency of feedings will decrease and may be scheduled further apart. Once the chicks begin self-feeding, they may begin refusing feedings at any point during the hand-rearing process. The fecal consistency will indicate whether the chick is processing formula or pellet diet.

## Weaning

Early weaning saves labor and limited resources. No significant differences in weight gains occurred with early weaning while rearing nearly 50 chicks over a 20-year period. In zoological habitats, flamingo chicks and juveniles will chase parents and solicit feedings for a year or more. Wild chicks are fed by the adults up to 2–3 months (Shannon 2007). Weigh chicks to monitor weight gains and do not feed more than 60 ml of hand-rearing diet per feeding while offering the pellets. Hand-reared flamingos often continue to beg for feedings long after they have learned to forage and self-feed. Healthy chicks will begin to eat if you limit the volume to 60 ml and allow chicks access to food in a water source.

The chicks naturally begin the weaning process as they increase their pellet intake. Reduce hand-rearing diet feedings from four to three to two to one time daily and then offer adult diet only. The chick crop capacity quickly increases to hold up to 180 ml of fluid, but feeding larger volumes will lead to a longer weaning period. Chicks will continue feeding from a syringe for 6 months or longer if the formula is not reduced. Capping formula feedings at 60 ml while encouraging self-feeding results in earlier weaning and natural foraging behaviors.

Each chick weans at an individual pace and while some American Flamingos will wean as early as 21 days, others may take 60 days or more. There are also differences among species in the weaning period. Lesser Flamingos wean more slowly than American Flamingos. Chicks continue to grow in stature and need to continue gaining weight at this stage. Offer pellets at all times and change feed often until they are eating independently. As chicks ingest more pellets and water, fecal output appearance will also change and may be watery. This is normal as long as some solids are processed. Medical treatment or illness may necessitate modifications to the rearing process.

Plastic paint roller trays provide a sloped, nonslip, and shallow surface that functions perfectly as a water element in a small enclosure once the chick can easily walk in and out of the tray. Offer food in the tray and remove and replace the food and water every hour (Figure 11.4). Provide plastic bus trays as feed pans once the chick outgrows the paint tray. Transition birds to feed from pans that visually resemble the feeder type that will be offered in permanent housing. Wild released birds should forage from troughs and be given a large, clean water source to bathe in. Do not allow birds to bathe in food trays. Plastic gutters or narrow plastic planters can be used as troughs. Provide plastic children's pools or another large, shallow water source for the birds to bathe in separately from food. By 60 days, chicks should live outside in an adult sized enclosure unless prevented by predator activity or weather. Provide juveniles with supplemental heat in temperatures below 55 °F (13 °C). Many zoos house adult flamingos indoors when temperatures are 32 °F (0 °C) or below. Chilean flamingos can tolerate slightly cooler temperatures and are moved to indoor holding at temperatures below 20 °F (−6.5 °C) or if conditions are icy, to prevent falls (Nelson and Lynch 2018).

## Expected Weight Gain

It is typical for chicks to lose weight for the first 3 days. On day 4, a small weight gain may occur and it takes until day 6 to reach hatch weight following the guidelines outlined in this chapter. Anticipate ~7–10% weight gain per day (Figure 11.5). Weight gains may be smaller the day after a feeding is dropped. Usually, the chick will consume additional pellets to make up the deficit in the hand-rearing diet. Keeping the weight gains consistent at 10% or less per day will help to avoid leg

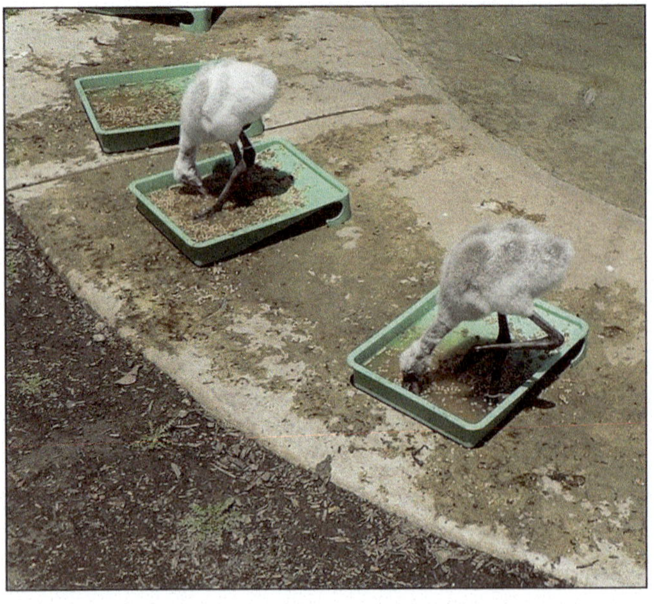

Figure 11.4 Flamingo chicks self-feeding from plastic trays.

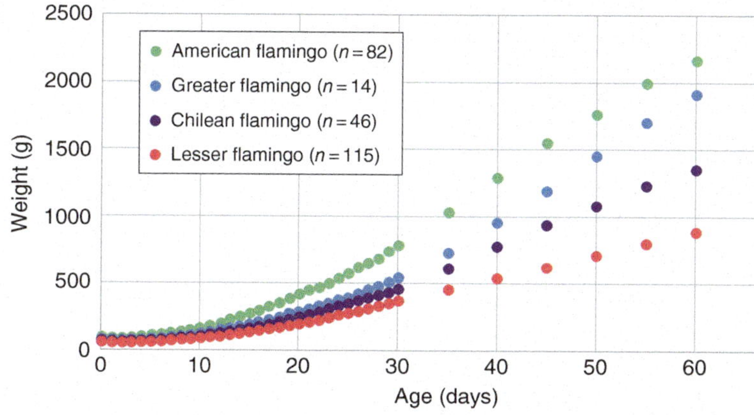


| Age (days) | American flamingo | Greater flamingo | Chilean flamingo | Lesser flamingo |
|---|---|---|---|---|
| 0 | 94 | 97 | 77 | 63 |
| 1 | 87 | 88 | 72 | 57 |
| 2 | 86 | 83 | 70 | 57 |
| 3 | 90 | 80 | 73 | 60 |
| 4 | 96 | 82 | 76 | 63 |
| 5 | 104 | 85 | 79 | 66 |
| 6 | 113 | 92 | 83 | 70 |
| 7 | 123 | 97 | 88 | 74 |
| 8 | 134 | 104 | 93 | 79 |
| 9 | 148 | 114 | 100 | 85 |
| 10 | 163 | 125 | 108 | 91 |
| 11 | 179 | 135 | 116 | 98 |
| 12 | 198 | 146 | 125 | 106 |
| 13 | 221 | 158 | 136 | 115 |
| 14 | 243 | 173 | 147 | 124 |
| 15 | 267 | 190 | 160 | 134 |
| 16 | 296 | 205 | 174 | 146 |
| 17 | 326 | 223 | 188 | 158 |
| 18 | 354 | 239 | 205 | 170 |
| 19 | 383 | 268 | 221 | 183 |
| 20 | 412 | 279 | 240 | 198 |
| 22 | 467 | 324 | 279 | 228 |
| 24 | 533 | 365 | 315 | 260 |
| 26 | 618 | 412 | 360 | 290 |
| 28 | 686 | 470 | 408 | 329 |
| 30 | 782 | 540 | 458 | 368 |

Figure 11.5 Growth chart for four species of hand-reared flamingo chicks.

problems. If weight gains are too high, formula can be diluted or a feeding can be dropped so that leg growth is even on each side of both legs. Uneven growth leads to joint issues, curved bones, and an uneven gait or limping. Growth plates will be open and the legs continue to grow for at least 3 months after hatch. Underfeeding can lead to dehydration. Weight gains should be monitored daily until the chick has weaned. Flamingos will approach adult weight between 2 and 3 months old, at fledging. When managing large numbers of chicks, it may be more stressful to catch and weigh individuals. Select small, thin appearing birds and weigh a sample group. Check flamingo crops after food trays are filled to evaluate appetites. Watch for competition and food trays and provide additional food areas as needed. Additional food should be added to food sources immediately after they empty so that the less-dominant birds can feed. If a bird is noted with an empty crop after a feeding, it should be monitored through observations and weighing.

## Housing

Chicks are housed in a forced-air brooder, such as an Animal Intensive Care Unit (AICU, Lyon Technologies), for the first 10–12 days after hatching. The brooder should be set at 96–97 °F (35.6–36.1 °C) and 55–60% relative humidity (RH), reducing the temperature 1 °F (0.6 °C) per day as tolerated by the chick. Flamingo chicks may require supplemental ambient humidity that can be provided by adding mesh-covered bowls of water or damp washcloths that are changed daily inside the brooder.

Similarly to ibis, hydration and temperature are critical to hand-rearing flamingos (see Chapter 18). Large fluctuations in temperature over the first few days may lead to illness or refusal to eat. Sometimes, overcorrection of temperature leads to overheating or chilling of the chick. Gradual corrections allow the chick to thermoregulate, although it may shiver for a few minutes. The most common problem is overheating and underhydrating during the first 2 weeks of life. Once hatched, turn the hatcher down 1–2 °F (0.6–1.2 °C) to ease the acclimation to the brooder. The chick hatches at 98.0 °F (36.7 °C) and should be brooded at a slightly cooler temperature when moved out of the hatcher. Maintaining a stable temperature within the brooder can be difficult if there are room temperature variations. Check the room conditions and adjust any HVAC vents to prevent drafts. Brooders next to windows and doors may also be subjected to fluctuations in temperature.

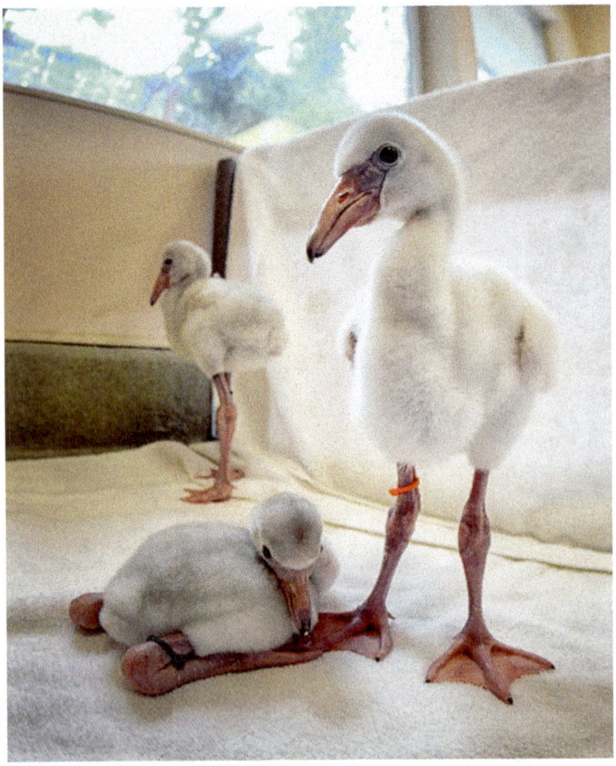

Figure 11.6 Chick floor housing and exercise bin with temporary dividers. *Source:* photo credit: Mike Aguilera/SeaWorld San Diego.

Sometimes chicks can be housed together if they are the same size, regardless of species. Larger chicks tend to pick on younger chicks resulting in bite marks on legs or refusal to feed. Larger species such as American Flamingos may outgrow smaller species such as Lesser Flamingos so it is necessary to watch for aggression when they are housed together. Divider panels to separate chicks provide housing flexibility. Exposing chicks to water early in the hand-rearing process helps them learn to feed and bathe rather than avoiding the water.

Move chicks to a larger floor "corral" or open box brooder between 10 and 12 days old (Figure 11.6). Continue to provide a heat lamp. Remove the heat gradually: turn heat lamps off during the day and on at night until the chick appears to be acclimated. Assess the chick's ability to thermoregulate once moved into the cooler enclosure and prior to removing heat at night. Temperature changes should be gradual and chicks should not be moved to areas with temperatures changes over 5 °F (2.8 °C).

At day 30 chicks may be moved to a larger enclosure and may need heat during the day and night – adjust the heat lamps gradually. Move chicks to an outdoor pen (weather permitting) during the day and back inside at night. Provide a plastic paint roller tray with water for the chick to dabble in. Do not use metal feeding trays because they can be too sharp and the bottom too slippery. Bus trays or plastic storage containers work well as feeders for older chicks. Always provide a ramp or other method that allows the chick to easily exit the water if housed near a pool. Additional details for housing can be found in the *Flamingo Husbandry Guidelines* (Brown and King 2001).

## Substrate

Substrate influences successful growth and development of bird limbs. In addition to proper diet and exercise, housing materials may cause or prevent developmental issues. Flamingos require a flat, nonslip surface to walk on during rearing. Rubber shelf liner or 3M Nomad matting works well as a substrate for young chicks in brooders. A washable material that can be cleaned and disinfected is recommended. Cedar or pine shavings are not recommended because flamingos filter-feed and naturally put their heads down in an attempt to kick up food and filter the water. When flamingos attempt to filter the shavings, their nares may clog which affects breathing, and if ingested will likely cause impaction. Newspaper is also not appropriate bedding for flamingos because it is too slippery. Similarly, all pool access should have a ramp free of rocks with a grade less than 20° for easy entrance and exit.

## Exercise and Sun Exposure

As with chicks of all long-legged bird species, daily exercise is essential for normal leg development. Encourage chicks to stand and walk beginning at 3 days of age. Chicks will readily follow caregivers for walks twice daily, increasing time and distance as they grow. Provide an outdoor exercise area if weather permits. Offer supplemental heat in outdoor areas until chicks are capable of thermoregulation and tolerate ambient temperatures.

Although the hand-feeding diet provides the required vitamin D, exposure to sunlight is important for vitamin D and calcium metabolism. Provide chicks supervised access to direct sunlight for at least 30 minutes daily beginning at 3 days of age, taking care to avoid overheating.

Lesser Flamingos will seek out sunny areas to loaf after feeding. The pen should have a large enough area for juvenile birds that weigh 1 kg or more to run and begin practicing flight (Figure 11.7). Pool and food bowl/trough placement should be carefully considered to allow birds a clear runway. The size of the enclosure and pool increases with the number of enclosed birds and they should have an area to run with wings outstretched.

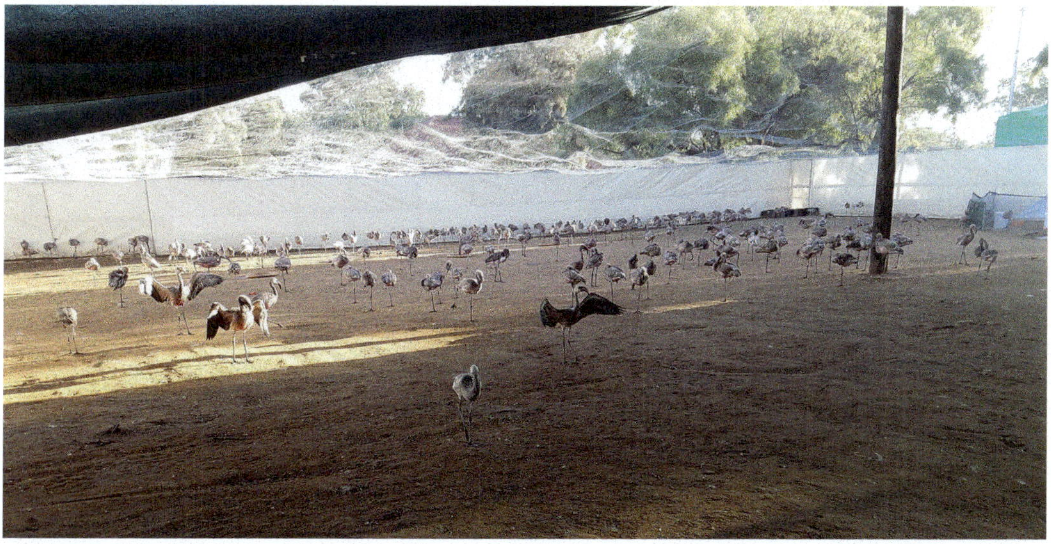

Figure 11.7 Large yard with shade and netting cover to allow ample room for exercise pre-release.

### Introduction to the Colony

Hand-reared chicks should be introduced to the zoological colony in open enclosures after they reach 3 months of age and are banded with an identification number. Chicks will continue to grow, but will be large enough to defend themselves against aggression from other flamingos and small predators. Ideally, chicks should be introduced as a group to reduce the attention on an individual and the chicks can crèche. There is safety in numbers. If introducing a group of chicks to the habitat, it is best to do this in the morning when they can be monitored over the rest of the day. The introduction will likely be successful if they are fully weaned, adjusted to ambient temperatures, and are able to recognize available food sources. If a single juvenile is introduced, it is advisable to only introduce it early in the day so that it can be carefully monitored. It may be necessary to pull the juvenile back for a few nights before it fully integrates into the flock. All chicks should be visually monitored to make sure that they are eating and behaving normally.

### Wild Release

The same principles should be applied to flamingos returned to wild colonies. Many scientific references discuss hard versus soft release for birds and other animals. Flamingos should be released using a "hard release" technique. The IUCN Conservation Translocation Specialist Group recommends health screening and quarantine prior to wild reintroductions (IUCN/SSC 2013). Taxa specific guidelines should be referenced and followed prior to release of the birds. Body condition and weight, feather condition, behavior, and overall physical health are evaluated by a veterinarian in addition to the recommended health screening prior to release. Once flamingos meet established release criteria they should be transported as close to the colony as possible. Flamingos will join the colony once they can see and hear the other birds. Juveniles should be released as close to the wild crèche as possible. Soft release is not recommended for flamingos.

## Acknowledgments

Thank you to Sherry Branch, Stephanie Costelow, Mike Mace, Christy Simeone, and past and present IUCN Specialist Group, AZA, and EAZA TAG members that have shared their knowledge and experiences to build upon and continue to improve animal care standards. And many thanks to the institutions who agreed to share their records and the individuals who painstakingly compiled the data. They are Shelly Collinsworth at Fort Worth Zoo, Justin Brackett at SeaWorld California, and Rose Legato at Los Angeles Zoo.

## Recommended Reading

The *Flamingo Husbandry Guidelines* compilation details many aspects of general flamingo care and rearing (Brown and King 2001). Some information has been updated since 2001; however, the information contained in the husbandry guidelines was written and compiled by the top experts in flamingo care and husbandry and continues to be an excellent source of information. For additional information, contact current European Association of Zoos and Aquaria (EAZA) or Association of Zoos and Aquariums (AZA) Flamingo Taxon Advisory Group (TAG) chairs for current contacts in flamingo care at www.eaza.net or www.aza.org.

## Sources for Products Mentioned

3M™ Nomad™ Unbacked Scraper Matting 8100: http://matsinc.com/3m-nomad-unbacked-scraper-8100, 1-800–628-7462.

Animal Genetics, Inc., 1336 Timberlane Road, Tallahassee, Florida 32312–1766, Int: (850) 386–1145, US: (800) 514–9672, www.animalgenetics.us.

AVID Identification Systems, Inc., 3185 Hamner Avenue, Norco, CA 92860–1983, (800) 336–2843, www.avidid.com.

Kinesio Tex Gold FP Kinesiology Tape: Kinesio USA Corp Limited, 4001 Masthead Street NE, Albuquerque, NM 87109, (888) 320–8273, https://kinesiotaping.com.

Mazuri Flamingo Maintenance # 5572: Mazuri Mazuri, PMI Nutrition International, LLC, PO Box 66812, St. Louis, MO 63166, (800) 227–8941, www.mazuri.com.

Krill and Fish Source: McRoberts® Sales Co., Inc., PO Box 489, Ruskin, FL 33575, (813) 645–2561.

Animal Intensive Care Units: Lyon Technologies, Inc., 1690 Brandywine Avenue, Chula Vista, CA 91911, (888) 596–6872, https://lyonusa.com.

Nolvasan Solution: Zoetis, Inc., 10 Sylvan Way, Parsippany, New Jersey 07054, (888) 963–8471.

## References

Brown, C. and King, C. (eds.). (2001). Flamingo Husbandry Guidelines. A joint effort of the Association of Zoos and Aquariums and European Association of Zoos and Aquaria in cooperation with the Wildfowl and Wetlands Trust. http://aviansag.org/Husbandry/Unlocked/Care_Manuals/Flamingo%20Husbandry%20Guidelines.pdf

Burch, L. and Gailband, C. (2000). Comparison of hand-reared Caribbean Flamingos and Lesser Flamingos at Seaworld California. *Waterbirds* 23: 193–197. https://doi.org/10.2307/1522165.

Collinsworth, S. (2014). Unique medical and management techniques used in working with Chilean (Phoenicopterus chilensis), Caribbean (Phoenicopterus ruber), and Lesser Flamingos (Phoeniconaias minor). 3rd International Flamingo Symposium, San Diego, CA.

Gehrmann, W.H. (1987). Ultraviolet irradiances of various lamps used in animal husbandry. *Zoo Biology* 6: 117–127.

IUCN/SSC (2013). *Guidelines for Reintroductions and Other Conservation Translocations. Version 1.0*, viiii + 57 pp. Gland, Switzerland: IUCN Species Survival Commission.

Shannon, P. (2007). Flamingos. In: *Hand-Rearing Birds* (eds. L. Gage and R. Duerr), 97–102. Ames, Iowa: Wiley Blackwell.

## Further Reading

Kear, J. (1974). Notes on keeping flamingos in captivity. *International Zoo Yearbook* 14: 142–144.

Kunneman, F. and Perry, J. (1990). Hand-rearing the Caribbean Flamingo *Phoenicopterus r. ruber* at the San Antonio Zoo. *International Zoo Yearbook* 29: 95–99.

Ward, A.M., Hunt, A., Maslanka, M., and Brown, C. (2001). Nutrient composition of American flamingo crop milk. In: *Proceedings of the Fourth Conference on Zoo and Wildlife Nutrition* (eds. M. Edwards, K.J. Lisi, M.L. Schlegel, et al.), 189–195. Lake Buena Vista, FL: AZA Nutrition Advisory Group.

# 12

# Penguins

*Linda Henry*

## Natural History

Penguins comprise 18 species that collectively rank among the most endangered seabirds (Crawford et al. 2017). Penguins are restricted to the Southern Hemisphere, spanning tropical, temperate, sub-Antarctic, and high-Antarctic regions. They are the most highly adapted marine birds: flightless, with flippers, solid bones, and a fusiform body shape. Species differ in size, feather ornaments, and forage habits.

Penguins forage on fishes, krill, and squid. Diets vary based on seasonal prey availability, species preference, and reproductive demands. Penguins spend most of their time at sea but must come on land for reproduction and molt. Breeding and molt cycles are species-specific. Life expectancy is ~20 years but penguins in human care can live beyond 30 years. Williams (1995) and Borboroglu and Boersma (2015) provide comprehensive species life history and conservation information.

In 1972, the National Science Foundation approached SeaWorld® and Hubbs-SeaWorld Research Institute to ask for help in establishing an ex situ colony of high-Antarctic penguins (Todd 1987a). The ensuing Penguin Encounters have led to a decades-long commitment to penguin care and the development of incubation and hand-rearing protocols that have been shared worldwide (Todd 1987b; Henry and Twohy 1990; Turner and Plutchak 1998; Henry and Sirpenski 2005; AZA Penguin Taxon Advisory Group 2014) including recommendations regarding overall penguin reproductive management in the *Penguin (Spheniscidae) Care Manual* (AZA Penguin Taxon Advisory Group 2014).

## Criteria for Intervention

Parent-rearing is preferred over hand-rearing but some assistance may be needed. Interventions should be customized to nest type, location, and birds' response to disturbance. Parental inexperience or behavior, a medical emergency, environmental conditions, and species-specific traits may influence management decisions. For example, *Eudyptes* are obligate brood reducers whereby A-eggs are at higher risk of loss and are recommended for removal for artificial incubation at lay. And while some species may be able to rear two chicks successfully, it is advisable to retain one fertile egg per nest to avoid overtaxing parents.

*Hand-Rearing Birds*, Second Edition. Edited by Rebecca S. Duerr and Laurie J. Gage.

Any time an egg is removed, it should be replaced with a dummy egg to prevent re-clutching, to assess parental behavior, or to provide options for later egg fostering. *Eudyptes* A-eggs are not replaced with a dummy. Dummy eggs should be removed at the end of the incubation period or by 2 weeks post-lay, based on the breeding season plan. When the first (A) egg is dummied with the intention of later parental incubation of the second (B) egg in any species, remove the dummy egg after the second egg is laid.

Eggs under parents should be monitored during incubation and hatching. Parents lift the brood patch more frequently near hatching when a pip hole may be observed for size and progression. It is prudent to avoid disturbing a pipped egg under parents until the maximum estimated pip-to-hatch interval has been exceeded. However, pipping eggs in the hatcher should be closely monitored.

Most penguin chicks will hatch normally over 24–48 hours. Chicks will be vocal in the egg starting with internal pip until hatching. Chicks in destress will have increased frequency and pitch of vocalizations and may require assistance. For eggs under parents, a vigorous, but stuck chick may be partially released then returned to the nest. During a prolonged pip-to-hatch period, chicks that become weak, still, and quiet will require support to hatch.

The most common hatching problem is poor pip-to-hatch progression due to malpositioning of the chick or dried, sticky membranes that prevent hatching rotation. Associated conditions include residual albumen, an open umbilicus, or incomplete yolk sac retraction. In penguins, it is advisable to assist hatching gradually over several hours, working to release the head so the chick can move the muscles that will trigger yolk retraction and encourage chick hatching behavior. See Chapter 3 for detailed assisted-hatch procedures.

Chicks under parents will be tightly brooded immediately following a normal hatch, with eyes somewhat closed. Their eyes will open fully by 4–6 days of age. Chicks will appear sleepy for the first 12–24 hours and few parental feedings may be observed. Thereafter, parental feedings should be more frequent. Parents should be fed by keepers away from the nest to reduce disturbance, and to encourage species-appropriate nest bout exchanges. However, a parent on the nest may be given one or two smaller fish (e.g. capelin) at the nest in the morning so that begging chicks can be fed without delay.

If a chick fails to thrive, managers should evaluate intervention options. Where parent behavior allows, and when a chick is still relatively alert and responsive, it might remain in the nest during treatment. The chick can be removed, examined, weighed, fed or medicated, and then returned. For example, excessive regurgitant observed around the nest suggests interrupted feedings, inexperienced parents, or a chick that is unable to eat. Once a serious medical condition is ruled out, chick care at the nest may be appropriate.

Whenever chicks are removed for later return, returns should be immediate or within 12–24 hours to avoid parental nest abandonment. If at any time a chick is unresponsive or unable to stand, it should be taken into care for hand-rearing and isolated from other chicks until medically evaluated.

There are times when interventions may be part of an overall egg/chick management strategy to maximize parent-rearing success, such as egg removal to determine fertility, during chick health and weight monitoring, or when habituating chicks to hand-feeding.

## Record Keeping

Systematic record keeping is essential to incubation and rearing decisions and to improvement of practices. Records should include individual adult histories, observations and maps of nests/pairs, egg logs, incubation notes, and chick rearing logs. See Chapter 3 for details on egg and incubation records. Penguin egg logs should also include documentation of fostered eggs (foster date, foster pair identification) and dummy placement and removal dates.

Good records begin with individual bird identification. Adult penguins are typically identified by a band placed at the proximal end of one or both flippers. Types of flipper bands include: cable ties, metal, plastic, and silicone. Chicks should be banded when more than one chick is hand-reared together or by 21 days of age for multiple chicks under parents. Colored cable ties are used for short-term identification but must be monitored for constriction and replaced as chicks grow. Subcutaneous transponders implanted at fledging assure continuity of identification if bands are lost.

Chick records must include parent IDs and nest location; egg ID (and weight when available), incubation type and duration; chick ID, hatch date and time; reason if removed, rearing type including parent-feeding observations or hand-rearing records. Chicks in the nest can be removed briefly for weekly weights and returned. Hand-reared chicks are weighed daily with food intake recorded along with ambient room and brooder temperatures. For all chicks, observations of chick behavioral responses and developmental stages should be recorded.

## Incubation of Eggs

Review Chapter 3 for general guidance on hatchery setup, egg handling, and incubation procedures. Incubators and hatchers should be set up 2 weeks prior to the expected first egg of the season and monitored for temperature and humidity stability.

An egg management plan should be defined as pairs are identified and likely interventions are anticipated. Apart from necessary interventions, eggs in nests need not be disturbed. However, candling eggs under parents 10–15 days prior to expected-hatch may enhance outcomes through the removal of infertile eggs and the return or fostering of fertile eggs. Eggs can also be transferred between zoos and aquariums at this time (Branch 2009).

Incubation parameters for penguins were established in the 1980s (Todd 1987b) and have since been refined (Table 12.1). SeaWorld uses the Humidaire Model 21 for incubation and the Grumbach Model S84 for hatching. Petersime and Rcom have also been used. Due to the relatively large size and weight of penguin eggs, incubator turning mechanisms may be inadequate. Turners on Humidaire incubators can be disabled with the racks secured in a level position to facilitate hand-turning.

Natural incubation, where feasible, improves hatchability. SeaWorld analyzed hatchability results over more than 20 years and found that viable eggs under parents for as little as 7–10 days had better hatching success when compared to full-term artificial incubation (SeaWorld San Diego, unpublished data).

If eggs are removed, they are labeled with the egg log number and turning arrows using an indelible marker. Eggs kept back for artificial incubation are immediately placed in the incubator on their sides, for hand-rotation seven times daily over 12 hours. Abandoned eggs in cold habitats may become chilled. If not frozen, these eggs should be set out at room temperature to warm prior to examination for damage and setting in the incubator as appropriate.

Eggs in the incubator are candled weekly to assess developmental progress. Penguin eggs are thick-shelled such that even a strong light source is insufficient to visualize structures in some species. These eggs are treated as fertile.

Pipped eggs are moved to the hatcher and rotation is discontinued. If multiple eggs are hatching simultaneously, eggs are partitioned to maintain egg-to-chick ID. A small rubber-mesh-covered reservoir of warm water (95.5 °F/35.8 °C) is placed in the hatcher 24 hours later. This procedure

Table 12.1 Penguin egg incubation and hatching parameters for the most common species.

| Species | Incubation Temperature (°F/°C) | Incubation Humidity (%RH) | Hatcher Temperature (°F/°C) | Hatcher Humidity (%RH) | Median Incubation Period (days) | Range Incubation Period (days) | Pip to Hatch Interval (hours) |
|---|---|---|---|---|---|---|---|
| Emperor | 96.5/35.8 | 51–54 | 95.5/35.3 | 74 | 64 | 62–65 | 24–48 |
| King | 96.5/35.8 | 51–54 | 95.5/35.3 | 74 | 54 | 52–56 | 24–48 |
| Adélie | 96.5/35.8 | 51–54 | 95.5/35.3 | 74 | 37 | 34–40 | 24–72 |
| Chinstrap | 96.5/35.8 | 51–54 | 95.5/35.3 | 74 | 35 | 33–36 | 24–48 |
| Gentoo | 97.5/36.4 | 52–54 | 96.5/35.8 | 74 | 38 | 36–42 | 24–48 |
| Macaroni | 97.5/36.4 | 52–54 | 96.5/35.8 | 74 | 37 | 36–42 | 24–72 |
| Northern Rockhopper | 96.5/35.8 | 51–54 | 95.5/35.3 | 74 | 35 | 32–36 | 24–48 |
| Southern Rockhopper | 96.5/35.8 | 51–54 | 95.5/35.3 | 74 | DD | 32–34 | 24–48 |
| Magellanic | 97.5/36.4 (93.2/34 measured at Punto Tombo) | 52–54 | 96.5/35.8 | 74 | 41 | 38–44 | 24–48 |
| Humboldt | 96.5/35.8 | 51–54 | 95.5/35.3 | 74 | 41 | 38–42 | 36–60 |
| African | 96.5/35.8 | 55 | 96.5/35.8 | >80 | 38 | 38–42 | 24–48 |
| Little | 97.7 | 50–60 | 97.7 | 60 | 36 | 33–37 | 24–72 |

Borboroglu and Boersma (2015), including data from Steve Sarro, Seana Flossic and Heather Urquhart (pers. comm.), and merged with SeaWorld data. DD = data deficient.

temporarily increases hatcher humidity to maintain supple shell membranes without altering machine settings. Once chicks hatch, the reservoir is removed and disinfected prior to the next use. Newly hatched chicks remain in the hatcher until dry (~12–24 hours).

## Initial Care and Stabilization

Chicks entering the nursery should be housed at a temperature consistent with age and stage; Table 12.3 shows temperature by age ranges. Penguin chicks are semi-altricial, progressing through two stages: the guard and the post-guard (crèche) phase. The guard stage is when chicks are closely brooded by the parents and dependent on them for warmth. The duration of this stage varies by species, transitioning to the post-guard phase as chicks grow, developing a second down. Chicks hatch with primary down then develop secondary down over several weeks concurrent with progression toward homeothermy at crèche age. These stages affect chicks' daily thermoregulatory needs. It is important to recognize that chick down has a higher insulating capacity than adult feathers and their feet aid in thermoregulation (Wilson et al. 1998).

Chicks from the hatcher should be evaluated for vitality, weighed, and the umbilical seal dabbed with a dilute iodine-based disinfectant before moving to the brooder.

Neonates entering the nursery from parental care should be evaluated for dehydration, seal-closure, and a cloacal swab taken for cytology. Sick chicks in the post-guard phase may need access to warmth based on medical evaluation. However, use care in applying heat and ensure chicks have access to a temperature gradient. Healthy chicks removed for habituation to hand-feeding should be housed consistent with penguin habitat temperatures and will normally refuse food for up to 3 days.

## Common Medical Problems

Problems encountered when hand-rearing penguins often occur as a consequence of overheating or overfeeding. Maintaining age-specific brooder temperatures and clean food-handling procedures and adherence to feeding protocols are essential to preventing heat-induced or food-borne illness.

Chick fecal output should be monitored for changes indicative of illness. Normal droppings should project 3–4 in. (7.6–10.2 cm) or more; thick, pasty feces suggest dehydration. Formula-like feces indicate a lack of normal digestive function. Chronically overheated chicks may present with foul smelling or dark-colored diarrhea, including a tight abdomen, lethargy, and dehydration. The risk of *Clostridium* overgrowth (determined via fecal cytology), or a yolk sac or gastrointestinal infection is possible. Antibiotics (metronidazole, amikacin, Tribrissen®) and subcutaneous lactated Ringer's solution (at ~5–10% of body weight per day) can support recovery.

Chicks may also present anemic in association with an infection or heart murmur. Thiamine deficiency is rare with sufficient dietary supplementation. West Nile virus and avian malaria are risk factors in outdoor habitats. Curled toes, splayed legs, and bumblefoot can be avoided by providing appropriate substrates. Rock ingestion, while not necessarily a medical concern, is observed in chicks at crèche stage. Rocks are usually regurgitated; rarely, retained rocks may cause gut irritation. Other conditions reported in the literature include gastrointestinal obstruction (Perpiñán and Curro 2009), septicemia (Nimmervoll et al. 2011), *Pseudomonas* (Widmer et al. 2016); traumatic injury (Emerson et al. 1990), and valvular dysplasia and congestive heart failure (McNaughton et al. 2014).

Medications given to adult females during egg-forming may cause birth defects, e.g. Daraprim® and Voriconazole should be discontinued 2 weeks prior to the estimated first egg.

*Aspergillus* spp. infection is always a risk in penguins. It may present as a secondary infection during medical treatment, or as a consequence of environmental conditions, such as high humidity coupled with still indoor air.

If illness is caught early, sick chicks can be maintained at age-specific temperatures. Very ill chicks may not be able to thermoregulate and require additional heat; however, monitor the temperature to avoid overheating. As health is restored, chicks should be returned to a temperature consistent with age/stage. Health evaluations and blood sampling are recommended for post-fledged chicks prior to their introduction into the colony.

## Diet Recipes

The SeaWorld Hand Rearing Formula consists of equal portions herring and krill blended with water and vitamins (Tables 12.2 and 12.3). Formula components are prepared when still partially frozen. Herring is prepared whole minus skin, head, tail, and fins to reduce syringe-clogging pieces; krill is squeezed of moisture. After blending, the formula is pressed through a sieve to assure a smooth consistency. Herring filets are used for the introduction of fish. Fillets are prepared in the morning with smaller portions cut and weighed just prior to feeding.

Prepare fish components while still very cold or partially frozen to preserve food temperature during preparation. Blend all ingredients thoroughly. Press through a sieve to ensure a smooth consistency. Transfer to a suitable refrigerator storage container and mark with the date and time of preparation for use within 24 hours. This recipe makes approximately 850 ml of formula. While this recipe may be doubled as needed, cutting the recipe in half may affect the ratio of nutritional components due to division of supplements. SeaWorld uses Pacific Herring and Superba Krill.

The best fish source is herring, or a fish with a comparable caloric content and similar percent fat, moisture, and protein. When krill is unavailable, fish-only formula has been used. The variable nutrient content of substituted fishes may alter chick growth rate expectations.

Fish lots should be analyzed for caloric content and nutrient levels. Alpha-tocopherol (vitamin E) degrades in stored fish and thiamine (B-1) is lost through thiaminase activity in some fishes (e.g. herring and capelin). These are the primary supplements recommended for penguins (Slifka et al. 2002; Bos et al. 2018). Mazuri® Vita-Zu Large Bird Tablets, without vitamin A, are used in the for-

Table 12.2 SeaWorld Penguin hand-rearing formula recipe.

| | |
|---|---|
| **220 g** | **Whole herring**, with head, tail, fins, and skin removed |
| **220 g** | **Krill**, squeezed of water prior to weighing |
| **600 ml** | Filtered tap **water** |
| **8 tablets** | **Brewer's Yeast** (7 grain tablets) |
| **550 mg** | **Thiamine** (B-1) |
| **2 tablets** | Mazuri Vita-Zu Large Bird Tablet **5TLB** |
| **4 tablets** | **Calcium carbonate** 10 grain (648 mg Ca) tablets (2600 mg elemental calcium total) |
| **1200 IU** | **Vitamin E** (squeezed from capsule) |
| **2 ml** | **Pedia Poly-Vite Children's Multivitamins Drops WITH IRON** |

Table 12.3 SeaWorld penguin vitamin guidelines by genus (weights refer to chick morning weight).

| **PARENT-REARED:** | | | | | |
|---|---|---|---|---|---|
| **To parents with >3 day old chicks twice/day** | **To parents with >14 day old chicks twice/day** | **To chicks in habituation >2 kg until fledge** | **To juveniles until 4 months post-fledge once/day** | | |
| ***Eudyptes, Spheniscus,* and *Pygoscelis*** | | | | | |
| • 2 tabs **5TLC**<br>• 1/2 tab B-Comp | • 1 tab 5TLB<br>• 1/2 tab B-Comp | • 1 tab **5TLB a.m.**<br>• 1/2 tab B-comp **a.m.**<br>• 1/8 tab $CaCO_3$ **a.m.**<br>• 1 Flintstones **p.m.** | • 1 tab **5TLB**<br>• 1/2 tab B-comp | | |
| ***Aptenodytes*** | | | | | |
| • 2 tabs **5TLC**<br>• 1/2 tab B-Comp | • 1 tab **5TLB**<br>• 1/2 tab B-Comp | • 1 tab **5TLB a.m.**<br>• ½ tab B-comp **a.m.**<br>• 1/8 tab $CaCO_3$ **a.m.**<br>• 1 Flintstones **p.m.** | • 1 tab **5TLA**<br>• 1 tab B-comp | | |
| **HAND-REARED:** | | | | | |
| **When chick starts receiving full strength formula** | **>4 days until 250 g** | **251–400 g** | **400–500 g** | **501–750 g** | **751–1000 g** |
| ***Eudyptes, Spheniscus,* and *Pygoscelis*** | | | | | |
| Pinch each of ground B-1 (100 mg) and B-comp-50 per 100 cc warmed formula prior to feeding | • Pinch B-1 and B-comp/formula<br>• 0.1 cc Poly-Vite **a.m.** | • Pinch B-1 and B-comp/formula<br>• 0.15 cc Poly-Vite **a.m.** | • 0.15 cc Poly-Vite **a.m.**<br>• 1/4 tab B-1 **a.m./ p.m.**<br>• 1/8 B-comp **a.m./ p.m.** | • 0.2 cc Poly-Vite **a.m.**<br>• 1/4 tab B-1 **a.m./ p.m.**<br>• 1/8 B-comp **a.m./ p.m.** | • 0.25 cc Poly-Vite **a.m.**<br>• 1/4 tab B-1 **a.m./ p.m.**<br>• 1/8 B-comp **a.m./ p.m.** |

*(Continued)*

Table 12.3 (Continued)

| **>1000 g or at twice/day formula** | **>2000 g or at twice/day formula until fledge** | | | | |
|---|---|---|---|---|---|
| • 1 tab **5TLC a.m.**<br>• ½ tab B-comp **a.m.**<br>• 1/8 tab CaCO3 **a.m.**<br>• 1/2 Flintstones **p.m.** | • 1 tab **5TLB a.m.**<br>• ½ tab B-comp **a.m.**<br>• 1/8 tab CaCO3 **a.m.**<br>• 1 Flintstones **p.m.** | | | | |
| ***Aptenodytes*** | | | | | |
| **When chick starts receiving full strength formula** | **>4 days until 400 g** | **400–500 g** | **501–750 g** | **750–1000 g** | **>1000 g** |
| Pinch each of ground B-1 (100 mg) and B-comp-50 per 100 cc warmed formula prior to feeding | • Pinch B-1 and B-comp/ formula<br>• 0.15 cc Poly-Vite **a.m.** | • 0.15 cc Poly-Vite **a.m.**<br>• 1/4 tab B-1 **a.m./ p.m.**<br>• 1/8 B-comp **a.m./ p.m.** | • 0.2 cc Poly-Vite **a.m.**<br>• 1/4 tab B-1 **a.m./ p.m.**<br>• 1/8 B-comp **a.m./ p.m.** | • 0.2 cc Poly-Vite **a.m.**<br>• 1/4 tab B-1 **a.m./ p.m.**<br>• 1/8 B-comp **a.m./ p.m.** | • 1 tab **5TLC a.m.**<br>• ½ tab B-comp **a.m.**<br>• 1/8 tab CaCO3 **a.m.**<br>• 1/2 Flintstones **p.m.** |
| ***Aptenodytes*** | | | | | |
| **>2000 g morning weight** | **>3000 g morning weight** | **>6000 g morning weight** | **>12 kg morning weight to fledge** | | |
| • 1 tab **5TLB a.m.**<br>• ½ tab B-comp **a.m.**<br>• 1/8 tab CaCO3 **a.m.**<br>• 1 Flintstones **p.m.** | • 1 tab **5TLB a.m.**<br>• ½ tab B-comp **a.m.**<br>• 1/8 tab CaCO3 **a.m.**<br>• 1 Flintstones **p.m.**<br>• 1/8 tab CaCO3 **p.m.** | • 1 tab **5TLB a.m.**<br>• ½ tab B-comp **a.m.**<br>• 1/8 tab CaCO3 **a.m.**<br>• 1 Flintstones **p.m.**<br>• 1/8 tab CaCO3 **p.m.** | • 1 tab **5TLA a.m.**<br>• ½ tab B-comp **a.m.**<br>• 1/8 tab CaCO3 **a.m.**<br>• 1 Flintstones **p.m.**<br>• 1/8 tab CaCO3 **p.m.** | | |

B-1 = 100 mg; B-Comp = B-Complex-50 mg; Calcium Carbonate (CaCO3) =10 grain; Flintstones = Flintstones Toddler Chewable; 5TLA, 5TLB and 5TLC = Mazuri Vita Zu Tablets; Poly-Vite = Pedia Poly-Vite Drops Children's Multivitamin.

mula, and are given to chicks along with other supplements. Consult a nutritionist for appropriate supplementation based on the types or lot of fish used.

Good quality fish with proper storage, thawing, and food-handling is fundamental to an effective penguin rearing diet. Whole fish is air-thawed overnight in a refrigerator, then briefly rinsed prior to use. Formula is prepared fresh daily, labeled with the preparation date/time; formula not fed within 24 hours is discarded. Fillets are made fresh daily. All food items are refrigerated until use; unused portions are discarded.

## Feeding Procedure

Chick rearing is a relationship between chick and feeder, involving observations and response. Penguin chicks should not be overfed or overheated. Hand-feeding equipment consists of a small heat-tolerant formula container and a feeding syringe. Formula is warmed via a hot-water bath (110 °F/43.3 °C), stirring constantly until the formula reaches 95–100 °F (35.0–37.7 °C). Formula should be kept warm during feeding in the water bath. Do not microwave and do not overheat formula. Chicks will refuse formula below 90 °F/32.2 °C. Formula exceeding 105 °F/40.5 °C should be discarded, as should warmed formula that is not fed. Guard-stage chicks are fed in the brooder or an alternate warmed area.

Parental feeding behavior is simulated by making an inverted "V"-formation over the chick's bill with the fingers, then wiggling them to induce the chick's feeding response (Figures 12.1 and 12.2). It is important for feeders to lift their feeding hand slightly, while wiggling the fingers, to encourage chicks to reach up into the "V." The syringe is then directed toward one side of the bill and the formula delivered. Feed 1–3-day old chicks small aliquots of 0.5–1 cc each, while continuing to wiggle fingers, and watching the back of the throat to see that the formula is being accepted. When the aliquot is delivered, continue to elicit the response until the chick finishes before slowly releasing the chick to rest before feeding the next aliquot, until the full allotment is fed.

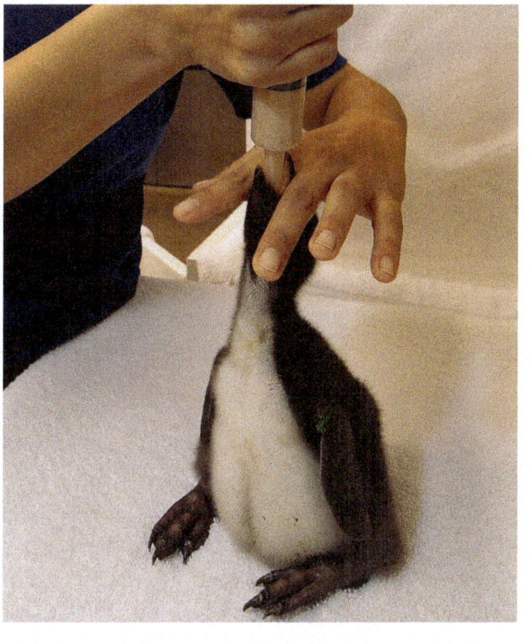

Figure 12.1 Penguin chick being syringe-fed using inverted "V." *Source:* photo credit: Mike Aguilera/SeaWorld San Diego.

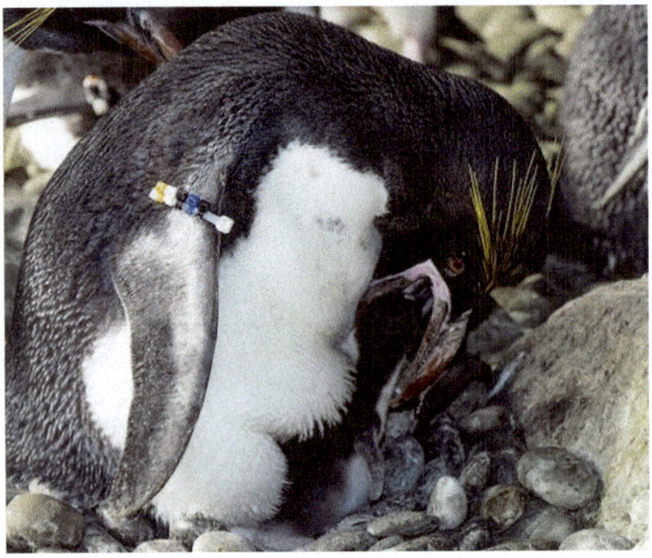

Figure 12.2 Adult penguin feeding a chick. *Source:* photo credit: Mike Aguilera/SeaWorld San Diego.

Feed slowly and observe chick responses. Common mistakes which increase the risk for aspiration are: failure to raise the "V" causing the chick to slouch or bend its neck, continuing to deliver formula after the chick stops swallowing, feeding too rapidly, and releasing the chick too quickly from the feeding response. Supporting the head allows chicks to expel formula sitting on the glottis. Chicks 1–4 days old are fed using a 1 cc syringe; thereafter, syringe sizes and aliquot amounts increase gradually concurrent with intake.

Warm water is given initially on the first day, transitioning through formula dilutions until full-strength formula is fed (Table 12.4). Undiluted formula can be attempted sooner than outlined but gradual introduction has been successful. When fish is introduced at day 7 (following at least 1 day on undiluted formula), fillets are warmed just prior to feeding by dipping in the water bath. Small amounts of warm water can be given between feedings, and/or 30 minutes after the last feeding, to offset the effects of chick overheating combined with fish introduction. Fecals may appear darker with increasing fish intake but should never smell sour or be thickened or pasty.

The guideline for chick total intake per feeding (formula plus fish) should not exceed 10% of the chick's morning weight. Chicks receive about half of their diet in fish by 17–21 days of age. As the maximum formula volume per feeding is met (usually 30–40 cc), the proportion of fish in the diet increases concomitantly; thereafter, whole-fish segments are then introduced, and formula decreased gradually.

As chicks grow and intake increases, the time between feedings should also increase to avoid overfeeding. Chicks should always demonstrate a sustained and vigorous feeding behavior. If a chick refuses food repeatedly, or fails to eat all recommended food amounts, check for overheating, a readiness to increase feed interval, or a medical condition. At about 30 days of age chicks may show some head-shy behavior when feeding responses are solicited. Chicks may be experiencing a normal predator-response behavior (crèche phase), may be overheated (reduce temperature), or overfed (increase feed interval).

By day 50–60, chicks are fed larger whole fishes, cautiously, to satiation twice daily. Continue to weigh and monitor intake through introduction to the colony. It is normal for chicks approaching fledging to self-regulate food intake intermittently.

Parent-reared chicks removed for hand -earing should be transitioned to the diet based on weight and health status. Chicks >21 days old may not need formula and may be fed initially with small whole fish. For chicks receiving formula, it is advisable to test syringe-feeding with warm water, then transition briefly through formula dilutions prior to giving undiluted formula per feeding guidelines.

## Expected Weight Gain

Penguin chick weight gain expectations vary with age and stage. Growth rates for hand-reared chicks are slightly slower than those of parent-reared chicks. Hand-reared chicks typically lose weight for the first 1–3 days or until undiluted formula is introduced, then gain 5–15% of their body weight daily thereafter. Weight gains escalate after 7 days until about 21–30 days (species dependent) when weight gains slow to 5–10% daily. Growth rate graphs for several species are available in Appendix I of the *Penguin Husbandry Manual* (Henry and Sirpenski 2005).

Most parent-reared chicks will double their hatch weight within the first 5–7 days, and weekly weights taken through 21 days reflect weights 1.5–2 times the previous week's weight. Thereafter, weight gains slow slightly until fledging. Hand-reared and parent-reared chicks share similar fledging and 1-year weight trends.

## Housing

Housing should be set up 2 weeks prior to the expected first chick and monitored for temperature stability. Penguins do best in a low-humidity, moving-air environment. Open-top brooders with heat lamps or Animal Intensive Care units (AICU) without water added are recommended. Substrate for neonates should be irregular, such as toweling set over a bed of river rocks or upside-down Dri-Dek tile. Later, bins or floor areas lined with river rock (2.5–3 in./5.1–7.6 cm size) are appropriate for chicks in the post-guard stage. Where feasible, chicks removed for habituation and hand-reared chicks aged >21–30 days should be housed separately within the main penguin habitat, within visual and vocal proximity of the colony.

Temperature regulation is vital to penguin chick-rearing success. While 1–3-day old chicks may need to be kept very warm, chick access to a temperature gradient in the brooder by days 5–7 will improve outcomes. Temperature needs of chicks change daily. Vigilance is necessary to avoid illness resulting from overheating. Signs of overheating include outspread extremities, difficulty waking up, weak or absent feeding response, lethargy, and/or panting. Moderately overheated chicks may show no behavioral signs other than refusing to finish all food offered. Shivering does not necessarily indicate a need for additional heat. Chicks use shivering to maintain and develop thermoregulation and it may also be observed immediately following a feeding. Penguin chicks tolerate cooling better than overheating; however, young chicks can become chilled. Rearing two to four chicks together will allow them to huddle for warmth.

A small, warmed rice bag may serve to provide temporary warmth for guard-stage chicks without modifying brooder temperatures. Overheated crèche-phase chicks can benefit from standing on a towel-covered frozen BlueIce® block.

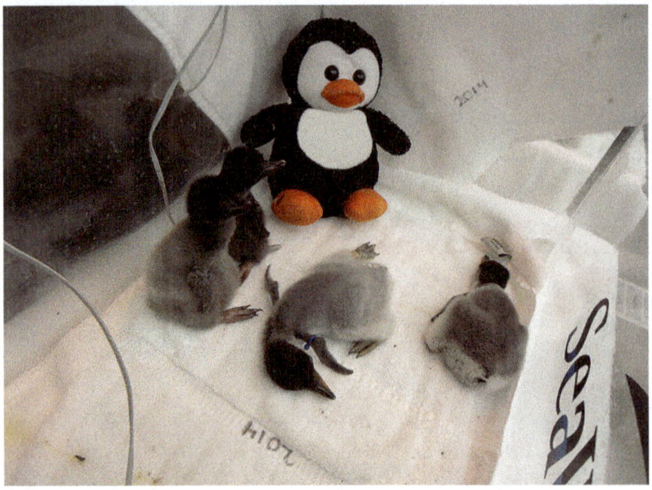

Figure 12.3 Young penguin chicks in plexiglass enclosure.

## Weaning

Weaning begins during rearing when the formula proportion reaches 30–40 cc per feeding and then is maintained at that amount while the fish component increases to equal 10% of the first morning weight in the guideline (Table 12.4). As chicks transition fully into the post-guard phase, feeding frequencies reduce and whole fish segments are introduced. As a consequence of this ongoing transition, formula is gradually discontinued and whole fishes are fed. The use of the "V"-feeding response is discontinued to encourage chicks to take fish on their own. Chicks are then fed commensurate with colony schedules as they grow into their adult feathers.

Parent-reared birds are weaned via habituation to hand-feeding whereby chicks are separated from the parents at crèche age and fed exclusively by animal care specialists.

## Preparation for Introduction to Captive Flock

Once juveniles have developed waterproof feathers, introductions can begin. Juveniles can be housed in an area inside the habitat and/or they can be taken into the colony during feedings for supervised visits. Aggression from conspecifics is likely; caretakers can monitor interactions and intervene as needed. Hand-reared chicks may have difficulty transitioning into the social structure if they have been imprinted on people. Penguin managers are discouraged from overly interacting with chicks during hand-rearing to ease later introductions.

Chicks can be introduced to the main habitat pool or tested in a smaller pool. Chicks supervised near the pool often enter the water on their own. For the first few days following introduction, chicks should be closely monitored, then returned to a separate area at night, away from pool access, until they have demonstrated that they are able manage within the colony social structure and are able enter and exit the pool on their own. Some species, such as Gentoo Penguins, practice extended parental care resulting in some parent-reared juveniles returning to the nest following habituation to hand-feeding.

Table 12.4 SeaWorld penguin hand-rearing guidelines (consult Table 12.3 for supplements).

| *Eudyptes, Pygoscelis, Spheniscus* | | | | | | | |
|---|---|---|---|---|---|---|---|
| | *Spheniscus* | *Eudyptes* and *Pygoscelis* | | | | | |
| **Age** | **Temp (°F/°C)** | **Temp (°F/°C)** | **Formula/feeding 1 cc = 1 g** | **~Fish/feeding** | **Feeding frequency** | **Housing** | **Other** |
| 0 | 96 (35.5) | 96 (35.5) | None | | | Hatcher x12–24 hrs | Primary down |
| 1 | 90 (32.2) | 86–93 (30–33.9) | 1–5 cc, diluted 50 : 50 | | Every 3 hours x5 | AICU or brooder/ heat lamp | |
| 2 | 84(28.9) | 86 (30) | 4–8 cc, diluted 75 : 25 | | | | |
| 3 | 82 (27.8) | 82 (27.8) | 4–10 cc undiluted | | | | 1–2 cc water between feedings |
| 4 | 82 (27.8) | 81 (27.2) | 10% a.m. weight | | | | |
| 7 | 79 (26.1) | 77 (25) | 10% a.m. weight[a] | 3 g fillets, 2nd feeding | | | ~2nd down phase begins |
| 8 | 76 (24.4) | 73–75 (22.8–23.9) | | 3–5 g fillets, 1st and 3rd feeding | | | |
| 9 | 75 (23.9) | 73–75 (22.8–23.9) | | 3–5 g, 1st, 3rd and 5th feeding | | | |
| 10 | 74 (23.3) | 72–74 (22.2–23.3) | | 3–5 g | | | |
| ~11[b] | 73 (22.8) | 71 (21.7) | | 5–7 g | | | |
| ~12 | 72 (22.2) | 70 (21.1) | | 7–10 g | | | |
| ~13 | 71 (21.7) | 67–68 (19.4–20) | | 10–15 g | | Reduced or no heat | |
| ~15 | 70 (21.1) | 60–65 (15.6–18.3) | | 15–20 g | | Bin/floor, no heat | |
| ~17 | 65 (18.3) | 60–63 (15.6–17.2) | 5% AM weight | 5% a.m. weight | Every 4 hours x4 | | |

(Continued)

Table 12.4 (Continued)

| *Eudyptes, Pygoscelis, Spheniscus* | | | | | | | |
|---|---|---|---|---|---|---|---|
| | *Spheniscus* | *Eudyptes* and *Pygoscelis* | | | | | |
| **Age** | **Temp (°F/°C)** | **Temp (°F/°C)** | **Formula/feeding 1 cc = 1 g** | **~Fish/feeding** | **Feeding frequency** | **Housing** | **Other** |
| ~19 | | 53–56 (11.7–13.3) | 30 cc/feeding max | +fish to =10%, introduce whole fish segments | | | Second down ~complete |
| ~24 | | 47–51 (8.3–10.6) | 30 cc formula x1 | | | | |
| ~29 | | 37–40 (2.8–4.4) | | Small whole fishes | | | |
| ~31 | | 34 (1.1) | | | Every 6 hours x3 | Corral/habitat | |
| ~35 | | 26 (−3.3) | Discontinue | | | | |
| ~50 | | | | Cautiously to satiation | Twice daily | | Adult feather growth starts |

| ***Aptenodytes*** | | | | | | | |
|---|---|---|---|---|---|---|---|
| | **King** | **Emperor** | | | | | |
| **Age** | **Temp (°F/°C)** | **Temp (°F/°C)** | **Formula/feeding** | **~Fish/Feeding** | **Feeding Frequency** | **Housing** | **Other** |
| 0 | 95 (35) | 95 (35) | None | | | Hatcher | Primary down |
| 1 | 90 (32.2) | 90 (32.2) | 5–15 cc, diluted 50 : 50 | | Every 3 hours x6 | AICU or brooder/heat lamp | |
| 2 | 85 (29.4) | 85 (29.4) | 14–17 cc, diluted 75 : 25 | | | | |
| 3 | 82 (27.8) | 82 (27.8) | 12–17 cc undiluted | | | | 1–4 cc water between feedings |

|  |  |  |  |  |  |  |  |
|---|---|---|---|---|---|---|---|
| 4 | 80 (26.7) | 80 (26.7) | 10% a.m. weight |  |  |  |  |
| 7 | 75 (23.8) | 75 (23.8) | 10% a.m. weight[a] | Herring filets 5–10 g at 2nd feeding |  |  | ~2nd down phase |
| 8 | 71 (21.7) | 71 (21.7) |  | 5–10 g at 1st and 3rd feeding |  |  |  |
| 9 | 70 (21.1) | 70 (21.1) |  | 10 g at 1st, 3rd, 5th feeding |  |  |  |
| 10 |  |  |  | 10–15 g/feeding |  |  |  |
| 11 |  |  |  | 15 g/feeding |  |  |  |
| 12 |  |  |  |  |  |  |  |
| ~13[b] | 65 (18.3) | 65 (18.3) |  | 20 g/feeding |  |  |  |
| ~14 |  |  | 40 cc/feeding max | fillets = 10%[a] | Every 4 hours x4 | No heat |  |
| ~16 |  |  |  |  |  |  |  |
| ~17 |  |  |  |  |  |  |  |
| ~18 | 55 (12.8) | 55 (12.8) |  | Introduce whole fish segments[a] |  |  |  |
| ~19 |  |  |  |  |  | Bin/floor |  |
| ~21 | 50 (10) | 50 (10) | Twice daily |  |  |  |  |
| ~24 |  |  |  |  |  |  |  |
| ~29 | 45 (7.2) | 37 (2.8) |  |  | Every 6 hours x3 |  | 2nd down ~complete |
| ~31 | 40 (4.4) | 34 (1.1) |  |  |  | Corral/habitat |  |
| ~34 | 40 (4.4) | 26 (−3.3) | Once daily | Small whole fishes |  |  |  |
| ~50 | Habitat | 26 (−3.3) | Discontinue | Cautiously to satiation |  |  | May refuse full amounts |

Chicks are weighed in the morning (a.m.) before feeding.

[a] Combined formula and fish per feeding should not exceed 10% of a chick's first a.m. weight.

[b] Age at transition to increased feeding amounts is approximate; assess chick readiness at all stages.

## Acknowledgments

Thank you to Steve Sarro, Seana Flossic, Heather Urquhart, and Justin Brackett for providing supplemental information for this chapter, to Stephanie Costelow and Laurie Conrad for supporting this work, and to my colleagues at SeaWorld and beyond for their dedication to penguin care. Special thanks to Frank Todd who achieved an impossible dream.

## Sources for Products Mentioned

Reusable BlueIce Block by RubberMaid® www.rubbermaid.com.

Animal Intensive Care Unit: Lyon Technologies, Inc., 1690 Brandywine Avenue, Chula Vista, CA. 91 911, https://lyonvet.com.

Dri-Dek Tile: Kendall Products, PO Box 8656 Naples, FL 34101 USA, (239) 643–0448, https://www.dri-dek.com.

Mazuri Vita-Zu Large (5TLB) and Small (5TLC) Bird and Marine Mammal (5TLA) tablets, no vitamin A added, www.mazuri.com.

Flintstones Toddler Chewable Tablets https://www.flintstonesvitamins.com/products/toddler-chewable-vitamins.

Pedia Poly-Vite Drops Children's Multivitamins, Bayshore Pharmaceuticals, Tampa, FL 33619.

## References

AZA Penguin Taxon Advisory Group (2014). *Penguin (Spheniscidae) Care Manual*. Association of Zoos and Aquariums: Silver Spring, MD https://www.aza.org/animal-care-manuals.

Borboroglu, P.G. and Boersma, P.D. (eds.) (2015). *Penguins: Natural History and Conservation*. Seattle: University of Washington Press.

Bos, J.H., Klip, F.C., and Kik, M.J. (2018). Plasma concentrations of vitamin A1, B1, D3, and E in Humboldt penguins (*Spheniscus humboldti*) before and after dietary vitamin supplementation of their fish diet. *Journal of Zoo and Wildlife Medicine* 49 (3): 732–737.

Branch, S. (2009). *Moving Birds In-Huevo*. Avian Scientific Advisory Group, American Zoo and Aquarium Association http://www.aviansag.org/ASAG_Documents/Egg_Transport.pdf.

Crawford, R., Ellenberg, U., Frere, E. et al. (2017). Tangled and drowned: a global review of penguin bycatch in fisheries. *Endangered Species Research* 34: 373–396.

Emerson, C.L., Eurell, J.A.C., Brown, M.D. et al. (1990). Ruptured intervertebral disc in a juvenile king penguin (*Aptenodytes patagonica*). *Journal of Zoo and Wildlife Medicine* 21 (3): 345–350.

Henry, L. and Sirpenski G. (2005). *Penguin Husbandry Manual*, 3. Penguin Taxon Advisory Group, American Zoo and Aquarium Association, 141 pp. http://www.aviansag.org/Husbandry/Unlocked/Care_Manuals/Penguin_HB.pdf.

Henry, L.M. and Twohy, F. (1990). Hand-rearing guidelines for the Humboldt penguin (*Spheniscus humboldti*) with special emphasis on common hand-rearing concerns. AAZPA Regional Conference Proceedings, AAZPA, Washington, DC.

McNaughton, A., Frasca, S. Jr., Mishra, N., and Tuttle, A.D. (2014). Valvular dysplasia and congestive heart failure in a juvenile African penguin (*Spheniscus demersus*). *Journal of Zoo and Wildlife Medicine* 45 (4): 987–990.

Nimmervoll, H., Wenker, C., Robert, N., and Albini, S. (2011). Septicaemia caused by *Edwardsiella tarda* and *Plesiomonas shigelloides* in captive penguin chicks. *Schweizer Archiv fur Tierheilkunde* 153 (3): 117.

Perpiñán, D. and Curro, T.G. (2009). Gastrointestinal obstruction in penguin chicks. *Journal of Avian Medicine and Surgery* 23 (4): 290–293.

Slifka, K.A., Crissey, S.D., and McGill, P. (2002). Penguins: nutrition and dietary husbandry. *Nutrition Advisory Group Handbook Fact Sheet 012.*

Todd, F.S. (1987a). The Penguin Encounter at Sea World, San Diego. *International Zoo Yearbook* 26 (1): 104–109.

Todd, F.S. (1987b). Techniques for propagating King and Emperor penguins *Aptenodytes patagonica* and *A. forsteri* at Sea World, San Diego. *International Zoo Yearbook* 26 (1): 110–124.

Turner, W.A. and Plutchak, L. (1998). SeaWorld California penguin hand-rearing guidelines. *Penguin Conservation* 11 (2): 2–9. http://www.aviansag.org/Newsletters/Penguin_TAG.

Widmer, D., Ziemssen, E., Schade, B. et al. (2016). *Pseudomonas aeruginosa* infection in a group of captive Humboldt penguins (*Spheniscus humboldti*). *Journal of Avian Medicine and Surgery* 30 (2): 187–195.

Williams, T.D. (1995). *The Penguins: Spheniscidae*, vol. 2. USA: Oxford University Press.

Wilson, R.P., Adelung, D., and Latorre, L. (1998). Radiative heat loss in gentoo penguin (*Pygoscelis papua*) adults and chicks and the importance of warm feet. *Physiological Zoology* 71 (5): 524-533.

# 13

# African Penguins

*Nicky Stander and Romy Klusener*

## Natural History

The African Penguin is endemic to the greater Benguela upwelling ecosystem off south-western Africa (Crawford et al. 2011). It breeds at 28 localities (Kemper et al. 2007a) from Hollams Bird Island, central Namibia, to Bird Island in South Africa's Eastern Cape Province (Hockey et al. 2005). In 2015, South Africa supported 77% of the overall breeding population of the species (BirdLife International 2019).

The overall (Namibian and South African) population in the 1920s was probably in the order of millions. By 1956–57 it had decreased to about 141 000 pairs. It fell further to about 69 000 pairs in 1979–80, 63 000 pairs in 2001, 57 000 pairs in 2004–05, to 36 000 pairs in 2006–07 (Kemper et al. 2007a). Due to the continuous decline, the IUCN reclassified the African Penguin from Vulnerable to Endangered in 2010; this trend has continued with declines to 25 000 pairs in 2015 (BirdLife International 2019) and 16 000 pairs in 2017 (DEA, unpubl.).

African Penguin colonies vary widely in their habitat, from islands with little or no cover to well-vegetated environments. Historically, nests were mainly burrows in guano, but the large-scale collection of guano deposits along the coasts of southern Africa since the mid-nineteenth century has removed much of the breeding habitat, resulting in these birds breeding in a variety of suboptimal habitats (Frost et al. 1976; Wilson and Wilson 1989). Today, nests are built where available in burrows in guano or sand but, more often, in clefts between rocks, or on the surface in the shade (preferably), in disused buildings, or artificial nests provided to replace lost habitat (Shelton et al. 1984; Crawford et al. 1995; Sherley et al. 2012). Nesting material includes seaweed, pieces of vegetation, rocks, shells, bones, and feathers, but some nests have no lining at all.

African Penguins usually breed for the first time between 4 and 6 years of age (Whittington et al. 2005a). Once they have bred, adults show strong fidelity to colonies and mates as well as some nest-site fidelity (e.g. La Cock and Hänel 1987; Randall et al. 1987; La Cock and Cooper 1988; Crawford et al. 1995; Whittington et al. 2005b; Barham 2017).

The clutch is usually two eggs, sometimes one, rarely three (Crawford et al. 1999). Eggs are white rounded ovals, becoming stained as incubation proceeds. The laying interval is 3–3.2 days (Williams 1981; Williams and Cooper 1984). Double clutching in one season is not unusual; both clutches may fail, or one or both succeed (Randall and Randall 1981; La Cock and Cooper 1988; Crawford et al. 1999; Barham 2017). Incubation starts with the first-laid egg, lasts 38–41 days (37–38 days/egg) and is shared by both sexes (Rand 1960; Williams and Cooper 1984; Randall 1989).

*Hand-Rearing Birds*, Second Edition. Edited by Rebecca S. Duerr and Laurie J. Gage.

Chicks generally hatch asynchronously, usually about 2 days apart (Williams and Cooper 1984; Seddon and van Heezik 1991). Chicks are closely attended by adults until about 26–30 days old, when they are mostly left unguarded and may form crèches of up to 25 chicks (Erasmus and Smith 1974; Seddon and Van Heezik 1993). Chicks fledge at 55–130 days old (Seddon and Van Heezik 1993; Kemper 2006). Often, both chicks will fledge from two chick broods, but survival from hatching to fledging is variable and influenced by a multitude of factors such as burrow collapse, drowning, predation by Kelp Gulls (*Larus dominicanus*), starvation, or heat stress (Seddon and Van Heezik 1991; Barham et al. 2007; Kemper et al. 2007b; Sherley 2010).

Molt in birds is energetically expensive (Hoye and Buttemer 2011). Molt in penguins is unique, since they replace all their feathers in a relatively short period of time compared to that of other birds, ranging from 13 to 40 days depending on the species (Stonehouse 1967). Molt in penguins is essential to them being able to remain waterproof and thus insulated in cold waters while foraging (Stonehouse 1967; Payne 1972). Penguins become hyperphagic during the pre-molt period (Otsuka et al. 2000) and are dependent on high and predictable food availability during the pre-molt fattening and post-molt recovery phases. The acquisition of sufficient body reserves during pre-molt foraging can be considered a greater priority than at any other time in the annual cycle (Croxall and Davis 1999; Wolfaardt et al. 2008, 2009).

African Penguins feed solitarily or in small to large groups of up to >150 birds (Rand 1960; Wilson and Wilson 1990; Ryan et al. 2012). They may dive to 130 m but usually forage at depths <80 m, with dives lasting 1–2 minutes on average. They may hunt cooperatively, swimming rapidly round a school of fish to compress it (Wilson 1985b; Wilson and Wilson 1990; Ryan et al. 2012) and this improves their catch per unit effort (McInnes et al. 2017). Most food is caught between 10:00 a.m. and 6:00 p.m., with a lull in feeding activity around midday (Wilson and Wilson 1995; Petersen et al. 2006; Ludynia 2007; Waller 2011). Birds generally do not feed at night (Wilson 1985a). When breeding, most foraging trips last <24 hours and adult penguins generally remain within 40 km of colonies (Heath and Randall 1989; Petersen et al. 2006; Ludynia 2007; Pichegru et al. 2010; Waller 2011), performing 200–400 dives in a foraging trip (Ryan et al. 2007). Foraging effort increases as chicks grow, and parents brooding large chicks can forage for 3–5 days (Ludynia, Waller unpubl. data). Outside the breeding season, birds may travel up to 350 km to feed (Ludynia 2007; Waller 2011). African Penguins feed mainly on active, free-swimming prey, usually schooling pelagic fish, which they may locate using their olfactory sense (Wright et al. 2011). Especially important are anchovy, sardine, and, in Namibia, Pelagic Goby (*Sufflogobius bibarbatus*) (Hockey et al. 2005; Ludynia et al. 2010; Crawford et al. 2011). Other prey includes cephalopods (Randall and Randall 1986; Connan et al. 2016), Horse Mackerel (*Trachurus capensis*), and juvenile hake (*Merluccius* sp.) (Hockey et al. 2005).

## Criteria for Intervention

Due to the conservation status of the African Penguin, there are circumstances that warrant an intervention that will benefit the species. In the wild, conservation authorities will remove eggs or chicks for hand-rearing when the parents have abandoned the nest (e.g. there are no parents present on the nest and eggs feel cool to the touch), when the parents have nested in an unsafe area (e.g. a public area such as a car park or at the side of a busy road, or if nesting has occurred in a residential garden where the chances of human disturbance or predation is high and therefore chick abandonment may occur), or if chicks or parents have suffered disease or injuries. Intervention may also occur during extreme weather events, such as extremely hot weather or during heavy rain and high sea swells.

The utmost care should be taken when handling eggs for any form of transportation. Any unnatural movements to the egg may damage or even kill the developing embryo within the egg. The Southern African Foundation for the Conservation of Coastal Birds' (SANCCOB) full protocol for hand-rearing African Penguins is available in Klusener et al. (2018).

## Record Keeping

Accurate record keeping is an integral aspect of the hand-rearing of African Penguin chicks, allowing the hand-rearer as well as the veterinary team insight into the progress of each individual bird. Keeping accurate and consistent records allows for Standard Operating Procedures to be developed, hand-rearing protocols to be designed and refined, and for research to take place if necessary.

It is recommended that each individual egg is issued an Egg Number; this number is written with pencil onto the eggshell. The egg is assigned an Egg Sheet where more detailed information is recorded. Daily weight, turning of eggs, candling, and humidity should be recorded (Table 13.1). Whether from the wild or captivity, other information that should be obtained when eggs are transferred includes parental identity, age of parents, reproductive experience, environmental and social conditions, date egg(s) were laid, and which egg is an "A" egg or "B" egg, reflecting the lay order. For chicks, minimum records should include where the chick originated from, the ID number assigned to that individual, the reason for admission, weight, body condition, and hydration. Figure 13.1 shows a sample admission record for a chick.

During hand-rearing, daily record keeping is essential for understanding the health and development of each individual chick and should include the first morning weight before feeding, the percentage increase or decrease in chick's weight, amount of food offered and consumed at each feed, plus administration of vitamin supplementation and any prescribed medication.

## Artificial Incubation and Egg Management

Egg incubators should always be thoroughly cleaned before placing any penguin eggs inside; a high-quality disinfectant should be used to ensure all potential pathogens are killed. In addition, a multipurpose disinfectant aerosol fogger can be used to clean out the incubators as well as the incubation room. A chlorine detergent disinfectant may be used to clean the egg incubators on a more regular basis. It is important that while cleaning, the egg incubators are switched off, allowed to cool, and the distilled water used to create humidity is drained out. Fresh distilled water may be added to the reservoir of the incubator after cleaning. To ensure a constant temperature, the incubation room should be kept at a steady temperature. Setting the room temperature using an air conditioning unit at 69.8 °F/21 °C (dry air) seems to be an ideal environment for the incubators to function optimally at the SANCCOB facility in South Africa. The temperature of the egg incubator is set at 97.7° F/36.5 °C and 45% humidity; however, this may differ depending on the geographic locality, humidity, and season.

African Penguin eggs brought in from the wild are naturally soiled and dirty; there is no need to clean or disinfect the eggs. Egg shells are porous and disinfectant agents can seep through the shell and affect the developing embryo.

The incubation period of the African Penguin is between 38 and 42 days; in captive institutions, knowing the exact hatching date is easily determined as the laying date is known. Eggs that are artificially incubated due to abandonment or unsafe nesting in the wild may be admitted at different

Table 13.1 Example of an egg sheet.

| | |
|---|---|
| **Name:**<br>**Egg number:**<br>**Sibling egg/chick no:**<br>**Date: Time:**<br>**Where egg came from:**<br>**Why was egg removed:**<br>**How egg was handled/transported prior to arrival:**<br><br>**Length: Width:**<br>**Temperature set at:**<br>**Incubator used**<br>**Estimated hatching date**<br>**Estimated hatching weight** | **Date and time starred:**<br><br>**Moved to:**<br><br>**Date and time pipped**<br><br><br>**Date hatched:**<br>**Chick number:**<br>**Hatching weight:** |

| DATE | TURN EGGS | WEIGHT | HUMIDITY | EGG BUDDY | CANDLING/ OTHER COMMENTS |
|---|---|---|---|---|---|
| | | | | | |
| | | | | | |
| | | | | | |
| | | | | | |
| | | | | | |
| | | | | | |
| | | | | | |
| | | | | | |
| | | | | | |
| | | | | | |

stages of development, making determining the hatching day not as accurate. It is normal for eggs to lose weight as the embryo develops. The rate of weight loss should remain the same no matter the stage of development (as long as the egg has no cracks), this is usually 13–15% of its laying weight over the entire course of incubation. See Chapter 3 for more information.

African Penguin eggs are laid flat (width ways) inside the egg incubator along set rollers which are spaced apart to allow the egg to sit carefully between the two rollers. It is recommended to choose an incubator with automatic temperature and humidity. To ensure healthy embryonic development, the eggs are set to mechanically turn every two hours; in addition, each egg is manually rotated 180° once daily to aid in the vascularization of the embryo.

Candling is an important tool used during egg management to determine the fertility and developmental age of the embryo, any abnormalities to the shell (such as hairline cracks or thickened

Admitted by:

AFRICAN PENGUIN

ADULT ☐ JUVENILE ☐ BLUE ☐

CLASS ☐

CHECK: P0 ☐ P1 ☐ P2 ☐ P3 ☐ P4 ☐

EGG: ☐

SANCCOB NUMBER ______________

RECAPTURE? Y / N

SAFRING NUMBER ______________________

TRANSPONDER NUMBER___________________

| ARRIVAL | |
|---|---|
| DATE: ___________ TIME: _______ | HM: ☐ |
| AREA: _______________________ | BL: ☐ |
| ORGANISATION: _______________ | |
| WEIGHT: __________ | BD: ☐ |

| RELEASE | |
|---|---|
| DATE: ___________ TIME: __________ | |
| AREA: _______________________ | HM: ☐ |
| WEIGHT: __________ | |
| BOAT ☐ BEACH ☐ COLONY ☐ | |

HYDRATION: N ☐ 5% ☐ 7% ☐ 10% ☐

DARROWS: ☐ RINGERS: ☐

HABITUS: 1 ☐ 2 ☐ 3 ☐ 4 ☐ BLOOD VALUES: PCV ☐ BC ☐ TP ☐

DEWORM: ☐

RFA

TREATMENT & FEEDING REGIME

| | | | | | |
|---|---|---|---|---|---|
| EYES: WNL | ☐ | REMARKS<br>EYE TREATMENT: ☐ | MUSCULUSKELETAL: WNL | ☐ | REMARKS |
| EARS: WNL | ☐ | REMARKS | ABDOMEN: WNL | ☐ | REMARKS |
| BEAK: WNL | ☐ | REMARKS | TAIL/PREEN GLAND: WNL | ☐ | REMARKS |
| NOSTRILS /NARES: WNL | ☐ | REMARKS | CLOACA: WNL | ☐ | REMARKS |
| MOUTH: WNL | ☐ | REMARKS | GUANO: WNL | ☐ | REMARKS |
| RESPIRATION: WNL | ☐ | REMARKS | SKIN: WNL | ☐ | REMARKS |
| FEATHERS: WNL | ☐ | REMARKS<br>OILED % ☐ FEATHER SAMPLE ☐ | FEET: WNL | ☐ | REMARKS |
| ECTOPARASITES: WNL | ☐ | REMARKS<br>KARBADUST ☐ | NEUROLOGICAL: WNL | ☐ | REMARKS |

**Figure 13.1** Example of a bird card for an African Penguin.

areas), size of the air cell, and whether there is embryo movement. It is good practice to candle eggs weekly, and after 2 weeks of candling it is often possible to determine the hatching day of the egg.

Candling is done on the blunt end of the egg at first, and as the embryo further develops candling can also be done on the pointed end. Care must be taken to prevent cooling the egg during candling, or burning with the light source. Each egg must be handled carefully and slowly, as any sudden movements or jarring can affect the viability of the embryo. There are numerous commercial brands of candlers available; however, a LED flashlight is an ideal substitution; with a bright white light and minimal heat discharged, it can work just as well as a candler.

## Hatching

Once the chick has internally pipped (pierced through the air cell), it is taken off the rollers and placed in a container with paper toweling; this container is still kept in the incubator; however, the turning has now stopped.

Once the chick has externally pipped/starred (pierced through the egg shell) the egg is removed from the egg incubator and placed into a hatcher, where the humidity is set at 60%, and the temperature is lowered slightly to 96.1 °F/35.6 °C. A higher humidity ensures the membrane does not dry and stick to the chick inhibiting the hatching process or blocking the nares. The hatching process takes 48–50 hours, African Penguin chicks hatch out of their shell in an anti-clockwise direction, and are positioned with their head under their right flipper and beak facing up toward the shell. A hatching egg should be checked on frequently to ensure the chick is still correctly positioned. If the chick has not shown progress after 50 hours has lapsed, an assisted hatch must be considered as the chick may be now fatigued or possibly malpositioned. By using the candler to shine into the external pip site, an evaluation can be made of the problem.

There are several reasons why a chick may not hatch successfully on its own, which is why it is so critical to monitor the pip to hatch interval carefully. If a chick has made internal pip but has failed to progress for over 12–15 hours, is well beyond expected incubation period, or if a chick has rotated inside the egg without further chipping such that the bill is no longer visible at the pip hole, this is a good indicator that something is wrong. However, the most common hatching difficulty for penguin chicks is malpositioning of the chick inside the egg. This may or may not be accompanied by unabsorbed yolk and/or residual albumen. Once a chick is determined to be having hatching difficulty, the egg should be removed for assistance.

When performing an assisted hatch, care should be taken not to introduce bacteria to the chick. Hands should be washed and gloved and all instruments sterilized. The pip should be examined and an evaluation of the problem should be made before beginning to assist the chick to hatch. The egg should be candled to assess vascularization and pip location (above or below the air cell), and a small flashlight can be used to look inside the pipped hole to look for unabsorbed yolk, residual albumen, or other problems. Once these steps are completed, carefully hold the egg in one hand and slowly peel away small portions of the shell from the pip site with sterile forceps. This must be performed under a heat lamp to keep the egg warm.

After the pip area has been further exposed, the membrane should be moistened with warm sterile water on a swab to check for active vessels. If no vessels are present, the membrane can be peeled back to expose the chick. Be sure that the membrane does not stick to the nares and occlude breathing. Efforts should be made to expose the head first. In extreme cases, it may be necessary to manipulate the head out from under the flipper. If the membranes are active, they will bleed when disturbed. Try another section of the egg to avoid active blood vessels. Throughout this process, monitor the chick's temperature; it may be necessary to place the chick back in the incubator to warm up before continuing the assisted hatch.

Very often, it is sufficient to expose the head and increase the size of the chipped shell and the chick will be able to complete the hatching process on its own. This will need to be monitored closely as sometimes chicks are too fatigued and will need full assistance. Remember to record that the chick was an assisted hatch and any other additional comments that may be relevant.

## Initial Care and Stabilization

The first 10 days after hatching are the most critical: the chicks are immunocompromised, cannot thermoregulate, and require intensive care. After finishing hatching, move the chick back to the egg incubator (97.7° F/36.5 °C and 45% humidity) to allow it to "fluff" out for about 12 hours, then transfer to a human baby incubator. At this young age chicks are kept in individual containers; these containers are placed inside the human baby incubator, which regulates the required temperature and humidity. Any sick chicks are kept in their own separate incubator to prevent the spread of infection to other chicks. Care must be taken with newly hatched chicks as they cannot hold their heads up on their own; feeding should be carried out slowly and gently to ensure the chick is swallowing.

As these chicks are intended for wild release, it is crucial to minimize handling of chicks and to aim for group feedings along with health checks. It is very important to stimulate chicks before feeding by "preening" their fluffy downy feathers to mimic what the parents would do. Initiating a feeding response by creating a "V" with the index finger and middle finger around the chick's beak (Figure 13.2) will often encourage the chick to beg for its food as opposed to needing to be force-fed. During initial care, note whether the chick is vocal and giving a feeding response, whether there is guano in the container, and, if so, what the consistency is, whether the abdomen is palpably bloated, and whether the chick appears normally hydrated.

### Chick Handling

Care should be taken when handling small chicks or hatchlings up to 550g. Place your index finger and middle finger over the shoulders of the chick, place your thumb and ring finger under each flipper, and support the chick's back with the palm of your hand – your index finger and middle finger act as a "seat belt" over the shoulder; using this handling method you are able to support the spine of the chick as well as keeping the head upright.

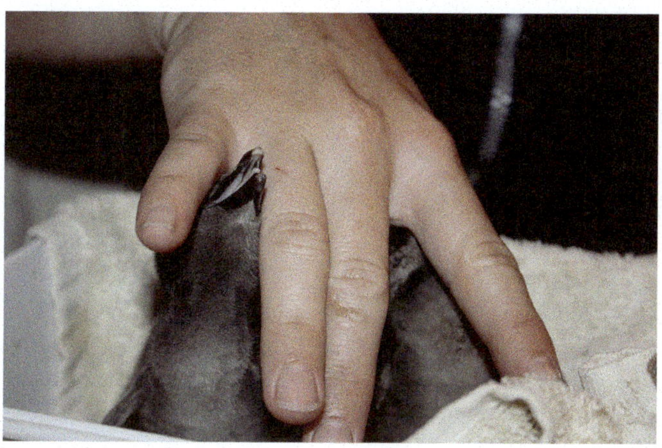

Figure 13.2 Stimulating a chick to feed by forming a "V" between fingers, while supporting the head.

When handling larger chicks (over 1 kg), place your dominant hand behind the eyes to firmly, but not roughly, hold the skull. Place the free hand around the abdomen to support the body. The chick should be held close to the handler's body. Larger more docile chicks may be picked up under the flippers, with both handlers' hands supporting the chick.

## Common Medical Problems and Solutions

### Hypo and Hyperthermia

The human incubator and brooder temperature should always be carefully monitored. Chicks should be observed closely for signs of heat or cold stress. The symptoms most frequently observed in overheated chicks include lethargy, inappetence, panting, and extension of feet and flippers, or restlessness when other chicks are sleeping or at rest. Overheating can be problematic for chicks of any age but can quickly become life threatening in very young chicks unless corrective measures are taken. Hypothermic chicks may be observed shivering or huddled against the side of the brooder and their feet will be cold to the touch. Chicks in this state will be slow to respond to feeding stimuli. Adjust housing temperatures accordingly.

### Overfeeding and Bloat

This problem can be avoided by carefully evaluating each chick's weight gain on a daily basis. Even when strictly following feeding protocols, problems from overfeeding can arise. It is always in the best interest of the chicks to address their needs individually. What may be an appropriate amount for one chick may be excessive for another. Generally, a 10–15% daily weight gain is expected during the first few weeks. Behavior associated with overfeeding includes lethargy, regurgitation, and disinterest in food at one or more feeds. Food should be withheld until the chick appears hungry. A dark, grainy stool may be indicative of improper digestion; thus, the veterinarian should be notified. Always gently palpate the chick's abdomen before feeds, as this can determine whether the chick has digested its previous meal and can help to determine what quantities to feed for the following meal.

### Dehydration

Throughout development, hydration should be carefully monitored; this is particularly important when solid fish is introduced to the diet. Symptoms of dehydration include dry-looking eyes, shriveled appearance of the skin on the feet, or thick, pasty feces. The skin along the back will remain "molded" up if the chick is inadequately hydrated (skin tent test). Oral electrolyte fluids and water will improve this condition. Subcutaneous fluids may be required in severely dehydrated chicks regularly throughout the day. The amount of subcutaneous fluids will vary depending on the size of the chick and severity of dehydration.

### Splayed Legs

Aptly named, this condition describes the outward turned position of the chick's legs. Although not often seen in penguins, this condition can result in serious and long-term complications; therefore, early detection is important. The brooder or nest substrate should be textured enough so the chick's feet do not slip out from underneath it.

### Respiratory Infections

Symptoms that are likely to be indications of chest infections in chicks include labored breathing (open mouth breathing), struggling to breath (dyspnea), coughing, mucus as sputum or in mouth, regurgitation, sneezing, lethargy, and separation from the group.

If any of these symptoms are identified, the veterinarian must be notified, and blood and fecal samples should be collected. Treatment will depend on whether the infection is bacterial, fungal, or viral, but nebulization is often useful to assist clearing the airways. It is important to isolate a sick chick away from the healthy chicks to prevent spreading an infection.

### Feather Loss Disorder

Abnormal feather loss may occur around the perineum and shoulders of the chick (mild cases) or the entire chick may lose all its feathers. As soon as this is detected, record keeping should describe the loss of feathers as a percentage. Supplementing the diet with zinc and omega fatty acids seems to promote feather regrowth.

### Neurological Abnormalities

Nervous system abnormalities can be described as twitching, head rolling back, falling over, lopsidedness, falling onto back, and seizures. The causes are variable from head trauma, avian malaria or other infections, emaciation, dehydration, and poisoning. If the cause is diagnosed, then treatment should be initiated. Treating seabirds undergoing rehabilitation with thiamine tablets once daily is recommended since the thiamine in frozen fish is depleted during the thawing process. Treating neurologically abnormal penguins with thiamine may be curative if this was the problem, and informative if treatment is not helpful.

## Diets

### Hand-rearing Diet Formula for African Penguin Chicks

- 880 g fish, removing the tail and fins
- 600 ml cold tap water
- 5 Edelweiss Large Fish Eater capsules (squeeze out the powder from the capsules)
- 10 Brewer's yeast 300 mg tablets
- 6 Vitamin B1 (Thiamine) 100 mg tablets
- 1 teaspoon cod liver oil (5 ml)
- 2 level teaspoons Kyron Protexin (5 g)
- 2 level teaspoons Kyron Cani-Cal (5 g)
- 1 level teaspoon calcium gluconate powder (2.5 g)
- 3 capsules vitamin E 400 IU (cut capsule and squeeze out oil)

Place into blender and blend thoroughly, for 5 minutes. Check that the consistency is like drinking yogurt; if it is not smooth, it can be blended for longer. Strain the mixture twice through sieves. Label the container with the date and time and place into the refrigerator. Refrigerate unused portions and discard within 12 hours for young chicks and 24 hours for older chicks. Warm refrigerated formula in a warm-water bath until it is body temperature prior to feeding. The Kyron Protexin is a probiotic product, and Cani-Cal is a vitamin and mineral supplement.

## Feeding Procedures

A feeding response can be initiated in a small penguin chick by forming a "V" with the middle and index fingers, then placing the "V" on the top of a chick's beak and wiggling the fingers. The chick should respond by pushing up into the crook of the fingers. If the chick does not display this feeding response, the beak should be opened gently using the thumb and index finger (Figure 13.2). The palm of the "holding" hand should face the ceiling, the chick's head sliding in between the little finger and the ring finger.

Prior to feeding, it is important to palpate the chick's abdomen to ensure that it has digested its fish from the previous feed. The syringe of fish formula should be shaken to evenly distribute the heat. The temperature of the formula can be tested on the wrist. Do not feed formula to chicks that is hot or cold; it should be at body temperature.

The feeding tube can be lubricated with cod liver oil. Insert the tube into the throat avoiding the trachea and ensuring that you can see clearly into the chick's mouth and that the windpipe is not obstructed. For older chicks, always feed formula first, and then fish pieces or tails; the fish can be dipped into water for lubrication before feeding it to the chick. Once feeding is complete, gently clean around the beak with warm water and gauze. A separate piece of gauze is used to clean the vent with warm water. Finally, use a piece of gauze and (10% diluted) betadine (povidone-iodine) to clean the umbilicus area. This is cleaned until the chick reaches 500 g.

### Hatchlings

Five hours after hatching, offer the chick 1–2 ml of probiotics and water every 3 hours. On day 1, 24 hours after hatching, begin giving formula diluted with tap water according to the schedule shown on Table 13.2. Work the chick onto full-strength formula in increasing proportions over days 1–3. On day 4, give full-strength formula, working up to 10% body weight in volume. When a chick reaches 100 g, it can begin to receive solid fish in addition to its formula. Introduce fish slowly using fish fillets cut into appropriately small sizes. Introducing fish can be done on the schedule shown in Table 13.2.

Hatchlings up to 500 g receive 6 feeds a day at 3-hour intervals. Feeding begins at 6:00 a.m. where the initial weighing and checking of its feeding regime is carried out. The last feed of the day for chicks of this age is 9:00 p.m. For the first 3 days after hatching, a predetermined amount of formula is given; after this, all chicks less than 1 kg receive 10% of their body weight at each feed (100 ml formula/kg) (Table 13.2). Feeding tubes for the youngest chicks must be small 6-French size, with size increased to 8-, 10-, 12-, and finally, 16-French as the chicks grow to over 500 g.

### Older Chicks

By the time chicks reach 400 g, fish should make up 50% of the diet, with the balance of 10% body weight per meal in formula. At 500 g, regardless of how much a chick solicits feeding, continue the 10% rule as a guide for food intake. It is common for chicks at this stage to take less than 10%; this is often no cause for alarm, and the chick will likely eat well at subsequent feedings. It is at this age that they tend to go through their "first phase" of being difficult. At this stage, vitamin supplementation

Table 13.2 Feeding schedule for African Penguins.

| Fluid and Feeding Times | | | | Hour of Day | | | | | | | | | | | | | | | |
|---|---|---|---|---|---|---|---|---|---|---|---|---|---|---|---|---|---|---|---|
| | Meal size | Formula (ml) | Fish (g) | 6 | 7 | 8 | 9 | 10 | 11 | 12 | 13 | 14 | 15 | 16 | 17 | 18 | 19 | 20 | 21 |
| Hatch Day | 1 ml max | Water + probiotics | 0 | Start 5 hours after hatch, then every 3 hours | | | | | | | | | | | | | | | |
| Day 1 | 1 ml max | 50 : 50 (formula: water) | 0 | F | | | F | | | F | | | F | | | F | | | F |
| Day 2 | 3 ml max | 75 : 25 (formula: water) | 0 | F | | | F | | | F | | | F | | | F | | | F |
| Day 3 | 5 ml max | Formula | 0 | F | | | F | | | F | | | F | | | F | | | F |
| Up to 100 g | 10% BW | Formula | 0 | F | | | F | | | F | | | F | | | F | | | F |
| Day 1 on fish | Y | Formula minus 3 g | 3 g fillet | F&F | | | F | | | F | | | F | | | F | | | F |
| Day 2 on fish | Y | Formula minus 5 g | 5 g fillet | F&F | | | F | | | F | | | F&F | | | F | | | F |
| Day 3 on fish | Y | Formula minus 5 g | 5 g fillet | F&F | | | F | | | F&F | | | F | | | F&F | | | F |
| Day 4 on fish | Y | Formula minus 5 g | 5 g fillet | F&F | | | F&F | | | F&F | | | F&F | | | F&F | | | F |
| Day 5 on fish | Y | Formula minus 7 g | 7 g fillet | F&F | | | F&F | | | F&F | | | F&F | | | F&F | | | F |
| Day 6 on fish | Y | Formula minus 10 g | 10 g fillet | F&F | | | F&F | | | F&F | | | F&F | | | F&F | | | F |
| 300–400 g | Y | Formula minus 15 g | 15 g fillet | F&F | | | F&F | | | F&F | | | F&F | | | F&F | | | F |
| 400–500 g | Y | Formula 50% | 50% | F&F | | | F&F | | | F&F | | | F&F | | | F&F | | | F |
| 500–600 g | Y | Formula 30 ml | Fish minus 30 ml | F&F | | | | F&F | | | | F&F | | | | F&F | | | F&F |
| 600–1 kg | Y | Formula 30 ml | Fish minus 30 ml | F&F | | | | F&F | | | | F&F | | | | F&F | | | |
| 1–1.5 kg | x | Formula 60 ml | 2–3 fish | | | Fish | | F | | D | | Fish | | F | | Fish | | | F |
| 1.5–2 kg | x | Formula 60 ml | 3–4 fish | | | Fish | | F | | D | | | | Fish | | W | | | F |
| 2–2.5 kg | x | Formula 60 ml | 4–5 fish | | | Fish | | F | | D | | | | Fish | | W | | | |

F&F = fish and formula feed.
F = formula only.
D = Darrow's solution (isotonic electrolytes).
W = Tap water.
BW = body weight.

may begin (Table 13.3). At 600 g, if the chick is doing well on a diet of half fish and half formula, the proportion of fish in the diet can be increased to two thirds of the total intake. It is increasingly important to stick to the 10% rule. Some chicks may require less than 10% of their first daily weight at each feeding. At above 600 g, begin reducing the number of daily feedings while increasing proportions of fish fed as shown in the feeding chart.

There are two stages at which most chicks become fussy: at around the 500 g mark for a day or two; and at 1 kg for several days. At these weights, they may refuse food at one feeding or not eat full amounts at each feed. At around 500 g, chicks generally become more skittish to any movements and often wrigglier to handle. Wrapping them in a towel helps during feeds. At 500 g, the chicks are moved into larger crates, as the brooders are now too small for them and the crates allow more movement for the chicks.

## Expected Weight Gain

Whether hand- or parent-reared, African Penguin chicks reach adult weight at about 2 months of age (Figure 13.3). At 60 days of age, they are more than 50% done molting their wooly down.

## Housing

African Penguins may stay in a room with temperature of 64.4–69.8 °F (18–21 °C) with a fan to circulate the air. At approximately 1 kg, the ambient temperature is reduced further as needed. As chicks lose their fluff, they are transferred to an outdoor enclosure and given access to the swimming pool at >45 days of age and 1.5–3 kg, when more than 50% of downy plumage has molted.

### Hatchlings

Newly hatched chicks up to 8 days old are housed in human baby incubators at 91.4 °F (33 °C) and 44–55% humidity. The hatchlings are placed in individual pots lined with soft paper towel, which absorbs the guano effectively and should be replaced during each feed (Figure 13.4). The temperature in the human baby incubator is lowered to 86 °F (30 °C) if chicks appear hot (panting/uncomfortable). While the chicks are in the human incubators, they should look comfortable and will sleep most of the time, unless it is almost feeding time, in which case they normally become vocal. It is important to monitor their behavior as each chick has individual needs and some may become uncomfortable if it is too hot, others may not be warm enough, and the temperature may need to be adjusted for individual needs.

Table 13.3 Daily vitamin regime.

| Monday | Fish eater tablet |
|---|---|
| Wednesday | Multivitamin |
| Friday | Thiamine |
| Sunday | Cani-vit in a gel cap |

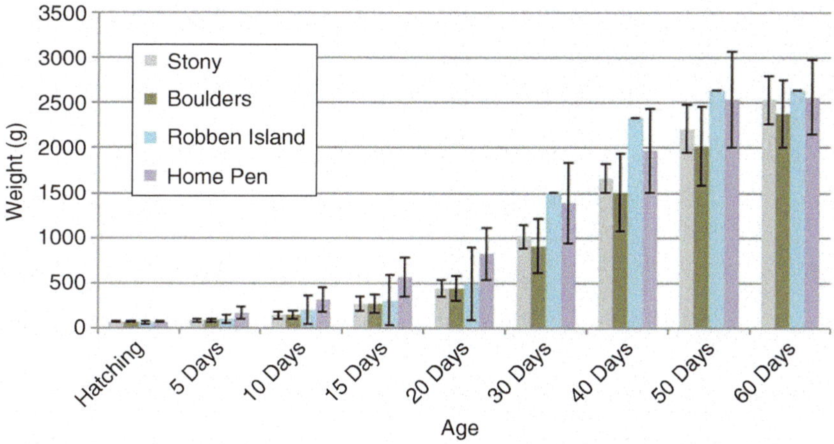


**Figure 13.3** Growth of hatchlings in the Chick Rearing Unit from nearby penguin colonies of Stony Point in Bettys Bay (34.3742° S, 18.8953° E), Boulders colony in Simonstown (34.1957° S, 18.4494° E), Robben Island (33.8076° S, 18.3712° E), as well as the growth of parent-reared chicks that were fostered to the resident birds of Southern African Foundation for the Conservation of Coastal Birds (SANCCOB) Table View (Home Pen).

**Figure 13.4** Small downy chick with eyes open.

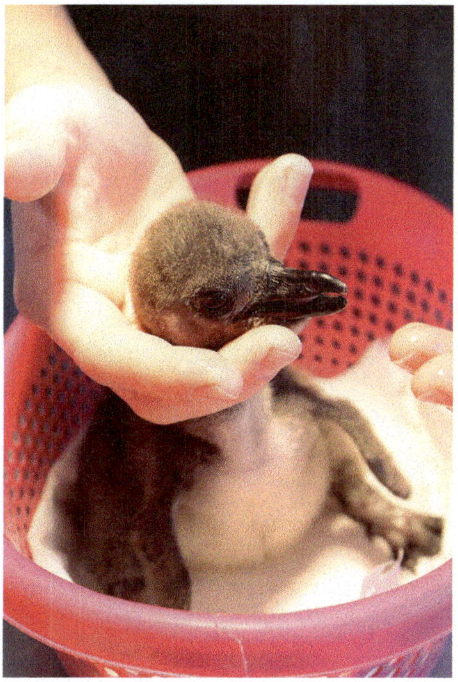

After 8 days in the human baby incubator, the chicks are transferred to open brooders (Figure 13.5), with an affixed heat source (175-W infrared bulb) and a temperature probe. It is advisable to have protective brooder grid covers to protect chicks from anything falling into the brooder. There should be sufficient air circulation; penguin chicks require a dry environment, as high humidity environments may cause respiratory issues.

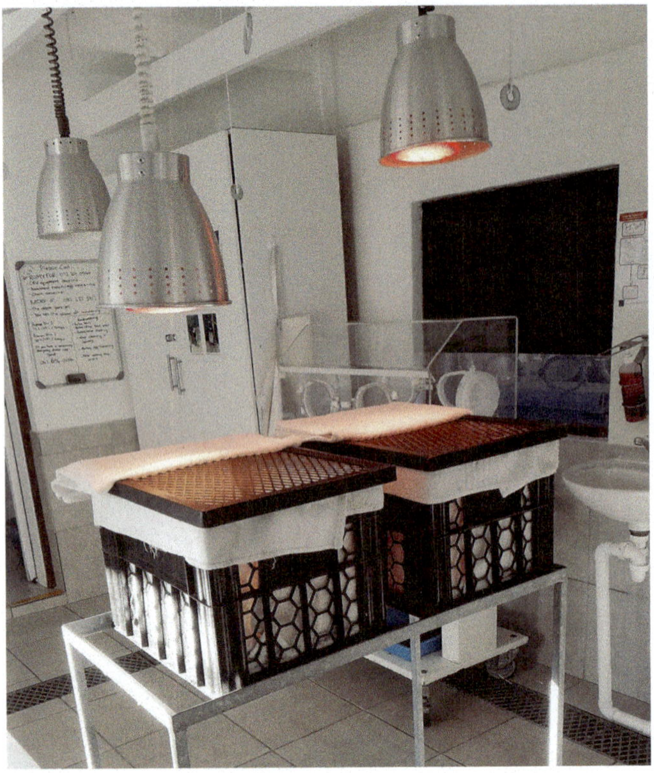

Figure 13.5 Bird crate appropriate for housing larger chicks.

Brooder crates need to be large enough to allow an approximate 9 °F (5 °C) temperature difference from one side of the brooder to the other to allow the chick to adjust its behavior to meet its own thermoregulatory requirements. However, if the brooder is too large, chicks may venture too far from the heat source and suffer serious cooling. It is recommended that no more than two chicks should be reared in a single brooder; overcrowding can lead to overheating and also increase the likelihood of transferring disease. Stuffed animals are used for companionship and comfort for single chicks.

Cloth toweling is the most commonly used substrate in the brooder and crates. Towels are easily available and can be easily cleaned. Roughly textured, holey, or frayed towels should not be used because of the risk of injuries resulting from snagged toenails or necks getting twisted in the frayed towels. It is equally important that the substrate is not smooth to prevent the chick's feet from sliding out underneath it. Temporary or permanent damage to muscles, tendons, and joints can result from improper footing.

## Older Chicks

As chicks reach 500 g, they are moved into larger crates (29.2 × 21.3 × 16.3 in./ 74.1 × 54 × 41.5 cm) and, weather permitting, may stay outside during the day. As chicks grow older and more timid, it is useful to provide an "air-kennel" with towels covering half of the crate so that the chicks may hide. This is usually the stage at which chicks go through their "first phase"; at this weight, they may refuse food at one feeding or not eat full amounts at each feed, they are more skittish to any

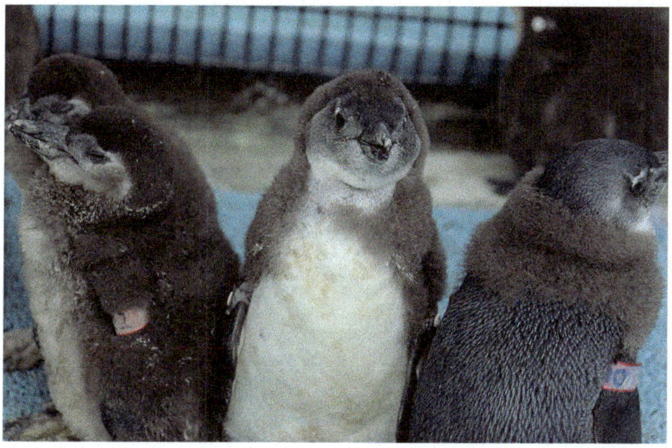

Figure 13.6 African Penguin chicks socializing, showing wooly down on the left and birds molting into mature contour feathers on the right

movements, and often wrigglier to handle. Chicks over 1.5 kg may be housed together in a small enclosure, this allows for socializing and gives a larger area for movement (Figure 13.6). Burrows may be placed in the pen for the chicks to retreat into.

Nomad matting (3M) is an ideal substrate to be used in an enclosure where larger chicks are housed together; it is a combination of fine and course tufted loop fibers which absorb water and guano, and minimize development of bumblefoot. These mats can easily be cleaned by hosing them down with water.

## Preparation for Wild Release

When penguin chicks lose their fluff, they can be housed outdoors with pool access in large groups. Over the course of several weeks, the penguins are introduced to a progressive swimming schedule, depending on their feather grading and overall physical health. Feather grading should be performed weekly by force-swimming the penguins for 10–20 minutes, then verifying the waterproofing of their plumage in order to evaluate their progress and to group them with penguins at a similar stage of the conditioning process. When the penguins are approved for other release criteria (apparently healthy, good body condition, normal behaviour, waterproof plumage after swimming for 60 minutes, and clear blood results), a more comprehensive feather grading should be conducted after force-swimming them for 60 minutes to ensure that only waterproof penguins are released back to the wild. African Penguins that meet the release criteria are microchipped and released during the morning, with good weather and a sea swell of no more then 8.2–9.8 ft. (2.5–3 m), with a gentle breeze under 12.4 mph (20 km/h).

## Acknowledgments

Thank you to the staff, interns, and volunteers at SANCCOB who contribute to the work of hand-rearing penguin chicks to release back into the wild. The African Penguin Chick Bolstering Project is a collaboration between SANCCOB, Bristol Zoological Society, the Animal Demography Unit

(University of Cape Town), South African Department of Environmental Affairs – Oceans and Coasts, Cape Nature, Robben Island Museum, City of Cape Town, and South African National Parks. Thank you to the various institutions around the world who have advised and assisted with incubation and hand-rearing advice over the years.

## Sources for Products Mentioned

3M™ Nomad™ Unbacked Scraper Matting 8100: http://matsinc.com/3m-nomad-unbacked-scraper-8100, (800) 628–7462.
Edelweiss Pharmaceuticals, PO Box 307, Steenberg 7947, South Africa, www.ewlabs.co.za.
Kyron Laboratories, 29 Barney Road, Johannesburg, Benrose 2094, South Africa, http://compfusionpreview.co.za.

## References

Barham, B.J. (2017). *Nest site fidelity of the African penguin (Spheniscus demersus) on Robben Island.* M.Sc: Thesis, University of Bristol.

Barham, P.J., Underhill, L.G., Crawford, R.J.M. et al. (2007). Differences in breeding success between African penguins (*Spheniscus demersus*) that were and were not oiled in the MV Treasure oil-spill in 2000. *Emu* 107: 7–13.

BirdLife International. (2019). Species factsheet: Spheniscus demersus. Downloaded from www.birdlife.org.

Connan, M., Hofmeyr, G.J.G., and Pistorius, P.A. (2016). Reappraisal of the trophic ecology of one of the world's most threatened Spheniscids, the African Penguin. *PLoS One* 11 (7): e0159402. https://doi.org/10.1371/journal.pone.0159402.

Crawford, R.J.M., Williams, A.J., Hofmeyr, J.H. et al. (1995). Trends of African penguin *Spheniscus demersus* populations in the 20th century. *South African Journal of Marine Science* 16: 101–118.

Crawford, R.J.M., Shannon, L.J., and Whittington, P.A. (1999). Population dynamics of the African Penguin *Spheniscus demersus* at Robben Island. *South Africa. Marine Ornithology* 27: 139–147.

Crawford, R.J.M., Altwegg, R., Barham, B.J. et al. (2011). Collapse of South Africa's penguins in the early 21st century: a consideration of the possible influence of food and fishing. *African Journal of Marine Science* 33: 139–156.

Croxall, J.P. and Davis, L.S. (1999). Penguins: paradoxes and patterns. *Marine Ornithology* 27: 1–12.

Erasmus, T. and Smith, D. (1974). Temperature regulation of young jackass penguins, *Spheniscus demersus. African Zoology* 9 (2): 195–203.

Frost, P.G.H., Siegfried, W.R., and Cooper, J. (1976). Conservation of the jackass penguin (*Spheniscus demersus* (L.). *Biological Conservation* 9: 79–99.

Heath, R.G.M. and Randall, R.M. (1989). Foraging ranges and movements of jackass penguins (*Spheniscus demersus*) established through radio telemetry. *Journal of Zoology* 217: 367–379.

Hockey, P.A.R., Dean, W.R.J., and Ryan, P.G. (eds.) (2005). *Roberts Birds of Southern Africa*, 7e. Cape Town, South Africa: John Voelcker Bird Book Fund.

Hoye, B.J. and Buttemer, W.A. (2011). Inexplicable inefficiency of avian molt? Insights from an opportunistically breeding arid-zone species, *Lichenostomus penicillatus. PLoS One* 6 (2): e16230. https://doi.org/10.1371/journal.pone.0016230.

Kemper, J. (2006). Heading towards extinction? Demography of the African Penguin in Namibia. Ph.D. dissertation, University of Cape Town, Cape Town, South Africa.

Kemper, J., Underhill, L.G., Crawford, R.J.M., and Roux, J.-P. (2007a). Revision of the conservation status of seabirds and seals in the Benguela Ecosystem. In: *Final Report of the BCLME (Benguela Current Large Marine Ecosystem) Project on Top Predators as Biological Indicators of Ecosystem Change in the BCLME* (ed. S.P. Kirkman), 325–342. Cape Town, South Africa: Avian Demography Unit.

Kemper, J., Underhill, L.G., Roux, J.-P. et al. (2007b). Breeding patterns and factors influencing breeding success of African Penguins *Spheniscus demersus* in Namibia. In: *Final Report of the BCLME (Benguela Current Large Marine Ecosystem) Project on Top Predators as Biological Indicators of Ecosystem Change in the BCLME* (ed. S.P. Kirkman), 89–99. Cape Town, South Africa: Avian Demography Unit.

Klusener, R., Hurtado, R., Parsons, N. et al. (2018). From incubation to release: Hand-rearing as a tool for the conservation of the endangered African penguin. *PLoS One* 13(11): e0205126. doi:10.1371/journal.pone.0205126.

La Cock, G.D. and Hänel, C. (1987). Survival of African Penguins *Spheniscus demersus* at Dyer Island, southern Cape, South Africa. *Journal of Field Ornithology* 58: 284–287.

La Cock, G.D. and Cooper, J. (1988). The breeding frequency of Jackass Penguins on the west coast of South Africa. *Journal of Field Ornithology* 59: 155–156.

Ludynia, K. (2007). Identification and characterisation of foraging areas of seabirds in upwelling systems: Biological and hydrographic implications for foraging at sea. Ph.D. dissertation, University of Kiel.

Ludynia, K., Roux, J.P., Jones, R. et al. (2010). Surviving off junk: Low-energy prey dominates the diet of African penguins *Spheniscus demersus* at Mercury Island, Namibia, between 1996 and 2009. *African Journal of Marine Science* 32: 563–572.

McInnes, A.M., McGeorge, C., Ginsberg, S. et al. (2017). Group foraging increases foraging efficiency in a piscivorous diver, the African Penguin. *Royal Society Open Science* 4: 170918. http://dx.doi.org/10.1098/rsos.170918.

Otsuka, R., Machida, T., and Wada, M. (2000). Hormonal correlations at transition from reproduction to molting in an annual life cycle of Humboldt penguins (*Spheniscus humboldti*). *General and Comparative Endocrinology* 135: 175–185.

Payne, R.B. (1972). Mechanisms and control of molt. In: *Avian Biology*, vol. Vol. 2 (eds. D.S. Farner and J.R. King), 103–155. New York: Academic Press.

Petersen, S.L., Ryan, P.G., and Gremillet, D. (2006). Is food availability limiting African Penguins *Spheniscus demersus* at Boulders? A comparison of foraging effort at mainland and island colonies. *Ibis* 148: 14–26.

Pichegru, L., Grémillet, D., Crawford, R.J.M., and Ryan, P.G. (2010). Marine no-take zone rapidly benefits endangered penguin. *Biology Letters* https://doi.org/10.1098/rsbl.2009.0913.

Rand, R.W. (1960). The biology of guano-producing seabirds. 2. The distribution, abundance and feeding habits of the Cape penguin, *Spheniscus demersus*, off the south-western coast of the Cape Province. *Investigational Report Sea Fisheries Research Institute South Africa 41*:1–28.

Randall, R.M. (1989). Jackass penguins. In: *Oceans of Life of Southern Africa* (eds. A.I.L. Payne, R.J.M. Crawford and A.P. van Dalsen), 244–256. Cape Town, South Africa: Vlaeberg.

Randall, R.M., and Randall, B.M. 1981. The annual cycle of the Jackass Penguin *Spheniscus demersus* at St. Croix Island, South Africa. Proceedings of the Symposium on Birds of the Sea and Shore, Cape Town, South Africa, pp. 427–450.

Randall, R.M. and Randall, B.M. (1986). The diet of jackass penguins *Spheniscus demersus* in Algoa Bay, South Africa, and its bearing on population declines elsewhere. *Biological Conservation* 37: 119–134.

Randall, R.M., Randall, B.M., Cooper, J. et al. (1987). Jackass penguin *Spheniscus demersus* movements, inter-island visits, and settlement. *Journal of Field Ornithology* 58: 445–455.

Ryan, P.G., Petersen, S.L., Simeone, A., and Grémillet, D. (2007). Diving behaviour of African Penguins: do they differ from other *Spheniscus* penguins? *African Journal of Marine Science* 29: 153–160.

Ryan, P.G., Edwards, L., and Pichegru, L. (2012). African Penguins *Spheniscus demersus*, bait balls and the Allee effect. *Ardea* 100: 89–94.

Seddon, P.J. and van Heezik, Y.M. (1991). Hatching asynchrony and brood reduction in the Jackass Penguin: an experimental study. *Animal Behaviour* 42: 347–356.

Seddon, P.J. and van Heezik, Y.M. (1993). Behaviour of the jackass penguin chick. *Ostrich* 64: 8–12.

Shelton, P.A., Crawford, R.J.M., Cooper, J. et al. (1984). Distribution, population size and conservation of the Jackass Penguin *Spheniscus demersus*. *South African Journal of Marine Science* 2: 217–257.

Sherley, R.B. 2010. Factors influencing the demography of endangered seabirds at Robben Island, South Africa: implications and approaches for management and conservation. Ph.D. thesis, University of Bristol.

Sherley, R.B., Barham, B.J., Barham, P.J. et al. (2012). Artificial nests enhance the breeding productivity of African Penguins (*Spheniscus demersus*) on Robben Island, South Africa. *Emu*: 97: 97–97: 106.

Sherley, R.B., Waller, L.J., Strauss, V. et al. (2014). Hand-rearing, release and survival of African Penguin chicks abandoned before independence by molting parents. *PLoS One* 9 (10): e110794. https://doi.org/10.1371/journal.pone.0110794.

Stonehouse, B. (1967). The general biology and thermal balance of penguins. In: *Advances in Ecological Research IV* (ed. J.B. Cragg), 131–196. London: Academic Press.

Waller, L.J. (2011). The African Penguin Spheniscus demersus: conservation and management issues. Ph.D. thesis, University of Cape Town.

Whittington, P.A., Klages, N.T.W., Crawford, R.J.M. et al. (2005a). Age at first breeding of the African Penguin. *Ostrich* 76: 14–20.

Whittington, P.A., Randall, R.M., Crawford, R.J.M. et al. (2005b). Patterns of immigration to and emigration from breeding colonies by African Penguins. *African Journal of Marine Science* 27: 205–213.

Williams, A.J. (1981). Why do penguins have long laying intervals? *Ibis* 123 (2): 202–204.

Williams, A.J. and Cooper, J. (1984). Aspects of the breeding biology of the jackass penguin *Spheniscus demersus*. In: *Proceedings of the 5th Pan-African Ornithological Congress* (ed. J.A. Ledger), 841–853. Johannesburg, South Africa: Southern African Ornithological Society.

Wilson, R.P. (1985a). Diurnal foraging behaviour of the Jackass Penguin. *Spheniscus demersus. Ostrich* 56: 212–214.

Wilson, R.P. (1985b). The jackass penguin (*Spheniscus demersus*) as a pelagic predator. *Marine Ecology Progress Series* 25: 219–227.

Wilson, R.P. and Wilson, M.-P.T. (1989). Substitute burrows for penguins on guano-free islands. *Gerfaut* 79: 125–131.

Wilson, R.P. and Wilson, M.-P.T. (1990). Foraging ecology of breeding *Spheniscus* penguins. In: *Penguin Biology* (eds. L.S. Davis and J.T. Darby), 181–206. San Diego, CA: Academic Press.

Wilson, R.P. and Wilson, M.-P.T. (1995). The foraging behaviour of the African Penguin *Spheniscus demersus*. In: *The Penguins: Ecology and Management* (eds. P. Dann, I. Norman and P. Reilly), 244–265. Chipping Norton, Australia: Surrey Beatty & Sons Pty Limited.

Wolfaardt, A.C., Underhill, L.G., Nel, D.C. et al. (2008). Breeding success of African Penguins *Spheniscus demersus* at Dassen Island, especially after oiling following the *Apollo Sea* spill. *African Journal of Marine Science* 30: 565–580.

Wolfaardt, A.C., Williams, A.J., Underhill, L.G. et al. (2009). Review of the rescue, rehabilitation and restoration of oiled seabirds in South Africa, especially African Penguins *Spheniscus demersus* and Cape gannets *Morus capensis*, 1983–2005. *African Journal of Marine Science* 31: 31–54.

Wright, K.L.B., Pichegru, L., and Ryan, P.G. (2011). Penguins are attracted to dimethyl sulphide at sea. *The Journal of Experimental Biology* 214: 2509–2511.

# 14

# Shearwaters and Petrels

*Tracy Anderson*

## Natural History

Shearwaters are part of the family Procellariidae that includes shearwaters and petrels, which are in turn a part of the order Procellariiformes that includes the "tubenoses" – albatross, fulmars, petrels, and storm-petrels. This chapter was written using knowledge and experience from the raising of Wedge-tailed Shearwaters (*Ardenna pacifica*) and Newell's Shearwaters (*Puffinus newelli*) and the post-fledging care of Hawaiian Petrels (*Pterodroma sandwichensis*) at Save our Shearwaters (SOS) in Hawaii, USA.

Shearwaters and petrels are long-lived species that reproduce slowly. It takes 3 to 6 years to reach breeding maturity. They then lay a single egg and it takes both parents to raise the chick to fledging age. Fledging takes place at night, and shearwaters and petrels provide no post-fledge parental care. During the first week or so post-hatch, they go through a "guard phase" when at least one parent is present and brooding the chick. Following that, the chick is able to thermoregulate and both parents go to sea to forage, leaving the chick unattended in the burrow during the day. Foraging strategies during chick rearing differ from species to species and can even differ between populations of the same species, depending on food availability. Generally, Procellariiforms have a bimodal foraging strategy that has one parent doing shorter feeding trips closer to the colony and the other doing a lengthier trip to more productive waters. Hawaiian Petrels do a short/long trip where one parent can be at sea for 21 days or so and fly nearly to Alaska and back to take advantage of the rich feeding areas in the North Pacific. The other parent does shorter feeding trips closer to the main Hawaiian Islands (Raine et al. 2017). Wedge-tailed Shearwater's foraging strategy appears to depend on the colony's proximity to productive waters, with birds adopting a bimodal (or dual) strategy when areas of high productivity are "at-distance" (Congdon et al. 2005) and a unimodal strategy when productive waters are close by (Baduini 2002). Due to the different strategies and the distances the parents must fly to find food, Procellariiform chicks may go without provisioning for several days and then receive meals from both parents on the same night. In one study it was determined that Hawaiian Petrels were fed 70% of their total food during the first half of the nesting period (Simons 1985). There is conflicting evidence regarding the "desertion period" just prior to the chick's fledge. Some parents desert entirely 1 to 2 weeks prior, while others continue to provide food up to when the chick leaves (Simons 1985). There is evidence that this is determined by the chick itself, as some will start to refuse food while others will continue to beg, which may correspond

*Hand-Rearing Birds*, Second Edition. Edited by Rebecca S. Duerr and Laurie J. Gage.

to parental provisioning ability, yearly food availability, and the body condition of the chick and how much fat it was able to store.

## Criteria for Intervention

### Chick-napping

Shearwaters nest on the ground in burrows that they excavate into soft soils such as sand, or utilize already-present crevices. Newell's Shearwaters and Hawaiian Petrels nest at higher elevations in the mountains, while Wedge-tailed Shearwaters nest on the periphery of the island close to the ocean. Some species such as Wedge-taileds may also forego a burrow altogether under crowded conditions (Whittow 1997) and place the egg in a depression or the crux of a tree root. In most areas where these species nest, they have evolved with no, or very few, terrestrial predators and thus do not recognize them as a threat. This also means that they are relatively naïve to people and will often allow a person to pick them up. Additionally, once past the initial guard phase, both parents generally leave the chick during the day to forage at sea and this can lead well-meaning people to mistake a perfectly healthy nestling for an orphan and pick the chick up for care. If a chick cannot be returned to its own burrow or the area right around it, then it cannot be put back as the adults will not be able to find the chick to feed it (Figure 14.1).

### Predation

Free-roaming dogs and cats are a problem for ground-nesting species that evolved in the absence of mammalian predators. With the introduction of such predators (free-roaming and feral domestic cats, free-roaming dogs, feral pigs, rats, and mongoose) large-scale predation events can happen at colonies and chicks may become orphaned from these predation events.

### Natural Disasters

Colonies can be located in areas that are unstable. Landslips at colony sites happen, especially during heavy rains. Members of the public may then find chicks at the base of a cliff in the rubble from the colony above.

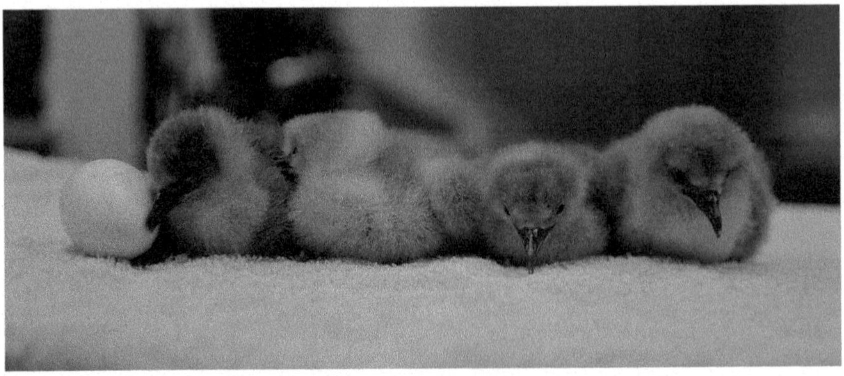

Figure 14.1 Orphaned Wedge-tailed Shearwater chicks and viable egg.

### Light Attraction

The procellarids provide no parental care or guidance once the young fledge the nest/burrow. Most shearwater and petrel species fledge at night. Unfortunately, these species are prone to light-attraction and when they fledge they are attracted to human-generated light sources which have altered natural light levels in the environment (Rodriguez et al. 2017). The naïve young birds become disoriented and come to the ground in a phenomenon known as "fall-out." Once on the ground, they are easy prey for dogs and cats, can get run over by vehicles, or stuck in areas and situations that they cannot escape. Because of their anatomy, these birds are unable to perform a takeoff from the ground unless they have some forward momentum, which can be achieved by dropping from a height, a strong headwind, or a runway. If they cannot take off again, they will die.

## Record Keeping

Each chick should have an individual identity to facilitate tracking progress, and a medical record. Many of the species in this taxonomic group are highly endangered and regulatory agencies may have special record-keeping requirements. If your program has the ability to band the birds prior the release, this is advisable. Note, however, that the bands used should be stainless steel or incoloy as the marine environment will degrade an aluminum band and these birds have a relatively lengthy life expectancy of 30+ years.

### Chick Identification

When very young and their legs are still small, strips of colored Vetrap™ (3M) wrapped loosely on their legs to identify individual chicks works well. These must be checked daily to ensure that the Vetrap does not become too tight as the chicks grow. As their tarsi reach adult diameters, colored zip ties can be employed in unique combinations. Alternatively, use Tyvek® (Dupont) wristbands, which come in multiple colors, are waterproof, can be cut down to size, and have the additional bonus of being able to be written upon with the chick's identification number.

## Initial Care and Stabilization

### Nestlings

Nestlings can be rescued from a variety of situations and the first thing, as with all neonates, is to get them warm. An incubator is the best method, but a heating pad set on low with towels between the chick and the pad can also suffice. Once the chick is warm and dry, a thorough exam can be performed and fluids and nutrition provided (Figure 14.2).

### Fledglings from "Fall-Out"

As noted above, these species are highly prone to light attraction. This is especially so with the young naïve fledglings. During their initial flight out to sea, they can become disoriented by anthropogenic light sources and come to the ground. This is especially problematic on nights

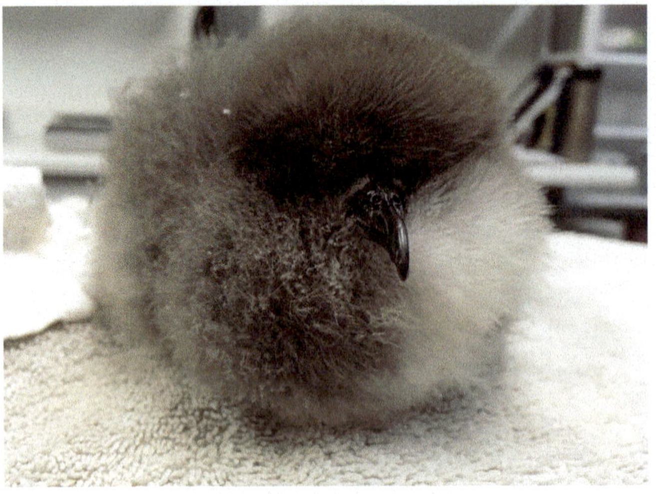

Figure 14.2 Newell's Shearwater chick.

where there is little light from the moon or it is very overcast. On Kauai (Hawaii, USA), members of the public find these birds and hand them into aid stations set up by the SOS program. These birds are given a physical examination to check for any injuries and/or contamination of feathers. Many of these downed birds have no detectable injuries and are banded and released at appropriate ocean-side sites – often on the same day. Birds that do not pass the initial exam are brought back to the facility for further care.

An intake exam consists of a full physical examination which also includes a "flap-test" wherein the bird's body is held securely aloft with the wings free to assess the symmetry of the flap. Blood is taken to look at packed cell volume (PCV), total protein (TP), and buffy coat. Body condition is assessed and scored. Plumage is evaluated with the knowledge that when birds come down on roads or crawl into garages, they can become contaminated with petrochemical oils. The shearwaters and petrels that this program works with tend toward lower body temperatures (99–100 °F/37.2–37.8 °C is normal), especially in the morning, but that can change rapidly when handling the stressier Wedge-taileds.

Birds that pass the more thorough intake exam and are not contaminated with oils are placed in the conditioning pools right away to assess their waterproofing and behavior. Remember, despite the fact that these birds are pelagic, this will be the first time that these birds have been in water. It is stressful and many will initially panic and try to get out. SOS does not leave birds in the pools overnight. The birds are housed off water on net-bottomed enclosures. Care must be taken if the birds are held in drying pens or tall-sided enclosures as many of these species are very good climbers and will get out if given half a chance. Also, if they are constantly trying to get out, they can do damage to their tail feathers and primaries as they reach to get a hold of the edge of the enclosure with their bill. When birds are not on the pools or being dried, they are housed in modified hard-plastic crates with mesh-bottom frame inserts (Figure 14.3).

The already fledged young shearwaters and petrels are rehabilitated the same way as any adults that are received by SOS, although more attention is paid to their pre-release body condition. Young seabirds have a much higher survival rate when they have a good body condition and fat reserves.

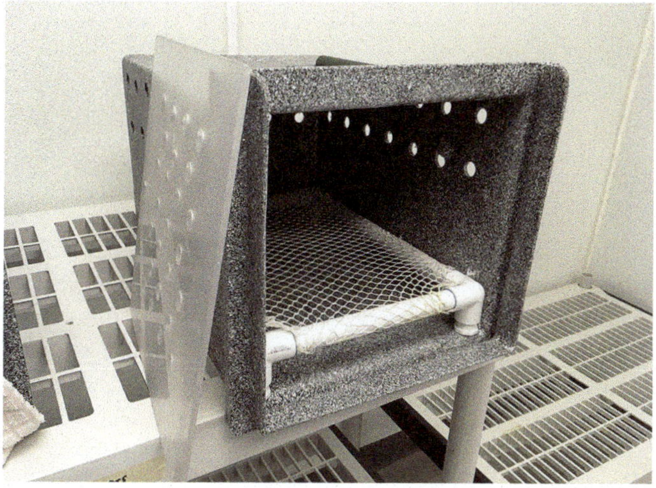

Figure 14.3 Fall-out fledgling crate with mesh-bottom frame insert.

## Common Medical Problems and Solutions

### Avian Pox

Avian pox is a concern in these species. Birds may come in with it or develop it while in care. Birds can survive the virus but sometimes end up with scarring from the healed lesions that can inhibit their chances of survival post-release; deformed bills, blindness, and misshapen nostrils can all result from pox healing poorly. The virus must run its course and supportive care is the only option. If there are large lesions that become infected, then a course of antibiotics may be recommended. Consult with your veterinarian. It is advisable to keep any afflicted chicks away from the rest and practice good quarantine and sanitation while caring for them. Mosquitos can also spread the virus, so mosquito control around the area in which the chicks are being raised is recommended. Mosquito netting over a sand-bottom or burrow enclosure can serve to protect chicks from mosquito-borne diseases such as avian malaria and avian pox.

### Endoparasites

Coccidia is not often seen in chicks raised from young nestlings, but we do see it in fledglings that have become grounded post-fledge. It is opportunistic and will affect chicks that are stressed. Treatment with ponazuril (or toltrazuril) at 20 mg/kg orally once daily for 3 days (Hawkins et al. 2018) following intake is standard for birds that will be in care for more than 2 to 3 days. Regular fecal sampling is suggested.

Roundworms are found as well on occasion and are treated with either panacur or ivermectin. Panacur is avoided if the bird is still growing feathers.

### Ectoparasites

Chicks may arrive with lice and/or mites. Treatment will depend on what type of parasite the bird has. Treatment of the burrow and substrate with a spray (pyrethrin) may be necessary to control mites. Following the instructions on the label, wipe the bird down with a spray-impregnated cloth and, while the bird is out of the burrow area, spray the burrow and the substrate. Let the area dry and then place the bird back into its pen.

### Injuries

SOS rarely receives very young shearwaters with injuries. However, as with most bird species, leg fractures can be splinted relatively easily and bones heal rapidly when very young. Wings are more problematic, as they will need to heal so that the bird will be able to fly once they fledge. Many of these birds must make immediate post-fledging migrations to their feeding grounds of hundreds, if not thousands, of kilometers and, if they cannot make it, they will perish. In addition to this, shearwaters are named for the dynamic soaring they use to traverse these distances. These facts should be kept under consideration when deciding to take on the care of a bird that will take several months to raise to fledging only to find that the wing has not healed sufficiently for the bird to be able to fly.

Grounded fledglings can come into care with a variety of injuries resulting from a truncated flight to the sea. Impact injuries are the most common. Head trauma in a Newell's Shearwater is extremely problematic and they do not tend to recover well enough for release. Hawaiian Petrels, on the other hand, can and have recovered well from head trauma. Missing feathers are also a problem with these birds, as when they hit power lines and other stationary objects, they can often remove a swath of body feathers from the head or neck areas. These birds do not re-grow feathers quickly and a decision must be made whether to release "as is." Often, they are waterproof in the conditioning pools even with a number of contour feathers missing. However, water pressure when diving to depths will exacerbate any leakage caused by imperfections in the feathers. This decision should include consideration of the natural history and feeding strategy of the species. We know that an adult Hawaiian Petrel, a primarily surface-feeding species, can survive with a large patch of feathers missing from its head. However, birds that dive deep for prey, such as Newell's Shearwaters, may not be able to overcome such a handicap.

### Emaciation/Failure to Thrive

This is seen when chicks have either become separated from their natal burrow, such as falling/rolling down a hill, or when parents have been killed or have abandoned the breeding attempt. Dog and cat predation is very prevalent in Hawaii and there has been wholesale slaughter of adults at colonies. A very young chick can bounce back from a period of poor or no nutrition relatively easily. The older they are and the longer away from parental support, the farther behind the growth curve and the more catching up they need to do. Once the feathers start growing, the periods of poor nutrition can be seen by way of fault/stress bars. There is evidence that when food becomes scarce, the chicks put all of their energy into growing their flight feathers so that they can leave the nest (David Hyrenbach, pers. comm.). The most problematic situation is when chicks are received that have obviously attempted to fledge prematurely from desperation. They are often less than half the weight that they should be at the time of fledging and have no fat reserves and little to no muscle. Blood values (PCV and TP) in these chicks will invariably be normal or near normal, which is astounding in an animal that is so obviously starving and undernourished. These chicks should be closely monitored for problems arising from long-term nutritional deprivation, as they can develop issues with digestion or have metabolic problems. Feathers can also have long-term damage in the form of stress/fault bars. Finally, since these birds will be in care for much longer in order to build them back up to a condition that is favorable to their survival, their natural migration patterns must be taken into consideration.

### Medications

Standard antibiotics are utilized for these species when indicated. Prophylactic antifungal medications are often used in seabird rehabilitation; however, with proper hygiene and airflow, we have found that aspergillosis infections are very rare in the shearwater and petrel species in care. Antifungals are used only as a necessary treatment rather than as a prophylactic. The SOS program does use meloxicam with shearwaters and petrels, but hydration is considered of top importance.

## Diets

Our chick slurry diet consists of more than three different types of fish, vitamins, and salmon oil. The added liquid is 0.9% saline, which we gradually increase to 2% saline as the chicks get older. We do not give them additional fluids unless the chick is showing signs of dehydration. These birds are very good at extracting fluids from the food that is provided. Thiamine added to fish slurry may break down rapidly once blended into the diet; however, we have not seen any problems attributable to thiamine deficiency. Fish species used include: lake smelt (*Osmerus mordax*), capelin (*Mallotus villosus*), pond smelt/arctic silversides (*Hypomesus olidus*), sardines (*Sardinella aurita*), Pacific herring (*Clupea pallasi*), silversides (*Menidia menidia*), and squid. The vitamins are Mazuri® Vita-Zu® Small Bird Tablets without Vitamin A, Centrum® multivitamin, and powdered calcium carbonate. At around 3–4 weeks of age, whole small fish are added to the diet (smelt or silversides when available). A small portion of Mazuri (about a 1/3 of a tablet) is placed in the gills of one of the fish once per day. The fish are always offered post-gavage.

### Young Chick Diet

- 700 g assorted fish
- 4 Mazuri tablets
- 1 Centrum tablet
- 1 cup (237 ml) 0.9% NaCl (saline) solution
- ½ teaspoon (2.5 g) calcium carbonate powder
- ¼ cup (60 ml) of fish oil (Grizzly Omega Health or Wild Alaskan Fish Oil)

The fish should be weighed on a scale minus any chunks of ice. Rinse the fish in water, drain, and re-weigh. Partially defrost the fish in water and drain well prior to blending. Crush the vitamins with mortar and pestle. Blend saline, vitamins, and salmon oil first, then add fish and blend to "high." Do not blend for too long as this will warm the mixture and start to cook the fish.

If necessary, add 1/8 cup (30 ml) more saline if the slurry is too thick and is not blending (this can depend on the fish species being used). Tip: if the slurry is still chunky and will not go through a gavage tube after blending, then the whole blender carafe can be put in refrigerator to cool down. Once cool, it can be blended again. The purchase of a good blender is worth its weight in gold!

### Fledgling Diet

- 700 g fish (50% capelin and 50% smelt)
- 4 Mazuri tablets

- 1 Centrum tablet
- 1 ½ cup of cold water
- 1 cup of Emeraid® IC Carnivore powder

This diet does not have additional salmon oil nor the fattier fish added. This is so that when these birds are pooled, they are not potentially excreting undigested fats. Any regurgitation on the pool is less likely to affect waterproofing.

Fish quality is important. Using fresh frozen fish that has been stored correctly and safely ensures that the birds are getting the most nutrition out of the feedings provided. Fish that is old and/or freezer burned lowers the nutritional quality, and fish that has been stored incorrectly can harbor bacteria or rancid fats that are bad for the birds.

## Feeding Procedures

### Frequency

When a nestling chick first arrives and it is warm and in good condition, it is initially gavaged a watery solution consisting of water, salmon oil, and a small amount of slurry. If the chick is very young (within the first week of hatching), feed it three to four times a day for approximately a week and then drop the feedings to twice daily.

### Methods

For young chicks, use a 14- or 18-French red feeding tube cut off so that it is approximately 12 cm long with a 35 ml catheter tip syringe. Round or burn the ends of the cut-off tubing to smooth sharp edges. As the chick grows, care must be taken that the shortened tube does not come off during exuberant feedings, as they will swallow it. When the chick reaches an age where the tube could potentially be swallowed, move to using a full-length tube for safety's sake.

Pre-warm the slurry in the syringes and tubes using a warm-water bath. Ensure that the slurry is warmed all the way through (approximately 10 minutes), but do not allow it to sit in the warm-water bath for an extended period of time. The raw fish will start to grow harmful bacteria that can make the chicks sick and potentially kill them.

Very young chicks, first admitted, are fed a very diluted mixture with more oil (salmon oil) and water than fish slurry. Procellarids produce a proventriculus oil that is very high in fat and calories (Pettit et al. 1984) and are fed small amounts frequently during the first week or so of life during the guard phase.

At about 3–4 weeks of age, always following the gavage feed, the chicks are offered small whole fish. The chicks learn very quickly how to take the fish when it is held alongside the bill. Take care not to feed messy fish – the fish juices and oils will compromise a chick's waterproofing. Wipe the bill with a cloth or paper towel once finished to remove any remnants of fish that could be preened into the developing plumage. Any gavage feeding should be done first and then the whole fish offered afterward.

Open the bill and insert the tube into the chick's mouth, taking care not to injure the growing bill. Place the tube at the back of the mouth/partially in the throat behind the glottis. Start to depress the plunger. As soon as the chick feels the food at the back of the mouth, it should stop struggling and start "gulping" and open its throat for the feeding (Figure 14.4). Depress the plunger firmly and steadily. Feeding should only take a few seconds once the tube is in place. Chicks that

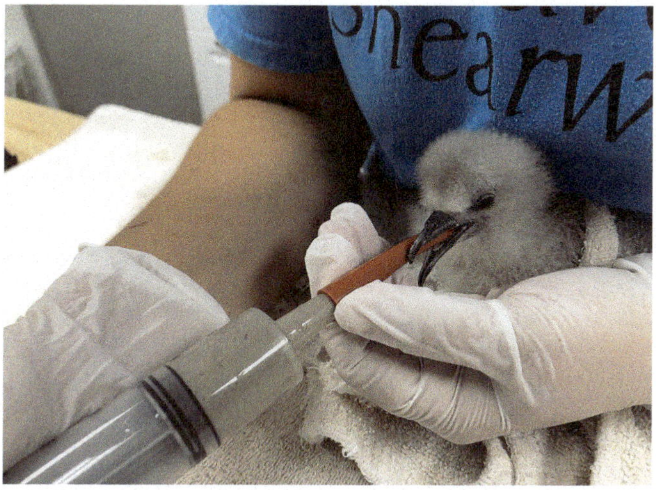

Figure 14.4 Feeding a Wedge-tailed Shearwater chick with a shortened gavage tube.

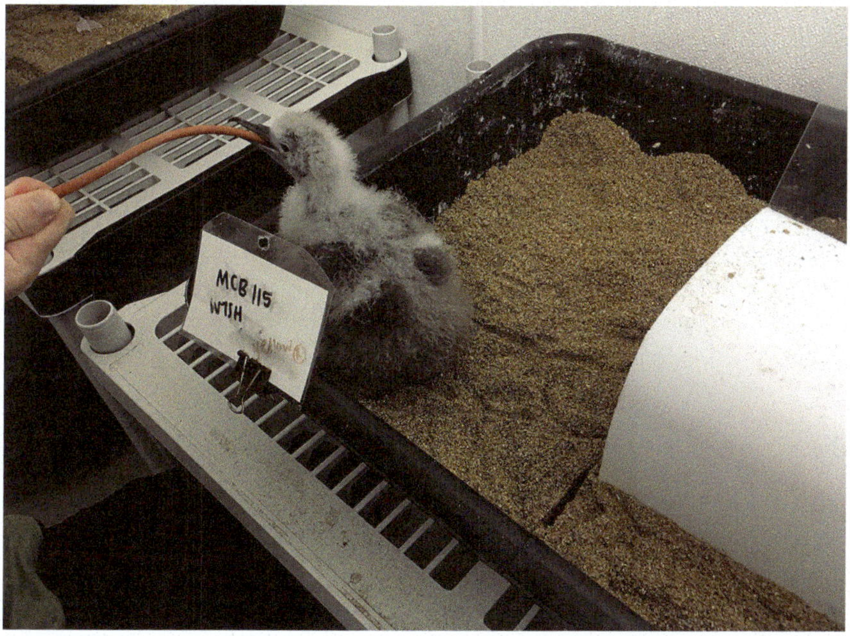


Figure 14.5 Feeding an older Wedge-tailed Shearwater with a full-length tube without restraint. Note the sand tray with plastic burrow.

are received at a later stage may always fight the feeding but willingly take the food once the tube is in place. As chicks mature, they may take the tubing with no restraint (Figure 14.5).

At SOS, chicks are fed twice daily until they are about 6 weeks of age and then the frequency is dropped to once daily. They still receive about the same amount as when they are fed twice a day (seabird stomachs are able to handle a good size bolus of fish). At once daily, the amount is roughly 15–20% of their body weight (150–200 ml/kg). A chick that needs to "catch up" should be introduced to the captive diet gradually but then fed twice per day for a longer period in order to get more calories into the bird than if it were fed only once.

Once they start the home run to fledging, they naturally lose body mass and become fussy to feed. They will start refusing their whole fish and previously easy-to-feed chicks will become more difficult. Reduce the amount fed and fast the chicks every few days. Smell their breath – it should not have a powerful or rancid smell.

## Expected Weight Gain

Healthy chicks should have a consistent weight gain. In the case of Wedge-tailed Shearwaters, they naturally hit their peak mass at around 80–87 days and then will gradually reduce weight until they fledge at around 109 days of age (Pettit et al. 1984). It has been documented in other shearwater species – such as Sooty Shearwaters (*Puffinus griseus*), Manx Shearwaters (*Puffinus puffinus*), and Cory Shearwaters (*Calonectris diomedea*) – that chicks with greater mass at fledging have a better survival rate (Sagar and Horning 1998; Mougin et al. 2000). Ensuring that the chicks are in the best possible body condition with plenty of fat reserves will give them the best possible chance of survival post-fledge (Figure 14.6).

## Housing

SOS has tried several substrates for raising shearwaters, including towels, net-bottom cages, and sand. The substrate that has worked best and promoted the best feather and foot health is sand based. The chicks like to create their own nest cups and the best substrate to allow them to do this is sand. The sand should be clean and dry. When they are very young and still in the guard phase, toweling and a heat pad or an incubator is acceptable. Once they are past the guard phase and are able to thermoregulate appropriately, then they can be moved to a sand-bottomed enclosure. SOS uses concrete mixing bins filled with a couple of inches of sand. The chicks also get a "burrow" made out of waste paper bins cut in half (Figure 14.5), but this can be made out of any readily cleanable material. The chicks quickly adapt to their new homes.

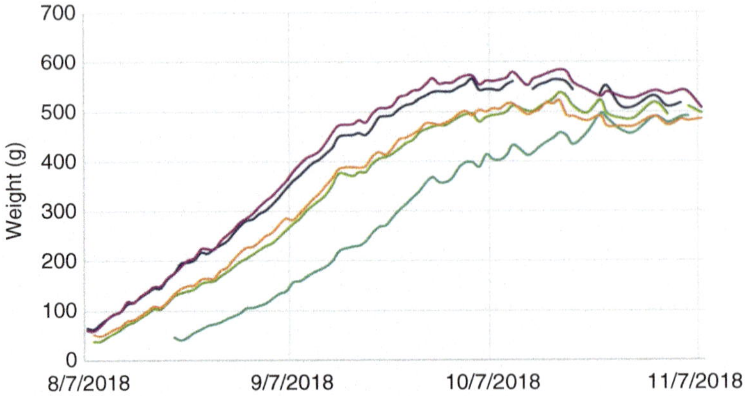


Figure 14.6 Weight gains of five Wedge-tailed Shearwater chicks.

In the wild, chicks will start venturing outside of their burrows and stretching their wings a few weeks before they first fledge, although this timing depends on the species. First emergence is thought to be at or around the point at which a chick imprints on its natal colony site. Some species, such as Wedge-tailed Shearwaters, dig variable burrow depths and some may not have as deep a burrow as others. This part of their natural history must be considered because if a colony of seabirds permanently taking up residence at the facility is not desirable, then steps must be taken to deter the imprint process. That being said, there is some elasticity in new birds returning to breed, and whereas they are most likely driven to return to where they hatched and grew up (hence the reason why translocation programs for petrels and shearwaters work), they also can get drawn into another colony by social attraction to the sounds and presence of other birds. Additionally, if the species normally breeds near to the ocean and the facility is inland, then the likelihood of birds returning to the facility to set up housekeeping is fairly remote.

This secondary step of using the concrete mixing bins may be skipped if there is an outside enclosure that is fully protected and rat-proof. Once the chicks are large enough and are starting to be more adventurous in their explorations, they can be moved to a larger enclosure. SOS uses a chain link dog run/kennel that is covered with a tarp and lined with shade cloth. Chicks are very territorial regarding their burrows and space, so they must be housed separately, otherwise the more dominant chick will force the weaker or more submissive one out of its burrow (Figure 14.7). SOS has implemented a system of stalls in an outdoor pen that give the chicks a bit of room to explore while keeping them separated from each other. Cleaning can be accomplished with a clean cat litter scoop and "spot cleaning." The sand absorbs any liquid and the chick's developing plumage stays clean.

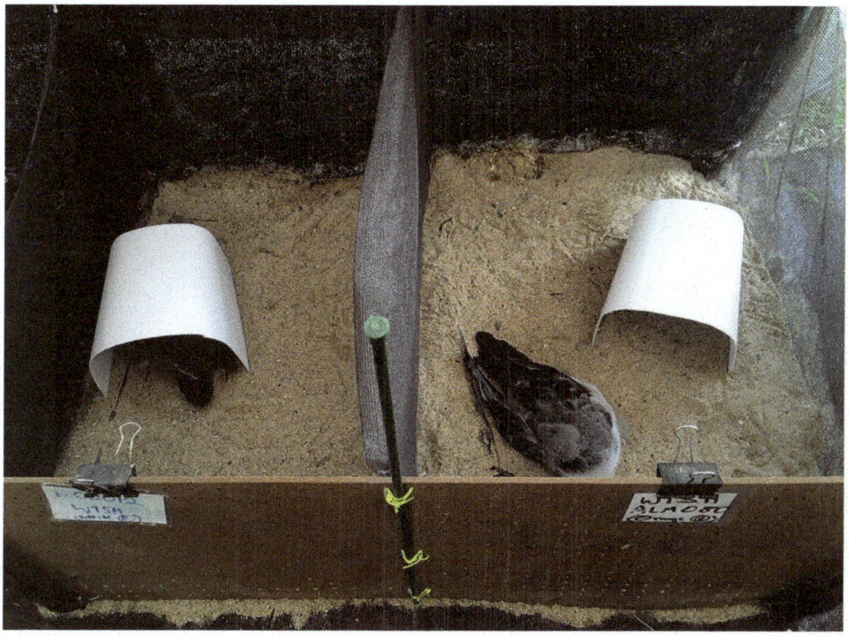

Figure 14.7 Older chicks housed outside with separate sand-bottom enclosures with burrows.

### Enrichment

To encourage exploration, scatter items in the enclosures that birds would naturally encounter around their burrows in the wild (e.g. rocks, leaves etc.). The chicks are mouthy; hence, to be on the safe side, do not give things that would cause digestive damage if swallowed. Naupaka (*Scaevola taccada*) leaves, scattered in their enclosures, have proved the most appealing as the older Wedge-tailed chicks gather them and use them to line their nest cups.

If handling and feeding have been done correctly and carefully, the chicks should all have perfect plumage at fledging. SOS starts giving chicks time in pools when their wing-chords are within a few millimeters of adult length. This gives them the opportunity to exercise and stretch their wings and become accustomed to water, which will shortly become a major part of their lives. We test their waterproofing at this time, although, as mentioned, if they have been handled and fed correctly, they should be waterproof from the first time on the pool (Figure 14.8).

## Release

Most shearwater and petrel species take their inaugural flight to sea at night. If the facility is fortunate enough to be situated on or very near the ocean, then, ideally, an area could be fenced off with a predator-proof fence and artificial burrows installed. The chicks can then be raised in the burrows and when they are ready to fledge, they may do it on their own time when they are ready. Because there is a high likelihood that these chicks will return to that spot when they are ready to breed, this might not be a good idea unless you are planning on starting a colony.

Barring that ideal situation, one is left with estimating when the bird is ready to fly. Down coverage is not a reliable indicator of readiness to fledge as some birds will fledge with a substantial amount of down still attached, while others will have none at all. At SOS, when the chicks' wing-chord is at adult length and they have demonstrated that they are waterproof on the pools, we take the birds on field trips to the beach. They are placed on the sand while other birds are being released to allow them to see and smell the ocean. Wedge-tailed Shearwaters can become overwhelmed and attempt to find a place to hide, so choose release locations wisely. Ideally, pick an area with open space, sloping sand, and nowhere for the bird to hide and not be retrievable if the release is

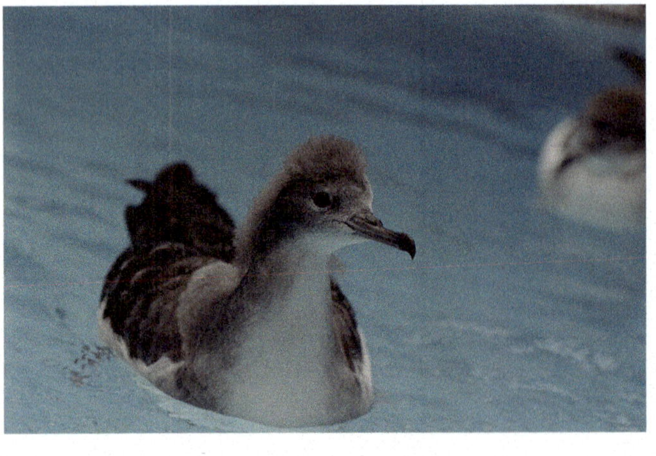

Figure 14.8 A Wedge-tailed Shearwater fledgling having pool time in the lead-up to release.

unsuccessful. The first time out they are not actively encouraged to fly, although if they do, then that is great. Newell's Shearwaters and Hawaiian Petrels (most of which are found following their maiden flight from montane burrows, having not quite made it to the sea) are quick to leave. Place them on elevated rocks several feet off the ground or near sea cliffs. If there are no injuries and the bird is in good condition and there is a good wind (3–4 on the Beaufort scale) they will leave very quickly. If the wind is coming from a poor direction (offshore) or there is very little wind, then the birds may refuse to take off or take much longer to do so. Wedge-tailed Shearwaters often take encouragement to get airborne. If a chick is not ready to go, return it to the facility for another attempt on a later date. Following repeated trips to the beach with refusal to become airborne, hold them aloft and directed into the wind and encourage them to flap and use their wings. This will generally encourage reticent fledglings to fly off. We release all of our young shearwaters and petrels during the day with enough time between release and sunset to ensure that the birds get a good distance offshore to not get drawn back in by lights, usually no later than 4:00 p.m. Birds slated for release (or a release attempt) that day are not fed in the morning. They have an unfortunate tendency to regurgitate any fresh food in their stomachs prior to taking off.

Despite the fact that most of these species make their maiden flight at night, releasing them during the day appears to have no negative consequences. In places where there may be aerial diurnal predators, you should look around the area carefully prior to release. Iwa (Great Frigatebirds) will dive on a young shearwater or petrel and force the inexperienced flier into the water, so also check for species that practice kleptoparasitism. Releasing during the day has the added benefit of being able to watch the bird fly and ensure that it has flown in the direction intended (out to sea) and made it out past the breakers.

As long as it is not pouring with rain or blowing a gale, most weather is fine for releasing these birds. We've watched released birds (via satellite track) fly straight through hurricanes and out the other side. Ideally though, weather should be fair.

### Translocation Considerations

Generally, birds that are part of a translocation program are taken from their natal colony just prior to first emergence from the burrow, as it is suggested that this is the point at which they imprint on their colony site (Miskelly et al. 2009). If the bird(s) being raised are intended to be a part of a new colony or to be integrated into an existing one, care must be taken to avoid them imprinting on an improper location. There are several successful shearwater and petrel translocation programs happening in various places in the world and if this is the route that is chosen, it would be beneficial to speak to people involved in these programs to see what methods have worked.

## Acknowledgments

Many mahalos (thanks!) to Molly Bache, Madelyn Jacobs, Jacqueline Nelson, Christa McLeod, and all of the SOS seasonal technicians and volunteers over the past several years who have helped raise these birds to fledging; the Kauai Island Utility Cooperative for funding the SOS program; and residents of and visitors to Kauai who rescue downed and distressed shearwaters and petrels. And to these amazing oceanic wanderers who, if it were not for the needs of the egg, could eschew dry land and its hazards altogether.

## Sources for Products Mentioned

Centrum: PCH Product Information, Pfizer Inc., PO Box 1043, Kings Mountain, NC 28086, (877) 236-8786, https://www.centrum.com.

Emeraid IC Carnivore: Lafeber Company, 24981 N 1400 East Road, Cornell, IL 61319, https://lafeber.com.

Fish: Bionic Bait (Bionic Zoo and Aquarium), 95 NW 13th Ave, Pompano Beach, FL 33069. 866-848-9289, www.bionicbait.com.

Mazuri products: Mazuri, PMI Nutrition International, LLC, PO Box 66812, St. Louis, MO 63166, www.mazuri.com.

## References

Baduini, C.L. (2002). Parental provisioning patterns of wedge-tailed shearwaters and their relation to chick body condition. *The Condor* 104 (4): 823–831.

Congdon, B.C., Krockenberger, A.K., and Smithers, B.V. (2005). Dual-foraging and co-ordinated provisioning in a tropical Procellariiform, the wedge-tailed shearwater. *Marine Ecology Progress Series* 301: 293–301.

Hawkins, M.G., Sanchez-Migallon Guzman, D., Beaufrere, H. et al. (2018). Birds. In: *Exotic Animal Formulary*, 5e (eds. J.W. Carpenter and C.J. Marion), 167–375. St. Louis, MO: Elsevier.

Miskelly, C.M., Taylor, G.A., Gummer, H. et al. (2009). Translocations of eight species of burrow-nesting seabirds (genera *Pterodroma, Pelecanoides, Pachyptila* and *Puffinus*: family Procellariidae). *Biological Conservation* 142 (10): 1965–1980.

Mougin, J.-L., Jouanin, C., Roux, F., and Zino, F. (2000). Fledging weight and juvenile survival of Cory's shearwaters *Calonectris diomedea* on Selvagem Grande. *Ringing & Migration* 20 (2): 107–110.

Pettit, T.N., Byrd, G.V., Whittow, G.C., and Seki, M.P. (1984). Growth of the wedge-tailed shearwater in the Hawaiian Islands. *The Auk* 101 (1): 103–109.

Raine, A.F, Vynne, M. Driskill, S., et al. (2017). Study of daily movement patterns of NESH and HAPE in relation to power line collisions. Year Three Report. Kaua'i Endangered Seabird Recovery Project, Hanapepe, Hawai'i.

Rodriguez, A., Holmes, N.D., Ryan, P.G. et al. (2017). Seabird mortality induced by land-based artificial lights. *Conservation Biology* 31 (5): 986–1001.

Sagar, P.M. and Horning, D.S. (1998). Mass-related survival of fledgling sooty shearwaters *Puffinus griseus* at the snares, New Zealand. *Ibis* 140: 329–339.

Simons, T.R. (1985). Biology and behavior of the endangered Hawaiian dark-rumped petrel. *The Condor* 87: 229–245.

Whittow, G.C. (1997). Wedge-tailed shearwater (*Ardenna pacifica*), version 2.0. In: *The Birds of North America* (eds. A.F. Poole and F.B. Gill). Ithaca, NY, USA: Cornell Lab of Ornithology https://doi.org/10.2173/bna.305.

# 15

# Cormorants

*Michelle Bellizzi, Isabel Luevano, and Jennifer Linander*

## Natural History

Cormorants – aquatic birds known commonly as cormorants and shags – are found on every continent except Antarctica. In North America, there are six species of cormorants, and their habitats span the continent: Double-crested Cormorant (*Phalacrocorax auritus*), Brandt's Cormorant (*Phalacrocorax penicillatus*), Red-faced Cormorant (*Phalacrocorax urile*), Pelagic Cormorant (*Phalacrocorax pelagicus*), Great Cormorant (*Phalacrocorax carbo*), and Neotropic Cormorant (*Phalacrocorax brasilianus*). While most of these species occupy near-shore areas exclusively on U.S. coasts, Double-crested Cormorants, the most numerous of the species, are found in both coastal environments and throughout the country's midland (Dorr et al. 2014).

Cormorants are formidable, opportunistic predators within their niches. Prey items mainly consist of slower-moving or schooling fish ranging in size from 3 to 40 cm, but the most commonly caught prey are in the <15 cm range. Cormorants feed on different species of fish, depending on location and season; they also feed, though less frequently, on insects, crustaceans, eels, and amphibians. Known for being somewhat clumsy appearing when ambulating on land and requiring long water runways to achieve flight, cormorants are extraordinarily agile under water, where they pursue their prey by propelling themselves with their feet. Cormorants have been observed foraging at depths of 75 m, although most commonly they forage in shallower waters of less than 10 m. Cormorants have also been observed forming foraging flocks in crescents to corral fish in clear waters. An adult Double-crested Cormorant's average daily consumption of fish ranges from 436 g/day during nonbreeding season, to 542 g/day during breeding season (Dorr et al. 2014). Cormorants cast indigestible food pellets encased in a pale, white mucous "shell." Captive birds generally produce one pellet/day, but may cast fewer than one per day or none if being fed soft-bodied fish; and captive cormorants regurgitate readily if agitated or disturbed.

Sexual maturity for most cormorant species occurs at 2–3 years of age. Cormorants nest in a variety of locations in communal settings or rookeries. Nests may be constructed in trees or on cliffs, artificial nest structures, transmission lines, or wharves and bridges. Colonies of breeding cormorants nesting in trees are likely to kill the trees over time. Ground-nesting cormorant colonies are generally on low-lying rocky islands or reefs with no vegetation. Nests are composed of twigs, sticks, grasses, and other readily available materials, and are loosely constructed. Ground-nesting cormorant nests are re-used seasonally and may become built-up tussocks at a well-established colony.

*Hand-Rearing Birds*, Second Edition. Edited by Rebecca S. Duerr and Laurie J. Gage.

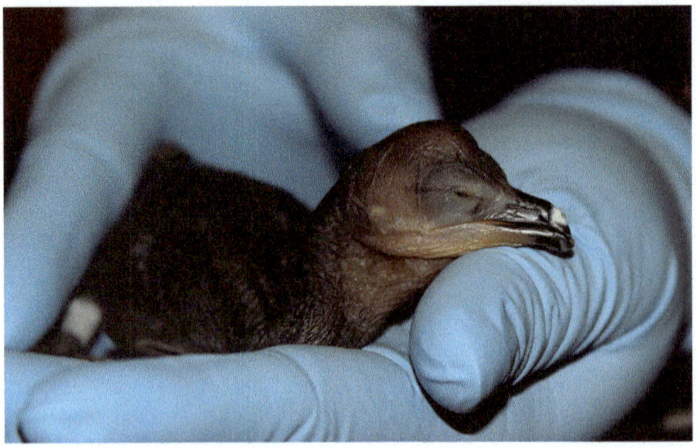

Figure 15.1 Hatchling Double-crested Cormorant, note closed eyes and egg tooth. *Source:* photo courtesy of International Bird Rescue.

Normal clutch sizes range from one to seven eggs, with an average clutch size of four. The eggs are generally laid every day over a period of several days, but some cormorant species may take 2–3 days between eggs. Both parents sit on the eggs throughout the incubation period, which averages 30 days across cormorant species. The smallest chicks often do not survive due to sibling competition for food (Dorr et al. 2014); if larger clutches survive, all chicks may experience slower growth (Hobson 2013).

Cormorants are altricial, hatching without feathers and with eyes closed (Figure 15.1). The chicks open their eyes approximately 3 days after hatching and take approximately 12–15 days to grow a wooly coat of down feathers, which remains until approximately 4 weeks of age. Chicks are typically able to thermoregulate once down growth is complete. They are cared for by their parents for approximately 6–8 weeks (Wallace and Wallace 1998; Hobson 2013; Dorr et al. 2014). Chicks at ground-nesting cormorant colonies may form nurseries or crèches once they are downy and old enough to venture from the nest. Adults will seek out their own young to feed within a crèche, and will rebuff chicks that are not their own. Cormorant chicks voluntarily seek out water when their plumage is complete, generally at 6–7 weeks of age.

## Criteria for Intervention

Because of their communal nesting proclivities, nestling and pre-fledgling cormorant chicks likely require intervention only if an active colony is devastated or disturbed – for example, by an oil spill, man-made interference (e.g. construction), or a weather event. While it is always in a chick's best interest to be raised by its parents, lone chicks may require intervention near such urban rookery sites as bridges, barges, and pier systems.

Intervention by putting healthy, uninjured, orphaned chicks less than 2 weeks of age to foster with wild adult parents at ground-nesting colonies may be successful, but care must be taken to match chick age and not overburden the parents with more than three total chicks or the smallest will likely starve. As with any wild foster placement, careful observation before, during, and after introducing chicks to prospective parents is recommended, and fostering should only be considered if reintroducing the chick will not disrupt the colony.

## Record Keeping

In the United States, it is the responsibility of every wildlife rehabilitator to keep accurate records of each admission to a rehabilitation facility and to report that information to regulatory agencies annually. Generally, the information requested by these agencies includes the date of admission, species, final disposition, and date of disposition. This information provides trustees with valuable data about human–wildlife interactions. Responsible rehabilitators also collect as much information as possible about each animal, not only to help guide the individual animal's care, but also to advance knowledge about the species. This information includes capture date and location, physical examination findings on arrival, treatments prescribed and performed, and detailed notes on continuing care and progress.

## Initial Care and Stabilization

As with any injured bird, cormorant chicks must first be warmed before any treatment or examination. Naked or cold chicks can be placed in a warming incubator set to approximately 100 °F (37.8 °C) with humidity of 50–60% (Lyon Technologies). To help warm a cold chick more rapidly, a heating pad set to low can be placed under the substrate in the incubator. If a chick that is downy and not in need of an incubator requires additional heat, a box with a heating pad on low under half of the box and a towel nest may suffice until the chick is warm and alert.

Once the chick is warm, dehydration must be addressed. Dehydration is detrimental to any animal, but cormorant hatchlings and nestlings are especially prone to its effects. Fluids may be administered by any usual route for birds; oral or subcutaneous (SQ) delivery generally works well. However, extremely young chicks' skin may become excessively perforated with repeated SQ boluses even when given with small gauge needles; hence, delivery of only a small number of administrations by this route may be best. Oral or SQ isotonic electrolytes should be delivered at normal body temperature (103–108 °F/39.3–42.2 °C) in order to avoid cooling the chick. Give oral fluids at 3–5% of body weight (30–50 ml/kg) every 60 minutes until the chick is well-hydrated. Sterile SQ isotonic fluids may be given up to 5% of body weight once or twice daily. If needed, oral and subcutaneous fluids can be given concurrently, with the caveat that one should be sure the chick is processing what has already been given before giving more. Passage of clear urine and white urates are good indicators that the chick is processing its fluids well.

## Common Medical Problems and Solutions

### Dehydration

As previously mentioned, cormorants are particularly susceptible to dehydration. Monitoring their hydration is vital to the successful raising of young cormorants. When a cormorant chick is naked, its skin should appear shiny and smooth with wrinkles only where limbs articulate. If the skin starts becoming dry or flaky or develops wrinkles in other areas, additional hydration is needed. Dehydration becomes less problematic as the birds mature. Monitor droppings carefully as an indicator of hydration; dehydrated chicks may become bloated or constipated.

### Metabolic Bone Disease (MBD)

Metabolic bone disease (MBD) (secondary nutritional hyperparathyroidism) is caused by an imbalance of calcium, phosphorus, and vitamin $D_3$. In growing birds, MBD, which typically manifests as a malformation of growing long bones, is almost always caused by a deficiency of dietary calcium during the rapid growth phase. Once a bird is identified as having MBD (i.e. bones palpate soft or rubbery, bird has trouble standing when old enough to do so, folding fractures are found on radiographs), it is considered to be a medical patient whose bones and ambulation need to be closely monitored and whose diet needs to be re-assessed. Administration of additional amounts of calcium or a vitamin D supplement may be needed. Some fish species used to feed piscivores in captivity have been found to have low calcium to phosphorus ratios (McRoberts Fish Company, unpubl. data) and/or to be deficient in vitamin $D_3$ (Hoopes and Clauss 2016). There is a likely role of contaminants such as mercury and PCBs in the development of skeletal abnormalities (Ludwig et al. 1996).

### Aspergillosis

Cormorants, like many seabirds, are susceptible to aspergillosis, an infection caused by *Aspergillus fumigatus,* a ubiquitous fungus found in decomposing organic matter. Aspergillosis is caused by fungal spores invading the respiratory system of immune-compromised animals, including those suffering from another illness, malnutrition, or stress. Diagnosis is commonly achieved at necropsy, although symptoms include anorexia, labored breathing, depressed activity, reduced preening, and chronic anemia. Healthy cormorant chicks are typically not treated prophylactically with antifungal medication, but if a chick is being treated with other medications, such as antibiotics for a wound, addition of an antifungal (such as itraconazole or voriconazole) is prudent.

### Disease

Some geographic areas may see fledgling Double-crested Cormorants presented for care with neurologic clinical signs due to infection with Newcastle disease. This disease is caused by avian paramyxovirus-1 and is quite deadly to affected chicks while also being highly contagious and of concern to regulatory agencies due to its deadliness to poultry (White et al. 2015). Suspected infected chicks should be quarantined away from other patients, humanely euthanized, and submitted to a diagnostic lab for necropsy and testing. Areas and caging that were in contact with the chick should be thoroughly disinfected with bleach.

## Avoiding Imprinting and Habituation

Double-crested Cormorants are highly susceptible to imprinting (if they have been hatched in captivity) and habituation (if they have lived some time with their parents). Knowing about this high susceptibility, it is important to plan ahead to avoid these problems, since they are very difficult to correct. The following techniques have resulted in fledglings that appropriately fear humans and fly off at release without looking back.

The first technique is to stage cormorant decoys (Knutsons Decoys) in each enclosure to ensure that all visual stimuli are related to cormorants, not people. It is important to conceal all human shapes and sounds during every encounter with the chicks (Figures 15.2 and 15.3). This can be

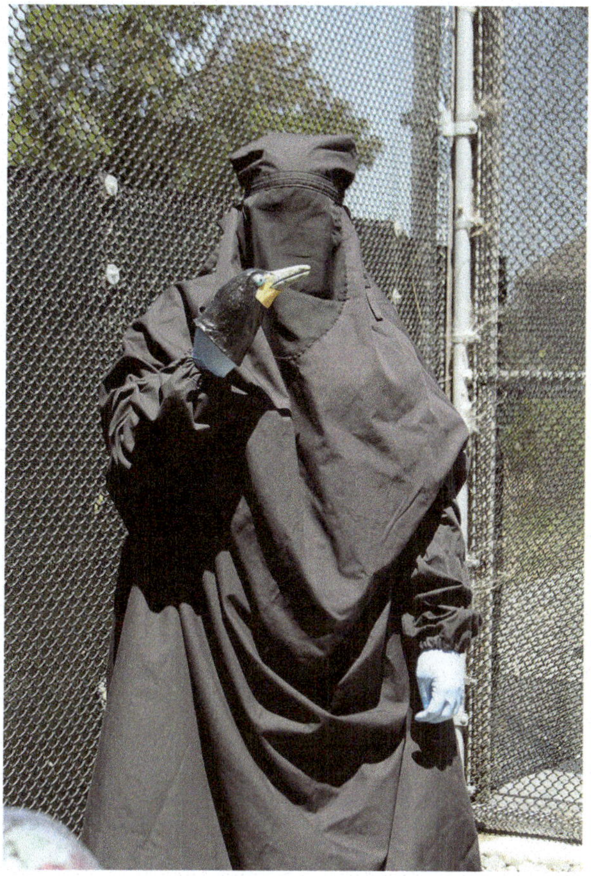

Figure 15.2 Using a full costume with adult cormorant head puppet is recommended with these species to avoid human imprinting or habituation. *Source:* photo courtesy of International Bird Rescue.

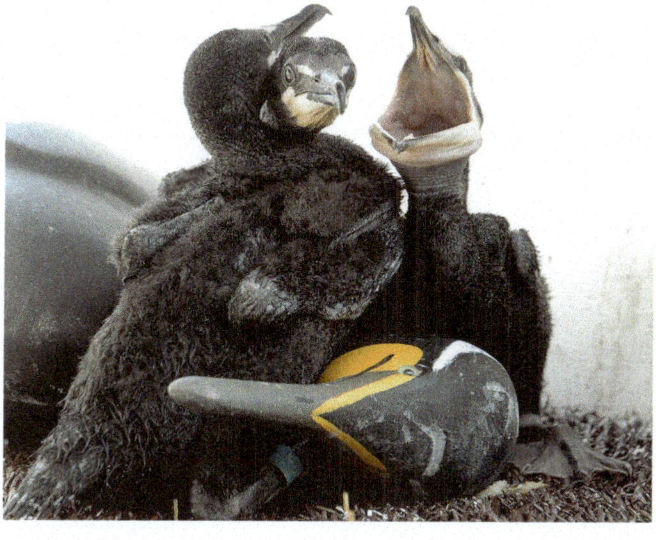

Figure 15.3 Three downy nestlings with an adult cormorant decoy. Note the very large mouth of cormorant chicks. *Source:* photo courtesy of International Bird Rescue.

accomplished by creating and using special costumes, with everyone involved dressing from head to toe whenever interacting with chicks, making sure to also always keep hands covered. In addition, audio tracks of cormorant colonies and vocalizations can be used to provide young birds with auditory stimulation and to help cover up anthropogenic sounds associated with their care. These tracks can be played on a loop throughout the day and turned off at night, when chicks normally sleep. Feeding puppets specially painted to replicate a cormorant adult are helpful for feeding times. If a chick has to be alone for any amount of time, a mirror should be provided such that the chick can always see "another cormorant." Regardless of how long or short the human–bird interaction, the human should always be completely costumed. The greater the use of puppets, decoys, and colony sounds, the less likely the birds are to habituate or imprint.

## Diet

In the wild, cormorants feed on a wide variety of fish specific to the areas they inhabit. In captivity, rehabilitators often need to rely on sporadic fish availability. Options for commercially available fish include night smelt (*Spirinchus starrski*), peruvian smelt (*Atherinella panamensis*), capelin (*Mallotus villosus*), and various minnows, sardines, anchovies, menhaden, and mullet species. Fish that may be too large for newly hatched cormorants to ingest may be cut or sliced into smaller, more size-appropriate pieces. It is good practice to cut these into pieces that are long and slender (fish-shaped) to best simulate smaller fish and allow for easy swallowing. The nutritional content of these fish depends on season, freshness, alive versus dead, and whether they have been frozen. Husbandry may need to be adjusted if feeding fattier fish, such as anchovies or sardines, to avoid contaminating the bird's feathers or substrate with fish oil from feedings or feces.

All cormorant chicks should receive vitamin and mineral supplements while in care to support healthy growth, unless being fed strictly fresh, unfrozen fish with an excellent calcium to phosphorus ratio. Nutrients of concern in piscivores fed frozen–thawed, small-bodied fish include thiamin, vitamin E, vitamin D, and calcium. Commonly-used supplements for piscivores include #5M2G Mazuri® Auklet Vitamin Tablets (www.Mazuri.com) or SeaTabs (Pacific Labs) and 500–600 mg calcium (from calcium carbonate) tablets. When needed, vitamin $D_3$ gelcaps intended for humans work well. Capelin, in particular, has been found to be deficient in vitamin D (Hoopes and Clauss 2016). Supplement doses are intended to be administered per kilogram of fish consumed; but in practice, it is best to dose on a regular schedule of every other day while a chick is having frequent interactions with caregivers (Table 15.1). Once a bird is living in an outdoor enclosure and no longer requires assisted feeding, the frequency of handling and supplementation decreases.

## Feeding Procedures

Emaciated chicks often need to be further stabilized prior to receiving solid foods. A critical care formula, such as Emeraid Piscivore (EP, Lafeber Company, fed at 11% fat from added salmon oil), works well for this purpose. When chicks are debilitated, a slow transition from fluids to the critical care formula can be beneficial. For example, start with 2-hourly tubings of 100% fluids, and then move to two tubings of 75% fluids/25% EP, two tubings of 50% fluids/50% EP, and so on until the chick is receiving 100% EP. Once the chick is more stable, it can be transitioned to eating solid foods.

Table 15.1 Supplement schedule and housing by chick weight, based on feeding small-bodied fish with unknown or low calcium to phosphorus ratio.

| Chick weight | Auklet Tab amount and frequency | Calcium amount and frequency | Housing location |
|---|---|---|---|
| <150 g | 1/8–1/4 tab EOD | 75–150 mg SID | Incubator with nest |
| 150–255 g | 1/4–1/2 tab EOD | 150–300 mg SID | Wood-sided pen with heat |
| 255–900 g | 1/2–1 tab EOD | 300–600 mg SID | Large "pelican box" with gradual heat reduction, days in play pen outdoors |
| 900–1500 g | 1 tab EOD | 600–1200 mg SID | Large "pelican box" with gradual heat reduction, days in play pen outdoors |
| >1500 g | 1 tab EOD-q7d | 1200 mg SID-q7d | Outdoors, free-roaming in large aviary |

EOD = Every Other Day.
SID = Once Daily.

Cormorant parents begin feeding their young within hours of hatching by forcing tiny particles of partially digested food into the mouths of the blind and helpless chicks. By 3 days old, chicks place their heads into the adult's mouth and bob excitedly to encourage the adult to feed them. Chicks signal for food by tapping on a parent's beak, drooping and quivering their wings, flailing their heads, and uttering high-pitched squeaks. This behavior becomes more exaggerated as the birds grow. In the wild, parents feed the chicks 3 times a day for the first several days after hatching, and then increase the frequency to up to 10 times a day for days 6–25. After that, the parents gradually decrease the number of feedings until the chicks fledge at about 10 weeks of age (Dorr et al. 2014).

Chicks should not be fed fish with long and/or sharp bones or spines that could perforate their esophagus or gut, regardless of their age. For young, down-less chicks, offer slivers of fish (with heads, tails, fins, and large bones removed) by forceps or puppet. It may be necessary to use one hand to steady the bird's head, and the other, puppeted or holding forceps, to offer the fish (Figure 15.4). Chicks may need encouragement to open their mouths to feed; this can be achieved by gently touching or pinching both sides of the base of the bill using the hand steadying the head. Table 15.2 shows a feeding schedule for Double-crested Cormorant chicks by age and weight.

Increasingly larger slivers of fish should be offered to birds until they are large enough to consume whole fish. Continue to hand-feed the birds as they grow, but also encourage them to self-feed using two methods: fish school and assist-feeding (Figure 15.5). Fish school consists of splashing fish in the feeding dish or tossing fish at the bird's feet to use the movement of the fish to encourage self-feeding. Assist-feeding, which acts as a bridge between hand-feeding and self-feeding, entails partially placing the fish into the bird's mouth and giving it a chance to manipulate the fish and swallow it on its own. An adult cormorant decoy used as a large puppet is very useful for inspiring a chick's interest in fish. For chicks at older ages, live fish can be used to encourage self-feeding, although it should be remembered that cormorant chicks in the wild do not encounter live fish until hunting on their own (unless a fish is still alive after being regurgitated by the parent).

After about 3–4 weeks of age, when chicks begin to stand on their own, whole small (<6 in., <15 cm) fish may be dropped on the floor of the cage or in a dish and pointed to by a puppet or decoy to encourage birds to self-feed. When feeding groups consist of three or more birds, the

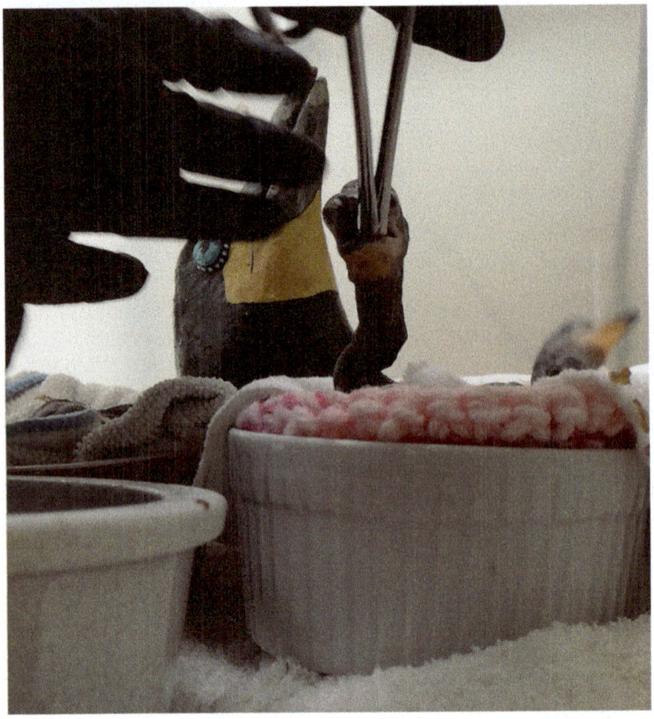

Figure 15.4 Hemostat feeding a very young cormorant, note the puppet head set up next to the nest. *Source:* photo courtesy of International Bird Rescue.

Table 15.2 Feeding and hydration schedule by age and weight for Double-crested Cormorant chicks.

| Age | Weight | Feeding interval | Hydration frequency |
|---|---|---|---|
| 0–2 weeks | 33–500 g | Every hour | q8–12h |
| 3–4 weeks | 500–1300 g | Every 2.5 hours | q8–12h |
| 5–6 weeks | 1400–1800 g | Assist-feed 5–7x/day | None[a] |
| 6+ weeks | 1800–2000 + g | Assist-feed 3–4x/day | None |

[a] Continue hydration checks through week 5, but likely none needed.

chicks frequently stimulate themselves into frenzied begging behavior, so leaving dropped fish close to chicks not being actively fed may encourage them to self-feed.

## Expected Weight Gain

A cormorant chick's weight should increase consistently until it reaches its adult weight at around 5 weeks of age, when weight gain will level off (Figure 15.6). It is recommended that nestling chicks be weighed daily until they are covered in down, reliably self-feeding whole food items, and gaining or maintaining weight according to age class. Thereafter, chicks are weighed as part of their routine health checks at least once or twice weekly to ensure no problems have developed and each chick is doing well.

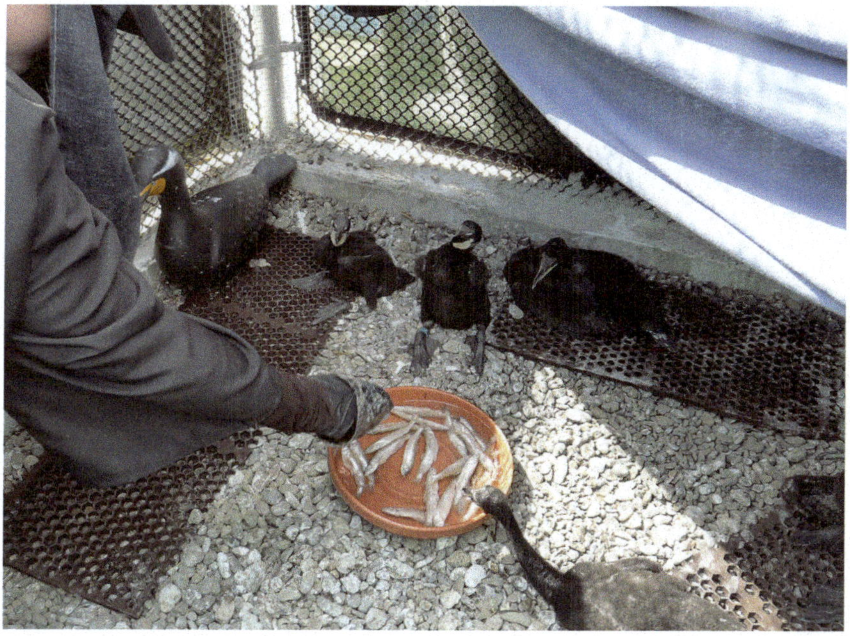

Figure 15.5 Fish school followed by assist-feeding, while obscuring the human form with costume. *Source:* photo courtesy of International Bird Rescue.

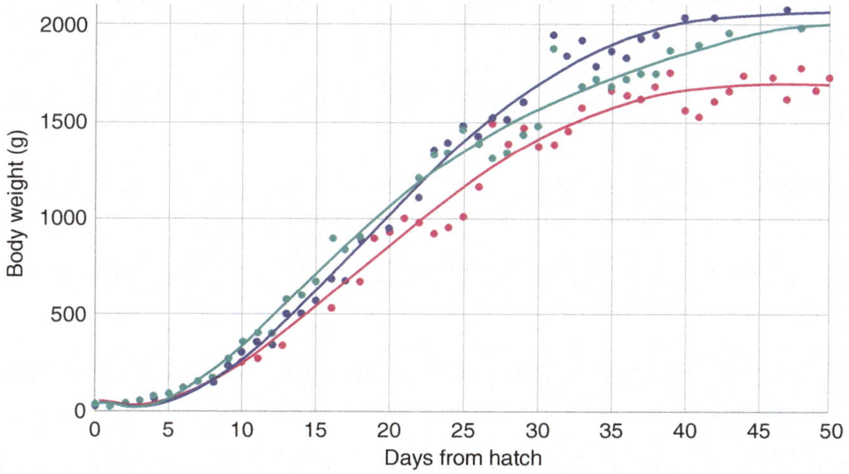


Figure 15.6 Weight gain of three Double-crested Cormorants. *Source:* data courtesy of International Bird Rescue.

## Housing

All housing should be cleaned every day, in some cases before feeding or exams, to remove large quantities of feces and any leftover food. Nests need to be cleaned frequently, up to four times/day, while the incubator itself needs to be cleaned and disinfected at least once daily. Birds should be removed from enclosures during cleaning, which provides an opportune time for weighing, examining, and administering nutritional supplements. If their housing is not yet ready after their exam, or if chicks need to be removed from their housing for any length of time, it is important to have a temporary housing area for them that has the appropriate level of heat support so they do not get cold. For the smaller single chicks, feather dusters can act as surrogate cohorts; for other single chicks, mirrors and decoys can be used.

Cormorants are communal nesters, thus chicks can be housed with other healthy cormorant chicks of similar size and demeanor. Down-less chicks should be housed in an incubator, such as an Animal Intensive Care Unit (Lyon Technologies), at 100 °F (37.8 °C) with 50–60% humidity, and there should be a makeshift nest consisting of a small bowl lined with towels/tissue and, preferably, sticks that mimic natural nest materials. The same type of caging environment is adequate for the first 10–14 days post-hatch until the chicks are down-covered, although the ambient temperature should be lowered if birds begin to show signs of hyperthermia (i.e. gular fluttering). Nest size needs to increase as the chicks grow to afford them some freedom of movement, but the nest should not be so large that the birds cannot easily travel from one side to the other.

Once the birds outgrow the incubator, they can be housed in a hard-sided cage with a makeshift nest and one of three types of heat support: a heating pad on medium beneath half the nest, a heating pad on low beneath the entire nest, or a ceramic heat emitter hung above the nest. All nest bowls should be lined with towels or tissue to help absorb feces and create padding. Small sticks may be placed at the bottom of the nest to help birds practice grabbing and gripping and to ensure normal foot and leg development.

When the birds are beginning to stand in their nests, the ambient temperature can be lowered and heat support can be confined to a small area in the enclosure by placing a heating pad under the nest or similar area. As birds grow larger, nests are modified into flat, padded areas or completely removed, and enclosure size is increased to encourage birds to roam. Birds will start to become curious about their surroundings and venture farther away from the nest to explore their enclosure. Older chicks that have begun to explore should be offered some enrichment items to discover, such as feathers, sticks, grass, and fish. These items should be replaced or cleaned daily. Vinyl mesh mat or rubber matting works well for maintaining foot health and for ease of cleaning once chicks are old enough to stand and walk.

Once birds are walking well and utilizing the space in their cage, advance them to a large indoor cage, for example a tarp-sided, wooden-frame cage with netted ceiling 7 ft. deep × 5 ft. wide × 7 ft. tall (2.1 × 1.5 × 2.1 m). By this age, heat support should not be needed but can be offered via a heating pad on the ground or a ceramic heating element hanging from a stand or from the enclosure ceiling (placed so as to not be a fire hazard). Offer flat nests to give birds the option of using them, but note that they may choose to use them only rarely or just for sleeping. The floor should be padded with towels or similar, which should be changed two to three times a day to remove excess feces. As the chicks start to become more active, introduce them to the outdoors using a play pen during the day in an outdoor aviary (Figure 15.7). The play pen is a small fenced area 5 × 3 ft. (1.5 × 1 m) inside a large outdoor aviary. This gives the young birds time in the sunshine as well as time to start interacting with other species in care that they may interact with in the wild (e.g. pelicans, gulls, other cormorants). Throughout these housing graduations, weight checks and exams should be performed regularly, and nutritional/fluid support should be provided as needed.

Cormorants can have access to water at around 5 weeks of age, when most of their body contour feathers have grown in. It is important to note that in the wild, cormorants that nest on piers/rooftops/bridges/etc. fledge directly into the water. While they may have great success with this type of fledging in the wild, it is recommended that captive-raised cormorants be introduced to water in a more controlled fashion, by allowing them access to a pool of clean water with either gently sloping banks or ramps that allow the birds to easily get in and out. When introducing chicks to water,

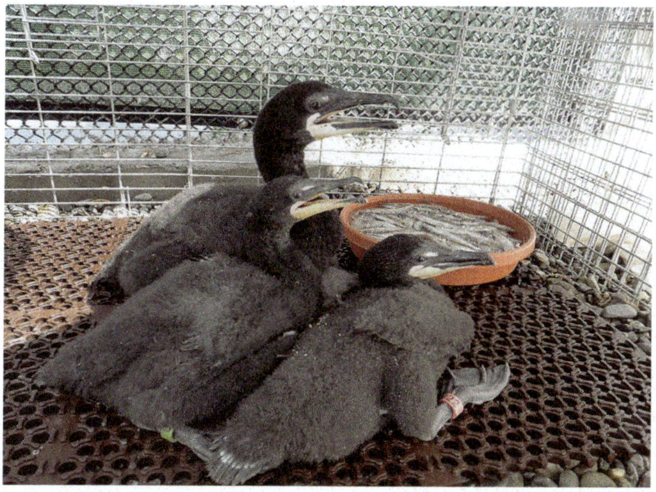

Figure 15.7 Play-pen-style fenced off area in a larger aviary that allows chicks to have exposure to other aviary residents and the outside world during the day. *Source:* photo courtesy of International Bird Rescue.

careful attention should be paid to pool water quality and its effects on plumage waterproofing, particularly if the birds are eating an oily species of fish.

Use caution when introducing young birds to potential foster parents or other adult birds. Adults may not accept begging behavior from chicks that are not their own, so it is important to monitor the situation to ensure the chicks continue to thrive.

## Preparation for Wild Release

Pre-release housing should be a large aviary with access to water for swimming and diving (Figure 15.8); this is where birds are weaned and learn to dive, swim, and fly. In the U.S., caging must conform to USFWS standards found in Minimum Standards for Wildlife Rehabilitation (Miller 2012); however, it is highly recommended that these standards be exceeded to allow plenty of room for birds to practice life skills. For cormorants, the minimum recommended housing for unlimited activity is an 8 ft. (2.4 m) diameter × 2 ft. (0.6 m) deep pool in an 8 × 20 × 10 ft. (2.4 × 6 × 3 m) aviary. Pools must have an overflow system to allow surface contaminants to run off so that the birds' waterproofing will not become compromised.

Cormorant chicks should be thoroughly evaluated for signs of habituation or imprinting at all stages of rearing, especially when considering release. Since cormorants' ranges include many populated areas, birds that are habituated or imprinted carry a significant risk to humans and vice versa if they show no fear of humans upon release.

When juvenile cormorants are living in an aviary, unobtrusive monitoring should occur to determine whether the birds are interacting normally with cohorts and are able to navigate their environment (i.e. enter and leave pool areas) with ease. Live or dead fish may be tossed into pools in pre-release enclosures to encourage natural hunting behavior.

Juvenile cormorants may take short flights in a large aviary, but they need not perform adroit maneuvers in a captive setting to be released. Release criteria include no physical or mental abnormalities, any previous injuries resolved, flight feathers completely emerged, plumage perfectly waterproof, well-fleshed body condition, and packed cell volume >40% and total solids >4.0 g/dl.

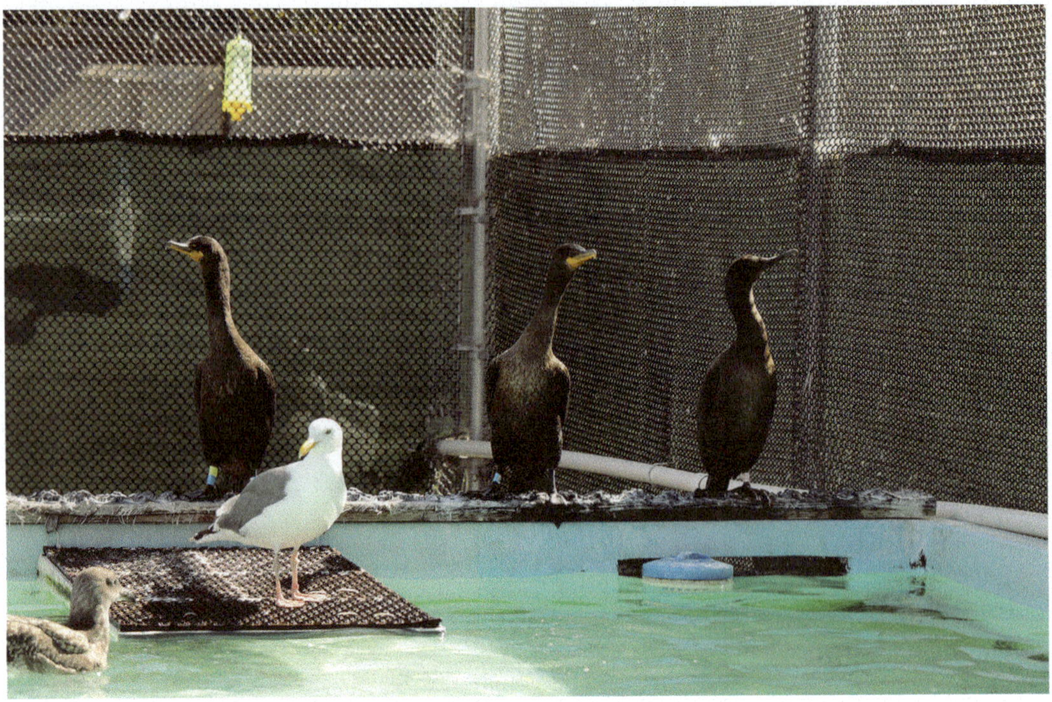

Figure 15.8 Fledging Double-crested Cormorants in a mixed species aviary with ramps for easy entry and exit from water. *Source:* photo courtesy of International Bird Rescue.

Ideally, cormorants are released into or near an existing colony. Since cormorants may nest in inaccessible locations, it is recommended that they be released in small groups, early in the day during a period of good weather, with an adult if possible, near the same species' loafing or nesting area. When possible, federally band (i.e. ring) all birds before release. Rehabilitators without a banding permit may form a partnership with a local bird bander if they are interested in collecting further data on the birds' success once released.

## Acknowledgments

Many thanks to staff, volunteers, and supporters of International Bird Rescue for caring for these birds, and to the many wildlife biologists who have assisted in the rescue of chicks in hazardous areas. Thanks also to SeaWorld, San Diego, for assistance with the development of protocols for these species, and to Jeri O'Donnell for editorial assistance.

## Sources for Products Mentioned

SeaTabs: Pacific Research Labs, Inc., 730 Saddlebrook Dr., Ramona, CA 92065, www.prlvitamins.com.

Emeraid Piscivore: Lafeber Company, 24981 N 1400 East Road, Cornell, IL 61319, https://lafeber.com.

Mazuri products: Mazuri, PMI Nutrition International, LLC, PO Box 66812, St. Louis, MO 63166, www.mazuri.com.

Knutson's Decoys: Knutson's Recreational Sales Inc., 164 Wamplers Lake Road, Brooklyn, Michigan 49230-0457, www.knutsondecoys.com.

Animal Intensive Care Unit: Lyon Technologies, Inc., 1690 Brandywine Avenue, Chula Vista, CA. 91911, https://lyonvet.com.

## References


Dorr, B., Hatch, J., and Weseloh, D.V. (2014). Double-crested cormorants (*Phalacrocorax auritus*) version 2.0. In: *The Birds of North America* (eds. A. Poole and F. Gill). Ithaca, NY, USA: Cornell Lab of Ornithology https://doi.org/10.2173/bna.441.

Hobson, K. (2013). Pelagic cormorant (*Phalacrocorax pelagicus*) version 2.0. In: *The Birds of North America* (eds. A. Poole and F. Gill). Ithaca, NY, USA: Cornell Lab of Ornithology https://doi.org/10.2173/bna.282.

Hoopes, L.A. and Clauss, T. (2016). Investigation of a potential vitamin D deficiency in an African Penguin (Spheniscus demersus) collection. International Association for Aquatic Animal Medicine, Proceedings of the 47$^{th}$ Annual Conference, Virginia Beach, VA.

Ludwig, J.P., Kurita-Matsuba, H., Auman, H.J. et al. (1996). Deformities, PCBs, and TCDD-equivalents in double-crested cormorants (*Phalacrocorax auritus*) and Caspian terns (*Hydroprogne caspia*) of the upper Great Lakes 1986–1991: testing a cause-effect hypothesis. *Journal of Great Lakes Research* 22 (2): 172–197.

Miller, E.A. (ed.) (2012). *Minimum Standards for Wildlife Rehabilitation*, 4e, 116 pages. St. Cloud, MN: National Wildlife Rehabilitators Association https://theiwrc.org/wp-content/uploads/2011/05/Standards-4th-Ed-2012-final.pdf.

Wallace, E. and Wallace, G. (1998). Brandt's cormorant (*Phalacrocorax penicillatus*) version 2.0. In: *The Birds of North America* (eds. A. Poole and F. Gill). Ithaca, NY, USA: Cornell Lab of Ornithology https://doi.org/10.2173/bna.362.

White, C.L., Ip, H.S., Meteyer, C.U. et al. (2015). Spatial and temporal patterns of avian paramyxovirus-1 outbreaks in double-crested cormorants (*Phalacrocorax auritus*) in the USA. *Journal of Wildlife Disease* 51 (1): 101–112.

# 16

# Brown Pelicans

*Yaritza Acosta*

## Natural History

In the United States, there are three subspecies of the Brown Pelican occidentalis group. *Pelecanus occidentalis occidentalis* is found throughout the Gulf Coast, from Mexico to both coasts of Florida. *Pelecanus occidentalis carolinensis* breeds from Maryland, around Florida and through the Gulf Coast to Central America. *Pelecanus occidentalis californicus* ranges from British Columbia down the Pacific coast, typically breeding from California into Mexico (Shields 2014).

Sexual maturity is reached between 3 and 5 years of age. Pelicans nest colonially, on the ground or in trees such as mangroves. The male selects the site and after attracting the female, the male begins gathering sticks, which the female arranges. Ground-nesting sites may be no more than a depression in the ground.

A normal clutch size is three eggs laid over a period of several days, normally with a 2-day interval between eggs; both parents incubate the eggs and share parenting duties. The incubation period varies by subspecies and region but appears to be between 30 and 35 days. Hatchlings are completely altricial. A high mortality rate may be observed with two or more chicks, especially if food is scarce. There is a higher survivability rate for single chicks than for two chicks, due to less competition for food presented by the parents (Shields 2014).

## Criteria for Intervention

Reasons for human intervention are most likely to involve a mass event caused by disruption or devastation to a rookery site, such as an oil spill or hurricane. Although it is unusual for members of the public to find and bring baby pelicans to a wildlife rehabilitation facility, as humans continue to encroach on coastal areas the chance increases. Pelicans prefer to nest on small coastal islands or on dredge islands in intracoastal waterways, many of which are easily accessible to recreational boaters and fishermen.

It is always in the best interests of the chick to be raised by its own parents or at a wildlife facility where foster parents are available. Not all eventualities can be dealt with in this chapter, and it is cruel and inappropriate (and illegal) for wild birds to be raised incorrectly or by inexperienced individuals and then released into the wild. Young pelicans easily imprint and habituate to people; hence, every effort must be made to keep wild pelicans wild.

*Hand-Rearing Birds*, Second Edition. Edited by Rebecca S. Duerr and Laurie J. Gage.

## Record Keeping

Wildlife rehabilitators and others handling migratory birds must hold state and federal rehabilitation permits requiring an annual report on each bird treated. Information required is as follows: date of admission, species, disposition, and date of disposition.

In addition, it is recommended that the following information be collected to ensure the best continuity of care for the bird: the location the bird was found (because it is hoped that the bird can be returned to the same location), the general condition and weight of the bird on intake, the location of any injuries on intake and follow-up treatment, records of fluids and any medications given, a feeding schedule, and notes pertinent to whether the chick is eating unassisted or whether it needs help. Young healthy pelicans should increase in weight every day until reaching adult weight; if they are merely maintaining weight or it is declining, it may mean there is a parasite infestation or other health problem.

## Initial Care and Stabilization

It is critical that the chicks be warmed first and then hydrated before taking any other action. Place the chick in a warm, quiet area in a towel nest. Baby pelicans feed from the nest floor, so it is recommended that paper, especially shredded paper, not be used as a nesting material, because it will be ingested. For approximately the first 3 weeks of life, until they are covered in down, pelican chicks have trouble thermoregulating and are constantly attended by a parent (Figure 16.1). At Pelican Harbor Seabird Station (PHSS), it has been observed that the runt or weaker sibling is often infested with ectoparasites and needs treatment during initial care and stabilization.

Hydration may be given orally, subcutaneously, or by IV bolus. Many different hydration fluids are available, and the choice should be made based on your wildlife veterinarian's recommendation. Fluid therapy charts are available for wildlife (Miller 2006). Once the chick has been warmed and rehydrated, feeding may begin.

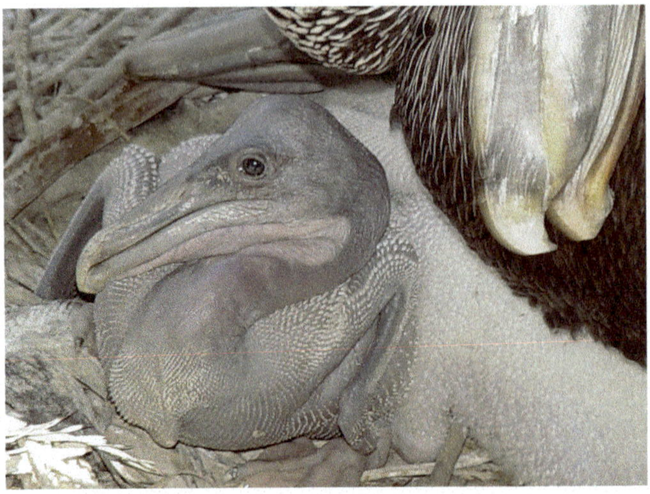

Figure 16.1 Nestling pelican: skin color is purplish before down grows in.

## Common Medical Problems and Solutions

Minor skin lacerations are not uncommon. Make sure the affected area is kept clean; this type of minor skin nick normally heals quickly. More serious wounds may occur if a chick is or has been attacked by older siblings in the nest. Another problem can occur during weaning. Juveniles may try to feed from any available adult, becoming quite aggressive in their attempts to force the adult's beak open. The adult will on occasion retaliate by biting the juvenile around the head, sometimes resulting in head injuries. Most injuries are superficial and will scab over and heal quickly. At this age the beak is still soft and is damaged easily. Normally, the injuries are located caudally on the bill. Scabbing can be quite severe, and the beak may take several weeks to fully heal. Birds with scratches to the eyes and birds exhibiting neurological symptoms should be seen by an experienced wildlife veterinarian. Hematological and biochemical reference values can be found in Zaias et al. (2000).

It is normal for Brown Pelicans to have what appears to be subcutaneous emphysema under the skin. This assists with buoyancy. When palpated, it will feel like bubble wrap and may make a crackling sound. If an air sac is ruptured there will be an obvious, larger outpouching of the skin. If a ruptured air sac is suspected, the bird should be referred to a wildlife veterinarian. The air sac may need draining, and the bird may also require ventilatory assistance as well as medication.

## Diet

In the wild, Brown Pelicans feed by plunge diving and bringing up to three gallons of water to the surface which is drained out to leave fish behind in their pouches. Brown Pelicans will also catch fish while floating on the surface if large, dense schools of small bait fish are available. In captivity, smelt, minnows, and anchovies are useful in small chicks, increasing in size to small threadfin herring, sardines, mullet, menhaden, capelin, and other small whole bait fish for juveniles. The nutritional value of fish varies depending on fish type, season, and whether the fish is alive or dead. Fish with a higher fat content will have a higher caloric density. Very oily fish, such as mackerel or capelin, can cause fish oil to adhere around the pelican's beak and will eventually end up on the feathers, causing waterproofing problems. Although fish are normally a good source of vitamins, changes can occur in dead or frozen fish. Birds fed dead or frozen–thawed fish should receive thiamine and vitamin E supplements and a good general vitamin supplement. Even birds being fed live fish in captivity will benefit from an appropriate good-quality vitamin supplement. Dosage is by weight and will depend on the diet given and combination of supplements used. Choices include Auklet or Vita-Zu Tablets (Mazuri®), and SeaTabs, which are formulated for fish-eating birds and mammals (Pacific Research Laboratories). Current recommendations for piscivores are 25–30 mg thiamine and 100 mg vitamin E per kg fish fed (Hawkins et al. 2018).

A general rule would be to use a variety of seasonal, locally available fish if possible, because the best diet should closely resemble what would be available to the birds in the wild during nesting season. Chunks of large fish or fish with large bones, gill plates, or skulls are not appropriate, because the bones are difficult and sometimes impossible for the pelican to digest. Large, sharp bones can perforate the stomach causing peritonitis or become lodged in the esophagus, making it difficult for the bird to swallow.

## Feeding Procedures

In the wild, feeding begins within hours of hatching. The parent regurgitates partially digested fish into the nest for chicks to pick up. This behavior lasts for approximately 3 weeks. The transition to a different feeding method coincides with the chicks becoming completely down covered. At about 2–3 weeks of age, the chicks begin feeding by reaching into the parent's throat for fish. This behavior lasts until the chick is ready to fledge. Once the chick can fly, the parent limits the number of feedings. PHSS is located on a flyway in Biscayne Bay, Florida, near a pelican nesting site. The author frequently sees young pelicans chasing adult birds both on land and water. Normal behavior is for the fledgling to waggle its wings, bob the head, and snap at its own wings to attract the parent's attention. More aggressive behavior includes trying to force the adult's beak open.

For small chicks without down, offer slivers of fish or small whole fish, such as small smelt, on the cage or nest floor. Leave the area, because the chick may become distracted and not eat while humans are present. It is important to count the number of fish placed with the chick so eating habits can be monitored. Introduce the chick to foster parents as soon as possible if available (Figure 16.2).

Older down-covered chicks may be more of a challenge as they have become used to eating from the pouch (Figure 16.3). If they will not pick fish off the floor, try presenting fish on the end of a hemostat or pair of scissors. They will learn quickly. Chicks that are standing well and developing feathers can be introduced to fish in a bowl of shallow water.

If foster parents are not available, it is in the chick's best interests to be transferred to a facility with foster parents and experience in raising pelicans. Foster parents are normally nonreleasable pelicans used for fostering or education purposes. Permits are required. Adults undergoing rehabilitation should not be used as foster parents.

When placing chicks with foster parents, it is normally readily apparent if the chick will be accepted or not. Normal behavior is for the adult to circle the chick, with head swaying and open

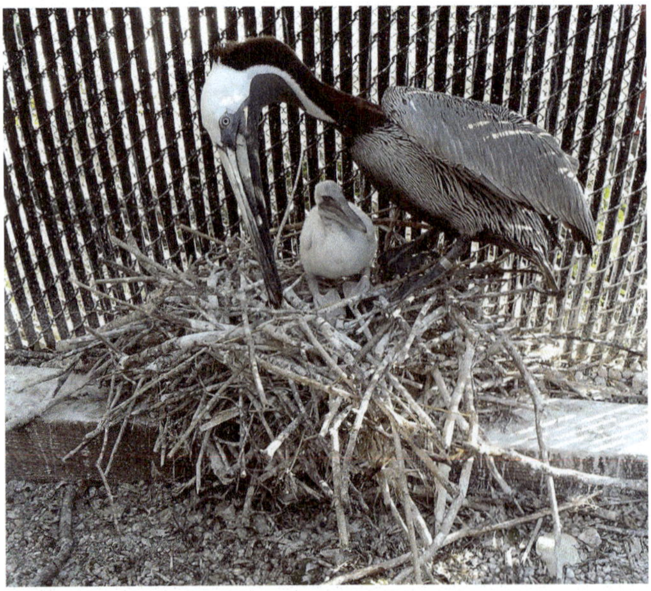

Figure 16.2 Downy chick with foster parent.

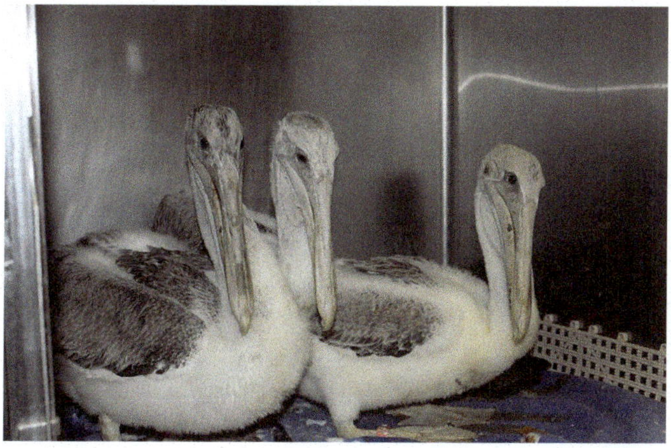

Figure 16.3 Three downy chicks beginning to grow contour feathers.

beak; "hissing" may also occur. The adult will settle over the chick fairly quickly. Pairs or single adults will foster.

Older chicks are best kept in groups with adult foster parents as role models. The number in each group depends on aviary size. In addition, be aware that young pelicans can become quite aggressive in their feeding techniques, often overwhelming adults or older juveniles with their anxiety to feed. This is a dangerous situation for both the chicks and adults, and is a reason to not use debilitated adults in rehabilitation as foster parents.

A slow introduction technique through a joint aviary fence needs to be used when introducing large groups of displaced pelican chicks, such as when a rookery island is destroyed after a hurricane. These pelicans tend to be traumatized by rescue and transportation issues and may have been in a large group for at least several days. After Hurricane Dennis in 2004, fifty 6–10-week-old pelican chicks were raised. The chicks were divided into three age-specific groups in aviaries that shared a common fence with foster adults. As night approached at the end of the first day, the chicks settled down to sleep against the common fence and the adults settled down next to the chicks on their side of the fence. By the next day, a calm and successful introduction was possible (Figure 16.4).

If no foster care is available: try to find a sibling. This reduces the chance of imprinting or habituation; if none are available, strict guidelines and protocols should be put into place. See Chapter 15 for additional ideas regarding how to keep wild chicks wild.

- *Limit handling:* Set a feeding schedule and have very limited personnel work with the chicks.
- *Wear a costume and mask:* Head and body should be covered when changing and feeding. Most pelicans self-feed when fish is placed on the ground if over 3 weeks of age, so interactions can be minimal. Set fish on a plate (count or weigh) to be changed out at each feeding.
- *Feed with puppets:* PHSS has used pelican stuffed toys or handmade puppets to put with nestlings if no other siblings were available and also to feed. One trick used was to cut open the mouth of the stuffed toy and put a small bowl of fish in it and sometimes chicks would eat from it. Take care the chick doesn't ingest any stuffed animal parts.
- *Keep in a group:* A singleton habituates to humans very easily. PHSS has had success (without foster parents) in raising orphaned pelicans for release.

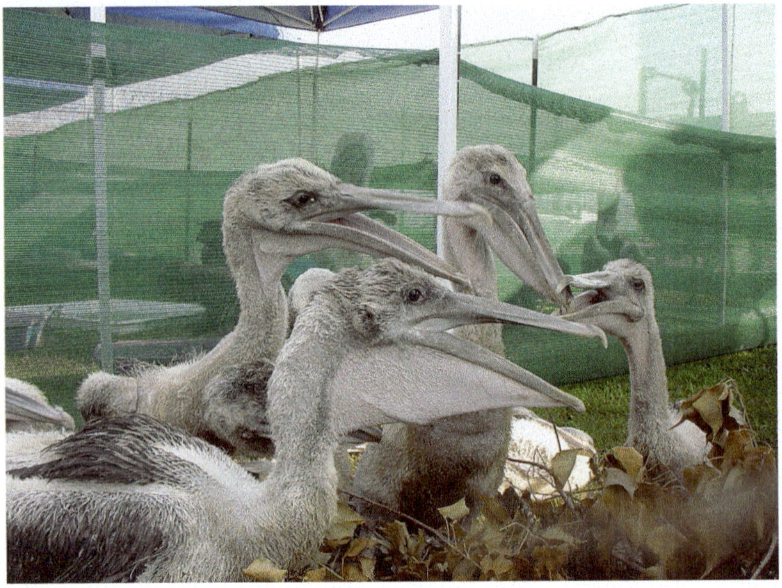

Figure 16.4 Chicks in care due to an oil spill, with adult birds visible behind the shared wall. *Source:* photo courtesy of International Bird Rescue.

Once a chick is less downy and around 2 months old, they are moved outside to adjust to enclosures with other rehabilitating pelicans, most often older juveniles. It is important to get orphans outside around other pelicans as soon as possible for their social development.

## Expected Development

Weight gain is rapid during the first 3 weeks. After 3 weeks, a steady, but not as rapid, weight gain will occur. Because pelicans vary greatly in size (particularly by sex, males are larger), weight gain should not be the only indicator of successful growth. Daily checks should show an increasingly active chick, well-hydrated with a well-rounded body and plump breast.

Chicks hatch with bare purplish skin for about 7 days, before white down begins to appear on the rump area first. The chick will be completely covered in white wooly down at about 3 weeks. Contour feathers begin to appear at about 4–5 weeks, beginning in the scapula area and extending onto the humerus.

Nestlings begin holding their heads up at 2–4 days. By 10–14 days they are moving in the nest and are able to hold themselves upright. At 3–4 weeks they sit or stand for prolonged periods of time, and after that, ground-nesting chicks become very mobile. They will leave the nest and begin to explore, closely watched over by their parents, although sometimes from a distance. Chicks in tree nests will move to perches next to the nest. First flight normally occurs between 12 and 14 weeks.

## Flight Cages and Pools

Caging standards for rehabilitating wild birds in the US are regulated by the United States Fish and Wildlife Service and by state wildlife agencies. In many states, Miller (2000) is cited as the guideline for caging sizes, although more recent revisions are available. Although the guidelines call for an aviary 12 × 30 × 10 ft. high (3.6 × 9 × 3 m high), the author believes that pelicans needing flight conditioning or fledglings being prepared for the wild receive better conditioning in a cage approximately 24 × 30 × 14 ft. high (7.3 × 9 × 4.3 m high) or even larger. This allows for turning while in flight. Different height perches should be made available. Pool size is also specified and should be at least 2 ft. deep (Figure 16.5). Saltwater pools are ideal. It is recommended that all pools have an intake on one side and outlet on the other side. This overflow arrangement allows for good water circulation and in particular keeps the surface of the water free of fish oil, feces, and other contaminants. Before release, all waterbirds' feathers must be waterproof and in top condition. This is essential to their success in the wild.

## Preparation for Wild Release

It is crucial to their success in the wild that pelicans are raised to avoid imprinting or habituation to people. Pelicans are naturally fairly curious, naturally fairly friendly, and will do just about anything for a fish. Sadly, at PHSS in Miami, over 90% of the injuries seen are caused by recreational fishing. Pelicans cannot tell the difference between a handout and a fish with a hook in it that is being used as bait. If, as chicks, they learn to associate people with food they will continue this behavior into adulthood making them even more vulnerable to injury and possible death. When raised in the appropriate caging with foster parents or in a group setting with other pelicans, they will have a much better chance of success in the wild. Although it is very difficult to teach plunge diving in a rehabilitation setting, with the appropriate type pool, caging, foster parents, and other pelicans to serve as role models, the chicks will quickly learn that fish come out of water. It is

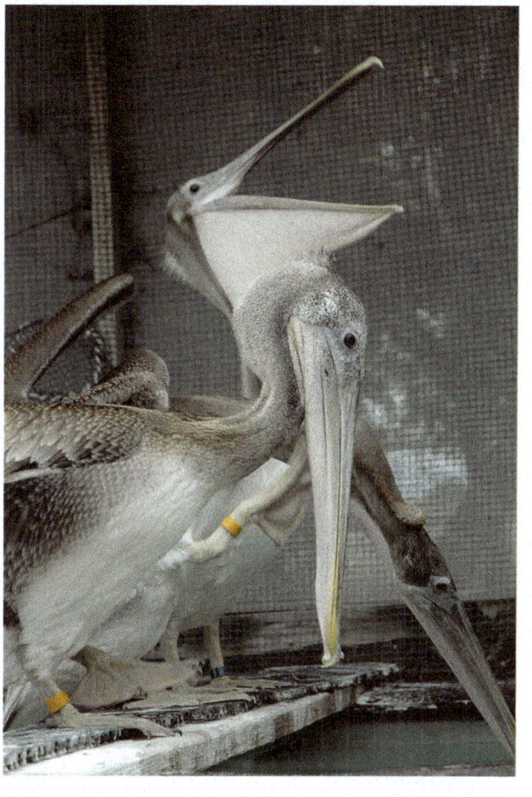

Figure 16.5 Three juvenile pelicans stretching and preening while perched on the edge of aviary pool. *Source:* photo courtesy of International Bird Rescue.

important to present them with live fish so that they experience catching live fish in their pouch, draining the water, and swallowing the fish without losing it. At PHSS, fish is delivered once a week from local fishermen for rehabilitation pelicans and enrichment for permanent residents.

A soft release is preferable if possible. It is also recommended that juveniles are released in groups in the vicinity of flocks of adult pelicans and, if possible, near a rookery site. At PHSS, rehabilitated and wild pelicans are banded with USGS metal bands. Juvenile pelicans released from the facility are often seen swimming and flying in the bay with wild adults. They leave with these wild groups of adults for the spring migration north. An avid birder has been active in reporting sightings and sending photographs of a rookery site 200 miles north of Miami. These reports show captive-raised and/or rehabilitated juveniles interacting in the wild with adults and other juveniles.

## Acknowledgments

Thanks to Linda Gregard DVM and Beth Hirschfeld DVM for their input, and many thanks to the late Wendy Fox who wrote the first version of this chapter, much of which remains here. Thanks to current and former staff and volunteers of PHSS, Miami, Florida, for caring for the birds.

## Sources for Products Mentioned

SeaTabs: Pacific Research Labs, Inc., 730 Saddlebrook Dr., Ramona, CA 92065, www.prlvitamins.com.

Auklet or Vita-Zu Tablets: Mazuri, PMI Nutrition International, LLC, PO Box 66812, St. Louis, MO 63166, www.mazuri.com.

## References

Hawkins, M.G., Sanchez-Migallon Guzman, D., Beaufrere, H. et al. (2018). Birds. In: *Exotic Animal Formulary*, 5e (eds. J.W. Carpenter and C.J. Marion), 167–375. St. Louis, MO: Elsevier.

Miller, E.A. (ed.) (2000). *Minimum Standards for Wildlife Rehabilitation*, 3e, 77 pp. St. Cloud, MN: National Wildlife Rehabilitation Association http://www.nwrawildlife.org/documents/Standards3rdEdition.pdf.

Miller, E.A. (ed.) (2006). *Quick Reference*, 3e, 148 pp. St Cloud, MN: National Wildlife Rehabilitators Association.

Shields, M. 2014. Brown pelican (*Pelecanus occidentalis*), version 2.0. In: *The Birds of North America*. A.F. Poole (ed.), Cornell Lab of Ornithology, Ithaca, NY, USA. https://doi.org/ 10.2173/bna.609.

Zaias, J., Fox, W., Cray, C., and Altman, N. (2000). Hematologic, plasma protein, and biochemical profiles of Brown pelicans. *American Journal of Veterinary Research* 61 (7): 771–774.

# 17

# Herons, Egrets, and Bitterns

*Megan Shaw Prelinger, Jennifer Linander, and Rebecca S. Duerr*

## Natural History

There are 65 species of herons, egrets, and bitterns in the family Ardeidae within the order Pelecaniformes, and 10 species of herons and egrets are found in North America. All species of herons and egrets nest in trees, although some may occasionally nest on the ground in treeless areas. All species have semi-altricial, downy chicks that hatch with their eyes open. Herons and egrets are colonial nesters and typically hatch groups of nestlings at the rate of two to four per nest. Incubation lasts 17–28 days, depending on the size of the species, and young are fully flighted by 7–8 weeks. Some species may continue to support fledglings for a short period after they have left the nest (Parsons and Master 2000; Hothem et al. 2010; McCrimmon et al. 2011; Vennesland and Butler 2011).

Herons and egrets have anisodactyl feet, with three long toes pointing forward and one pointing back, with partial webbing between digits 3 and 4. Each toe is furnished with a sharp and pointed claw. The remarkable length and hensile strength of their toes and the sharpness of their claws enable them to firmly grip tree branches of varying thicknesses.

Adult diets are adaptable to available food stocks. Small fish and aquatic invertebrates are preferred foods, although all herons and egrets rely additionally in varying measures on small rodents and insects. Young are fed a regurgitated diet for their first few days of life, but they readily learn to pick up foods left for them on the floors of their nests.

## Criteria for Intervention

Herons and egrets are gregarious colonial nesters that are less sensitive to human population density than some other families of birds. Many young fall from nests in their early days or weeks of life. Fallen young hatched in colonies that are situated in remote environments may climb back up to nests or be fed on the ground by their parents while they hide in surrounding grasses, and slowly learn to feed themselves. Fallen chicks hatched in urban or suburban colonies, however, are extremely vulnerable to predators such as birds of prey, cars, cats, and dogs, because such colonies tend to be situated above cropped grass or pavement rather than above tall natural undergrowth. Fallen nestlings are thus left entirely exposed, and may be miles away from an appropriate habitat. Some species normally fledge from the nest prior to being capable of flight, but this may be

*Hand-Rearing Birds*, Second Edition. Edited by Rebecca S. Duerr and Laurie J. Gage.

impossible in an urban colony; fledged chicks may find themselves running in traffic rather than foraging in a wetland. They are also subject to being harassed or "rescued" by passing children or adults. Such interventions are likely to end a young bird's life unless a subsequent intervention is made by a rehabilitator. Placing healthy and alert individuals back in their nests is often impossible due to the heights at which tree-nesting colonies are located and potential disturbance of the whole colony, which could cause more chicks to fall. Nestlings and fledglings that fall from high branches are prone to skeletal and soft tissue injuries. Chicks also may be targets for human neighbors upset about the noise and smell of the colony, and may present with gunshot wounds. Urban colony management is an ongoing challenge in many cities. Any chick found running in traffic, hiding under cars, or obviously injured or in distress on the ground is in need of rescue. Fledglings moving normally and foraging in an appropriate habitat should be left alone.

## Record Keeping

It is important to keep records on individual orphaned and injured herons and egrets, both due to regulatory agency reporting requirements and so that developmentally similar individuals can be housed and cared for together. It is also important to track and note each chick's progress in injury recovery as well as key developmental stages as birds advance from rescue to release. Rescue events tend to be clustered around specific locations and seasons, so rehabilitators are more often faced with hand-rearing groups of animals rather than individuals. For an example of an animal care record please see Appendix 1; also see Chapter 1 for information on record keeping.

It is important to keep detailed notes on the progress of feather coverage on young birds' bodies, because as the plumage develops, so does the bird's ability to thermoregulate. This is the most important criterion by which healthy chicks are graduated from stage to stage within the orphan-rearing process. Careful tracking will also allow age-appropriate clustering of patients, which will facilitate peer group socialization and insulate individuals from peer-to-peer aggression that may occur when young at different developmental stages are housed together.

## Initial Care and Stabilization

The importance of addressing hypothermia in young herons and egrets cannot be overstated. Rehabilitators expecting the arrival of young herons and egrets should keep a pre-warmed incubator or cage with heat lamp ready, set to maintain an ambient temperature of 100 °F (37.7 °C) and 40–50% humidity. Young birds should be placed within such an environment immediately upon arrival, even if they are alert (Figure 17.1). Older patients may be placed in a warm (85 °F/29.4 °C) room on top of a heating pad set to low if they are bright and alert. New patients should be allowed 30–60 minutes to rest and warm up prior to any examination. If birds seem sleepy or unresponsive, a cloacal temperature should be taken using a digital human quick read thermometer to determine necessary heat supplementation. Normal body temperature is 103–106 °F (39.5–41.1 °C). Be careful to insert only the tip of the thermometer into the bird's vent, as trauma to delicate tissue is a risk. If a bird's temperature is less than 98 °F (36.7 °C), it should be immediately placed into a 100 °F environment with a towel-wrapped heat pad beneath and gently folded over them like a cave. Check temperature approximately every 45 minutes until temp is at least 98 °F (36.7 °C). For chicks with temperatures of 98–101 °F (36.7–38.3 °C), very warm fluids (105 °F/40.5 °C), such as an

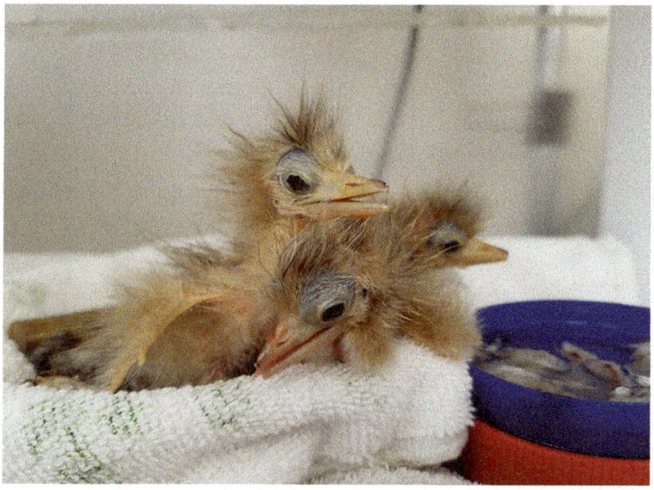

Figure 17.1 American Bittern chicks in a 100 °F (37.8 °C) animal intensive care unit, note the diversity of sticks for toes to grab and fish offered in shallow dish. *Source:* photo courtesy of International Bird Rescue.

electrolyte solution, may be given orally at 5% (50 ml/kg) of body weight. This helps hydrate and warm them internally and promotes gastrointestinal motility. Subsequent hydrations and all nutrition should be withheld until after a complete examination has been performed after giving the chick 30 minutes to absorb its tubing. Oral fluids may be given with size 8–12 French red rubber tube attached to an appropriately-sized syringe.

Alert young herons and egrets are poor candidates for oral hydration. The ability to expand the throat and mouth very wide is required for young to ingest the sometimes-large fish, insects, and rodents that parents may deliver to the nest. However, the ability to gape wide enough to swallow a whole 15 g fish provides these birds with an easy mechanism for rejecting oral hydration: they simply open their throats in a gape following fluid administration and the fluids fall right out of their proventriculus onto the floor of the cage in front of them. This scenario creates unnecessary risks of aspiration and can be avoided by administering pre-warmed sterile isotonic fluids, such as lactated Ringer's solution, subcutaneously at 5% body weight (50 ml/kg).

Extremely young hatchlings arriving with only downy feathers may be placed in a shallow dish lined with cloth to support their bodies in an upright position. Place small sticks or grasses in the nest to give their large feet something to grasp, which aids in foot development. Herons and egrets that are old enough to begin developing contour or flight feathers on their bodies are generally able to hold their bodies up independently and look around. Do not use terrycloth with older chicks as they may catch their toenails in the loops.

When warm and alert, new arrivals should be given a thorough initial examination, consisting of a cloacal temperature check followed by a beak-to-toe physical exam (see Chapter 1).

## Common Medical Problems and Solutions

### Metabolic Bone Disease

Metabolic bone disease (secondary nutritional hyperparathyroidism) (MBD) is caused by an imbalance of calcium, phosphorus, and vitamin $D_3$. Young herons and egrets are vulnerable to skeletal problems at all stages of rearing, and may enter care with MBD or develop it during care. In growing wild birds, MBD typically manifests as a malformation of growing long bones and is almost always caused by a deficiency of dietary calcium during the rapid growth phase. In affected chicks, the bones may palpate soft or rubbery, the chick may have trouble standing when old enough to do so, or it may develop folding fractures of the long bones. Radiographs are helpful to ascertain whether the problem is limited to one long bone or to the entire body. Chicks with only one or two affected bones may recover well but chicks with multiple or all long bones affected hold a poor prognosis. Chicks with spinal deformities also hold a poor prognosis; those not able to normally ambulate or fly when old enough to do so should be humanely euthanized. For mild to moderately MBD-affected chicks, administration of additional amounts of calcium or a vitamin D supplement may be helpful in assisting the chick with rapid mineralization of the skeleton. If a chick enters care with the problem, feeding a diet with a calcium-to-phosphorus ration of 3:1 during the rest of growth will provide additional calcium to help make up the deficit. Some fish species used to feed piscivores in captivity have been found to have low calcium to phosphorus ratios (Table 17.1) or to be deficient in vitamin $D_3$ (Hoopes and Clauss 2016).

For chicks with questionable (e.g. rubbery) bone quality at arrival, supplemental calcium is recommended in the form of calcium carbonate ($CaCO_3$) pills, usually 500–600 mg tablets, being sure to avoid those containing vitamin $D_3$, unless the primary food items are known or suspected to be deficient (e.g. capelin, Hoopes and Clauss 2016). Vitamin D may be given separately orally or intramuscularly to assist with uptake of the calcium supplementation if the diet is known or suspected to be deficient. Consult your avian veterinarian for species-appropriate doses and combinations of supplements to assist bone development. Excessive vitamin D supplementation can result in mineralization of soft tissues and other problems; hence, it is prudent to know the content of foods before assuming more is better.

Table 17.1 Calcium and phosphorus content of commercially available feeder fish, with calcium supplement amounts needed to support skeletal growth of piscivorous chicks.

| Species | Calcium (mg/100 g fish) | Phosphorus (mg/100 g fish) | Calcium Phosphorus ratio | Calcium supp. needed (mg/100g fish) to have Ca : P = 1.5 : 1 |
|---|---|---|---|---|
| Atlantic Herring | 392 | 389 | 1.01 | 191.5 |
| Atlantic Mackerel | 137 | 255 | 0.54 | 245.5 |
| Capelin | 352 | 400 | 0.88 | 248 |
| Finger Mullet | 1040 | 764 | 1.36 | 106 |
| Lake Smelt | 301 | 202 | 1.49 | 2 |
| Night Smelt | 557 | 473 | 1.18 | 152.5 |
| Pacific Herring | 644 | 528 | 1.22 | 148 |
| Peruvian Smelt | 479 | 393 | 1.22 | 110.5 |
| Pink Salmon | 280 | 364 | 0.77 | 266 |
| Silversides | 752 | 510 | 1.47 | 13 |

*Source:* data from McRoberts Sales Inc., 2015–2016 catch analyses.

Throughout the orphan-rearing process, heron chicks should be checked regularly for any signs of limping, unwillingness/reluctance to stand if old enough to do so, or drooping wings that could indicate hairline fractures or folding fractures. Bone injuries are often subtle enough in their beginning stages that they may not be observable on a tabletop exam, but with practice, the presence of small lumps or angular deformities toward either end of long bones can be detected. If more than one chick is affected, especially if the chicks are unrelated, the diet and supplement regimen should be reassessed. Chicks with mild MBD may benefit from lightweight splints that do not impede use of the limb and help keep the bone straight while it finishes growing.

### Fractures

Heron and egret chicks from urban rookeries may be struck by cars if they fall from nests into a street, or if they become confused and run into traffic. If a limp or a wing droop is detected on intake or at any time during the orphan-rearing process, radiographs should be taken. However, young herons often stand with their wings drooped, and this must be differentiated from abnormal droops where something is wrong with the wing. They also sometimes sleep flat-out in a posture that looks disturbingly abnormal, rather like a dinosaur fossil (as if dead). This also may be normal.

Fractured limbs require stabilization with a supportive wrap or splint. Management of fractures in these species is covered in Duerr (2017). Heron and egret chicks tend to develop joint contractures, especially of the carpus (wrist), when the wing is immobilized during growth; hence, wing wraps should be applied cautiously and only when truly necessary. They also must be applied so as to avoid damaging or impeding growing flight feathers. Some chicks land on their faces when they fall and may fracture the tip of their mandible. If the mandible tip bends sideways when the mouth opens, it should be splinted immediately to prevent it from becoming an open fracture. It is difficult to get adhesives to stick to the bill of these species, but self-adhesive hydrocolloid blister bandages stick well for temporary stabilization and may incorporate a tiny splint. This type of fracture typically requires pinning by a veterinarian. Instructions for this procedure can be found in Duerr (2017). Additional splinting techniques applicable to herons and egrets can be found in the Small-bodied Birds chapter in that resource.

Chicks with orthopedic injuries under treatment should be housed to allow as much normal activity as possible given the injury, to reduce stress and allow normal behaviors; however, some injured chicks may be stressed or bullied by uninjured conspecifics. Conversely, some temporarily disabled chicks may bully others. A quiet, nonstressful housing situation with a single calm companion, where the chick can calmly eat and heal, is ideal.

### Wounds

Many nestlings sustain bruising or lacerations during falls from their nests. In some cases, these falls can result in organ damage or internal hemorrhage that is life-threatening. Bright light shown against the skin of the abdomen can reveal hemorrhage in the coelomic cavity. Subcutaneous emphysema (air under the skin) is common in chicks that have sustained traumatic injuries, and usually resolves on its own unless severe.

Superficial skin injuries should be cleaned daily with a dilute solution of chlorhexidine or betadine. If lacerations are small, clean, and have already begun to heal through secondary intention, daily cleaning is generally adequate to result in quick resolution. Fresh lacerations, and larger or deeper lacerations, should be cleaned and temporarily covered with a topical dressing such as

Tegaderm (3M). Lacerations that involve exposed muscle, bone, or tendon heal quickly when closed with sutures. When evaluating lacerations on admission, special care should be taken to identify all wounds that may be present. Patients with bite wounds from mammalian predators should be treated with an antibiotic such as amoxicillin with clavulanic acid (125 mg/kg q12 h) until the wound has fully healed (Hawkins et al. 2018).

Young birds that are rescued from rookeries situated near or over water are also susceptible to any of the injuries that generally befall waterbirds: fish hook and fishing line injuries, oiling, and boat collisions. Although these conditions are less likely to be seen in hatch-year birds than in adults of the same species, they should not be forgotten if a young bird has been rescued from an aquatic environment.

## Endoparasites

Herons and egrets are vulnerable to debilitation due to heavy parasite loads. Routine deworming with ivermectin (0.2–0.4 mg/kg orally once, repeated in 10 days) and fenbendazole (100 mg/kg orally once, repeated in 10 days) may be useful in areas where moderate or severe endoparasitism is common (see Hawkins et al. 2018 for dosing information). Consult your veterinarian for a deworming protocol tailored to local conditions.

Every intake exam of a young bird should include an oral examination, to look for parasites in subcutaneous mouth tissues, and a gentle but thorough palpation of the abdomen to feel for abnormal lumpy areas. Common oral parasites include flukes, which look like small leeches attached inside the mouth and under the tongue, and *Avioserpens taiwana* (Kinsella 2008), a nematode that resides subcutaneously, looking rather like vermicelli within the floor of the mouth. Swellings from severe Avioserpens infections may become infected or cause tissue necrosis in the floor of the mouth (Figure 17.2). At International Bird Rescue, affected chicks are treated with fenbendazole at 100 mg/kg once, with a repeat dose 10 days later. Lower doses of fenbendazole were ineffective, as was ivermectin, both orally to the bird and injected directly into the worms. No toxicities or plumage effects of fenbendazole have been encountered at this dose in many hundreds of chicks. If the worms are killed, they begin to slowly dissolve within the tissue and disappear within a few

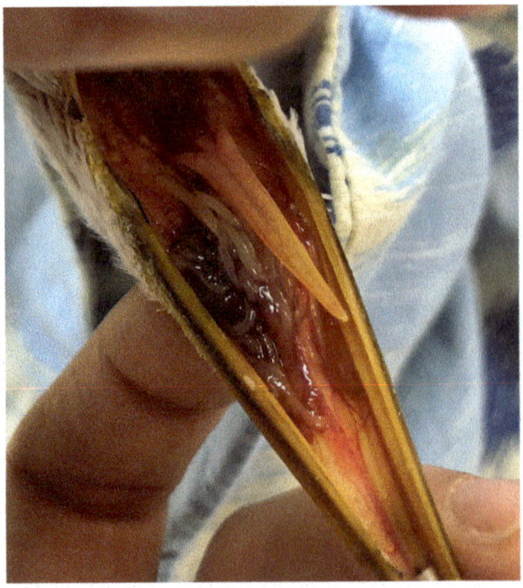

Figure 17.2 Severe avioserpens infestation in the floor of the mouth of a Snowy Egret chick. *Source:* photo courtesy of International Bird Rescue.

weeks or become an inspissated mass of dead tissue that may need debridement. However, if the worm mass begins to look more swollen and yellowish, it has become infected and a course of antibiotics such as amoxicillin with clavulanic acid (125 mg/kg q12 h) may be needed.

Verminous coelomitis resulting from infestations with *Eustrongylides ignotus* can often be identified by wormy ridges crisscrossing a firm, lumpy abdomen (Figure 17.3). This bean sprout-sized worm pokes holes in the bird's stomach and causes abdominal abscesses and adhesions that can affect peristalsis and organ function and causes significant mortality in young wading birds (Spalding and Forrester 2008). This can be differentiated from fish in the stomach by palpating the bird's abdomen when both empty and with a full meal on board. Monitor the shape and size of the mass, and how the chick is doing. At International Bird Rescue, it has been noted that birds with these masses affecting more than half of their abdominal volume, or those where the worm mass feels like it is penetrating the body wall, tend to do very poorly. In California, this problem is seen commonly in Green Heron (*Butorides virescens*) and Great Egret (*Ardea alba*) chicks, and less commonly in Black-crowned Night-Heron (*Nycticorax nycticorax*) chicks.

## Diets

Young herons and egrets in the wild eat a diverse diet that is based on fish but also includes small rodents, crustaceans, and large insects. Great Blue Herons eat more small mammals than do smaller herons and egrets. Cattle Egrets are less oriented toward water than other egrets. Black-crowned Night-Herons rely more exclusively on fish than other species. Within and across these

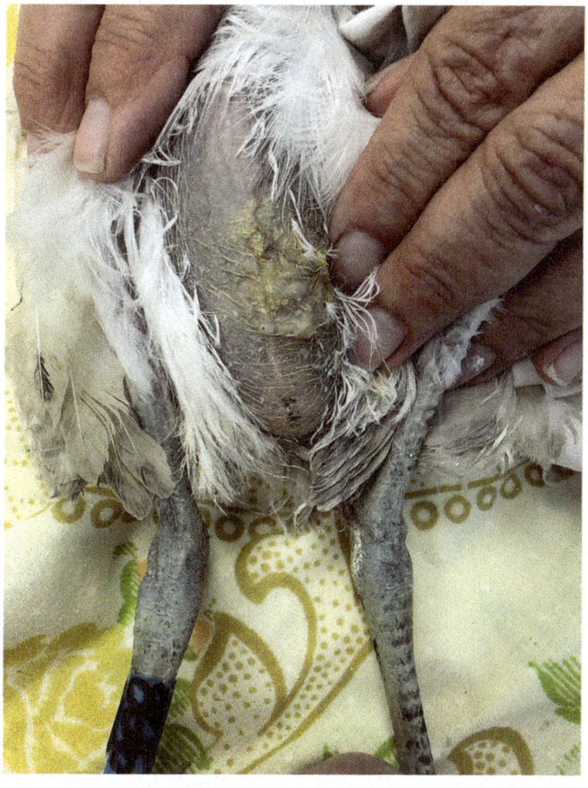

Figure 17.3 Abdominal mass due to infestation with *Eustrongylides ignotus*, coelomic worms, in a Snowy Egret chick. Chicks with this problem often have a palpable firm lumpy mass occupying space in the abdomen, but the mass does not always visibly affect the external contour of the body like in this bird. *Source:* photo courtesy of International Bird Rescue.

generalities and specificities, a basic set of diet supplies can be stocked that will satisfy the nutritional needs of all herons and egrets. This basic set must include an adequate stock of frozen blocks of small fish (smelt or herring, in the 5–20 g size range), which comprise the basic captive diet, and stocks of frozen mice and live insects. If only larger fish are available (30–40 g size range), the fish can be cut diagonally into smaller strips so that both ends are pointed, simulating smaller fish. Mealworms (*Tenebrio molitor*), mature mealworm beetles, and crickets provide more options for diet diversity. The beetles make excellent live forage practice for birds in pre-release flight aviaries. Because young herons and egrets can eat their own body weight each day, it may be impractical to rely on live food for the bulk of their diet. Live fish are useful, however, especially for getting reluctant eaters to start eating. At all stages of orphan rearing, food should be sprinkled with crushed calcium carbonate tablets or pills can be administered orally to improve calcium to phosphorus ratios.

Thawed, quartered mice should be introduced into the diets of all herons and egrets as a complement to the basic diet of fish: one mouse per bird per day will give the birds a chance to sample these nonfish foodstuffs. Rehabilitators can assess additional quantities based on species preferences and local species wild diets. Snails, lizards, and crayfish may form substantial portions of wild diets.

### Supplements

All chicks should receive vitamin and mineral supplements while in care to support healthy growth, unless being fed strictly fresh, unfrozen fish with an excellent calcium-to-phosphorus ratio. Nutrients of concern in piscivores fed frozen–thawed, or certain small-bodied fish include thiamin, vitamin E, vitamin D, and calcium. Commonly-used vitamin supplements for piscivores include #5M2G Mazuri® Auklet Vitamin Tablets (www.Mazuri.com) or SeaTabs (Pacific Labs) and 500–600 mg calcium (from calcium carbonate) tablets. When needed, vitamin $D_3$ gelcaps intended for humans work well.

Supplement doses are intended to be administered per kilogram of fish consumed; but in practice, food intake may be hard to determine in a busy clinic. When heron and egret chicks are growing rapidly, they may eat their own body weight in fish daily; hence, a good rule of thumb for multivitamins is one tab per kg of bird for hatchlings and nestlings, with reduced frequency as chicks' growth and food intake slows as they reach adult size. Although variation in nutritional content of fish is seen seasonally and from year-to-year, as shown in Table 17.1 different fish species vary widely in mineral profiles and require different amounts of calcium supplementation to support chick growth. In poultry, calcium-to-phosphorus ratios of 1.6–2.7 are needed for growth (Klasing 1999). Capelin has been found to be deficient in vitamin D compared to other fish as well (Hoopes and Clauss 2016). If skeletal maturation problems are seen in multiple chicks, reconsider supplementation regimens. Laboratory analysis of food composition may be informative if problems are persistent.

## Feeding Procedures

Dead fish should always be kept well-refrigerated or frozen until immediately before being fed out, and thawed–frozen fish should be fed within 24 hours of thawing. Uneaten fish in heated environments, such as presented for self-feeding in an incubator, should be changed frequently because hot temperatures encourage bacterial growth and spoilage. All chicks that are not yet self-feeding should be considered for twice daily, 5% body weight (50 ml/kg), pre-warmed, sterile, isotonic, subcutaneous fluid injections, which may be discontinued when the bird is eating well.

## Hatchlings

Hatchling birds should be offered small pieces of fish that have been soaked in water or electrolyte solution and sprinkled with powdered calcium. It is very important for the fish to be sliced diagonally, so that each sliver has two pointed ends. Young birds learn to navigate food in their mouths by instinctively finding "head" and "tail" ends of food items, and only diagonally-sliced fish slivers can substitute effectively for whole small fish. Hands should be disguised in a sock or puppet of appropriate appearance to discourage habituation to humans. Herons and egrets are less vulnerable to imprinting than many other species of birds, but they are capable of it, so it is always best to err on the side of caution. Avoid chicks seeing human hands associated with food. Birds should be offered food hourly throughout the day until they begin self-feeding.

The size of the fish pieces offered should correspond to the size of the hatchling. Small hatchlings should be offered small fish slivers, about the size of a 10 g smelt, sliced into four to six pieces. At the other end of the size spectrum, Great Blue Heron and Great Egret chicks can eat whole 10 g fish even at the hatchling stage. Snowy Egrets and the Black-crowned Night-Herons may be fed 5 g fish halves at the hatchling stage and, as nestlings, will progress quickly to whole fish.

Hatchling herons and egrets do not gape and must have their mouths opened in order to be fed. Often their mouths can be opened by the suggestive tap of a fish on the side of the beak. Weaker, less active individuals may need to be force-fed at first until they learn to respond to the sight of fish.

As they become aware of their surroundings, nestlings will look to the cage floor for food left for them by their parents. A food dish should therefore be left in the cage with young birds, to familiarize them with the appearance of the food presentation. At feeding time, every effort should be made to entice young birds to notice the fish dish that is in front of them and encourage them to self-feed. Fish slivers left in cages for free-feeding should be presented in dishes 0.5 in. (1 cm) deep, submerged in fresh water and covered with a light "snowfall" of calcium powder (Figure 17.4). Young herons and egrets may begin self-feeding at a remarkably early age, before their bodies are covered with down. Do not underestimate the amounts they can eat – Black-crowned Night-Herons in particular are voracious eaters that can eat their body weight per day in fish, distributed across several feedings.

## Nestlings and Fledglings

Partially and fully feathered herons and egrets should be able to self-feed. Nestlings can be introduced to self-feeding by having fish splashed in the dish in front of them (using a hemostat or puppet), and by having fish tapped on the side of their beak and then splash-dropped into the dish when they open their mouths for it. Fish dishes should be checked frequently and refilled when empty. There is no need to hesitate to graduate newly self-feeding birds to whole fish as soon as they will accept them.

It is important to perform follow-up checks of a birds' temperature if they ever appear sleepy or fluffed up. Self-feeding birds given a large meal of recently refrigerated fish may result in a drop in body temperature as the bird warms up the meal it has just consumed, thus potentially increasing the need for heat supplementation.

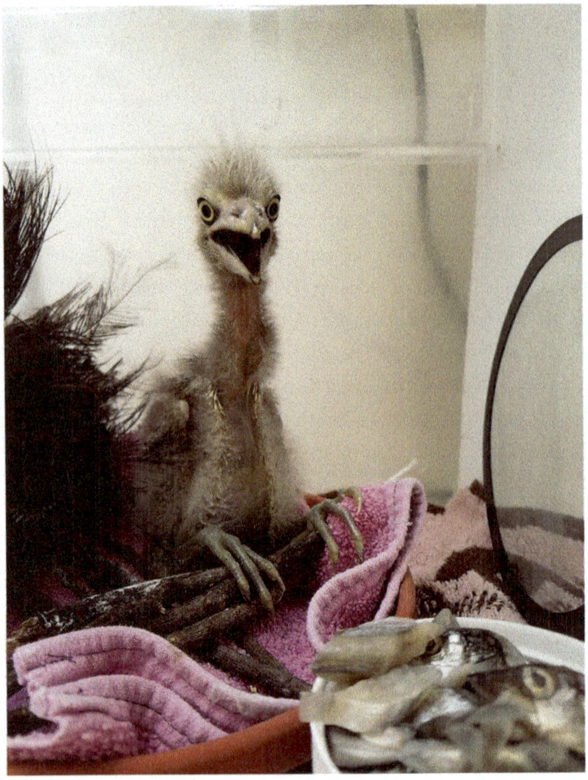

**Figure 17.4** Solitary Black-crowned Night-Heron chick in an animal intensive care unit, furnished with a clean feather duster and mirror for company, sticks for toes to grab, and diagonally sliced fish. *Source:* photo courtesy of International Bird Rescue.

## Expected Weight Gain

Birds should be weighed daily and weights recorded in each bird's record until eating reliably in each stage of housing. New additions to a group of chicks should be monitored closely to ensure they are finding the food and getting enough. Weight gains and losses within 10% of a bird's weight are normal on a daily basis, but any series of weight measures that shows a failure to increase as expected, or a trend toward decrease over two to three days, should be addressed directly. Hydration also needs to be monitored and addressed, especially in birds that require nutritional support. Weights should be measured first thing in the morning to reduce variation due to ingested food, because young herons and egrets may eat as much as 20% of their body weight in a single meal. Additionally, individuals at the same development stage, as measured by feather growth, may vary considerably in size. Males tend to be larger and heavier than females in many species.

## Expected Thermoregulation Progress

The development of thermoregulatory ability is the central benchmark in the hand-rearing of orphaned herons and egrets. They are extremely vulnerable to hypothermia throughout their first 8–12 days of life. Their normal body temperature is 103–106 °F (39.5–41.1 °C). It is not unusual for newly arrived hatchlings and fledglings to register significantly lower body temperatures prior to stabilization. For this reason, pre-warmed stabilization environments should be kept standing ready throughout the season.

Housing plans should allow for four main stages of thermoregulatory support:

- *Stage one:* 100 °F (37.8 °C) with 40–50% humidity environment for initial stabilization of hypothermic birds of all ages, and housing for hatchlings and young nestlings.
- *Stage two:* 85 °F (30 °C) environment for fledglings in early stages of feather growth.
- *Stage three:* 70–75 °F (21–24 °C) environment (ambient indoor temperature) for fledglings that are developing feather growth throughout their backs, axillary regions, sides, hocks, and chests.
- *Stage four:* Variable outdoor ambient environment for fledglings that have contour feathers covering their backs, axillary regions, sides, hocks, and chests.

Caging in the first three stages should have heating pads and heat lamps available as accessories that can be added and removed as needed to create transitional stages of thermal support within the basic stages. At every transition point, birds should be monitored closely to ensure that they are comfortable in their new heat environment. Cloacal temperatures should be taken daily while birds are housed in stage one and stage two environments. When moved to stage three, birds should be provided with a heating pad or heat lamp in one corner of the cage for the first day, and they should have their temperatures checked daily for the first 2 days in the new environment, or every day until stable. Behavior changes such as anorexia, hunching, and sitting quietly are all indicators of possible thermoregulatory distress. Any bird that exhibits these signs or has a body temperature below 102 °F (39 °C) should be regressed one step and reevaluated for progress in 24–48 hours.

After birds have demonstrated consistent thermoregulatory ability over 2–3 days at stage three, daily temperature checks can be discontinued, and thermoregulatory progress can be monitored visually on the basis of behavior changes. Warm birds will be alert, active, vocal, and self-feeding.

Before young birds are moved to variable outdoor ambient environments, they should have contour feather growth covering their axillary areas and backs. The axillae are the last part to become covered, and this is necessary to protect birds from ambient temperatures below 65 °F (18.3 °C). Birds raised in climates where it remains warm at night may be able to be housed outdoors without thermal support at younger ages.

At no point in time will young birds' abdomens become fully feathered. A fringe of powder down feathers will grow underneath coverts at the perimeters of the abdomen, but this area remains bare through adulthood.

## Housing

Whenever possible, young herons and egrets should be housed together in groups matched by developmental age and species. They are gregarious in hatchling and nestling stages and will be especially well-supported to develop self-feeding habits if housed in a casually competitive caging environment. Cages should be monitored for aggressive competition, and aggressive individuals should be moved in with birds of like demeanor.

For birds at the first stage of thermoregulatory support, appropriate housing may consist of an Animal Intensive Care Unit (Lyon Technologies). This is a clear acrylic box with a sliding front door and hinged roof (Figure 17.1). Its side-mounted electric powered heating unit is adjusted by an exterior control panel. It also has a removable water trough that keeps the environment hydrated and an automatic alarm that sounds if the temperature diverges from the level that has been set. Such incubators can be set to 100 °F (37.8 °C). Interior measurements of such units are typically 24 × 12 × 12 in. (61 × 30 × 30 cm).

Where such a pre-made device is not available, heat lamps and heating pads can be furnished in other forms of caging to create a 100 °F (37.8 °C) environment. In such cases, a thermometer should be placed inside the cage where it is easily visible from outside and monitored several times per day to check for temperature fluctuations.

Standard veterinary animal cages are well-suited for housing fledgling herons and egrets at stage two, and also at stage three when indoor flight caging is not available (Figure 17.5). Suggested cage sizes include interior measurements of 24 × 23 × 23 in. (61 × 59 × 59 cm) for up to three individuals of smaller species, or 43 × 23 × 36 in. (109 × 58 × 91 cm) for up to six individuals of smaller species. Cages should be furnished with branches to enable birds to practice grasping and balancing. Cage bottom inserts should be plastic-coated metal with no sharp edges and should easily allow droppings to fall through to the cage bottom below. Cage bottoms should be lined with newspaper or towels for easy cleaning. Cages should be cleaned daily and disinfected with an agent such as dilute bleach or accelerated hydrogen peroxide.

When possible, indoor flight housing should be provided to enable young birds to practice flying in advance of their thermoregulatory capacity allowing them to be moved outside. An example of indoor flight housing is a cage constructed of a wood plank frame with walls of canvas or tarpaulin, a net ceiling that allows maximum light and air exchange, and a hinged door of canvas or tarpaulin that has a small window cut in it covered with fishing net to allow for visual checks of the animals (Figure 17.6). A good size for such a cage is 6 × 6.5 × 7.5 ft. (1.5 × 2 × 2.25 m). Such caging can be built on wheels with no flooring, to be rolled over whatever area of floor is convenient for its location. Flooring can then be covered with one or two layers of sheets, newspapers, or towels for easy cleaning. Ample perches should be provided to allow every individual housed to perch up off the floor. Up to 10 individuals can be housed in such a box, depending on species size. Provide numerous perches of similar heights from the floor, as chicks may have dominance disputes over the highest perches. Swinging branches are a great perch option within housing that allows birds to practice balancing on unstable perches and navigating short distances between floors and perches.

Outdoor flight aviaries should be located in a shady area and provide ample free-hanging branches or other swinging perches of varying thicknesses to allow young herons and egrets to

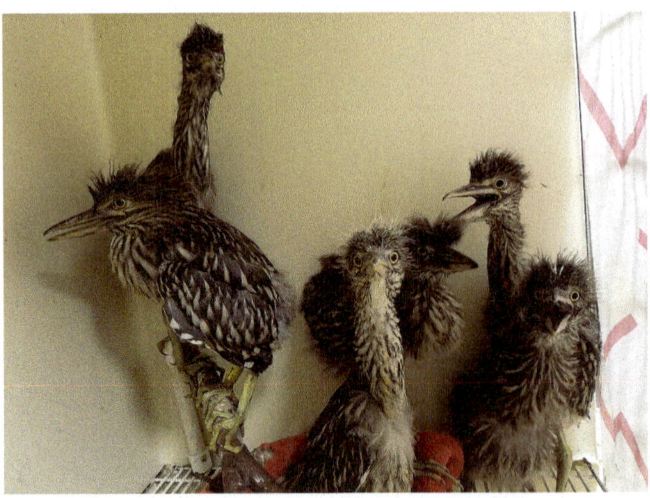

Figure 17.5 Black-crowned Night-heron chicks in a wall cage. Note stick perches, coated wire floor, and light-colored fabric covering the inside of the wire door. *Source:* Photo courtesy of International Bird Rescue.

practice perching, balancing, launching, and alighting from waving branches. One good size for an outdoor flight aviary for up to 20 birds, depending on species size, is 8×16×12 ft. (2.5×5×3.5 m). Flooring may be of deep gravel or removable rubber textured mats. Aviaries can be constructed of wood or aluminum frame, with hardware cloth or nylon fishnet walls and ceiling, with shade cloth, plywood boarding, or other screen type surrounding the lower 5 ft. (1.5 m) of wall area, to diminish animals' visual stress. Aviaries not situated in naturally shady locations should have shadecloth drapes over at least 50% of their ceiling area. It is essential that outdoor aviaries have hardware cloth flooring that is firmly attached to the walls at their bases. Otherwise, young birds may be exposed to tunneling predators.

In the pre-release aviary, young birds will be acclimating to outdoor ambient temperatures, developing their ability to balance on swaying branches, and learning to forage live food from the cage floor and in water (Figure 17.7). The most economical live food is ambiently available aquatic fauna gathered from the outdoor environment. These can be supplemented by mealworm beetles, live minnows or other feeder fish, frozen–thawed fish, pond bugs, and rodents.

Birds should be evaluated for release from the aviary on a regularly scheduled basis, usually once or twice per week. During the evaluation, it will become apparent which birds are strong, competent flyers, skilled at balancing on swaying branches, and extremely alert and active. New arrivals

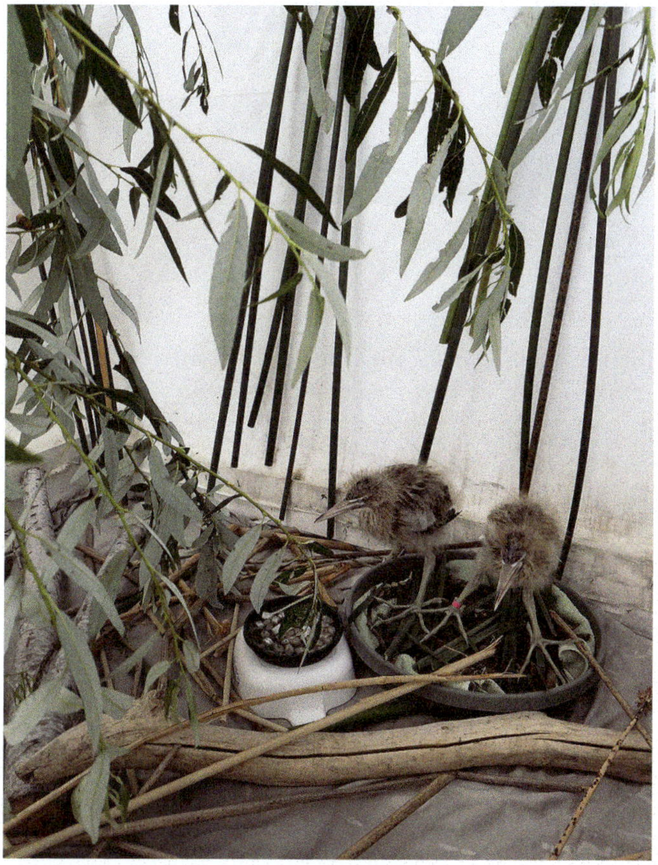

Figure 17.6 Large indoor cage setup for American Bittern chicks with a nest area and vegetation for privacy. *Source:* photo courtesy of International Bird Rescue.

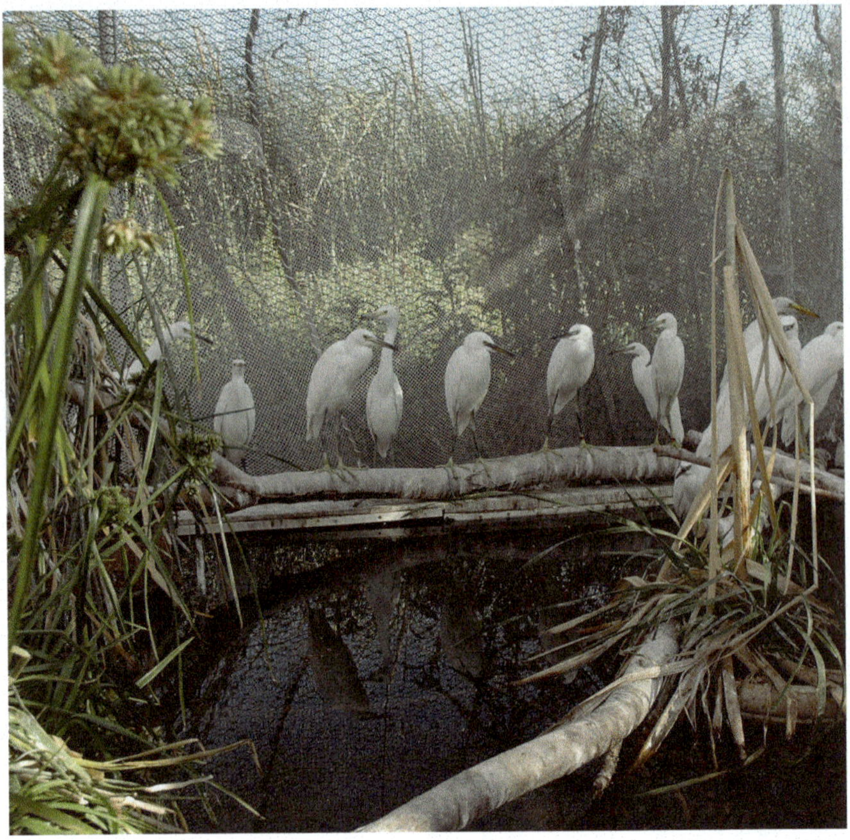

Figure 17.7 Snowy Egrets in an aviary with vegetation and a shallow pool. *Source:* photo courtesy of International Bird Rescue.

will contrast with releasable birds by their relative clumsiness and uncertainty in the flight aviary environment. Be aware that these species can be somewhat fragile during capture. When managing large numbers of these chicks, it may be less disruptive to quickly capture the whole aviary for evaluations, rather than searching for specific individuals while frightening all the birds. Release candidates should be organized in groups of three or more, due to these species' gregarious nature. Young herons and egrets can be soft released into a semi-supported environment where food is provided to them for a brief transitional period, usually 1 to 2 weeks. However, young herons and egrets are vulnerable to habituation and certain individuals may become dependent on caregiver foods and fail to transition to foraging on their own.

## Release

Most herons and egrets are not broadly migratory. Northern colonies may migrate south in the winter within North America; colonies in temperate regions may not migrate at all. Individuals do range over wide swaths of land and are not territorial. Great Blue Herons and Great Egrets are solitary as adults outside the breeding season, and young can be released singly. Smaller species are more gregarious and should be released in groups whenever possible. They can be released into any territory that is not already overcrowded with conspecifics, and where there is ample food available. The smaller the number of individuals to be released together on a given day, the more important it is to identify a release location where conspecifics are present to provide young birds with community upon release. Releases of most species are best done in the morning, and during clear weather, to allow young birds maximum daylight hours and weather advantages to orient themselves to their new environment.

## Acknowledgments

Thanks to Jay Holcomb, Michelle Bellizzi, Marie Travers, and Molly Horgan for contributing to the knowledge base on which this chapter is founded, and to International Bird Rescue's current and past staff and volunteers for caring for these birds.

## Sources for Products Mentioned

Incubators: Lyon Technologies, Inc., 1690 Brandywine Avenue, Chula Vista, CA 91911, (888) 596-6872.

Mazuri products: Mazuri, PMI Nutrition International, LLC, PO Box 66812, St. Louis, MO 63166, www.mazuri.com.

SeaTabs: Pacific Research Labs, Inc., 730 Saddlebrook Dr., Ramona, CA 92065, www.prlvitamins.com.

Vetrap and Tegaderm: 3M Corporate Headquarters, 3M Center, St. Paul, MN 55144-1000, (888) 364-3577.

## References

Duerr, R.S. (2017). Wading birds (herons, egrets, ibis, others). In: *Topics in Wildlife Medicine, Vol. 4: Orthopedics* (eds. R.S. Duerr and G.J. Purdin), 84–98. St. Cloud, MN: National Wildlife Rehabilitators Association.

Hawkins, M.G., Barron, H.W., Speer, B.L. et al. (2018). Birds. In: *Exotic Animal Formulary*, 5e (eds. J.W. Carpenter and C.J. Marion), 167–375. St. Louis, MO: Elsevier.

Hoopes, L.A. and Clauss, T. (2016). Investigation of a potential vitamin D deficiency in an African Penguin (Spheniscus demersus) collection. International Association for Aquatic Animal Medicine, Proceedings of the 47th Annual Conference, Virginia Beach, VA.

Hothem, R.L., Brussee, B.E., and Davis, W.E. Jr. (2010). Black-crowned night-heron (*Nycticorax nycticorax*), version 2.0. In: *The Birds of North America* (ed. A.F. Poole). Ithaca, NY, USA: Cornell Lab of Ornithology https://doi.org/10.2173/bna.74.

Kinsella, J.M. (2008). Avioserpensosis. In: *Parasitic Diseases of Wild Birds* (eds. C.T. Atkinson, N.J. Thomas and D.B. Hunter), 384–387. Ames, IA: Wiley-Blackwell.

Klasing, K. (1999). *Comparative Avian Nutrition*, 245. Cambridge, MA: CAB International.

McCrimmon, D.A. Jr., Ogden, J.C., and Bancroft, G.T. (2011). Great egret (*Ardea alba*), version 2.0. In: *The Birds of North America* (ed. A.F. Poole). Ithaca, NY, USA: Cornell Lab of Ornithology https://doi.org10.2173/bna.570.

Parsons, K.C. and Master, T.L. (2000). Snowy egret (*Egretta thula*), version 2.0. In: *The Birds of North America*. (eds. A.F. Poole and F.B. Gill). Ithaca, NY, USA: Cornell Lab of Ornithology https://doi.org/10.2173/bna.489.

Spalding, M.G. and Forrester, D.J. (2008). Eustrongylidosis. In: *Parasitic Diseases of Wild Birds* (eds. C.T. Atkinson, N.J. Thomas and D.B. Hunter), 289–315. Ames, IA: Wiley-Blackwell.

Vennesland, R.G. and Butler, R.W. (2011). Great blue heron (Ardea herodias), version 2.0. In: *The Birds of North America* (ed. A.F. Poole). Ithaca, NY, USA: Cornell Lab of Ornithology https://doi.org/10.2173/bna.25.

# 18

# Ibis

*Laurie Conrad*

## Natural History

Ibis are of the order Ciconiiformes, although discussions about reclassifying the order to Pelecaniformes have taken place. The Threskiornithidae family includes 28 species of ibis. All ibis have long legs and down-curved bills used for probing for food items (Ryder and Manry 1994). Many ibis species inhabit wetlands, marshes, and agricultural fields. They feed in large flocks and forage on a variety of insects, fish, and amphibians found in the soil. They also visually locate food items and pick them up from the surface of the water. Prey is swallowed whole after being tossed back into their throat. Other ibis live in arid, wooded areas and grasslands. The terrestrial ibis diet consists mainly of insects and other invertebrates, and small mammals and reptiles (Birdlife International 2016). Many ibis frequent grasslands and fields, but also live near inlets in many parts of the world

Population threats for the various ibis species vary. While some species have stable wild populations, others are listed as Least Concern by the International Union for Conservation of Nature (IUCN). The Association for Zoos and Aquariums (AZA) supports several species of ibis classified as endangered or critically endangered, including Cape and Madagascar Crested Ibis that face serious threats to their habitats and populations. The experience gained from husbandry of species held in zoological institutions can be transferred to conservation work with similar species with endangered status and sick or injured rescued birds from wild populations.

## Criteria for Intervention

Egg abandonment, nest disturbance, injury or illness, population management, or habitat disruption may necessitate artificial incubation or hand-rearing. New and Old-World ibis respond similarly to egg incubation, chick rearing diets, and housing guidelines. When hand-reared, chicks are fed formula, transitioned to solids, and weaned at 3–4 weeks of age.

## Record Keeping

Mark eggs with a number using a nontoxic Sharpie®. Record incubation start date, sire/dam identification, incubation parameters and fertility, and hatching information in an egg log or data sheet

*Hand-Rearing Birds*, Second Edition. Edited by Rebecca S. Duerr and Laurie J. Gage.

to track eggs for genetic management of the population. Band and weigh each chick and assign a number for identification if one was not acquired when an egg. Record egg data and chick identification and tie all future records to the chick identification number. Thorough record keeping is necessary to ensure each chick is progressing as expected and to track any interventions that are needed. Wild birds undergoing rehabilitation also need appropriate record keeping as required by regulatory agencies and to manage the progress of each chick.

## Initial Care and Stabilization

### Eggs

If parental incubation is interrupted or circumstances prevent parent-rearing, pull eggs directly from the nest to an incubator because parents begin incubation immediately when eggs are laid. Do not store eggs as part of the management of these species due to this natural reproductive behavior of the birds.

There are many ways to safely transport ibis eggs. One simple method requires transfer of eggs safely into a container filled with millet warmed to 99.0 °F (37.2 °C) to cushion the delicate eggs and keep them warm. Ensure that there are no hot spots in the millet. Continually monitor the temperature of the millet with a thermometer during transit. Weigh and candle eggs prior to transferring to an incubator. Candle eggs using a Marsh Farm's Hi-Intensity Candler, an LED flashlight, or a focused light source that does not put off heat to determine fertility and check eggs for damage. Confirm fertility and viability by looking at the developing vessels and embryo. Repair any cracks in eggs as needed. See Chapter 3 for more information.

Incubate eggs at 99.5 °F (37.5 °C) dry bulb, 80–82 °F (26.7–27.8 °C) wet bulb (WB) for White-faced Ibis (WFI) and 99.0 °F (37.2 °C) dry bulb, 84–86 °F (28.9–30.0 °C) WB for Scarlet, Bald, and Madagascar Crested Ibis. WFI (*Plegadis chihi*) incubation period ranges from 17 to 21 days (Ryder and Manry 1994). WFI eggs are smaller than the other ibis species mentioned. A percentage of WFI eggs incubated at the parameters used for other ibis species have hatched; however, hatchability improved and eggs hatched closer to the predicted hatch dates when dry bulb parameters were changed. Manually turn eggs 180° by hand, seven times a day rather than the more typical five times per day (SeaWorld CA, unpubl. data). Weigh and graph the results to monitor percent weight loss. Adjust the humidity in the incubator as needed to keep the eggs within a 10–15% egg weight loss range. Mark each egg with two arrows, each pointing opposite directions 180° apart from each other, to indicate the turning direction and prevent constant rotation in the same direction.

Egg turning stops once the chick pips through the exterior eggshell. At this time, move the chick to a hatcher such as a Grumbach Hatcher™. Decrease the dry temperature in the hatcher by 1 °F and increase the humidity for hatching. Place the hatching egg on a bar mat-lined (nonslip) tray with the air cell tilted slightly upwards during the 24–48 hours pip to hatch interval. Calculate the chick's time interval from pip to hatch.

### Hatchlings

Once the chick hatches; lower the temperature of the hatcher to 97 °F (36.1 °C) and reduce the humidity. Ibis chicks are semi-altricial and require attention after hatching. They hatch with their downy feathers matted to their skin (Figure 18.1). The newly hatched chick will appear wet but will dry with a fluffy appearance. Chicks have long skinny legs and may have a bald head. Swab the chick's umbilicus with a sterile povidone iodine swab. The umbilicus should be closed and appear clean. Inspect the eyes, legs, feet/toes, wings, and abdomen. The abdomen will appear distended or

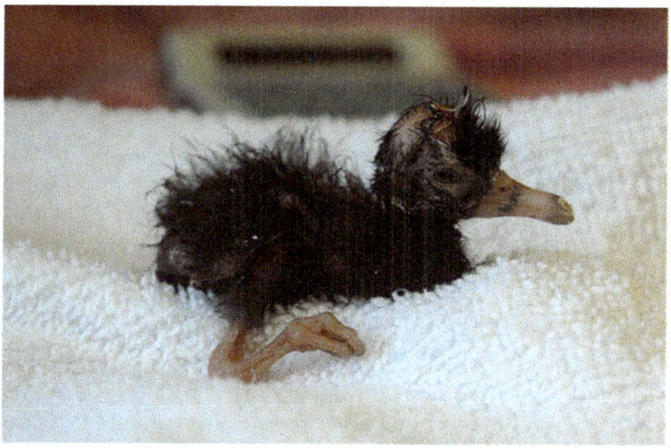

Figure 18.1 Hatchling White-faced Ibis (WFI) chick, still wet from hatching. *Source:* photo courtesy of International Bird Rescue.

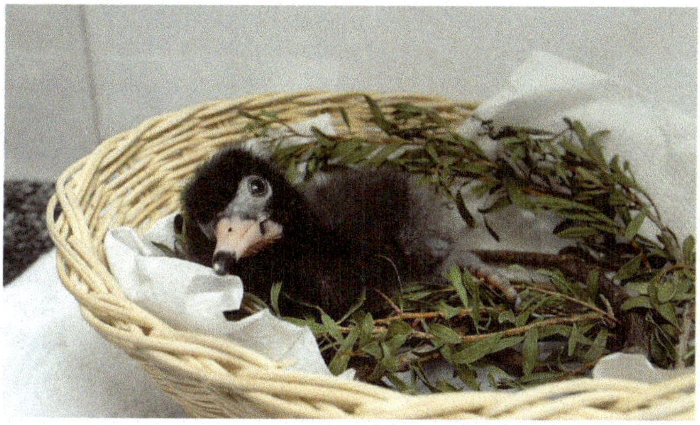

Figure 18.2 Ibis nest with sticks as substrate inside an Animal Intensive Care Unit (AICU).

rounded at hatch and will decrease as the chick uses the internal yolk after hatching. Many yolk sac infections are noticed up to a week after hatch and need quick medical attention. Seek veterinary care if the chick appears to be lethargic or if the umbilicus is open or discolored.

### Older Chicks

Chicks acquired at older ages may be injured and have medical issues that require treatment. As with all chicks of any species, initial care involves warmth, then hydration, then beginning a feeding plan (Figure 18.2).

## Common Medical Problems

### Hydration and Thermoregulation

Environmental conditions largely determine the hand-rearing outcome for ibis. Maintenance of normal hydration is important during the hand-rearing process and critical during the first 2 weeks of life. Thermoregulation is equally important. Maintaining a stable temperature within the brooder can be difficult if there are room temperature variations. Sometimes, overcorrection of temperature leads to overheating or chilling of the chick. Gradual corrections allow the chick to adjust, although the chick may shiver for a few minutes. The most common problem is overheating during the first 2 weeks of life. If the brooder is not holding a stable temperature prior to moving a chick in, check the room conditions and adjust any vents as needed. Brooders next to windows and doors may be subjected to fluctuations in temperature.

### Feces and Pathogens

Assess fecal output regularly. Expect to see the fecal color change during the first few days. Yellow colored feces after hatch are common as the chick is using its yolk. Fecal color may change to a dark green color as it transitions from the yolk to water to formula. The recommended diet in the chapter will produce light brown feces. Feces may look red or oily when krill in the diet is processed. Feces should be a quick "projectile squirt." If a chick is seen straining or produces thick and small droppings, skip the next schedule feeding and replace with oral water feedings until hydration is improved. Establishing hydration is more important than calories, which may mean missing a couple of scheduled feedings and substituting water feedings. Consult your veterinarian for a health assessment. Dehydration or GI upset may require subcutaneous fluids, antibiotics, or other treatment as determined by the veterinarian. If diarrhea or "smelly" feces are noticed, consult with a veterinarian immediately. Overheating, overfeeding, dehydration, or combinations thereof can lead to clostridium or other intestinal pathogen overgrowth. Separate ill chicks from healthy chicks.

### Feather Condition

Crowding can affect the condition of feathers. Birds that perch over one another and defecate on their cagemates can lead to poor feather grooming and waterproofing. Be aware of the placement of perching. There should be adequate space for each bird to roost on a horizontal perch without crowding. Substitution of diet items and lack of bathing areas also contributes to changes in feather condition. Remember that if oily fish such as salmon are substituted in the chick formula, the feces will contain more oil and this can lead to greasy appearing feathers. Ibis will wade in shallow pools and bathe and should have access to water area. The birds will also bring food items over to the water and "wash" their food. Keep the water source clean. When possible, allow the water surface to skim into a standpipe or a drain. If water can only be supplied in a small pool or tray, change often (two to three times daily). Providing a fine mist for the birds to bathe in will also help with grooming.

### Crooked Toes and Angel Wing

Adequate nest and habitat substrate are crucial for normal growth and development. Failure to provide the proper substrate in the nest may result in crooked toes or splayed legs. Carefully select and place sticks in the basket so that the chick is able to grasp the twigs. Select perching that provides a varied surface; avoid smooth branches. The initial perching should be relatively flat to the ground. Be aware of gaps in the branches where chicks could become stuck or injure a leg when learning to perch. Attach perches horizontally and allow chicks to perch without their feathers touching wire or walls. Raise the perches as chicks develop confidence and begin exploring larger areas.

Allow chicks to walk around their housing as soon as they are old enough to do so. Adequate space to exercise is needed for normal bone growth and feather development. Simply changing perching and substrate might be enough to correct crooked toes; however, toes can be taped into correct position if the problem is caught early and will straighten as they grow. If wings begin to turn outwards when the primary wing feathers are emerging, a figure-of-eight wrap may be used to correct the position by keeping the primary flight feathers folded underneath the secondaries. Be careful to apply any wraps so as to not disturb the growth of flight feathers. Check the wrap daily, and remove it every day or two to check whether or not the wrap is still needed. Consult with a veterinarian if growth abnormalities are noted.

### Imprinting and Habituation

Ibis imprint on humans and habituate to human presence easily, particularly when reared as single chicks. This should be stringently avoided if chicks are intended for wild release or captive breeding. Puppet-rearing and ghost-rearing (where the human form is disguised) minimize imprinting, and puppet-rearing is recommended for single chicks. Recordings of nature or wetland sounds help disguise ambient noise in the environment. Take care not to talk to or around chicks during the rearing process. Offering food without interacting with the chicks is recommended. Imprinting may not be recognized until the chick is nearly fledged and can be difficult to reverse; the best solution for imprinting is prevention. See Chapter 15 for more information on avoiding imprinting and habituation.

## Diets

In zoological situations, most ibis are fed dog food or an extruded feed, plus live insects, fresh frozen crustaceans and fish, and/or rodents and meat. Choose the protein source by researching the natural history of the species. Aquatic species should receive a higher proportion of fish or crustaceans and terrestrial ibis should receive animal protein such as neonate mice or geckos in addition to insect protein. Only offer items that are small enough to be easily swallowed whole.

Good nutrition begins with proper sanitation, food handling, and storage. Inspect all food upon receipt. Do not use any food items that appear freezer burnt, rotten, have peculiar odors, or that have not stayed within food handling guidelines. The freezing process breaks down tissues and makes fish and meat products more susceptible to bacterial growth after thawing. Do not air-thaw potentially hazardous foods. Thawing under running water can leach out soluble nutrients, hence this is a less desirable method. Once thawed, meat must be used within the next 24 hours. Discard all thawed and unused meat and fish products at the end of each day as thawed meat products are known to rapidly grow pathogenic bacteria (Crissey et al. 2001). *Salmonella* spp., *Staphylococcus aureus, Clostridium perfringens, Campylobacter jejuni, Clostridium botulinum, Listeria monocytogenes, Escherichia coli,* and *Yersinia enterocolitica* are pathogens that can be transmitted during food handling (Richter and al-Sheddy 1990). Thorough handwashing also reduces the risk of food contamination with other pathogens (Rehe 1990).

USDA cites a refrigerator temperature of less than 40–43 °F (4–6 °C) as optimal. Maintain meat stored for prolonged periods (up to 1 year) in a freezer with temperatures at −10 °F (−23 °C) or lower (Crissey et al. 2001). Separate all meat and fish products from fruit diets if in a shared refrigerator. Cover and date all food containers. Chick gruel can be made in large batches and stored in the freezer. Track all temperatures on a log sheet daily. Clean and disinfect food handling room and areas daily. Disinfect counters, utensils, or other contact surfaces after each use. Wash hands after handling potentially hazardous food items, birds, or used bird housing supplies.

## Ibis Hand-feeding Formula (SeaWorld, San Diego)

### Pre-soaked Dog Food

Thoroughly soak dog food in water for 8–12 hours beginning the evening before blending, refrigerate overnight.

- 50 g Purina ONE® Smart Blend Lamb and Rice
- 100 ml Water

### Mixing Formula

Make fresh formula every morning for use that day. Alternatively, freeze in ice cube trays and thaw prior to feeding. Blend the following ingredients well:

- 50 g Silversides (fish), heads, and. tails removed
- 250 mg Calcium from calcium carbonate (ground from 250 mg tablets)
- 50 mg Vitamin $B_1$ (thiamine)
- 150 g Purina ONE Smart Blend Lamb and Rice dog food, pre-soaked
- 200 ml Water

Strain formula after blending. Place formula in a closed container marked with the preparation date and time. Refrigerate the formula immediately. Warm the diet to body temperature using a warm-water bath prior to feeding and add a pinch of powdered vitamin $B_1$ to the formula immediately before feeding. Throw away excess formula after feeding; do not reheat.

This diet is appropriate for White-faced, Scarlet, Sacred, Madagascar Crested, and Cape Ibis, and is likely appropriate for additional ibis species. Research the natural history of each species to make adjustments based on the requirements of the species. Feed chicks a dog food (lamb and rice) based formula and then slowly transition to an adult diet (Table 18.1). Chicks may become impacted if they are fed exoskeletons (such as found in insects or crustaceans) too fast or in too high concentrations. Watch fecal output to ensure that digestion is appropriate and regular defecation is occurring. See Dierenfeld et al. (2002), Finke (2015), Chapter 41, and individual food supplier websites for nutritional information of diet ingredients.

## Feeding Procedures

### Hatchlings

A long pip-to-hatch interval may mean that a chick is ready for feedings earlier than a chick that has a short interval. Wait 12 hours after hatch before feeding water or food items. There may exceptions to this guideline based on chick activity. Table 18.2 shows feeding intervals, amounts, and details about housing by age.

Evaluate the chick and offer water at the end of the day if the pip-to-hatch interval was less than 12 hours. Begin the feeding schedule the following morning. Evaluate the chick's vitality, hydration, and fecal output prior to each feeding. Feed up to 10% of the chick's morning weight at each feeding. Always increase volumes in small increments

Chicks should be bright, alert, and vocal. Do not force-feed healthy chicks. Feed formula using a 1 cc syringe, with a feeding tube extension if needed (see Figure 6.1). A feeding response is elicited by holding a forefinger and middle finger over the chick's mouth in the shape of a "V" (Figure 18.3).

Table 18.1 Example ibis adult maintenance diets, per each bird per day.

| Terrestrial Ibis: Southern Bald (Cape) Ibis (*Geronticus calvus*) | |
|---|---|
| **Amount** | **Diet Items** |
| 1 ½ tsp. | Nebraska® Carnivore Feline Premium (shaped into balls) |
| 3/4 cup (180 ml) | Dog food, soaked |
| 4 | Neonate mice, whole |
| 1 | Mouse (cut into ¼s) |
| 2 | Whole smelt or capelin |
| 5 | Crickets |
| 5 | Mealworms |
| 1 | 50 mg thiamine tablet |
| 1 | 100 IU vitamin E every other day |
| **Aquatic Ibis: White-faced Ibis (WFI) (*Plegadis chihi*)** | |
| **Amount** | **Diet Items** |
| ¼ cup (60 ml) | Dog food, soaked |
| 1 cup (240 ml) | Mazuri Flamingo Complete, extruded pellet |
| ¼ cup (60 ml) | Krill |
| 2 | Silversides |
| 5 | Crickets |
| 5 | Mealworms |
| 1 | 50 mg thiamine tablet |
| 1 | 100 IU Vitamin E every other day |

Fingers may be wiggled, but care should be taken not to push the chick down. Allow the chick to stretch up to meet the feeder's hand as if the parent were placing its bill over the chick's mouth prior to regurgitating. Support the chick's head until it becomes strong enough to support itself. Initial feeding responses will be short in duration and chicks will initially tire easily during feedings. Feed in the brooder or set up a nearby counter supplemented by heat. Do not allow chicks to become chilled during feedings. Chicks may be housed together but may need to be separated during feedings if they are causing disruption while other chicks are fed.

Feed the 50 : 50 ratio of formula : water for five feedings before transitioning to 100% formula on day 1 of feeding. Feed 100% water if the chick hatched under the parents. Supplement water as needed between feedings and continue feeding dilute feedings until fecal output looks well hydrated. Ambient humidity and temperature combined with formula variations may increase the need for supplemental fluids.

Begin the transition from 50 : 50 to 100% formula on the second day of feeding. If the chick shows any sign of dehydration while transitioning to 100%, move to 75 : 25 formula : water until well-hydrated before trying to transition to full-strength formula. Do not ignore signs of dehydration – this is critical – if chicks refuse feedings, check the temperature and hydration of the chick, plus check for anything awry regarding housing or formula. The most common reason for a chick refusing to eat is dehydration.

Table 18.2 Feeding schedule by days of age for ibis chicks.

| Day of Age | Temperature, Housing, and Humidity | Feeding Frequency | Diet | Volume | Comments |
|---|---|---|---|---|---|
| 0 | 96–97 °F (35.6–36.1 °C) Hatcher, small bowl lined with tissue. | SID | Do not feed for 12–24 hours | 1–2 cc water if chick hatches in the afternoon. | Chick will dry off in hatcher and use yolk sac. |
| 1 | 95 °F (35 °C) in Animal Intensive Care Unit (AICU)<br>80–82 °F Wet bulb (WB).<br>Nest cup w/ Nomad matting or Excelsior.<br>Decrease temperature 1 °F every day. | Every 2.5 hours (6x/day) spread over 12 hours. Do not crowd feedings. | 50 : 50 Formula : water; Warm food via hot-water bath. | 10% AM body weight, fed with 1 cc syringe | Feed slowly – aspiration is a concern with this species. |
| 2 | 94 °F (34.4 °C)<br>80–82 °F WB.<br>In nest cup w/Nomad mat in AICU w/ water pan for extra humidity. | Every 2.5 hours (6x/day) spread over 12 hours. Do not crowd feedings. | 75 : 25 Formula : water;<br>Warm food via hot-water bath. | 10% a.m. body weight, fed with 1 cc syringe | Do not overheat chick – most common issue with new ibis hatches. |
| 3–4 | 92–93 °F (33.3–33.9 °C)<br>80–82 °F WB.<br>Add sticks to nest cup in AICU. | Every 3 hours (4x/day) | 100% formula Supplement 1–2 cc water in between feedings as needed | 10% a.m. body weight, fed with 1 cc syringe. Day 4 add 1 g of well-soaked dog food in addition to the formula at two (1st and 3rd) feedings. | Begin exposure to sun, no less than 15–30 min/ day (weather permitting). Check legs/toes daily. |
| 5–6 | 90–91 °F (32.2–32.8 °C).<br>Ambient humidity. | Every 3 hours (4x/day) | 100% formula Supplement water in between feedings as needed. | 10% a.m. body weight, plus 1–2 g soaked dog food and soaked Mazuri Flamingo Pellets, Day 4 raise to 4 g solids per meal. | Standing on hocks. If leg issues are noted, consult veterinarian immediately and check substrates of bird habitat. |
| 7–10 | 86–89 °F (30–31.7 °C)<br>Nest tub w/ sticks in entire brooder area.<br>Outside during the day, provide shade and supplemental heat – return inside at night each day. | Every 3 hours (4x/day) | Leave soaked food in a flat dish between feedings and encourage self-feeding with puppet.<br>Discontinue supplemental water feedings. | Feed 6–8 g of solids at each feeding in addition to formula (25% pellet, 25% krill, 50% neonate mouse). In aquatic species use a 50 : 50 ratio of pellet: krill. | Begin increasing solids and reducing formula once the chick begins to eat on its own. |

| | | | | | |
|---|---|---|---|---|---|
| 11–13 | 83–85 °F (28.3–29.4 °C). | Every 3 hours (4x/day) | Add silversides.<br>Sprinkle CaCo3 on food and add 25 mg $B_1$ daily SID. Offer water in a bowl. | Feed 15 cc formula at this point forward plus 9–10 g of solids at each feeding in addition to formula (25% pellet, 25% krill/silversides, 50% neonate mouse). | Watch for chick to refuse formula; feed solids ad lib when chick refuses. Watch weight, fecal output, and hydration. |
| 14–20 | 76–82 °F (24.4–27.8 °C). | Every 3 hours (4x/day) | Day 14 add 2 live crickets. Day 15 add quartered mouse (terrestrial spp. only). Day 16 add mealworms. | 15 cc formula plus solids 25% dog food and flamingo pellet, 25% fish/krill, 50% quartered mouse, 2 crickets, 5 mealworms. | Able to stand up completely for very brief periods by Day 18. |
| 21–30 | Ambient temperature during the day (70–80 °F) (21.1–26.7 °C).<br>Heat lamp off during day, on during night. In outside run, on mat (remove nest tub). | Every 3 hours (4x/day) | Consider not exceeding 15% wt gains | | Should be able to stay outside in temps 55 °F (12.8 °C) and above. |
| 31–36 | Floor pen with low branches on the floor for perching at night; heat.<br>Outside in brooder bin during the day with heat. | 2x/day | | Soaked dog food, mouse-halved, krill, 1 chopped capelin, 5 crickets, 5 mealworms per day – reduce krill for terrestrial species. | Starting to stand on feet, not just hock sitting. |
| 37–41 | Discontinue heat inside at night. | 2x/day | | Eliminate krill for terrestrial species. | |
| 42+ | Outside at night with heat, discontinue heat when fully feathered and thermoregulating. | 2x/day | | | Weigh weekly (can stop daily weights earlier if needed). |

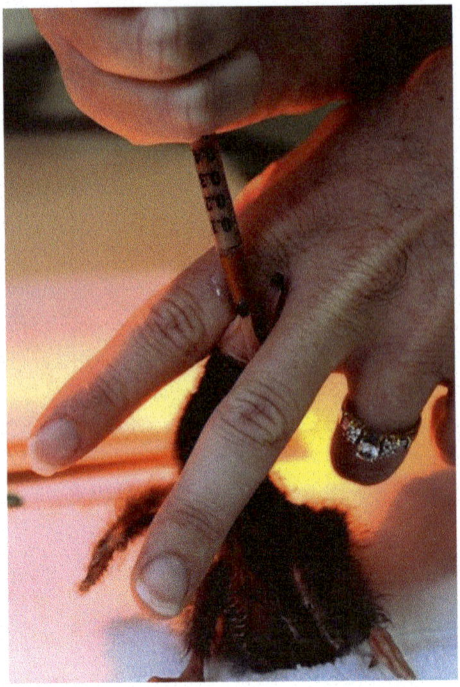

Figure 18.3 Two-day old Scarlet Ibis chick stretching up to eat during syringe-feeding.

On day 3 (or once the chick has transitioned to 100% formula for one full day of feeding), introduce solids at two feedings. The solids are fed in addition to the formula (10% of morning weight) in 1 g increments. Introduce easily-digested soaked dog food first by eliciting a feeding response and dropping half a piece of soaked dog kibble into the chick's up-stretched mouth. Dog food needs to be well-soaked or may lead to dehydration and will be more difficult to swallow. Supplement a few drops of water after feeding if needed. Gradually increase the size of the items as the chick develops. Eventually, an adult can swallow a whole mouse.

Continue to feed the chick 10% of its morning weight in formula and slowly increase the amount of solids as shown in Table 18.1. The chick should settle down (rest and stop begging) between feedings. Evaluate the amount fed and consider increasing the amount of solids if the chick constantly vocalizes in between feedings.

Leave solid food items in a small, flat dish once the chick is eating solids at each feeding. Add food items to the tray as they are introduced while hand-feeding. Change the dish at each feeding to ensure food items are always fresh. For example, if the chick is being hand-fed 5 g of a mix of soaked dog food, chopped krill, and soaked flamingo pellets, then leave those same items in a dish so that the chick is stimulated to begin to eat those same items independently. By day 10–12, ibis may eat 5–10% solids on their own in addition to 10% of body weight in formula.

Ibis should receive soaked extruded pellet feed diets plus animal and insect protein until they are eating independently. Adjust the animal protein so that it is consistent with the species' foraging habits in the wild. Aquatic ibis receive chopped fish and krill and terrestrial ibis feed consists of neonate mice in place of a percentage of the fish offered. Shed mealworms and crickets are added to both diets as insect protein. Introduce a commercial meat product such as Nebraska Brand Feline Carnivore Premium to terrestrial species diets once the chick is full sized. Flamingo-Fare and horse meat products are not recommended for young ibis chicks due to risks of impaction, and should only be introduced once the chicks have been self-feeding for some time.

The chick should move to four feedings a day by 8–10 days of age. Feed at regular intervals and continue to spread the feedings out evenly throughout a 12-hour day. Feeding during an 8-hour day is generally sufficient for chicks over 8–10 days of age. Continue to monitor the hydration and activity of the chick. The chick should begin to eat from the tray on its own. Encourage the chick to eat by holding the dish up to the chick and tapping on it with your finger. The chick will begin to refuse formula as the volume of solids increases. Once 15 cc of formula is reached (10% of the chick's morning weight), discontinue increasing the formula volume and increase solids only. At this stage, the chick will begin to refuse formula. Discontinue formula feedings if the chick is gaining weight and eating solids, but refusing formula. Chicks are usually eating solids independently by 3 weeks of age.

Self-feeding aquatic ibis intended for wild release may be offered natural prey items, such as krill, small or chopped fish, or invertebrates in narrow trays filled with mud or sand, or live small fish in shallow water trays, to simulate wild foraging (Figure 18.4). Terrestrial species should be offered foraging that closely mimics what the birds will need to do to feed themselves after release. Avoid chicks associating people with food at all ages, as human imprinted or habituated chicks will not be releasable.

## Nutrients of Concern for Fish and Meat Eaters

Very little research has been conducted specifically related to ibis nutritional requirements. Most nutritional studies used for current bird diet formulation are based on poultry, pet bird, and marine mammal and penguin research. The following recommendations are based on those, as well as zoological experiences, including the work conducted at SeaWorld California and personal communications with Elizabeth Koutsos, a nutritionist.

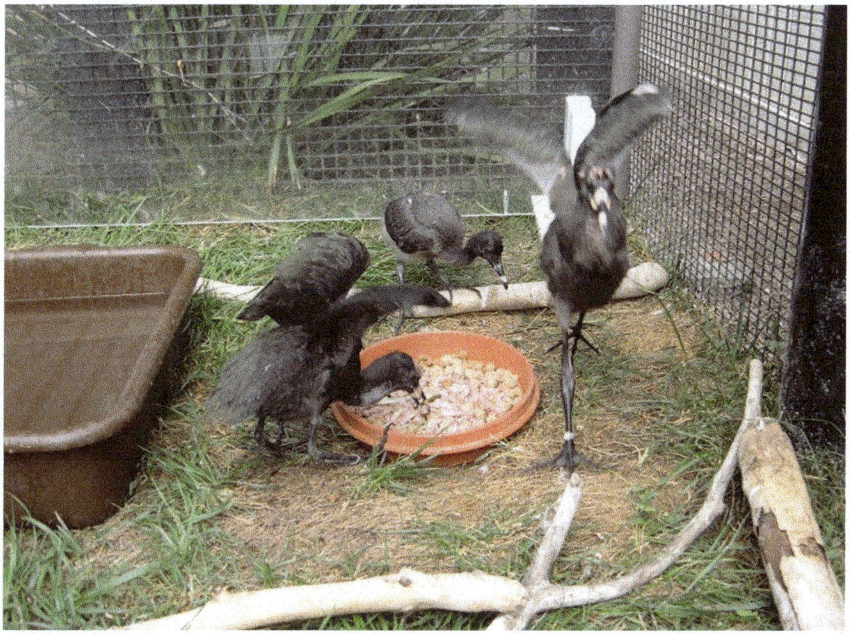

Figure 18.4 Ibis eating in a portion of outdoor housing setup.

Table 18.3 Recommended nutritional supplements for fish eaters.

| Nutrient | Indoors | Outdoor Exposure |
|---|---|---|
| Vitamin A | No supplement | No supplement |
| Vitamin E | 100 IU/kg of fish | 100 IU/kg of fish |
| Vitamin D | 15–20 min/day of sunlight or UV full-spectrum lights during daylight hours | No supplement |
| Thiamine | 25–35 mg/kg of fish | 25–35/kg of fish |
| Calcium | In chick formula | In chick formula |

Ibis are nomadic species that forage on a variety of animal and insects. A variety of protein sources are beneficial as a nutritional source because these sources vary in their fatty acid, vitamin, and carbohydrate contents. Nutritional values vary in feeder prey based on the age, species, and season caught, among other variables. For piscivorous feeders, the main nutrients of concern are vitamin E, vitamin B (thiamine), vitamin D, and calcium in growing chicks (Table 18.3).

Vitamin A is the most toxic of the fat-soluble vitamins and is already found in high concentrations in fish livers. Vitamin A levels are very high in some commercial nutritional supplements. Additionally, high doses of vitamin A have been shown to decrease vitamin E absorption in many species including humans and chickens, suggesting the need for vitamin interaction awareness. Birds ingesting whole fish probably do not need Vitamin A supplementation.

Vitamin E is of concern in fish-eaters and supplementation is recommended to prevent deficiencies. Vitamin E oxidizes easily (peroxidation) and may be lost prior to the thawing process (Bernard and Allen 1997); 100 IU vitamin E/kg of fish is recommended (Geraci 1972). Vitamin E deficiency may lead to electrolyte imbalances, irregular molts, steatitis, muscular degeneration, liver necrosis, or anemia (Geraci and St. Aubin 1980).

Thiamine ($B_1$) supplementation is critical in birds with diets largely composed of fish. The process of thawing fish in running water depletes the fish of water-soluble vitamins. In addition, many fish species contain thiaminase, an enzyme that destroys thiamine ($B_1$). Thiaminase is not destroyed by the freezing process and thiamine continues to break down while frozen. Thiamine is important for the nervous system and also for conversion of carbohydrates to glucose. Feeding a variety of fish and limiting the consumption of fish containing thiaminase prevents thiamine deficiency syndrome. Syndrome symptoms manifest in paralysis, anorexia, "star-gazing," or death. Star-gazing is often one of the first recognized symptoms. Take immediate action if neurological issues are noted. When recognized early, thiamine deficiency can be reversed with supplementation of $B_{1.}$ The recommended routine supplementation is 25–30 mg of thiamin per kg of fish (wet basis) (Bernard and Allen 1997).

Vitamin D supplementation is not usually needed for ibis with access to direct sunlight. Windows interfere with UV light and do not provide adequate intensity. It is recommended to provide a full-spectrum UVB artificial light source during daylight hours if ibis cannot be housed with natural lighting.

Calcium concentrations in whole fish and krill are typically 0.9–6.4% of dry matter, and may need supplementation as growing chicks need a calcium to phosphorus ratio of 2 : 1 to support rapid skeletal growth (Klasing 1998). The concentrations of calcium, phosphorus, and vitamin D in dietary items and the calcium : phosphorus ratio can negatively affect metabolism when out of balance (Bernard and Allen 1997). Ibis likely need calcium supplementation during growth stages.

Mealworms and crickets are nutritionally beneficial additions to faunivore diets, particularly when they are enhanced through gut-loading or sprinkling with calcium (Finke 2015; also see Chapter 41). The calcium level in crickets, mealworms, and waxworms is low compared to higher phosphorous levels, indicating that the insects need to be supplemented with calcium to maintain balance. Vitamin A levels are typically below recommended levels for poultry. Vitamin D levels also fall below recommended levels, but Vitamin D can be addressed through full-spectrum UV lighting or access to sunlight. Commercial diets for feeder insects are readily available. An alternative is to provide a commercial poultry starter diet sprinkled with calcium carbonate in a shallow dish or to use it as a substrate. Sliced apples provide moisture for mealworms. Provide crickets with access to a shallow water dish. Provide pebbles or another substrate to prevent drowning as needed. Waxworms do not need to be fed; store at 55–60 °F. Store mealworms and crickets at room temperature in a container covered with a screen.

## Expected Weight Gain

Chicks should gain weight daily until they reach their adult weight at 6–8 weeks of age. Weight gains of four species of ibis chicks are shown in Figure 18.5. Incomplete data are shown for White-faced and Scarlet Ibis; these species adult weights are typically in the 550–700 g range (Dunning 2018).

## Housing

### Brooder

Many zoos use commercial brooders such as the Animal Intensive Care Unit (AICU) (Lyons Technology, Inc.), which was developed specifically to maintain stable temperature and humidity; it is also easy to clean (Figure 18.6). Set the AICU temperature to 95 °F (35 °C) and monitor for

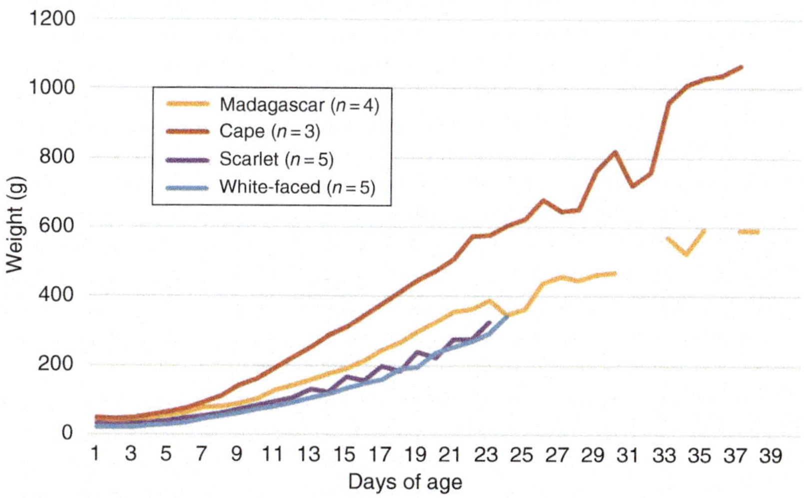


**Figure 18.5** Growth of four species of ibis chicks.

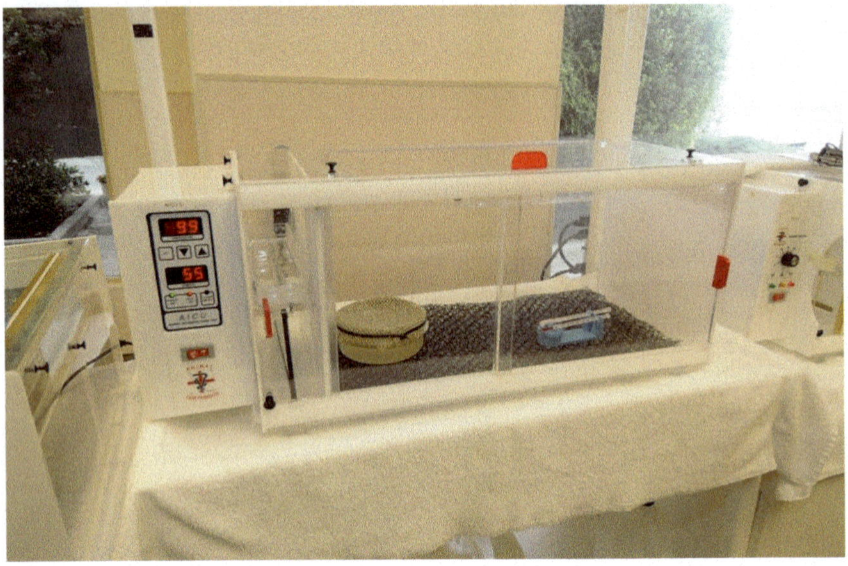


Figure 18.6 Animal Intensive Care Unit (AICU) set up for chick.

several days to ensure temperature stability before the chick hatches. Adjust the AICU down by a degree each day and as indicated by the chick's behavior.

When access to an AICU is limited, a 60-quart (57-l) polypropylene container with a heat lamp can function as a brooder. Attach a heat lamp to a stable and fixed location. Secure the heat lamp so that cords are not touching the lamp. Do not direct the lamp closer than 3 ft. (0.9 m) to chicks or other surfaces so that chicks are not burned or overheated. Monitor the temperature at the level of the chicks to guide placement of the heat source. Stabilize the temperature in a brooder for at least several hours before putting a chick into an area with a newly installed heat lamp. Gradually reduce the heat supplemented to the brooder each day by moving the heat source away from the chick.

Place the chick in a small plastic tissue-lined bowl at hatch. Cover the chick with a small, tented piece of material to simulate parental brooding for the first few days. On day 2, line the bowl with tissue and place natural excelsior (wood shavings) or a piece of Nomad™ matting (3M) cut to fit in the bottom of the bowl over the tissue. By day 3, small sticks replace the mat in the bottom of the basket. Ibis are open nesters. Use pliable, nontoxic branches to create an artificial nest by bending and weaving branches into a circle. Provide small diameter branches so that the chick is able to grasp onto the nest. It is important to wedge the branches into the nest so that they do not roll. Do not remove all of the leaves from the branches to fill the gaps in the branches. Change and clean the nest bowl at every feeding. Continue to use twigs as the chick develops; graduate to larger sticks to increase the perching diameter (Figure 18.7). These grabbable substrates allow for proper toe and foot development. Supply a nest until the chick begins walking around the brooder. Line the brooder with bar mat or shelf liner atop a clean towel free of holes or frays. Ibis chicks are easily tangled in loose threads; thus, it is important to check towels daily.

Clutchmates or chicks of similar size can be housed together. Chicks are not usually aggressive and will stimulate each other to eat independently as they mature. Monitor the environment and feces carefully. Excessive vocalizations or movement may be an indication of a chick in distress. Monitor and maintain stable brooder temperatures. Feather dusters may pose a risk of entanglement when used as a "brooder buddy," stuffed animals may provide safer companionship when housing solitary chicks.

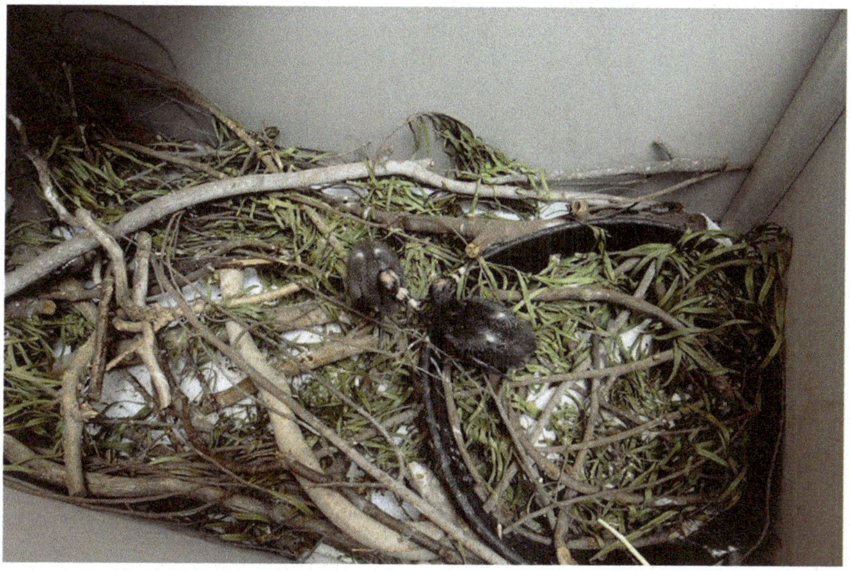

Figure 18.7 Open bin with room to walk around and learn to perch.

## Brooder Bin

At 7–8 days of age, transfer the chick to a larger bin set up in a similar fashion as the brooder. Provide supplemental heat so that the chick's housing temperature is not lowered more than a couple of degrees. A 42×42×22 in. high (107×107×56 cm) brooder provides additional space that encourages the chick to move around, which is important for leg and foot development (Figure 18.8). The chick will begin to grow in flight feathers so the bin needs a cover, such as a PVC or wooden frame with netting stretched across the bin perimeter, which allows air circulation and light. Expose the chick to indirect sunlight outside for several hours during the day. Providing separate outdoor housing simplifies care requirements and the chick can be transferred outside while housing is cleaned indoors. Monitor the temperature of the chick and provide heat or shade to match the temperature outside to that of the inside housing. Clean and disinfect all housing daily. Ibis food invariably attracts ants – one method to ant proof brooders is to use raised bins with water pans under each leg. Change the water frequently as evaporation or accumulated dust or debris may quickly allow ant access.

## Outdoor Housing

Each housing transition should be gradual so that sudden temperature extremes are avoided. Do not house juveniles out in open pens overnight until they are thermoregulating and have reached adult weight, usually at about 3 months of age. Feather condition and waterproofing should be assessed and deemed sufficient for thermoregulation without supplemental heat. Housing must provide shade, heat, food, and water as required by each species.

Aviaries for ibis intended for wild release should provide adequate space for flight practice and exercise, naturalistic foraging opportunities, and protection from local predators. Miller (2012), which provides guidelines for housing birds undergoing wildlife rehabilitation and is an accepted standard by many regulatory agencies in the U.S., suggests an aviary a minimum of 10×25×10 ft. (3×7.6×3 m) high with a wading pool 5–6 ft. (1.5–2 m) in diameter and 6–10 in. (15–25 cm) deep. Water in pools must be maintained with excellent water quality to avoid adversely impacting birds' waterproofing.

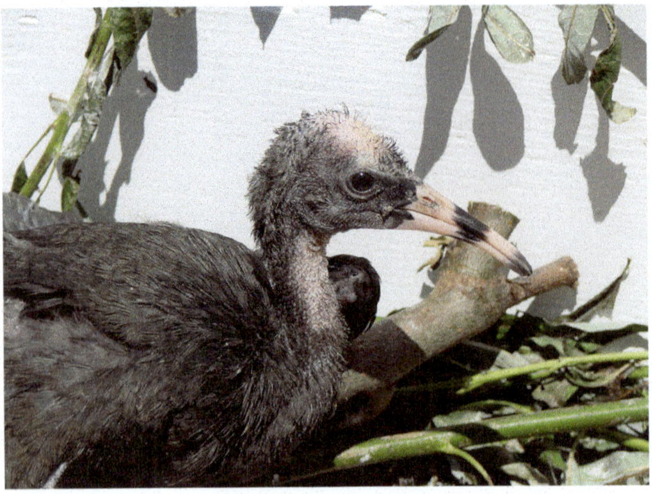

Figure 18.8 White-faced Ibis (WFI) chick in indoor housing that allows movement and exposure to natural substrates. *Source:* photo courtesy of International Bird Rescue.

## Preparation for Release and Release Criteria

Ibis should not be directly interacted with other than during routine health checks once self-feeding. All supplemental heat should be discontinued for several weeks prior to release. Once chicks are living outside and eating independently, they should maintain weight and be within the species norm. Ibis have a prominent keel and may feel thin subjectively, but should have palpable muscle mass on each side of the keel. Ibis propagated or rescued with the intent to release into wild habitats should meet established release criteria for the species, such as flight feathers fully grown in, plumage in good condition and waterproof, behavior appropriately wary of people, and blood parameters within normal limits. Birds should be healthy and free of injury prior to release. Birds with poor waterproofing should not be released without addressing plumage issues. Birds should be able to fly and demonstrate the ability to forage and feed unassisted and without soliciting caregivers for food by begging as a chick would to its parents. Ibis should have reached their asymptotic weight and then lost weight as they fledged. As colonial birds, they may learn additional behaviors, such as predator avoidance and breeding behaviors, from adult birds in wild colonies. Release ibis into appropriate habitat with established colonies or in the vicinity of other ibis when possible.

Many American AZA accredited institutions support field conservation programs related to species recovery and have established guidelines or taxon advisory groups eager to share information and experiences regarding this complex aspect of propagation (Association of Zoos and Aquariums (AZA®) 2018).

## Acknowledgments

Thank you to Christine Simeone, Linda Henry, Stephanie Costelow, Wendy A. Turner, Hannah Bailey, Christopher Holmes, and Susie Kasielke for their insights into hand-rearing birds. Thank you to Elizabeth Koutsos for sharing her knowledge about nutrition in fish-eating birds. Thank you to Justin Brackett for compiling weight loss data. Thank you also to SeaWorld San Diego for sharing unpublished hand-rearing data. Last, but not least, thank you to my SeaWorld editor, Dr. Judy St. Leger.

## Sources of Products Listed

Animal Intensive Care Unit™ and Grumbach Hatcher: Lyon Technologies, Inc., 1690 Brandywine Avenue, Chula Vista, CA. 91 911, (619) 216-3400, https://lyonvet.com.

Feeder insects: Grubco, 7995 North Gilmore Rd., Fairfield, OH 45014, (800) 222-3563, www.grubco.com.

Frozen feeder rodents: Layne Laboratories, Inc. (805) 474-1354, www.Laynelabs.com.

Frozen fish and krill: McRoberts Sales Co.®, Inc. PO Box 489, Ruskin, FL 33575, (813) 645-2561, http://www.mcrobertssales.com.

Flamingo Maintenance # 5572 Mazuri®, Mazuri, PMI Nutrition International, LLC, PO Box 66 812, St. Louis, MO 63166, (800) 227-8941, www.mazuri.com.

Nebraska Brand Premium Feline Carnivore®: Central Nebraska Packing, Inc. PO Box 550, 2800 East 8th Street, North Platte, NE 69103-0550 1 800 445 2881.

3M™ Nomad Unbacked Scraper Matting 8100 Unbacked: 3M, St. Paul, MN, (800) 628--7462, https://www.3m.com/3M/en_US/company-us/all-3m-products.

Purina ONE Smart Blend Lamb and Rice dog food: Nestlé Purina PetCare Company, 1 Checkerboard Square, St. Louis, MO 63164, https://www.purinaone.com/dogs.

## References


Association of Zoos and Aquariums (AZA®). (2018). Field Conservation. http://www.aza.org/field-conservation (accessed 13 January 2019).

Bernard, J.B. and Allen, M.E. (1997). *Feeding Captive Piscivorous Animals: Nutritional Aspects of Fish as Food*. Nutrition Advisory Group Handbook Fact Sheet 005. Brookfield Zoo, Brookfield, IL: Chicago Zoological Society.

BirdLife International. (2016). Geronticus calvus. The IUCN Red List of Threatened Species 2016: e. T22697496A93617026 (accessed 13 January 2019).

Crissey, S.D., Slifka, K.A., Shumway, P., and Spencer, S.B. (2001). Handling Frozen/Thawed Meat and Prey Items Fed to Captive Exotic Animals: A Manual of Standard Operating Procedures. U.S. Department of Agriculture, Agricultural Research Service, National Agricultural Library.

Dierenfeld, E.S., Alcom, H.L., and Jacobson, K.L. (2002). Nutrient Composition of Whole Vertebrate Prey. http://wildpro.twycrosszoo.org/000ADOBES/Bears/D317WholePreyFinal02May29.pdf (accessed 13 January 2019).

Dunning, J.B. (2018). *Body Masses of North American Birds* (ed. M. Ghadrdan), 117 pp. Eugene, OR: The International Wildlife Rehabilitation Council.

Finke, M.D. (2015). *Complete nutrient content of four species of commercially available feeder insects fed enhanced diets during growth. Zoo Biology* 34: 554–564.

Geraci, J.R. (1972). Experimental thiamine deficiency in captive harp seals, *Phoca groenlandica*, induced by eating herring, *Clupea harengus*, and smelts, *Osmerus mordax. Canadian Journal of Zoology* 50: 179–195.

Geraci, J.R. and St. Aubin, D.J. (1980). Nutritional disorders of captive fish-eating animals. In: *The Comparative Pathology of Zoo Animals* (eds. R.J. Montali and G. Migaki), 41–49. Washington DC: Smithsonian National Press.

Klasing, K. (1998). *Comparative Avian Nutrition*, 352 pp. Cambridge, MA: CAB International.

Miller, E.A. (2012). *Minimum Standards for Wildlife Rehabilitation*, 4e. St. Cloud, MN: National Wildlife Rehabilitators Association.

Rehe, S. (1990). Preventing food-borne illness, a guide to safe food handling. *U.S. Department of Agriculture, Home and Garden Bulletin No. 247.*

Richter, E.R. and al-Sheddy, I. (1990). Microbiological quality and safety of zoo food. *Applied and Environmental Microbiology* 56: 877–880.

Ryder, R.A. and Manry, D.E. (1994). White-faced Ibis (*Plegadis chihi*) version 2.0. In: *The Birds of North America* (eds. A.F. Poole and F.B. Gill). Ithaca, NY, USA: Cornell Lab of Ornithology https://doi.org/10.2173/bna.130.

## Further Reading

Allen, M.E., Baer, D.J., and Bernard, J.B. (1989). Fat-soluble vitamin concentrations in fish commonly fed to zoo animals. Proceedings of the American Association of Zoo Veterinarians, Greensboro, NC, p. 104.

# 19

# Vultures

*Susie Kasielke*

## Natural History

The Old World vultures are classified in the family Accipitridae, now in the order Accipitriformes, while the New World vultures are classified in the family Cathartidae, now in the order Cathartiformes (Table 19.1). Both families were formerly included in the order Falconiformes but have recently been reclassified based on genetic and morphological characteristics (Gill and Donsker 2019). Their natural history strategies are the result of convergent evolution as the families are not closely related.

Both Cathartid and Accipitrid vultures are obligate scavengers, spending much of their time soaring at great heights to watch for activity on the ground that might indicate a feeding opportunity. They often feed together in large numbers in a guild of avian scavengers that may include other vultures, eagles, storks, and/or corvids. They also compete with mammalian scavengers such as coyote, jackal, fox, hyena, and bear. Their foraging strategy relies on a high degree of learned behavior, with young birds remaining with their parents for a year or more as they absorb the foraging traditions of the population.

These large vultures are long-lived, with both species of condor as well as the King Vulture often living more than 50 years in captivity. Andean Condors have been recorded to have lived as long as 70 years and males have produced offspring as late as 50 years. For both families, age-related disease and reproductive senescence have been documented infrequently and primarily in birds taken from the wild at unknown ages.

In Cathartid vultures, males are slightly larger than females and all but the Andean Condor are essentially monomorphic, although there are subtle differences in adult coloration between genders. All are primarily cliff nesting, utilizing sheltered ledges and caves, or occasionally open hollows in large trees, with no added nest material.

The California Condor is critically endangered due largely to habitat loss and lead poisoning. Thanks to captive propagation and other intensive management efforts, there are now over 500 birds, more than half living in the wild with many pairs breeding. The Andean Condor is listed as near-threatened. Detailed census data are lacking, but the population continues to decline due to multiple factors including human persecution. The remaining Cathartid species are currently listed as least concern for conservation.

As with all Accipitriformes species, female Accipitrid vultures are somewhat larger than males. All species are otherwise monomorphic and all build large stick nests, either on cliffs and ledges or

*Hand-Rearing Birds*, Second Edition. Edited by Rebecca S. Duerr and Laurie J. Gage.

Table 19.1 Vulture species.

| Species | Conservation status (IUCN Red List) | Adult weight (g) | Clutch size | Incubation period, days | Fledging age, days |
|---|---|---|---|---|---|
| **Cathartidae** | | | | | |
| California Condor, *Gymnogyps californianus* | Critically endangered | 8000–11 500 | 1 | 57 ± 1 | 165–180 |
| Andean Condor, *Vultur gryphus* | Near threatened | 8000–15 000 | 1 | 60 ± 2 | 180–210 |
| King Vulture, *Sarcoramphus papa* | Least concern | 3000–4500 | 1 | 55 ± 1 | 120–150 |
| Black Vulture, *Coragyps atratus* | Least concern | 1100–1200 | 2 | 42 ± 3 | ~90 |
| Turkey Vulture, *Cathartes aura* | Least concern | 850–2000 | 2 | 40 ± 1 | ~90 |
| Greater Yellow-headed Vulture, *Cathartes melambrotus* | Least concern | | | | |
| Lesser Yellow-headed Vulture, *Cathartes burrovianus* | Least concern | | | | |
| **Accipitridae** | | | | | |
| Griffon Vulture, *Gyps fulvus* | Least concern | 6000–10 000 | 1 | 56 ± 2 | 120–135 |
| White-backed Vulture, *Gyps africanus* | Critically endangered | 4150–7200 | 1 | 54 ± 1 | 120–135 |
| Rüppell's Vulture, *Gyps rueppelli* | Critically endangered | 6800–9000 | 1 | 55 ± 1 | 120–135 |
| Cape Vulture, *Gyps coprotheres* | Endangered | 7070–10 900 | 1 | 55 ± 1 | 135–165 |
| Himalayan Vulture, *Gyps himalayensis* | Near threatened | 8000–12 000 | 1 | 55 ± 1 | 150–180 |
| White-rumped Vulture, *Gyps bengalensis* | Critically endangered | 3500–6000 | 1 | ~55 ± 2 | ~120–135 |
| Indian Vulture, *Gyps indicus* | Critically endangered | 5500–6300 | 1 | ~55 ± 2 | ~120–135 |
| Slender-billed Vulture, *Gyps tenuirostris* | Critically endangered | ~4500 | 1 | ~55 ± 2 | ~120–135 |
| Red-headed Vulture, *Sarcogyps calvus* | Critically endangered | 3600–5400 | 1 | 45 ± 2 | unknown |
| Cinereous Vulture, *Aegypius monachus* | Near threatened | 7000–11 500 | 1 | 55 ± 1 | 120–135 |
| Egyptian Vulture, *Neophron percnopterus* | Endangered | 1600–2400 | 1–3 | 42 ± 3 | 75–90 |
| Bearded Vulture, *Gypaetus barbatus* | Near threatened | 4500–7100 | 1–2 | 54 ± 2 | 135–165 |
| Lappet-faced Vulture, *Torgos tracheliotos* | Endangered | 5400–9400 | 1 | 55 ± 1 | 120–135 |
| White-headed Vulture, *Trigonoceps occipitalis* | Critically endangered | 3300–5300 | 1 | 54 ± 2 | 135–150 |
| Hooded Vulture, *Necrosyrtes monachus* | Critically endangered | 1500–2600 | 1 | 50 ± 3 | 90–135 |
| Palm-nut Vulture, *Gypohierax angolensis* | Least concern | 1200–1800 | 1 | 42 ± 3 | ≥120 |

in trees. Most cliff-nesting species nest colonially while pairs of tree-nesting species usually maintain individual territories, although some are loosely colonial.

Four Asian vulture species, the White-rumped, Indian, Slender-billed, and Red-headed are now critically endangered and the Egyptian Vulture is endangered. In South Asia, vultures feed largely on carcasses of cattle, many of which had been treated with the NSAID diclofenac, now known to be extremely toxic to vultures. Although veterinary use of this drug has been prohibited, it is still easily available as a human medicine drug and is very inexpensive. Nearly all other NSAIDs have proven to be similarly toxic. Vulture-safe zones that provide drug-free carcasses are helping to slow the decline and captive propagation of assurance populations of the three *Gyps* species is ongoing in India.

In Africa, four vulture species – the White-backed, Ruppell's, White-headed, and Hooded – have recently been classified as critically endangered and three – the Cape, Lappet-faced, and Egyptian – as endangered. This precipitous decline has been primarily due to widespread direct poisoning by poachers. Collisions with power lines and ritual use of vulture parts are contributing to the decline.

Although protocols in this chapter are based on experience with California and Andean Condors, King Vultures and *Gyps* vultures specifically, the methods described should work equally well with other vulture species with adjustments for incubation and rearing periods and proportionate feeding and weight gain amounts. See Chapter 20 for more information specific to hand-rearing American Black and Turkey Vultures.

## Criteria for Intervention

Eggs or chicks that are neglected or compromised and cannot be returned to the parents – whether due to poor parenting, interference by enclosure mates, accident, or weather extremes – are candidates for hand-rearing. It is generally not advisable to hand-rear vultures to produce handleable animals for educational programs as these birds invariably become quite aggressive when they reach sexual maturity, greatly limiting their usefulness and diminishing their breeding potential. Whether the choice to hand-rear is intentional or as a result of rescue, use of the strict isolation rearing methods described below will prevent malimprinting on humans and produce behaviorally healthy adults.

Determining that an egg or chick requires intervention is usually straightforward, but the need for this can often be avoided through good husbandry and subtle management techniques. If given an appropriate, private nesting area, most vultures will prove to be excellent parents. Even so, it may be desirable to artificially hatch and rear chicks, allowing multiple clutching to increase production, as in the case of endangered species being reared for release to the wild. Occasionally, parent birds are not able to care for the egg or chick. This is more often the case with inexperienced, young parent birds and those that were hand-reared without adequate socialization with conspecifics. Individual birds, usually males, may be overly aggressive with their mates, despite proper rearing and experience. In any of these situations, birds may fail to incubate consistently or brood and feed chicks adequately. They may also fight over these duties, risking egg breakage or cannibalization of the chick. Tensions are highest and the risk of injury is greatest around the times of egg laying and chick hatching. Parent birds that feel they must defend their nest site will be more aggressive with each other in general and are more likely to break eggs or injure chicks.

A good nest box or platform design will allow close monitoring of eggs and chicks, through one-way glass or closed-circuit television, while ensuring a sense of privacy and security for the parents. Adults can be accustomed to feeding in a specific area at a specific time, ideally one in which they can be secured and that is out of view of the nest area, thereby allowing eggs and chicks to be checked directly without the parents' awareness of this activity. This can facilitate removing eggs and replacement with dummy eggs, fostering eggs or chicks to more reliable parents, monitoring eggs and chicks, and providing supportive care to chicks until parents can fully care for them. For example, these techniques allowed a male–male pair of Cape griffon vultures that had built and defended a nest to foster hatch and rear a chick. The chick was given supplemental feedings for 3 weeks before morning and evening weights demonstrated that the parents were feeding it adequately. After that, no further intervention was needed.

## Record Keeping

Detailed records are essential to ongoing improvement of rearing methods and future successes. Careful recording of quantitative data will facilitate later analysis. Key data can be captured easily with an efficient record-keeping system. Active records should be kept in the rearing area so that information is captured while it is fresh in one's mind. Recording data directly to the computer is most efficient and will facilitate later analyses.

Chicks are considered to be 0 days old on the day of hatch. Daily weights, diet and amounts consumed, feeding frequency, type of enclosure, enclosure mates (if any), and brooder temperature and humidity are the most essential data to record. Weights should be taken each morning before the first morning feeding. It is useful to record the percent gained each day and/or to track weights graphically. Diet ingredients, including supplements and size of pieces offered, should be noted and the actual amount consumed recorded. This may be complicated by the fact that water or other fluids are usually added, but solids and liquids offered should be weighed separately, both to guide others in the future and to allow nutritional analysis. After each feeding, the weight of any remaining food is subtracted from the total offered, giving the amount consumed. An alternative way to determine the amount consumed is to weigh the chick before and after each feeding. This second method is less easily done when isolation rearing methods are being used. The brooder temperature and humidity, or those of the room or chamber once the chick is no longer brooded, should be recorded at each feeding and when the chick is handled for other reasons, such as a veterinary check.

Other quantitative information recorded at each feeding includes an estimate of crop fullness (0–100%) before and after feeding, duration of feeding/puppeting session, and feeding response. A scale of 0–4 is used for the feeding response, with 0 defined as no feeding response and 4 as lunging eagerly and eating very quickly. Even if separate medical records exist elsewhere, including basic information about examination, treatment, and/or medication (including method of administration and acceptance) ensures that the chick-rearing record provides a complete picture.

In addition, narrative comments, especially detailed descriptions of behavior and developmental stages, as well as both successful and unsuccessful feeding and handling techniques, are particularly useful for future chick rearing and for training new staff. Comments should be more detailed than "looks good" or "ate well." Photo and video documentation of California Condor chicks at all stages of development is proving especially valuable for determining whether chicks being reared by condors in the wild are developing normally.

## Incubation of Eggs

California Condor eggs are incubated at 98.0 °F (36.7 °C). Humidity is set at 45–55% relative humidity (RH) to start. As with all artificially incubated eggs, eggs should be weighed on a regular schedule to monitor egg weight loss, adjusting incubator humidity to increase or decrease weight loss (see Chapter 3). Eggs from this species, particularly from older females, may have difficulty losing sufficient weight even in a dry incubator running at 30% RH or less. If left under the incubating parent for 7–14 days before being removed for artificial incubation, such eggs usually establish an appropriate weight loss trend that can be maintained in the incubator with sufficient care. Rarely, eggs that have not received parental incubation or otherwise do not lose sufficient weight may require drastic measures such as sanding or drilling a small hole in the shell over the air cell. In addition to machine turning every 2 hours, eggs are hand turned through ~180° twice daily in opposite directions to ensure optimal membrane development.

Signs the hatching process has begun may be observed on candling as early as day 49 but more typically on day 50–51 with the air cell beginning to draw down. Between this stage and the internal pip, the egg is transferred to a separate hatcher set at 97.5 °F (36.4 °C) and 50% RH and is no longer turned. It is important to use a soft but nonslip substrate, such as Grip Liner (Con-Tact®), to prevent abrasions and leg splaying after hatching. Internal pip usually occurs on day 53 and external pip on day 54. Once the egg is externally pipped, humidity is increased to 80% RH or more to prevent the shell membranes and extraembryonic membranes from drying out during the protracted hatching process. Hatching usually occurs on day 57. Healthy self-hatches have occurred in as little as 45 hours after external pip or as long as 96 hours. Condor eggs are easily candled, which facilitates frequent monitoring during the entire hatching process at intervals of 2–6 hours depending on the stage and progress of the egg. Chorioallantoic vessels can be seen gradually receding and yellowing. Unlike most bird species, California Condor embryos typically defecate in the shell shortly before hatching. The small amount of dark green feces may also be visible on candling and, along with absence of active vessels, is a good indicator that hatching should be imminent. The embryo will respond to tapping and vocalization as it would to the parent during this stage. This can encourage the embryo to make progress toward hatching. Embryos that do not make sufficient progress at this stage may require assistance.

Andean Condor eggs are also incubated at 98.0 °F (36.7 °C) and started at 45–55% RH; and hatched at 97.5 °F (36.4 °C) and ≥70% RH. Because this species has been reared at many different facilities, incubation temperatures of 97.5–99.5 °F (36.4–37.5 °C) have been used with success, but incubating at 98.0 °F (36.7 °C) gives the most consistently healthy hatches. Their incubation term is 60 days ±2 days with a similar pattern of internal pip 4 days prior to hatching and external pip 3 days prior. The incubation term for eggs from specific females is usually consistent from egg to egg. In other words, a female whose egg hatches at 59 days of incubation will likely have future eggs that hatch on day 59.

King Vulture eggs are incubated at 98.5 °F (36.9 °C) and started at 50–60% RH and hatched at 98.0 °F (36.7 °C) and ≥70% RH. Their incubation term is 55 days ±1 day with a similar pattern of internal pip 4 days prior to hatching and external pip 3 days prior. Both Andean Condor and King Vulture eggs are also easily candled.

Eggs of *Gyps* species, as well as those of other large Accipitrid vultures (Red-headed, Cinereous, Bearded, Lappet-faced, and White-headed), are incubated at 98.5 °F (36.9 °C) and started at 45–55% RH and hatched at 98.0 °F (36.7 °C) and ≥70% RH. Their incubation term is 54–56 days, depending on species, ±1 day, with a similar pattern of internal pip 4 days prior to hatching and external pip 3 days prior. Accipitrid vulture eggs, like all eggs from species in this family, are difficult to candle. *Gyps* vulture eggs are white-shelled and typically unmarked, so early embryonic development can be readily observed, although this will appear less distinct than in Cathartid eggs. By ¼–⅓ of incubation, the progression of the chorioallantoic membrane lining the inside of the shell will make the egg virtually opaque below the air cell. It is difficult to assess viability after this. One method, for eggs past mid-incubation, is to place the egg on a hard, flat surface, guarding it carefully to prevent rolling, and watch for movement. This may take up to 2 minutes. Another option is the use of a heartbeat monitor made for eggs, such as the Egg Buddy (Avitronics). A negative result from either of these tests cannot confirm mortality, so eggs should be left in the incubator at least to full term unless obvious signs of death are present. Lastly, eggs of any species can be radiographed to confirm a full-term embryo and determine whether it is in the correct hatching position (see Chapter 3).

There is limited information available on successful artificial incubation of eggs of smaller vulture species (American Black, Turkey, Egyptian, Hooded, and Palm-nut). Their incubation period is 40–42 days, ±1 day. Based on successful guidelines for all species based on egg size and incubation period, an incubation temperature of 99.0 °F (37.2 °C) and initial humidity of 45–55% RH should work well for these species.

Andean Condor and Accipitrid vulture eggs, like those of California Condors, may have difficulty losing sufficient weight and should be treated similarly. King Vulture eggs, however, rarely present this challenge, perhaps because they come from a climate with much higher humidity.

Once the chick has hatched, any pieces of membrane adhering to the chick, as well as feces or urates, should be gently removed with a moistened cotton swab or gauze sponge while the chick is still wet as they are nearly impossible to remove without damaging down or skin once dry. Residual umbilical vessels, if present, may be cut to a length of 1 cm. The umbilical seal should be swabbed with a povidone-iodine solution. This is repeated about every 8 hours for the first 72 hours. Betadine ointment, which is water-based, may be used instead of solution after the first swabbing as it stays longer without keeping the area too moist as would a petroleum-based ointment.

The newly hatched chick is allowed to rest and dry off in the hatcher on the shelf liner material with a piece of sterile gauze under the belly. Once it is able to maintain sternal posture, has given a feeding response, and hopefully has defecated, it will be moved to the brooder.

## Initial Care and Stabilization

Artificially hatched chicks that have met the above criteria for moving to the brooder may be fed 6–12 hours after hatching. Feeding may be delayed longer for chicks that have a particularly large yolk reserve. Meals are initially kept small, dilute, and frequent to allow the digestive tract to adapt gradually to processing food along with the remaining yolk reserve. Chicks fed too much too soon are at risk of yolk sac stasis, which usually requires surgical removal.

Chicks pulled due to parental neglect, illness, or injury may be chilled and/or dehydrated. Most chicks can be warmed in a pre-heated brooder set at 96.0–97.0 °F (35.5–36.1 °C), but severely hypothermic chicks may benefit from additional contact heat from a hot-water bottle or similar mild heat source. As with any hypothermic animal, care must be taken to warm it gradually to ensure the core temperature rises along with that of the extremities. Dehydrated chicks should be given fluids subcutaneously, usually in the inguinal web. Injectable antibiotics may be given to treat or prevent infection in wounds or systemically. Rocephin (Roche) has been preferred for use with chicks, particularly since it is less likely than some other products to damage immature kidneys.

Compromised chicks may have difficulty feeding and may suffer from GI stasis. Small, dilute meals given more frequently are safest in this situation. Mouse pinks can be minced finely enough and mixed with distilled water to pass through a standard syringe if necessary. Oral feeding is preferred whenever possible, but gavage feeding is also an option. For dehydrated chicks, an electrolyte solution, such as unflavored Pedialyte (Abbott) or lactated Ringer's solution, may be used instead of distilled water to moisten and dilute the diet. Ensure the chick is swallowing well when feeding a very liquid diet or supplemental fluids so that the chick does not aspirate these into its lungs. This is especially true of weak chicks. If the chick does not swallow readily, it is better to continue injectable fluids and/or gavage feeding until it can safely be fed by mouth.

## Common Medical Problems and Solutions

Vulture chicks are exceptionally hardy and resilient. Given appropriate rearing conditions and diet, illness is rare. Of 40 California Condor chicks artificially hatched and hand-reared over a 10-year period, during the first 30 days after hatch, morbidity was 10% and mortality was 5%. A chick whose un-retracted yolk sac was amputated at hatch was given extensive supportive care and successfully treated for star-gazing (opisthotonos). Another chick developed sour crop and was also successfully treated. Six chicks that required hatching assistance were treated prophylactically with antibiotics but were never clinically ill. One chick was euthanized due to congenital deformities and neurological problems and another due to a severely infected yolk sac.

### Hatching Difficulties

Chicks that require hatching assistance are at higher risk of infection. They may have been unable to self-hatch due to pre-existing infection, edema, or dehydration. Eggs of these large vulture species that are assisted to hatch may have been opened to the air 3 or more days before hatching, with the exposed extraembryonic membranes and open umbilical seal being ideal substrates for opportunistic microbial growth. It may be useful to treat such embryos prophylactically with antibiotics. An antibiotic least likely to cause kidney damage, such as Rocephin (Roche), is given to the embryo *in ovo* if an injection site is accessible or, if not, dripped onto the inner surface of the chorioallantoic membrane. The dosage for a California Condor embryo, which will weigh on average 183 g at hatch, is 12.5 mg twice daily. If the chick is normal and vigorous, with a good umbilical seal at hatching, antibiotics are discontinued. If the chick has an open seal, exposed yolk sac, or is otherwise compromised, the antibiotics are continued until the condition resolves.

### Yolk Sac Infection/Omphalophlebitis

Although unusual, the most common illness and potential cause of death in any chick is umbilical and/or yolk sac infection. Symptoms may include diarrhea, GI stasis, redness/inflammation around the seal, discoloration of the yolk sac visible through the skin, lethargy, and/or swelling of the limb joints. When some or all of these symptoms are present, the prognosis is likely to be poor, but some chicks may recover with antibiotic therapy and supportive care.

One California Condor chick whose yolk sac was completely unretracted and partially necrotic at hatch required complete removal of the yolk sac as part of the assisted hatching procedure. Immediately following the procedure, the chick weighed 99 g, 84 g lighter than the average hatch weight of 183 g of a healthy California Condor chick. This chick was given frequent, fluid meals as described above and treated with antibiotics. Within 8 days it was indistinguishable from other chicks of the same age and was eventually released to the wild.

### Edema

Edema due to insufficient egg weight loss may severely compromise the chick's mobility initially, particularly when the head is very edematous and difficult for the chick to lift. Although this usually dissipates through pulmonary respiration within 24–48 hours, special care and feeding assistance will likely be required during this period. Administration of a diuretic, such as furosemide, may be necessary if the edema is severe. The chick may need to have its head slightly elevated and supported to ensure normal respiration while at rest and during feeding. If the edema in the head is such that creases are formed on the neck, frequent, gentle massage of these folds seems to help reduce the swelling more rapidly.

### Star-gazing

Three unrelated California Condor chicks presented with opisthotonos, or star-gazing, immediately following hatching. Their heads were pulling sharply backward at rest and occasionally chicks would flip over onto their backs. Most of the time, chicks could bring their heads into a normal posture for a few seconds to a minute, such as for feeding, but would immediately revert to the head-back position when the effort ended. This condition may be caused by thiamine deficiency in the egg. Each of these chicks was treated with both injectable and oral thiamine in varying doses within the first 24 hours and all made a full recovery, one within 15 hours and the other two within a few days. They were able to feed relatively normally during treatment with some steadying of their heads. Although the cause of the thiamine-deficient eggs could not be determined, a simple diet change seems to have eliminated the problem. Prior to producing these affected chicks, adult birds were fed frozen, thawed trout once every 2 weeks. Because condors tear up their food rather than swallowing it whole, the fish could not be adequately supplemented to compensate for the deficiency of vitamin E and thiamine, and the presence of thiaminase that is well documented in frozen, thawed fish (Bernard and Allen 1997). The small proportion of fish in the overall diet was not harmful to the adults, but the effect on egg formation was not anticipated. Since the fish was removed from the diet of breeding birds, no further incidences of star-gazing in chicks have occurred.

### Sour Crop

Sour crop is more common in true raptors, but has occurred in large vulture chicks. It may be evident immediately by a strong, sour odor coming from the chick, or the chick may regurgitate its malodorous crop contents. The feces are also likely to be strong-smelling. The smell of sour crop is much stronger than that of normal castings or other regurgitant and is almost unmistakable. It may be a side effect of systemic infection in which the digestion is otherwise slowed, or it may result from overfeeding or feeding of spoiled food. Left untreated, crop and gut stasis may follow. Treatment may be as simple as emptying the crop contents and flushing it with normal saline solution (Heidenreich 1997). Great care must be taken with these procedures to prevent aspiration of fluid into the lungs. Additional treatment for systemic infection may also be indicated.

### Splayed Legs

Splayed legs can be caused by the chick slipping on a substrate that does not provide enough traction, such as toweling that is laid flat and smooth. In a normally developing chick, the knee joints should be vertically aligned with the hock joints and the feet hip-width apart. Failure to promptly correct splaying will result in permanently deviated legs. An early, mild tendency to splay may be corrected by keeping the chick tucked into snug folds of the toweling or in a towel-lined, straight-sided nest bowl for a few days. More severe cases require hobbling the legs in the normal posture.

The hobbles can be made with a nonflexible bandaging tape that is doubled over to prevent it sticking to the chick's skin at any point. Hobbles are placed just below the hocks, around the tarsometatarsi, and should be loose enough that circulation is not compromised, but not so loose as to allow the hobbles to slip over the hock or foot or allow toes to get caught. They must be changed daily or every other day as the chick grows.

### Toe Constrictions

King Vulture chicks may develop constriction bands around the toes. This syndrome is also seen in parrot chicks but has not been documented in other Cathartid or in Accipitrid vultures. The cause remains unclear, but the constriction can be so severe as to restrict blood flow and cause necrosis of the distal part of the affected toe(s). Ensuring that the humidity in the brooder remains high (≥50–60% RH) will usually prevent this condition. If detected early, immediately increasing the humidity, maintaining a very light coating of an oil-based lubricant – such as triple antibiotic ointment – and frequent massage of the toes, can prevent permanent damage. If the condition is advanced, surgical intervention may be indicated (Romagnano 2003).

### West Nile Virus (WNV)

Cathartid vultures are not as susceptible to WNV as many other species of birds but a few California Condors, both adults and chicks, have died from the disease. In addition, two adult Andean Condors became severely ill but recovered from WNV infection and some California Condors are showing titers far too high to have been vaccine-induced. There have been no reports of WNV morbidity or mortality in Accipitrid vultures in the U.S., but the majority of them, along with most birds in potentially affected taxa in zoological collections, have been vaccinated with the equine vaccine (Fort Dodge). California Condors were included in the DNA vaccine testing program conducted by the Centers for Disease Control and have continued to receive this vaccine. The product has not been made available commercially at the time of writing. Regardless of species, chicks are vaccinated beginning as early as 30 days and definitely before being placed in outdoor environments. Parent-reared birds are vaccinated at 30 days.

### Other Conditions

Condor and King Vulture chicks usually develop flaky skin on the head during the brooder stage. This appears to be a normal process and not a result of low humidity or nutritional deficiency. It resolves without intervention. Condors have an extensive system of air sacs that extend under the skin of the neck and head, allowing inflation for dramatic effect. A few California Condor chicks have developed a large, persistent air "bubble" along one side of the head which is not considered problematic and disappears by 6–8 weeks of age.

## Diet and Weaning

While this chapter is based primarily on experience with Cathartid and *Gyps* vultures, the methods, including the following diet protocol, have worked well for other Accipitrid vulture species. The only exceptions may be the Bearded Vulture, whose adult diet is at least 70% bone, and the Palm-nut Vulture, whose adult diet includes more than 50% oily palm fruit. Bearded Vultures feed their youngest chicks soft animal tissue rather than bone. Up to 30% bone may be included after 4 weeks (Frey and Llopis 2015). There is limited information on chick rearing for the Palm-nut Vulture, but it is likely that parents feed primarily digestible animal protein for optimal growth. The following protocol may work well for Palm-nut Vultures, but additional information should be sought.

For the first 72 hours, chicks are fed mouse pinks (newborn mouse pups), well minced and moistened with distilled water. Typical amounts and feeding frequencies for California Condors are shown in Table 19.2. Over the next 72 hours, the diet is converted from pinks to fuzzies (partly furred mouse pups), and then from fuzzies to adult mice (skinned, with heads, tails, and feet removed), so that by day 9, chicks are receiving 100% skinned mouse torsos (SMTs), chopped more coarsely. The ratio of solids to liquids is 2 : 1 and the mixture is warmed to body temperature before feeding.

This initial diet, without supplementation of calcium or vitamin D, works well for these slow-growing vultures, but might result in metabolic bone disease if used for true raptors and other faster growing species. Accipitrid vulture and small Cathartid vulture chick diets have been supplemented with a multivitamin product, such as Vita Hawk, and/or taken outdoors for exposure to direct sunlight for 30 minutes per day to ensure adequate vitamin D metabolism.

By day 12, some fur is left on the mice, which will help chicks to cast properly. Chicks will not cast every day, especially early on, and there is considerable variability in frequency, quantity, and consistency. Casts will not be pelleted as with raptors, but should be moist and semi-formed. Some will produce small balls of material or may pass indigestible material in the feces. Wet, pasty castings and those with a sour odor indicate that chicks are not receiving sufficient casting material to cast as often as they should. At 2 weeks, chicks are often able to consume 100% furred mice, chopped but including some of the heads, tails, and feet. By 4 weeks, condor chicks can usually consume mice cut in quarters or halves and by 6 weeks may easily swallow whole mice. Although parent-reared chicks would have little or no exposure to whole carcasses until fledging, hand-reared chicks at this age will also begin to eat from rat carcasses that have been cut open for them and presented when other food is not available. Encouraging this ability to self-feed makes food preparation more efficient and less costly for the remainder of the rearing period and helps the chick master feeding skills at an early age.

By 12 weeks, if chicks are feeding well on rats, leaving little but the skins and heads, mice can be gradually eliminated from the diet and other adult items gradually introduced. During the nestling period, this includes adult rabbits once per week and horsemeat (or beef), cut in strips and supplemented with calcium carbonate ($CaCO_3$) at 6 g $CaCO_3$ per 1 kg of meat, also once per week. The latter would be a poor diet alone, but in combination with whole prey items, it is economical and ensures birds will eat this readily available product in case of interruption in the supply of rats or rabbits. Ground meat bird of prey diets are avoided during the nestling phase due to the potential for rapid spoilage and potential quality control issues.

By fledging, nestlings should be established on the adult diet. The diet for one California Condor would include one rabbit one day per week, 600 g (1.25 lb) chunk horsemeat (unsupplemented) or bird of prey diet one day per week, and four to five rats daily for 3–5 days per week. Adults feeding chicks and recently fledged, hand-reared juveniles are fed daily until the youngest bird is 9–10 months old, when 1–2 fast days per week are implemented.

Protocols must be adapted to available materials and foods. At the breeding facilities for the critically endangered vultures in India, the only readily available meat is goat. Chicks are reared exclusively on this food, supplemented with 6 g $CaCO_3$ per 1 kg of meat. They are limited to no more than 10% of body weight per feeding to reduce the potential for crop stasis, metabolic bone disease, and other problems. The growth rate is slower than chicks reared on the more varied diet with the

Table 19.2 Los Angeles Zoo California Condor chick rearing guidelines.

| Age in days | Diet | Supplements | Solids, amount per feeding, g (average) | Liquids, amount per feeding, g (average) | Number of feedings per day and feed interval (hours) | Brooder temperature | Other |
|---|---|---|---|---|---|---|---|
| 0 | Pinks (finely minced) | — | 4 | 2 | 7–2½ h | 95 °F (35 °C) | Distilled water in diet, sterile towel substrate, Betadine ointment to seal q6 h x 72 h |
| 1 | Pinks (finely minced) | — | 4 | 2 | 7–2½ h | 94 °F (34.4 °C) | Introduce puppet |
| 2 | Pinks (finely minced) | — | 6 | 3 | 7–2½ h | 93 °F (33.9 °C) | Full isolation |
| 3 | Pinks 2 : 1 fuzzies (minced) | — | 7 | 3 | 6–3 h | 92 °F (33.3 °C) | |
| 4 | Pinks 1 : 2 fuzzies (¼" pieces) | — | 8 | 4 | 6–3 h | 91 °F (32.8 °C) | |
| 5 | Fuzzies (¼" pieces) | — | 9 | 4 | 6–3 h | 90 °F (32.2 °C) | |
| 6 | Fuzzies 2 : 1 skinned mouse torsos (SMT) (¼-½") | — | 10 | 5 | 5–3½ h | 89 °F (31.7 °C) | |
| 7 | Fuzzies 1 : 2 SMT (¼-½") | — | 11 | 5 | 5–3½ h | 88 °F (31.1 °C) | |
| 8 | SMT (½ in. pieces) | — | 13–14 | 6 | 4–4 h | 87 °F (30.6 °C) | |
| 9 | SMT (½ in. pieces) | — | 15–16 | 6 | 4–4 h | 86 °F (30.0 °C) | |
| 10 | SMT 1 : 1 mice (furred, quartered) | — | 29–30 | 12 | 3–5 h | 85 °F (29.4 °C) | |
| 11 | SMT 1 : 1 mice (furred, quartered) | — | 30–38 | 12 | 3–5 h | 84 °F (28.9 °C) | |
| 12 | Mice, adult (quarters & halves) | — | 33–45 | 12–13 | 3–5 h | 83 °F (28.3 °C) | |
| 13 | Mice, adult (quarters & halves) | — | 37–52 | 12–13 | 3–5 h | 82 °F (27.8 °C) | |
| 14 | Mice, adult (quarters & halves) | — | 43–62 | 13–17 | 3–5 h | 81 °F (27.2 °C) | |
| 15 | Mice, adult (quarters & halves) | — | 58–90 | 13–17 | 2–10 h | 80 °F (26.7 °C) | |

*(Continued)*

Table 19.2 (Continued)

| Age in days | Diet | Supplements | Solids, amount per feeding, g (average) | Liquids, amount per feeding, g (average) | Number of feedings per day and feed interval (hours) | Brooder temperature | Other |
|---|---|---|---|---|---|---|---|
| 16 | Mice, adult (halves) | — | 66–106 | 18–24 | 2–10 h | 79 °F (26.1 °C) | |
| 17 | Mice, adult (halves) | — | 72–102 | 18–24 | 2–10 h | 78 °F (25.6 °C) | |
| 18 | Mice, adult (halves) | — | 80–124 | 20–26 | 2–10 h | 77 °F (25.0 °C) | |
| 19 | Mice, adult (halves) | — | 88–130 | 20–30 | 2–10 h | 76 °F (24.4 °C) | |
| 20 | Mice, adult (halves) | — | 98–138 | 22–30 | 2–10 h | 75 °F (23.9 °C) | |
| 21 | Mice, adult (halves) | — | 110–160 | 26–30 | 2–10 h | 75 °F (room) | Move to tub (18–21 days) |
| 35 | Rat, adult slit open – a.m. | — | 1 each | — | 2–10 h | 75 °F (room) | |
| | Mice, adult (halves) – p.m. | | 265 g | 30–38 | | | |
| 42 | Rat, adult slit open – a.m. | — | 1 each | — | 2–10 h | Outdoor w/ heat lamp | |
| | Mice, adult (whole) – p.m. | | 265 g | 30–38 | | | |
| 60 | Rats, adult (whole) | — | 4–5 each | — | 1 | Outdoor w/ heat lamp | Move to outdoor rearing chamber |
| 75–80 | Su·M·Tu·Th·F·Sa: rats, adult (whole) | — | 4–5 each | — | 1 | Outdoor | |
| | W: horsemeat (cut in strips) | 0.60 g $CaCO_3$/ 100 g meat | 125 g | | | | |
| 150–180 | M: feline diet | — | 500 g | — | 1 | outdoor | fledge |
| | Tu: rabbit, adult | | 1 each | | | | |
| | W: horsemeat (chunk) | | 570 g | | | | |
| | Su·Th·F·Sa: rats, adult (whole) | | 4–5 each | | | | |

SMT = skinned mouse torso

protocol above. At 60 days of age, Indian Vultures have reached 35% of adult body weight and White-rumped Vultures have reached 40% (J. Parry-Jones and N. Prakash, pers. comm.). California Condors and Cape Vultures reach 55–70% at the same age, even though their nestling period is longer. The Asian species do eventually achieve normal adult size.

## Feeding Procedures

To elicit feeding by the parent, the chick will reach upward toward the parent's beak, wing begging by pumping its wings rapidly up and down. The parent then regurgitates partially digested food, which is very liquid for a new chick but more solid later on, and the chick may reach part-way into the parent's mouth to feed. For hand-reared chicks, this feeding response can be elicited by placing the thumb and forefinger alongside the beak. Initial feedings are best delivered using a small, flexible plastic spoon to slowly slide the diet into the chick's mouth. It is important to get all the fluid into the chick to ensure good hydration. Most new chicks will stop feeding and turn away if they bite down on anything hard, such as the spoon or a bone fragment, so care should be taken to avoid this. Some prefer using their fingers to using a spoon, but it is difficult to get all the liquid into the chick by this method. Coordination of this process with an eager but uncoordinated chick takes practice. Chicks may eat so fast that they expel fluid from their nares, which should be promptly blotted away. As long as the chick is feeding voluntarily, aspiration of fluids into the lungs is rare, but the chick should be monitored for a few minutes to ensure this has not occurred.

Chicks can learn to self-feed from a small cup as early as the first day, but most will take 2–3 days to master this. It is essential that chicks are able to do this by about 72 hours of age in order to implement an effective isolation rearing protocol at this stage. A shallow, light-colored, plastic measuring cup of 50–75 ml (¼–⅓ cup) capacity works well. Chicks are naturally attracted to the red color of the food and will quickly reach for it when the cup is held at just the right angle (Figure 19.1). This takes practice for both chick and feeder. Ensure the fluids are consumed, using the spoon at the end of the feeding if necessary.

Amounts fed are not limited to a prescribed amount or percentage of body weight since excessive weight gain has not been a problem with these species. Records from healthy chicks provide a guide for expected intake. The chick's crop should empty to no more than 5–10% fullness between feedings and should empty completely overnight. If this does not occur, the scheduled feeding

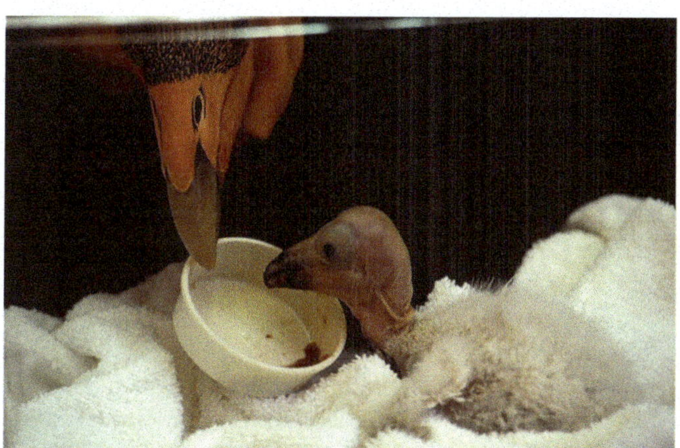

**Figure 19.1** Feeding a 36-hour-old California Condor chick with a puppet. *Source:* photo by Mike Wallace, courtesy of the Los Angeles Zoo.

should be delayed or skipped until the crop clears. Chicks that are overfed or are slow to process may develop sour crop and subsequent crop stasis, requiring intervention.

Once chicks are out of the brooder and housed in a tub, food is presented in a small, shallow ceramic crock. Water is offered in a deeper crock with supervision initially. Plastic crocks have also been used but are more lightweight and easily spilled by the chick. Beginning at about 5 weeks, chicks are offered larger whole prey items, such as rats and rabbits, which provides exercise and develops skills for feeding on carcasses. The size of these items is not crucial as lot of waste is expected at first. When chicks have moved and adjusted to an outdoor nest box chamber, food and water are delivered in larger crocks placed in a shallow tray, such as a small cat litter box. The tray slides into a custom-made, fixed plywood box with a sliding lid. This allows food and water to be changed from outside the enclosure without human contact. This system also minimizes the chicks' ability to remove the crocks to out-of-reach areas of the chamber.

After fledging, juveniles and adults are usually fed only in the holding enclosure, which is about 6×12×8 ft. (2×4× 2.5 m) high and attached to the main flight enclosure. This conditions birds to routinely enter this enclosure, the door of which can be closed from the outside, allowing staff to capture birds easily for physical exams and moves. Food is delivered by way of a chute, made from a section of 8 in. (20 cm) diameter PVC pipe, painted black and mounted through the fence on a downward angle at a height of 6 ft. (2 m). The tube is covered with a PVC cap when not in use. The holding area and adjacent enclosure walls are covered with solid material, such as corrugated metal sheets, to provide a sight barrier. This virtually eliminates the birds' associating humans with food, as long as staff members are especially quiet and stay out of view when feeding.

## Expected Weight Gain

Weigh chicks daily before the first morning feeding to provide the most consistent basis for comparison. This is easily done while chicks are still housed in brooders or in open "tubs" indoors. Chicks usually do not gain weight the first day and in fact lose 1% of their hatch weight on average. Initial weight gain is slow, from 3 to 5% daily for days 2–5, but jumps dramatically to an average of 12% ±5% for days 6–18. From day 19–35, weight gain averages 7% daily but varies from 2 to 16% each day (Figure 19.2).

Once they have been moved to outdoor rearing chambers or nest boxes, weighing is more difficult as chicks are no longer handled directly on a daily basis. Weights may be taken opportunistically during this period, such as when chicks are vaccinated. Once they are old enough to jump up on a low perch, 12–15 in. (30–40 cm) high, a sturdy spring scale (Pelouze model 10B60 heavy-duty receiving scale, 27 kg/60 lb capacity), on which a protective plywood box housing is attached to replace the weighing platform, may be mounted inside the rearing chamber. Placed where it is likely to be a favored perch and facing the camera or observation window, this scale can provide weights on a fairly consistent basis without the need to handle the chick. Scales can also be placed in outdoor flight enclosures, mounted high on a sturdy post to serve as a preferred perch, to provide weight information on fledged juveniles and adults. Because the birds tend to bounce heavily on the scale, the plywood box housing should be mounted to the scale platform brackets using nuts and bolts designed for aircraft. Hang gliding shops and light aircraft mechanics are good places to find these. Similarly, the lightweight metal ferrule that secures the clear cover over the face of the scale must be secured with screws to prevent the birds from systematically tearing it off and destroying the face of the scale. Electronic scales have been tried with condors but have not proven to be practical as both the birds and the environment are too hard on the scales.

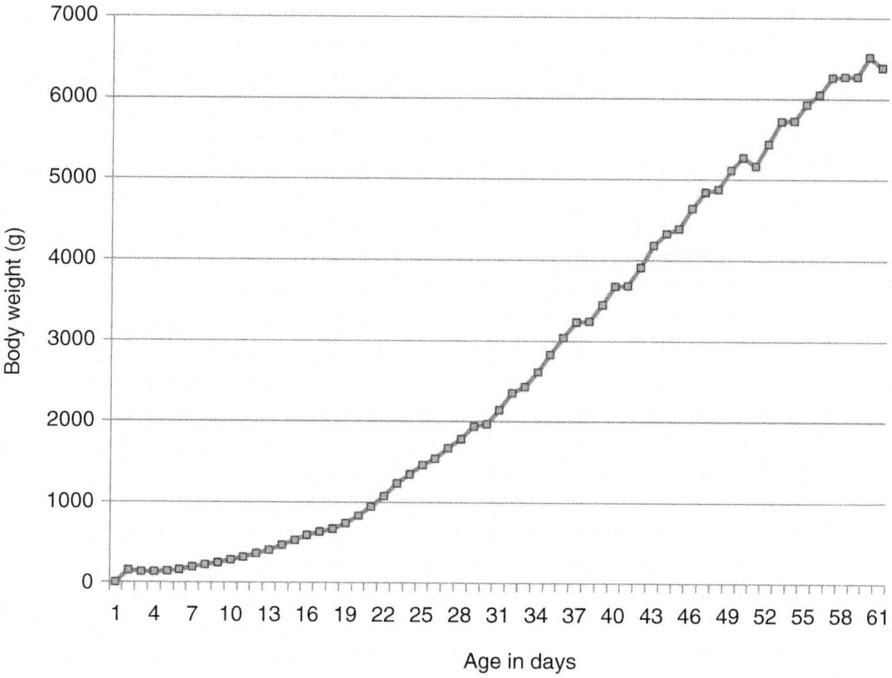


| Age in days | Body weight (g) |
|---|---|
| 1 | 147 |
| 2 | 137 |
| 3 | 134 |
| 4 | 144 |
| 5 | 161 |
| 6 | 195 |
| 7 | 220 |
| 8 | 248 |
| 9 | 283 |
| 10 | 320 |
| 11 | 364 |
| 12 | 406 |
| 13 | 468 |
| 14 | 525 |
| 15 | 592 |
| 16 | 630 |
| 17 | 664 |
| 18 | 735 |
| 19 | 832 |
| 20 | 942 |
| 21 | 1075 |
| 28 | 1940 |
| 35 | 3040 |
| 42 | 4180 |
| 60 | 6390 |

Figure 19.2 Weight gain – Cape Vulture, *Gyps coprotheres*, chick hatched 2013. *Source:* data courtesy of the Los Angeles Zoo.

Unlike many smaller bird species, Cathartid and Accipitrid vulture chicks may not achieve or exceed adult weight before fledging and, although they are essentially at adult stature when fledged, they will continue to increase bone mass and overall bulk for more than a year.

## Housing

The Animal Intensive Care Unit (AICU) brooder (Lyon Technologies) has been used most frequently for rearing condors and other vultures. Other types of forced air brooders, such as Rcom or human infant incubators, may also be used as long as stable temperature and humidity can be maintained, and the design does not present a physical hazard to these large, active chicks. Chicks that are healthy and vigorous at hatching, whether hatched by parents or in an incubator, are placed in the brooder set at 95.0 °F ± 1 °F (35.0 °C ± 0.5 °C) and 35–40% RH. This level of humidity is achieved at this temperature in the AICU when the water reservoir tray is kept full of distilled water. Although low, it has proven appropriate for both species of condor and *Gyps* vultures. King Vultures will require higher humidity, at least 50% RH. Until the temperature begins to approach room temperature, when ambient humidity will be adequate, using a second reservoir inside the brooding chamber helps to increase humidity. A straight-sided, plastic food container, about 6–8 in. (15–20 cm) square, partly filled with distilled water and paper or cloth towels (bunched up to increase the evaporative surface area), and securely covered with wire or plastic mesh, works well. Towels in this container should be changed daily to limit microbial growth.

As with egg incubators, prior to placing a chick in a brooder, take temperature readings in all parts of the chamber to ensure there are no hot or cool areas and, if there are, to compensate for them. A digital thermometer or remote sensing probe should be placed as close to the chick as is possible and safe. AICU brooders run at temperatures over 86 °F (30 °C) will maintain more consistent and stable temperatures if a folded bath towel is placed on top for insulation and multiple layers of towel substrate are used under the chick.

Larger, more vigorous chicks may require slightly lower initial temperatures, while small or compromised chicks tend to need a higher temperature. Chicks that are too hot will be sprawled or listless, may develop white salt accumulation around their nares (Cathartid species), and may become dehydrated. Cold chicks will huddle tightly, have grayish mouth and skin color, and may even shiver or feel cool to the touch. Their appetite and digestion will slow, potentially resulting in crop stasis and/or sour crop.

The brooder is bedded thickly with white terrycloth towels, with the top layer thoroughly rumpled in small, snug folds to prevent the chick from slipping and splaying its legs. Initially, towels may be sterilized by autoclaving and the chick placed on a square of sterile gauze as a precaution against umbilical infection. Care must be taken to remove all loose threads from towels to prevent injury due to entanglement of the chick's extremities. Towels should be changed as soon as they become soiled.

Brooder temperature is reduced approximately 1.0 °F (0.5 °C) daily, adjusting as indicated by the individual chick. By 3 weeks, the brooder temperature will be about 75 °F (24 °C) and the chick can be moved to an open, deep-sided tub. At this age, the brooder becomes too small and difficult to clean for a chick that may now weigh 1 kg (2.2 lb). The tub may be the bottom half of a plastic animal shipping crate, such as Vari Kennel (Pet Mate), modified by covering the door opening with plywood or mesh, a large, plastic storage tub, or a deep, rubber feeding tub (Fortex). The tub may be lined only with towels or may have a 3–4 in. (8–10 cm) layer of substrate such as decomposed granite or sand lightly covered with towels. If a substrate is used, it must be changed at least weekly to prevent the buildup of ammonia from urates. This is most easily done by having duplicate tubs to swap out. Chicks should be monitored to ensure that they do not drag food through the substrate and ingest it. Accipitrid vultures are reared in stick nests in the wild, so a stable arrangement of sturdy sticks under older hand-reared chicks may help with foot development. Chicks from this stage onwards spend a lot of time manipulating objects in their immediate environment. Clean, molted feathers from adult birds and rocks or sturdy sticks too big to swallow make good nest "toys."

It is also possible to house chicks in open tubs a few days earlier if a contact heat source is provided. Towels should be the only substrate for these younger chicks. A heating pad set under half of the tub allows chicks that are able to move around to self-regulate their need for warmth. Heating pads should never be placed directly inside the chick's enclosure due to the risk of burns or of electrocution should the wiring become exposed. Chicks under 2 weeks of age are not mobile enough to self-regulate their temperature needs and should be kept in a forced-air brooder.

At 6–8 weeks of age, chicks may be transferred to an outdoor rearing chamber that allows them to see and hear adult birds, weather permitting. This may be an enclosure designed especially for this purpose or an unused nest box. Nest boxes for condors are usually 6 × 6 × 6 ft. (2 × 2 × 2 m) high, while dedicated rearing chambers may be only 2/3 this width, or smaller for King Vultures. Chambers should be large enough to allow chicks to vigorously exercise their wings. Enclosure materials are plywood, plastic, or fiberglass on all sides with a sturdy wire mesh covered opening, 1.5–3 ft. (0.5–1 m) square, on the side adjacent to the flight enclosure. The bottom of this opening is about 2 ft. (0.6 m) above the floor with a sturdy shelf perch just underneath that allows the chick to directly view the adult enclosure at will when it is old enough to jump up on the shelf. As with nest boxes for condors and King Vultures, the chamber floor should be covered with clean sand 4–6 in. (10–15 cm) deep. When chicks are first transferred from the indoor tub to the outdoor rearing chamber, a few of the terrycloth towels are also placed in the chamber as familiar things that help ease the transition. These are eventually removed and not replaced. If temperatures will drop below 65 °F (18 °C), supplemental heat should be provided by a heat lamp or other radiant heat source placed over one section of the chamber and protected by a wire mesh cover to prevent older chicks from having direct contact with it. Ventilation should be provided by an exhaust fan and/or mesh-covered windows around the top of the chamber.

A dark blind, made of plywood or dark, opaque tarp over a PVC pipe frame is attached to the outside of the rearing chamber and all chick care is provided through small doors accessed through this blind. A small window, 4 × 12 in. (10 × 30 cm) covered with dark automotive window tinting film to create one-way glass and installed above the access door (about 4 × 8 in. [10 × 20 cm]) allows staff members to continue to use the puppet surrogate to interact with the chick. Initially, food and water crocks can be put in and removed through this port, but chicks will soon begin dragging crocks out of reach. When chicks have adjusted to their new enclosure and are large enough to reach, a feeding box (described under "Diet" above) can be used.

Closed-circuit video systems are used to monitor chicks remotely from hatching through fledging and beyond. This may be a sophisticated, commercial system or a simple, inexpensive home security system.

## Preparation for Wild Release

Vulture chicks that will be hand-reared and later released to the wild must be carefully managed in strict isolation from human contact and socialized with adult conspecifics in order to have the best chance of survival and long-term success in the wild. Unlike most raptors, such as hawks, eagles, and falcons, vultures do not have a discrete, hard-wired window of imprintation as young chicks in which they form their species identity. With the high capacity for learned behavior and innate inquisitiveness required of these scavenging species, vultures very readily malimprint on humans. This tendency persists well beyond a year of age and disappears entirely only by the age of sexual maturity.

Visual and auditory isolation from human contact is implemented with chicks no later than 72 hours after hatching. No talking or whispering of any kind is permitted near chicks or juvenile birds and a recording of nature sounds is played continuously in the brooder room to mask the sounds of people working. All feeding and other care is provided with the caregiver in a dark blind and the chick, whether in a brooder or later in a tub, in a well-lighted area. The blind is constructed using dark, opaque fabric curtains with openings at arm height and a shaded viewing window. The fabric of the armholes is overlapped to prevent gaps. The window, about 8 × 12 in. (20 × 30 cm), is made of two or more layers of window screen or shade cloth and is covered with a dark fabric flap when not in use. The curtains are suspended from cables anchored to the walls or attached to PVC pipe frames. Dark fabric is also used for the ceiling of the blind.

A lifelike condor (or other vulture species) hand puppet is used to interact with the chick (see Figure 19.3). The puppet is made with an acrylic molded skull, glass taxidermy eyes, and elk hide skin, attached to an artificial fur sleeve that reaches the caregiver's upper arm. The puppet rarely offers food to the chick but rather functions in social interactions, behaving and responding as much like a parent condor as possible, including preening the chick, chastising it when it is too assertive, and reacting to external noises. The caregiver's other arm is covered with a loose, closed-ended lightweight black fabric sleeve of equal length. This allows good dexterity for handling the chick and materials around it. To remove the chick from the brooder for daily weighing and

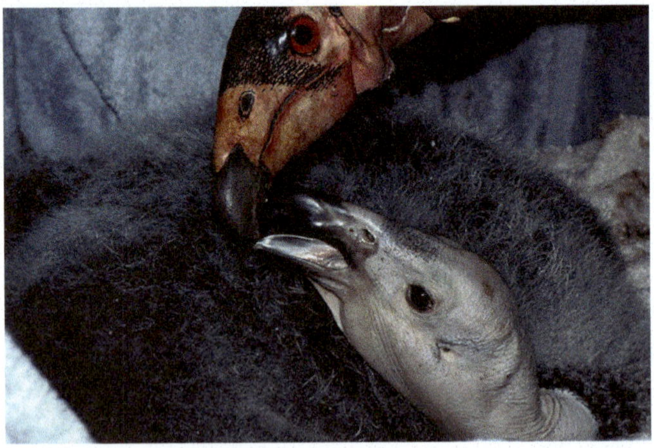

Figure 19.3 California Condor chick at 46 days interacting with a condor puppet. *Source:* photo by Mike Wallace, courtesy of the Los Angeles Zoo.

cleaning or for medical procedures, a dark drape is first loosely placed over the chick by the puppet and sleeve. The caregiver can then move the curtain aside and place the covered chick in a deep container for weighing. It is very important to ensure adequate ventilation for these young chicks that have a naturally low carrying capacity for oxygen in the blood. Isolation can be maintained if the weighing container has numerous ventilation holes on one side that is always kept facing away from the caregiver and the drape is placed loosely over the top of the container.

A newer method of maintaining visual isolation during routine procedures is to use the loose sleeve as a hood. Chicks will naturally probe and push, so the caregiver uses the sleeved hand to gently cover the chick's head and then inverts the entire sleeve over the chick's neck. The open end is gathered with a soft elastic insert which helps secure it. As with a drape, the time a chick is hooded should be kept brief and adequate ventilation must be ensured. As long as the fabric is lightweight and the elastic end is slightly loose, and the chick is not agitated, ventilation should be adequate. Chicks that are draped or hooded behave much as they do when brooded or when it is dark, remaining very relaxed. They will, however, continue to probe and poke their heads out from under a drape or through a curtain if given the opportunity. This might seem like a minor problem, but chicks very rapidly become habituated with just this limited exposure to humans, so caregivers must be vigilant to prevent this.

Even with good isolation, chicks can become habituated to change of all sorts if they are handled too much or desensitized to many new experiences. Because of this, moves and other changes in the chick's environment, incidences of physical restraint and exposure to other chicks are kept to an absolute minimum. For older chicks and juveniles, moves and exams are best done at night when the birds are less alert and there is no association with routine, daytime activities.

As chicks get older and are moved to outdoor chambers, the puppet becomes less suitable to fill the role of an adult condor, so its use is decreased over time. Chicks may become overly aggressive with this surrogate parent, which is not appropriate chick-to-adult behavior. At this stage, visual and auditory access to one or more adult condors provides more appropriate role modeling for the chick. For California Condors, a single adult male mentor is housed adjacent to the hand-reared chicks and they are later fledged, one at a time, into the enclosure with him. Males have proven more tolerant with chicks than females who are often far too aggressive with them, especially if there is an adult male nearby. Females have been good mentors for juveniles over 1 year of age.

Mentors are chosen for their appropriate behavior in response to human activity, primarily avoidance or at least lack of interest. Birds that are inquisitive about human activity and novel events are not suitable mentors even if they have previously been in a flock situation or have been good parents. The goal is for young birds to be wary of new things and to develop the skills and confidence necessary for social interaction in a competitive, hierarchical population (Clark et al. 2007).

This rearing method, conscientiously carried out, produces chicks that are as wild as their wild-reared counterparts, but it requires careful management during the remainder of their time in human care. A fledged juvenile that is suddenly frightened may fly into the enclosure mesh, attempting to climb it to gain height, but eventually putting so much pressure on its beak that it cracks or breaks, requiring major repair. To prevent this, the beak tips of chicks are blunted by filing with an emery board or rotary tool with an abrasive bit before fledging.

California Condor juveniles, whether hand-reared or parent-reared, remain with their initial adult mentor until they are about 14–18 months old. Once all juveniles in the cohort have developed appropriate confidence and social behavior, they are ready to be transferred to the pre-release enclosure in the field. This enclosure is similar to the captive-breeding enclosures. The juvenile cohort stays in this facility with the adult mentor for several weeks to months, adjusting to the diet and environment they will find after release. Once released, biologists continue to place carcasses in or near the enclosure, ensuring the birds find food while they are adapting to the wild and providing a ready means of recapture.

## Preparation for Introduction to Captive Flock

Birds that are hand-reared for captive-breeding or display purposes should also be reared by the above methods but require less stringent precautions to avoid exposure to human activity after fledging. The primary consideration should be to avoid the chick developing a strong association with humans as a food source as this will lead to aggression. It is not necessary to deliberately habituate juveniles to any particular aspect of captive life. If staff members conduct routine activities, such as cleaning and maintaining enclosures, without encouraging interaction with the birds and discouraging their approaches, juveniles will not feel rewarded by human attention and will naturally acclimate to the captive environment.

## Behavioral Training for Educational Programs

Birds intended to work in educational programs ideally should be parent-reared or isolation-reared up to the age of fledging. Hand-reared birds with which no isolation precautions have been taken are very affectionate and relaxed with human caregivers well into their juvenile stage. As these birds approach sexual maturity, however, they will become increasingly aggressive, particularly with people they don't recognize other than those who reared them. Even parent- or isolation-reared birds, especially males, tend to become increasingly challenging to work with at this age. These large vultures are best prepared for educational programs by individuals with a strong animal training background, ideally in both falconry methods and general operant conditioning with a variety of species. Vultures used in educational programs can also become good breeding birds later on if socialized with conspecifics as juveniles and managed consistently well. Adult birds that were not handled properly when young may become unmanageable and dangerous, necessitating their removal from programs. They are likely to be poor display birds, lacking the social skills to integrate with other vultures, and will be unlikely to be good parents. Given the long lifespans of these species, careful and informed management from the beginning is essential.

## Acknowledgments

The California Condor Recovery Program would not be possible without the selfless dedication and collaboration of the many people working in captivity and in the wild to recover this magnificent species. The staff at the Los Angeles Zoo has worked tirelessly over the years to continually improve all aspects of how California Condors and all our vultures are reared and prepared for their future. Their abilities are amazing and their passion inspiring. Our work together with California Condors and many other vultures is the foundation of this chapter.

## Sources for Products Mentioned

Abbott Nutrition, Department 107089, 3300 Stelzer Road, Columbus, Ohio 43219–3034, (800) 227–5767, https://pedialyte.com.

Animal Intensive Care Units: Lyon Technologies, Inc., 1690 Brandywine Avenue, Chula Vista, CA 91911, (888) 596–6872. https://lyonusa.com.

Avitronics, Rose in Valley, Lower Hugus Road, Threemilestone, TRURO, TR3 6BD, Cornwall UK, 0044(0)1209–212 775, www.avitronics.co.uk, info@avitronics.co.uk.

Con-Tact Brand Beaded Grip Liner: Kittrich Corporation, 1585 W Mission Boulevard, Pomona, CA 91766, (714) 736–1000, https://contactbrand.com.

Fort Dodge Animal Health, West Nile Vaccine Product Manager, P.O. Box 25945, Overland Park, Kansas 66225–5945, (800) 477–1365 (U.S.), 800-267–1777 (Canada).

Pelouze Scales, Rubbermaid Commercial Products, 125 High Rock Avenue, First Floor, Saratoga Springs, NY 12866, (800) 810–7847, https://www.rubbermaidcommercialproducts.com, service@rubbermaidcommercialproducts.com.

Rcom Company, P. O. Box 780 871, Wichita, Kansas 67278–1038, (912) 239–5612, (888) 504–1113, http://www.r-com-hatcher.com, info@R-com-Hatcher.com.

Rubber tubs: Fortex® Fortiflex®, (800) 468–4460, http://www.fortexfortiflex.com/index.php/products/category/rubber-pans-tubs, info@fortexfortiflex.com.

Vari-kennel: Petmate, 2300 East Randol Mill Road, Arlington, Texas USA 76011, (877) 738–6283, https://www.petmate.com/petmate-vari-kennel/product/21790, customerservices1@petmate.com.

VitaHawk, 2063 Main Street, PMB 406, Oakley, California 94 561, Fax: (406) 567–2449, www.vitahawk.com, vitahawk@gmail.com.

## References

Bernard, J.B. and Allen, M.E. 1997. Feeding captive piscivorous animals: nutritional aspects of fish as food. In: *Nutrition Advisory Group Handbook, Fact Sheet 005*. Association of Zoos and Aquariums. Silver Spring, Maryland. 12 pp. https://nagonline.net/wp-content/uploads/2014/01/NAG-FS005-97-Fish-JONI-FEB-24-2002-MODIFIED.pdf.

Clark, M., Wallace, M., and David, C. (2007). Rearing California Condors for release using a modified puppet-rearing technique. In: *California Condors in the 21st Century* (eds. A. Mee and L.S. Hall), 213–226. Washington, DC: American Ornithologists Union and Nuttall Ornithological Club.

Frey, H. and Llopis, A. (2015). Bearded Vulture European Endangered Species Programme (EEP): Guidelines for Feeding Bearded Vultures in Captivity. European Association of Zoos and Aquaria. Vulture Conservation Foundation, https://www.4vultures.org/our-work/captive-breeding/bearded-vulture.

Gill, F. and D. Donsker (eds.). (2019). IOC World Bird List (v9.1). doi: 10.14344/IOC.ML.9.1.

Heidenreich, M. (1997). *Birds of Prey: Medicine and Management*. Oxford: Blackwell Science.

Romagnano, A. (2003). Avian pediatrics. Proceedings of the International Aviculturists Society.

## Further Reading

del Hoyo, J., Elliott, A., and Sargatal, J. (eds.) (1994). *Handbook of the Birds of the World, Volume 2, New World Vultures to Guineafowl*. Barcelona: Lynx Editions.

Ferguson-Lees, J. and Christie, D.A. (2001). *Raptors of the World*. New York: Houghton Mifflin Co.

Kasielke, S. (2010). When good eggs go bad: hatching assistance and egg necropsy. Proceedings of the American Association of Zoo Veterinarians Annual Conference, South Padre Island, TX, pp. 126–131.

Koford, C.B. (1953). *The California Condor*. New York: Dover Publications, Inc.

Kuehler, C.M., Sterner, D.J., Jones, D.S. et al. (1991). Report on the captive hatches of California Condors (*Gymnogyps californianus*): 1983–1990. *Zoo Biology* 10: 65–68.

Ritchie, B.W., Harrison, G.J., and Harrison, L.R. (1994). *Avian Medicine: Principles and Application*. Lake Worth, Florida: Wingers Publishing, Inc.

SAVE: Saving Asia's Vultures from Extinction, http://www.save-vultures.org.

The IUCN Red List of Threatened Species, www.iucnredlist.org.

The Peregrine Fund, www.peregrinefund.org.

VulPro, www.vulpro.com.

# 20

# Diurnal Raptors

*Louise Shimmel*

## Natural History

There are several types of birds that make up the very large diurnal (daytime-active) raptor group: 313 species worldwide of hawks, harriers, eagles, falcons, kites, osprey, and vultures. Although this classification changes from time to time, especially with DNA analysis rather than morphological attributes, generally accepted categories are as follows: the order Accipitriformes includes osprey (1 species in its own family), kites (23 species), Old World vultures (16 species), harriers (15 species), hawks (120 species), and eagles (68 species covered in a separate chapter). The order Falconiformes includes the falcons (54 species), caracaras (9 species), and Secretary Bird (1 species).

The seven species of New World vultures, briefly classified in the order Ciconiiformes (with storks) due to some physiological and behavioral attributes, are now – based on recent DNA analysis – currently classified in their own avian order: Cathartiformes (Chesser et al. 2018). California Condors are discussed in Chapter 19; the two species that commonly enter rehabilitation in North America, Turkey Vultures (*Cathartes aura*) and Black Vultures (*Coragyps atratus*), are covered here.

Raptors are obligate or absolute carnivores that (except for the scavengers) typically catch their food with their well-adapted feet, which have long, sharp, curved talons and strong toes. Their hooked beak is designed for ripping and tearing flesh, whether it's a small animal they have caught alive or a carcass into which they are tearing as scavengers. The vultures and many of the buteonine hawks and eagles scavenge already-dead animals as at least part of what they eat. All or part of the diet of any one species may be insects, reptiles, amphibians, fish, birds, small rodents and other mammals, or carrion of any animal.

However, there are lots of other avian species not considered raptors that are obligate carnivores and eat the same type of prey items as do the raptors. Thus, it is actually anatomy rather than diet that determines which species are considered raptors or birds of prey. Like any rule, there are often exceptions, and although vulture feet do not carry the same equipment as a typical raptor, their powerful hooked beak and diet do match those aspects of the raptor profile.

*Hand-Rearing Birds*, Second Edition. Edited by Rebecca S. Duerr and Laurie J. Gage.

### Hawks

Among the hawks, there are two general, distinctively different types. The "true" hawks or *accipiters* tend to be long-legged, long-toed, long-tailed, short-winged birds whose sprint-like speed and maneuverability in a typically wooded habitat allows them to make other birds a high percentage of their diet. The soaring hawks or *buteos* (typically called "buzzards" outside the Americas) are birds whose long, broad wings allow them to be relatively hefty, in a bird sense, because they are built for gliding and soaring, but otherwise tend to be perch-and-pounce predators rather than chasers.

In North America north of Mexico, the hawks routinely found include three species of *accipiters:* Sharp-shinned Hawk, Cooper's Hawk, and Northern Goshawk. There are also 11 species of *buteos:* Red-tailed Hawk (having the largest range), Rough-legged Hawk, Red-shouldered Hawk, Broad-winged Hawk, Ferruginous Hawk, Swainson's Hawk (the next most widespread, at least during certain times of the year), plus Short-tailed Hawk, Zone-tailed Hawk, White-tailed Hawk, Black Hawk, and Road-side Hawk, all of which have ranges that barely extend into the southern United States. Harris' Hawks are a *parabuteo* hawk found in the South western U.S. and down into Central and South America.

Hawks are typically tree-nesting birds that build nests of sticks, in trees, cliff edges, or even on a slight promontory on the ground, if that's all that is available. Harris' Hawks are fascinating communal raptors that build stick nests on cactus. Where hawks re-use nests in subsequent seasons, the nests are typically well-constructed and are refurbished as needed. Orphaned hatchlings or nestlings come in most often because of windstorms blowing whole nests down or breaking branches, or from logging or landscaping that takes out trees.

### Harriers

Harriers are long-winged, slender birds that typically course back and forth over fields searching for food using their owl-like facial disks, it is thought, to help locate their prey by sound. The one representative of this group of birds in North America is the Northern Harrier (previously known as the Marsh Hawk). This bird nests on the ground, making a rough nest with trampled grass and some sticks, in tall grass or under a small shrub. Most eggs, hatchlings, or nestlings come in from accidents with mowers, as the field is hayed or mown by someone not knowing that this secretive bird has a nest there. Even food exchanges, where the male is bringing food to his mate and offspring, take place away from the hidden nest.

### Osprey

Osprey are found worldwide, always near water, and their diets are almost exclusively fish. Though remains of a wide range of other prey items have been found in nests, such nonfish prey typically represent a very small percentage of their diet. Osprey nests can be very bulky affairs, placed on the very top of dead trees, power poles, or platforms introduced specifically for their nesting. Awkward birds, except in the air, they seem to require clear access to their nests, rather than hiding them down in the branches as most other raptors make some effort to do. Hatchlings or young nestlings are sometimes blown down with a nest; and returning them can sometimes be difficult when the nest is at the very top of a snag whose overall condition may make it dangerous to climb. If it does not overburden a nest or place a nestling with much younger or much older adoptive siblings, fostering into nests of a different pair placed on lower, often man-made platforms is a viable alternative to returning them to their own nest. In captivity, this species is particularly difficult to condition for release, so maximal efforts should be made to reunite uninjured fallen chicks with their parents. Because their nests are high, and their wings are long and heavy, chicks blown from nests are frequently badly injured, usually suffering fractures of the wings. Unless they are found promptly, the fracture is midshaft and repaired promptly and perfectly, the prognosis of full return to function for these birds is poor.

### Kites

Kites are most typically found in the southern states in the U.S., although the White-tailed Kite has recently expanded its range north into Oregon and Washington from California. In North America north of Mexico are Mississippi Kites, Swallow-tailed Kites, the White-tailed Kite (with the widest distribution); and the Snail Kite and Hook-billed Kite whose ranges barely touch Florida and the southernmost tip of Texas, respectively. As tree or woody vegetation nesters, young kites are most likely to be presented for care due to windstorms, landscaping, or other nest disruption.

### Falcons

Falcons found in North America north of Mexico consist of the Gyrfalcon, Peregrine Falcon, Prairie Falcon, Merlin, and American Kestrel primarily, with the Aplomado Falcon the subject of re-introduction efforts in south Texas. Falcons are typically open-country or edge habitat birds that do not make a nest; they are either cliff- or cavity-nesters, or will take over an old corvid nest (Merlins). Kestrels and Peregrines have adapted to human habitats, with Peregrines found in many cities nesting on tall buildings, industrial towers, or bridges where suitable platforms can be found or are placed. Kestrels opportunistically use any cavity of a suitable size, and very young birds present typically from human disruption of a nest site or because of a fall from a poorly chosen nest site.

### New World Vultures

New World Vultures found in North America north of Mexico are the Black Vulture, Turkey Vulture, and California Condor. California Condors are covered in Chapter 19, but are realistically unlikely to be presented for hand-rearing outside a small number of specialized institutions. However, if the population continues to grow in the wild, it may eventually become possible that a juvenile condor would be presented for temporary care, such as if an injured fledgling was found by a member of the public.

Turkey and Black Vultures often nest on the ground, under windfalls or in caves, and occasionally in broken top snags or hollow stumps. Eggs or young birds may be brought into care due to logging or development, or other type of nest disturbance. It is strongly encouraged that Turkey Vultures, of all birds, be reunited with parents or placed in wild foster nests, if at all possible, because they are extremely difficult to raise in captivity without excessive socialization to people. Given their highly developed sense of smell, it is very difficult to avoid having them associate humans with food.

## Criteria for Intervention

As with many other species of wild birds, both parents are actively involved in rearing young. The loss of one parent may or may not be cause for intervention. The death of a brooding female could lead to the death of hatchlings or nestlings, because males of many species will not brood.

In cold weather the death of a male while the female is incubating or brooding may lead to the death of the young, because the female could certainly provide food for the young but not also keep them warm.

Young found on the ground that are cold, injured, dehydrated, caught by a cat or dog, or emaciated should be presented for human care. If the condition can be corrected quickly (e.g. cold or dehydrated), the nest location is known and reachable, and the parents are obviously still present, the young can often be replaced in the nest within a day or two. If other young are known to be in the nest and the chick can be replaced in or near the nest at fledging age, a delayed reunion with the natural parents remains a possibility even after treatment for a more severe condition, such as a broken bone or wound.

Long-term human care due to the loss of the whole nest or even the nest tree may at times be avoided by placing the nestlings in a replacement nest, such as a basket or an open-topped wooden box with drainage holes. The young need to be old enough to thermoregulate and vocalize and thus be found by the parents. Nest boxes for kestrels can also be put up. Kestrels are the most likely to require intervention due to inappropriate nesting sites, such as in an old barn about to be torn down. If, however, the nest or nest tree is lost due to larger scale destruction at a logging site or new development or mowed field, intervention may be necessary. Even though both parents are still present, continuous disturbance or lack of a nearby tree or other appropriate nest site may preclude the return of the nestlings.

Healthy fledglings of any species found on the ground should be left alone or perhaps put nearby, somewhere safe from domestic predators. Though essentially full grown, they cannot yet fly. Their parents will continue to feed them wherever they are.

Some birds may come in through regulatory agency action when, occasionally, due to extremely aggressive parents nesting close to human activity, governmental authorities authorize taking eggs or young from the nest, sometimes even killing the parents. This seems to happen most often with Red-shouldered Hawks. This should obviously be an absolute last resort and working with the public on how to avoid injury to themselves and the birds is critical, before authorities are asked to intervene.

## Record Keeping

Detailed information on the location where the bird was found should be recorded. This will serve as a guide for suitable habitat for release and also will place the bird back with its relatives, which may still recognize the young bird.

Wildlife regulatory agencies have minimum standards for record keeping that require tracking of individual animals undergoing rehabilitation. Check with your regulating agencies for further information. As a minimum, the following information should be kept: species, age, location found, reason brought into care, medical problems, final disposition, and release location. Each nestling in care can be given a unique log number and its leg banded with temporary materials in order to track its growth. To avoid placing sticky tape directly on the bird's leg, the lower tarsus can be wrapped first with a layer of nonsticky elastic bandaging material, and then with a white cloth tape on which the log number can be written with permanent marker. There are also plastic poultry bands available in different colors or with distinct numbers or blanks on which numbers can be written. Care should be taken, however, that the hard edges of such bands will not cut into the bird's skin when the nestling is back on its hocks or will not trap inquisitive beaks while preening.

All bands, cloth or otherwise, need to be checked daily as the bird is growing quickly, and all such identification bands must be removed before release.

A detailed medical record should be kept on each animal, with results of the initial examination recorded and any updated information added as it happens. This should include daily body weights taken at the same time each day, whether the bird has cast (regurgitated a pellet of indigestible materials such as hair and bones), any unusual droppings, whether the crop is emptying, what has been fed at what times and how much was eaten, and any medications given, as well as progress of treatments and pertinent notes on behavior.

## Initial Care and Stabilization

The main rule of initial baby bird care for any species is warmth, rehydration, and feeding, in that order. Warm chicks before giving fluids, and then hydrate them until they start passing droppings. Only then is it safe to commence feedings. Feeding a cold or dehydrated baby bird before it is warm and hydrated could kill it as it might not be able to process the food.

New patients should be allowed to rest for 15–20 minutes in a warm, dark, quiet container before examination. If the bird is not able to stand, it should be placed in a soft support structure such as a rolled cloth "donut" or paper nest not much larger than the bird's body. For larger species, an upside-down cloth toilet seat cover with a towel rolled and placed under the elastic edges makes a good substitute nest. The whole thing can be covered with another towel to minimize how many towels need to be changed at each feeding. This provides the legs with the necessary support to avoid splaying.

Do not allow the bird to lie on its side or other abnormal positions. Hatchlings and nestlings should be placed in a climate-controlled incubator if available. When the animal is warm and calm, it may be hydrated orally and/or subcutaneously (SQ). If there is any sign of blood in the mouth or droppings, or extensive bruising of the abdomen, any of which might signal injuries from the fall from the nest, SQ administration of fluids is advised. A gentle palpation of the abdomen will indicate whether there is food or casting material in the ventriculus.

Warm sterile fluids, such as 2.5% dextrose in 0.45% sodium chloride or lactated Ringer's solution, may be administered SQ at 5% (50 ml/kg) of body weight once, although repeated administrations every 2 or 3 hours may be needed for extremely dehydrated birds.

Because raptors do not gape, active hatchlings or nestlings should be orally hydrated via gavage until they produce droppings. Human infant electrolyte fluids (unflavored) are excellent for oral rehydration of baby birds. Again, ensure that the bird is warm before administering fluids, and that the bird is both warm and well-hydrated before receiving food. Start the bird on a small piece of clean meat dipped in warm water after it begins passing droppings.

If the bird is depressed or not swallowing well, oral rehydration must be done especially carefully, because there is a greater risk of aspiration of fluids into the respiratory system. It may be better in this circumstance to use SQ fluids, rather than to give oral fluids. If SQ fluids are not an option, give tiny amounts of oral fluids deep into the mouth by tube (into the crop if possible) and ensure that the bird swallows everything before giving more.

If a young bird does not begin passing droppings within 3 hours of having been given the fluids, begin feeding the appropriate diet. However, keep the diet very moist and the meal size small until droppings are seen.

## Common Medical Problems

### Metabolic Bone Disease

Metabolic bone disease is seen unfortunately often in young birds that have been in the hands of the public for even a few days on an inadequate diet. Though recognizing a young raptor as a meat-eater, people fail to understand that a diet of hamburger, organ meat, or muscle meat creates a severe imbalance of calcium and phosphorus at a very vulnerable time when young birds are growing at an astronomical rate. The severely unbalanced calcium-to-phosphorus (Ca : P) ratio in such meats causes stripping of available calcium from the bones, leading to deformities such as bowing of the long bones, greenstick or outright fractures. When these birds come into care, often because the finders finally realize that something is wrong, this situation can only sometimes be corrected. Providing a diet with the correct Ca : P ratio of 2 : 1 plus oral calcium supplementation for as long as the inadequate diet was fed can sometimes overcome the problem if the birds do not yet have any fractures or major deformities. A veterinarian should be consulted for help in such cases. Once fractures have occurred, little can be done because the cortices of the bones are usually so thin that they will break somewhere else if an attempt is made to immobilize or pin the fracture site. Feather development will usually be severely compromised in these cases as well.

### Head Injuries

Do not overheat a bird with a head injury because this may aggravate bleeding/swelling in the brain. Steroids or nonsteroidal anti-inflammatory drugs (NSAIDs) may be of use in treating head injuries, although steroid use is controversial; using dexamethasone for head injuries raises concerns over the steroids causing a depression of immune system function. Many wildlife veterinarians prefer NSAIDs in these cases, although there is a large amount of variation in safety and effectiveness between species. Extrapolate between species cautiously. Dosing for some raptor species has been published (Hawkins et al. 2018) and is an area of current research. Each new edition of the *Exotic Animal Formulary* (Hawkins et al. 2018) reviews current published papers and it is prudent to stay informed with new knowledge.

### Other Injuries

Young birds without wing feathers to slow their fall can be badly bruised in a drop from a high nest. If very young, their abdomen tends to be the center of gravity, and bruising there can lead to impactions of pellet material. Fecal matter in droppings may look like a string of small beads rather than a typical fried egg appearance. Appetite may be low and a hard mass may be palpated between the legs in the abdomen. Fluids and a small amount of Metamucil can help correct this over time. Clean meat (i.e. no casting material) supplemented to correct the Ca : P ratio can also be dipped in Metamucil and then fed. This will provide nutrition without adding to the casting burden. This condition sometimes takes up to 3 days to resolve.

Wounds can be treated as in adult birds but if antibiotics are deemed necessary for, say, a cat bite, check with an avian veterinarian. Broad-spectrum antibiotics frequently used in injured raptors include penicillins such as amoxicillin/clavulanic acid at 125 mg/kg orally (PO) every 12 hours or amoxicillin at 100–150 mg/kg PO every 12 hours, or cephalosporins such as cephalexin at 40–100 mg/kg PO or intramuscularly (IM) every 6–8 hours, or cefazolin at 50–100 mg/kg PO or IM every 12 hours. Open fractures are most often treated with clindamycin at 25–50 mg/kg PO every

8–12 hours to prevent osteomyelitis (Hawkins et al. 2018). See Ponder and Willette (2017) for information regarding management of orthopedic injuries in raptors, including chicks.

### Parasitism

Severe infestations of external or internal parasites are sometimes found in young raptors. Pale mucus membranes or emaciation should lead to further diagnostics such as a blood smear or fecal analysis, if not done routinely. Coccidia infections may be severe enough to cause anemia and a failure to thrive, as can leucocytozoonosis, especially in older post-fledging birds. Coccidiosis is best treated with ponazuril (various brand names) compounded into a liquid of 50–100 mg/ml and dosed at 20 mg/kg once a day for a week. Coccidia is one parasite that keeps evolving resistance, and sometimes different antiparasitic drugs need to be used in progression to remove all signs. Treatment can also involve a week-on, week-off, week-on regimen to get all life stages of this parasite. Another common drug to use for coccidia is Toltrazuril (Baycox, Bayer) at 10 mg/kg once every other day for three treatments (Hawkins et al. 2018). Leucocytozoon infection is treated with both Primaquine given once PO at 0.75–1.0 mg/kg and then Chloroquine at 25 mg/kg at 0 hour, and thereafter 15 mg/kg at hours 12, 24, and 48 (Hawkins et al. 2018). Ectoparasites, which may also lead to severe anemia or feather damage if not controlled, can be treated with a pyrethrin-based powder. Treating all birds for external parasites upon admission is a good practice to help limit disease and blood parasite transmission between birds.

### Imprinting and Habituation

Young raptors in the hands of the public are frequently malimprinted on humans, which, though not a medical problem, nevertheless leads to a nonreleasable bird. This may become a lethal problem if placement in permanent care is not available. Euthanasia may be the only option in such cases, because these birds cannot be released.

## Re-nesting

Usually, the best choice for an uninjured, displaced wild raptor is returning it to its nest. Local tree services, arborists, utilities, and state or federal forest service offices may have tree climbers willing to assist in returning youngsters to nests.

## Fostering

Placing uninjured, displaced hatchling or nestling raptors in a foster nest is also an option preferable to being raised by humans. Care should be taken in regard to the following: that the orphan and his surrogate nestmates are old enough to thermoregulate in case the brooding adult female is flushed from the nest for a prolonged period of time by the activity of adding a new youngster; that a nest is not overloaded, jeopardizing the ability of the parents to care for the expanded number of young; that nestmates are neither so much older nor so much younger than the introduced youngster that it would either outcompete the natural young or be outcompeted. Maximum number per nest is dependent on the normal number of young for each species. A kestrel nest might do well with four to five chicks, whereas two to three would be maximum for an osprey nest.

Prey availability in each given season should be taken into account as well. If local raptors are having a tough year, fewer young per nest is warranted. Consult local natural history sources to find out the normal clutch size of each species.

## Captive Fostering

Using captive, nonreleasable adults as foster parents is also an option to be considered before hand-rearing. Some adults, either male or female, will foster any young of their own species that makes an appropriate sound; the only way to find out whether an adult will foster is to test it. To keep the young safe during the initial introduction, it is recommended that they be in sight of the adult but protected. For example, the nestling can be placed inside the captive adult's mew in a box or airline kennel with wire front, so that the adult can see the young and vice versa. Ideally, the box could have a rear door through which the human caretakers can feed the young without entering the enclosure. If the adult starts sitting near the nestlings, or tries to shove food through the wire in response to the begging calls, access can be provided (Figure 20.1).

If the adult takes no interest in the young, it can still fulfill the important role of a visual model. Once the youngsters are eating cut-up food off a plate, food can be placed in the box or kennel through a slot, while the young have 24-hour visual contact with the adult. Once at branching or fledging age, the two can be put together. If introducing them into the adult's territory gives rise to aggression, consider moving them both to neutral territory while taking the young through live-prey training.

### Re-nesting and Fostering Caveat

When re-nesting or fostering, the introduction of the young to the adults should be done as soon as possible, and all precautions to avoid imprinting on humans (e.g. use of feeding puppets, ghost costumes, feeding through a chute or slot) should be taken in the meantime. If, on introduction, the young bird reacts inappropriately to the adult by showing fear or aggression, it may be killed. If the youngster has been presented for care and it is not known how long the finder has had the bird, safely testing the youngster with a captive adult or conspecifics could be critical.

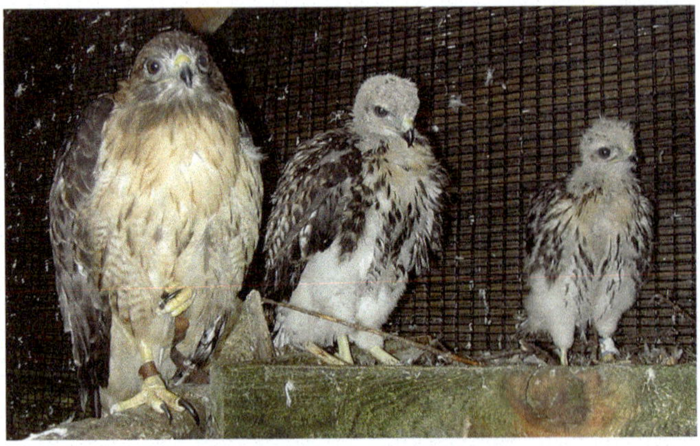

Figure 20.1 Education Red-tailed Hawk acting as a foster parent for two orphans.

## Hacking

Hacking is an appropriate technique, especially for a lone nestling at high risk of malimprinting and for young, bird-catching falcons and *accipiters,* for which it is really impossible to provide adequate live-prey training in a cage. A hackbox is a wooden box, the size of which varies depending on the type of bird for which it is designed. The front of the box is a door that is opened when the bird is old enough to begin exploring its environment, when it reaches "branching" age. The primary considerations are: (i) that the box be mounted such that the bird has a wide view of its surroundings (which should be habitat appropriate for the species, obviously, because the bird will be released there); (ii) that the bird be protected from the elements and predators; and (iii) that the back of the box must be solid except for a feeding slot so that the bird does not associate humans with food. For example, to meet the first criterion, the front and half the roof and sides can be slatted. For the second, the remaining part of the roof and sides would be made of solid wood for shade and protection from rain, and consideration should be given, depending on the location of the box, to add predator barriers such as wire on the outside of the slats or flashing around the base of the tree to prevent climbing. For the third, human access to the hackbox and the entire approach to the box should be from the back or blind side to avoid even a conditioned response that the approach of a human means food (Figure 20.2).

The young bird must be placed in the hackbox at nestling age, as soon as it is thermoregulating and eating cut up food from a plate. The hackbox is its nest, and it must have the opportunity to branch and fledge from there. It is of little use to place an older brancher or fledgling in a hackbox. There is typically not enough room to give it the exercise needed for flight and as soon as the door is opened, the bird may just disappear as there has been insufficient developmental time for it to

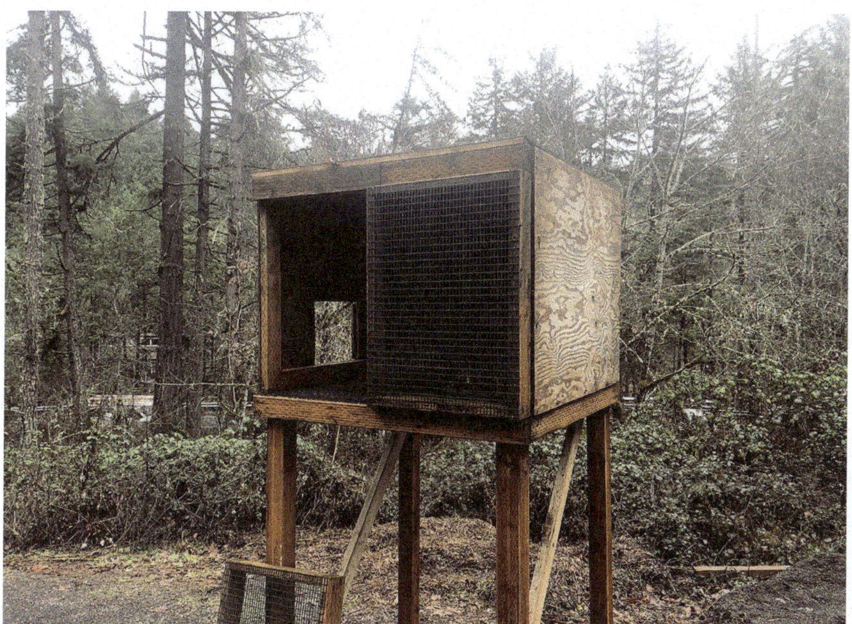

Figure 20.2 Hackbox with half of the front removed. Note the feeding slot that allows food delivery without chicks seeing humans. Once the front is permanently left open, the chick may return for supplemental feeding as it learns to hunt.

imprint on the hackbox as its nest. A bird that is imprinted on the box as its home nest will continue to return for food while exploring the area and attempting to hunt on its own. To this end, a *hackboard* or consistent feeding tray is used. Whether it is white or black or a plastic plate or board, it is important that it be something consistent and recognizable that the young bird will associate with food, even after the hackbox is opened. The bird will come back less and less as it becomes competent at hunting

## Conspecifics and Feeding Puppets

In the unfortunate event that none of the above is possible (for example, the nestling is injured and needs daily medication or bandage changes, there is no way to return the bird to its own or another nest, or no hackbox is available), hand-rearing will be necessary. Wherever possible through networking with others in the area, babies should be placed with conspecifics, because it will help limit the risk of human imprinting to be with other young of their own kind (Figure 20.3). These conspecifics can be older, if the single youngster can at least have visual contact with them, even when actually placing them together would put the nestling at risk. Care should be taken with *accipiters,* however, as the much smaller male is at risk of being killed and eaten if placed with even a slightly older female.

If feeding puppets are available, their use can make a huge difference when used as the youngsters' eyes are opening and beginning to focus. Providing 24-hour visual access to the puppet or to a study skin placed over a bottle of water, or taxidermy mount of an adult, can also be an important aid in appropriate imprinting (Figure 20.4). Human voices should be kept to a minimum, especially at feeding time. Even without puppets, "ghost" costumes (shapeless white or camouflage coverings to hide the human face and form) should be worn for feeding, as well as carefully facing the very young birds away from the person feeding. See Chapter 15 for more information on avoiding imprinting and habituation, and Chapter 19 for images of feeding puppets.

## Diet Recipes

With raptors, there is no substitute for a whole small animal diet. The age of the bird will determine how much, if any, casting material (bones, fur, feathers) should be given. The species of bird and its natural diet can help determine a substitute food while in care, but typically quail or mice

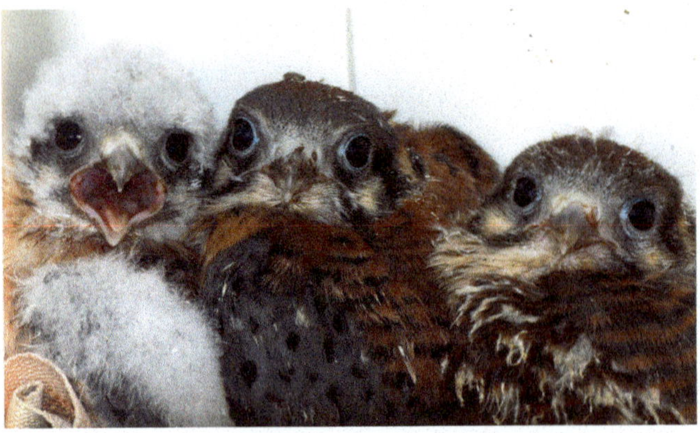

Figure 20.3 Young kestrels, and other orphans, benefit from being with conspecifics, despite an age difference.

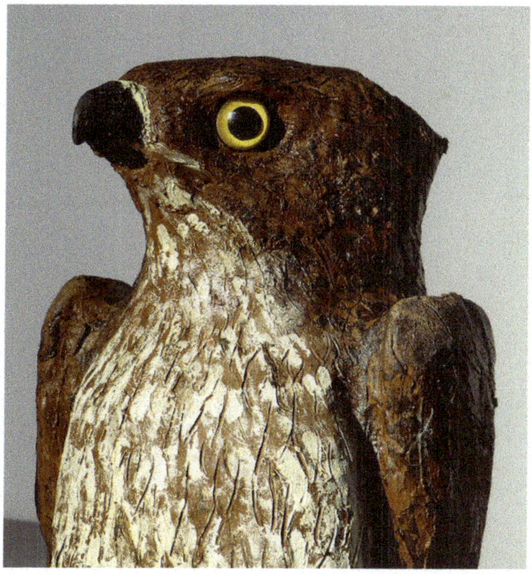

Figure 20.4 Hawk puppet that allows hemostat feeding through the mouth.

are a good place to start with very young birds that do not yet have, or need, a search image of what appropriate food for their species looks like. Day-old chickens can be fed to young raptors if the Ca : P ratio of the chicks is augmented. It is generally felt that the undeveloped bones of such young chickens are not sufficiently mineralized to provide enough calcium or phosphorus, even if what is there is in a low but balanced ratio (Ca : P of 1 : 1 is the typical ratio of a day-old chick).

If large numbers of young birds need to be fed, quail can be plucked; head, feet, wings, and lower intestine removed; and the remains then placed through a meat grinder. The resulting paste can be made into patties and frozen in a thin layer between sheets of waxed paper for later thawing as needed. Mice, too, can be easily skinned and ground. Remove heads prior to grinding. Leave the tails because they form an excellent source of calcium and, indeed, may be one of the first casting materials fed to chicks, because they are not as sharp as other bones. Using whole adult animals as food allows the nestling raptors to get the minerals from the bones they would otherwise be too young to handle whole.

## Feeding Procedures

### Hatchlings

Blunt forceps or hemostats can be used to pick up very small pieces of warm, clean meat (e.g. quail breast meat) dipped in warm water. The hemostat should touch the beak to elicit a feeding response: the hatchling will grab the food from the instrument as it would from the tip of its mother's beak, even before its eyes are open. It will be quickly obvious if a piece is too large or an awkward shape. Four or five very small pieces are probably all a hatchling can handle at a feeding before it falls back asleep. It is easy to see the food in the crop and easy to see or palpate when the crop is empty. Hatchlings should be fed every 2 hours or so during daylight hours, if the crop has emptied, the bird is hungry, and droppings have been passed. Very small bits of bone, carefully broken or ground can be included by 3 days of age, casting material by day 5. The food should be warmed to approximately body temperature by placing it in a container that is then placed in or above hot water. Dipping the individual pieces of food in the warm water as they are fed provides the extra moisture needed by hatchlings.

### Nestlings and Fledglings

Blunt forceps or hemostats may continue to be used to feed, until the nestling recognizes cut-up food on a small plate or lid and starts to pick it up on its own. This can be encouraged by placing the lid or small plate of food directly in front of the nestlings and picking the food up from the lid while they watch. Typically, younger nestlings dropping food seem to think it has simply disappeared; once they start to discover the food that has fallen to their feet, they are often ready to start picking it up themselves from a plate. The sooner they eat on their own, the less the risk of socialization to humans. Picking up small pieces of food from a plate should be expected by at least 2 weeks of age, usually before they can stand, though holding food down with their feet and ripping it up takes quite a bit longer, of course.

Once the birds' eyes are open and focusing, a puppet should be used for feeding, "ghost" costumes to disguise human caregivers should be worn, and the babies carefully faced away from the human feeder during meals. If at all possible, do not house a baby alone. Place it with or in sight of conspecifics or in sight of adult surrogates, if an actual foster parent is not available.

## Expected Weight Gain

It is important to chart weights daily, weighing them at the same time each day, preferably before their first meal. Weight gain in the first few days after hatching can be expected to be slow but should be steady. Hatch weight should double within 5–7 days, and will rise very rapidly after those first few days. With smaller species like the kestrel, approximate adult weight can be reached before they are even off their hocks and have much of their feather tips out of the sheath, at around 2 weeks of age. With the larger species, like the Red-tailed Hawk or Turkey Vulture, it may take 5–7 weeks to reach adult weight. Again, each species varies, but they should be able to pick up cut-up food from a plate or lid on their own within 10–14 days and should be placed in a hackbox at that point, if that is the method of choice.

## Housing

Hatchlings should be kept at 85–90 °F (29–32 °C) and around 40% humidity; however, more important than an absolute temperature and humidity level is watching the comfort of the birds. A cold baby will be reluctant to eat; a hot one may pant or be splayed out in the nest. These birds all have some natal down but cannot usually maintain their own body temperature until the secondary down comes in. This secondary down is very wooly in texture and provides excellent insulation.

For young chicks, towels (without holes or stringy edges) provide the best substrate. The towels should be arranged to surround them, as in a nest, giving them something to grip with their feet and to support them in an upright position with their legs tucked under (Figure 20.5). The hawks, osprey, harriers, and young kestrels *slice* their droppings: that is, shoot them either out or up or both. This creates an obvious challenge to keeping their enclosure clean! Caging should be cleaned thoroughly at least once a day, wiped down with a disinfectant such as dilute chlorhexidine, towels or papers changed, or the chicks moved to new housing as necessary to maintain a hygienic environment. It is critical that the young, growing feathers be kept clean, including those around the mouth, which can be soiled during feeding. Whereas adult birds that slice are usually given a tail

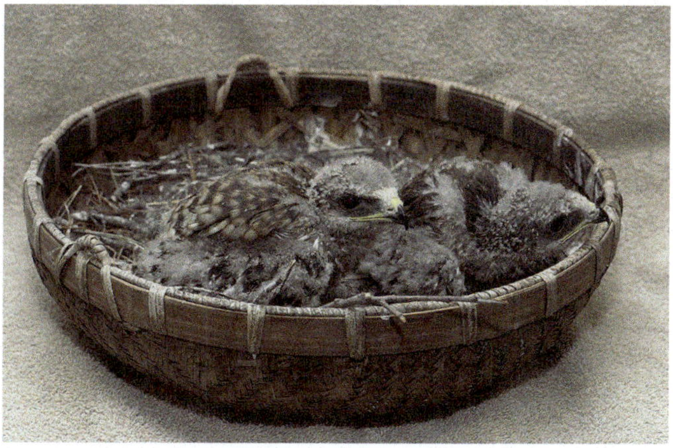

Figure 20.5 White-tailed Kite chicks in a nest. *Source:* photo courtesy of Lindsay Wildlife Experience.

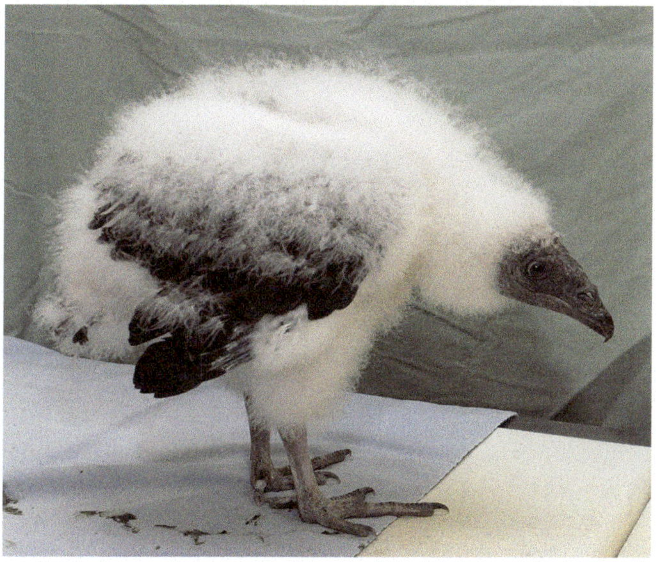

Figure 20.6 Turkey Vulture chick with white down and flight feathers emerging. *Source:* photo courtesy of Lindsay Wildlife Experience.

sheath while in hospital cages, this is not possible when the feathers are growing in, because the birds need to be able to preen the feather sheaths off.

As the birds come off their hocks (Figure 20.6) and start to flap their wings in practice flight, they should be allowed to *branch,* i.e. leave the nest and move around a safe environment. If thermoregulating and eating on their own, being outside with access to ambient temperatures and correct photoperiods, as well as sunlight, is important.

Minimum required cage sizes for pre-release conditioning can be found in Miller 2012. Recommendations vary widely in relation to the size and needs of the species, from 8×16×8 ft. high (2.4×4.9×2.4 m high) for kestrels, small kites, and merlins, to 20×100×16 ft. high (6.1×30.5×4.9 m high) for Turkey and Black Vultures, Ferruginous Hawks, Osprey, and Peregrine and Prairie Falcons. Walls should be constructed of wood or narrowly spaced wood slats, with no chain link or wire used anywhere the birds have access for clinging or climbing. Ample clean drinking and bathing water must be available at all times. Plastic artificial turf or indoor–outdoor carpeting must be used to pad round dowel or plastic pipe perches to help prevent pododermatitis (bumblefoot). Natural branches with textured bark make excellent perches. Provide at least two perches of varying heights and angles. Many rehabilitation centers suspend perches from pulleys such that when raised they form a "swing," which provides excellent exercise and practice landing on moving objects, and when lowered they allow easier cleaning or capturing of birds.

## Weaning

For most raptors, catching live prey is obviously a critical skill. Presentation of whole food items should begin as soon as the birds learn to hold food down and tear it up. Darkly colored mice make an excellent starting point for most species. With kestrels and the insectivorous kites, mealworms make a good starting food because their movement attracts the birds' attention. Adding live crickets is often the second step, then young mice, then older mice, and then providing the mice with hiding places. There is no way to really provide sufficient experience in captivity to prepare them for the real-world difficulties of wild prey, so releasing them at a time when, and in a place where, naïve young prey are available is critical.

## Preparation for Wild Release

A kestrel or harrier, possibly a merlin, and most of the *buteos* can probably receive adequate tuition in a large flight cage with a live-prey arena. Live-prey arenas are typically large, secure, open-topped containers placed within the aviary, where live prey is presented to the birds for hunting practice. These can be set into the ground or placed on the surface. These can be constructed of plywood with a secure bottom that cannot be dug through, or be a large pre-made container such as horse trough. Important aspects are that they must be rodent escape-proof and must be large enough for the birds to maneuver to capture their dinner.

For several species, however, live-prey arenas are not sufficient. Assuming re-nesting or wild fostering was not an option, hacking is the method of choice for *accipiters,* large falcons, and osprey. The latter should also be released in an area with other osprey, so as to provide models for fishing. The larger falcons and *accipiters* are best transferred to licensed falconers, if they cannot be hacked. The amount of practice, experience, and skill needed to catch birds on the wing needs to be learned with a backup system in place that can really be provided only by one of these two systems.

## Release

Besides flight conditioning and live-prey training, finding an appropriate release site is critical. A cavity-nester like a kestrel is best released into a nest box rather than simply allowed to fly off. Being hidden in a box adds a level of security and provides extra time for birds to recover from the stress of transport and handling. They can then look out of the box and get used to their surroundings rather than simply taking off for the horizon.

The timing of release is also critical. Ideally, release would coincide with the independence of wild young in the area, because that is designed to be optimal. If a migratory species, release must precede the earliest migration dates by at least 2 or 3 weeks for the bird to orient itself and practice hunting in a familiar place, before linking up with others of its species.

## Acknowledgments

Thanks to Carol Lee, South Plains Wildlife Rehabilitation Center, Lubbock Texas, for information on kites; to members of RaptorCare for generously sharing information, trials, and tribulations over the last 15 years; and to the great team of volunteers and staff at Cascades Raptor Center for tolerating me in all my moods.

## References

Chesser, R.T., Burns, K.J., Cicero, C. et al. (2018). *Check-List of North American Birds (Online).* American Ornithological Society http://checklist.aou.org/taxa.

Hawkins, M.G., Barron, H.W., Speer, B.L. et al. (2018). Birds. In: *Exotic Animal Formulary*, 4e (eds. J.W. Carpenter and C.J. Marion), 167–375. St. Louis, MO: Elsevier.

Miller, E.A. (ed.) (2012). *Minimum Standards for Wildlife Rehabilitation*, 4e, 116 pp. St. Cloud, MN: National Wildlife Rehabilitation Association.

Ponder, J. and Willette, M. (2017). Raptors. In: *Topics in Wildlife Medicine, Vol. 4: Orthopedics* (eds. R.S. Duerr and G.J. Purdin), 27–52. St. Cloud, MN: National Wildlife Rehabilitators Association.

## Further Reading

Brown, L. and Amadon, D. (1968). *Eagles, Hawks and Falcons of the World*, 945 pp. New York: McGraw-Hill, Inc.

Ehrlich, P.R., Dobkin, D.S., and Wheye, D. (1988). *The Birder's Handbook: A Field Guide to the Natural History of North American Birds*, 785 pp. New York: Simon and Schuster, Inc.

Ferguson-Lees, J. and Christie, D.A. (2001). *Raptors of the World*, 992 pp. New York: Houghton Mifflin.

Fox, N. (2000). *Nutrition, The Bird of Prey Management Series.* Faraway Films Productions.

International Wildlife Rehabilitation Council (2000). *Basic Wildlife Rehabilitation 1A/B, An Interpretation of Existing Biological and Veterinary Literature for the Wildlife Rehabilitator.* San Jose, California: International Wildlife Rehabilitation Council.

Johnsgard, P.A. (1990). *Hawks, Eagles & Falcons of North America.* 403 pp. Smithsonian Press.

Palmer, R.S. (ed.) (1988). *Handbook of North American Birds, Volumes 4 and 5: Diurnal Raptors.* 898 pp. New Haven, Connecticut: Yale University Press.

Poole, A. and Gill, F. (eds.) (1992–2004). *The Birds of North America.* Philadelphia: The Academy of Natural Sciences Washington, DC: The American Ornithologists' Union.

Weidensaul, S. (1996). *Raptors: The Birds of Prey*, 382 pp. New York: Lyons & Burford.

# 21

# Eagles

*Marjorie Cahak Gibson*

## Natural History

Eagles are a charismatic group of raptors. There are over 60 eagle species in the world; however, many are not even closely related. Eagles are categorized as "eagles" as much because of their large size and power as their genetic kinship with each other. They hold a great deal of fascination for the public; that interest can be both beneficial to eagle conservation, as well as problematic. Some of the allure of eagles is simply based on the elegant raptors' beauty, large size, strength, and the intrigue created by their very existence. Some fascination over eagles is centered on the myriad myths and legends that depict eagles and follow the huge birds throughout every culture since the recorded history of man began on the walls of cave (Bahn 2016).

This is an exciting time in the history of the Bald Eagle in the United States. With the help of the banning of DDT in 1972 and passage of the Endangered Species Act in 1973 (Baur and Irwin 2010) the eagle population has recovered well. No one alive today has seen the population of Bald Eagles in the U.S. as high as it is at this time in history. The eagles themselves are making changes as they adapt to the stronger eagle population and the challenges that come with it. Once, not long ago, remote habitat available for hunting and breeding was plentiful. Now the big birds are feeling the squeeze to find adequate nesting and hunting territories that fulfill their needs. At the same time, the human population is growing and increasingly encroaching on wilderness areas in which to live and recreate. Areas that were previously difficult for people to access are now fully accessible with all-terrain vehicles and even snowmobiles. Human disturbance is becoming a part of life for Bald Eagles in populated areas. Large nesting trees are needed to support the eagle's massive nests that can weigh over a thousand pounds. Safe, abundant prey that has not been exposed to toxins such pesticides, rodent poisons, or lead fragments is vital for eagles to successfully raise a family. Eagle rehabilitators in areas of high density report territorial disputes that cause death or serious injury to one or both participants are at an all-time high. As the eagles adapt to their new normal of a higher population and increased stressors associated with living closer to the human population, so too must we as wildlife rehabilitators. For instance, release protocols have had to change to keep up with the eagles' responses to changes in their population and other stressors such as habitat loss. Spring, summer, and fall releases in areas of the country that enjoy a near-saturated Bald Eagle population are no longer possible without the threat of endangering an entire nest due to a territorial dispute. In wildlife rehabilitation, the wild population must take precedence over the

*Hand-Rearing Birds*, Second Edition. Edited by Rebecca S. Duerr and Laurie J. Gage.

release of a rehabilitated bird. If the release may cause a negative response in a wild nesting pair, it is not ethical to release in that area or at that time.

### Species Considerations

The natural history of each species and other members of its genus provides vital guidance for captive care, and may show regional variation. Legal guidelines and laws that govern the handling and captive care of eagles may vary in each state, province, or country. Most eagle species of the world are found in Africa, Europe, or Asia (Clark 1999; Steyn et al. 2001). North America has two native eagle species (Dunne and Karlson 2017), whereas three species are native to Australia (Hollands 2004), and nine are found in Mexico, Central, and South America (Clark and Schmitt 2017). Be aware that species may vary greatly in terms of behavior of both the adults and youngsters, tolerance for disturbance at the nest, and parental care post-fledging. Behavior varies greatly between individuals as well as species. These aspects must be considered before intervening or removing an eaglet from the nest area. Consult with local or regional wildlife professionals when possible to obtain history and information regarding the specific nest site and adult birds in residence at the nest before interacting with it.

## Criteria for Intervention

Eaglets are always best reared by their natural parents whenever possible. After an examination, if an eaglet is found to be healthy, has no serious injuries, and can eat and digest food well, it is possible to return it to the nest. If the natural nest has been destroyed, an artificial structure should be considered if it can be installed at or very near the original nest site. When using an artificial nest or nest platform, or fostering an eaglet into a different wild nest of the same species with a single same-age chick, it is not ethical practice to overburden and therefore jeopardize a natural wild nest. The natural wild nestlings must take precedence over those already in rehabilitation as they hold a higher likelihood of successfully becoming a reproductive adult.

### Questions to Ask the Public

Questioning the individual that has found an eaglet is important to make sure the chick is truly injured or in need of care. Ask that photos be taken of the eaglet and its surroundings and sent to the center. In this way the rehabilitators and veterinarians can evaluate the chick before it is moved or removed from the nest area.

- Are the parents in attendance? A single parent can finish rearing an older chick.
- Is blood or obvious traumatic injury visible?
- Is the chick in immediate danger from dogs or other predators?
- Are weather conditions in the area a risk for the chick (forest fire, floods etc.)?

Most eaglets admitted to wildlife rehabilitation centers are youngsters that are not yet flighted, have been found on the ground, and do not have parents in attendance. Situations causing a chick to leave or be ejected from the nest include a predator at the nest or storms that cause nest trees to be toppled or youngsters to be blown out. Territorial aggression by sparring adults at the nest can oust an eaglet accidentally and cause failure of the nest structure. Loud sounds near a nest, particularly those at night – such as fireworks – may cause a chick to bolt and flee the nest. This scenario is particularly true as a chick nears fledging. Occasionally, low prey availability either from loss of one or both parents or failure of a prey source will cause a chick to abandon its nest.

No matter the cause, a young eagle that is on the ground after a fall from a great height may have suffered serious injury, including fractured bones, head injury, or internal injuries. It is also very possible for an eaglet to survive such a fall in miraculous fashion, with few if any injuries. The chick should be carefully evaluated in the field. Photos taken in the field and sent to the wildlife rehabilitator play an important role in evaluating the eaglet and making a choice to bring it into captive care or simply replace it in the nest.

### Mortality in the Wild

The mortality of raptors is high in the first year of life, even in the best of circumstances with natural nests and wild parents. Sources suggest over 50% of Bald Eagles in wild nests die in their first year of life. Causes of mortality at the nest vary greatly and include siblicide, weather events, low prey availability, hazardous material such as fishing line in the nest, or even ingestion of tainted food delivered by the parent. Post-fledging causes of mortality include that of a weak individual unable to hunt adequately or compete with their counterparts, injuries due to disputes with other eagles, vehicle collisions, illegal shootings, encountering other obstacles such as wind turbines, or toxin ingestion. Rearing an eagle in captivity without the advantage of a species-specific foster parent to teach it hunting, vocalizations, cues for social behavior, and survival techniques, reduces its chance of success.

## Re-nesting and Fostering

### Return to Natural Nest

This option can be used if the original nest and supporting structures are stable. After a physical examination, if an eaglet that has not yet fledged is found to be healthy, with no serious injuries, and can eat and digest food, the best option for the eaglet and its family is to return it to its own nest. The temptation to remove an otherwise healthy eaglet from his nest area for captive care should be avoided.

Adult eagles will accept a returned chick if it is behaving and vocalizing normally. Siblings of the same nest will accept the chick, if the food supply is adequate for all nestmates and the age of the chicks is within a few days of each other. Rejection occurs when a chick is not well or unable to compete with the siblings. A nonviable chick at the nest may endanger the eagle family. When returning a chick to its nest, take a light towel (not frayed) or similar weight material with you. After replacing a chick in the nest, place the towel over it and the sibling for a few minutes and back out of the nest bowl. The weight of the towel is important as it allows the chicks to feel "brooded." They will settle and the panicked "fight or flight" response to danger will abate. After a few moments, slowly remove the towel and continue your descent.

Do not attempt to replace a chick if it or the siblings are near fledging. The disturbance created by climbing the nest tree and approaching the nest may cause the eaglets in the nest to bolt and leave the nest prematurely. An option for a nearly-fledged chick is to place it on a sturdy adjacent tree. This technique allows an older chick to vocalize to the adults alerting them to its presence, as well as allow it to return to or near the nest on its own. Leave the area immediately or the eagles may not be comfortable approaching the youngster. Monitoring can be carried out if necessary, using a spotting scope at a distance.

## Artificial Nest Platforms

The use of an artificial nest is useful if chicks were ejected from their nest and the natural nest was either destroyed or inaccessible. An artificial structure should be considered if it can be installed at or very near the original nest site. Raptors have defined territories that they defend vigorously. The nest should be a strong and stable structure approximately 4×4×1 ft. (1.2×1.2×0.3 m). The nest should be installed high enough that the parents feel comfortable to return and resume caring for the youngsters. Generally, it is best to aim for a height of 25 ft. (7.6 m) at a minimum. There should be enough cover to protect the youngster from weather and predation. The type of artificial platform used will depend on the species, local habitat, and age of the chick. It can be as simple as a box type platform with sturdy sides and drainage holes drilled in the bottom. Keep in mind the structure must be large and stable enough to accommodate the eaglets as they grow and reach full size, as well as their parents. Edges should be sturdy and extend 10–12 in. above the platform material to protect eaglets from falling. Sides will also serve as a perch for the youngsters as they grow. Place newly cut pine boughs or similar material native to the surrounding habitat in the nest to cushion the eaglets, provide familiar surroundings, and allow the chick to begin using its legs and feet for perching.

## Wild Fostering

This technique involves placing a chick in an existing, same-species, wild nest with parents other than their own. Wild fostering can be used with many species of raptors, including eagles, if the species is amenable. When considering this technique, be certain the wild family is the same species with a single same-age chick. Different age chicks in the same nest may result in siblicide of either the fostered or natural chick. It is not ethical to place chicks in a natural nest already at capacity. The result will overburden the parents and jeopardize the success of the wild nest.

## Foster Parent Reared at Wildlife Facility

No one can raise an eaglet as well an eagle. A wildlife rehabilitator may try their best, but the fact is we are humans not eagles and they are not humans. Experience has taught us that the life of any species, including our own, is far more complicated than being supplied food and a clean space in which to grow. We cannot teach an eaglet the social cues, vocalizations, and other vital behaviors that will make them successful with their own species. If a chick is to be raised in captivity for release to the wild, it is important the facility rehabilitating the chick have a foster parent of the same species to raise the chick or immediately transfer the eaglet to a facility that does. This is the only way to assure the young eagle has a future in the wild. Delay in transfer of even a few days may affect the outcome of the eaglet in terms of being releasable to the wild.

The foster parent or parents should be nonreleasable wild adults, and preferably have reared chicks in the wild. The sex of the foster parent is not important other than males seem to be more at ease with chicks than females; however, that varies with individuals. Human imprints are not an option as a foster parent. Human imprinted eagles are not "normal" and therefore cannot teach the chicks normal behavior or vocalizations. The chances of an imprinted adult killing the chick is great. Education birds are acceptable; however, they must remain in the rearing chamber with the eaglets with no interruption until the youngsters are fledged and ready to begin the flight conditioning process.

### Puppet Rearing

Puppets have been used to rear young raptors and prevent human imprinting. Along with the puppet, the caretaker is gowned in a costume meant to both change the outline of a human form as well as to offer a rough visual depiction including appropriate colors of the parent bird of the species. In some cases, the disguised appearance of the human caregiver has been considered adequate to rear orphaned chicks. While those techniques still play an important role in caring for chicks while in critical care and rearing some species, especially those that are rare or endangered, it is labor intensive and has some problems including the lack of socialization and species confusion in the offspring reared in this manner. Puppet rearing continues to be successful for birds that will remain in a zoo situation or other captive care (Wallace 2000; Finkelstein et al. 2015). Foster parents of the same species are key to the rearing and release of normal, well-adjusted wild eagles.

## Initial Care and Stabilization

Normal body temperature for avian species is between 104 and 106 °F (40–41 °C.). Eaglets are covered with very light-brown down at hatch until they are about 10 days old. At this first stage of life, they are unable to thermoregulate or control their own body temperature. The ability to thermoregulate begins to develop gradually about the same time that the eaglet's down changes to a dark gray color, or when the eaglet is about 2 weeks old. Before that time, the body temperature of the young eaglet reflects that of their surroundings and, consequently, they must have a supplemented heat source to support their body temperature, unless their parents or foster parents are brooding them.

Eaglets admitted from dire situations in the wild, such as fallen nests or flooding, will often be in shock, hypothermic, and dehydrated upon admission (Figure 21.1). They will present huddled, shivering, lethargic, and uncoordinated, and have a slowed heart rate and slowed respirations. It is vital to warm them quickly during evaluation. This is best done in an incubator or a cardboard box version of an incubator described below. When examining the patient, do so on a heated

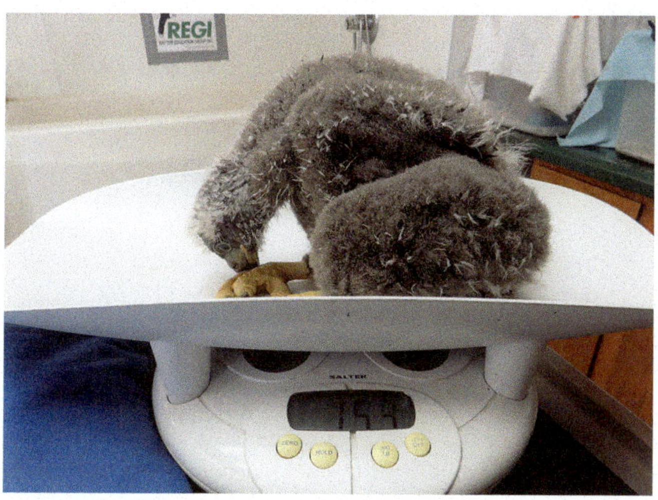


Figure 21.1 Eaglet being weighed. Cold, dehydrated chicks will appear droopy and poorly responsive.

examination table or a heating pad on low, with towels between the heat source and the patient to prevent burns and overheating. Rehydration with warmed fluids is important to bring the core body temperature up to normal range before extensive handling and examination. If the chick is alert, rehydration can be accomplished orally with warmed fluids tubed into the crop or proventriculus with a red rubber or silicon catheter. Warmed subcutaneous (SQ) fluids are important as well if sterile fluids, syringes, and needles are available. Place the eaglet in a heated "box" incubator at 95–99 °F (35–38 °C), without disturbance, for several hours until the body temperature returns to normal. At that time, begin to treat any injuries or reason for admission.

In the case of an eaglet presenting with hyperthermia, over 109 °F (42.7 °C), methods to bring down the body temperature must be implemented immediately along with fluid therapy. Depending on the age of the patient, cool/ice packs can be used under their wings as well. Refrain from handling the young patient as handling can raise the body temperature. Monitor your patient closely through both physical signs of recovery (increased activity and mental awareness, etc.) and body temperature. If the patient is conscious, cool, not cold, water can be tubed into the patients crop.

Both body temperature extremes of hypothermia and hyperthermia are emergencies that can cause patient death quickly even in the absence of injury or disease. They must be recognized immediately on admission and treated to stabilize the patient before evaluating most injuries or other reasons of admission. Both hypothermia and hyperthermia cause combinations of brain dysfunction, heart irregularities, cellular death, and organ failure.

Towel and blow drying a wet eaglet before putting it into a warming area will speed the warming process. If using a blow dryer, take care not to burn the eaglet's delicate skin, face, feather follicles, and emerging feathers with excessive heat. It is helpful to use your own ungloved hand when evaluating the temperature of a blow dryer before using it on a patient.

Traditional clear incubators that allow full vision of the chick should be avoided as they add stress to the young bird and present an opportunity for human imprinting. If these are used, cover the incubator with a towel or attach solid paper to the exterior. Traditional heat lamps should be avoided as intense temperature is directed into a small area and can cause severe burns. The author uses a low-tech incubator that consists of a clean cardboard box with towels in the bottom and a heating element under the box itself. A heating pad on low or other appropriate heating element placed under one-half of the box to reach 95–99 °F (35–38 °C) creates gentle, consistent warming. This method allows the eaglet to rest and recover without the visual stimulation of lights or humans, or the sounds of a clinic (Figure 21.2). Mirrors can provide chicks with companionship (Figure 21.3). Secure mirrors well to the box or carrier to prevent accidental injury to the patient.

## Diet

The regular diet of a healthy young eagles in rehabilitation or captive care is based on the age of the chick and species. The diet should be as natural as possible, if the bird is able to digest food normally. A good basic diet for young eaglets in captive care is pinkie mice, rats, and muscle meat from rabbit or other natural prey items other than fish. Vitamin supplements such as Nekton-Biotic Bird and Nekton-Calcium should be used as well as an additional calcium supplement until the patient is on a full normal prey diet. The diet should continue to evolve as the young eagle grows until finally opened whole prey is presented. Prey items can be supplemented with beef heart or whatever nonfatty unprocessed muscle meat is available.

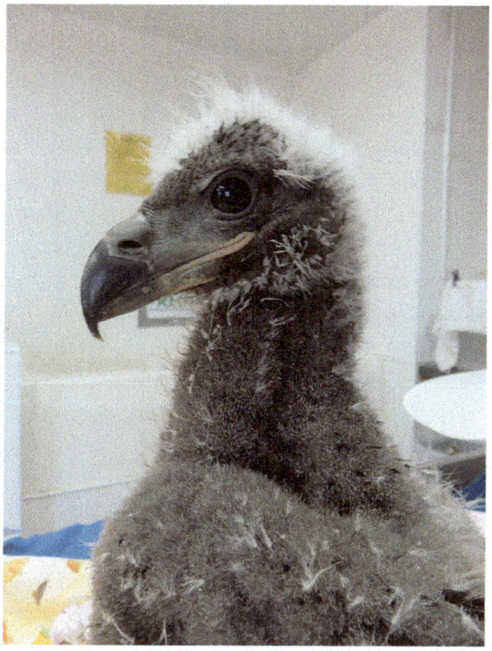

Figure 21.2 Warm and well-hydrated chicks will appear alert and responsive.

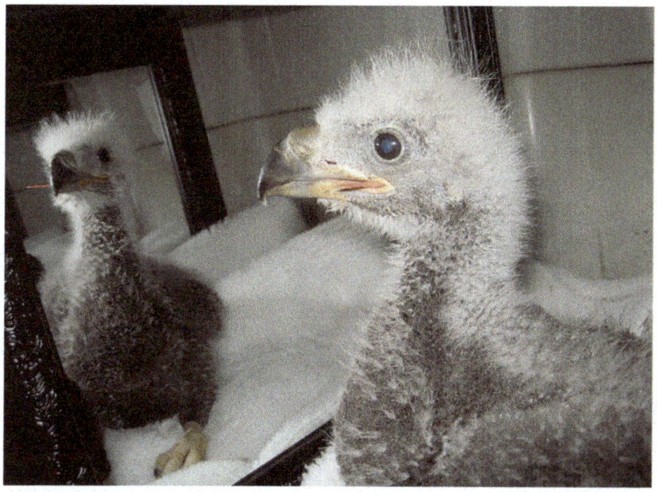

Figure 21.3 Small housing with eaglet provided with mirror as companionship and to prevent the chick from focusing on human caregivers. Secure the mirror well to the box or carrier to prevent accidental injury.

## Re-feeding Process for Emaciated or Debilitated Patients

Feeding a whole diet to an emaciated bird can have fatal results. Emaciated or debilitated birds must go through a process of "re-feeding." Re-feeding is an important step in the recovery of the bird's metabolism and digestive systems after a period of starvation.

During the hand-feeding and critical care process, care should be taken to not imprint the bird to the human handler. The critical care area should be quiet, without human voices. Visuals should be limited to a mirror for the chick and natural habitat images. Some rehabilitators suggest that the use of nature sounds is helpful to young birds and gives the chicks a distraction to the otherwise unstimulating atmosphere of a critical care room. The caregiver should use a gown or costume, mask, and gloves to disguise the human form. If a puppet is available for the species, it is wise to use it for food delivery while the chick is in critical care.

Eaglets that are severely emaciated or debilitated when admitted should be tube-fed a warmed, not hot, liquid emaciation diet for obligate carnivores such as Carnivore Care (Oxbow Animal Health) or Emeraid IC Carnivore (Lafeber Company). The author often uses human chicken baby food as a first food during recovery. Use either a luer-lock syringe and stainless-steel feeding needle to deliver smaller amounts of diet to a younger eaglet, or a catheter-tipped syringe and red rubber catheter tube for larger eaglets of 4 weeks and older. Tube-feed the emaciation diet for 1–3 days until the chick begins to digest fully and easily. If they are not digesting well in that time frame, continue with the liquid diet until they do. Amounts fed will depend on the eaglet's age, development, and degree of emaciation. During any one feeding the crop should be not be more than one-third full until digestion is occurring at a normal rate. As a rule of thumb, feed every 3–4 hours during daylight hours (7:00 a.m.–9:00 p.m.). Small pieces of muscle meat and skinned chopped pinky mice may be added to the diet once the crop is emptying normally. Feed small easily digestible meals four times a day while continuing supportive tube-feeding of the liquid diet. This slow return to a normal diet allows the digestive system to re-engage and begin functioning again. Resist the urge to overfeed the youngster that is undergoing the re-feeding process. If the crop has not emptied a few hours after a feeding session, skip the meat diet for a few feedings. The re-feeding process may have to be restarted more than once with extremely fragile emaciation cases. Once the chick is clinically recovered and is digesting well, add natural diet items gradually while reducing tube-feedings until the chick is eating normally.

Very young eagles, in their first few days of life, eat only the muscle meat from an animal with no bones. Quail breast or other pure muscle meat cut into small bite-sized pieces and moistened with Nekton-Biotic-Bird, which contains probiotics to aid digestion normally transferred by the adult bird mouth to food items fed to the chick, is a good first meat meal. Calcium supplement should also be sprinkled on the meat meals. Young eagles up to about 2 weeks of age do not self-feed and will have to be hand-fed small bite-sized pieces and cut-up pinkie mice and rats with the use of feeding tongs or forceps. By 10 days of age, eaglets are eating small amounts of finely crushed bone (no sharp edges) as well as the muscle. As the young bird reaches 3 weeks, it will begin to try to take meat from a carcass. Do not offer whole fish at this age as fish bones easily penetrate the thin walls of the digestive tract of a developing bird. The chick will not be able to totally self-feed in this way, and small pieces of meat with finely crushed bones and calcium supplements must continue to be provided. The act of pulling at its food helps the chick develop strong neck and back muscles. Meat supplied to chicks at this age should have calcium carbonate with vitamin D pills crushed and liberally sprinkled on it.

Once the eaglet is out of critical care, eating and digesting well, it should be allowed to eat as much as it wants with no restrictions on amount. Chicks do not overeat, ingesting only what their growing bodies require. As with any young bird, eaglets will eat more, up to three times the amount of a healthy adult, until they are fully developed. Some food should always be left over in the box after feeding to assure the eaglet is getting enough. Weighing amounts is good practice for documentation; however, the metabolism varies in each individual patient: hence, it is hard to know exactly in terms of weight how much an eaglet should eat in any given day. The eaglet's food demands are the best guide.

Once the chick is active, eating and digesting normally, can pick food up by itself, is thermoregulating and vocalizing, it can be placed in a rearing chamber with other eaglets of similar age.

## Common Medical Problems

### Lead Poisoning

Once the patient is stable it is advisable to get an x-ray to ensure there are no lead fragments or hooks in the digestive system. Lead fragments as well as hooks, sinkers, and fishing line are regularly found in eaglets still in the nest. It is good practice to do a blood lead test on admission of all eagles including eaglets as they may have seen exposed to lead in the food fed to them by the parent on the nest. Lead exposure causes neurological problems as well as other nonspecific symptoms that may be misinterpreted as injury from fall from a nest or other incident.

### Imprinting

Imprinting is a learning process by which a newborn or very young animal establishes a behavior pattern of recognition and attraction to its own species. It is a permanent learning process and alters the animal for its lifetime. Imprinting cannot be reversed or changed. Imprinted eagles and other raptor species are not suitable for release to the wild. They have very little option for life in captivity. The harsh reality is, because they become aggressive to humans, dogs, or whatever crosses their path, most imprints are killed either by their wild counterparts or by humans they encounter. When we hear of an eagle or raptor acting aggressively toward a human, outside of a nesting situation, it is likely a human imprint. The window of imprinting begins at hatch and in large species like eagles, condors, and vultures, the period of imprinting continues to some degree past fledging. The author has found that in situations of serious injury or trauma, a fledged eaglet can revert and once again be susceptible to malimprinting to humans. In the case of an injured fledged eaglet, it is important to limit human contact and place them with other eagles as soon as possible, even as they continue to recover from their injuries. The presence of other eagles of any age will reinforce their natural behavior and avoid malimprinting. Isolation of the young eagle does not replace contact with its own species.

A great deal of information is transferred to the chick by a parent bird including appropriate body language, vocal cues, and behaviors. This information in totality allows the young bird to be accepted by its counterparts in wild society (Wilson 2001). The society of birds is more complicated than previously understood. We continue to learn as we gain experience with these species. New methods including nest cams allow us to observe and better understand natural behaviors at the nest and social requirements as never before (see Box 21.1 Webcams). Social behaviors, including proper vocalization and knowing how to interact with all age groups of other eagles, is key to the young bird being successful in the wild.

### Habituation

Habituation is the process of people or animals becoming comfortable with something or a situation, so that they no longer find it unpleasant or think it is a threat. It does not affect the identity of the species and is not a permanent condition. Habituation is essentially taming, and can

**Box 21.1 Nest Cams**

***Jean Pichler***

The popularity of nest cameras has played a major role in piquing interest in many avian species, including eagles. Remote viewing cameras were originally used by scientists to document behaviors and aid in data collection for sensitive, protected, or difficult to access species. Both live streaming and video recorded Bald Eagle nest cams revealed new data and information that could not be collected from ground observations alone. The educational aspects of these nest cam observations for researchers, classroom students, citizen scientists, and nature enthusiasts were soon realized, and remote viewing opportunities are now available to anyone with Internet access and a webcam for 24-hour a day nest views of an eagle family during their most intimate moments. With advances in camera technology, throughout the breeding season the eagle family can be observed and heard in real time engaging in courting, bonding, laying, and hatching eggs, and rearing tiny, helpless chicks that weigh merely ounces until 10–12 weeks later when they are as large as their parents and ready to fledge. While under observation by a wide range of people from the comfort of their computers, the activities of these protected birds can be documented and enjoyed by professionals and the general population alike, resulting in greater understanding and appreciation of the eagles' behaviors and natural history. For some avian species, such as Bald Eagles and condors, whose populations are recovering from near extinction, this newly acquired information is rewriting previously held knowledge that was based on very limited populations and even more limited access to the birds' actual natural history surrounding nesting habits and nest successes and failures.

It follows naturally that with this manner of exposure, viewing an eagle's home life, creates an emotional response. The public can relate to what they observe, interpreting for themselves the activities they witness. They develop a greater awareness not only of the birds' life cycle but also the interactions between adults, and adults and chicks. People are beginning to consider questions such as whether eagles are intelligent beings involved with their own life, family, and survival. Or are they, as some would suggest, mere feathered objects that respond only by instinct, without the capacity to recognize each other or their family? Emotional responses by the public can be beneficial to wildlife conservation. This often encourages the public's interest in birds, raises awareness of the challenges wild birds face, and promotes personal relationships and actions that aid wildlife conservation – including volunteerism and financial support. People understand as never before that wildlife and the natural world matter to them and that help may be needed, especially when humans are responsible for negative impacts upon wildlife.

Because of this increased exposure to wildlife, education regarding legal and ethical issues, conservation, and rehabilitation is paramount especially for the general public. Overly emotional reactions to natural occurrences – such as eaglets' failure to thrive, attacks by nonmates, invasive nest encounters with other species, and calls for immediate intervention or rescues – expose negative consequences of publicly viewed nest cams. While often well-intentioned, individuals sometimes assume they must interfere with or even possess wildlife, including eagles, in inappropriate or destructive ways. Overly emotional and potentially harmful engagement by the public may be countered by fostering a more genuine understanding and appreciation for wild species through increased educational opportunities and appropriate exposure to wildlife, including to nonreleasable ambassador animals.

be reversed as circumstances change. It is not beneficial for a wild bird to be habituated, particularly in the habit of seeking out people when it is hungry. Habituated birds are rarely aggressive; however, if an eagle approaches people or domestic animals, its intentions may be mistaken as an attack.

To prevent the patient from becoming habituated, in the months prior to release, cease any personal interaction such as focused food delivery or special attention. It is important that a wild patient also not interact with domestic pets including dogs, cats, or farm animals in a casual manner. They may become habituated to dogs and incorrectly perceive them not to be a danger, or approach farm animals they see as companions. That behavior is not looked on kindly by the public and may be interpreted as an attack, which can lead to the eagle being killed due to the misunderstanding between species. It is important for their life in the wild to remain wild in every aspect from seeking food to the company that they keep.

## Expected Weight Gain and Feather Development

Eaglets grow quickly. At hatch, a Bald Eagle weighs just 70–100 g, but 10–12 weeks later when they are ready to fly and leave their nest, they weigh in at 2.7–6.8 kg depending on gender (females are larger) and the area of the country in which they are native. The rapid growth rate requires a constant food supply always available to the young eagles in the nest. While in captive care, food should not be withheld or limited if the youngsters are healthy and appear alert. Good quality and quantity of nutritious food items supports the growth of bones, organs, connective tissue, and feathers. If the young eagle's food intake suddenly stops or is compromised due to parental loss, storms that prohibit a parent from hunting, or lack of prey availability, the eaglets growing body suffers. One of the most visible indicators is reflected in the feather growth. When a chick suffers either physiological or nutritional stress, the feathers that were developing at the time of the stress will develop stress bars across the feathers. There are times when the stress bars are so extreme that the tail feathers break off, leaving the young eagle with a short tail. In these cases, the remaining feather shaft may be too weak to allow successful imping of tail feathers. The full tail is important to flight. The tail feathers are longer in a chick than an adult and play a vital role in successful flight and maneuverability. It is not advisable to release an eagle that does not have full-length tail feathers.

## Housing

### Rearing Chamber

The rearing chamber should be a large area 40 × 60 × 20 ft. (12.2 × 18.6 × 6.1 m) that contains natural logs and perches. It should have limited sound of human interaction or activity. Nature soundtracks played during daylight hours may help provide a natural ambiance to the chamber and mask human sound in the area. The rearing chamber should have cameras to allow the rehabilitation staff to observe the eaglet's growth and development remotely. In this way, the health and behavior of the eaglets, as well as their interaction with the adults and each other, can be documented without entry to the chamber. A constructed nest 4 × 4 × 1 ft. (1.2 × 1.2 × 3 m) lined with fresh pine boughs and elevated at least 2 ft. (0.6 m) from the floor will be needed to accommodate up to three eaglets. Additional nests and foster parents can use the same rearing chamber (Figures 21.4 and 21.5). A "hatch" or "food drop" door should be used to deliver food to the foster

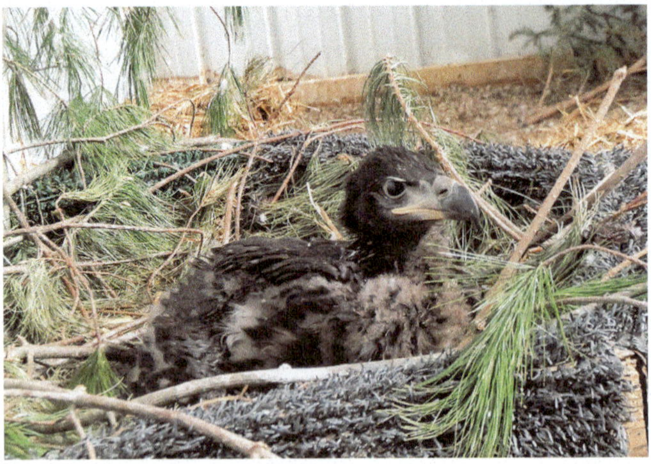

Figure 21.4 Eaglets in an artificial nest.

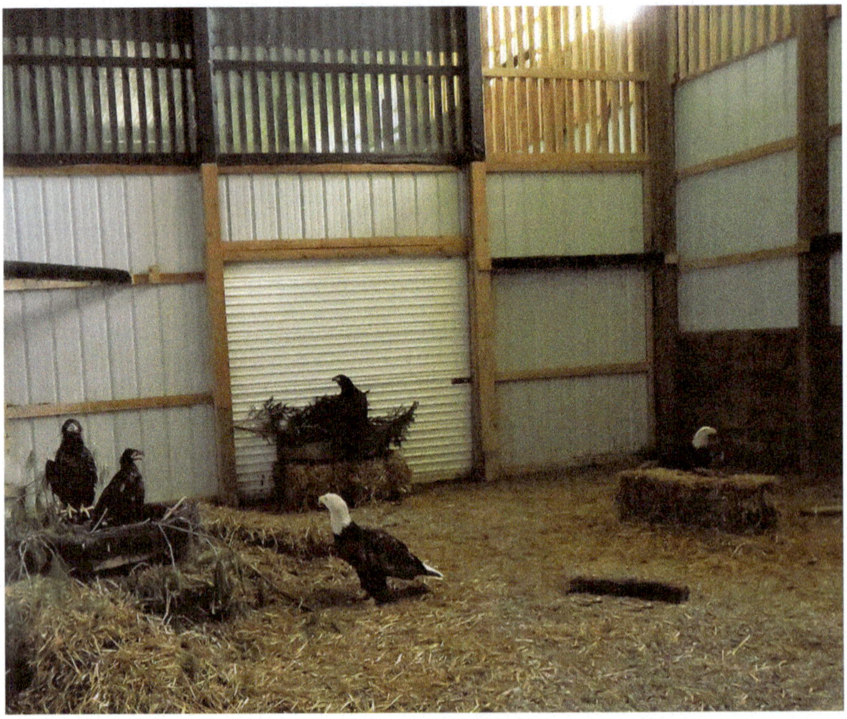

Figure 21.5 Foster parents and eaglets in a large aviary rearing chamber.

nest rearing chamber. Two separate food delivery drop doors or hatches should be used. One hatch delivers food to the nest that is age appropriate for the eaglets. The second food drop is used primarily to deliver food to the foster parents. This system allows for separation of the diet of the adult fosters and the diet and amounts fed to the eaglets.

Cleaning in the rearing chamber should be done quickly no more than once a week and less if possible, unless there are special circumstances that affect the health of the family. The eaglets may be weighed and evaluated at the same time. In the wild, eagle nests contain food past its prime that is not sanitized. It is important that the eaglets are exposed to the bacteria they will encounter in the wild. In doing so they will develop the strong immune system needed for a life in the wild.

Several eaglets can be reared together without danger if they are all well-adjusted (not imprinted) and adequate food is supplied. The large chamber allows the eaglets to exercise and begin flying when ready. Ideally, the eaglets should remain with the foster parent in the rearing chamber for a month or more past the time they fledged. This time will give them additional behavioral information and confidence which will be important when they are put into a flight enclosure with other eagles to begin conditioning for release to the wild.

### Flight Aviary

The conditioning flight is a large enclosure 110 × 35 × 28 ft. (33.5 × 10.7 × 8.5 m) (Figure 21.6) that allows the young eagles to develop their flight muscles and hone flight maneuvers while learning to interact with other eagles of all age groups. The building should be free of support structures that could cause injury to birds in flight. Perches on each side of the structure should be padded and covered in artificial turf or loop-free pile carpet to protect the eagles' feet from injury. Food is

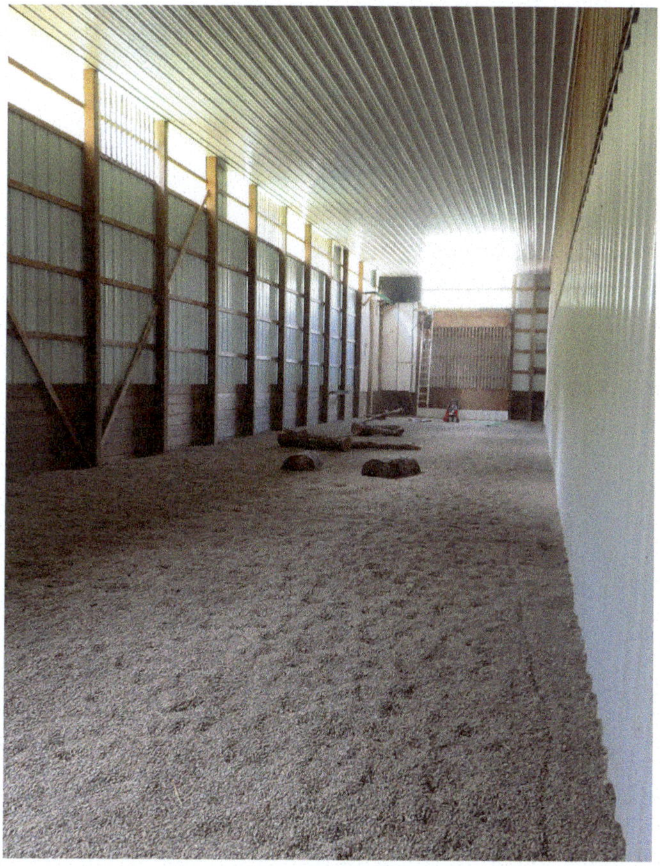

Figure 21.6 Eagles require a very large flight conditioning enclosure in order to develop flight muscles and practice flight maneuvers while socializing with other eagles.

placed on the floor or on logs accessible to the eagles. Food items including opened carcasses of deer (donated from deer farms or car hit and pre-evaluated for lead fragments by radiographs), rabbits, rats, salmon and other fish, or other natural prey items that the eagles will encounter in the wild. Domestic animals including road-killed dogs, cats, or whole chickens should never be fed to young eagles, as those items will become incorporated as part of their search image as natural prey choices. Natural prey items may be augmented with trimmed commercially purchased beef heart or other lean meats. A large part of an eagles' diet in the wild consists of carrion. Exposure to natural prey is an important aspect of training for young eagles, not only teaching them to recognize carrion in the wild, but also providing the experience of gaining confidence while being competitive during interactions with other eagles around food. A young eagle that has not been exposed to these conditions will not be prepared for life in the wild.

Bald Eaglets leave the nest between 10 and 14 weeks of age depending in part on the individual and geographic location of the nest site; however, adults continue to provide support for the youngsters post-fledgling. The adults act as a safety net when the youngsters are learning how to maneuver, how to fish, and whenever they need assistance. Usually, youngsters stay relatively close to their parents, but not always. Releasing a young eagle because it can fly is akin to letting a human toddler live alone. The use of a conditioning flight where young eagles can experience and learn from other aged eagles including other adults is important. It has been documented through banding and satellite tracking that immature Bald Eagles return to their natal area in the years following fledging and occasionally until they become sub-adults (Gibson et al. 2005)

## Preparation for Wild Release

### Flight Conditioning

Flight conditioning is imperative to develop the muscles needed for flight as well as agility. Conditioning is vital to the successful release of any bird, including eagles. No eagle should be released unless it has been actively flying and has demonstrated the ability to turn and maneuver well in flight.

The most successful way to exercise an eagle is in a large flight aviary. This technique has many advantages including the fact that the bird can self-exercise and interact with others of its own species, gaining socialization experience as well as flight training. Free flight is recommended for at least several weeks to a month or more in the case of body trauma or wing injuries to ensure the birds' muscles are back to full use.

### Creance Flying

Creance flying is a falconry technique used to exercise birds with the use of a line attached to the leg jesses. It is used when exercising raptors for release in situations where no conditioning flight is available; however, creance flying has its limitations. It is a labor-intensive process for the handler, stressful for the bird, and has limited ability to demonstrate ability in flight.

The bird must be 100% capable of flight, maneuvering, and landing. A bird's feathers serve many purposes. They are its means with which to fly and provide waterproofing and insulation from the elements. Birds that come into rehabilitation often present with feather damage either from a trauma incident or nutritional deficit. Flight and tail feathers must be present and full length. Imping feathers into the tail is possible if only a few are damaged and the remaining feather shafts are strong (Scott 2016) and have excellent feather quality, or the bird is not a candidate for release to the wild. The bird may need more time in the conditioning flight or may need to complete a molt before it is ready to succeed as a wild bird.

## Release

The release of a patient is the final stage of rehabilitation. The release must be planned and carefully considered as seriously as every other aspect of care from admission through flight conditioning. The best option for the release of a young eagle is to find a wintering area where eagles of all ages congregate. Wintering areas are chosen by eagles because the site is habitat that can support a large congregation of eagles with a reliable and abundant prey source, while having limited human disturbance. Wintering eagles are not defending their own territory and aggressive disputes are rare. Adult eagles are cooperative with immature birds and will often assist a youngster.

Networking with other rehabilitators, birding clubs, and wildlife professionals will ensure an appropriate site for successful release. Traditional thought was that a bird should be released at the site where it was found. That was sound advice in the past and still is for many species and some circumstances. However, in some parts of the U.S. where the Bald Eagle population has reached near saturation levels, release at the same site is simply no longer possible without endangering or causing the death of both the released patient and their wild counterparts. Where once territorial disputes were skirmishes that ended with the loser leaving the area, in recent years a dispute may well end in the death of one or both birds. As our population of Bald Eagles has recovered in the U.S.' lower 48 states, eagle behavior is changing. We can expect it will continue to evolve in response to population pressure, habitat loss, prey availability, and toxic events such as lead exposure. These changes require rehabilitators to pay close attention to the eagles' behavior and alter our protocols, especially those surrounding the release of patients. Currently, many parts of the country have reached what biologists feel may be a saturated population. Eagles are increasingly reluctant to accept newcomers moving through their territory. While this example is of Bald Eagle recovery in the United States, that scenario may be true of any population of eagles anywhere in the world that has faced population change, habitat loss, or other stressors.

It is well documented through the banding and tracking of released eagles that no matter where they are released, Bald Eagles naturally return to their natal sites and to their territory on their own. Convincing an anxious property owner that wants "their" eagle back of that fact can be difficult. It is, however, the responsibility of the wildlife rehabilitator to educate and make certain the patient is released safely and has a chance to continue to recover or adjust to the wild without being attacked, reinjured, or killed. When it eventually returns to the natal area or its former territory, it will be on its own terms and in its own time. A dispute may occur, but the bird will have a choice to participate in a dispute or not, rather than being tossed into a bad situation where it has no choice.

There are parts of the country where the Bald Eagle population is not as robust and habitat loss not as evident. In these regions, the rehabilitator can still return a bird to its site; however, that should be done carefully and with the advice of local biologists. The population is changing quickly in some regions. Keeping pace with the behavior of the local birds is not an exact science. It is far better to err on the side of safety for your patient as you educate the public on the new normal for eagle rehabilitation.

## Acknowledgments

My thanks and gratitude to Pete Bloom for sharing the wonderful world of raptor research –along with his passion for the natural history of everything – with me so long ago. My parents and sister for loving their strange little bird girl despite my tunnel vision, and my dear family for their love and support as I continue to dedicate my life to eagles and all wild birds. My thoughts are of the thousands of birds that have passed through my hands over the past 50 years; it has been my honor to know each one.

## Sources of Products Mentioned

Carnivore Care: Oxbow Animal Health, 11 902 South 150th Street, Omaha, NE 68138, (800) 249-0366, info@oxbowanimalhealth.com.

Emeraid IC Carnivore Diet: Lafeber Company, 24981 N 1400 East Road, Cornell, IL 61319, (800) 842-6445, https://lafeber.com, for international inquiries, please call +1–815–466–8040.

Feeding Tongs: Trans American Medical, 7633 W. 100th Place, Bridgeview, IL 60455, (708) 430-7777.

Nekton-Calcium-Plus and Nekton-Biotic-Bird: Nekton USA, 600 F Street, Arcata, CA 95521, (707) 822-2417, www.nekton.net.

Red Rubber Catheter/French Silicone Catheters and 60 ml Catheter Tip Syringes: Vitality Medical, 7910 South 3500 East Suite C, Salt Lake City, Utah 84121, (800) 397-5899, https://www.vitalitymedical.com/guides/urinary/catheter-product-comparison-and-sizing-guide.

Stainless Steel Feeding Tubes and Luer Lock Syringes: Veterinary Specialty Products, 10 504 W 79th St, Overland Park, KS 66214, (913) 268-3108, www.vetspecialtyproducts.com.

## References

Bahn, P. (2016). *Images of the Ice Age*. Oxford University Press.

Baur, D.C. and Irwin, W.R. (eds.) (2010). *Endangered Species Act: Law, Policy, and Perspectives*. American Bar Association.

Clark, W.S. (1999). *A Field Guide to the Raptors of Europe, the Middle East, and North Africa*. Oxford Press.

Clark, W.S. and Schmitt, N.J. (2017). *Raptors of Mexico and Central America*. Princeton University Press.

Dunne, P. and Karlson, K.T. (2017). *Birds of Prey: Hawks, Eagles, Falcons, and Vultures of North America*. Houghton Mifflin Harcourt.

Finkelstein, M., Kuspa, Z., Snyder, N., and Schmitt, N.J. (2015). California Condor (*Gymnogyps californianus*), version 2.0. In: *The Birds of North America* (ed. P.G. Rodewald). Ithaca, NY, USA: Cornell Lab of Ornithology. https://doi.org/10.2173/bna.610.

Gibson, M.J., Papp, J., and Murray, D. (2005). Bald Eagle (Haliaeetus leucocephalus) natal dispersal in the Upper Peninsula of Michigan. Raptor Research Foundation Conference, Green Bay, WI.

Hollands, D. (2004). *Eagles, Hawks and Falcons of Australia*, 2e. Nelson.

Scott, D. (2016). *Raptor Medicine, Surgery and Rehabilitation*, 2e, 212–293. CAB International.

Steyn, P., Kemp, A., and Knobel, J. (2001). *Eagles of Africa*. Sunbird Publishers.

Wallace, M.P. (2000). Retaining natural behavior in captivity for re-introduction programs. In: *Behavior and Conservation* (eds. L.M. Gosling and W.J. Sutherland), 300–314. Cambridge, UK: Cambridge University Press.

Wilson, E.O. (2001). *Sociobiology*, 2e, 175–255. Belknap Press: Harvard University Press.

## Further Reading

Bird, D.M., Seymour, N.R., and Gerrard, J.M. (1983). Biology and management of Bald Eagles and Ospreys. Proceedings of 1st International Symposium on Bald Eagles and Ospreys, McGill University, Quebec, pp. 325.

Bortolotti, G.R. (1984). Criteria for determining age and sex of nestling bald eagles. *Journal of Field Ornithology* 55 (4): 467–481.

Brown, L. and Amadon, D. (1989). *Eagles, Hawks and Falcons of the World*. Wellfleet Press.

Carpenter, G.P. (1990). *Illustrated Guide for Identifying Nestling Bald Eagles in the Field*, 31. San Francisco, CA: San Francisco Zoological Society.

Christie, D.A. and Ferguson-Lees, J. (2010). *Raptors of the World*. Bloomsbury Publishing 992 pp.

Garcelon, D. and Schwemm, C.A. (eds.) (2005). *Proceedings of the Sixth California Islands Symposium, Ventura, California, December 1–3, 2003*. Arcata, CA: Institute for Wildlife Studies.

Gill, F.B. (2006). *Ornithology*, 3e, 748. W.H. Freeman.

Jackman, R. and Jenkins, J. (2004). Protocol for evaluating Bald Eagle habitat and populations in California. Prepared for U.S. Fish and Wildlife Service, Sacramento, CA. pp. 1–23. https://nrm.dfg.ca.gov/FileHandler.ashx?DocumentID=83707&inline.

Kiff, L.F., Wallace, M.P., and Gale, N.B. (1989). Eggs of captive crested eagles. *Journal of Raptor Research* 23: 107–108.

McLaughlin, G.S., Beheler, K.A., Sileo, L., et al. (2004). Winter mortality of Bald Eagles along the Lower Wisconsin River. Proceedings of the American Association of Wildlife Veterinarians and Wildlife Disease Association Joint Conference, San Diego, CA, pp. 312–313.

USFWS. (2007). Bald Eagle (Haliaeetus leucocephalus) fact sheet. https://www.fws.gov/pacific/ecoservices/documents/bald_eagle_fact_sheet.pdf.

Wallace, M.P. (1994). Control of behavioral development in the context of reintroduction programs for birds. *Zoo Biology* 13: 491–499.

# 22

# Coots, Gallinules, and Rails

*Marie Travers and Isabel Luevano*

## Natural History

Coots, gallinules, and rails belong to order Gruiformes and the family Rallidae. They are generally shy wetland species that build floating nests, and their chicks are semi-precocial or precocial at hatching. All birds in the family Rallidae are small to medium sized and have short, rounded wings and short tails. They all also have large feet with long toes adapted to walking on marshy land and aquatic plants, except for coot species, which have lobed toes that enable them to swim better than the rest of the rallids. The most variable feature within this family is the bill. In some species (e.g. coots), the bill is short and somewhat wide; in other species (e.g. the Clapper Rail), the bill is longer than the head and slightly decurved.

Rallids are opportunistic omnivores whose diet depends on the seasonal and local availability of a wide variety of plant matter, invertebrates, seeds, fruits, small vertebrates, and sometimes carrion. Once hatched, chicks are able to leave the nest within 6–48 hours, depending on the species, although most are fed and brooded by their parents for the first few weeks. Rails, coots, and gallinules are considered sub-/semi-precocial, meaning that once hatched, they can leave the nest and walk, swim, and forage (Conway 1995; Bannor and Kiviat 2002; Brisbin Jr. and Mowbray 2002).

Chicks of these species typically have blackish down covering much of their bodies, plus several species have sharply contrasting head coloration known as "chick ornaments" consisting of bright reddish-orange feathers. American Coot chicks have a reddish-orange, bald-appearing head with fringes of these brightly colored plumes (Figure 22.1), while Sora hatchlings are covered with black down with a bright reddish-orange bill ornament and fringe at the base of the bill.

### Coots and Gallinules

Compared with rails, coots and gallinules are outgoing and easily seen. Whereas gallinules are generally solitary species, coots often flock like ducks, swimming in open water and waddling conspicuously on shore. Gallinules, often called moorhens (or "marsh hens"), comprise 10 species worldwide, 2 of which, the Common Gallinule and the Purple Gallinule, are native to North America. These birds are more shy and more solitary than American Coots, but share the coots' duck-like appearance, although not the specialized semi-lobate toes that enable coots to quickly move across water surfaces (Bannor and Kiviat 2002). See Figure 22.2a and b for a comparison of toe morphology.

*Hand-Rearing Birds*, Second Edition. Edited by Rebecca S. Duerr and Laurie J. Gage.

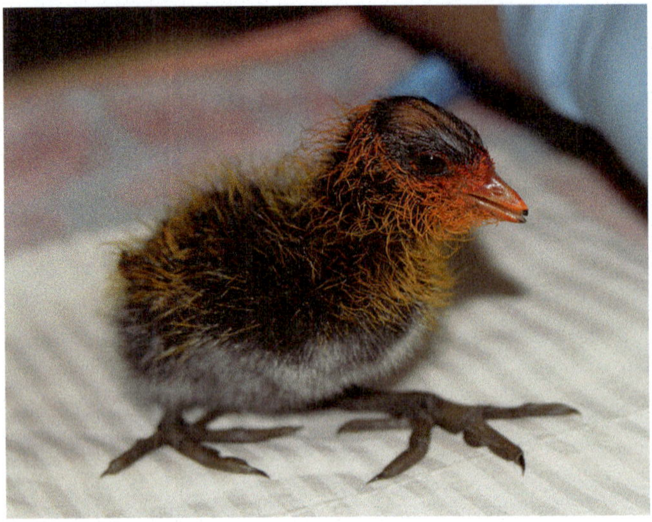

Figure 22.1 American Coot chick, note semi-bald head with bright colorful plumage. *Source:* photo courtesy of International Bird Rescue.

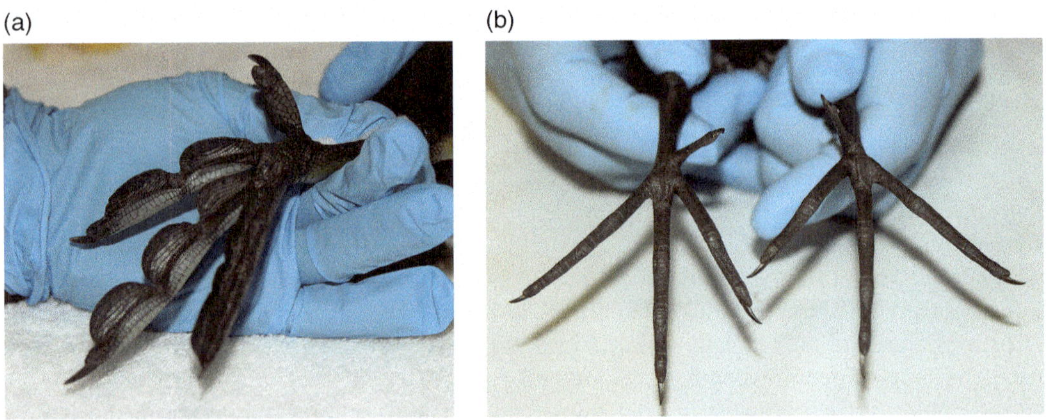

Figure 22.2 (a) Semi-lobate toes of an American Coot. *Source:* photo courtesy of International Bird Rescue. (b) Non-semi-lobate toes of a Common Gallinule chick. *Source:* photo courtesy of International Bird Rescue.

Coots occupy a variety of habitats, ranging from shallow freshwater wetlands with cattails, to prairie potholes, to swamps and marshes, to suburban park and sewage ponds, to the edges of large lakes. They prefer areas of standing water with a muddy bottom. They are common in wetlands having a mixed coverage of tall, exposed vegetation along with open water, mudflats, and areas with matted vegetation. Although often found in shallow freshwater areas, they can also occupy deeper wetlands and saltmarshes.

American Coots mainly eat aquatic plants and insects, such as algae, duckweed, and eelgrass. When on land, they pick at terrestrial plants and sometimes eat seeds, beetles, snails, spiders, flies, small fish, slugs, crayfish, and frogs. Typically, they probe the surface of muddy and silty-bottomed wetlands for prey at dawn and dusk (Brisbin Jr. and Mowbray 2002).

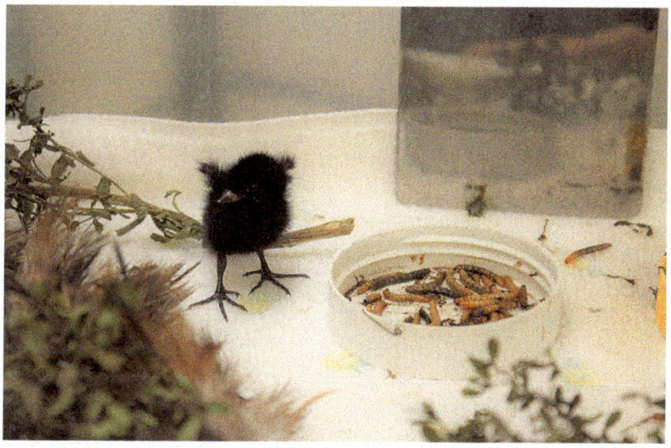

Figure 22.3 Black Rail chick in heated brooder with mirror, vegetation for privacy, and shallow dishes of various invertebrate foods. *Source:* photo courtesy of International Bird Rescue.

### Rails

In contrast to other rallids, rails are shy, secretive birds, with cryptic, irregular coloration that enables them to hide among reeds at the water's edge by day. There are 127 species of rails distributed throughout the world except for at high latitudes. They vary in length from about 4–18 in. (11 to 45 cm) and have laterally compressed bodies that allow them to move furtively in dense vegetation. While many rails are very rarely seen, their loud calls can reveal their presence in dense, marshy areas, often at night.

The young of all rail species have black down and are about the same size as the adult Black Rail, which is the smallest rail, and which has the smallest chicks, a mere 2–3 g at hatch (Figure 22.3). These semi-precocial chicks are capable of leaving the nest as early as 6 hours after hatching but typically stay on the nest for up to 2 days. The parents feed chicks from their bill until the chicks are about 2–3 weeks of age. Most rails leave their family unit after 4 weeks (Conway 1995).

## Criteria for Intervention

Human disturbance of nesting sites is one of the main causes for intervention for baby coots, gallinules, and rails. Disruption of their habitat creates a situation in which both the adults and their young can be stressed and scared, leading to separation of the adult from its young. Many of these birds, especially the smaller rail species, come into care because of being caught by a predator such as a cat, and predation of parents may also result in an orphaned chick that needs help. Fledged chicks and adults that enter the rehabilitation setting often present with head trauma caused by being flushed out of their environment, chased by a predator, or striking a car or window.

## Record Keeping

Detailed records are vital to bird care and continual improvement of rearing techniques. Until the bird is eating well and gaining weight on its own, its weight should be checked daily, and detailed care notes should be recorded. Each time the chick is handled for a weight check, notes should be made about hydration, bone growth, feather condition, and enclosure. Until the chick is reliably self-feeding, a quick (no longer than a few minutes) but thorough physical exam should be completed daily to monitor growth and check for any medical issues.

It is also important to note behaviors, vocalizations, and ambulation to ensure the bird is growing at a normal pace and showing signs of normal behavior. Temporary banding of patients is ideal when multiples of the same species are in care; this ensures individual birds are tracked, and key behavioral and physiological changes are monitored. Temporary leg bands should also be checked regularly to ensure they do not become tight as the chick grows. Electronic or paper records should be kept in a well-organized location where all caregivers can easily access them and record notes. When working with an unfamiliar species, photographic documentation of milestones is useful for informing future care.

## Initial Care and Stabilization

### Special Considerations

Coots, gallinules, and rails are secretive and easily stressed, so contact with humans should be kept to a minimum. Whenever possible, these birds, especially rails and gallinules, should be housed in a very quiet, calm environment, since an increased stress level can inhibit growth, reduce feeding, and slow the healing process. A stressed bird that is struggling to hide from view or to avoid capture can easily injure itself. A video baby monitor mounted within an enclosure can limit the number of entries needed and allow easy observation. In addition to being easily stressed, these birds are incredibly fast, so care should be taken during handling – for instance, covering a bird's head and body with a cloth to help reduce visual stress and the risk of escape or injury. Use a non-looped fabric, such as a pillowcase, during handling to avoid catching these birds' long toes and nails. In addition, flighted coots, gallinules, and rails are talented escape artists, so housing needs to be specially prepared to limit escapes.

As with all baby birds, treatment should begin with heat, fluids, and feeding, in that order. Chicks should be warmed before they are given fluids, and fluids should be given until they are hydrated and pass normal droppings. All new patients should be given at least 15–20 minutes to rest in a warm, dark, quiet location before being examined. This allows the bird time to de-stress and normalize. Immediately on arrival, chicks should be placed in an incubator at 92–99 °F (33.3–37.2 °C) and left to rest and get warm. A heating pad or other removable heating element can be added temporarily for critically cold chicks until they become warm and active. The initial rest period also allows time for the examiner to gather supplies for the exam and to set up an appropriate enclosure into which the bird can be moved following the exam. Very small chicks that are not yet self-feeding can be offered fluids by drawing a warmed droplet of rehydration solution (such as lactated Ringer's solution or other isotonic electrolyte solution) along the side of the closed bill. If the droplet does not wick in or if the bird is not seen to swallow, the bill can be very gently turned up so that gravity encourages the solution inward. Chicks should be offered as much as they will drink, one drop at a time. The offering of fluids should be repeated every 30 minutes, alternating between the rehydration solution and a 50% dextrose solution, until the bird becomes active. The purpose of the dextrose solution is to raise the bird's blood glucose level so that the bird will become active, alert, and hungry. The best starting point for housing for young chicks is a 90–100 °F (32.2–37.8 °C) incubator with 70–80% humidity.

Once the bird becomes alert and active, live food can be offered in shallow dishes. Birds that are not alert are at risk for aspirating or lying in their food and becoming dirty. Live food items (such as tubifex and small mealworms) are helpful in that their movement stimulates the bird to start pecking and self-feeding. Because many rails, gallinules, and coots are semi-precocial, their food may have to be gently dangled on the tips of hemostats until they are reliably self-feeding. This replicates an adult offering food. However, if the bird is not alert or active enough to respond to food items offered in these ways, the rehydrating process of offering fluids every 20–30 minutes should be restarted.

Chicks should be housed in a warmed environment until they are reliably self-feeding. Raising rail chicks with conspecifics may help encourage eating behaviors, decrease stress, and decrease the chance of habituation. Rallid chicks can become habituated, so human contact, especially in the case of coots, should be limited. Disguise human faces and hands when interacting with chicks, especially when coots are fed by hemostat or offered food.

## Common Medical Problems and Solutions

### Pododermatitis

Coots, gallinules, and rails are highly susceptible to foot issues such as pododermatitis (bumblefoot), which is classified as dry, cracked bottoms of feet that may become infected. Monitoring the feet of birds in care is vital. Foot issues can be treated or minimized by providing proper substrate and cleanliness throughout care. It is vital to offer access to water and keep pool water clean to keep feet healthy and free from lesions.

### Metabolic Bone Disease

Metabolic bone disease (MBD) may occur in rallid chicks and may manifest as ambulation issues or rubbery soft bones, so it is important to palpate birds' bones and monitor their ambulation daily to detect the presence of this problem. This disease is often caused by a vitamin D deficiency or insufficient dietary calcium intake. Vitamin D and calcium supplements can be given on a regular schedule for all young, growing birds, with additional calcium given to chicks with fractures or skeletal development problems.

### Caught by Predator

Chicks often arrive into care because of predator (e.g. cat) capture. In this case – whether or not there are injuries found – the bird should be started on a prophylactic antibiotic course, such as amoxicillin with clavulanic acid at 125 mg/kg every 12 hours for at least 5 days or until wounds have healed (Hawkins et al. 2018).

### Head Trauma

Head trauma is another common problem, often seen in older fledglings in the form of neurologic issues, vision impairment, and/or head wounds. Depending on the severity of the neurologic issues, birds can often benefit from being put in a quiet environment with food and shelter in order to recuperate. Offering anti-inflammatory medications, such as meloxicam at 0.5 mg/kg orally every 12–24 hours (Hawkins et al. 2018), can help reduce pain and swelling from head trauma. It is important to note that access to heat should be limited for patients with head trauma because warmth can increase swelling.

## Diets

Coots, gallinules, and rails are omnivorous and thus should be offered a wide variety of food items while in care. Their diets naturally vary by season, location, and availability of food items, so it is important to provide a smorgasbord of food for them. As is true for many species of birds, rallid parents feed their young a diet high in protein during the first 2 weeks of life, so that is what chicks will need in care. Appropriate live food items include mealworms (small or medium), tubifex worms, and minnows (generally found at aquarium or pet stores or bait shops). Nonlive food items that can be offered are seed, frozen–thawed bloodworms, brine shrimp, and krill, duckweed, or other greens, small slivers of fish (cut to fit the chick's bill size), and a small amount of soaked waterfowl starter (a high-protein and nutrient-dense diet supporting health and growth of adolescent waterfowl). All food items should be sprinkled with vitamin $B_1$ and calcium carbonate powder at each feeding.

Food items should be placed in shallow, size-appropriate dishes in which birds can wade and feed without risk of drowning or other harm. It is important to observe chicks to ensure that all food dishes are safe and allow the bird to get in and out easily and to feed properly. A tiny chick can easily drown in a dish that is too deep. Small jar lids, ashtrays, small platters or trays, and other shallow types of dishes work well for presenting food (Figures 22.3–22.5). Dishes can be elevated if there is concern that chicks will lie in them and get food on their feathers. All food should be checked three to four times per day and refreshed as needed, but caregivers should always be mindful of the fact that any disturbance is stressful for these birds. One way to cut down on food-related disturbances is to notice whether birds are eating all of their food quickly or are eating

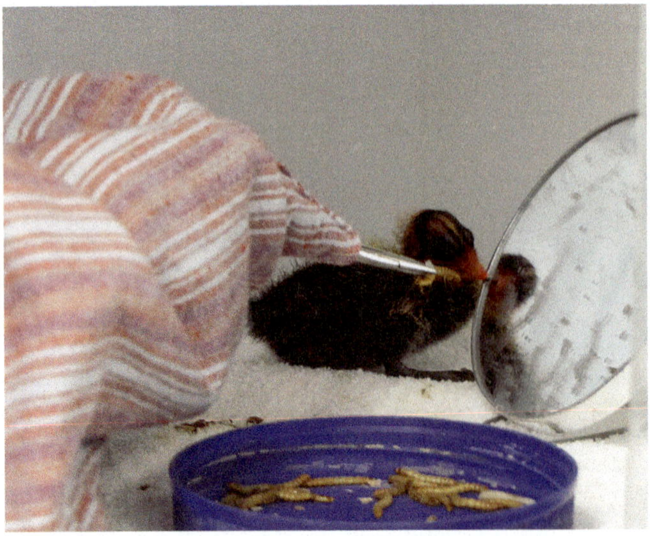

Figure 22.4 American Coot chick being hemostat-fed by a disguised human arm. *Source:* photo courtesy of International Bird Rescue.

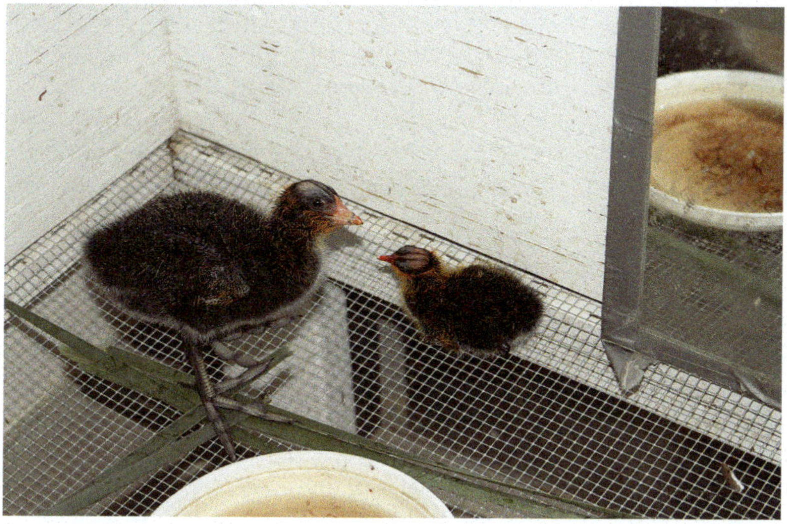

Figure 22.5 Coot chicks of different ages typically get along well. Note the shallow dish of water with bloodworms, and the mirror. *Source:* photo courtesy of International Bird Rescue.

mostly certain items, and then making sure to offer larger quantities of those items. Food that is being offered in a heated environment should be changed several times through the day to prevent feeding chicks spoiled food.

Frozen food items need to be thawed before they are presented, and food items must be sized for the birds being fed – small, young birds will only be able to eat what fits into their mouths. Very young birds may be more inclined to eat live food, because they will be attracted to the movement, which will usually stimulate foraging and eating. For chicks less than a week old, large mealworms can be cut into smaller pieces so they can easily be eaten.

As birds grow, increasingly large food dishes can be offered so that birds get used to foraging in larger areas. Once birds are active and alert, a shallow bathing dish should be put in all enclosures so that birds can maintain clean and healthy plumage.

## Feeding Procedures

Coots, gallinules, and rails are extremely secretive birds, so providing a quiet environment with hiding places and a normal photoperiod is key to successful self-feeding. Housing should be set up to simulate a natural environment, should contain shallow feeding dishes (such as small lids or platters), and should be away from humans, since gallinules and rails become too stressed to eat when disturbed or frightened. Coots and gallinules can be raised together if similar in age, which helps decrease the chance of habituation; and most rail species can be raised together because they do not show much aggression toward each other. Raising rails with coots or with gallinules is not ideal, however, given the differences in size, growth rates, and stress levels.

The key to determining when a bird is able to self-feed is to monitor and record all feeding behaviors. Use of a remote camera can provide critical information. Once birds are self-feeding, they should be weaned off hemostat-feeding, and weight should be closely monitored to ensure that it is no longer needed.

Food items that could contaminate the birds' feathers should be offered in shallow dishes, such as jar lids, ashtrays, or shallow pans/serving trays, and should be made to look as natural as possible. Food items that will not contaminate feathers (such as greens) can be offered in a pool or bathing water. All food and water dishes should be changed on a regular basis. Ensure that the dishes used are the proper size so that all birds housed together, even if of different ages and sizes, can get in and out of dishes safely. For all birds in care, calcium powder should be added to their food items to grow strong, healthy bones.

### Rails

As semi-precocial birds, most rails stay on their nests for at least 1–3 days, depending on species and disturbance by humans/predators. Immediately upon hatching, chicks are weak and wet; once dry and active, their parents will feed them for 1–2 weeks, until the hatchlings can reliably forage and feed themselves. When in care, any chick less than 2 weeks of age should be hemostat-fed every 30 minutes until it is reliably eating on its own. Determining a rail chick's age by weight is difficult since many rail species vary in size. It is necessary to research each species to identify hatchling versus fledgling weights. As hatchlings, most rails will be downy and fluffy; as fledglings, most will have some adult feather growth.

Rail diets vary with species' primary food source, so it is important to identify the species in order to offer the proper food options. It is best to offer a wide variety of live and frozen invertebrates, as well as seeds and aquatic greens. All wet food can be combined in a small shallow container that is suitably sized to allow the bird to easily wade into the container to access the food. This mimics their normal eating situation – finding food in shallow, moist, wet, marshy areas.

### Coots and Gallinules

Coots and gallinules can leave the nest 6 hours after hatching, but they usually remain on the nest for up to 2 days unless disturbed by humans or a predator. Once they leave the nest, they begin to pick at food items but continue to rely on parental feedings until they are 25–30 days old. In care, coot and gallinule hatchlings should be offered a wide variety of live and frozen food items, as well as seed and aquatic greens. These can be placed in shallow, size-appropriate dishes (or other, similarly shallow containers) that allow the birds to easily step into and out of them. For birds from 1 day to 2–3 weeks old, hemostat-feeding may be necessary every 30 minutes or until the bird is reliably self-feeding. Coots and gallinules are *highly* susceptible to habituation, so humans who care for and feed them must cover their hands (and faces, if need be) during all feedings. See Chapter 19 for more information regarding methods of reducing habituation.

### Hatchlings

Hatchlings and birds younger than 2–3 weeks generally need to be offered food items with a hemostat (Figure 22.4). With birds this young, it is important to carefully observe feeding behaviors and back off on hemostat-feedings as the bird learns to self-feed. This will encourage more self-feeding and potentially lower the bird's disturbance-caused stress level. Monitor the bird's self-feeding behavior by observing the bird quietly and discreetly. Also, when you begin to cut back on the hemostat-feedings, keep an eye on the bird's weight, measuring it daily or even twice a day (a.m. and p.m.), to ensure it is increasing. The goal is to wean the bird off hemostat-feeding and get it self-feeding as soon as possible to limit its exposure to human interactions and disturbances.

Gallinule chicks may respond better to hemostats with red/orange tips, likely because their parents display red frontal shields that may be used to get chicks' attention for feeding.

### Fledglings

Older coot, gallinule, and rail chicks – those 3 weeks of age or more – usually self-feed when food is presented properly and there are hiding places and appropriate lighting in their enclosure. Offering fledglings live food can inspire self-feeding more quickly. Weight must be monitored the first few days that a fledgling is in care to be sure it is eating and gaining weight. Wet food items (thawed frozen food, live food) should be offered in separate, appropriately sized (for safety) shallow dishes from dry food items. A dish of clean water that contains aquatic plants can serve for bathing if the bird is alert enough to easily climb in and out.

Rail parents have been known to feed their chicks for up to 3 weeks, and up to 30 days in coots/gallinules, but there have been cases in which chicks started to eat on their own sooner. Due to this variability, it is critical that the eating behaviors of rallids in care be monitored until self-feeding occurs reliably and the bird is thriving.

### Supplementation

While in care, coots, gallinules, and rails must be supplemented to ensure they get the vitamins and nutrients they would ingest in the wild. The supplementation schedule used differs in terms of frequency and dose depending on the bird's diet, medical issues, and housing. For birds housed indoors, the dosage is Mazuri® Auklet Vitamin Tablets or SeaTabs (Pacific Research Labs), ½ tab/kg, once every or every other day; for those housed outdoors, it is every other day to every 4–7 days. For small hatchlings, a slurry can be compounded from one Auklet tablet ground with mortar and pestle and mixed with 1 ml suspension liquid such as OraPlus® to be delivered at 0.5 ml/kg. Calcium carbonate should be given every or every other day orally to birds housed indoors and sprinkled on all foods offered to them. Once a bird is living outdoors and almost grown, it can receive calcium carbonate supplements every other day, transitioning to every 4–7 days as the chick matures. Any chicks with evidence of abnormal bone growth, unwillingness to stand and walk, or fractures should be supplemented with extra calcium. A calcium carbonate slurry can be made to allow the small dosages needed for small birds by mixing 5 g calcium carbonate powder (2000 mg Ca) with 10 ml OraPlus and 10 ml tap water to create a calcium slurry of approximately 100 mg/ml. Small pieces of 500–600 mg calcium carbonate tablets can be given orally to larger, fledgling birds. The more calcium-deficient foods a chick is eating (e.g. mealworms, some small-bodied fish), the more calcium supplementation they will need for proper bone growth. See Chapter 41 for more information on the nutritional composition of invertebrates.

## Expected Weight Gain

Chicks should steadily gain weight from the time they hatch until they are fledglings (Figure 22.6). If a chick is not gaining weight or loses weight for more than 2 days in a row, the chick should be carefully assessed. Lack of weight gain can result from medical issues, being outcompeted for food, stress, abnormal light or photoperiod, or lack of cover. Daily weight monitoring is critical for the first 2 weeks of care or until the bird has proven it is reliably self-feeding. Once birds are

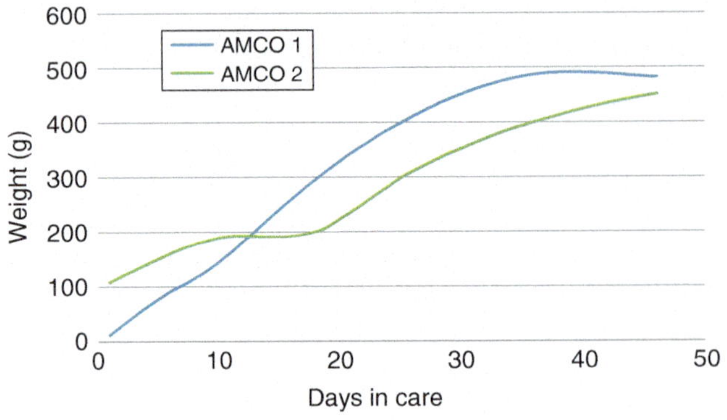


Figure 22.6 Weight gain of two American Coot chicks.

self-feeding, weight checks can be done every 2–7 days, starting with every 2 days and expanding the number of days between checks as the bird continues to prove it is self-feeding. Care should be taken to monitor and document food consumption as well.

## Housing

Because coots, gallinules, and rails are very susceptible to foot problems, attention should be paid to their feet at all stages of care. To reduce the possibility of foot lesions, birds must be provided with varied substrates to walk on. Materials that can be used include daisy mat, anti-fatigue mat, clean sand, reeds, and ¼–⅛ in. (3–6 mm) hardware cloth, which has the added benefit of letting food and feces fall through. While it seems counterintuitive to house these small birds on hardware cloth, these authors have not seen any problems resulting from its use.

### Hatchlings and Nestlings

Rallid parents brood their chicks for warmth at night during the first 1–2 weeks of life, depending on the species, so a supplemental source of heat must be provided when nestlings and hatchlings are in care. An incubator at 99–100 °F with or without an additional heat pad on low may be needed, depending on the age and alertness of the bird.

The youngest chicks should be kept in a 100 °F (37.8 °C) incubator such as an Animal Intensive Care Unit (AICU, Lyon Technologies). Set up the cooler side of the incubator for food presentation, and the warm side for hiding and resting. Many parents will continue to brood their chicks 1–3 weeks after hatching, especially at night. The AICU works well to maintain a warm and humid environment. Incubators, brooders, and aquariums can also work in this manner with the additional heat support of heating pads on low or heat lamps/emitters if necessary. Using an air thermometer can help to ensure the proper temperature is reached. If the entire enclosure cannot hold heat, it is important that at least one section has adequate heat so the mobile chick can choose to be in a warm area. It is important to monitor young chicks for signs of lethargy, shivering, or fluffed feathers, which could indicate hypothermia. Hyperthermia is also a risk if the enclosure is too hot; signs of hyperthermia include panting, open mouth breathing, or panicked behavior, trying to escape the enclosure. Substrate inside an incubator, brooder, or aquarium can be a lightweight cotton towel or flannel pillowcase, which will absorb any spilled liquids or feces into the material but create enough traction for the chick to walk and run comfortably. Using a material that is absorbent and smooth is ideal as these species have toenails that can easily get caught in textured fabrics. Substrates should be changed daily and coordinated with weight checks and exams to limit human interaction and handling.

If a chick is housed alone, add a clean feather duster (exercise caution with placement under heat lamps as this may be a fire hazard) and mirrors to help provide a sense of companionship and relieve the stress of being alone. This will also help keep the bird from becoming habituated. Adding small areas with greenery and sand or shallow water access can be used, but it is critical that birds are closely monitored until assured the chick is not having issues navigating vegetation, becoming wet or chilled, or at risk of drowning due to being unable to exit the water. These items can be added a few days after care begins to ensure young chicks are alert and coordinated enough to navigate their enclosure.

### Fledgling

Fledgling rallids are typically 4–8 weeks of age, with larger-sized species tending to have later fledging ages. The goal of creating a housing environment for these older chicks is to gradually acclimate them to ambient outdoor temperatures and the type of wild environment they will experience after release. Heat support should be gradually reduced, and greater access to water given.

As with any patient in care, birds should be closely monitored for the first 24 hours in a new enclosure, especially if moving to a substantially larger cage, to ensure the bird is not having difficulty navigating a new environment. As secretive birds, young coots, rails, and gallinules must be provided with hiding places such as plants, reeds, and other vegetation to hide behind in all enclosures. Feather dusters are no longer needed, as chicks would no longer be brooded at night.

Once the chick is known to be able to thermoregulate, it can be moved to an environment that is half water and half land. Wide shallow pans can be used as pools (Figure 22.7), as can deeper water containers. A sloping, marshy, beach-like water border is ideal. Other suggestions for housing include a wooden-sided pen that allows for half land with a mesh bottom raised a little above a tub

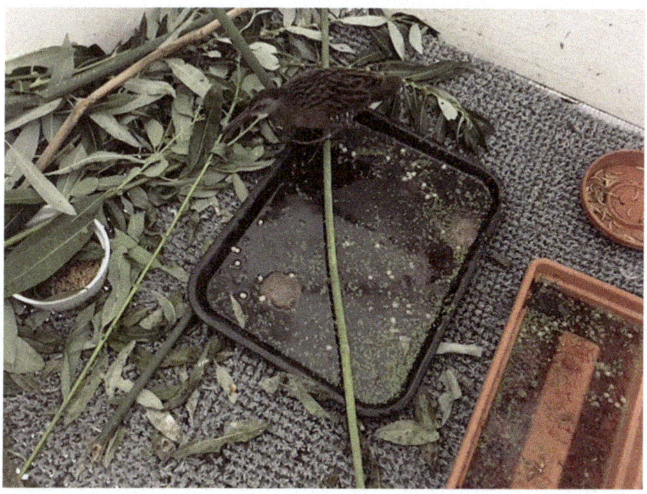

Figure 22.7 Virginia Rail in a wood-sided pen with daisy matting, greenery, and shallow food platters, wet and dry. *Source:* photo courtesy of International Bird Rescue.

for water access. Another option is a wood-sided pen with a raised ⅛ in. (3 mm) mesh floor, with shallow pans for water access.

Chicks should be monitored closely when first introduced to water to make sure they do not get wet and hypothermic. A heat lamp over the land area of their enclosure will help with thermoregulation and with drying after swimming. The land area can be mesh-bottomed, which allows dropped food and feces to fall through, keeping the area clean. Otherwise, a fabric-covered land area can also be used, ensuring the area stays clean by regular changes. Use of towels can be dangerous due to long toenails, so pillowcases or a nonfabric substrate will help minimize the risk of their nails becoming injured in the enclosure.

All birds must have an opportunity to swim and bathe to become waterproof. Duckweed can be added to the pool so they can forage in the water. Water in enclosures should be changed daily or have constant surface runoff to ensure excellent water quality for healthy plumage.

## Preparation for Wild Release

Pre-release conditioning aviary sizes for these species for unrestricted activity are recommended in Miller (2012) as 4×8×8 ft. (1.2×2.4×2.4 m) with a 45 in. (114 cm) diameter ×8 in. (20 cm) deep pool. Birds should spend at least 7–14 days in such an adequately-sized aviary to practice flight and prove to be a strong flyer before release (Figure 22.8). Birds should be comfortable in ambient outdoor temperatures, and should have had plenty of time with water access and be able to swim, float, and stay waterproof. Each bird should be of normal adult weight with all known medical

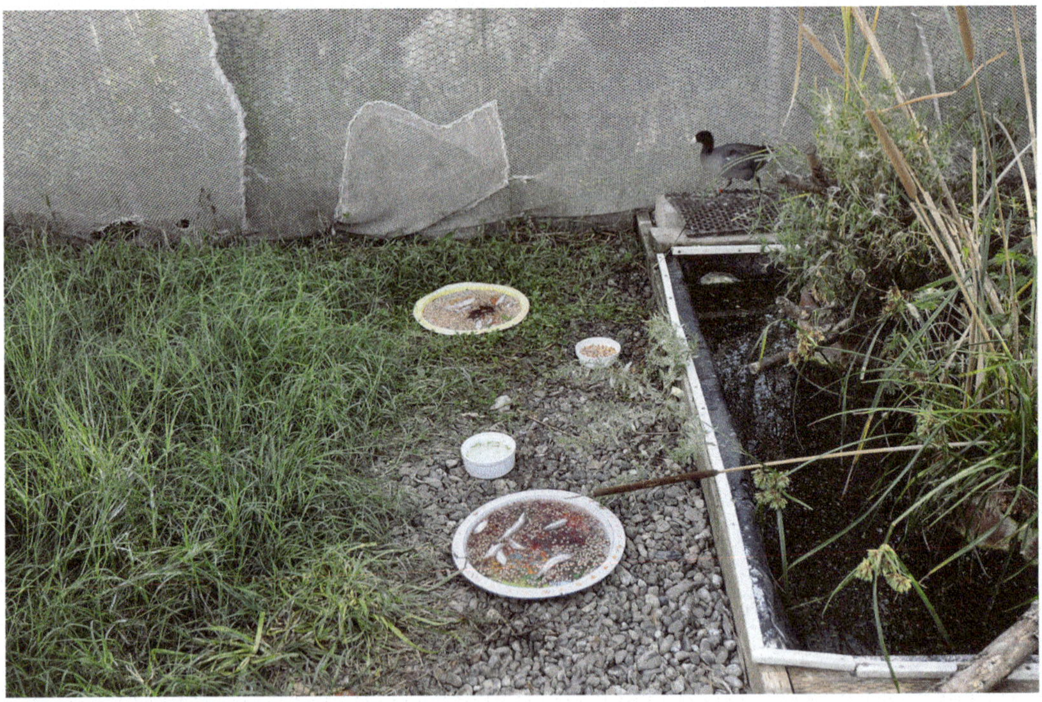

Figure 22.8 American Coot pre-release enclosure with water access, shallow food dishes, greenery, and adequate flying space. *Source:* photo courtesy of International Bird Rescue.

issues completely resolved. A thorough physical exam should be completed prior to release, identifying full growth of all primaries to ensure capable flight to evade predators, plus good body condition and muscle mass. Birds should show capable hunting and foraging skills, and show no signs of human interest.

## Release

Whenever possible, birds should be released to an appropriate environment at or near where they were found, in an area with conspecifics. Coots and gallinules are gregarious and can be released into or near a wild flock. Rails are more solitary and secretive species that do not migrate widely, which makes it especially important to release them near where they were found. While some rail species are territorial, warnings from others are generally vocal, not physical. It is best to release birds in the morning during a period of calm weather; this will allow them maximum time to explore and adjust to their new environment before nightfall or bad weather.

Birds should be transported to release in an enclosure they can walk out of, such as a sky kennel. Upon arrival at the release site, the enclosure door should be opened, all humans should stand behind enclosure and allow the birds to walk out when they are ready. There is no need to rush this important moment by poking or prodding the bird. Under no circumstance should rails or coots (and most other birds) be thrown in the air when released. In addition to causing stress from handling, it also gives the bird no time to adjust to its environment and scan for predators.

## Acknowledgments

Thank you to the awesome coots and rails who grace us with their beauty. Thank you to the 3-g Black Rail for giving us the experience of learning how to care for and raise such a unique species, and for being a cooperative patient. Getting to release you back to your Pickleweed Marsh was one of the most rewarding experiences of all.

## Sources for Products Mentioned

Calcium carbonate powder and 1 cc syringes: Chris's Squirrels and More, LLC., 304 Turnpike Rd., Somers, Ct. 06071, (860) 749–1129, www.squirrelsandmore.com.

Incubators: Lyon Technologies, Inc., 1690 Brandywine Avenue, Chula Vista, CA 91911, (888) 596–6872.

Mazuri products: Mazuri, PMI Nutrition International, LLC, PO Box 66812, St. Louis, MO 63166, www.mazuri.com.

Mealworms and other feeder insects: Rainbow Mealworms, PO Box 4907, Compton, CA 90220, (800) 777–9676, www.rainbowmealworms.net.

OraPlus: Perrigo Company PLC, North American offices, 515 Eastern Avenue, Allegan, Michigan 49010, (269) 673–8451, https://www.perrigo.com/business/product.aspx?ID=173&cat=comp.

SeaTabs: Pacific Research Labs, Inc., 730 Saddlebrook Dr., Ramona, CA 92065, www.prlvitamins.com.

Tyvek leg bands: TabBand 7150 West Roosevelt Street, C113, Phoenix, Arizona 85043, (602) 257–0141, http://Tabband.com.

## References

Bannor, B.K. and Kiviat, E. (2002). Common Gallinule (*Gallinula galeata*), version 2.0. In: *The Birds of North America* (eds. A.F. Poole and F.B. Gill). Ithaca, NY, USA: Cornell Lab of Ornithology. https://doi.org/10.2173/bna.685.

Brisbin, I.L. Jr. and Mowbray, T.B. (2002). American coot (*Fulica americana*), version 2.0. In: *The Birds of North America* (eds. A.F. Poole and F.B. Gill). Ithaca, NY, USA: Cornell Lab of Ornithology. https://doi.org/10.2173/bna.697a.

Conway, C.J. (1995). Virginia rail (*Rallus limicola*), version 2.0. In: *The Birds of North America* (eds. A.F. Poole and F.B. Gill). Ithaca, NY, USA: Cornell Lab of Ornithology. https://doi.org/10.2173/bna.173.

Hawkins, M.G., Barron, H.W., Speer, B.L. et al. (2018). Birds. In: *Exotic Animal Formulary*, 5e (eds. J.W. Carpenter and C.J. Marion), 167–375. St. Louis, MO: Elsevier.

Miller, E.A. (ed.) (2012). *Minimum Standards for Wildlife Rehabilitation*, 4e. St. Cloud, MN: National Wildlife Rehabilitation Association.

# 23

# Cranes

*Marjorie Cahak Gibson*

## Natural History

Cranes are classed among the oldest families of birds. Of the 15 species in the Gruidae family worldwide, 9 are threatened or endangered. Cranes are tall, stately birds with long necks and legs and heavy bills. They have distinctive silhouettes with the tertial feathers drooping over the rump in a bustle. Cranes are best known for strong mate fidelity, intricate "mating dances," and the practice of siblicide.

Two species are found in North America, with another species, the Common Crane (*Grus grus*) of Eurasia, being sighted occasionally. The Sandhill Crane (*Grus Canadensis*) has six subspecies, including Canadian, Greater, Lesser, Florida, Mississippi, and Cuban. The Whooping Crane (*Grus Americana*) is endangered in North America.

Sandhill Cranes are 34–48 in. (0.8–1.2 m) tall with wingspans of 73–90 in. (1.8–2.3 m), with variation in size depending on the subspecies. Whooping Cranes are 52 in. (1.3 m) tall with wingspans of 87 in. (2.2 m). Successful captive-breeding programs for Whooping Cranes have been established, and these birds are currently being reintroduced to regions within the U.S. With continued success of captive-breeding and reintroduction, it may be possible to encounter wild Whooping Cranes in need of rehabilitation within the next decade.

Cranes are long-lived and monogamous. They nest in marshy areas and build simple nests of vegetation gathered from around the nest site. The gathering of nesting material plays an important role in nesting because a watery barrier must be created around the nest site. This act may contribute to the reproductive success of cranes. Both male and female incubate the two eggs, which hatch asynchronously in 28–36 days.

Young cranes are called *colts*. Crane colts can be very aggressive to each other and siblicide is common. Asynchronous hatching gives the older chick an advantage but leaves the second egg and resulting chick as a "backup" if the first colt should perish. If both chicks survive past hatch, they are generally separated, with each adult taking one chick and acting as its primary parent. In this way, the young are physically separated until tolerance is attained.

Crane colts are precocial at hatch. They are covered with thick, rusty brown-colored down. They are active after hatch and can leave the nest the same day. Young cranes follow their parent, often walking underneath the abdomen of the adult as they move through the marsh. They can swim short distances. There is a wide variety of vocalizations that occur between adult cranes and their young. Sounds can change from a soft pumping noise to an aggressive trumpet when danger is near.

*Hand-Rearing Birds*, Second Edition. Edited by Rebecca S. Duerr and Laurie J. Gage.

The young vocalize a soft purring sound, almost constantly, to maintain contact with the adult as they walk. Adult cranes feed the young by killing prey such as crustaceans, frogs, snakes, or mice, and thrashing it to bits for the youngster. They also teach chicks to secure their own food by turning over mud or soil in upland areas to expose insects or aquatic invertebrates. Crane colts are naturally attracted to movement and shiny objects and learn to feed themselves quickly.

Cranes in the wild eat a wide variety of plant material plus insects, aquatic invertebrates, frogs, small animals, and even small birds if the opportunity presents itself. Hence, do not house them with song-birds or young ducklings. Although plant material is ingested in small amounts, most of the diet in the first 6–8 weeks of life consists of insects, invertebrates, and larger vertebrates that have been killed and ripped apart by the adults.

### Captive-breeding Facilities

Husbandry of captive and breeding cranes has been researched extensively by scientists at Patuxent Wildlife Research Center in Laurel, Maryland, and The International Crane Foundation in Baraboo, Wisconsin. Through these excellent sources, wildlife rehabilitators have access to a wide variety of information on the various aspects of captive crane care. One of the best reference books and a must for every rehabilitator considering cranes is *Cranes: Their Biology, Husbandry and Conservation* by David Ellis, George Gee, and Claire Mirande (Ellis et al. 1996).

Although information on long-term captive care of cranes is excellent, it must be kept in mind that the rehabilitation of cranes will have a different approach when compared to permanent captive and breeding care. Those differences focus on preparing for life in the wild in the case of a colt, and for return to the wild in that of an adult. The captive care of birds in rehabilitation is a short period, rather than their entire life. Some of those differences will be discussed in this chapter.

## Criteria for Intervention

Cranes' large size, interesting behavior, and considerable folklore draw the interest of the public when nest sites are close to human activity.

### Adults

Most calls received by wildlife centers concerning adult cranes will be those hit by cars, shot, trapped, accidentally poisoned from overspray or runoff in agricultural areas, or contact with other poisons placed for animals in depredation situations. Large die-offs of cranes have been reported due to mycotoxins. These are produced by fungi that grow on crops that have been left unharvested. Crane species may be hypersensitive to mycotoxins (Ellis et al. 1996; Altman et al. 1997). Lead poisoning and ingestion of items such as screws or staples can also occur. For this reason, the crane patient with digestive problems should be x-rayed to determine whether ingested material is the source. Gruidae as a family tend to be temperature-hardy. However, individuals exposed to extreme cold without protection may suffer frostbite to the toes. Patients with frostbite are usually birds that have been unable to migrate for some reason and are forced to remain in extreme winter temperatures.

### Colts

Very young crane colts are often hypothermic when found. Colts hatched during very cold temperatures have a poor chance of survival. Although able to thermoregulate to some degree, circumstances require youngsters to follow their parent through wet, marshy habitat soon after hatch. Periods of cold temperatures, particularly when prolonged, often prove to be too harsh for survival. Colts admitted in this situation will be hypothermic, cold to the touch, and have delayed or minimal response to stimulation. In serious cases, they can be mistaken for being dead. Young cranes with hypothermia can be revived, even when there is lack of movement, with application of heat.

The appearance of a crane colt, with the long neck, legs, and soft coloring, is attractive to the public, and once spotted, they are often victims of kidnapping from the wild. Dogs, cats, and wild predators are also a threat. The incidence of these kidnappings increases when nest sites border parks, agricultural, or other recreational areas. Advice given to the public plays an important role in assuring normal, uninjured youngsters stay in the wild with their parents.

Questions to ask the public when answering calls:

Is the crane standing or lying down?
Is there blood visible?
Is the youngster running and active?
Can the youngster hear an adult crane vocalizing or see an adult in the immediate area?
Is the youngster in immediate danger? (If dogs or children are chasing it, for example, a chick can be temporarily captured and placed back in the area when the danger is gone.)

Young cranes, although very mobile, can be easily captured. Colts can suffer heat exhaustion, capture myopathy, or injury when chased. In most cases, parent birds are near. Adults can become aggressive in defense of their young. Initially, the adult response is to become vocal. The vocalizations increase in volume and tone to warn the youngster of the approaching danger and "predator" of the adult presence. The stout and heavy beak of an adult crane can be dangerous.

Parents occasionally abandon newly hatched cranes. This phenomenon may occur if the weather at hatch is extreme. Siblicide can and does occur with cranes. Although siblicide occurs more often in captive situations, it also occurs in the wild. Care must be taken when housing even very young or debilitated cranes together. Colts injured by siblings or other cranes may present with penetrating injuries to the head and neck (Figure 23.1).

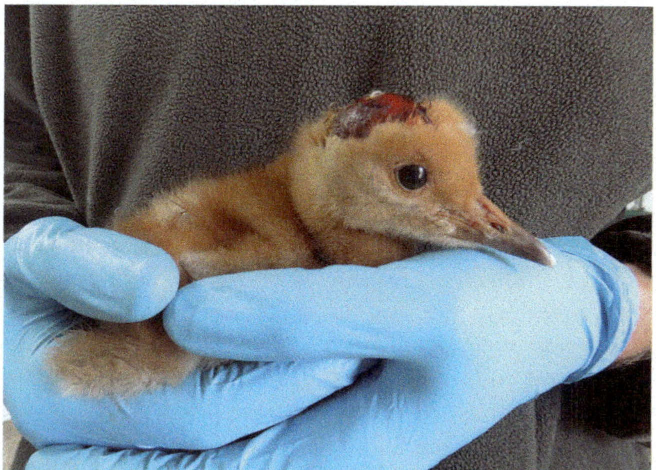

Figure 23.1 Crane colt with a severe scalp injury. Cranes may injure or kill each other in territorial disputes or siblicide by stabs to the head and neck.

### Transportation to Wildlife Facility

The colt should be transported as soon as possible. Instruct the transporter that the youngster should kept quiet, and away from dogs, cats, and children before and during transport. A transport box no more than twice the size of the colt, but that allows it to stand, will lower stress and keep the youngster secure. A cardboard box with air holes works well. A clean towel on the bottom of the box will prevent chicks from sliding and possible splaying of legs. Do not transport with a food or water, as spilled water will wet the chick and cause hypothermia. Provide supplemental heat during transport. Warmed rice bags, hot-water bottles, or an equivalent work well. Pad the heat source with towels so the colt is not directly in contact with it. A stuffed animal, feather duster, or calmly and gently holding the colt in a towel during transport may provide comfort.

### Networking Is a Vital Link to Successful Rehabilitation

Networking with others is the most valuable tool available to wildlife rehabilitators. Networking is, in part, how we gain information concerning the regional nuances of animal behavior and needs. This information can make all the difference in the welfare of your wild patient. Local agency biologists, university researchers, veterinarians, avid birders, or land-owners – all make great networking partners. It is only through the help and advice of others that wildlife rehabilitation can be done successfully. This is particularly true with sensitive species that have exacting requirements for success. As professional wildlife rehabilitators it is our responsibility to make certain the animal in our care has the best possible chance of recovery and survival after release.

## Initial Care and Stabilization

If the colt is cold to the touch but responsive, put it in a dark, quiet box on heat of 90–95 °F (32–34 °C) until the core body temperature returns to normal and is stable (104–108 °F, 40–42 °C). The patient should be gently massaged with a warmed towel to stimulate response. When the youngster is warm, an exam can be done.

Do not give oral fluids or food to a colt that is nonresponsive. Oral fluids can be given only when the colt is able to hold its head up for at least brief periods on its own. An oral emaciation diet should be the first food for colts coming out of hypothermia, or those in critical condition (see the section "Diet," later in this chapter).

Give subcutaneous fluids warmed to 100.4–102.2 °F (38–39 °C) to chicks that are weak or poorly responsive. Oral fluids can be given via gavage tube to strong chicks. The author prefers to be conservative in fluid amounts given, giving 5% of body weight (50 ml/kg) at a maximum to avoid overhydrating crane chicks. Fluid therapy is important in cases of starvation or other conditions where dehydration is present. Dehydration will be an element in starvation cases and should be addressed immediately.

Handle colts as little as possible. This is important both for keeping the stress level low, in consideration of injury that may result due to handling, and limiting the opportunity for human imprinting. The body structure of members of the crane family is conducive to injury at the smallest provocation. A heightened awareness of possible injury must be built into the handling protocol of members of the *Grus* genus. When handling is necessary, care must be taken to protect the legs. A towel can be used to hold and gently restrain young cranes. If the patient is a youngster, one hand should always be securely under the feet (Figure 23.2 and 23.3). Joints and legs are very delicate in cranes. Inappropriate handling can cause permanent damage to the integrity of the legs, pelvis, or joints.

If the chick is thin and has not been eating, give emaciation diet via a gavage tube into the crop following initial subcutaneous (SQ) fluids. A stainless steel feeding tube or French catheter tube of appropriate size may be used. Use minimal amounts at first (2–5 ml) to make sure the digestive system is moving before offering solid food. Once the young patient is stable, a full exam and additional medical intervention can be carried out.

## Common Medical Problems

Cranes are subject to several viral diseases, fungal diseases, and a host of bacterial and parasitic conditions (Olsen et al. 1997; Candelora et al. 2010; Bertram et al. 2015). Cranes in the wild have, and tolerate, many parasites. It is not necessary to evaluate every patient unless secondary problems are apparent. If the patient presents with or develops diarrhea, has poor weight gain, or is lethargic, a workup should be done to identify the problem. Good sanitation, pen rotation, fresh food, and clean water are the best means with which to prevent disease.

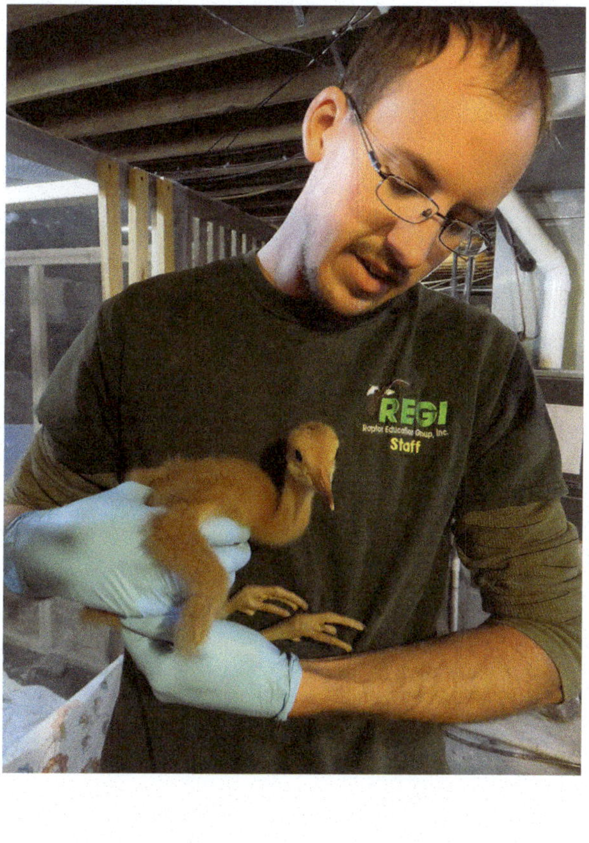


Figure 23.2 It is important to support the legs of a young colt gently under it to prevent leg injury.

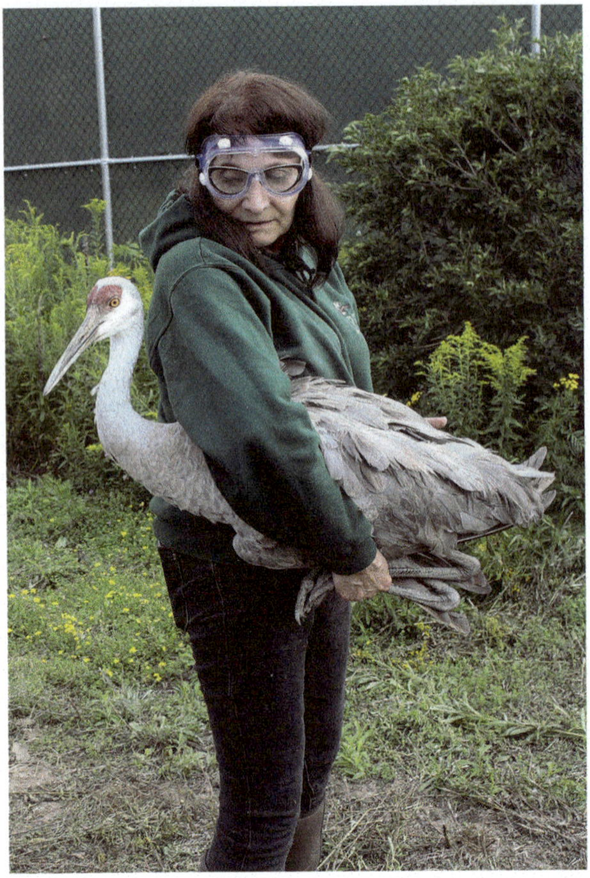

Figure 23.3 Restraining an adult crane involves holding the bird facing backward with the legs and feet restrained. Safety glasses are prudent.

## Respiratory Disease

Respiratory disease is common in crane colts. General symptoms include pale mucous membranes and lethargy in the early stages of any respiratory condition. Chicks exhibiting signs of illness should be given supplemental heat (90–97 °F, 32–36 °C) and supportive care immediately. Raspy or open-mouthed breathing requires immediate intervention. In very young chicks, the problem is generally bacterial in nature; however, after 2 weeks of age, fungal disease including aspergillosis and coccidioidomycosis should be considered with appropriate medical care (Altman et al. 1997).

## Parasites

Parasites such as *Syngamus trachea* (gapeworm) occur in cranes and create respiratory symptoms. Earthworms serve as an intermediate host. This parasite should be considered in young cranes, particularly those that have been fed or have had access to earthworms early in their life. Gapeworm produces many symptoms, including head shaking, raspy sounding respirations, open-mouth breathing, and coughing. In some cases, the worms are easily visible as red threadlike strands on the wall of the trachea when viewed down the glottis from inside the mouth. Eggs can be detected in the feces. This parasite can cause death in young cranes from anemia, asphyxiation from mucous production, or even tracheal ulceration (Ritchie et al. 1994; Rupley 1997). Treatment once diagnosed is ivermectin or thiabendazole.

### Heatstroke

Heatstroke can occur in cranes, particularly on hot summer days. This can be prevented with a few simple measures. Provide a shelter or shaded area in the compound. Only emergency handling should be done on hot days. If handling cannot be avoided, do it in the cooler early morning hours. Provide an adequate water supply. Be certain the crane can drink from the water container. The long beak requires a deep dish or pail. Cranes cannot drink from a shallow dish.

Heatstroke is demonstrated with gasping, panting, rapid breathing, staggering, and wings held away from the body of the crane or drooping. If the body temperature remains elevated, death may result. If heatstroke is suspected, cool the bird immediately by placing its body or parts of its body in cool water. Cold packs may be placed under the wings to facilitate more rapid cooling. For birds that are conscious, alert, and capable, a swimming pool may be used to allow the bird to cool itself.

### Injuries to Bones and Beaks

This section covers only injuries that can result in the full recovery and wild release of a crane. Many orthopedic procedures have been developed that work well for captive cranes, including leg prosthesis. Information for these procedures is available in many excellent textbooks, many of which are listed in this chapter's reference section. One of the best resources on avian medicine which includes wild species is Altman et al. (1997). Serious (e.g. open, comminuted, or close to a joint) fractures should be evaluated and repaired by your avian veterinarian. Management of orthopedic injuries in wild birds, utilizing various technologic levels from simple wraps and splints to surgical repair, are covered in Duerr (2017).

Cranes often present to rehabilitation facilities with damage to the beak. Beak injury can be caused by a collision with an object or defensive maneuvers by the crane itself. In most cases, a broken tip of the beak needs little intervention unless it is bleeding or interferes with the ability of the bird to eat or drink. Some filing of the broken area, either with a hand file or Dremel tool, is recommended to create a smooth surface.

Serious fractures of the beak can be repaired with self-curing dental acrylics reinforced with Kirshner wires. Most healing takes place in 4–6 weeks with the wires being removed at that time. In young cranes, the splint must be changed frequently to accommodate the growth of the beak.

Broken wings can be successfully repaired by a variety of methods. Bandaging, splinting, and surgical repair are all valid methods of response to a wing fracture. Which technique is used will depend on the age of the patient, how recent the fracture is, which bone is fractured, and whether the fracture is a closed or open fracture; see Duerr (2017).

Broken legs, although difficult to repair, can be attempted with the use of a sling to hold the body in a natural upright position. Due to the weight-bearing exercise need of young cranes during their accelerated growth period, this method is generally reserved only for adults or juveniles that have achieve full height. If a sling is used, the caregiver must be certain it is stable, and the vent area is uncovered and allows the bird to defecate.

### Angel Wing

A diet too rich in protein, carbohydrates, and sulfur-containing amino acids can cause deformities of the wings and legs. An excess of calories and carbohydrates can cause the primaries in a colt to grow too fast, compromising the muscles and support tissue of the wing. This condition is commonly known as *angel wing* or *airplane wing*. The name comes from the visual effect of the condition in which the tip of the wing turns up in an unnatural position. It is a permanent disability, and results in the bird being unable to fly, if not caught when a slight change in the wing feather growth is noticed. Angel wing can usually be corrected if caught very early, by bandaging the wing in a natural position for 2 days. Wing wraps must not be left on longer than 2 days due to the fast growth rate of a crane colt. Usually, one treatment is effective to correct the condition (Ellis et al. 1996).

Angel wing is commonly caused by feeding white bread to young colts or waterfowl. Wild crane colts hatched near parks or other recreational areas that bring humans into contact with young wild cranes can be affected by the human need to feed bread to birds.

### Feather Problems

Quality of feathers is often underestimated in evaluating suitability for release of both captive-raised cranes and those that have been rehabilitated. Attention to feather quality (stress bars, dull or dirty, broken feathers, and issues such as barb defects) is essential. Feathers are responsible for maintaining waterproofing to prevent hypothermia, as well as for flight. Feathers directly affect the survival of a bird living in the wild. Malnutrition or other conditions can cause feather changes and indicate that the bird is not ready for release. Birds that fit this description should be retained and given supportive nutritional care. Feather damage can be so severe as to delay the release of an otherwise releasable crane until molting occurs.

Broken primaries can occur with injury, or because of a viral infection. Feathers can also be broken or in poor condition due to even a short time period in inadequate or inappropriate housing. Primaries can be *imped,* a process by which replacement feathers are fixed artificially into existing feather shafts, with the same methods as those used for raptors.

## Imprinting and Habituation

Imprinting and habituation are very different behaviors. Imprinting is the permanent alteration of sexual identity and species orientation. Imprinted birds can be imprinted to humans, objects, or even another species when cross-fostering techniques are used. During early efforts to save the Whooping Crane from extinction, Sandhill Cranes were used to cross-foster Whooping Crane colts. The result was that the young Whooping Cranes never learned the courtship behavior expected of a Whooping Crane and were rejected by them. Sandhill Cranes also rejected the young Whooping Cranes, likely due to vocalization variations (Ritchie et al. 1994; Baughman 2003).

The process of imprinting begins soon after hatch and continues at least through the first month of life. Recent evidence suggests that imprinting can occur in birds with a long lifespan and slow maturity post-fledge. Imprinting is thought to be associated with food delivery during the first days or weeks of life. It is at this time that the young bird incorporates and retains important sounds and behavior clues that become a permanent part of its identity. Imprinting aids natural reproduction in terms of recognizing or attracting a mate. Vocalization development of imprinted birds may be impaired, with chick calls being retained for a lifetime. Aggression often occurs in imprinted birds, particularly when they reach breeding age. Imprint aggression can be extreme. Imprinted birds should be considered dangerous and unpredictable. Human-imprinted birds can pose a danger to humans and should never be released to the wild or used in wildlife petting zoos due to the unpredictable nature of this aggression. If they are maintained in captivity, they should be handled by only the most experienced handlers.

Habituated cranes do not respond with appropriate caution or fear to humans, dogs, or situations to which they have been repeatedly exposed without consequence. Release of a habituated bird may create a variety of problematic scenarios, none of which are healthy for the crane. There are methods that can retrain a habituated crane and help incorporate it into the wild population. Housing habituated cranes with normal cranes is very important to success. Restrict contact with humans as soon as possible. Aversion techniques, such as noise-making, may encourage the habituated bird to reconsider its level of comfort with things that will prove dangerous to it in the wild.

Consider a crane that has been reared in contact with a family dog. Although that dog may not cause the crane harm, other dogs likely will once the bird has been released. The bird must have the correct fear response to survive. Habituation can be reversed; imprinting cannot.

Cranes are curious by nature and both imprint and habituate easily to human caretakers. There are several successful methods by which to raise wild crane colts without imprinting them to humans:

- Pair each chick with a nonreleasable crane foster parent. This is the least labor-intensive and produces the best results if an appropriate adult is located. The limiting factor is that each adult can generally rear only one colt at a time due to sibling rivalry when others are introduced. Adult cranes may be aggressive to colts. If this is a problem with a bird that is available to use as a foster, install a see-through wall or screening that will allow the adult to be in sight and hearing of the colt. This way it can still serve as a role model.
- Raise colts in visual and auditory contact with other cranes of the same species.
- Play audio recordings of wild cranes with young.
- Rear in a sheltered area with a taxidermized adult crane mounted in the head-down position if a live foster is not available.

As a last resort, if captive fostering is not an option, use costume rearing, with the human caregivers dressed as cranes or covered in material similar in color to the adult crane, and a puppet that mimics the adult crane closely in size, shape, and coloration. Sounds are important to a youngster, so human voices must be kept to a minimum. Recordings of breeding cranes should be used.

## Diet

While in captivity, a very young crane colt can be encouraged to eat from a bowl if a red item, simulating the tip of the parent's beak, is placed into the food dish. Care should be taken that the simulated beak is sturdy and not an ingestion danger to the colt. The diet of cranes varies with age. It is important to remember that while the adult diet includes vegetation and grain, the diet of a young crane, for the first 45–60 days, consists almost entirely of killed insects, invertebrates, and aquatic vertebrates.

Feeding live insects or animals to a very young crane is dangerous and not recommended. Young birds do not have the experience, skill, or digestive enzymes to kill and digest live prey. The parent kills all but the smallest insects for the first weeks of life and continues to kill larger prey for several weeks.

Offer as much natural food, such as insects and aquatic invertebrates, as the colt will eat. Fresh food should always be available. Cranes reared in captivity but destined to go back into the wild need a natural diet. This is not only for nutritional support, but to develop their normal intestinal flora and gain experience foraging as well. Cranes grow at a rapid rate and ingest large amounts of food to provide the calories, minerals, and other nutrients to support their metabolic needs.

When augmented with natural foods, a successful basic diet can consist of Science Diet Feline or Canine Growth pellets saturated in water overnight in a refrigerator. Do not feed pellets before they are fully saturated. Care must be taken to ensure the pellets remain refrigerated before use and are changed once a day at room temperature or more frequently in warm conditions. Once soaked in water, do not keep pellets more than 3 days in the refrigerator before using, as they will sour and spoil with age. Allow the colt to eat as much as it wants during the day. Grain can be added once the young crane is more than 45 days old. This regime must be accompanied by substantial exercise for the growing colt.

After 30 days of age, small live crustaceans should be offered along with mayfly larva, moths, mealworms, waxworms, and other invertebrate prey. The colt may play with the new food items for several days before it successfully kills and eats them. It is important to offer a variety of items because each provides elements needed in the diet. It is best if the young crane has access to an enclosed natural area so it can graze and select a wide range of natural insects and vegetation on its own. After 60 days of age, crayfish, frogs, and mice can be added to the colt's diet.

Commercial starter diets such as Zeigler Crane Breeder (Zeigler) or Mazuri® Crane Diet are easily obtained and can be used to supplement a natural prey diet. It is important to note the difference in a maintenance diet used for adult birds and the starter diet used for the active growing stage. The type of protein used in the diet of a colt is important.

Diets with a high percentage of sulfur-containing amino acids must be avoided because they contribute to developmental abnormalities, such as leg and wing problems. For instance, fish should be fed in very small quantities because they contain a higher percentage of these amino acids. Breeders suggest a diet with 24% protein, 1.4% calcium, 0.90% phosphorus, 0.7% methionine and cystine, and 1.3% lysine. The kcal/kg is higher in starter or chick diets than those developed for adult birds. Maintenance diets have lower protein levels and can be used once the crane is over 2 months of age (Ellis et al. 1996).

A crane in rehabilitation should be not be fed exclusively an artificial or commercial formula. If commercial diet is the only food offered, intake should be limited to prevent weight gain too quickly. Natural diet, however, may be difficult to provide daily in quantities large enough for captive crane patients. Most cranes will eat commercial diet once it is introduced. Sprinkling corn or insects on top of commercial diet will encourage first-time investigation. An adult crane will do well on a commercial maintenance diet containing about 19% protein. Introduce breeder formula if an adult patient is held to early spring or the breeding season. Breeding formulas offer higher protein, calcium, and metabolizable energy. The importance of maintaining dry or pelleted commercial foods in a dry and fresh condition cannot be overemphasized.

Observe the wild rehabilitation patient from a remote location, or by a video camera located within its enclosure, to make certain it is eating. If the bird is not eating, tube-feeding should be initiated within 24 hours.

### Emaciation Diet for Crane Colts

The following is a recommended diet for emaciated crane colts:

2 oz (56 g) human baby mixed grain cereal, such as Gerber's brand
One 2.5 oz (71 g) jar of Gerber's baby meat food (beef, chicken, turkey or veal)
One 2.5 oz (71 g) jar water
One 2.5 oz (71 g) jar human infant electrolyte replacer such as Pedialyte®

Whip ingredients together, adding more water if needed until the diet will pass through a size 14 French red rubber feeding tube (catheter tube). Make the diet thinner for very weak patients.

The diet should be prepared fresh for each feeding in the amount required. Start newly hatched colts with 5 ml and monitor how fast the crop empties. Increase the quantity fed as the chick successfully empties its crop. Feed the amount that fills the crop and can be moved out of the crop in an hour. If the chick regurgitates or fluid comes up, cut back the quantity given. Continue tube-feedings until the chick is eating on its own. Offer food items when the chick can stand. The diet must be warmed to 90 °F (32 °C) when administered but it should not be hot or crop burns will result. Microwave heating is not recommended due to the uneven heating of the food particles. Feeding a cold diet may push a fragile patient into shock and result in death.

If the bird has diarrhea or is losing fluid, add extra isotonic electrolytes to replace those lost. In most cases of simple starvation or emaciation, the kidneys and most organs are functioning at a low level and plain water is sufficient.

If prepared baby meats are not available, steam pure fresh meat (no fat) until it is fully cooked. Purée the meat using a blender. The mixture may need blending before each feeding to maintain a liquid fine enough to pass through a feeding tube.

This is not meant to be an all-inclusive balanced diet. It is used only to get a bird to a place where it can digest whole or natural food again. Very emaciated birds need the process of "re-feeding," which gives them a small amount of simple food to get their digestive system moving and calories coming in, but does not overload a body that is in a fragile condition. Digestive enzymes or probiotics such as lactobacillus are useful to aid digestion in severely emaciated patients.

## Expected Weight Gain

Sandhill Crane chicks typically grow rapidly from a tiny 6 in. (15 cm) high hatchling to adult height in 56–64 days. By 3 months they should have attained adult weight, including muscle weight if able to fly. Weighing the bird frequently carries the risk of habituation and damage to the delicate legs, hence monitoring each chick's attitude and appetite is a better indication of progress. The body weight of North American cranes may also vary considerably by geographic region.

## Housing

### Young Colts

Housing for a stable colt can be a simple cardboard box approximately 36 × 24 × 30 in. (90 × 60 × 75 cm) with a securely fixed reflector lamp. The lamp should be in one corner, safely attached, so it does not come into contact with the chick. One part of the box must be maintained at 95–99 °F (35–37 °C) for a hatchling. Older colts need less heat, but they require supplemental heat until they begin to feather out or have regained health. Decrease the temperature in 5 °F (2–3 °C) increments each week or more rapidly if the youngster shows signs of being too warm, such as moving to the opposite side of the box.

Substrate for the bottom of the box should provide firm leg placement without slipping (Ellis et al. 1996). Pea gravel, soil, or towels can be used. Sand can be tried but may cause eye irritation with possible complications. If sand is used, the colt should be observed carefully for behaviors such as frequent rubbing of its face or head indicating eye irritation. Do not use wood shavings, kitty litter, or any material other than natural soil that can be ingested by the patient as intestinal blockage can result. Wet shavings or grasses harbor fungus and may result in respiratory infections. Whatever material is used, keep it dry and clean. Cranes walk in their food and bring feces from the substrate into their food.

Water pans for a very young crane should be of the nontip variety with a substrate in the bottom such as pea gravel that provides firm nonslip footing. Durable, nontoxic, flowerpot drip saucers come in a variety of sizes, are easily cleaned, and make good water dishes for very young birds. Cranes grow quickly, and their needs for drinking receptacles change with growth. Make certain the youngster can actually drink. Cranes' long beak necessitates deeper water pans than those provided for most bird species. It cannot be emphasized too much that if the colt can walk into the pan, it will. A sturdy substrate such as pea gravel should line the bottom of all pans or bowls for secure foot placement and to prevent leg injury or splaying.

Once a youngster can eat on its own, provide a raised bowl such as a cat or dog dish that cannot tip. If the bowl can be tipped, it will be, and it may cause injury to the colts' legs. Both water and food should be changed frequently to prevent bacterial growth.

In any housing, take care to check for any unnatural shiny objects, such as staples, bits of wire, or nails. As discussed previously, cranes are attracted to shiny objects, and ingestion can cause death (Ellis et al. 1996). It is good practice to use a commercial magnetic sweeper such as the Buffalo Magnetic Sweeper, to scan the entire ground area in the pen prior to cranes being housed or allowed to graze. This is particularly true when using new or recently remodeled construction.

Young cranes need adequate room to exercise. Joints and ligaments grow at a rapid rate along with the rest of the body. A youngster reared without significant exercise will be unable to support itself and cannot survive. If any swelling is noted in the ankle, or the colt sits down on its hocks frequently, begin a more aggressive exercise program immediately. Swimming is an excellent means of exercise for cranes in addition to walking (Ellis et al. 1996). A camouflaged gown, matching the landscape in color and design, can be used when walking or grazing crane chicks to prevent imprinting or habituation. The author uses gowns of fabric that appear to be tall grass, matching the habitat of our exercise area.

It may be helpful during the first few days of confinement to house the colt with a young waterfowl companion, such as a Canada gosling close in age. This may prevent stress and encourage eating. Some rehabilitators have had success using week-old baby chicks as companions. However, be aware of the possibility of infectious diseases that can be transferred in these cases. The urge to siblicide does not generally apply to other species companions large enough to not appear as prey.

A product made for human babies to simulate sounds of the womb is helpful with baby cranes and waterfowl. The Homedics® portable "on the go" sound spa is small, inexpensive, and available at most retail outlets. A windup alarm clock (alarm option turned off) and mirror with a feather duster may also be helpful to provide the youngster with a substitute parent figure. If using a feather duster, make certain no chemicals or preservatives have been used. Toxic fumes may result when feathers that are chemically preserved or treated become wet. Synthetic feathers may be the safest for this use.

### Colts over the Age of 30 Days

A large natural area fenced with 1 × 0.5 in. (2.5 × 1 cm) coated wire provides the most secure pen. A rectangular pen is the most versatile shape and allows for the most natural exercise for youngsters. Weasels or rodents can access larger-diameter wire and may kill young cranes. Cranes can also injure themselves by getting their heads or beaks caught in larger-diameter fencing.

Solid or opaque material 4–6 ft. (1–1.7 m) high attached to the inside of the fence is recommended. The solid barrier is necessary to prevent self-inflicted injury. Cranes may seriously injure themselves running into fencing when frightened, during escape attempts, or when reacting to sudden movement inside or outside the pen. A solid barrier is also helpful to lessen habituation by providing a visual barrier to human activity. The natural behavior of young cranes includes jumping into the air, simulating the adult mating dance. This behavior is done for various reasons, including greeting other cranes or as a stress reaction as well as the legendary mating ritual. The enclosure should be tall enough to allow this movement without causing injury to the bird or feathers. A 12–15 ft. (3–3.5 m) high perimeter fence is generally considered sufficient for all age cranes.

Enclosures should have natural shade areas that allow the birds to be sheltered from heat or other weather extremes. Privacy areas, either a building or area with solid roof and fencing, should be provided. Cranes love to bathe, and they benefit from a shallow pond with a nonslip bottom or firm substrate. Water must be flowing, changed often, or have a filtration system to prevent bacterial growth and algae. Until the age of 6 weeks, supplemental heat must be used if temperatures drop below 50 °F (10 °C). Sandhill colts can fly at 56 days. Anticipate the first flight in advance to prevent premature release.

### Predator Guards

Caging is more complex than just preventing captive birds from escaping. As important as keeping the birds in, is keeping undesirables out. Birds depend on caregivers to keep them safe while in captive care. Even those that when healthy can protect themselves need protection from physical injury or disease transference during rehabilitation. Predator guards are a must for all enclosures housing wildlife patients, and cranes are no exception. There are many successful fencing techniques to discourage predators. Multiple methods, including buried fencing, electric fencing, and humane trapping of persistent predators or other techniques may be required on a single enclosure to adequately protect wild patients. It will be necessary to customize the protection of your enclosures to the predators and type of soil native to the region. This information will be best obtained from wildlife agencies within the area.

One important approach to protecting your patients from predation is to take steps not to attract predators to your pens. This involves not leaving excess food around and spilled grain outside the pen. Solid barrier fences will block visual attraction. Trees near or bordering enclosures may allow avian predators to perch and climbing predators to use them as a launching platform to access the enclosure. Digging animals such as skunks can be discouraged with buried 1 × 0.5 in. (2.5 × 1 cm) galvanized wire hardware cloth. The wire should be buried 2 ft. (60 cm) straight into the ground and angled outward from the pen another 2 ft. (60 cm). The use of galvanized moderately heavy-gauge wire is wise because less substantial wire may require costly maintenance or replacement every few years. Some rehabilitators have had success using multiple strands of electric fencing on the outside of the perimeter fencing. This technique will discourage climbing predators, such as raccoons, mink, and fishers. Several strands of electrical fencing starting a few inches from the ground and going up approximately 5 ft. from the ground are generally adequate to discourage most predators. Check with local wildlife officials for a list of predators that frequent your area and for regulations on legal means to control them. Humane trapping using live traps or other methods may be needed for persistent predators. Local regulations will also affect the translocation of live-trapped predators. Under no circumstances should poison be used. The chance of poisoning non-target species is great, including the cranes being protected. For the most complete protection, the enclosure should be covered or enclosed to prevent avian predation, wild visitors that may bring parasites, and premature release.

## Preparation for Wild Release

By the time colts are several months old, at the end of summer, they should be introduced to each other to form pre-release "family groups." Once colts are this old, the urge to siblicide declines, but individuals should be monitored closely. Aggressive individuals should be placed in visual and auditory contact with other colts only. Some colts are sociable and others are not.

## Release

The release site should be well-researched to assure it is safe in terms of toxin use in the area, and without free roaming dogs or other dangers. Most crane species are migratory and migrate in flocks. During the winter months, even nonmigratory cranes gather in groups (Ellis et al. 1996).

Young cranes must be in excellent body and feather condition and comfortable with their natural diet, hunting techniques, and other cranes before they can be released into the wild. It is beneficial for young cranes to socialize with others prior to release. Captive-raised orphans that range freely in a large, fenced, natural area with little human contact are the best prepared for transition into the wild. Cranes can be aggressive to their own species; however, once they become juveniles, their tolerance for each other increases. By fall migration, youngsters, if allowed to socialize with others, will have formed a "family group." Releasing these juveniles in their family groups, into migratory flocks, in early fall, offers an excellent chance of survival.

Wild-reared colts may spend the first winter with their parents (Kaufman 1996). For a lone crane, release timed early in the spring after overwintering may increase survival. A *soft hack* release, where food and shelter continue to be provided after release, is the best release option for these birds. If soft hack is not an option, release in the early spring with a migratory flock if possible. The release area should be a natural habitat where prey is abundant, and it should not have nesting cranes in the area. Check the nesting dates in your region to ensure a safe, unchallenged release.

Rehabilitated adult cranes must have flight exercise pre-release. This is particularly important if the cranes are a migratory species and are released in the fall in areas other than wintering destinations. Whenever possible, band birds prior to release (Figure 23.4).

Release of adults should occur in the area in which they were found, if possible. Cranes are monogamous and may be aggressive to others in their territory. Adults can also be released into a migratory group. Locations of staging areas for migration or migratory groups of birds can be found by maintaining good communication with state biologists, local Audubon or birding clubs, or even landowners in the area.

## Acknowledgments

Thank you to Dr. Barry Hartup for his help and encouragement with this chapter; Arzelee Drown, for her love of cranes, inspiration, and photos; and to the cranes themselves from whom we continue to learn. Their time with us, spent in rehabilitation, is brief but invaluable in allowing us to better understand their species.

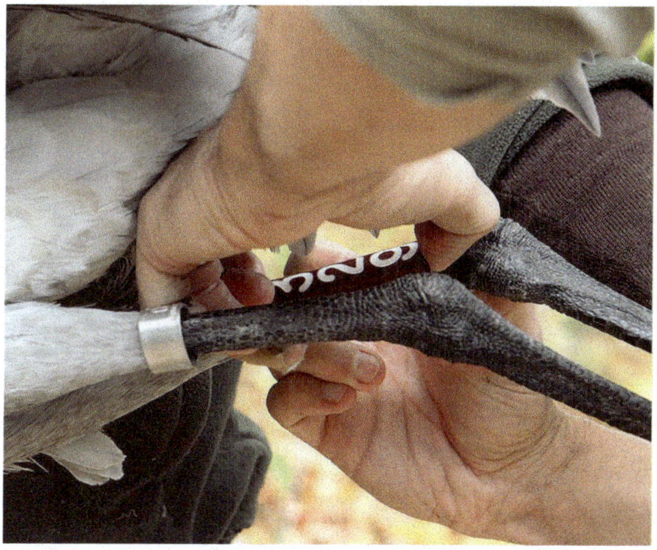

Figure 23.4 Crane being banded prior to release.

## Sources for Products Mentioned

Buffalo Tools Magnetic Sweeper: Buffalo Corporation, 950 Hoff Road, O'Fallon, MO 63366, (636) 532–9888, http://www.buffalotools.com/products/mpsweep.html.

Mazuri Exotic Animal Nutrition, PO Box 66812, St. Louis, MO 63166, https://www.mazuri.com/mazuri/outdoor-bird/waterfowl/crane-diet.

MyBaby On the Go Sound Spa Sound Machine: Homedics, 3000 N. Pontiac Trail, Commerce Township, MI 48390, https://www.homedics.com/soundspa-on-the-go-s115.html.

Zeigler crane feeds: Zeigler Bros, Inc. PO Box 95, Gardners, PA 17324, (800) 841–6800, http://zeiglerfeed.com/bird.htm.

## References


Altman, R.B., Clubb, S.L., Dorrestein, G.M., and Quesenberry, K.E. (1997). *Avian Medicine and Surgery*, 1070. Philadelphia, PA: W.B. Saunders Co.

Baughman, M. (ed.) (2003). *Reference Atlas to the Birds of North America*, 136–140. Washington DC: National Geographic Society.

Bertram, M.R., Hamer, G.L., Snowden, K.F. et al. (2015). Coccidian parasites and conservation implications for the endangered Whooping crane (*Grus americana*). *PLoS One* 10 (6): e0127679. https://doi.org/10.1371/journal.pone.0127679.

Candelora, K.L., Spalding, M.G., and Sellers, H.S. (2010). Survey for antibodies to infectious bursal disease virus serotype 2 in wild turkeys and Sandhill cranes of Florida, USA. *Journal of Wildlife Diseases* 46 (3): 742–752.

Duerr, R.S. (2017). Wading birds (herons, egrets, ibis, others). In: *Topics in Wildlife Medicine, Vol. 4: Orthopedics* (eds. R.S. Duerr and G.J. Purdin), 84–98. St. Cloud, MN: National Wildlife Rehabilitators Association.

Ellis, D.H., Gee, G.F., and Mirande, C.M. (eds.) (1996). *Cranes: Their Biology, Husbandry and Conservation*, 308. Baraboo, Wisconsin: U.S. Department of the Interior, National Biological Service, Washington DC and International Crane Foundation.

Kaufman, K. (1996). *Lives of North American Birds*, 173–175. Houghton Mifflin Harcourt.

Olsen, G.H., Turell, M.J., and Pagac, B.B. (1997). Efficacy of eastern equine encephalitis immunization in whooping cranes. *Journal of Wildlife Diseases* 33 (2): 312–316.

Ritchie, B.W., Harrison, G.J., and Harrison, L.R. (1994). *Avian Medicine: Principles and Application*, 842–849. Lake Worth, Florida: Wingers Publishing, Inc.

Rupley, A. (1997). *Manual of Avian Practice*, 265–291. Philadelphia PA: W.B. Saunders Co.

## Further Reading

Baicich, P.J. and Harrison, C.J.O. (2005). *Nest, Eggs, and Nestlings of North American Birds*, 2e, 347. Princeton, NJ: Princeton University Press.

Gibson, M. (1994). Natural history: the square one for wildlife rehabilitation. *Journal of Wildlife Rehabilitation* 17 (1): 3–16.

Gibson, M. (1996). The ABC's of housing raptors. *Journal of Wildlife Rehabilitation* 19 (3): 23–31.

Johnsgard, P.A. (2011). *Sandhill and Whooping Cranes: Ancient Voices over America's Wetlands*, 184. Lincoln, NE: University of Nebraska Press.

Rogers, L.J. and Kaplan, G. (2000). *Songs, Roars and Rituals*. Cambridge, MA: Harvard University Press pp. 70–89, 128–140.

# 24

# Shorebirds

*Libby Osnes Erie and Aimee Greenebaum*

## Natural History

Shorebirds are found on every continent except Antarctica. Numbering more than 214 species worldwide, about a third of these species touch down in North America on their intercontinental travels and, of these, 49 species breed here regularly. Five major shorebird families found in North America include Scolopacidae (sandpipers), Charadriidae (plovers), Haematopodidae (oystercatchers), Recurvirostridae (American Avocet and Black-necked Stilt), and Jacanidae (Northern Jacana). Shorebird migrations are among the most spectacular animal movements in the Western Hemisphere, spanning up to 15 000 miles (25 000 km), much of it over inhospitable oceans (Thurston 1996). Not all shorebirds are long-distance migrants. Many species winter in coastal and interior areas of the United States and Mexico. The majority, however, reach the Neotropics, in Central and South America.

Shorebirds usually occur near water but can be found in a wide variety of habitats, from tundra to grasslands to forests to open oceans. They spend two-thirds to three-quarters of their year on migration routes and wintering grounds, largely in tidal environments where they feed on marine invertebrates. The far-flung network of coastal and interior wetlands, rich in invertebrates, is critical to their ability to complete their annual cycle (Thurston 1996).

The variability in bill morphology of shorebirds results in a wide variety of feeding niches. Where a shorebird species is likely to be found feeding, in relation to the tide line and other birds, is determined by the length of its bill and, to a degree, the length of its legs (Thurston 1996). They generally feed by picking, probing, or scything.

Shorebirds are gregarious. On their migratory stopover sites and wintering grounds, they congregate in flocks varying in size from a few individuals to hundreds of thousands. During the breeding season, however, they disperse. These species display a great diversity of mating systems that seem to relate to the best use of available resources, including monogamy, polygyny, polyandry, and sequential polyandry (Thurston 1996).

The incubation period for most shorebirds is relatively brief (17–39 days, depending on the species). Shorebird chicks are extremely precocial; that is, they are capable of moving around on their own very soon after hatching. As soon as they dry, they stumble from the nest and begin pecking for insects. On day 1, the chicks preen, exercise their wings, and crouch when warned by parents. With the exception of oystercatchers, shorebird parents do not feed their young but rather lead them to foraging areas. Oystercatcher young are fed by their parents for up to 1 month or more and

*Hand-Rearing Birds*, Second Edition. Edited by Rebecca S. Duerr and Laurie J. Gage.

may stay with adults for up to 6 months, learning foraging skills before becoming fully independent (Petersen 2001a; Klusener et al. 2018).

Brooding is especially important during the first 2 weeks of life when the young cannot maintain a proper body temperature on their own (Petersen 2001b). In North American species, fledging can occur anywhere from 14 to 63 days after hatching and, in some cases, the young may remain with their parents for even longer.

## Criteria for Intervention

Human disturbance of nesting sites and severe weather conditions are the most common reasons for shorebird eggs and chicks to be brought into captivity. Shorebird parents may abandon their nests if humans or their pets remain in close proximity for an extended period of time. Nesting site conditions may change due to weather, with nests being temporarily flooded by extremely high tides or heavy rain or covered by sand, dirt, or debris in strong winds. Abandoned eggs may survive to hatching, even those moved by high tides, if found in time and incubated properly.

Shorebird chicks that become temporarily separated from their parents may be captured by well-meaning rescuers. If the chick is brought immediately to a wildlife rehabilitator and is in good condition, it may be possible to reunite it with the parents if the location where it was found is known. However, chicks are often kept by the rescuer for a day or more before being brought to a rehabilitator, in which case the bird will need immediate attention.

Orphans may be the product of asynchronous hatching if the last chick or egg is left behind by the parents. Predation or injury of parents also may create orphans.

## Record Keeping

Detailed information on the location where the bird was found should be recorded. This will serve as a guide for suitable habitat for release. Wildlife regulatory agencies have minimum standards for record keeping that require tracking of individual animals undergoing rehabilitation. Check with your regulating agencies for further information. As a minimum, the following information should be kept: species, age, location found, reason brought into captivity, medical problems, final disposition, and release location.

A detailed medical record should be kept on each animal, with results of the initial examination recorded and any updated information added as it happens. This should include regular body weights, progress of treatments, and pertinent notes on behavior.

Marking the top of their head with a sharpie marker or temporary plastic leg bands may be used to identify individual chicks (National Band and Tag Company). Leg bands used for identification should be regularly checked for correct fit, because many shorebirds have a substantial increase in leg size between hatching and fledging. The marker may need to be reapplied as it fades.

## Incubation and Hatching of Eggs

Proper incubation temperature is critical for ensuring the maximum hatchability of the eggs as well as the best physical condition of the chicks that hatch. For more detailed information on incubation of eggs, see Chapter 3.

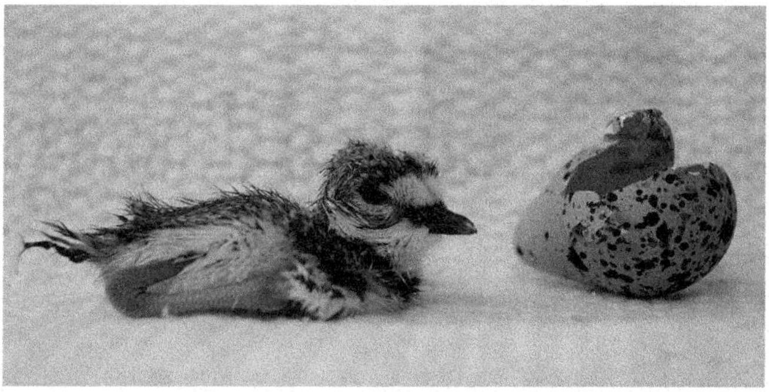

Figure 24.1 Killdeer hatchling. *Source:* photo courtesy of International Bird Rescue.

For most shorebirds, use the settings recommended for quail, which is 99.6–100 °F (37.6–37.8 °C). Moisture normally should be about 40–55% relative humidity. The eggs should be rotated 180° every two hours and, depending on the incubator used, may be set to turn eggs automatically. During the final 4–5 days of incubation, the eggs should not be rotated and the temperature should be lowered by 1 °F and humidity increased to about 65%. Make sure the inside of the hatcher used is safe for hatchlings. If the bottom of the hatcher has larger mesh that a leg could fall through, place some finer mesh on the bottom.

Fine cracks can appear at the large end of the egg up to 4–5 days before hatching (these cracks are difficult to see without magnification). Regular tapping can be heard 2 days before hatching and regular peeping can be heard 1–5 days before hatching. Eggs can hatch at any time of the day or night. Once they have externally pipped (can see a distinct hole), they can hatch within 20 minutes up to 48 hours later. If no progress is seen within 24 hours or it has pipped in the incorrect spot, assistance may be required. See Chapter 3 for more information on how to assist a hatch.

After hatching, swab the umbilicus area with betadine to help prevent infections. Briefly examine the chick once it is dry to make sure the yolk sac is retracted and there are no obvious deformities. Allow the chick to dry completely, fluff up, and gain strength inside the egg incubator (Figure 24.1). At this point, the chick may be moved to a brooder.

## Initial Care and Stabilization

Chicks should be placed in a climate-controlled intensive care unit or brooder on arrival. New patients should be allowed to rest for 15–20 minutes in a warm, dark, quiet container before examination. Depending on the age of the chick, the ICU could be set at around 95 °F (35 °C). Adjust the temperature based on the chicks' behavior. Warm chicks are mobile and very active. Cold or stressed chicks sit down and appear sleepy.

Once the bird is warm, if it is active, offer live food items in shallow dishes. The best first live prey to offer are tubifex worms (in water) and small fly larvae (*Musca domestica*). These food items are active and the movement attracts the chicks. Chicks should begin pecking at the food almost immediately. If they are not eating well, try sticking a hand in the brooder, with the remainder of yourself hidden, and try dropping the food at their feet and tapping at it with your finger.

After being warmed, if the bird appears too weak to eat or stand, consider rehydrating the bird orally. If the chick will not eat on its own after being warmed to normal body temperature, and appears too weak to eat on its own, it should be rehydrated orally. Place a drop of unflavored electrolyte solution (such as Pedialyte®) or lactated Ringer's solution (LRS) very carefully on the tip of the bill and allow it to roll down the bill for the chick to swallow. If needed, gently open the mouth slightly and insert a drop in the side of the bill. Be careful so that the chick does not aspirate. Repeat this a few times. Follow the drops of electrolyte solution with drops of 50% dextrose if the chick is still poorly responsive. If the chick is extremely young or has been chilled or is lethargic, see Box 24.1 on intensive care of hatchlings.

Most shorebirds are very easily stressed. A warm, quiet, environment and as minimal handling as possible are important to their success. Make sure new arrivals are warm and well hydrated before proceeding with a thorough physical exam. During their time in captivity, birds should be briefly examined each time they are weighed for feather condition, vent cleanliness, foot condition, injuries, or signs of illness. See Chapter 1 for information on performing a physical exam on chicks.

Always hold a bird by reaching around from the back. Birds must expand their chests to breathe and if they are held from the front their breathing may be restricted. Chicks are very fragile so be gentle, taking care that a chick does not suddenly jump out of your hand and fall to the floor. Because shorebird chicks must be able to run shortly after hatching, their legs are well developed from the start.

## Common Medical Problems and Solutions

### Metabolic Bone Disease

Due to rapid growth and often extremely long limbs, shorebirds may be susceptible to metabolic bone disease (MBD). High calcium, low-fat diets are very important in rearing long legged birds. See Chapter 17 for a discussion of this problem.

### Angel Wing

Wing abnormalities in the carpometacarpal area commonly called *slipped wing* or *angel wing* may occur for several reasons: deficiencies in one of several nutrients such as vitamin E, vitamin $D_3$, or manganese, excessive dietary protein, or overfeeding (Flinchum 2006). If this occurs, the chick should be moved into a larger enclosure to increase its activity level. Adjusting the diet so that a greater percentage is chitinous food, such as crickets and mealworms (waxworms and fly larvae are higher in fat), also may help. Food should be supplemented with powdered calcium carbonate and avian vitamins (Nekton-S). The wing should be wrapped into normal position and checked daily for improvement in its alignment. If attempts to correct this problem are made promptly, correction may occur within 3–5 days. Be careful to not damage growing flight feathers with wraps.

### Leg and Toe Abnormalities

Stilts and avocets seem to be particularly susceptible to foot problems, such as drying, cracking, and pressure sores. Keeping the substrate clean and soft and offering clean wading dishes and pools are important factors in preventing foot problems. Splayed legs and curled toes can also be an issue. The proper substrate is very important to prevent this. They need to have good traction and not slide around.

**Box 24.1 Hatchling Killdeer Intensive Care**

*Kappy Sprenger*

### Warmth

Almost all Killdeer chicks (*Charadrius vociferous*) are less than 5 days old when presented for care. Weighing around 10 g at hatch, these chicks are usually seen 1–3 days later at weights of 7–9 g. Many have become chilled. When cold, a precocial chick becomes inactive and lies down. Some Killdeer also lie down when frightened. However, within 15–20 minutes in a quiet, warmed place these birds should be up and running around. Chilled young take considerably longer to become active.

Immediately upon admittance, Killdeer chicks should be placed in a heated container or incubator and allowed to rest and get warm. If the chick is lying down or appears weak, the best temperature is 92–95 °F (33.3–35 °C). After warming, the chick can be weighed. Those that are weak or were chilled should remain at that temperature. Strong young up to 12 g can safely be kept at 90–92 °F (32.2–33.3 °C); those above 12 g, at 90 °F (32.2 °C). Until they are self-feeding, these temperatures should be maintained.

### Hydration and Liquid Nutrition

Until a chick has become warm and is strengthening, it should not be hydrated. The author generally uses lactated Ringer's solution or Pedialyte (Abbott), but any good hydrating solution will work. The warm fluid is offered from a 0.5 or 1.0 ml syringe, eyedropper, or a saturated cotton swab. This is much safer than attempting to gavage. One drop of fluid is drawn along the edges of the bill and repeated until drinking occurs. As it swallows, the bird's throat will move and the drop of liquid will disappear; however, the mouth will not appear to open. Each chick may be offered as much as it will drink, one drop at a time. Repeat every 30 minutes until definite strengthening is seen, and then hourly until the chick defecates. Defecations are quickly noticed if a white paper towel is used as a smooth-cover bedding. Next, warm liquid nutrition may be started using the same method. Formula V Enteral Care (High Protein) (PetAg) or another easily-assimilated critical diet for carnivores is suggested. Initially, alternate diluted liquid nutrition with hydrating solution every 1–1.5 hours. Do not mix hydrating solution with liquid nutrition. As the chick continues to strengthen, this routine should be maintained, with the liquid nutrition at full strength until the chick is reliably self-feeding.

### Monitoring

Be sure each chick's bottom is clean at all times. Until it is self-feeding and especially on a younger chick that has been chilled, a small bit of dark fecal matter may be noticed stuck to the white down just outside the vent. Remove this gently using a cotton swab dipped in warm water, carefully rolling the swab away from the vent area until it is clean, but not saturating the down. If the fecal matter appears again, clean it off. Left untended, this could build up and clog the vent, causing an obstruction and death.

### Getting Them to Start Eating

When a chick is steady on its feet and running around, a very shallow dish or lid with water may be provided. This should be less than 3 in. (1.2 cm) across, no more than 0.5 in. (1 cm) deep, and easily stepped into and out of without tripping. Sometimes a chick will drink from this dish, but it shouldn't be depended upon for hydration. Once warm and hydrated, Killdeer chicks quickly learn to feed themselves if they are offered live foods of appropriate sizes. As a chick wades and stands in the little water dish with live creatures wiggling around its toes, it can hardly resist eating them and will learn to feed itself much faster than if food is given separately. Tubifex worms are the right size, naturally live in water, and are very wiggly. Available in some aquarium shops, they are also nutritious and easily cared for until being fed. Tiny white mealworms (just having shed) are a good initial food as well. Although these may not live very long, if the water is just barely covering the bottom of the dish, they might remain active long enough to catch the chick's attention. They may also be placed in a small container immediately beside the shallow water dish. Do not risk using mealworms with hard, light brown skins. The skins are difficult to digest and can cause obstruction in debilitated, dehydrated, or very young birds. Live adult brine shrimp may be taken, as may very small earthworms. The diameter of any one item of food should not exceed the diameter of the bird's lower mandible. Once a plover chick starts feeding itself, it will quickly learn to eat nonliving foods as well.

Chicks seem to learn faster if small amounts of food are provided rather than large "clumps" where individual "bites" are not so readily noticed. Live guppies might be offered. Because the dish is shallow and temperatures high, the water will evaporate in just a couple hours. These shallow-water feeding dishes will need to be replenished several times a day. Calcium carbonate powder should be lightly sprinkled on a chick's food at least once a day.

Live food is not always available. Frozen or freeze-dried products available in aquarium shops or tropical fish departments of large pet shores may be used. Before feeding, frozen foods should be defrosted and freeze-dried products soaked a few minutes until saturated with water. Put a small amount of food in the shallow water dish. If the water is stirred gently for a moment causing the food bits to slowly swirl around, the chick's interest may be aroused. When it sees the movement of the bits of food it usually will pick at them and quickly learn to eat. A slow drip of water into the water dish from above also creates movement to catch attention. If neither of these tricks work, try gently opening the chick's mouth after it has been given liquid nutrition or hydrating solution, and put in one small piece of food. This step may be repeated a couple times at each feeding until the chick gets the idea. Once plover chicks have started eating, they are quite willing to take a variety of foods, and have surprisingly large appetites. Among the frozen foods, "bloodworms" (sometimes called "red mosquito larvae") are a favorite and nutritious starter food, as are adult brine shrimp. Of the freeze-dried products, tiny krill or ocean plankton, tubifex, and tiny shrimp may be taken. Soon, processed foods may be added to the diet. Cichlid minipellets are small enough for very young Killdeer, beginning with just a few placed in the shallow water dish, and later offered dry. It is usually only a day or two until the chicks that will recover are on their feet and running around, hungry and ready to grow.

## Diet

In the wild, it is the parent's job to lead the chicks to the food. Without their parents, they need help finding the food. Smaller chicks should be kept in smaller holdings and food should be made very obvious. As they grow, make food less obvious; scatter it around in dishes so they might have to look a little for it; and as they get close to fledging, all food should be scattered outside the dishes to promote good foraging behavior.

Most species of shorebirds do best with small, live, wiggly worms. They swallow their prey whole, so use small items for newly hatched chicks and larger items as they grow. Good examples are mini-mealworms, fly larvae, and blackworms or tubifex worms. Live adult brine shrimp may be used, as well as very small earthworms. Crickets and a few waxworms can also be offered to older chicks. Once a plover chick starts feeding itself, it will quickly learn to eat nonliving foods as well. See Box 24.1 for tips on feeding frozen and freeze-dried foods.

Use small jar lids or small, shallow dishes for food and water so that chicks can easily walk in and out of them and so, if chicks fall, they can easily get out of the dish (Figure 24.2). Larger chicks will need wider dishes. All food should be coated in powdered calcium carbonate. For species such as avocets, Nekton vitamins may also be needed. Oystercatchers require a specialized diet and require a different protocol, see Klusener et al. (2018).

Long-legged birds, such as avocets and stilts, do better with primarily extruded diets until fledging to help with getting enough calcium for their fast-growing bones. The following is a recommended diet protocol:

Approximate age 1–2 or 3 days old: In wide, shallow pans, 1 part Mazuri™ brand waterfowl starter pellets soaked in shallow water pan to 1 part blackworms soaked in water in a separate dish. Sprinkle a few mealworms and fly larvae on the pellets and around floor. All food is coated in 1 tbsp. of calcium carbonate powder per dish.

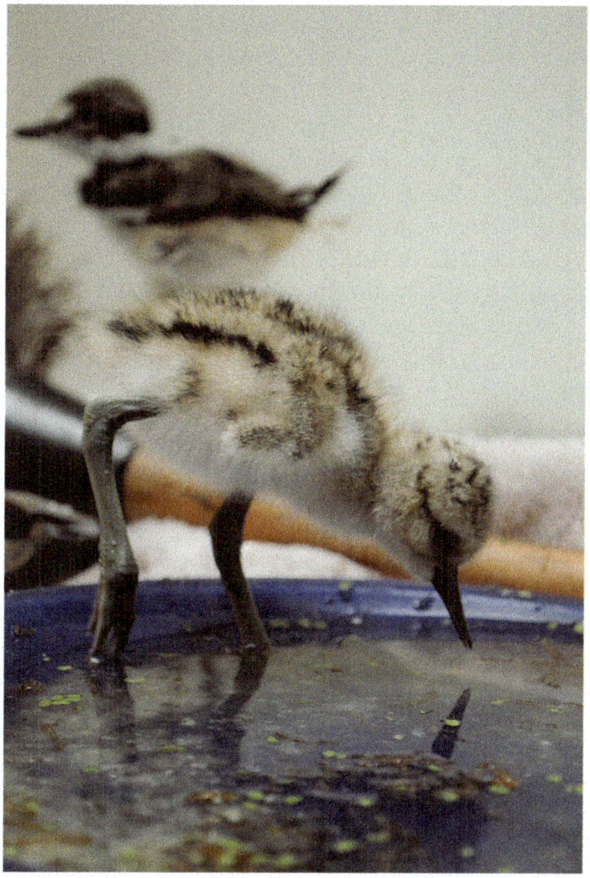

Figure 24.2 American Avocet chick housed with Killdeer chicks eating bloodworms from a shallow dish. *Source:* photo courtesy of International Bird Rescue.

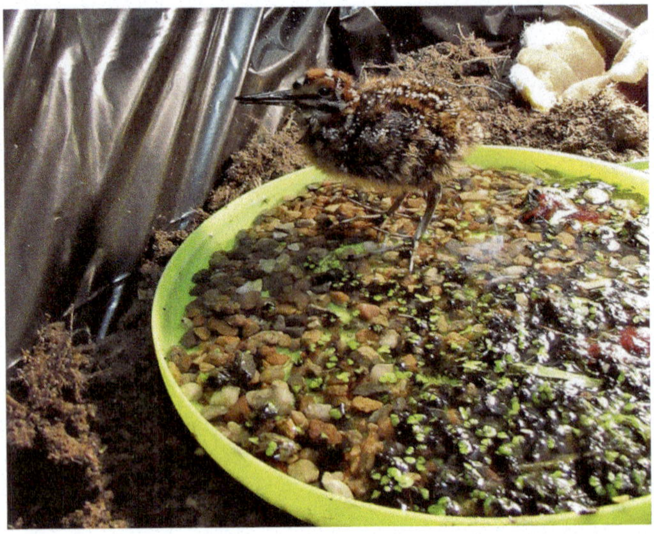

Figure 24.3 Wilson's Snipe chick offered invertebrates and duckweed in shallow dish of water with pebble substrate. *Source:* photo courtesy of Marjorie Cahak Gibson.

Age 2–5 or 6 days old: Use a large, shallow dish, such as a cafeteria tray. Use the same diet as above but start mixing some blackworms in with the pellets. Increase to ¼ cup of calcium carbonate powder and ½ tbsp. of Nekton scattered over each food dish. Can also introduce small crickets coated in calcium at this stage.

Age 6 days to fledge: Start a slow introduction of Mazuri brand sea duck pellets to the diet and decrease the amount of blackworms to an approximate ratio of 3 parts starter pellets: 2 parts blackworms: 0.5 part sea duck pellets. Continue sprinkling ¼ cup of calcium carbonate powder and ½ tbsp. of Nekton over each food dish. As they get older, increase the sea duck pellets and decrease the starter pellets until 100% sea duck pellets instead of the waterfowl starter close to fledging age. Continue with blackworms and other live insects.

While chicks are in brooders it is best to feed small amounts of food frequently (at least four times a day) because food will die from the heat after a few hours and shallow water will evaporate. Adding ice chips to the wet food (tubifex worms) may help. Open-top containers, such as aquariums or terrariums with a heat bulb, can be partially covered to create a shaded area where temperatures are somewhat cooler and the food stays alive longer. Do not place food dishes directly under the heat lamps. Depending on the number, age, and general temperament of the birds, multiple feeding stations and wading dishes should be provided (Figure 24.3).

## Expected Weight Gain

Chicks should steadily gain weight until close to fledging, when they approach adult weight. It is common to lose a gram or so from the day of hatching to the next day, but after that, it should be a pretty steady weight gain. If a chick is losing weight or not growing as rapidly as its cagemates, this may indicate a health problem, that the bird is not getting enough food, or that its access to food is being limited by larger birds. Weigh each chick regularly but care should be taken to not overly stress the bird through handling and, if the bird seems active, alert, and has been seen eating, do not feel like you need to get a weight. Weighing should always be coordinated with cleaning. See

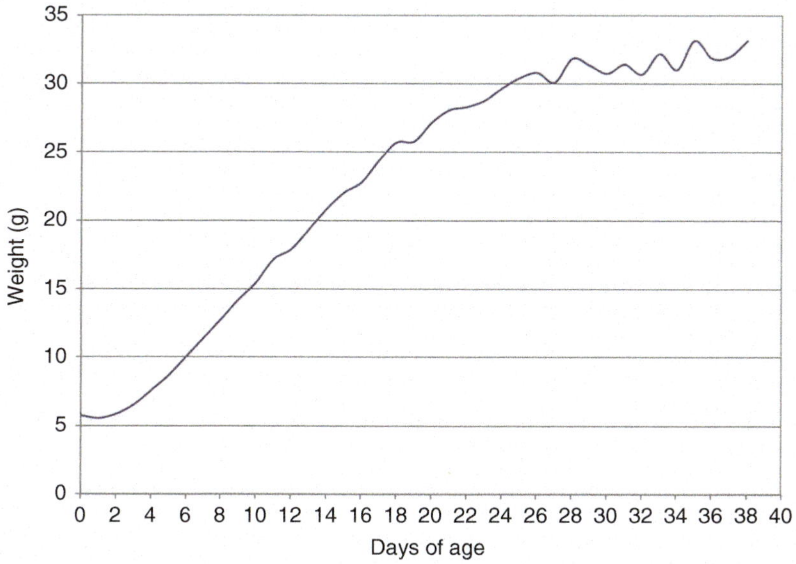


Figure 24.4 Average weight gain of Western Snowy Plover chicks.

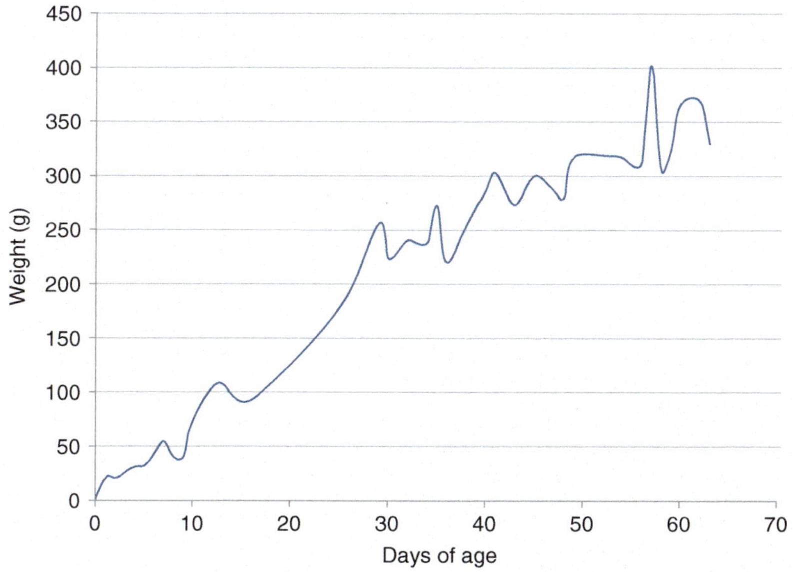


Figure 24.5 Average weight gain of American Avocet chicks.

Figures 24.4 and 24.5 (data courtesy of Monterey Bay Aquarium) for examples of weight gain in different species.

## Housing

It is important to limit human contact to prevent stress and habituation to people. Whenever possible, raise chicks with conspecifics of similar size. This may mean sending the chick to, or getting a chick from, another rehabilitator. If you are unable to match a chick with a conspecific, try putting it with other shorebirds of similar size so that it at least has another chick for companionship. Although aggression does not seem to be a problem between most shorebird chicks, when putting different chick species together it is important to be wary of larger chicks accidentally stepping on smaller chicks. It is not recommended to raise shorebird chicks with other precocial chicks, such as quail, because disease transmission, such as avian pox, may occur. Any bird that is kept by themselves should always have a mirror. Oystercatchers imprint on humans easily and special care and protocols may be needed.

There are many factors to consider that may influence how shorebirds are housed, such as the local ambient temperature, financial resources, and supplies and equipment available. At each step along the way, attention needs to be paid to each individual bird and how it is progressing in its development to determine when it is ready for the next step.

For hatchlings, start with a smaller enclosure, such as an Animal Intensive Care Unit (AICU, Lyon Technologies, Inc.), for the first few days. Other items that could work are brooders, aquabrooders, or aquarium/terrariums. The initial temperature of ICUs and incubators should be around 98–99 °F (36.6 °C–37.2 °C) and the temperature reduced by 1–2 °F each day, depending on the needs of the chick. Containers that are not fully enclosed should contain a heated section (warmed by a heat lamp) that is around 98–99 °F and an unheated section in case the chick gets too warm. Flannel pillowcases work very nicely for the top layer of cage substrate; they have some traction but are smooth so toenails do not catch. Use a thin towel, pillowcase, or something that provides some padding 1–2 in. (2.54–5.08 cm) thick underneath the top layer. Change the pillowcase daily and coordinate with weighing to keep handling at a minimum and chicks contained during cleaning.

Once they are eating readily and gaining weight, move them to a larger holding, such as a large aquarium/terrarium, long container, stock tank, or human infant playpen, depending on the size and activity level of the chicks. Sand substrate is recommended. Use clean, mesh #30 sand, at least 1 in. (2.54 cm) thick for smaller birds and at least 2 in. (5.08 cm) thick for larger birds, such as avocets and stilts (Figure 24.6). Monitor the temperature of the sand below the heat bulb to ensure that it does not become too hot. If sand is unavailable, use flannel sheets or smooth fabric with padding

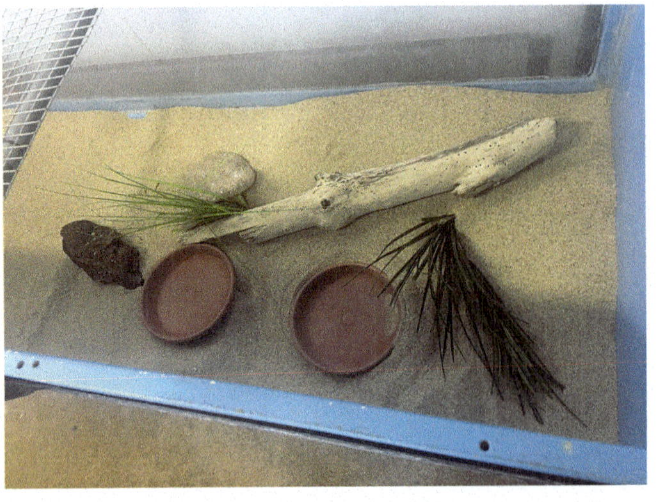

Figure 24.6 Indoor tank housing with naturalistic furnishings, shallow feeding dishes, heat support as needed, and full-spectrum lighting with natural day/night cycles.

underneath, such as towels or more sheets or soft nomad matting. It is important to keep the substrate clean. Use a small hand broom and dustpan to sweep the debris off the sand and into a bucket. Provide freshwater wading dishes daily. Clean the substrate several times a week, the frequency is dependent on the size of the enclosure and the number of birds in it. It is important to keep the disruption to a minimum. Coordinate the cleaning with weighing and have them caught up and placed in box while cleaning.

Another caging option would be to make an enclosure up on legs off the floor with plywood walls, mesh flooring, and light fabric sheeting covering the top. The mesh bottom allows feces and urates to pass through, but the mesh must be small enough to not risk entanglement of toes or feet.

A heat source around 95 °F (35 °C) should be offered in one area and ambient temperature in the other area. A variety of spot heat bulbs may be used to create a warm area, such as a 100–150-W spot incandescent nocturnal black heat lamp (e.g. ESU Reptile NightLight Spot). The distance the heat lamp is above the brooder will need to be determined by the individual setup. As the chicks get closer to fledge and they stop spending a lot of time under the heat lamp at night, the heat source can be removed.

Full-spectrum lights on a natural light cycle, such as Reptisun 5.0 UVB (ZooMed Laboratories), should also be provided for birds housed indoors. See the manufacturer's specifications regarding the proper distance for placement of bulbs above the chicks and the frequency that bulbs require replacement.

As chicks get older and are feeding well, they may be kept in an outdoor aviary, depending on ambient temperature and the size and activity level of the chicks. Aviaries range in size from 8 to 25 ft. long × 5.5–24 ft. wide × 6–16 ft. high, depending on the size of the species. For minimum recommended sizes for waterbirds, see Miller (2012). Aviaries should be designed as naturalistic enclosures, offering ample opportunity for birds to explore and forage (Figure 24.7). Sand substrate is preferred and must be at least 2 in. (5 cm) thick. The larger the shorebird species, the thicker the sand should be, at least 3 in. thick for stilts and avocets. Additional substrate can include small smooth stones, mud, grasses, and/or nomad matting.

All food and water dishes should be shallow and easy for birds to step in and out of. For newly hatched chicks, small plant saucer dishes work well, as do baby jar lids. For Killdeer chicks, a size that works well should be less than 3 in. (1.2 cm) across, no more than 0.5 in. (1 cm) deep and easily stepped into and out of without tripping. For older birds, medium-size planter saucer dishes work well. For long-legged birds, such as avocets and stilts, cafeteria trays work well. Sometimes a chick will drink from food dishes, but they shouldn't be depended upon for hydration.

All birds should always have access to water to wade in. It should be no deeper than just covering their feet for newly hatched chicks and a little past their feet for older birds. They should always be able to easily get in and out of the dishes. For birds such as avocets and stilts, larger, shallow plant saucer dishes work well for wading in water. The long-legged birds can easily slip, so care should be given to make sure the surface is not slippery. A shallow sloped bottom pool covering a portion of the floor would also be beneficial in the outdoor aviary.

Young chicks should be provided with a feather duster to brood under, and stuffed animals may provide companionship for solitary chicks. If outside, provide some short of shelter and a warm area with a heat lamp. As the birds approach fledging age, remove the shelter, heat source, and feather duster. Fake or real plants as well as driftwood can also be provided to give birds a sense of privacy. Care should be taken that the plants do not cause any entanglement or trip hazards.

Use a disinfectant footbath and rinse before entering and after exiting outdoor aviaries to decrease the chance of tracking contaminants from shoes into and out of aviaries. Clean and disinfect aviaries thoroughly after birds have been released before setting up for new birds.

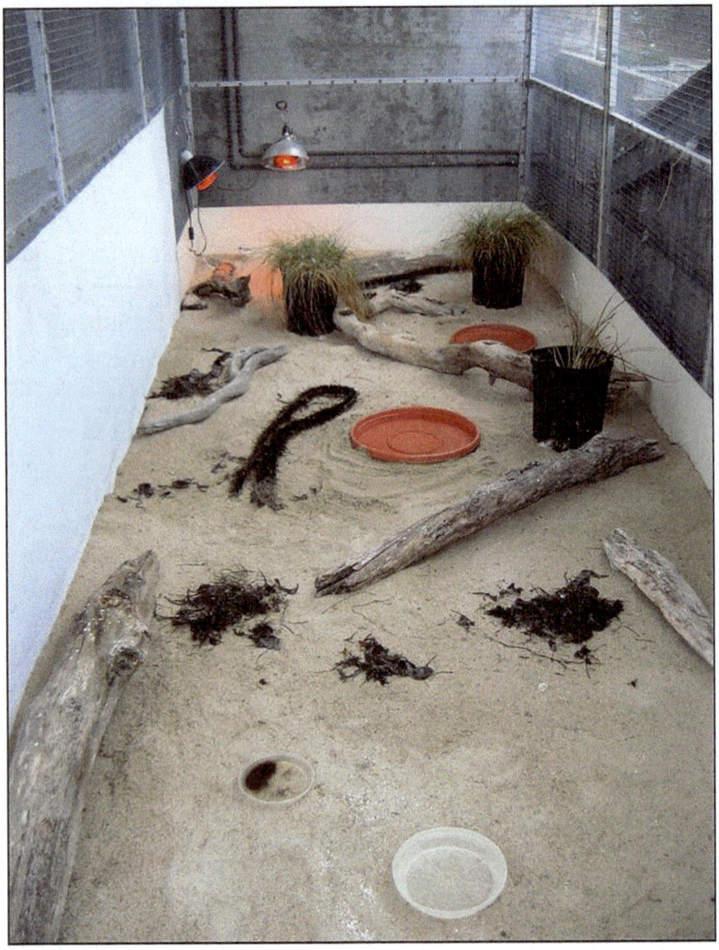

Figure 24.7 Pre-release aviary set up for shorebirds, with sand substrate, small, shallow feeding dishes, and vegetation for privacy.

## Preparation for Wild Release

Find out the local wild fledging age to get an approximate time frame for release. Release birds a week or so after the normal fledging age, when they are flying well. When they are starting to learn how to fly, care should be given to keep human disturbance to a minimum because injuries from birds hitting the walls can occur. Each bird should be in excellent health, waterproof, and an excellent flyer. Make sure each bird is well-muscled and can fly well enough to avoid predators and travel with conspecifics. Fledglings may not weigh as much as an adult, so find out what is normal for that species.

Birds should exhibit appropriate foraging behaviors and wariness of humans. Release birds in areas where there are conspecifics. They will do better if they can join a flock or groups of other fledglings. It is beneficial to work with researchers that may be studying shorebird species in the wild to gather post-release data; whenever possible, coordinate with permitted bird banders to apply federal leg bands prior to release. If a shorebird is nonreleasable, please consider captive placement in an AZA accredited zoo or aquarium.

## Acknowledgments

We would like to thank the many participants in the Snowy Plover Conservation Project, headed by Point Blue Conservation Science (PBCS), for their tireless efforts to monitor, protect, rescue, raise, and rehabilitate Snowy Plovers along the California coast. PBCS researchers also banded and monitored released chicks, which provided valuable post-release information. We also would like to thank the Monterey Bay Aquarium for their work with the rehabilitation of shorebird eggs and chicks which were instrumental in the development of the rehabilitation methods described in this chapter. A special thank you to "Snowy" (a.k.a. The Little General), a favorite Snowy Plover who was an ambassador for his species and a great dad to orphaned chicks.

## Sources for Products Mentioned

Animal Intensive Care Units: Lyon Technologies, Inc., 1690 Brandywine Avenue, Chula Vista, CA 91911, (888) 596-6872. https://lyonusa.com.

Crickets: Bassett's Cricket Ranch, Inc., 365 S. Mariposa, Visalia, CA 93292–9242, (800) 634-2445 or (559) 747-2728, Fax 559-747-3619, https://store.bcrcricket.com.

Feeder insects: Arbico Organics, PO Box 8910, Tucson, AZ 85738-0910, (800) 827-2847, https://www.arbico-organics.com.

Feeder insects: Grubco, 7995 North Gilmore Rd, Fairfield, OH 45014, (800) 222-3563, www.grubco.com.

Formula V Enteral Care (High Protein): PetAg, Inc., 255 Keyes Avenue, Hampshire, IL 60140, www.petag.com.

Full-spectrum lighting: Zoo Med Laboratories Inc., 3650 Sacramento Drive, San Luis Obispo, CA 93401, (888) 496-6633, https://zoomed.com.

Leg bands: National Band and Tag Company, 721 York St, Newport, KY 41072-0430, (800) 261-TAGS (8247).

Mazuri, PMI Nutrition International, LLC, PO Box 66812, St. Louis, MO 63166, www.mazuri.com.

Mealworms: Rainbow Mealworms, Inc., P.O. Box 4907, 126 East Spruce Street, Compton, CA 90220, (310) 635-1494, www.rainbowmealworms.net.

Nekton-S: Nekton USA, 600 F Street, Arcata, CA 95521, (707) 822-2417, www.nekton.net.

## References

Flinchum, G.B. (2006). Management of waterfowl. In: *Clinical Avian Medicine* (eds. G.J. Harrison and T.L. Lightfoot), 846. Palm Beach, FL: Spix Publishing.

Klusener, R., Hurtado, R., Stander, N., and Parsons, N.J. (2018). First report of a hatched, hand-reared, and released African oystercatcher. *Zoo Biology* 37 (1): 54–58.

Miller, E.A. (2012). *Minimum Standards for Wildlife Rehabilitation*, 4e. National Wildlife Rehabilitators Association: St. Cloud, MN.

Petersen, W.R. (2001a). Plovers and lapwings. In: *The Sibley Guide to Bird Life and Behavior* (eds. C. Elphick, J.B. Dunning Jr. and D.A. Sibley), 257–264. New York: Alfred A. Knopf.

Petersen, W.R. (2001b). Oystercatchers. In: *The Sibley Guide to Bird Life and Behavior* (eds. C. Elphick, J.B. Dunning Jr. and D.A. Sibley), 265–267. New York: Alfred A. Knopf.

Thurston, H. (1996). *The World of the Shorebirds*, 117 pp. San Francisco: Sierra Club Books.

# 25

# Alcids

*David A. Oehler*

## Natural History

The family Alcidae, or auk, is a group of marine, neritic, and pelagic birds with a circumpolar range, found exclusively in the Northern Hemisphere. The name *auk* was derived from the Norse word *ãlka,* given to describe the calls of these seabirds. Alcids have been divided into 11 genera represented by 22 species. These species are represented by six major species groups divided into two phyletic lines, one involving puffins and the other comprised of the auklets, murrelets, guillemots, Dovekie, and the auks. All members of this group are highly specialized, wing-propelled, diving birds with thickset, torpedo-shaped bodies and short wings and tails. Typical morphology consists of plumage that is mainly black or gray above and white below. Dramatic alterations of this plumage occur during the winter months, with certain species obtaining gray-and-white plumage. The specific diving abilities of particular species, coupled with variations in prey items from zooplankton to fish, alleviate competition among species. There is a close correlation between diet to body mass and bill type (del Hoyo et al. 1996).

Due to their prey selection, alcids are normally found in the waters of the continental shelf located in low and Arctic waters, with only members of the genus *Synthliboramphus* located in subtropical waters. Foraging entails remaining on the water for a majority of the year and coming to land only to nest and propagate. Alcids normally use islands and sea cliffs to establish breeding colonies of up to more than one million birds in size. Nests within these colonies usually are found within rocky substrates, earthen burrows, or inaccessible cavities, with only one species utilizing an arboreal platform nest. Adult feeding of chicks typically follows a pattern of increased provisions affected by the nutritional status of the chicks, followed by restricted amounts prior to fledging (Hudson 1979; Ashcroft 1979; Emms 1987; Harding et al. 2002).

## Criteria for Intervention

Very few alcid species' chicks are encountered by rehabilitation facilities, which may be due to the inaccessibility of most breeding colonies and nest sites. Logging activities have resulted in a small number of Marbled Murrelets (*Brachyramphus marmoratus*) requiring intervention, since this species nests on the branches of old-growth conifers (Hamer and Nelson 1995). Murres and Razorbills (*Alca torda*) have an intermediate developmental strategy, allowing the chicks to depart

*Hand-Rearing Birds*, Second Edition. Edited by Rebecca S. Duerr and Laurie J. Gage.

the colony at 2–3 weeks of age. Fed by the parents, these chicks then remain with the adults at sea for up to 8 weeks. Common Murre (aka Common Guillemot) (*Uria aalge*) chicks may become separated from their parents at sea and beach in sometimes large numbers. *Synthliboramphus* chicks depart the nest with the parents shortly after hatching. These strategies likely reduce the energetic costs of chick rearing (Sealy 1973). The majorities of alcids that need assistance are fledglings of the larger species and are found along the coastline. These puffins, murres, or guillemots are usually underweight and often have compromised plumage. Taking immediate action is critical in reducing the cold stress that may negatively impact the immune responses in these birds (Siegel 1985). Rearing of seabird chicks may contribute significantly to conservation efforts, particularly within threatened species (Montesdeoca et al. 2017; Morten et al. 2017).

## Record Keeping

The importance of maintaining detailed records for each bird cannot be emphasized enough. General background information is needed for reporting requirements, such as species, age, the locale of rescue, reason brought into captivity, medical information, final disposition, and/or release location. Monitoring each individual bird requires a systematic and consistent means of evaluation to ensure its health, and to provide data for future use. Recording environmental conditions, exposure to infectious agents or toxins, diet, feed intake, physical condition, and body mass are essential in the care of alcids in a captive situation. Weigh chicks each morning, prior to the first feeding, and record the volumes of feed, along with brooder temperature, the attitude of chick, and medical notations.

## Initial Care and Stabilization

Make every attempt to obtain a complete history of a bird upon arrival. This will assist in the evaluation of the bird and provide information designating proper release sites. Observe the bird and record the attitude, respiration, and plumage condition. A physical examination is required to ascertain body weight, general condition, and possible trauma. Conduct the examination and give suitable medical treatment as quickly as possible to reduce the stress to the bird.

Usually, alcids that arrive at rehabilitation centers are dehydrated, undernourished, and hypothermic. Arrange for supportive care as part of a standard protocol for incoming birds. Once warmed, begin rehydration of the bird by administering oral or subcutaneous fluids: 40–50 ml/kg of lactated Ringer's solution (LRS) or a similar balanced isotonic solution. Administer a broad-spectrum antibiotic if indicated after an initial examination or preliminary diagnostic testing. This therapy should be prescribed by a veterinarian and may be altered based on clinical signs, diagnostic tests, and culture and sensitivity results. Prophylactic antifungal therapies are often recommended for captive alcids because secondary fungal infections are common in seabirds. Some rehabilitators recommend the initiation of itraconazole therapy within 48 hours of arrival, although only after the bird has been rehydrated to minimize the risk of potential toxic effects on the kidneys. Vitamin B-complex, A, $D_3$, and E supplementation should also be provided (ASLC 2006b; Huckabee pers. comm.).

Complete blood collection and analysis to assist in the diagnosis of medical problems. If the chick is strong enough, collect a sufficient volume of blood for a packed cell volume (PCV) and total protein (TP). If indicated and feasible, more detailed bloodwork, such as white blood cell count and biochemistries, may be informative.

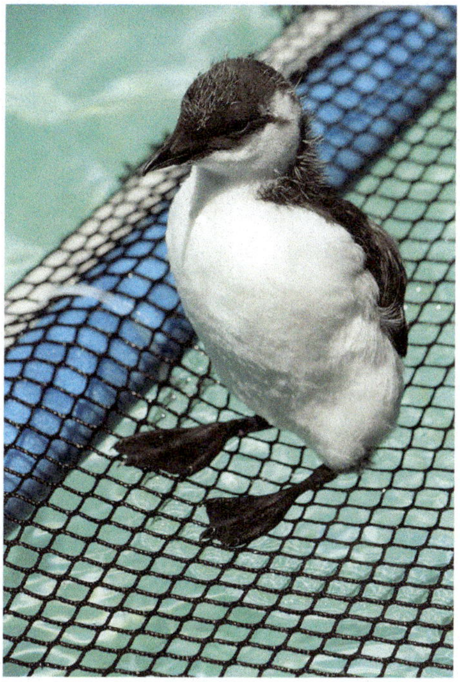

Figure 25.1 Common Murre chick standing on a pool haul-out. *Source:* photo courtesy of International Bird Rescue.

Evaluate the plumage of each chick to determine the level of waterproofing. Place birds with good plumage, which properly sheds water, directly into an enclosure with pool facilities (Figure 25.1). Never offer standing containers of water to any of the alcids since this results in compromised plumage and hypothermia. Plumage that is excessively worn, oiled, and/or absorbs water precludes the introduction of the bird to open water. Transfer these birds with compromised feathers to suitable holding areas and provide supplemental heat. Poor plumage may indicate underlying and/or long-term health problems that may be investigated further.

## Common Medical Problems

The duration of residence in a rehabilitation facility should be as short as possible to minimize the risk of medical issues (Molina-López et al. 2013). Wild-stranded chicks presented for rehabilitation may be extremely emaciated or anemic upon arrival and may require intensive care and thermoregulatory support.

### Parasitism

Ectoparasites, such as lice and ticks, adversely affect alcids, reducing growth rates and the condition of the plumage (Muzaffar and Jones 2004). Utilize a water-based pyrethrin spray to eliminate these infestations. Any spray or other substance used on the feathers must not damage or leave a residue on the plumage that will interfere with the waterproofing capabilities. Avoid oil- or petroleum-based products.

Perform a direct fecal analysis to evaluate for endoparasites; coccidia are common. Fledglings may also present with hemoparasites such as *Babesia uriae* (Yabsley et al. 2009). Screening birds by examination of a blood smear may be informative. Affected chicks may have greatly elevated TP values with or without concurrent anemia (R. Duerr pers. comm.).

### Fungal and Viral Infections

Alcids, along with other seabirds, are susceptible to a fungal infection, aspergillosis, especially when held indoors particularly in facilities inland (Burco et al. 2012; Burco et al. 2014). Inappetence may be one of the first clinical signs that this condition exists. Itraconazole therapy, maintaining a clean environment, fresh air, and proper ventilation (10–12 air exchanges per hour) are the best preventative measures that may be enacted. Recent trials involving *Aspergillus* vaccinations are underway and may have significant benefits to seabirds held in these captive situations. Avian pox has been identified in stranded juvenile Common Murres in California (International Bird Rescue, unpubl. data).

### Nutritional Deficiencies

Vitamin deficiencies occur regularly in piscivorous birds, due to loss of vitamins in the freezing and thawing process in the fish that are fed to these birds in a captive situation, and may result in a variety of morbidity and mortality events. Vitamin supplementation, mixing vitamin powder on smaller feed items, or placing tablets in feed fish prevents these deficiencies (Mejeur et al. 1988; Tocidlowski et al. 1997).

### Pododermatitis

Pododermatitis or *bumblefoot* is an inflammatory or degenerative condition, common in the feet of seabirds that are forced to stand on hard, smooth cement surfaces for extended periods of time. Incorporate preventative measures (see the section "Housing," later in this chapter) into any holding enclosure provided to alcids. Resolution of bumblefoot is slow and may require intense management. While on land, murres stand on tarsi or lower legs rather than on their feet. Monitor the hocks frequently for swelling or heat, and place birds demonstrating these clinical signs into pools for as long as possible. It is far better to prevent the development of foot lesions than to attempt treatment after they have progressed to the point of bumblefoot.

### Injuries

Some species of alcids have life histories that expose chicks to possible injuries. For example, Common Murre chicks must jump from their cliff-edge nests to join their father in the water below, and on the way down may bounce off rocks or be attacked by predators. Other species of Alcids must run to the ocean through forest while still quite young, or fly from forest to ocean without adult guidance. Fractures and wounds may be found in these chicks.

## Artificial Incubation

Artificial incubation of eggs is not required on a routine basis. Late-term incubation parameters indicate that a dry-bulb temperature of 99.5 °F (37.5 °C) with a relative humidity of 60% is sufficient to accomplish a successful hatch (see Chapter 3).

## Hatchlings

Although the dietary requirements for hatchlings vary between species, the brooder requirements may be interchanged based on the developmental rate of the species. ThermoCare Inc. Portable ICS Units and/or Dean's Model II Brooders have been used as brooders for chicks under 3 days of age. A thermoregulation pad, set at 98.0 °F (36.7 °C), is rolled into a cylinder and placed at one side of the brooder. Suspend a feather duster from the ceiling of the brooder, providing the chicks with an insulated, dark, and secure area next to the heat source. Cover each brooder with a towel to keep the interior darkened further. Although these high-tech brooders work well, we have been forced to improvise during excursions in the field. A shoebox, lined with lichens and moss, with heat supplied by refilling a water bottle with warm water, has been used successfully to rear day-old auklet and puffin chicks. Move chicks greater than three days of age to a cool room with an ambient temperature of 50 °F (10.0 °C). Although in the wild chicks may be brooded initially by the adults, after hatching we maintain a heat source for up to 2 weeks. A hot water heat source remains with the chicks and they are allowed access to the warmth and will self-regulate. Remove chicks at 21 days of age to an air-conditioned holding room with an ambient temperature of 55–60 °F (12.8–15.6 °C). Individuals remain separated from each other, using solid wall dividers between brooder sections to prevent aggression and to allow for monitoring of food intake (Figure 25.2). Furnish the wire- or net-bottomed brooders with a 1 × 1 × 1 ft. (30 cm × 30 cm × 30 cm) cardboard box, waxed on the outside, with a small opening approximately 4 × 5 in. (10 × 12 cm) cut in the front of the box.

Paper towels line the bottom of the boxes and are cleaned at each feeding. Monitor chicks for dehydration and overheating throughout the day. Dry eyes and pinched skin that remains tented are signs of dehydration, and increased fluids in the formula may be required. Labored respiration,

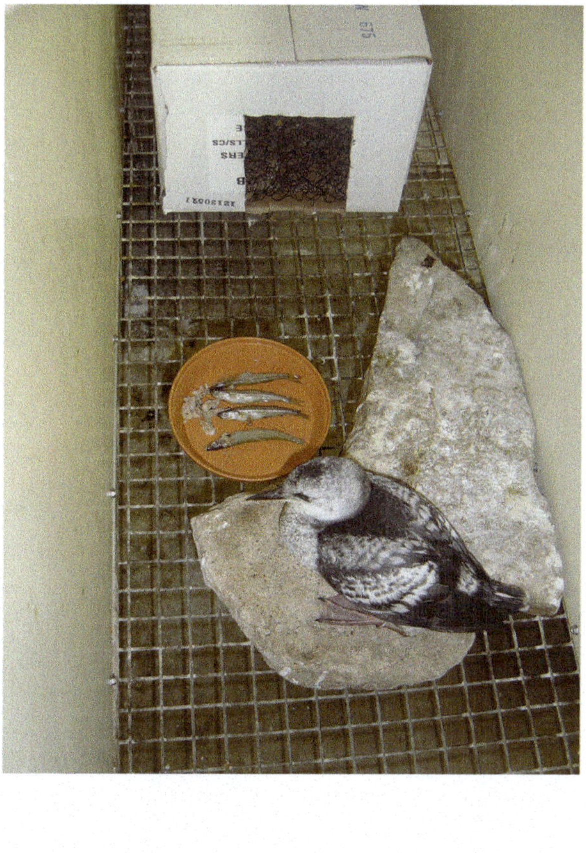

Figure 25.2 A 5-week-old Pigeon Guillemot fledgling is readied for transfer to open water. Note the use of a typical alcid brooder with solid wall dividers, cardboard box retreat area, and wire mesh substrate. *Source:* photo by David Oehler.

inappetence, or feet that radiate excess heat are clinical signs of heat distress and require a reduction in brooder or room temperature.

## Captive Fostering

If adult Common Murres are available in rehabilitation, many will allow murre chicks to approach and then exhibit protective behaviors, seeming to adopt the chicks. Others will ignore or rebuff the chick's requests for parenting behavior. Whenever possible, match chicks with an adoptive parent during care and release the birds together when both are ready. Adult birds recuperating from their own problems may be either stressed or enthused by the presence of a chick needing parenting; hence, thoughtful consideration of the match is needed (Figure 25.3).

## Diet Recipes

### Small Alcids

The base auklet formula consists of 85 g Cyclopeeze® (decapod microscopic crustaceans), 85 g Superba krill, 30 g mealworms, and 60 cc Pedialyte (Abbott), with 5 g of Mazuri Alcid vitamin supplement added (Mazuri). On short notice, substitute Mysis shrimp from your local freshwater and marine pet store for Cyclopeeze. Utilize additional Pedialyte (total of 100 cc) for chicks less than 3 days of age. Process all ingredients in a blender until smooth, taking care not to blend long enough to heat the mixture. Upon completion, refrigerate the formula and make a fresh supply daily. The formula must be able to pass easily through a modified syringe and 14 French catheter tube (Oehler et al. 2003).

Use a 50–60 ml catheter tip syringe. Attach a 14 French feeding tube or urethral catheter tube. Cut the tube to a length of approximately 4 in. (10 cm) at a 45° angle. Heat the cut end of the tube with an open flame to remove any sharp edges. One can find similar pet-quality feeding syringes

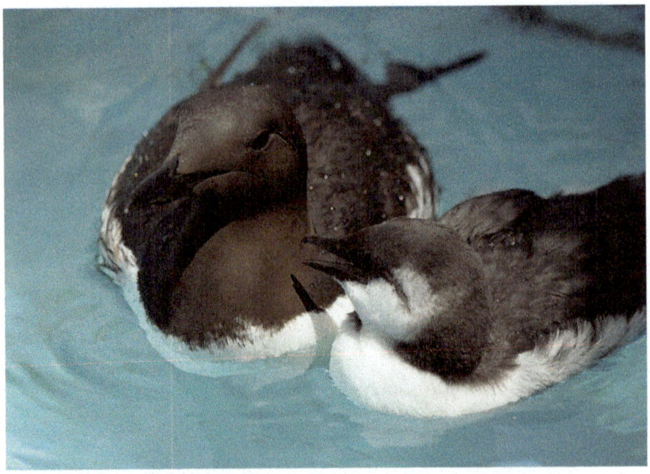

Figure 25.3 Common Murre adult exhibiting tolerance for an orphan while both are undergoing rehabilitation. *Source:* photo courtesy of International Bird Rescue.

and tubes at most larger pet stores. Secure the tube properly onto the syringe. This type of feeding tube has been used for thousands of feedings, and occasionally the tube will become separated from the syringe and is swallowed by the chick. With patience and some manipulation, the tube can be removed, but this adds unnecessary stress to the bird.

## Hand-rearing Diets and Feeding Procedures

Providing the proper nutrition to captive avifauna, even for commonly held taxa, is challenging. Feeder fish and krill are nutritionally diverse and care should be taken in choosing the proper food provisions for individual species of seabirds (Koutsos 2012). Improperly provided diets may lead to vitamin deficiency, fragile plumage, low bone density, and many other life-threatening problems. Commercially formulated diets are not available for alcids in general, and the difficulty of duplicating the diet of the various auklets compounds the challenges we face.

Current recommendations for alcid diets parallel the diet of their wild counterparts as closely as possible. Small alcids, such as Whiskered and Least Auklets, are exclusively planktivorous; Dovekies, the remaining auklets, and murrelets consume zooplankton and fish. Large alcids, the puffins, murres, and guillemots are mainly piscivorous, with nearly 95% of their diets consisting of fish, the remainder of invertebrates (Hatch and Sanger 1992; Ewins 1993; Hunt Jr. et al. 1993). The main difference between the diets of larger and small alcids is that the smaller birds feed on meals rich in wax esters (more than 60% of their total energy intake). This selection in prey items means that wax esters (long-chain fatty alcohols esterified to long-chain fatty acids) are the dominant dietary neutral lipid (Roby et al. 1986; Roby 1991). Many birds, especially seabirds, have a unique capacity for assimilating wax esters with higher efficiencies (greater than 90%) than that attainable by mammals (less than 50%) (Place 1992). Piscivorous species, the large alcids, rely on lipid-rich prey items, such as sand lances, Atlantic cod, Arctic cod, and pollock, to maintain their dietary requirements and in chick rearing (Ainley et al. 2002; Gaston and Hipfner 2002; Litzow et al. 2002; Piatt and Kitaysky 2002).

### Small Alcids

Alcid chicks demonstrate a rapid growth rate, given the short Arctic summer. As a result, these chicks need to take in a higher percentage of calories than many neonatal birds. Crop content of auklets in Alaska indicates that they forage for krill, small medusa, fish, and copepods, although this varies greatly for each species (Day and Byrd 1989; Harrison 1990). The more diminutive auklets rely more heavily on smaller zooplankton and do not take fish. Copepods appear to be a major dietary component of auklets in the wild, but the availability of copepods as feed for captive specimens is limited. Successfully incorporating frozen cultured copepods into the hand-rearing formula increases the calorie content per volume fed.

Using a warm-water bath, heat an appropriate amount of the small alcid formula required for one feeding and discard any unused portions. Feed chicks approximately 10% of their initial morning body weight for each feeding. Placing the tube to the side of the bill and extruding a small amount of formula onto the bill may elicit a feeding response. As the chick tastes the formula, place the tube into the chick's mouth and allow the chick to swallow the tube on its own. Depress the plunger of the syringe with a slow and constant pressure, ensuring the chick continues to swallow (Figure 25.4). If the chick stops swallowing or pulls away from the tube, discontinue the feeding. If the chick refuses to give a feeding response, do not force-feed, place the chick back in the

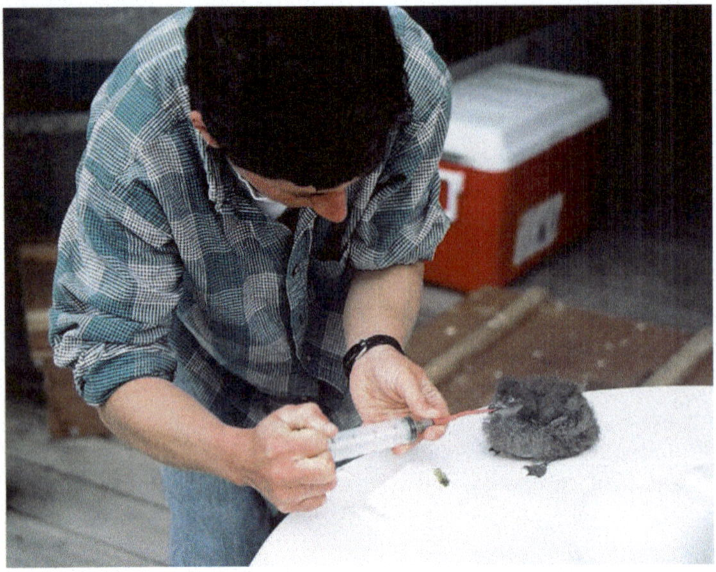

Figure 25.4 Aviculturist Sue Schmid, of the Cincinnati Zoo and Botanical Garden, hand-feeds a 25-day-old Whiskered Auklet. *Source:* photo by Mark Alexander.

brooder and try again in 1 hour. It cannot be stressed enough to allow the chick to dictate how much food it will take at each feeding (Oehler et al. 1995, 2001) (Table 25.1).

## Large Alcids

Larger alcid hatchlings, such as the guillemots, puffins, and murres, are hand-fed sand lances, silversides, herring, smelt, or capelin, whole or sliced fish, up to five times per day. Murrelets, which normally prey upon smaller fish and fish larvae, require small sand lances or thinly sliced fillets of larger fish. Soak each fish in Pedialyte prior to each feeding. Feed chicks less than 5 days of age approximately 40% of their initial morning body weight divided into five feedings over a 12-hour span. Elicit a feeding response by placing the fish to the side of the bill, although these birds quickly recognize feed and will move toward the fish when the brooder is opened. At 5 days of age, begin to offer whole fish on a plate instead of hand-feeding. Remove feed if not taken within the first 20–30 minutes. When chicks begin to consistently feed from the plates, larger amounts of fish may be placed upon the plates on beds of ice and left in the brooder. Feeding schedules will fluctuate between species, but as a general rule, reduce the number of feedings to three per day when chicks are 21 days of age (Thompson 1996; ASLC 2006a) (Table 25.1).

## Fledglings

Provide feed twice daily to mimic their natural foraging habits in the wild and to ensure that the feed items are fresh. To maintain a safe supply of feed, place these items in the water or on plates, with ice. Do not allow the feed to remain in the enclosure for extended periods. Because a majority of the feed items are stored frozen, vitamin supplementation is required. Provide these food items in clean, nontoxic, shallow bowls or plates. Offer water in a pool only and avoid the use of water bowls.

Table 25.1 Outline of the development of alcids in the wild and hand-rearing in captivity with suggested feeding schedules.

| Species | In-situ or Ex-situ | Hatch wt (g) | Feeding schedule: days 1–7 | Growth rate: days 1–7 | Feeding schedule: days 8–14 | Growth rate: days 8–14 | Feeding schedule: days 15–21 | Growth rate: days 15–21 | Fledge age (days) | Fledge wt (g) | Release wt (g) | Adult wt (g) |
|---|---|---|---|---|---|---|---|---|---|---|---|---|
| Common Puffin[a b c d] | In-situ | 48 | 4/day | 6 g/day | 10/day | 11–12 g/day | Up to 15/day | 11–12 g/day | 38–59 | 350 | | 460–490 |
| | Ex-situ | 41 | 5/day over 12 hours | 7 g/day | 5/day over 12 hours | 12 g/day | 5/day over 12 hours | 14 g/day | 32–45 | 280–440 | | |
| Horned Puffin[e] | In-situ | 59 | 3/day over 15 hours | 11 g/day | 3/day over 15 hours | 11 g/day | 6/day over 15 hours | — | 38–43 | 408 | | 581–648 |
| | Ex-situ | — | 5/day over 12 hours | 15%/day | 4/day over 12 hours | 10%/day | 4/day over 12 hours | 8%/day | — | — | >375 | |
| Tufted Puffin[f] | In-situ | 64 | 2–4/day over 15 hours | 16 g/day | 2–4/day over 15 hours | 16 g/day | 2–4/day over 15 hours | — | 44–55 | 496 | | 700–840 |
| | Ex-situ | | 5/day over 12 hours | 15%/day | 4/day over 12 hours | 10%/day | 4/day over 12 hours | 8%/day | — | — | >450 | — |
| Common Murre[g] | In-situ | 55–95 | 4–5/day over 15 hours | — | 4–5/day over 15 hours | — | — | 15 g/day | 14–21 | 200 | — | 945–1044 |
| | Ex-situ | — | — | — | — | — | 3/day over 15 hours | — | — | — | >700 | — |
| Thick-billed Murre[h] | In-situ | 65–70 | 2–6/day over 15 hours | 5–10 g/day | 10–15/day over 15 hours | 5–10 g/day | — | — | 18–21 | 200–250 | — | 810–1080 |
| | Ex-situ | — | — | — | — | — | 3/day over 15 hours | — | — | — | — | — |
| Pigeon Guillemot[i] | In-situ | 34–43 | — | 8–15 g/day | — | 10–20 g/day | — | — | 35–42 | 400–500 | — | 450–550 |
| | Ex-situ | — | 5/day over 12 hours | 15%/day | 4/day over 12 hours | 10%/day | 4/day over 12 hours | 8%/day | — | — | >400 | — |
| Marbled Murrelet[j k] | In-situ | 33 | — | — | — | — | 6/day over 12 hours | — | 27–40 | — | — | 220 |
| | Ex-situ | — | 5/day over 12 hours | — | 4/day over 12 hours | — | 4/day over 12 hours | — | — | — | — | — |

*(Continued)*

Table 25.1 (Continued)

| Species | In-situ or Ex-situ | Hatch wt (g) | Feeding schedule: days 1–7 | Growth rate: days 1–7 | Feeding schedule: days 8–14 | Growth rate: days 8–14 | Feeding schedule: days 15–21 | Growth rate: days 15–21 | Fledge age (days) | Fledge wt (g) | Release wt (g) | Adult wt (g) |
|---|---|---|---|---|---|---|---|---|---|---|---|---|
| Parakeet Auklet[l m] | In-situ | 27–32 | — | — | — | 9 g/day | — | — | 33–36 | 208–237 | — | 238–247 |
| | Ex-situ | 24 | 12/day over 22 hours | 25%/day | 8/day over 20 hours | 15%/day | 6/day over 12 hours | 8%/day | — | — | >200 | 273 |
| Crested Auklet[n] | In-situ | 25 | 1–4/day over 15 hours | — | 1–4/day over 15 hours | — | — | 11–13 g/day | 27–36 | 260 | — | 211–322 |
| | Ex-situ | | 12/day over 22 hours | 25%/day | 8/day over 20 hours | 15%/day | 6/day over 12 hours | 8%/day | — | — | >230 | 235 |
| Whiskered Auklet[o] | In-situ | 12–14 | | 4–5 g/day | — | 4–5 g/day | — | — | 39–42 | 106 | — | 99–136 |
| | Ex-situ | 14 | 12/day over 22 hours | 25%/day | 8/day over 20 hours | 15%/day | 6/day over 12 hours | 8%/day | — | — | >100 | 99 |
| Least Auklet[p q] | In-situ | 11–12 | 3/day over 15 hours | 5–6 g/day | 3/day over 15 hours | — | — | — | 26–31 | 82 | — | 85 |
| | Ex-situ | 11 | 12/day over 22 hours | 25%/day | 8/day over 20 hours | 15%/day | 6/day over 12 hours | 8%/day | — | — | >80 | 82 |

[a] D. Dial (pers. comm. 2018).
[b] Barrett (2002).
[c] Wickett (1999).
[d] Eilertsen (2008).
[e] Piatt and Kitaysky (2002).
[f] Wehle (1983).
[g] Ainley et al. (2002).
[h] Gaston and Kipfner (2000).
[i] Ewins (1993).
[j] del Hoya et al. (1996).
[k] Kappy Sprenger (pers. comm. 2006).
[l] Jones et al. (2001).
[m] Oehler et al. (1995).
[n] Jones (1993a).
[o] Byrd and Williams (1993).
[p] Jones (1993b).
[q] Wehle (1983).

Due to commercial availability, or unavailability, and given the specific requirements of each taxon, give careful examination to the choice of food items. Many of the alcids' food items are not commercially available, so choice in prey items is severely limited. Boiled Superba krill has been proven to maintain auklets in captivity and makes up the bulk of their diet. This diet is deficient in extra-long-chain fatty acids, a major component of their natural diet. Supplementation of live aquatic and nonaquatic invertebrates, along with cultured copepods, offsets this deficiency with success. The addition of live mealworms and Cyclopeeze has been effective in supplying the specimens with an abundance of medium- to extra-long-chain fatty acids and caloric intake. Shipping of Superba krill occurs in both boiled and raw forms; but the raw krill, being high in water content, spoils faster and tends to soil plumage. Because of its larger size, Superba krill must be cut down for smaller auklet species, such as the Least, *Aethia pusilla*, and Whiskered Auklets, *A. pygmaea*. Never offer sand lances to these auklets, because the high protein content and the high-energy requirements associated with the assimilation of these proteins places the individuals in a negative calorie situation. Boiled krill may be thawed overnight and stored in a refrigerator for 3–4 days. Never feed krill that has turned brown or that smells rancid, and remove food from the enclosure within 15 hours, or less if housed in an environment that is conducive to accelerating the decomposition processes. Sand lances are the preferred food item of puffins, murres, and guillemots, forming the bulk of the diet for these larger alcids, and they can be diced for the smaller taxa. In the absence of sand lances, silversides may be more easily purchased and are a suitable alternative.

During the freezing and thawing process, vitamins and nutrients naturally denature; therefore, add vitamin supplements daily. A multivitamin mix is essential to replace missing elements in the diet due to both the limited types of food available and the freezing and thawing process. Facilities housing birds in freshwater pools full time should provide salt supplementation at a suggested dosage of 250 mg NaCl /kg every 48–72 hours to assist in the regulating electrolyte balance in these birds (Frankfurter et al. 2012; R. Duerr, pers. comm.). Mazuri Auklet Blend (Mazuri) is a supplement containing essential vitamins and minerals, developed specifically for alcids. It is not always possible to have this type of vitamin mix available. A good quality multivitamin for birds, such as Quickon's Multivitamin or an equivalent, will supplement the birds' nutritional requirements while the birds are being held. Place these mixes on the food daily, in prescribed amounts. Vitamin supplementation for the smaller alcids can be challenging, due to the minute size of the items provided. To overcome this obstacle, supplements are produced or ordered in a powdered form. Place feed items in a clean feed bucket, in a predetermined quantity, and add a set amount of vitamin powder to the total supply of feed. The prescribed ratio of Mazuri Auklet Vitamin mix to feed has been determined to be 1.6 g of vitamin powder to 1.0 kg of feed. Mix the vitamins into the provisions to ensure a homogenous blend prior to placement in feed dishes.

Offer feed plates placed on ice to birds that have compromised plumage, such as oiled feathers, or do not have access to a pool. If providing a pool, toss fish and krill into the water to promote diving behavior. Discontinue tossing into the pools when the bird(s) are eating well from pool dishes.

In emergencies, you may substitute frozen shrimp and live baitfish as feed items for these alcids. Dice the shrimp into small pieces for the small alcids because they cannot break larger feed items apart. Live baitfish, placed in a small plastic pool, will provide larger alcids with food until alternative arrangements can be provided. Supply the pool with a source of fresh water that will create an overflow. This will remove any oils from the surface and maintain the condition of the birds' plumage.

## Weaning

Small alcids are more difficult to acclimate to feeding on their own than the larger alcids. Initial steps should be made to encourage these birds to feed from plates. Most of the smaller alcids will not begin to feed on their own until after fledging; larger alcids do so prior to fledging. Once they begin to feed off of plates, employ the same techniques to condition all alcids to forage in the water.

Toss appropriate feed items in front of the birds and into the pool throughout the day. Take measures to prevent the birds from seeing the person providing the feed so that released birds do not associate people with food. Once the feed has been placed in the water, continue tossing small amounts of feed in front of the bird. If the bird ignores the feed, discontinue this activity for an hour. When the bird begins to dive and eat the feed provided, continue feeding until the bird has had its fill. If possible, maintain like species of alcids together when conditioning them to forage and feed on their own. Once one bird becomes proficient in feeding, others follow quickly.

Feed problem birds by hanging or floating feed plates. Use live feed to stimulate foraging behavior. Easily obtained feed, such as brine shrimp and baitfish, will attract the attention of the bird.

## Expected Weight Gain

Small alcids should gain approximately 25% of their body mass each day during the first week after they hatch (Table 25.1). Daily growth rates slow to 15% at 7–14 days of age, 8% at 15–21, and 5% at 22–34. For example, a Least Auklet with a weight of 12.0 g at day 1 should gain approximately 3.1 g on day 2, 3.8 g on day 3, 4.7 g on day 4, and so forth, slowing to 15% of their daily body mass gain by about 7 days of age.

Large alcids vary, although approximate growth rates for the first week should be around 15%, slowing to 10% at 7–14 days of age, 8% at 15–21, and 2% as they reach 34 days of age (Table 25.1). Weight losses post-hatch and after fledging are not uncommon.

## Housing

As with other pelagic avifauna, alcids in a captive situation are colonial in nature and share the intricate behaviors of their wild counterparts. An assemblage of alcids must not only address their requirements for the congregation but also must respect their needs for spatial segregation (Figure 25.5).

Exacting environmental conditions are the first requirements in maintaining any alcid species. Vigilant monitoring of environmental conditions eliminates possible pathogens, environmental stresses, and physical sources of trauma that would endanger the health of the specimens held in any facility.

Facilities created for the housing of alcids indoors must condition the air to reduce the threat of overheating. Temperatures no greater than 40.0–50.0 °F (4.4–10.0 °C) are recommended for most alcids, although they are capable of withstanding temperatures well below these points. Medically compromised birds require supplemental heat and should be maintained at 72.0–80.0 °F (22.2–26.7 °C) to assist them in thermoregulation. Oiled birds require an ambient temperature at upwards of 80.0 °F (26.7 °C).

Pool areas should provide chilled water, a surface skimmer (either physical overflow or protein skimmer), a multifaceted filtration system, and an easy haul-out area (Figure 25.6). Maximum water temperatures of 40.0–50.0 °F (4.4–10.0 °C) provide a suitable aquatic environment. Due to

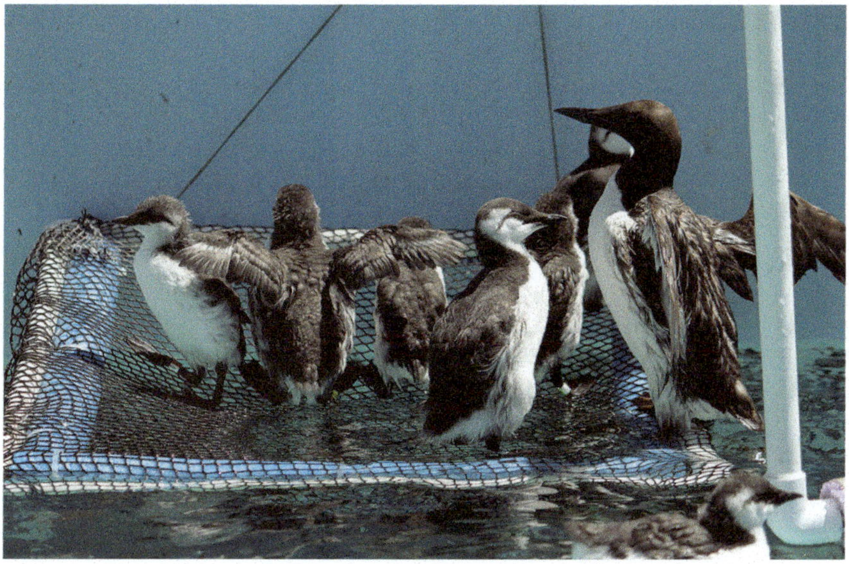

Figure 25.5 Multiple Common Murre chicks on a haul-out in a large pool, with an adult murre. Note the haul-out is constructed of a foam and PVC frame with soft netting. *Source:* photo courtesy of International Bird Rescue.

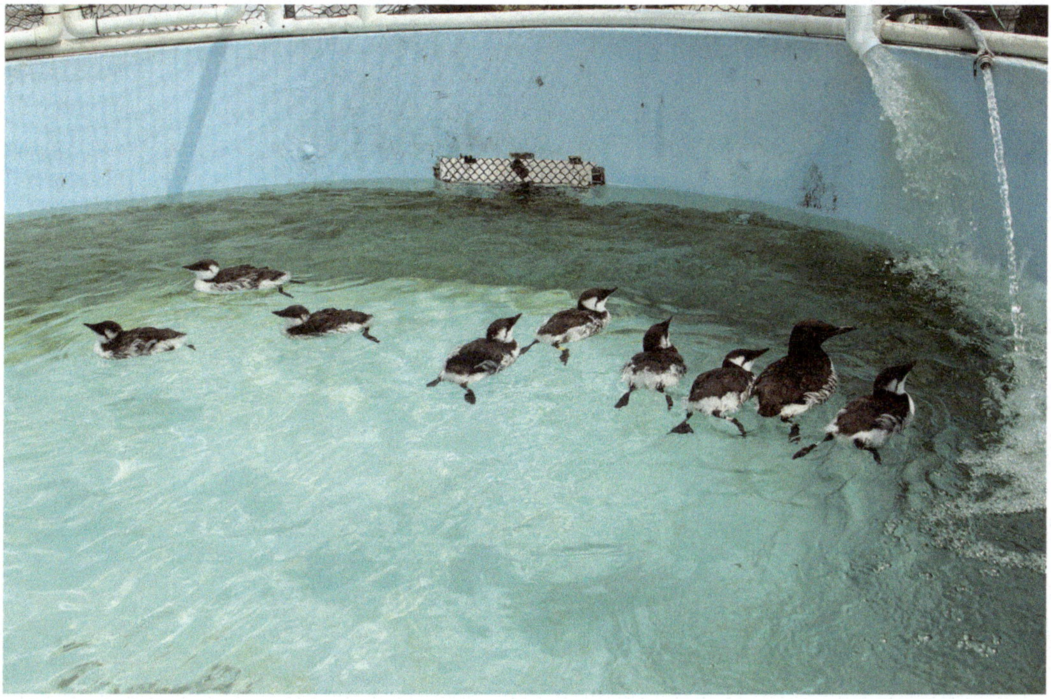

Figure 25.6 Large pre-release pool with surface-level drainage of water, filtration system, and constant inflow of clean water to maintain water quality. *Source:* photo courtesy of International Bird Rescue.

the delicate nature of the alcids' plumage and the diminutive body mass of specific taxa, it is imperative for these birds to be able to bathe and maintain perfect plumage to ensure thermoregulation. Quickly remove all oils on the surface of the water to prevent these contaminants from building up on the outer contour feathers. If oils cannot be properly removed, low-lipid fish must be provided to prevent loss of waterproofing. Water filtration may be achieved through various filtration methods, including sand and gravel filters, bag filters, UV filtration, and ozone filtration. Avoid the use of chlorination to prohibit degradation of the feathers that are in contact with the water.

Use of fiberglass, urethane, rock, and gravel substrates affords the birds with a solid surface that allows proper maintenance of plumage and prevents foot lesions. All deck areas should be well-drained in a manner to prevent contamination of pool and feeding areas. The abrasive alkaline nature of a cement deck is possibly the most detrimental surface that can be provided for alcids and seabirds in general. If an alternative substrate cannot be provided, the birds may benefit from the use of an antimicrobial mat such as Nomad™ on these hard surfaces to aid in the prevention of foot issues.

Pelagic avifauna, due to their access to an abundance of UV light in their natural environment, require greater amounts of supplemental lighting in a captive situation. Hypovitaminosis $D_3$ may occur in birds reared in indoor or shady enclosures, resulting in rickets. Augmentation of UV lighting, via an adequate lighting scheme, must be provided for any colony or individual alcid housed in an artificial environment.

## Preparation for Wild Release

Fully waterproof plumage is critical for alcid survival in the wild. Birds that have obtained proper plumage to survive in open water, are near adult weight, and are in good health, based on physical condition and blood parameters, are good candidates for release. Release sites should be determined by revisiting the original location of the rescue or known locations of like species in the area. All birds should be able to comfortably live in a water environment without haul-outs full time without becoming wet to skin at any areas or being stressed.

## Release

Whenever possible, release alcids at sea into a foraging group of conspecifics, as the capture beach may be an unknown distance from good foraging grounds or good forage may have moved. Once a release site has been chosen, make sure the weather conditions and the area are conducive to a successful release. The weather forecast should be for stable, clear weather for a 24-hour period. Alcids have difficulty becoming airborne and require long running starts to take flight, which precludes fully conditioning these birds for flight prior to release. Ensure the release site is open and free of immediate obstacles the birds may collide with and that there are no gulls or other predators in the vicinity. Use a boat to transport the released bird further from shore whenever possible. Sun-filled skies along open shorelines will give each bird ample opportunity to go out to sea, maintain good plumage, and with luck find birds of their own kind.

## Acknowledgments

Thanks to Barbara Callahan/International Bird Rescue, California (IBR); Debra Dial/National Aquarium, Maryland; Rebecca Duerr/IBR; Tasha DiMarzio/Alaska Sea Life Center, Alaska; Karen McElmurry/Center for Wildlife, Maine; Cindy Palmatier/Bird Treatment and Learning Center, Alabama; and Mark Russell/IBR for providing valuable insight into the rehabilitation aspects of alcids. In particular, I am grateful to Dr. John Huckabee, DVM/PAWS Wildlife Department, Washington, Kappy Sprenger, and Fritz Haas/Cincinnati Zoo, who critically read all or parts of the manuscript, providing information and improvements through their reviews.

## Sources for Products Mentioned

Cyclop-eeze®, Argent Chemical Laboratory, 8702 152nd Ave, N.E., Redmond, WA 98052, (800) 426–6258, www.argent-labs.com.

Mazuri Auklet Vitamin Mix (5M25-3M), Mazuri, 1050 Progress Dr., Richmond, IN 47374, (800) 227–8941, www.mazuri.com, http://www.mazuri.com/product_pdfs/5M2G.pdf.

3M™ Nomad Scraper Matting: Mats Inc., 179 Campanelli Parkway, Stoughton, MA 02072. (800) 628–7462, https://matsinc.com/commercial-flooring-brands/matting-branded/3m-matting.

Quiko Multivitamin: Orchid Tree Exotics, 2388 County Road EF, Swanton, OH 43558, (866) 412–5275, www.sunseed.com.

ThermoCare Portable ICS Units ThermoCare Inc., PO Box 6069, Incline Village, NV 89450, (800) 262–4020, www.thermocare.com.

Pedialyte: Abbott Laboratories, Columbus, OH 43215, www.abbott.com.

Portable Brooder: United Laboratory Plastics, PO Box 8585, St. Louis, MO 63126, (636) 343–2202, www.unitedlabplastics.com, www.unitedlabplastics.com (search mini-transportable-incubators).

## References

Ainley, G.G., Nettleship, D.N., Carter, H.R., and Storey, A.E. (2002). Common Murre (*Uria aalge*). In: *The Birds of North America, No. 666* (eds. A. Poole and F. Gill). Ithaca, NY, USA: Cornell Lab of Ornithology. https://doi.org/10.2173/bna.666.

Ashcroft, R.E. (1979). Survival rates and breeding biology of puffins on Skomer Island, Wales. *Ornis Scandinavica* 10: 100–110.

ASLC. (2006a). Alaska Sea Life Center, Seward, Alaska, ASLC Alcid Rearing Protocol (in-house publication).

ASLC. (2006b). Alaska Sea Life Center, Seward, Alaska, ASLC Marine Bird/Mammal Rehabilitation SOPAVIAN (in-house publication).

Burco, J.D., Etienne, K.A., Massey, J.G. et al. (2012). Molecular sub-typing suggest that the environment of rehabilitation centers may be a potential source of Aspergillus fumigatus infecting rehabilitating seabirds. *Medical Mycology* 50: 91–98.

Burco, J.D., Massey, J.G., Byrne, B.A. et al. (2014). Monitoring of fungal loads in seabird rehabilitation centers with comparison to natural seabird environments in northern California. *Journal of Zoo and Wildlife Medicine* 45 (1): 29–40.

Day, R.H. and Byrd, G.V. (1989). Food habits of the whiskered auklet at Buldir Island, Alaska. *The Condor* 91: 65–72.

Eilertsen, K., Barrett, R.T., and Pederson, T. (2008). Diet, growth and early survival of Atlantic puffin (*Fratercula arctica*) chicks in North Norway. *Waterbirds* 31 (1): 107–114.

Emms, S.K. (1987). The adaptive significance of pattern of nesting dispersion of the pigeon guillemot. M.Sc. thesis. Simon Fraser University, Burnaby.

Ewins, P.J. (1993). Pigeon Guillemot (*Cepphus columba*). In: *The Birds of North America, No 49* (eds. A. Poole and F. Gill). Ithaca, NY, USA: Cornell Lab of Ornithology. https://doi.org/10.2173/bna.49.

Frankfurter, G., Ziccardi, G., and Massey, J.G. (2012). Effects of freshwater housing and fluid types on aquatic bird serum electrolyte concentrations. *Journal of Zoo and Wildlife Medicine* 43 (4): 852–857.

Gaston, A.J. and Hipfner, J.M. (2000). Growth of nestling thick-billed Murres (*Uria lomvia*) in relation to parental experience and hatching date. *The Auk* 119 (3): 827–832.

Gaston, A.J. and Hipfner, J.M. (2002). Thick-billed Murre (Uria lomvia). In: *The Birds of North America, No. 497* (eds. A. Poole and F. Gill). Ithaca, NY, USA: Cornell Lab of Ornithology. https://doi.org/10.2173/bna.497.

Hamer, T.E. and Nelson, S.K. (1995). Characteristics of Marbled Murrelet nest trees and nesting stands. In: *Ecology and Conservation of Marbled Murrelet* (eds. C.J. Raphael and J.F. Piatt), 69–82. U.S. Department of Agriculture, Forest Service General Technical Report PSW-GTR-152.

Harding, A.M.A., Van Pelt, T.I. et al. (2002). Reduction of provisioning efforts in response to experimental manipulation of chick nutritional status in the horned puffin. *The Condor* 104: 842–847.

Harrison, N.M. (1990). Gelatinous zooplankton in the diet of the parakeet auklet: comparisons with other auklets. *Studies in Avian Biology* 14: 114–124.

Hatch, S.A. and Sanger, G.A. (1992). Puffins as samplers of juvenile Pollock and other forage fish in the Gulf of Alaska. *Marine Ecology Progress Series* 80: 1–14.

del Hoyo, J., Elliott, A., and Sargatal, J. (eds.) (1996). *Handbook of the Birds of the World*, vol. 3. Barcelona: Hoatzin to Auks. Lynx Edicions.

Hudson, P.J. (1979). The parent-chick fledging relationship of the puffin, *Fratercola arctica*. *Journal of Animal Ecology* 48: 889–898.

Hunt, G.L. Jr., Harrison, N.M., and Piatt, J.F. (1993). Foraging ecology as related to the distribution of planktivorous auklets in the Bering Sea. In: *The Status, Ecology and Conservation of Marine Birds of the North Pacific* (eds. K. Vermeer, K.T. Briggs, K.H. Morgan and D. Siegel-Causey), 18–26. Ottawa: Can. Wildl. Serv. Spec. Publ.

Jones, I.L., Konyukhov, N.B., Williams, J.C. et al. (2001). Parakeet Auklet (*Aethia psittacula*). In: *The Birds of North America, No. 594* (eds. A. Poole and F. Gill). Ithaca, NY, USA: Cornell Lab of Ornithology. https://doi.org/10.2173/bna.594.

Koutsos, E.A. (2012). General principles of nutrition for the newly hatched Chick. *Veterinary Clinics: Exotic Animal Practice* 15 (2): 195–204.

Litzow, M.A., Piatt, J.F., Prichard, A.K., and Roby, D.D. (2002). Response of pigeon guillemots to variable abundance of high-lipid and low-lipid prey. *Oecologia* 132: 286–295.

Mejeur, J.H., Dierenfeld, E.S., and Murtaugh, J.A. (1988). Development of a vitamin supplement for puffins and Other Alcids. American Association of Zoological Parks and Aquariums, Regional Proceedings, pp. 696–700.

Molina-López, R.A., Casal, J., and Darwich, L. (2013). Final disposition and quality auditing of the rehabilitation process in wild raptors admitted to a wildlife rehabilitation center in Catalonia, Spain, during a twelve year period (1995–2007). *PloS One* 8 (4): e60242.

Montesdeoca, N., Calabuig, P., Corbera, J.A., and Orós, J. (2017). A long-term retrospective study on rehabilitation of seabirds in gran Canaria Island, Spain (2003–2013). *PloS One* 12 (5): e0177366.

Morten, J.M., Parsons, N.J., Schwitzer, C. et al. (2017). Body condition as a quantitative tool to guide hand-rearing decisions in an endangered seabird. *Animal Conservation* 20 (5): 471–479.

Muzaffar, S.B. and Jones, I.L. (2004). Parasites and diseases of the auks (Alcidae) of the world and their ecology – a review. *Marine Ornithology* 32: 121–146.

Oehler, D.A., Schmid, S.C., and Miller, M.P. (1995). Maintaining parakeet auklets at the Cincinnati Zoo and Botanical Garden: Hand-rearing protocol with development and behavioral observations. *Avicultural Magazine* 101 (1): 3–12.

Oehler, D.A., Schmid, S.C., and Miller, M.P. (2001). Maintaining least auklet, *Aethia pusilla*, at the Cincinnati zoo and botanical garden: hand-rearing protocol with field, development and behavioral observations. *Zool Garten N.F.* 71: 316–334.

Oehler, D.A., Campbell, C., Edelen, C., et al. (2003). Auklet Husbandry Manual (in house publication; The Cincinnati Zoo and Botanical Garden).

Piatt, J.F. and Kitaysky, A.S. (2002). Horned puffin (*Fratercula corniculata*). In: *The Birds of North America, No. 603* (eds. A. Poole and F. Gill). Ithaca, NY, USA: Cornell Lab of Ornithology.

Place, A.R. (1992). Comparative aspects of lipid digestion and absorption physiological correlates of wax ester digestion. *American Journal of Physiology* 263 (3 Pt 2): R464–R471.

Roby, D.D. (1991). Diet and postnatal energetics in convergent taxa of plankton-feeding seabirds. *The Auk* 108: 131–146.

Roby, D.D., Place, A.R., and Ricklefs, R.E. (1986). Assimilation and deposition of wax esters in planktivorous seabirds. *The Journal of Experimental Zoology* 238: 29–41.

Sealy, S.G. (1973). The adaptive significance of posthatching developmental patterns and growth rates in the Alcidae. *Ornis Scand* 4: 113–121.

Siegel, H.S. (1985). Immunological responses as indicators of stress. *World's Poultry Science Journal* 41: 36–44.

Thompson, T. (1996). Hand rearing a tufted puffin chick. *Animal Keeper's Forum* 23.

Tocidlowski, M.E., Cornish, T.E., Loomis, M.R., and Stoskopf, M.K. (1997). Mortality in captive wild-caught horned puffin chicks (*Fratercula corniculata*). *Journal of Zoo and Wildlife Medicine* 28 (3): 298–306.

Yabsley, M.J., Greiner, E., Tseng, F.S. et al. (2009). Description of novel Babesia species and associated lesions from common Murres (*Uria aalge*) from California. *Journal of Parasitology* 95 (5): 1183–1188.

## Further Reading

Ainley, D.G., Manuwal, D.A., Adams, J. et al. (1993). Cassin's auklet (*Ptychoramphus aleuticus*). In: *The Birds of North America, No. 50* (eds. A. Poole and F. Gill). Ithaca, NY, USA: Cornell Lab of Ornithology. https://doi.org/10.2173/bna.5.

Barrett, R.T. (2002). Atlantic puffin *Fratercula arctica* and common guillemot *Uria aalge* chick diet and growth as indicators of fish stocks in the Barents Sea. *Marine Ecology Progress Series* 230: 275–287.

Byrd, G.V. and Williams, J.C. (1993). Whiskered auklet (*Aethia pygmaea*) version 2.0. In: *The Birds of North America, No. 76* (eds. A. Poole and F. Gill). Ithaca, NY, USA: Cornell Lab of Ornithology. https://doi.org/10.2173/bna.76.

Jones, I.L. (1993). Least Auklet (*Aethia pusilla*). In: *The Birds of North America, No. 69* (eds. A. Poole and F. Gill). Ithaca, NY, USA: Cornell Lab of Ornithology.

Jones, I.L., Konyukhov, N.B., Williams, J.C. et al. (2001). Crested auklet (*Aethia cristatella*), version 2.0. In: *The Birds of North America* (eds. A. Poole and F. Gill). Ithaca, NY, USA: Cornell Lab of Ornithology. https://doi.org/10.2173/bna.70.

Konyukhov, N.B., Zubakin, V.A., Williams, J., and Fischer, J. (2000). Breeding biology of the whiskered auklet (*Aethia pygmaea*): incubation, chick growth, and feather development. *Biology Bulletin* 27 (2): 164–170.

Wehle, D.H.S. (1983). The food, feeding and development of young tufted and horned puffins in Alaska. *Condor* 85: 427–442.

Wickett, M.R. (1999). Atlantic puffin/razorbill assessment. *Maine Department of Inland Fisheries and Wildlife Division*. https://www.maine.gov/ifw/docs/species_planning/birds/atlanticpuffinrazorbill/puffinrazorbillassesment.pdf.

# 26

# Gulls and Terns

*Meryl Faulkner*

## Natural History

Laridae (gulls and terns) are represented in North America by 25 species of gulls, including two called kittiwakes; and eighteen species of terns, including two called noddies. Gulls and terns are closely related to skuas, jaegers, and skimmers, and are grouped in the order Charadriiformes. Gulls and terns are colonial breeders nesting on the ground, on and around beaches, marshland, and abandoned salt works. Some gull species nest on rocky cliffs, but some species also may nest on manmade structures such as hotel, apartment, and office building roofs in many coastal cities. Nests may be a shallow scrape or structure lined with grass, twigs, pebbles, and debris. Incubation typically lasts 21–27 days, depending on species.

Gull and tern chicks are semi-precocial. They hatch with their eyes open, are covered with down and able to walk, but remain at or near the nest for the first 2 or 3 weeks. Depending on the species, chicks fledge at 21 days (Least Tern) to 42 days (Western Gull), but are fed by parents for additional time. In the case of Western Gulls, this may last for 11–12 weeks post-hatch.

Although both gulls and terns have webbed feet and have waterproof plumage, only gulls swim and float on the water for extended periods of time. Terns have shorter legs and smaller feet and do not spend any extended time paddling. Adult gulls and terns eat fish; however, gulls are more likely to take invertebrates and human refuse, particularly if not feeding young or if environmental conditions change and fish are scarce.

Gulls and terns range in weight from the 40 g Least Tern to more than a kilogram in larger gulls. Young terns and gulls are fed primarily fish of the appropriate size on the day of hatching by the parent. Least Terns feed their chicks fish approximately twice an hour. Western Gull males feed chicks every 2–3 hours, with females feeding every 3–4 hours by the fledging period. Fish is offered whole by terns, but gulls regurgitate a bolus of food such as small fish or shrimp into young chicks' mouths or drop larger fish onto the ground for chicks older than 10 days to pick up (Pierotti and Annett 1995; Thompson et al. 1997).

## Criteria for Intervention

Terns and gulls may be brought to rehabilitators by state or federal agencies in cases where endangered or threatened species have been disturbed at nesting sites and the young abandoned. In addition,

*Hand-Rearing Birds*, Second Edition. Edited by Rebecca S. Duerr and Laurie J. Gage.

in some areas gulls may nest inappropriately on the roofs of commercial or residential buildings and, because of aggressive behavior, the U.S. Fish and Wildlife Service (USFWS) or state agencies may give permission for removal of the chicks.

Fledglings may be presented when predators have attacked nest sites, or fledglings have fallen from nest sites on roofs. Least Terns nest on rooftops in Florida and have been successfully reunited with parents. Replacement may be attempted if access to the correct nest site on the rooftop is possible. Chicks should be checked for injuries before this is attempted, and parental care should be observed after return to the nest site before the chick is left there.

## Record Keeping

State agencies require record keeping, which may vary from state to state. Minimum requirements are species, age class, location found, name and address of finder, reason for removal from nest site, medical problem, final disposition, and release location. Endangered or threatened species may require additional detailed record keeping, which usually is mandated by the biologists managing the species' recovery.

## Initial Care and Stabilization

As with other avian species, young gulls and terns should be warmed, hydrated, and then fed. Fluids can be given orally (by gavage) or subcutaneously at 5% of body weight if the bird is thin, underweight, or injured. Small species such as the endangered California Least Tern have fragile skin and often struggle when the subcutaneous route is attempted. The author prefers giving small terns appropriate amounts of lactated Ringer's solution or Pedialyte orally for the first feeding, and then both large and small species can be given Multimilk (PetAg) diluted one part powder to two parts water, or, alternatively, Isocal (Mead Johnson) or Ensure (Abbott), for another two feedings if the birds are thin or unsteady. Multimilk contains milk proteins; however, it is low in the carbohydrates (e.g. lactose) which are not normally ingested by birds. Nonetheless, it is available in powdered form, and is tolerated well by sea and shorebirds. Other critical care diet options include Emeraid Piscivore (Lafeber Company) or Carnivore Care (Oxbow Animal Health). Warming the fluids helps raise the core body temperature in hypothermic chicks and adult birds.

Young gulls and terns should be placed in a warm container and kept in a quiet area. Hatchlings (downy young chicks that would still be brooded) should be kept in a climate-controlled incubator and be given fur, fabric, or some other "tented" product to hide under as a surrogate parent (Figure 26.1). If the chick is orphaned but healthy, one feeding of fluids can be followed by solid food. Fish should be offered to terns, and shrimp, cat food, or chopped fish to gulls. Gulls and terns can be fed on demand every 90 minutes to 3 hours depending on age and size.

Hatchlings and young chicks may be kept in homemade aquabrooders or commercial incubators on paper or cloth towels. An aquabrooder (Graboski 1995) is constructed of two plastic or rubber containers, one inside the other with water between, with an aquarium water heater providing warmed water to heat the dry chamber, with the inside of the second container set up as a comfortable habitat for very young chicks. A screen top with a heat lamp provides additional heat and light as needed (Figure 26.2). Older chicks of larger species may be kept in cardboard or plastic pet carriers placed on heating pads on "low" setting to keep the interior warm.

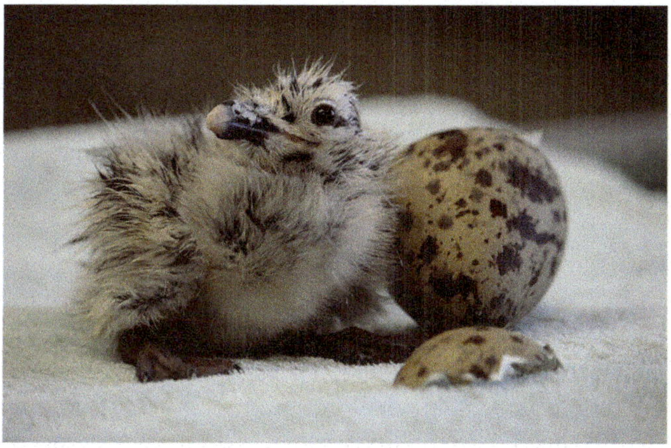

Figure 26.1 Western Gull hatchling. *Source:* photo courtesy of International Bird Rescue.

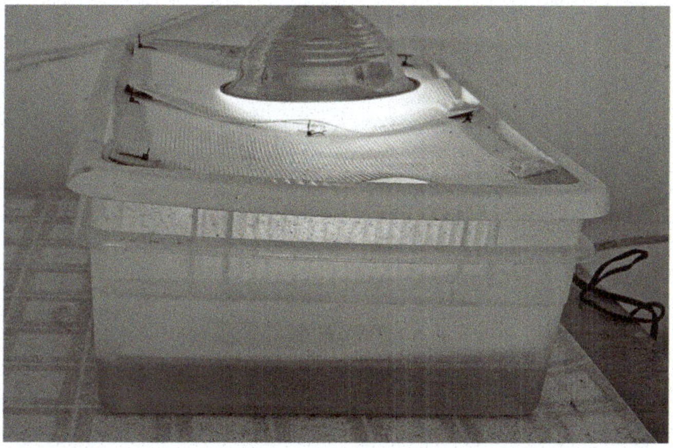

Figure 26.2 An aquabrooder constructed of two containers with heated water between, a screen top, and additional heat or light provided through the top screen.

## Common Medical Problems and Solutions

### Fishing Gear Injuries

Occasionally, adults feed chicks a bait fish with a hook attached, or may bring the chick a fish-shaped lure laden with deadly hooks. Juveniles that have literally swallowed the bait may present with a small length of line hanging from the bill. Usually because of emaciation of the chick and possible peritonitis, these birds may die before any treatment or surgery can be attempted. In older fledglings, lacerations and fractures of wing and leg can be caused by fishhooks and fishing line that causes constriction injuries.

### Other Injuries

Head wounds are seen in juvenile gulls and seem associated with sibling or adult attacks in crowded nesting conditions. Falls from rooftops may result in injured heads, legs, and wings. Tern species in San Diego (Least, Forster's, Elegant, Royal, and Caspian) nest and roost on beaches. Injuries are often caused by predators such as raptors, but coyotes and raccoons often invade beach and lagoon nesting sites and cause adults to trample and injure young in their haste to escape. Superficial wounds are treated by cleaning, disinfection, and the application of silver sulfadiazine cream or other dressings. Large scalp wounds should be surgically repaired for fastest recovery. Oil-based ointments are not recommended because they contaminate feathers and allow water to penetrate the feathers.

### Orthopedic Injuries

Wing and leg fractures may be lightly splinted with appropriate material and Micropore paper tape (3M) or a light stretch fabric wrap. Unlike in adult gulls with closed fractures of the humerus, downy Western Gull chicks with closed near-midshaft fractures heal well when the wing is splinted and wrapped, and they have a good prognosis for being able to fly post-recovery. Tern species with wing fractures should be assessed on the basis of post-release flying ability because perfect flight is necessary for foraging. See Duerr (2017) for information regarding management of fractures in these species.

Both juvenile gulls and terns with unilateral foot trauma (over half the foot missing) or an injured hock, knee, or hip joint may have a poor prognosis, depending on the nature of the injury. As the chicks or fledglings grow, increasing weight is borne on the uninjured leg or foot, and the healthy limb may develop pododermatitis or joint deformity. Early diagnosis and treatment of injuries improves outcomes, as these species must be able to run and walk comfortably as adults.

Because plumage has to be intact prior to release for waterproofing purposes, veterinarians should be aware that sticky or adhesive wraps directly on feathers are contraindicated in these species. The author prefers using nonadhesive materials such as Vetrap or Coban (3M) in a "figure of 8" format to wrap wings of larger species of terns and gulls. Small tern species' wings can be wrapped with light Micropore paper tape (3M), or narrow strips of nonadhesive materials. Do not damage growing flight feathers with wraps.

Small tern species are particularly prone to pododermatitis, which starts as reddening and swelling on the underside of the toes. This may occur when underweight or injured fledglings have to be maintained indoors on fabric or paper toweling. Foot lesions are difficult to treat and often result in systemic infections and death. Damp and wet conditions with debris (feces or dirt or gravel) on flooring increase the chances of damage to delicate feet (see the section "Housing," later in this chapter, for suggested substrates).

In captivity, beak damage may occur in older juvenile gulls when housed temporarily in kennels because they may abrade their beaks on the metal door. The lesions heal once the bird is placed in an aviary setting. Gulls may also damage their feathers when placed in wire cages for even short periods of time.

### Aspergillosis

Young gulls and terns treated with antibiotics should also be medicated with an appropriate antifungal medication, such as itraconazole (Janssen) at 15 mg/kg orally once daily to prevent opportunistic fungal infections. Healthy chicks are not generally treated with these drugs prophylactically.

## Diet

Small tern chicks (Least, Common, or Forster's) can be fed silversides (*Menidia*) or lance fish (*Ammodytes* spp.) (Figure 26.3). Many retail and online pet food suppliers carry these items frozen. Larger terns and Western Gull chicks can be fed small whitebait, lake smelt, or other whole fish. Gull chicks less than a week old can also be fed shrimp. Whole food items are better than chopped fish, because fish oils may sometimes remain on the beak, causing contamination of body plumage and the vent area when birds preen. Fish or shrimp or other food items should be offered fresh at each feeding. Older gulls can be offered dry cat food and cooked eggs as an introduction to the later miscellaneous diet that many gulls subsist on from humans. Least Terns and other small tern species will also eat large or giant mealworms when they are old enough for outdoor housing. For larger terns and gulls, whole lake smelt or night smelt (Canadian origin) are often available at local Asian markets fresh or frozen. Older gull chicks may enjoy picking apart fish carcasses that are too large to eat whole, and this provides great enrichment and foraging practice.

## Feeding Procedures

Gull and tern chicks can be fed within a few hours of hatching. Parent birds of these species feed chicks on the day of hatch, although the yolk sac can nourish the bird for the first 48 hours if necessary. Chicks sit quietly until they become hungry and then begin soliciting for food by vocalizing. Food items can be given to the bird using a pair of forceps or by hand. Juvenile gulls and terns advance toward the handler and grasp offered fish after calling and gaping. Do not allow beaks to become sticky or dirty with food. Clean the beak and nares if this should become necessary. Food should be freshly thawed the day of feeding and kept refrigerated until an hour or two before feeding. These species are susceptible to imprinting and habituation. See Chapter 15 for more information on avoiding these problems when raising susceptible chicks.

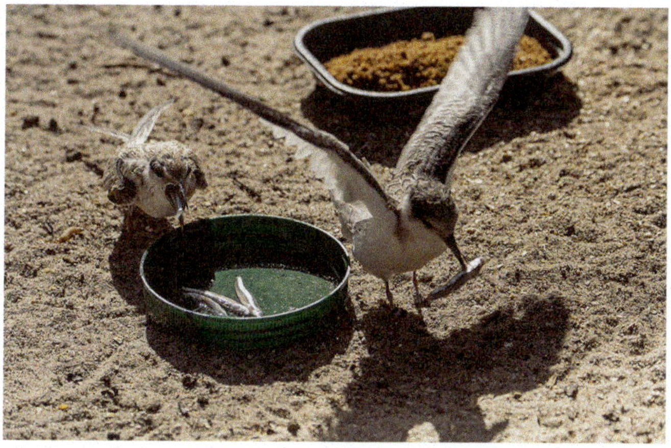

Figure 26.3 Two Least Tern fledglings in outdoor caging with a dish of fish. *Source:* photo courtesy of Mary F. Platter Rieger.

### Hatchlings

The feeding frequency of hatchlings will depend on the species and size of the hatched chick. Hatchling gulls and terns eat readily, but less frequently on the day of hatch. By the second day, chicks should eat approximately every 60–90 minutes. Feed every 90 minutes (9–10 times daily) until the chick is satiated, for 12–14 hours a day. If a chick seems reluctant to eat, it may be gently force-fed a moistened fish.

If the chick refuses to gape or beg for food, give fluids, skip the next feeding, and check that stool color and consistency are normal for the species and diet. Fish diets usually result in dark gray fecal material in a splash of white urates. Gray granular stools may indicate illness or dehydration. Birds that do not defecate regularly after every one or two feedings should be checked for cloacal impactions by inspecting the vent area for chalky or granular concretions. A gentle stream of warm water on the cloacal area may stimulate the bird to defecate. The bird should then have additional fluids added to its diet by tube-feeding fluids between solid feeding.

### Nestlings and Fledglings

Nestlings and fledglings can be fed about every 90 minutes for 12–14 hours a day (Figure 26.4). After the first week, time intervals can be lengthened to every 3–4 hours for gull species, and every 90 minutes to 2 hours for terns. Small terns may need feeding every 2 hours until they are picking up food items from a dish. Larger tern and gull species will start picking up food from a dish after about 1–2 weeks, and at that stage food dishes should be refilled with fresh food at least four times daily.

## Expected Weight Gain

After hatching, gull and tern chicks may remain at the same weight for the first 48 hours. After this time period, weight gain should be steady and fairly linear until about 2–3 weeks of age, at which point weight gain will slow, while feather growth continues (Figures 26.5 and 26.6). Individual

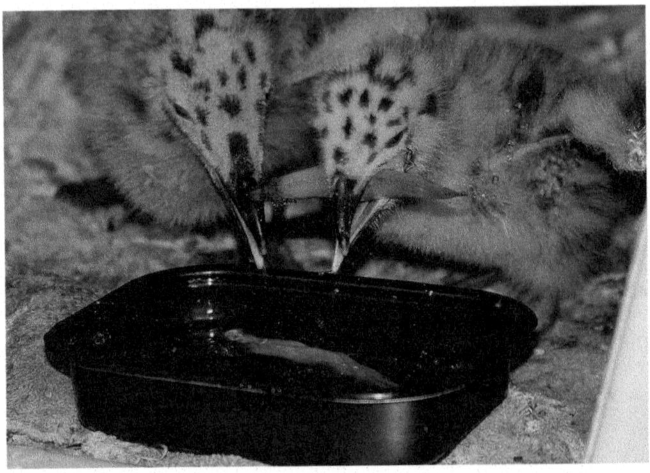

Figure 26.4 Two Western Gull chicks competing for lunch. *Source:* photo courtesy of Mary F. Platter Rieger.

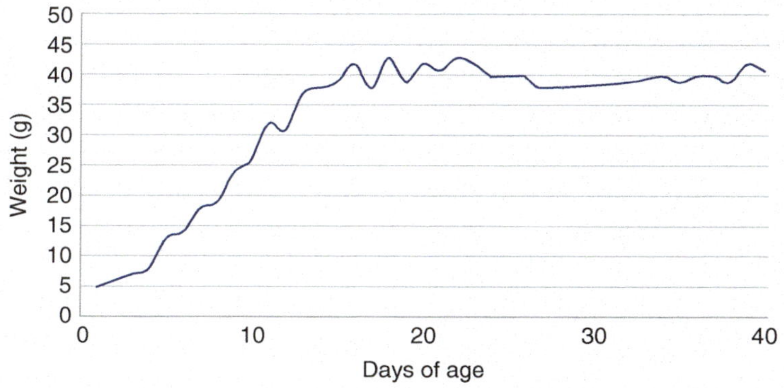


Figure 26.5 Average weight gain of 17 Least Tern chicks.

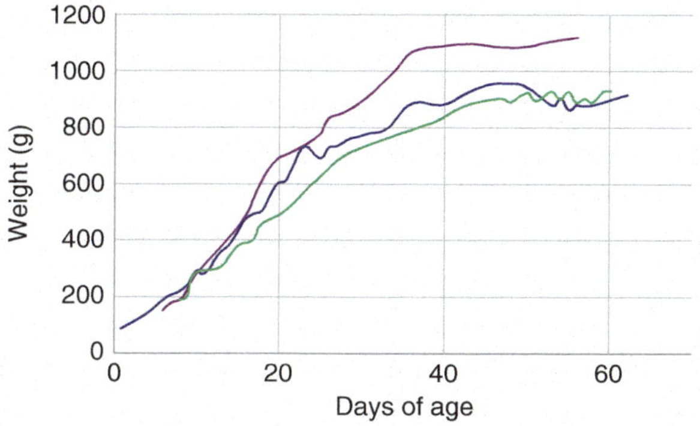


Figure 26.6 Weight gain of three Western Gull chicks. *Source:* data courtesy of International Bird Rescue.

variation is normal, but weights vary if taken fasted or nonfasted. Weigh birds at the same time each day because these species can hold a significant amount of their body weight in food within their digestive tract.

## Housing

Hatchlings should be kept between 90 and 100 °F (32–38 °C) on hatch. The incubator floor temperature should be approximately 93 °F (34 °C), with a 40-W light over one end of the incubator. A 4 in. (10 cm) square piece of synthetic fur fabric is placed at the lighted end in one corner for small tern chicks to huddle under or sit on. Clean feather dusters and mirrors can provide comfort to solitary chicks (Figure 26.7). The author uses an incubator (aquabrooder) for smaller terns and gull chicks less than 5 days old, which allows the chick to choose from a temperature gradient in the brooder. As the birds start to grow in size, smaller species can be kept in an incubator; larger species can be housed in a kennel with a heating pad under one end to maintain a temperature between 85 and 95 °F (29–35 °C).

Hatchlings of California Least Terns and Forster's Terns can be housed on several layers of paper towels or cotton velour towels, changing the towel or paper when soiled. Another option is to use sterilized play sand 0.25 in. (0.5 cm) deep, removing debris from the surface daily and changing the sand as needed.

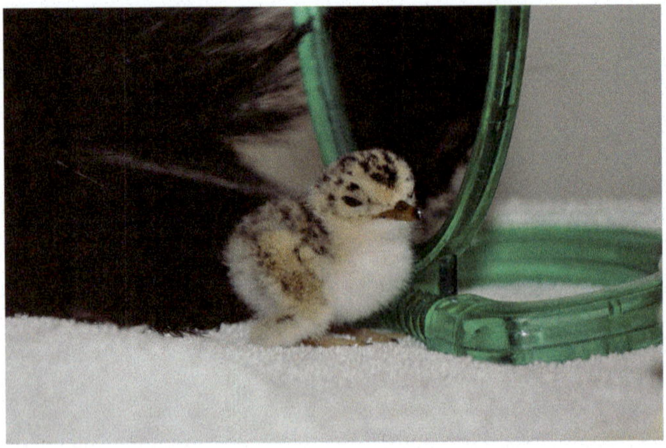

Figure 26.7 Least Tern chick in well-heated brooder with a clean feather duster and mirror to provide company. *Source:* photo courtesy of International Bird Rescue.

After the chicks are able to thermoregulate – at about 1 week of age for gulls, or 2 weeks for smaller tern species – the overhead tungsten light can be replaced with a full-spectrum light. In tern and gull species, metabolic bone disease is rare, but since the birds are reared indoors, full-spectrum lights over the incubator (or through the door of the kennels) are prudent to provide chicks with adequate vitamin D production.

Once chicks are able to thermoregulate, the ambient temperature in their enclosure can be decreased gradually, and they can be moved to a larger enclosure. At about 3 weeks of age for terns, or 4 weeks for gulls, the chicks should be near 80% of normal adult weight and have primary feathers at least half grown. Small terns will have lost most or all of the downy tufts on the head and back, larger gull species may still have some down. Gulls and terns at this stage of development are completely self-feeding, and can be transferred either to a small 6 × 8 ft. (1.8 × 2.4 m) enclosure with a sand floor and small pool or directly into the final flight aviary.

When first placed outdoors, birds should be monitored to check that they do not get wet or become hypothermic. Monitoring is especially important if the weather is cool or if any birds are not completely waterproof. Heat should be provided in a protected corner of the aviary until it's certain that all birds are doing well at ambient outdoor temperatures.

Flight cages should have sand floors that are swept of surface debris several times a week. Fresh sand should be added when necessary. Pools (either concrete or with PVC liners) within the aviary should have a gradual slope, and they should be drained daily and filled with fresh water or allowed to overflow to constantly remove any floating potential plumage contaminants. Pools should be of a size and slope that allows birds to walk in and out to bathe. The minimum access to water recommended for these species is one 45 in. diameter, 10–12 in. deep pool for every four to six birds (Miller 2012).

## Weaning

Most terns will start picking up food within 2 weeks of hatch. Some species (Western Gulls) will pick up dropped food at 3 days of age; some may take a little longer. Individuals may be slower to self-feed; several chicks grouped together will self-feed more rapidly and are less likely to become

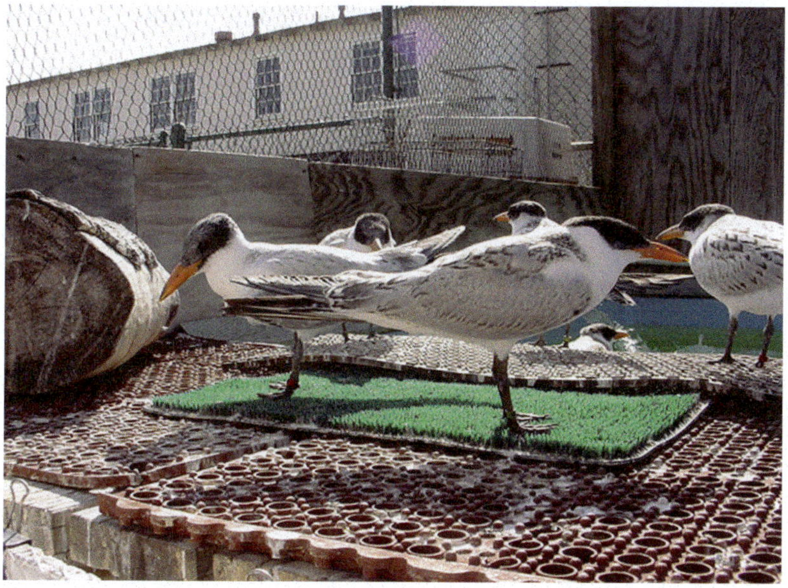

Figure 26.8 Caspian Terns in an outdoor aviary with a pool. *Source:* photo courtesy of International Bird Rescue.

habituated to a human caregiver (Figure 26.8). The caregiver should feed smaller, weaker individuals if older birds in the group are more aggressive. Older juvenile terns are less likely to attack younger birds housed with them than are gulls. Overcrowding (or simply aggressive personalities) can cause Western Gull chicks to peck at the heads of younger birds and cause feather loss and sometimes lacerations.

### Encouraging Foraging Skills

Western Gulls feed on land and water, but do not usually dive for food. These birds require no particular training to pick up food. For terns, first place the usual food dishes in the aviary near the pool. After a few days, place the fish at the edge of the sloping pool. The pool should be about 4 ft. (1.2 m) in diameter and 1 ft. (30 cm) deep in the center so that the birds are used to picking up fish in the shallow area. Then toss the fish in a little deeper, and encourage the birds to wade into the water. Terns will not jump into deep water, so the slope needs to be gradual. If birds are reluctant, feed at 8:00 a.m., and then withhold food until 3–4:00 p.m. After several more days the fish can be placed somewhat deeper, and the birds should wade and then fly in and pick them up. Finally, feeder (live) goldfish should be placed in the food dishes for a day or two so the birds are accustomed to catch the feeders, and then the live feeders placed in the pool itself. Sometimes the birds have to be left with the feeder fish all day before they will forage, but hunger will usually prove adequate to overcome the reluctance to enter the water.

## Preparation for Wild Release

Pre-release conditioning aviaries for small terns should minimally be 10 × 12 × 8 ft. high (3 × 3.6 × 2.4 m high) with predator proof plastic mesh netting (0.25 in./0.5 cm mesh) to prevent feather damage. Larger terns should be housed in an enclosure at least 10×16×8 ft. high (3×4.9×2.4 m high), but this is not really tall enough to provide practice plunging. Aviary size for large terns such as Caspian Terns should be at least 8 ft. (2.4 m) wide, 32–50 ft. (9.6–15 m) long and 12–25 ft. (3.6–7.5 m) high. Large gulls can be safely housed in 0.5 in. (1.25 cm) wire mesh "hardware cloth" enclosures. Flooring should be sterilized play sand to a depth of 1 in. (2.5 cm) and the surface brushed once weekly to remove debris. Wire mesh under the cage may be necessary to prevent burrowing predator attack. Birds should be held until they are able to make sustained flights, and in the case of gulls fly up to a perch 6 ft. (1.8 m) above the ground. Terns and gulls should be capable of sustained flight without panting for several circuits of the flight cage and land with wings folded.

Terns should walk or plunge into water to capture and swallow live feeder fish of appropriate size. Gulls should readily eat a variety of foods, including fish, bread, cat or dog food (dry or soaked), and human "refuse" (fast food leftovers). Gulls and terns reared in groups rarely become imprinted on humans; however, gulls reared with close human contact may never develop an appropriate fear of humans and may become a nuisance or a danger to the public.

In the case of Western Gulls and California Least Terns, it is the author's experience that fledglings of these two species can be safely housed with an adult conspecific in an aviary during the breeding season. Least Terns tolerate Least Tern chicks in a recovery cage or aviary; Western Gull adults have sometimes regurgitated food for Western Gull chicks when housed in an aviary. A recovered adult then can be released with a group of chicks. Some adults appear to welcome parenting duties during their own rehabilitation, but others may be stressed by the presence of chicks. Monitor the situation closely until certain all are doing well.

California Least and Forster's Terns raised from hatch or brought in for rehabilitation beg for food from the caregiver and may appear tame. However, once in the fledgling stage when food is no longer offered by hand, these birds lose their "tameness" and quickly become apprehensive of human contact if weighed and measured once or twice prior to release.

Chicks of varying ages can be housed together, but older gull chicks may show aggression to younger, smaller birds. This is manifested in aviaries by the appearance of reddened areas and missing feathers at the back of the head where they have been pecked. The younger bird should be separated into a younger group, or the aggressive bird detected and separated from the group. Adult terns of various species do not seem to attack juvenile conspecifics or other tern species but do vocalize during competition for food and give warning calls.

Chicks of most tern species remain with the parent and have been observed receiving supplemental food for extended periods of time. Little is known about the survival of hand-reared birds. However, Western Gull chicks released at 12 weeks of age have been observed surviving successfully 1 year post-release in San Diego. Banded Caspian Terns that were hand-reared as chicks at International Bird Rescue in Los Angeles have been re-sighted breeding at Bolsa Chica Ecological Reserve in Orange County, CA, more than 5 years after release (C. Collins, pers. comm.).

## Criteria for Release

Birds should be wary of humans, able to sustain flight without panting, bank and turn circles in an aviary, and land smoothly. The birds' primary, contour, and tail feathers should be full length, and the birds should be able to bathe and emerge from the water looking dry (i.e. are waterproof). Fledglings should achieve the minimum weight for their species, and have no foot or beak abnormalities. Birds should readily enter the water to bathe and pick up food.

### Release Sites

Terns and gulls reared in captivity must be released in an appropriate habitat where there are others of the same species. Because some tern and gull species migrate, if birds are reared or rehabilitated late in the season and the others of that species have already migrated, they may need to be overwintered in suitable rehabilitation facilities or transported to catch up with conspecifics. Release early in the day during a period of good weather. Always release young terns into a group of foraging conspecifics.

## Acknowledgments

Thanks to Mary F. Platter Rieger for her enthusiasm, interest, and support, and the generous use of her photographs. Thanks also to the many endangered species monitors working at California Least Tern breeding sites, in particular Elizabeth Copper, Brian Foster, Robert Patton, and Shauna Wolf. Many thanks to Project Wildlife in San Diego, its wonderful volunteers, and to my late husband Dr. John Faulkner, who always encouraged me to pass on my knowledge through publication. Thanks to Julie Skoglund for reviewing this chapter.

## Sources for Products Mentioned

Carnivore Care: Oxbow Animal Health, 11902 South 150th Street, Omaha, NE 68138, (531) 721-2300, http://www.oxbowanimalhealth.com.

Emeraid Piscivore: Lafeber Company, 24981 N 1400 East Road, Cornell, IL 61319, (800) 842-6445, https://lafeber.com.

Ensure: Abbott Laboratories, Abbott Park, IL, (800) 986-8501, https://ensure.com.

Multimilk: PetAg Inc., 255 Keyes Avenue, Hampshire, IL 60140, (800) 323-6878, https://www.petag.com.

Vetrap, Coban, and Micropore paper tape: 3M, St. Paul, MN, (800) 628-7462, https://www.3m.com/3M/en_US/company-us/all-3m-products.

## References

Duerr, R.S. (2017). Gulls, terns, and shorebirds. In: *Topics in Wildlife Medicine, Vol. 4: Orthopedics* (eds. R.S. Duerr and G.J. Purdin), 145–153. St. Cloud, MN: National Wildlife Rehabilitators Association.

Graboski, R. (1995). Simple things that make a difference: making water-based incubators. *Journal of Wildlife Rehabilitation* 18 (2): 16–17.

Miller, E.A. (ed.) (2012). *Minimum Standards for Wildlife Rehabilitation*, 4e. St. Cloud, MN: National Wildlife Rehabilitation Association.

Pierotti, R.J. and Annett, C.A. (1995). Western Gull (*Larus occidentalis*), version 2.0. In: *The Birds of North America* (eds. A.F. Poole and F.B. Gill). Ithaca, NY, USA: Cornell Lab of Ornithology https://doi.org/10.2173/bna.174.

Thompson, B.C., Jackson, J.A., Burger, J. et al. (1997). Least Tern (*Sternula antillarum*), version 2.0. In: *The Birds of North America* (eds. A.F. Poole and F.B. Gill). Ithaca, NY, USA: Cornell Lab of Ornithology https://doi.org/10.2173/bna.290.

# 27

# Pigeons and Doves

*Nancy Eilertsen and Guthrum Purdin*

## Natural History

The family Columbidae (order Columbiformes) comprises 313 species worldwide. Nine species of pigeons and doves are native to North America, including the Band-tailed Pigeon, Mourning Dove (so called because of its mournful coo), Inca Dove, and White-winged Dove. Nonindigenous species have been introduced, most notably the Rock (Common) Pigeon, and Eurasian Collared-Dove (Leahy 2004). For the purposes of this chapter, the family will be considered as a unit with specific differences noted where necessary. Columbids range in size from 6 to 30 in. (15–75 cm). They are plump with small heads and short legs and are generally drab-colored, though iridescent patches are common. The bills are slender with a cere, or operculum, at the base.

Pair bonds are formed for life; unfortunately, the high mortality rate of these nonaggressive birds means that new pairs are formed yearly. A common sight in cities and towns is a male Rock Pigeon doing a courtship "dance": fluffing up while strutting around and rotating in place while bobbing near the female. The Rock Pigeon chooses manmade ledges that mimic its native cliff nest sites; doves may select hanging baskets, intersecting phone wires, house gutters, or low bushes or trees. Dove nests are flimsy platforms of sticks, dried grass, and twigs, usually containing two eggs that range from white to pale blue. These birds may nest multiple times in a season. Eggs and chicks are often lost to predators and gravity. Hence, presentation of orphaned and injured wild chicks can occur at nearly any time of the year, although numbers peak in spring and early summer.

Incubation is 14–19 days, with parents sharing incubation and feeding duties. The altricial young hatch with pink or gray skin covered in long down and eyes closed. Feet are anisodactyl with three toes forward and one toe back. Chicks grow rapidly and attain near-adult weight by 3 weeks of age. The most common predators of columbids include Peregrine Falcons, Cooper's and Sharp-shinned Hawks, and the domestic cat. Native Band-tailed Pigeons may be differentiated from Rock Pigeons by legs that are yellow rather than red or pink, and bills that are yellow with a black tip.

Pigeons and doves feed largely on grains, seeds, and fruit, and are often seen on the ground in flocks. Features that set these birds apart from other birds are their ability to drink without raising their heads and the ability to feed their young with a secretion produced in the crop known as "crop milk." Crop milk is a cheese-like material composed of crop muscle cells that have been fortified with lipids and nutrients; composition is about half protein and half fat (Sales and Janssens 2003). Crop milk also contains beneficial flora and immunoglobulins that help the young chick with immune function (Engberg et al. 1992). Crop milk is typically fed to hatchlings for the first

*Hand-Rearing Birds*, Second Edition. Edited by Rebecca S. Duerr and Laurie J. Gage.

several days of life, then increasing amounts of adult diet are mixed in until weaning occurs (Vandeputte-Poma 1980). Dove and pigeon hatchlings, consequently, are appropriately fed a more carnivorous diet than would be expected from the adult birds' diets.

## Criteria for Intervention

Doves are frequent victims of cat attacks, window strikes, and car collisions. Young are often found on the ground after storms when heavy wind or rain causes the flimsy nest to collapse. Loss of parents to predators is very common as the dove is a favorite prey for hawks. Crows and jays will attack chicks as well. Pigeons are likely to present with pellet gun injuries, poisoning, car collision injuries, and feather damage from bird repellant substances. Their young are often orphaned due to nest removal by exterminators because the nests are frequently found on ledges and rooftops of business buildings.

Because of frequent nest damage, returning the young to the original nest is often not possible and orphaned doves and pigeons make up a large percentage of birds presented to rehabilitation centers. However, doves are one of the easiest birds to re-nest under the right conditions. The parents will follow the baby's cries for food and often a parent dove will try to continue caring for a grounded baby by feeding it and brooding it as much as possible. Grounded neonates will not survive, but if the chick is warm and alert and the parent birds are nearby, then re-nesting can be attempted and is often successful. Use a makeshift nest (small natural fiber basket lined with dried grass or the remains of the old nest) and attach it to a branch in a nearby tree. Make sure that the nest is protected from exposure, especially to afternoon sun. Observe the nest from a distance to make sure the parent birds are caring for the baby. It might take an hour or two for the parents to return.

Proper species identification is necessary to determine whether release or captivity is suitable. Rock Pigeons and other nonnative species in the U.S. are not protected by the Migratory Bird Treaty Act of 1918, so permits are not required to rehabilitate or keep them. Some breeds of domesticated pigeons are not suitable for wild release due to behavior or plumage.

## Record Keeping

To comply with Federal regulations, records should be kept per the Minimum Standards for Wildlife Rehabilitation (Miller 2012); contact state or regional wildlife agencies for additional requirements. As a minimum, the following information should be kept: species, date admitted, location found, approximate age, reason admitted for care, medical problems, admission weight, and final disposition including transfer, death, euthanasia, or release date and location. Contact information for the finder is useful in the event that more information is required.

A complete medical record should also be kept with each bird, detailing findings of the initial examination, medications administered, daily body weight, progress of treatment, and behavioral notes. A daily feed and care chart should be maintained throughout the birds' stay in captivity. It is particularly useful to note changes in weight as well as changes in appetite, temperature, hydration, crop clearance, and diet. Each bird should be assigned a patient number. If multiple birds are being cared for, small plastic numbered leg bands (National Band and Tag Company) available from avian and poultry suppliers can be used to track individual progress.

## Initial Care and Stabilization

As a general rule, when wild birds are presented for rehabilitation, they arrive under extreme stress – stress which arises from whatever initial traumatic event lead to their being found and captured, duration of time since the trauma, plus being handled for sometimes prolonged periods by the finders. This stress alone can be life threatening, especially in prey species like doves and pigeons; these birds may put all their energy into frantic attempts to escape a perceived deadly predator (the well-meaning rescuer). Doves, especially, have been known to die from stress in the hands of rehabilitators during treatment.

Birds often arrive cold and dehydrated, so a common rule is to keep the animal warm, dark, and quiet for at least 15–20 minutes after arrival before extensive handling. Place fully-feathered birds in a covered, padded container atop a heating pad set on "low." Be aware that a bird (especially an adult) that seemed lifeless on intake may become active and attempt escape once it reaches normal temperature. Higher temperatures are needed for hatchlings (90–100 °F, 32–38 °C) and nestlings (80–90 °F, 27–32 °C) depending on how fully feathered they are; they should never feel cold to the touch of a warm human hand.

Birds may also arrive hyperthermic due to high environmental temperatures or capture stress. Clinical signs may include rapid, shallow, or open-mouthed breathing, and weakness. These birds will feel hot to the touch. Place them in a cool, dark, and quiet place. A gentle breeze from an electric fan may help. If they don't cool down after 15 minutes, give room temperature subcutaneous (SQ) fluids at 5% of body weight (50 ml/kg).

At the end of this calming period, do a quick evaluation for injuries and disease. With these findings in mind, prepare all the materials and tools needed for post-stabilization treatment, thus reducing handling times. Providing fluids is crucial at this stage. This can be most quickly and efficiently done using pre-warmed (105 °F, 41 °C) lactated Ringers solution (LRS) given SQ at 5% of body weight (50 ml/kg). Give SQ fluids via a 25-gauge needle under the loose skin at the front (cranial aspect) of the knee, directing the syringe forward, parallel with the femur and at a very shallow angle. Create a small bleb of fluid under the skin, then re-position the needle as needed. Do not turn birds onto their backs to give fluids, or put pressure on their crop if it has anything in it. Allow the bird to absorb this for another 15–20 minutes at which point perform a full, thorough examination (see Chapter 1). An additional 5% body weight of fluids can be given after this exam if needed. Do not offer food until birds are warmed and begin to pass urates in droppings.

During periods of extreme heat and subsequent dehydration, multiple administrations of fluids may be necessary – continue hourly until the birds begin to pass urates. Do not continue giving SQ fluids unless the previous bolus has been absorbed. Fluids can also be given via gavage, but this should only be done in a bird that is alert and can hold its head up, lest the bird regurgitate and risk aspiration. A well-hydrated bird will be alert, with skin that snaps back easily, bright eyes, moist mucus membranes, and well-formed, moist feces. A moderately dehydrated bird will be less than fully alert and have dry, wrinkled skin, dull eyes, unformed feces, and tacky mucus membranes with stringy saliva. A severely dehydrated bird will be lethargic or unconscious, with skin that stays "tented" when slightly pinched, and will have sunken eyes, dry or absent feces, and dry mucus membranes.

One caveat regarding the initial rest period after arrival: always do a quick scan of the patient before placing it on the heating pad. Some injuries require immediate attention lest a treatable problem becomes a life threatening one. For example, if the tibiotarsus is broken and the bird tries to stand on it, a closed fracture can become a compound fracture or worse. This sort of fracture needs immediate care; be careful to move quickly and efficiently and reduce handling time as much as possible. At this stage, do only as much as necessary to stabilize an injury – a broken wing can often get a simple metacarpal wrap initially, and then a time-consuming splint and wing wrap later, after the patient is more stable. See Duerr et al. (2017) for information regarding treatment of orthopedic injuries in small birds.

Fecal matter may cake around the vent area, causing blockage. This can be caused by dehydration, improper diet, or illness. Gently wash the fecal matter away with warm water on a soft cloth. The bird should defecate once the blockage is gone. Check for dehydration and signs of inflammation around the vent.

## Common Medical Problems and Solutions

### Caught by Cat

One of the most common predators of both young and adult doves is the domestic cat. The cat's oral flora contains *Pasturella multocida,* a gram-negative rod that is highly infective and can kill a bird quickly if not treated. If a bird is admitted with any reported interaction with a cat, it should be put on antibiotics immediately even in the absence of confirmed puncture or laceration wounds. Regardless of origin, all open wounds should be treated with antibiotic such as Clavamox (amoxicillin plus clavulanic acid) at 125 mg/kg twice daily for 7–14 days (Hawkins et al. 2018). Continue antibiotic therapy until wounds have completely healed. Provide control for pain and inflammation using meloxicam orally at 0.5 mg/kg twice daily for 3–10 days, with an initial loading dose of 1 mg/kg.

### Miscellaneous Lacerations

All open wounds should be closed or covered. Whenever possible, closure of lacerations should be done with sutures and/or surgical glue. This is especially true of wounds at highly mobile areas like the knee, which usually need to be sutured. Peri-operative pain control can be provided by dripping a small amount of dilute lidocaine (a 2% solution further diluted into saline at 2:8, 0.2 ml 2% lidocaine with 0.8 ml 0.9% NaCl); this is less physiologically stressful and less time consuming than full anesthesia. These species, when stressed, can be poor anesthetic candidates and may have a better prognosis when wounds are treated intermittently over the course of a few hours. However, if a procedure is going to be prolonged or especially painful, isoflurane gas anesthesia is an option, when available. If sutures or glue are not possible, cover with an adhesive dressing after cleaning the wound. Self-adhesive hydrocolloid dressings work well to keep the wound moist and protected while allowing tissue to heal. Another option is a semi-permeable film dressing such as Tegaderm™ (3M™), which can be more easily shaped to the small, curved surfaces of these patients, but when used alone may tend to allow the wound to dry out and consequently prolong healing. Each type of dressing has its benefits and use is determined by the circumstances of the individual case.

Creams and ointments should never be used in conjunction with sutures. These greasy substances are notorious for causing the sutures to dehisce. In general, ointments should not be used on birds with open wounds because they rapidly make the surrounding feathers, and often the entire bird, increasingly greasy, thus damaging feathers and destroying waterproofing.

## Degloved Scalp

Scalp lacerations exposing large amounts of skull are common, and may occur during care when fledglings accidentally escape and fly frantically into light fixtures or windows. In such cases, suturing the wound is by far the best option. A small amount of surgical glue can help keep the suture from dehiscing. If this isn't possible, cover the wound with a moist hydrocolloid dressing. In cases where a very large amount of skull is exposed, apply a very small amount of silver sulfadiazine (SSD) cream and cover that with a shape-able, adhesive dressing like Tegaderm. The SSD cream keeps the wound moist and allows cell migration under the dressing; however, it makes keeping a dressing on extremely difficult. In these cases, use thin strips of paper tape (Micropore™, 3M™) or other feather-friendly tape to form a "bonnet" to keep the dressing in place. Change dressings every 2–3 days until healed. Columbids with head trauma should be given meloxicam for at least 5 days, longer if necessary. Those with scalp lacerations also should be treated with an antibiotic until the wound is healed (7–14 days).

## Crop Disorders

These species have a crop that holds approximately 10% of the bird's body weight. There are several potential crop problems in chicks. Failure of the crop to empty, termed crop stasis or sour crop, can occur in doves and pigeons of all ages. Causes include immunosuppression, crop infections, foreign bodies (such as bedding materials), inappropriate food items (such as earthworms or dry rice), poor feeding technique (overfeeding, cold or indigestible formula), and less commonly vitamin/mineral deficiencies (vitamin $B_1$ and copper). In severe cases, the crop may need to be emptied by a veterinarian and any underlying problems treated. *Candida albicans* (yeast) infections are a common cause of crop stasis and can be avoided by providing a clean, stress-free environment with proper nutrition. The most common source of candida infection comes from old, contaminated seed, expired formula powder, or by feeding formula that has been left out too long. It can be easily diagnosed by microscopic examination of a crop swab or fecal smear where high numbers of budding yeast is diagnostic. Treat with nystatin at 300 000 IU/kg (Hawkins et al. 2018) given orally, twice daily for 7 days. Extend another week if birds are still positive on day 8.

New birds presenting for rehabilitation should not be given formula feedings until the crop has fully emptied of parent food or crop stasis may occur. For these birds, allow the crop to empty normally. If the patient is dehydrated or the crop is slow to empty, gavage a small amount of warmed saline every hour until the crop has cleared before starting formula. Gentle massage may help break up an impacted food mass. Crop impaction, resulting from feeding large quantities of dehydrated food, can be treated as above, but if there is no movement after a few hours, consulting a veterinarian familiar with these species may be necessary.

Crop burns may occur when formula is fed too hot. A visible hole can appear over the crop and the surrounding area may become swollen and discolored with a foul odor and matted feathers. Most often these birds require euthanasia.

Crop punctures or lacerations may be caused by predator attacks or poor gavage technique. These can be successfully sutured by isolating the individual layers of crop and overlying skin. Use only absorbable sutures for the inner suture of the crop. Birds being treated for crop tears should be given meloxicam (0.5 mg/kg twice daily for 5–7 days) and Clavamox (125 mg/kg twice daily for 7–14 days).

## Trichomonas

Trichomonas is a flagellated protozoan parasite transmitted through mouth-to-mouth contact between parents or when adults feed chicks and is a serious threat to many dove and pigeon species (Girard et al. 2014). Shared water sources are common points of infection, as is wet, contaminated seed in bird feeders. Fortunately, this organism is not environmentally stable, does not have a cystic stage, and is effectively killed by drying or exposure to many disinfecting agents. Oral lesions consisting of cheesy, foul-smelling masses cause gagging, neck stretching, difficulty swallowing or breathing, and regurgitation. When the lesions begin to block the esophagus, the bird is unable to eat and a slimy discharge is produced from the beak. Birds with severe cases may present emaciated with obvious masses in the throat and seed spilling out (Figure 27.1). Mild cases may not be readily apparent on physical exam. Definitive diagnosis is made by identifying the flagellate on a wet smear taken from the mouth or crop. However, many experienced caregivers can often make a presumptive diagnosis based on the overall presentation of the case. Treatment with carnidazole dosed at 25 mg/kg orally once (Hawkins et al. 2018) is generally effective in cases before caseous plaques have formed. For more severe cases, carnidazole given once daily for 3–5 days is recommended. Metronidazole has been used by some rehabilitators, but the author (GP) has found this to have very poor efficacy for this parasite. In situations where "azole" antibiotics cannot be used, some treatment success may occur with daily crop washes using dilute chlorhexidine. Be aware that federal and state regulations can limit the administration of certain drugs in birds that might enter the human food chain.

If the esophagus is blocked such that a feeding tube cannot be inserted into the crop, if the bird is neurologically abnormal, if skeletal structures have been eroded by the infection, or if the crop has ruptured, euthanasia is indicated. Special care must be taken to disinfect dishes and feeding implements because trichomoniasis is highly contagious among many avian species and can quickly kill some passerines. It is prudent to house passerines away from columbids for this reason. All columbids can be given one dose of carnidazole on arrival at a shelter to avoid the rapid spread of this parasite through the patient population. In some high-volume shelters, it has proven necessary to re-dose susceptible species weekly.

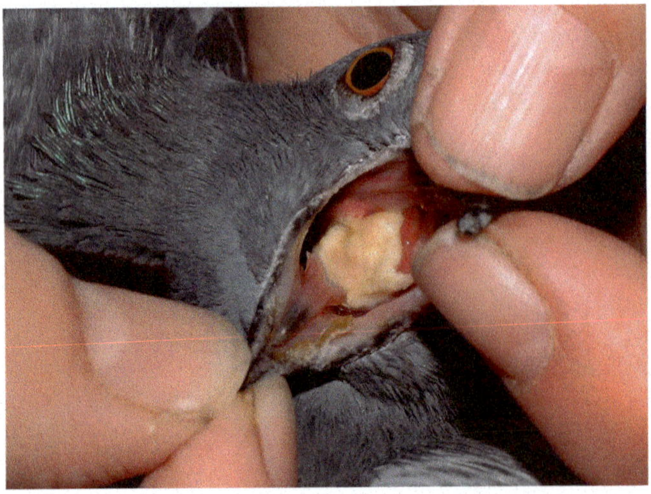

Figure 27.1 Severe trichomonas plaques blocking a pigeon's throat.

### Other Parasites

Pigeons often present with ectoparasites, such as feather lice and flat flies (*Hippoboscidae*). If these parasites are noted, spray the bird (while covering the head) with a topical anti-arthropod spray such as UltraCare Mite and Lice Bird Spray (8 in 1 Pet Products). Provide adequate ventilation during and after application to prevent inhalation of vapors. Columbids may have intestinal parasites, such as coccidia and nematodes (e.g. *Capillaria* spp.). Clinical signs include depression, emaciation, poor weight gain despite good appetite, and diarrhea. These organisms are diagnosed by fecal floatation and microscopic examination. *Capillaria* may be treated with fenbendazole at 50 mg/kg orally once daily for 5 days (Hawkins et al. 2018). Treatment may need to be repeated in 14 days. Coccidiosis can be treated orally with ponazuril at 20 mg/kg once daily (Hawkins et al. 2018), treating for 5 days clears almost all cases, continue to day 7 if still positive on day 6. Some rehabilitators use toltrazuril but this can be hard to find in the United States. Coccidia is a highly infectious, environmentally stable organism that can spread rapidly in crowded shelters and aviaries. It is very important to wear disposable gloves when handling infected birds and to wash all tools, bedding, caging, and cage furnishings thoroughly. Once an aviary has become contaminated, steam cleaning may be the only option to control the parasite.

### Avian Pox

Avian pox is a viral disease that can affect most or all birds with strains specific to related groups of species. It usually presents as wart-like nodules on unfeathered parts of the body, such as the feet and beak, but may be found on the wings and around the vent. This is also a highly contagious disease that spreads rapidly in shelters when the scabrous lesions begin to exfoliate. Patients may present with visible lesions on arrival or pox nodules can develop in care, especially if the animal is stressed. It transmits from bird to bird through direct contact or contact with fomites (e.g. dust from scab exfoliations, contaminated feeding utensils, bedding, caging, insects, or a caregiver's hands). The disease is environmentally stable for months to years. In high volume shelters, it is recommended that all affected birds are euthanized and exposed birds (that were in direct contact) be quarantined for 14 days. Affected birds can be treated, but only if they can be kept completely isolated from conspecifics or related species; ideally in a separate building with caregivers that only work with these individuals. Handlers of pox-infected birds should wear disposable gloves, wash hands and arms after handling, then change clothing and shoes before handling any other birds.

There is no specific treatment for pox other than supportive care. Lesions should be cleaned daily with dilute chlorhexidine or povidone-iodine solutions. Reduce stress as much as possible. It may be necessary to prevent secondary infections of severe lesions by using systemic antibiotics or antifungal medications. Large pox nodules can sometimes be removed by a veterinarian, which may shorten recovery times, but is not curative. Be aware that pox may take several months to resolve.

### Splayed Legs

Splayed legs can occur in developing birds when there is not enough support from the nest during joint development or a poor calcium-to-phosphorus ratio (Ca : P) in the diet. Slippery, flat substrates with poor traction (e.g. newspaper) and a lack of nest materials that growing toes can grab can cause splaying. At first, the hock appears flattened, widened, and swollen. As the condition worsens, the tendon at the hock may slip, or the tibiotarsus and tarsometatarsus become twisted or bowed. In early stages, an improved Ca : P in the diet and correction of nests and substrates may help. If the legs are flexible enough to be positioned correctly, they can be hobbled. Use a strap of Micropore paper tape (3M) attaching the tarsometatarsi (between the hock and the foot) to connect the legs and bring them into a normal standing position. Continue hobbles as long as needed, which is usually 1–2 weeks once the substrate and dietary deficiencies are corrected. Severe cases may require euthanasia.

### Curled Toes

A curled foot or toe may be caused by an injury to the leg or foot, as well as nutritional deficiencies. A "snowshoe" splint is often successful in guiding the foot/toes into the anatomically correct position as the chick matures. This can be made from plastic or thin foam cut in the form of a diamond shape, approximating normal foot shape. Use a glue-stick to attach soft padding, like nonadherent gauze dressing, to the shoe splint to pad and protect the underside of the foot, then tape the splint onto the foot, making sure the digits are in a normal position. Leave in place for 5–7 days, then remove the splint to check the positioning. If the digits still curl into a ball, then replace for another week. Do not use cardboard for the splint, which tends to get wet and bend, providing poor support for the foot. If only the first digit (the hallux) is reflected under the foot, then tape it to the tarsometatarsus in a normal position. Check positioning in 5–7 days after removing the tape. Monitor that the hallux doesn't become swollen.

### Constriction Injuries

Occasionally, human hair or fishing line gets into nesting material, which can wrap around a nestling's foot or leg causing deep wounds and ischemic necrosis. Remove the entire strand, being careful not to leave any fibers embedded in the wound. A jeweler's loop or other magnification may be helpful. Clean and dress the wound with a hydrocolloid dressing until healed. Clean away all necrotic debris initially, then again at each bandage change, which should be done every 2–3 days until healed. While the wound is open, keep the bird on a broad-spectrum antibiotic. Use meloxicam to control pain and inflammation. Necrosis due to restriction of blood flow may worsen for a while even after the fibers are removed. This can lead to loss of toes or deep necrosis of the foot. At each handling, assess prospects for survival, especially if the bird is intended for wild release. Euthanize if the prognosis for normal use of the foot becomes poor.

## Diet or Hand-feeding Recipes

There are several diets successfully used for neonate columbids, too many to cover in a single chapter. Of these, some are more conducive to good health and growth than others. Included here are two diets that have proven effective for the authors. The underlying principle is to mimic the natural diet as much as possible. For the first 2–3 days of life, columbids are fed crop milk, which is largely composed of partially-digested proteins and fat. At about day 3 or 4, small amounts of regurgitated seed are added to the milk. Crop milk production begins to drop off at about day 12 and regurgitated seed is fed throughout the balance of the fledging period (Vandeputte-Poma 1980). To approximate this shifting ratio of foods in wild chicks, the general idea is to feed two diets and shift their relative proportions over time. One diet approximates crop milk and one is similar to regurgitated adult diet.

**Two Crop Milk Replacer Options:**

1) Emeraid® IC Carnivore (Lafeber Company)
2) Baby food diet
   - 1 jar (71 g) Gerber's chicken and gravy human baby food
   - 1 tbsp. plain nonfat yogurt
   - 1 ml corn oil
   - 1/8 tbsp. Avi-Era avian vitamins (Lafeber Company)
   - 100–150 mg elemental calcium from 250 to 375 mg calcium carbonate

The most commonly used diet that approximates regurgitated adult diet for many of these species is Kaytee® exact® Hand Feeding Formula (Kaytee). In a busy shelter where gradual phasing of the crop milk replacer into the adult diet replacer is impractical, using a 50/50 mixture of exact Hand Feeding Formula and Emeraid IC Carnivore for the youngest chicks has been quite successful. Mix equal amounts of the two powdered diets, then use one part of the combined powder to two parts warm water, bringing the slurry to the consistency of apple sauce. The youngest hatchlings, or older birds with slower crop clearance, may need the diet further watered down until crop clearance normalizes. A pinch of BeneBac® Plus Bird and Reptile Powder (PetAg) or other avian probiotic can be added for those who seem to have trouble digesting. For individuals with persistently slow crop clearing, alternate feeding formula with warm water that includes a pinch of probiotic until crop clearance normalizes. When fed by the parent, hatchlings get a bolus of the adult's microflora. A newly arrived hatchling may benefit from a small bolus of fluid lavaged (transfaunated) from the crop of a healthy adult, especially if the chick is suspected to have never been fed by a parent.

Make diets fresh every feeding with warm water. Refrigerate powdered diet and do not store after being mixed with water so as to avoid overgrowth of yeast and bacteria. Once chicks reach species-specific target weights, switch to straight exact mixed at 1-part powder to 2-parts warm water to 90–100 °F (32.2–37.8 °C) (Tables 27.1–27.3). Feeding 100% exact to hatchlings and younger nestlings usually results in poor quality feathering, presumably due to the lower protein content of the diet.

When gradually shifting the diet from the crop milk replacer to the adult diet formula is feasible, after the fourth day of life, add 1 tsp. of exact and a small amount of extra water to the crop milk replacer. As each day goes by, add a little more exact and less crop milk replacer until the diet fed is 100% exact. If the diet becomes too thick or the chick's crop emptying slows, add more water.

## Food for Nestlings and Older Birds

A good quality seed mix is essential to continued optimal development and there is a variety available. A commercial dove diet can include white proso, German millet, milo, wheat, and safflower; while for pigeons, diets may include wheat, milo, safflower seed, oat groats, barley, vetch, and dehydrated peas. Finch seed mixes can be added to dove diets to provide more diversity. Some species also enjoy pieces of finely chopped greens such as parsley or fruits; research the natural history of the species to know what adult diet foods to offer as chicks mature. The seed in pigeon mixes tends to be too large for doves, but some pigeons prefer the smaller seeds in dove mixes. Experiment to find what works best for the species in hand. Note what types of seed are consistently ignored by the birds and adjust purchases accordingly. Offer seeds and water as soon as the birds are out of the nest. Pigeons will usually start eating seed as soon as they are old enough to walk. Offer ample seed

Table 27.1 Feeding schedule for Mourning Doves.

**Diet for chicks under 25 g Diet = 50/50 (Emeraid/Exact): Birds on this diet may not require as frequent feedings. Check crop and feed when nearly empty. Food expires after 1 hour. DO NOT FEED COLD 50/50.**

| Weight (g) | Amount (ml) | Hours between feeds |
|---|---|---|
| 10 | 1 | ½–1 |
| 15 | 1.5–2 | 1–1½ |
| 20 | 1.5–2.5 | 2 |
| **For chicks over 25 g, feed exact only: DO NOT FEED COLD EXACT** | | |
| 25 | 2–3 | 2 |
| 30 | 2.5–3.5 | 2 |
| 35 | 4 | 2 |
| 40–50 | 5 | 3 |
| 50–60 | 6 | 3 |
| 60 | 6–7 | 3 |
| Above 65 g, begin checking crop for seed before feeding. Do not tube if seed is present. | | |
| 65 | 6–7 | 3 ½ |
| Juvenile Mourning Doves over 70 g will usually self-feed unless debilitated. | | |
| 70–80 | 8 | 4 |
| At 90 g, do not tube unless bird is debilitated. Healthy juveniles will self-feed. | | |
| 90 | 9 | x3/day |
| 95 | 9–10 | x3/day |

*Source:* information courtesy of the Wildlife Care Association in Sacramento, CA.

in wide flat dishes. Check the crop for seed before every feeding. If a bird is starting to peck at food and has bunches of seed in its crop, skip the meal and check again at the next feeding interval. Once the bird has had seed in its crop for 48 hours and is of weight, consider the bird self-feeding. Continue checking its attitude and weight daily to ensure it is thriving.

In the wild, columbids ingest small caliber rocks as grit, facilitating grinding up food in the ventriculous (gizzard). In captivity, when using commercially available seed mixes, pigeons and doves do very well without grit, since the seed itself helps in grinding. If a caregiver chooses to add grit to a bird's diet, a small amount is sufficient. Beware of giving birds large amounts of grit, as birds may over-eat this non-nutritive material. Using ground oyster shells as grit can add calcium to the diet; a small amount is adequate. Beware crushed oyster shell that has sharp edges, as it can cause esophagus lacerations.

## Feeding Procedures

The most effective method used to feed juvenile doves and pigeons is by gavage, or "tubing" a nutritionally complete liquid ration directly into the bird's crop (Figure 27.2). This technique takes practice but is invaluable when feeding large numbers of individuals. Feeding syringes should be

Table 27.2 Feeding schedule for Rock Pigeons.

**Diet for chicks under 75 g Diet = 50/50 (Emeraid/Exact): Birds on this diet may not require as frequent feedings. Check crop and feed when nearly empty. Food expires after 1 hour. DO NOT FEED COLD 50/50.**

| Weight (g) | Amount (ml) | Hours between feeds |
|---|---|---|
| 20 | 1–2 | 1 |
| 30 | 2.5–3.5 | 1–2 |
| 40 | 3–5 | 2 |
| 50 | 4–6 | 2 |
| **For chicks over 75 g, feed exact only: DO NOT FEED COLD EXACT** | | |
| 75 | 5–8 | 2 |
| 100 | 8–10 | 2 |
| 125 | 11–13 | 2 |
| 150 | 14–16 | 2 |
| 175 | 17–18 | 3 |
| 200 | 18–20 | 3 |
| 225 | 18–20 | 3 |
| 250 | 18–20 | 4 |
| Birds over 250 g rarely require tube-feeding unless they are debilitated. | | |
| 300 | 18–20 | 4 |
| 350 | 18–20 | 4 |
| 400 | 18–20 | 4 |

*Source:* information courtesy of the Wildlife Care Association in Sacramento, CA.

constructed well ahead of time. The length of tubing required is that which reaches past the glottis and into the crop. Most doves require tubing of 3–4 in. (7.5–10 cm); pigeons may need tubing as long as 6 in. (15 cm). Intravenous extension set tubing cut to an appropriate length makes an excellent feeding tube. This tubing is typically 1/8 in. (3 mm) in diameter, which is sufficient to pass the diet. The tube should be cut straight across, never at an angle (which will produce a "spear" that can puncture a bird's crop). Lightly pass a flame (e.g. cigarette lighter) over the cut end of the tube so that the tube end develops a rounded edge, thus avoiding sharp edges and preventing internal crop lacerations. Steel feeding needles, originally intended for parrots, are also used by some rehabilitation centers, but are not necessary for Columbiformes because there is no risk of the bird biting off the tubing. An author (GP) has seen numerous cases of metal feeding needles rupturing crops, and even being forced through the back of a bird's neck, when used by inexperienced handlers.

Attach the flexible tubing to a feeding syringe and fill with warmed formula. Warm the formula to 100–105 °F (38–41 °C) and draw up into a syringe barrel. Remove any large air bubbles from the syringe and wipe the outside of the tubing clean of any excess liquid to keep feathers dry and avoid aspirating the patient. Wrap the bird securely in a soft cloth, and extend the neck to straighten the esophagus. Open the beak with a finger and introduce the tubing into the mouth, aiming toward the bird's right side at the back of the mouth. Pressing on the upper and lower bases of the beak

Table 27.3 Feeding schedule for Eurasian Collared Doves.

| Diet for chicks under 40 g Diet = 50/50 (Emeraid/Exact): Birds on this diet may not require as frequent feedings. Check crop and feed when nearly empty. Food expires after 1 hour. DO NOT FEED COLD 50/50. | | |
|---|---|---|
| **Weight (g)** | **Amount (CC)** | **Hours between feeds** |
| 15 | 1.5–2 | 1 |
| 25 | 2–3 | 1–2 |
| 35 | 4 | 2 |
| **For chicks over 40 g, feed exact only: DO NOT FEED COLD EXACT** | | |
| 40 | 4–5 | 2 |
| 45 | 4.5–5.5 | 2 |
| 50 | 5–6 | 2 |
| 55 | 5.5–6.5 | 2 |
| 60 | 6–7 | 3 |
| 65 | 6.5–7.5 | 3 |
| 70 | 7–8 | 3 |
| 75 | 8.5–9.5 | 3 |
| 80 | 9–10 | 3 |
| 85 | 9.5–10.5 | 3 |
| Juvenile birds over 90g will usually self-feed unless debilitated. | | |
| 90 | 10–11 | 3 |
| 100 | 11–12 | 3 |
| 110 | 12–13 | 3 |
| 120 | 13–14 | 3 |
| At 130g, do not tube unless bird is debilitated. Healthy juveniles will self-feed. | | |
| 130 | 14–15 | x3/day |
| 140 | 15 | x3/day |

*Source:* information courtesy of the Wildlife Care Association in Sacramento, CA.

will stimulate many young columbids to gape; this simulates the way adult birds feed their chicks. Advance the tube slowly until ruffling of the feathers over the crop is observed. If at any time there is resistance, stop and remove the tube. Once in the crop, the tip of the tube can be seen or felt through the skin. If the tube cannot be felt, or there is any uncertainty of position, remove it and try again. Malpositioning of the tube can cause the bird to inhale formula (aspiration) and is potentially fatal. When the tube is in place, deliver the formula steadily into the crop. Make sure the tube does not slip out from the crop and that there is no formula welling up in the mouth. If any food pools in the bird's mouth, pull the tube immediately and set the bird down to allow it to clear its glottis. If the bird cannot quickly do so, wipe the mouth out with a cotton-tip applicator and give it time to recover. If a bird aspirates such that formula reaches deeper respiratory structures and cannot be cleared, it should be started on antibiotics.

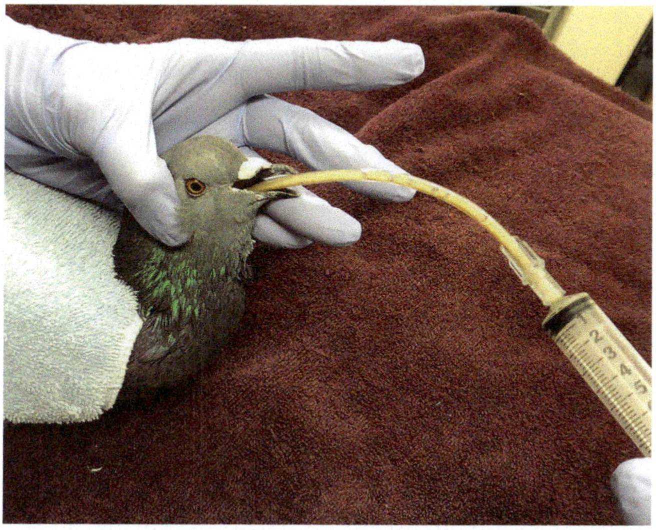

Figure 27.2 Tube-feeding a Rock Pigeon. Keep the neck extended during feeding. Wrapping snugly in a towel restrains fractious birds but is not necessary for habituated chicks.

Another method used by some caregivers simulates the natural feeding action of young doves, whereby they insert their heads into the parent's mouth and throat and eat as the parent regurgitates food from the crop. Load a syringe with formula and secure a cohesive bandage (e.g. Vetrap™, 3M) over the wide opening and cut a slit to accommodate the bird's beak. While the container is held, allow the bird to feed from the syringe. While in some ways a more natural feeding method, this can be very messy and time-consuming, poses an aspiration risk, and it is difficult to tell how much formula was consumed. Formula on feathers must be cleaned off immediately with a wet washcloth or paper towel and warm water. Formula allowed to dry on feathers quickly becomes hard and crusty, can lead to skin infections and feather damage, and is very hard to remove.

Perform any treatments and give medications before feeding to avoid squeezing a full crop and causing aspiration. Young columbids will beg frantically when they are hungry, and often when they are not. To avoid crop problems, do not feed again until the crop has emptied. If there is a delay in emptying, gavage a small amount of warm saline. If that is not effective, excess fluid can potentially be removed by "lavage," which is drawing fluid out in a procedure reversing the steps of gavage. An overstretched crop can sometimes be supported with a "crop bra," a piece of Vetrap wrapped around the bird's chest so the crop does not overhang the sternum. Chronically overfilled crops are susceptible to poor motility plus prone to yeast and bacterial infections, which can be diagnosed via microscopic examination of lavaged crop fluid and treated accordingly. Crop capacity of most columbids is 10% of body weight (100 ml/kg).

Another feeding technique involves putting seed in a small container, like a baby food jar, covering the opening with cohesive bandage, and cutting a small, beak-sized hole in it. Juvenile birds can quickly learn to swallow seeds when the jar is partially inverted and their beaks inserted in the hole. The young birds can get very excited feeding in this manner and it is likewise a fun way for caregivers to provide nourishment. However, many individuals seem to become "addicted" to this feeding style and become resistant to weaning. These birds need to have the jar held gradually closer and closer to the ground to get them to focus downward toward the flooring rather than upwards to the jar. Fledglings that are especially resistant to weaning from seed jars should be housed with older self-feeding birds that can provide better "role models" for independence. Hatchlings and younger nestlings should not be fed using seed jars because the seed is not nutritionally balanced for their age-specific needs. Individual birds who are otherwise ready to wean may be resistant to doing so when accustomed to being fed in this manner. Force feeding a few seeds can "jump start" them to eating whole seeds on their own.

## Expected Weight Gain

Pigeon and dove chicks typically reach adult weight by 3–4 weeks of age (Figure 27.3). Chicks should gain weight daily until they have finished growing. Weigh them before the first feed of the day to avoid confounding from the amount of food in the crop.

## Housing

To avoid habituation in orphaned birds intended for wild release, it is crucial to raise them in pairs or small groups of similar ages and sizes (Figure 27.4). If housed alone, add a mirror to the enclosure until a cagemate can be found. See Chapter 19 for numerous suggestions to avoid imprinting and habituation. Never combine doves and Rock Pigeons older than nestlings together because the larger, more aggressive pigeons may stress the doves. Band-tailed Pigeon fledglings may display extreme stress responses to handling. A calm, nonaggressive, self-feeding role model to show the bird how to eat seed may be useful, even if the role model is of a different, but similar-sized species. Housing should have visual barriers that block view of humans while providing adequate light.

For hatchlings and nestlings, nests can be made with a bowl or plastic berry basket covered with absorbent paper toweling and lined with facial or toilet tissues. White unscented paper products are preferred. If cloth is used, change it frequently, as soon as it gets soiled by feces, to avoid damage to skin and feathers. All hard surfaces must be covered. Plastic mesh must be completely covered with tissue; these species may injure themselves if placed in unlined berry baskets. Coiled tapered tissue at the bottom of the nest works well to prevent leg splaying and provides material

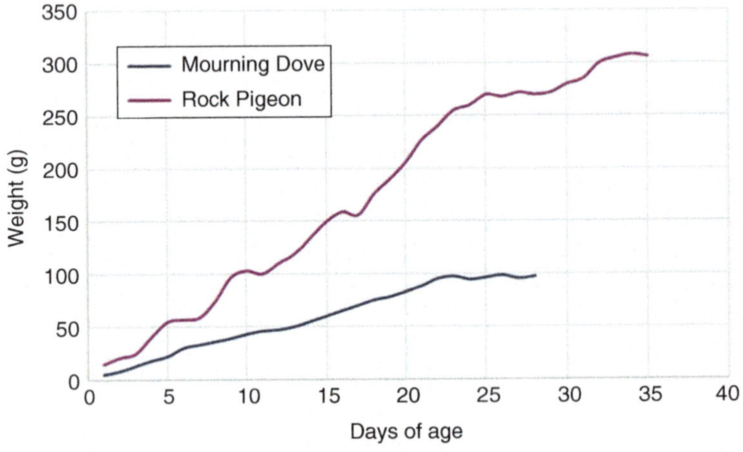


Figure 27.3 Expected weight gain of Mourning Dove and Rock Pigeon chicks.

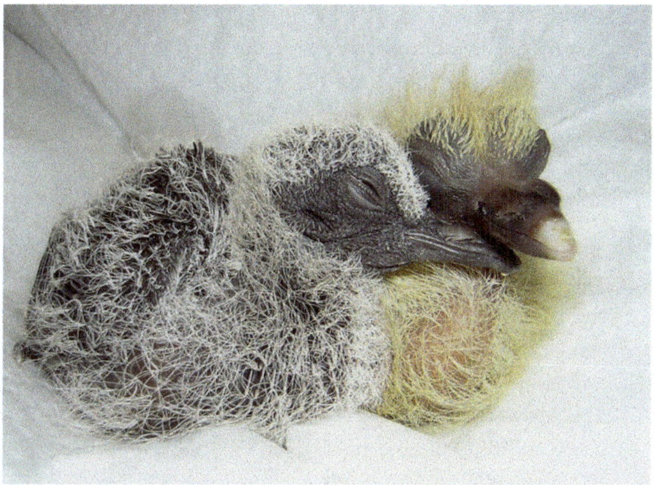

Figure 27.4 Newly hatched Rock Pigeon housed with a size-matched 5-day old Mourning Dove as a nest companion.

that tiny toes can grab. Nest size will be dependent on number and size of the birds; the birds should be able to shift comfortably but remain close together. Most dove and pigeon species have two chicks at a time, so keeping birds in pairs is ideal. Most are sociable and will accept higher numbers of chicks in groups without dominance issues. The rim of the nest should be low enough to allow the birds to defecate over the edge.

For hatchlings, poorly feathered nestlings, and debilitated chicks, housing should be fully environmentally controlled. One option is lining the bottom of an aquarium or incubator with paper towels and placing the nest inside. Add a small jar with cotton balls and water for humidity and include a thermometer inside the enclosure. Cover the top of the aquarium with cloth and monitor the temperature. The optimum temperature for unfeathered birds is 95–100 °F (35–38 °C); humidity should be approximately 50–60%. Heating pads can be used for warmth under a covered aquarium. Check the temperature frequently when setting up new housing. Do not use heating pads with automatic shutoffs, and beware of overheating the chicks. Animal Intensive Care Units (Lyons Technologies, Inc.) allow close regulation of both temperature and humidity and are relatively easy to clean.

Doves and pigeons grow rapidly. As the birds grow, they require less heat. Monitor for signs of overheating (gasping, dehydration) or chilling (fluffed feathers). Nestling temperature needs vary from 80 to 95 °F (27–35 °C). When they are fully feathered, they may be moved to the next stage of housing. A laundry basket that has been screened on the inside and lined with paper towels can be used for most birds. Cover the top with fiberglass screening or mesh and secure with clothespins. Ideally, baskets should be wide enough to allow the bird to extend its wings once old enough to do so. Cover the front of the basket with cloth so there is less exposure to human activity. Do not cover the top of the cage with cloth so the birds have enough light to see and forage. A perch can be made from a plastic brick wrapped in paper toweling, taping the ends underneath, which keeps the perch from absorbing fecal matter (a similar-sized wooden block can also be used, but should be wrapped in wax paper or plastic wrap under the paper towel to avoid spread of disease). The perch should be placed to keep the bird's tail from bending on the bottom or sides of the basket, while not having its head in contact with the ceiling. Having several perch sizes on hand will allow for growth. Clean or change perches daily and then as needed to remove fecal material.

Stick perches may be used (especially for tree-perching birds like Mourning Doves) but it is recommended that these be kept very close to the floor. Avoid stick perches with highly stressed birds because they may damage their flight feathers by hitting them on the perch. Use a stick slightly longer than the basket is wide so it can be wedged securely in place. The width of a stick perch should allow the bird to grip it comfortably; neither too small (toes overlap), nor too wide (toes do not wrap around the perch enough to grip). Special attention should be paid to hygiene with frequent cleaning and replacing of the stick perches.

Some species can be highly fractious and, as they approach adulthood, may exhibit frenzied attempts to escape the cage when people approach. The top of the basket may need to be covered with light-colored cloth, even if it makes the inside darker than normal. These baskets should be padded with light fabric on the walls and the bird transferred to an aviary as soon as possible.

Using branches with leaves can help provide a sense of security plus natural enrichment. Natural-looking plastic vegetation from craft stores can also be used. Clean and sanitize with a bleach solution as needed. Be careful not to add so many furnishings to the enclosure that the birds cannot move around easily. In this case, less is better than too much.

Wide, flat jar lids of various diameters can be used for seed. Pigeons and doves both will learn to eat faster with food presented in this manner rather than in a deep crock-style food dish. When weaning, scatter some seed around the floor of the cage to encourage self-feeding. Water should be provided in bowls at least as deep as the bird's beaks are long, but not so high that the bird cannot easily reach in. A rock can be added to water bowls to prevent tipping but make sure the rock is not so big that the bird cannot easily get to the water. For pigeons, use water dishes at least 1–1.5 in. (2.5–3.5 cm) deep. Place seed and water dishes at the opposite end of the basket from the perch to prevent contamination from droppings.

If possible, housing may be placed in a protected area to provide natural sunlight. If outside, patients will thus be better acclimated when it is time to go to aviary. Full-spectrum lighting can be purchased that provides both UVA and UVB light for times when natural light is not available. Transfer the bird to an outside flight cage when it has been self-feeding and maintaining weight for seven days without supplemental gavage. Never allow the bird to fly free inside a building.

## Weaning

Doves and pigeons can learn to pick up seeds at an early age (Figure 27.5). Housing weaning-age birds with slightly older birds that are self-feeding will usually speed the weaning process. The older bird should be close in size to the younger and not aggressive, especially when dealing with pigeons. Adult pigeons are often intolerant of younger birds that are not their own offspring and can do serious damage and even kill a youngster. Some young pigeons learn to self-feed as early as 2 weeks of age or as soon as they can walk, and the majority of doves and pigeons are enthusiastic about learning to eat on their own. Monitor weight and check crops carefully and frequently. Although some birds seem to be pecking, they may not be taking in sufficient food for growth.

A Mourning Dove of below 65 g should continue to get formula feedings even if there is a small amount of seed in the crop; this produces birds with better feathering that grow more quickly. At 65 g and above, don't gavage if there is any seed in the crop unless the bird is not sustaining its weight. Once a Mourning Dove is 70–80 g, they will usually be self-feeding unless debilitated. Once they reach 90 g, cut them off from formula feeding even if there is no seed in the crop; they usually start self-feeding immediately, but do monitor weight and crop contents. Rock Pigeons can be cut off from formula as soon as they have a significant amount of seed in the crop, and they will

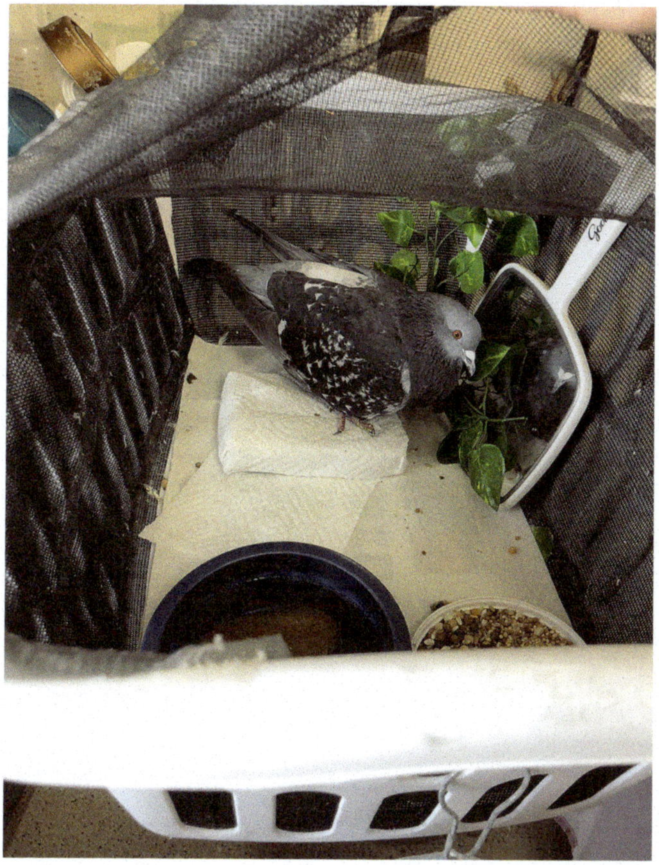

Figure 27.5 Basket set up for young pigeons or doves. Note the screened walls, flat perch, deep water crock, and flat seed dish. Mirrors are helpful for single birds.

continue to develop well. Here again, monitor condition and crop contents to watch for the rare bird that needs additional attention. See Tables 27.1–27.3 for tips on crucial weights that reflect developmental milestones in three species.

A crop with seed in it is usually described as feeling like a bean bag. Palpate the crop gently, rolling the skin between two fingers. A bird that is successfully feeding itself will have noticeable seed in the crop. If it does not, monitor droppings and continue to supplement the bird's diet with reduced volumes of formula until the crop is consistently full of seed. If added feedings are necessary, make one of the feedings in the late evening to ensure the bird has enough food to last through the night.

## Preparation for Wild Release

When the bird has been self-feeding and continuing to gain weight for at least 7 days inside, it can be transferred to an outside flight cage or aviary (Figure 27.6). Minimum aviary size for Columbiformes is 12×8×8 ft. (3.6×2.5×2.5 m) (Miller 2012). Plywood, fiberglass, or hardware (wire) cloth can be used for the sides of the cage. Having at least a portion of the ceiling solid allows

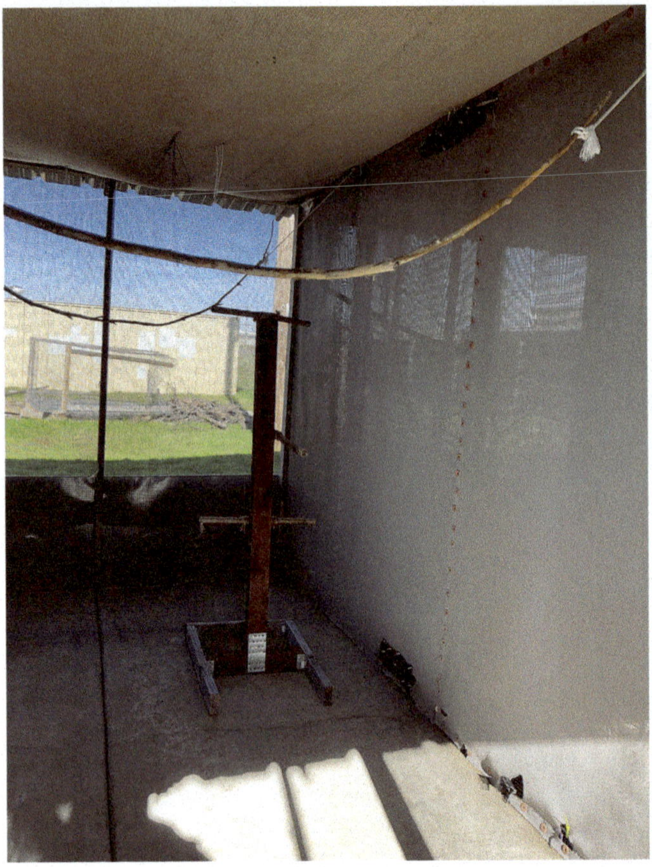

Figure 27.6 Aviary for Mourning Doves. Note the dropped fabric ceiling to prevent birds scalping themselves if startled.

occupants to shelter from bad weather. Flooring options include concrete or plywood treated with marine varnish, which are relatively easy to keep clean. If pea gravel flooring is used, plan to allow sifting and cleaning between occupants. Floors of dirt or sand are the hardest to decontaminate when environmentally-stable, disease-causing organisms like coccidia appear. Wire walls and the ceiling should be screened to prevent feather damage caused by panic flights. Doves may flush frantically when frightened in the aviary and are at risk of lacerating their heads on the ceiling. Ideally, dove aviaries should have a layer of soft screening between them and the roof to prevent scalping injuries and bumper trauma to the wings. Food and water should be on the ground and additional food can be provided in hanging feeders. Doves should have branch-style perches and feral pigeons should have shelf-style perches. In the wild, columbids live in complex environments and diverse perching opportunities will help prepare them for release.

Pigeons and doves are flocking birds and therefore should be released into a flock of their own species. Prior to release, the birds should be completely self-feeding outside for at least 1 week and have heavy muscling on the breast. In addition to acclimation to outdoor conditions, time in the aviary will demonstrate the bird's stamina; do not release if the bird appears winded by short flights. Feathers should be intact, waterproof, and free of parasites. Any bird that does not appear wary of humans or other animals is not suitable for release. If a bird has spent significant time without other birds, introducing additional birds of the same species may help a human-habituated bird to "wild up." Whenever possible, never raise a bird alone if it is intended for wild release. Alternatively, for those birds destined to be companion animals, the more they can be handled from an early age, the better adjusted they will be to perceiving humans as sources of comfort and safety.

Check weather forecasts and release only when weather is expected to be calm and dry, without temperature extremes, for 2–3 days. Early morning releases enable the bird to adjust to its surroundings before nightfall. If birds are to be released in areas that allow hunting, it is prudent to postpone release until the season is ended.

## Acknowledgments

Guthrum Purdin, DVM, offers his heart-felt thanks to the staff and volunteers at the Wildlife Care Association in Sacramento, CA, for their tireless dedication to the needs of the animals in their care. Nancy Eilertsen would like to thank Linda Hufford, who has been a continual source of moral support, knowledge, and sanity stabilization for many years.

## Sources for Products Mentioned

Ultracare Mite and Lice Bird Spray: 8 in 1 Pet Products, Hauppauge, NY, (800) 645-5154.

Leg bands: National Band and Tag Company, 721 York St, Newport, KY 41072-0430, (800) 261-TAGS (8247), https://nationalband.com.

Vetrap, Tegaderm, and Micropore paper tape: 3M, St. Paul, MN, (800) 628-7462, https://www.3m.com/3M/en_US/company-us/all-3m-products.

Kaytee products: 521 Clay St, PO Box 230, Chilton, WI 53014, (800) KAYTEE-1, https://www.kaytee.com.

Avi-Era Avian Vitamins and Emeraid products: Lafeber Company, Cornell, IL 61319, (800) 842-6445, http://www.lafeber.com.

BeneBac Plus Bird and Reptile Powder: PetAg, Inc., 255 Keyes Avenue, Hampshire, IL 60140, https://www.petag.com.

Animal Intensive Care Unit™ and Grumbach Hatcher™: Lyon Technologies, Inc., 1690, Brandywine Avenue, Chula Vista, CA. 91911, (619) 216-3400, https://lyonvet.com.

## References

Duerr, R.S., Purdin, G.J., and Bowers, V. (2017). Small-bodied birds: passerines, doves, woodpeckers, others. In: *Topics in Wildlife Medicine, Vol. 4: Orthopedics* (eds. R.S. Duerr and G.J. Purdin), 53–74. St. Cloud, MN: National Wildlife Rehabilitators Association.

Engberg, R.M., Kaspers, B., Schranner, I. et al. (1992). Quantification of the immunoglobulin classes IgG and IgA in the young and adult pigeon (Columba livia). *Avian Pathology* 21 (3): 409–420. https://doi.org/10.1080/03079459208418859.

Girard, Y.A., Rogers, K.H., Woods, L.W. et al. (2014). Dual-pathogen etiology of avian trichomonosis in a declining band-tailed pigeon population. *Infection, Genetics and Evolution* 24: 146–156.

Hawkins, M.G., Barron, H.W., Speer, B.L. et al. (2018). Birds. In: *Exotic Animal Formulary*, 5e (eds. J.W. Carpenter and C.J. Marion), 167–375. St. Louis, MO: Elsevier.

Leahy, C.W. (2004). *The Birdwatcher's Companion to North American Birdlife*, 223, 638. Princeton, New Jersey: Princeton University Press.

Miller, E.A. (ed.) (2012). *Minimum Standards for Wildlife Rehabilitation*, 4e. St. Cloud, MN: National Wildlife Rehabilitation Association.

Sales, J. and Janssens, G.P.J. (2003). Nutrition of the domestic pigeon (*Columba livia domestica*). *World's Poultry Science Journal* 59 (2): 221–232.

Vandeputte-Poma, J. (1980). Feeding, growth and metabolism of the pigeon, Columba livia domestica: duration and role of crop milk feeding. *Journal of Comparative Physiology* 135: 97–99.

# 28

# Turacos

*Kateri J. Davis*

## Natural History

The turacos of order Musophagiformes, are found solely in Africa south of the Sahara. There are 23 species of turacos in five genera, with several subspecies identified. Common names are many, including *plantain-eater, go-away bird, loury,* and *touraco,* although *turaco* is currently the most popular.

All species are about the size of a chicken with long tails, short rounded wings, zygodactyl toe arrangement, and strong legs for running along and bounding off branches. They have smooth plumage and crests, which most can erect at will. A unique characteristic is that the green and purple turaco species possess two actual copper-based feather pigments: turacoverdin (green) and turacin (red).

Although there are five genera, turacos can be grouped into four basic categories: the greens (genus *Tauraco*), purples (genus *Musophaga*), grays (genera *Corythaixoides* and *Crinifer*), and the blue (one species, the Great Blue Turaco, *Corythaeola cristata*). The purples tend to be called plantain-eaters and the grays tend to be called go-away birds. There is variation in habitat, diet, and behavior between the green/purple and gray groups.

Most species of turacos are found in pairs or small groups in the mid-canopy section of evergreen and rain forest environments, with the exception of the gray group which inhabits the drier savanna areas. Fruit is the main diet of most species, with the gray species taking more leafy fare. Occasional animal protein in the form of grubs or other insects is taken.

Turacos are monogamous and make a flat, insubstantial stick nest, much like a pigeon. They are semi-determinate layers of two to three white eggs. The young are fed by regurgitation. All species, except the White-bellied Go-away Bird, *Criniferoides leucogaster*, are sexually monomorphic.

## Criteria for Intervention

Because of their color and other display qualities, turacos are some of the more commonly kept softbill private avicultural subjects in the United States and Europe, as well as being popular in many zoological institutions.

*Hand-Rearing Birds*, Second Edition. Edited by Rebecca S. Duerr and Laurie J. Gage.

The Houston Zoo in Texas, U.S. has been a leader in turaco husbandry for years. The green turacos are the most commonly kept turacos in the U.S., followed by the purples and then the grays. The most popular avicultural species in the U.S. are White Cheek (*Tauraco leucotis*), Red Crest (*Tauraco erythrolophus*), Green (*Tauraco persa*), and Violet (*Musophaga violacea*) Turacos. The Great Blue Turaco is extremely rare in captivity in the U.S. The Houston Zoo has had success with raising this species, and a few pairs and individuals are in private hands due to small groups imported into the U.S. around 2015.

Hand-rearing of turacos is done usually to increase the productivity of a pair, for the safety of the chick, or to have a tame adult. Hand-rearing for household pet quality is becoming more popular despite the fact that turacos do not make the greatest pets in the average home.

## Record Keeping

At this time, no federal permits are required to keep and raise turacos. However, state laws vary and should be checked before attaining turacos.

Record keeping varies with each aviculturist but should include the basics, such as date hatched, parents and bloodline, sexing information, and any medical issues. Leg bands or microchipping is recommended to identify and track individuals. Traditionally in aviculture, the gender of sexed birds can be visually marked by bands placed on the right leg for a male and left for a female. Tattoos are used on the appropriately sided wingweb.

## Incubation of Eggs

In addition to cases of rescuing eggs that would be destroyed, turaco eggs are sometimes removed and artificially incubated to induce a pair of birds to lay again within a couple of weeks. It is much better for the parents to be able to raise the chicks on their own, but in certain cases, such as rare species, this is a valid technique as long as it is not overused and the female's health put at risk from excessive egg production.

Turaco eggs can be artificially incubated at a temperature of 99–100 °F (37.2–37.8 °C) and 45% relative humidity in a standard incubator unit. They should be turned 180° in opposite directions every 1–5 hours. Evidence of fertility can be seen by candling methods around days 7–10. See Chapter 3 for greater detail.

Incubation times vary between species and even individuals. Green turacos hatch in 19–23 days, and Great Blues take 31 days. Purple and gray turacos fall between these values. Hatching can take up to 48 hours.

Since turaco eggs are relatively easy to artificially incubate, it is often done if a pet bird and hand-rearing from day 1 is desired.

## Initial Care and Stabilization

Turaco chicks are semi-precocial, opening their eyes soon after hatching, and are very alert to their environment. Chicks in the nest will hiss, threaten an intruder with an open mouth, and defecate when handled. When incubator hatched, they will imprint on the human caregiver immediately and not show these reactions unless frightened.

The newly hatched chick can stay in the incubator for a few hours until it is dry. No food should be given the first 12–24 hours so that the yolk sac can be absorbed. The umbilicus may be swabbed with an iodine solution to help prevent infections. Watch behavior for insight into the comfort of the chick because turaco chicks will pant when too hot and will not gape or feed when too cold.

## Common Medical Problems and Solutions

Turacos, especially the greens, are hardy and typically have few health problems if environments are kept clean and food is fresh. They are a group that can be affected by iron storage disease, or hemachromatosis, which is a fatal dietary condition wherein the liver stores too much iron. Although they are not as prone to this as toucans or starlings, attention should be paid to a turaco's diet, thus avoiding animal-based iron foodstuffs and citrus fruits. Low-iron softbill pellets, such as Kaytee Exact® Mynah or Mazuri® Softbill diets, should be chosen.

The most common problem seen in hand-raised turacos is splay-leg due to improper substrate. From day 1 turacos must be kept on a substrate that can be gripped easily, such as wire/plastic mesh and fibrous grass or hay. If the chick is on a surface that is too slick, the legs will splay quickly and may be permanently damaged. In mild cases of splay-leg, the legs may be taped in position and allowed to heal for a few days. If applying tape in this manner, be sure not to cover the bird's vent with tape. Placing the chick in a small bowl to force his legs to stay under his body in proper position may sometimes be effective.

Hand-raising the Great Blue or gray turaco species is much more difficult. Chicks are quite susceptible to yeast and bacterial infections. Veterinary assistance is recommended at the first hint of trouble.

## Hand-Feeding Diet

The different groups of turacos require different diets. The greens and purples are the most commonly and successfully hand-raised, and they are more frugivorous. There is currently much variation in hand-rearing diets used for all species of turacos. Each successful aviculturist has their own preferred diet and feeding schedule. The grays and the Great Blue Turaco are more herbivorous as adults. Not as much is known about the nutritional needs of their chicks so rearing them is more problematic, although some people have been successful hand-raising them.

Feedings should start about 6:00 a.m. and continue until 10–11:00 p.m. Feeding throughout the night is unnecessary for healthy chicks. The regularity, appearance, and amount of feces should be recorded at each feeding time to ensure that the chick is not having problems. Turaco feces are soft, brownish, somewhat formed, and sometimes have a mucous layer. Runny or smelly stools may indicate a yeast or bacterial problem, and immediate medical care is advised. If the stools are too dry, add a little more water to the formula. If the chick is not defecating or is straining, stimulate the vent with a warm moist swab. If the chick is not gaping and the temperature is fine, it may mean that it is constipated or dehydrated, and may require fluid therapy.

## Hand-feeding Diet for Green and Purple Turacos

The following is a recommended diet for hand-feeding green and purple turacos:

- 2 parts commercial hand-feeding formula for parrots, such as Kaytee Exact Hand Feeding Formula, mixed with warm water to reconstitute as directed on package
- 1 part strained fruit human baby food, such as Gerber's pear, apple, papaya, or banana (Gerber Products Company)

Formula should be warm, but not hot, and should be made fresh for each meal. As the chick develops, the formula should be made with less water for a thicker pancake-batter consistency. Mashed watersoaked softbill pellets, such as Kaytee Exact Mynah, can be substituted for the hand-feeding formula in emergencies. As the chick grows, small chunks of fruit and water-soaked pellets should be fed and the amount of formula decreased.

### Suggested Feeding Schedule

Larger species such as Lady Ross can take slightly larger feedings (see Table 28.1). Feeding size gradually increases throughout the day; for example, the day 2 first feeding may be 0.3 ml but by the last feeding it is 0.5 ml. Weight gain will tell the hand-feeder whether the meals are the right size. Increase the amount of fruit and pellet pieces while reducing the amount of formula so that by day 10 or 11 the chick is eating only solid food.

## Alternate Hand-feeding Diet

The following list summarizes an alternate hand-feeding diet (See Table 28.2 for feeding schedule):

- 2 parts soaked Mazuri Parrot Breeder Pellets
- 1 part fruit: applesauce, papaya, or both
- 1 part greens: kale or endive

Add enough Pedialyte® (Abbott) or other pediatric electrolyte solution to moisten to a consistency that is from runny oatmeal to chunky peanut butter. The solid foods offered first are usually grape, papaya, banana, or soaked parrot pellets (see Table 28.1).

For Great Blue Turacos, the Houston Zoo includes additional vegetable or fruit baby food in the above gruel and increases the amount of greens in the mixture. For gray species, Mazuri Leaf-eater Primate Pellets and Mazuri Parrot Pellets are included. Chicks may seem insatiable, and no problems have been seen with allowing them to eat larger amounts than other turaco species. These diets are constantly under revision, because the ideal diets for these species have not as yet been

Table 28.1 Turaco feeding schedule.

| Age (days) | Meal Size (ml) | Frequency (min) |
|---|---|---|
| 2 | 0.3–0.5 | 30 |
| 3 | 0.6–0.8 | 30–60 |
| 4 | 1.0–1.2 | 60 |
| 5–6 | 1.3–2.5 with pieces of fruit, such as pear, papaya, melon, apple, and soaked pellets | 75 |

Table 28.2 Alternate turaco diet feeding schedule.

| Age (Days) | Diet |
|---|---|
| 0–10 | Gruel mixture: fed with plastic pipette or spoon |
| 10–18 | Whole pieces of fruit and parrot pellets mixed in with gruel, offered from forceps; gradually reduce gruel |
| 18–20 | Whole foods offered from spoon or forceps |
| 22–25 | Adult turaco diet – tray left with chicks |

developed. Many Great Blue and gray chicks require medication for gastrointestinal upset at some point during growth. Consult an avian veterinarian for medication information.

## Feeding Procedures

Turacos tend to be easy to hand-feed (Figure 28.1). They readily gape at the feeder, although older chicks that have been recently pulled from the nest take longer to adjust. Like mousebirds, they do not have a crop but have an expandable esophagus, so a swelling on the right side of the neck is normal when feeding.

Care must be taken not to overfeed to avoid aspiration. Most chicks will stop gaping when they are full, but some will continue to beg even when food can be visualized in the throat. It is best to feed slowly, allowing time for the chick to swallow, and not fill the esophagus to the point where food can be seen. Place the syringe on the right side of the beak while feeding to lessen the chance of aspiration. Start with a 1 ml syringe with a regular tip, and use larger syringe sizes as the chick requires more food. Some individuals will get frantic at feeding time, and the head may need to be gently corralled and held steady.

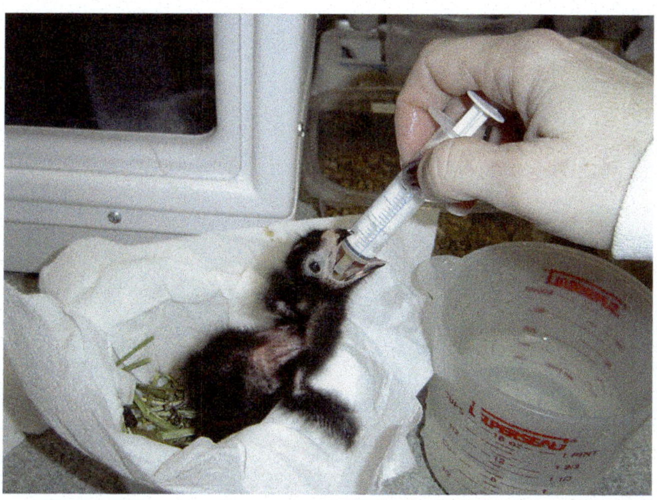

Figure 28.1 A turaco chick eagerly stands and balances with its wings as it is fed.

Wipe the beak and any other soiled areas of the body with a warm moist swab after each feeding to reduce the chance of infection from spoiled food. Do not allow spilled food to dry on developing feathers or get into the bird's eyes.

Some turaco species, such as Lady Ross (*Musophaga rossae*), have very prominent claws on their wrist joints resembling the Hoatzin (*Opisthocomus hoazin*). These claws disappear as the chick gets older. Also, Lady Ross and several other turaco species will use their wings like arms to bring their body forward and push themselves upright while begging.

## Expected Weight Gain

Turaco chicks grow quickly. Chicks should be weighed daily before the first feeding so that weight trends can be tracked. A 5–14% increase in weight daily, depending on species, is typical, although there can be some normal fluctuation. After day 18 or weaning, turaco chicks do not gain as much daily weight. A lack of weight gain or weight loss could mean problems, especially if it is consistent for 2 or more days. Consult your avian veterinarian if a chick becomes ill or is not progressing.

Different species of adult turacos and their chicks vary in size and weight slightly. The average hatchling weight of the green turaco species is 18–20g.

## Housing

After about 12hours in the incubator, a hatchling can be moved to a brooder (Figure 28.2). The brooder can be a professional one or as simple as a clear plastic critter container with an adjustable heat and humidity source. Place the chick in a small bowl with a substrate that can be gripped easily and will not move aside as the chick wiggles. Keep the chick and its area clean of feces and uneaten food. A clean tissue or lightweight cloth can be draped over the bowl to simulate being brooded by a parent. As the chick grows, it will become more active, and the bowl may need to be

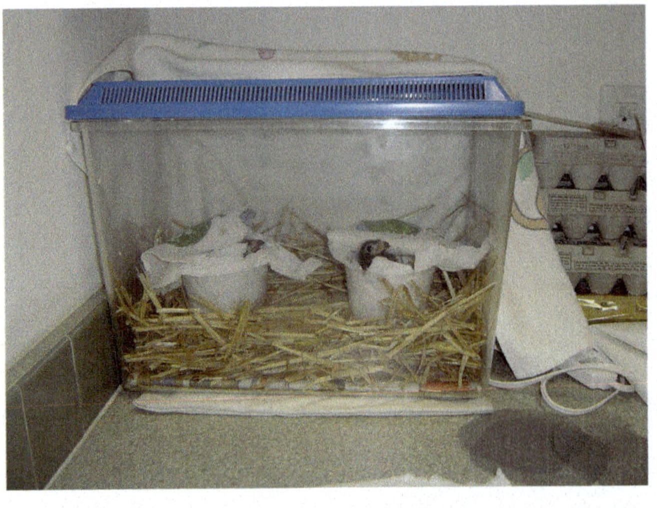

Figure 28.2 Simple brooder setup with a plastic tank with ventilated top, heating pad underneath, a towel over the top to adjust the interior temperature, straw bedding to protect the chicks from overheating and from splay-leg if or when they jump out of their cups.

larger so as not to tip when the chick begs. Around day 11–14, the chick will jump out of the bowl and start moving around the brooder.

Brooder temperature at day 1 should be at 96 °F (35.5 °C), and it should be lowered gradually, about a degree a day. Although not as crucial as temperature, humidity can be kept at 50–60% and can be gradually lowered to room humidity in the same way as the chick grows. By day 16–18, the chick can be moved to a cage without supplemental heat unless the room is colder than an average room temperature of 74–80 °F (23–27 °C). The cage should be supplied with heavy perches on which the chick can run and bounce off. It is normal for turacos to suddenly have periods of intense excitement where the chick will be very active, flapping, and running. Flight will occur at approximately 1 month of age.

## Weaning

Turaco chicks start to wean at day 18 and generally are completely weaned by day 30 or earlier (Figure 28.3). Shallow bowls of adult food and water should be offered at day 18, and the chicks usually investigate and wean themselves. Some weight fluctuations normally occur at this time. The chicks will also start to bathe in their drinking water so frequent changes may be needed. Young green turacos' plumage is dull, and it takes several months to acquire the adult sheen and color (Figure 28.4).

## Introduction to Captive Flock

Young turacos, even of mixed species, can be housed together safely for a while if they are all similar ages. Mature turacos tend to be aggressive toward each other, and it is recommended that they be housed separately or in bonded pairs. Species should be kept separately. Mate aggression and fatalities in all species are common, even after years of being together, and it can happen quickly

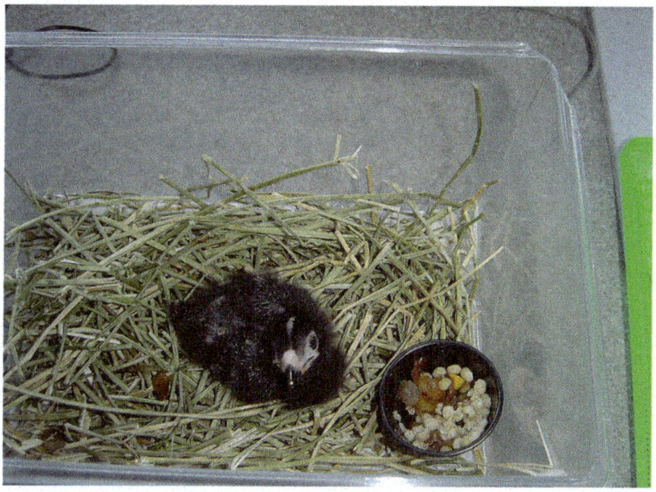

Figure 28.3 Turacos are so eager to feed that hand-raised turacos can often be weaned before they are even fully feathered, as in this chick.

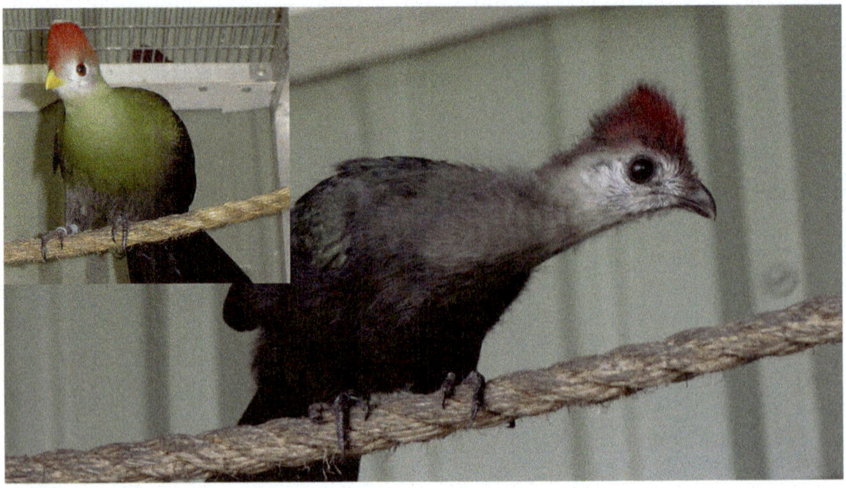

Figure 28.4 Juvenile Red Crest Turaco (*Tauraco erythrolophus*) halfway to adult plumage.

with little or no warning. Hiding places on the ground, such as appropriately sized hollow pipes, should always be available in turaco enclosures. Use of the "howdy cage" technique described in Chapter 35 is recommended when introducing turacos to one another.

Turacos of all ages are generally safe to house with other birds, even small finches, although they may start chasing other birds when in breeding condition. Turacos have very individual temperaments so there are many exceptions, but generally the green species, such as White Cheek Turacos, are more aggressive to mates and to other avian species in community aviaries.

## Behavioral Training for Pet Turacos

Turacos are not birds recommended as house pets for several reasons, but mainly because they require large amounts of space, are strong flyers and jumpers, and are very active. Most people who want a pet turaco tend to think that turacos can be treated as parrot-type pets, which is not the case. With very rare exceptions, turacos cannot be trained to stay out on shoulders, perches, or cage tops like most parrots. Although young turacos can be stroked and petted, adult turacos are not cuddly at all and do not like being touched, no matter how socialized to it when young. They will only endure, or usually avoid, physical touching interactions with their keepers. Tame turacos will interact with people by approaching the person, tugging at clothing, landing on heads, and eating out of hands.

However, tame birds, even in large aviaries, can be quite endearing because they will interact with people even after they mature. But beware, tame birds, especially when in breeding condition, have absolutely no fear of people and can be dangerously aggressive, pecking at and jumping on faces and heads.

Typically, turacos cannot be trained out of this behavior, so it is generally best to modify the keeper's behavior by learning to read the bird's mood and when necessary avoid direct eye contact (which is considered a challenge), keep interaction to a minimum, and wear protective headgear and glasses. Turacos will usually warn the person of these moods by approaching and displaying with open wings, head bowed, and loud calling or growling. Novice turaco owners and observers tend to be thrilled at this interaction by the bird and may feel inclined to display back by mimicking the bird's calls and actions. This just increases the bird's excitement and makes it more prone to attack.

## Author's Note

The author has written the only book strictly about turacos in aviculture appropriately called *Turacos in Aviculture* and published in 2012 by Birdhouse Publications. All species and subspecies are examined, with details of their life in the wild and aviculture. Extensive information about diet, care, parent-raising, and hand-rearing turacos is covered, including a chapter on hybridizing. A wealth of turaco information has been published in various magazines and journals. A great resource is The International Turaco Society, founded in Great Britain in the early 1990s.

The author owns Davis Lund Aviaries, which specializes in softbilled birds, and more pictures and information about turacos and other softbill birds can be found on the author's website, https://dlaviaries.wordpress.com. She would like to make contact with other people that are working with turacos and can be reached at 541–895–5149 or DLAviaries@ http://aol.com.

## Acknowledgments

I would like to thank all the softbill aviculturists, past and present, who have so generously shared their experiences throughout the years. Many thanks to Hannah Bailey from Houston Zoo for sharing turaco protocols and diets. Thanks also to Pat Witman for assistance with diet information.

## Sources for Products Mentioned

Kaytee Exact Hand Feeding Formula and Mynah Diet: Kaytee Products, Inc., 521 Clay St, P.O. Box 230, Chilton, WI 53014, (800) KAYTEE-1, https://www.kaytee.com.

Mazuri bird diets: Mazuri Products, PMI Nutrition International, (800) 227–8941, www.mazuri.com.

Gerber human baby food: Gerber Products Company, 445 Sate St, Fremont, MI, 49413–0001, (800) 4-GERBER.

## Further Reading

Davis, K. (2012). Turacos in Aviculture, 246 pp. Creswell, OR.: Birdhouse Publications.

Milne, L. (1994). Touracos. *AFA Watchbird* 21 (6): 40–43.

Peat, L. (2000). Touracos galore. *International Turaco Society Magazine* 13: 8–14.

Plasse, R. and Todd, W. (1994). Turaco husbandry at the Houston zoo. *AFA Watchbird* 21 (6): 34–39.

Todd, W. (1998). Turaco TAG Husbandry Manual, 30 pp. Houston.: Houston Zoological Gardens.

Vince, M. (1996). Softbills, Care, Breeding and Conservation, 278 pp. Blaine, Washington: Hancock House Publishers Ltd.

# 29

# Yellow-billed Cuckoos

*Maureen Eiger*

## Natural History

Yellow-billed Cuckoos (YBCUs) (*Coccyzus americanus*) are not often seen in the wild since they are fairly cryptic in the leaves of trees. Unless spotted flying from tree to tree, they are more often heard calling, especially when it is humid outside or about to rain. Their nickname is "rain crow" by some birders. Yellow-billed Cuckoos are something of an enigma because they are quite secretive. Reports written by various well-known observers when compared to each other have conflicting information or missing information on their breeding behavior and how their young develop. More research, record keeping, and observations are needed to clarify the conflicting observations about the YBCUs life cycle, breeding habits, and the effect that loss of habitat and man-made disturbances have on their survival.

Western YBCUs are generally listed as a species in steep decline, and the birds are listed as endangered or near threatened on several U.S. state bird lists. In October 2014, YBCUs were listed by U.S. Fish and Wildlife Service as "threatened," though this designation seems to have a lot of controversy behind it. According to the American Bird Conservancy (2019), this species has been reduced to fewer than 500 breeding pairs and is largely absent from most of its historical range.

Adult YBCU are slender-bodied and long-tailed birds about 12 in. (30.5 cm) long, with grayish brown contour feathers on their head, nape, back, and top surface of the tail and white feathers on their cheeks, throat, and belly. Adults weigh 50–65 g, and have short blueish-gray legs with zygodactyl toes. Their bills are slightly downward-curved toward the tip and the lower mandible is yellow-colored when mature. Rufous wing coloring is evident as soon as their chicks grow feathers. The birds also have large oval white spots against black on the undersurface of its grayish brown tail feathers.

Fledgling YBCUs look like miniature adult birds but with shorter beaks and tails. They have very fluffy (not sleek) feathers. It's easiest to identify a young YBCU when it opens its mouth. The bird has a black-tipped tongue and white bumps on the roof of its pinkish mouth. The "white bumps" are often mistaken for a fungus/yeast infection but are normal for the bird and may aid in swallowing spiny caterpillars or help lock onto the adult's beak when being fed. The easiest way to tell the difference between a young YBCU fledgling vs a Black-billed Cuckoo of similar age is by the rufous coloring on the YBCUs wings.

*Hand-Rearing Birds*, Second Edition. Edited by Rebecca S. Duerr and Laurie J. Gage.

## Cuckoo Breeding Habits

There are Old World and New World cuckoos. Many Old World cuckoos are considered to be true brood parasites. New World cuckoos, especially those breeding in North America, are not considered to be true brood parasites since they build their own nests and will raise their own young, at least most of the time. They are themselves occasionally parasitized by Brown-headed or Bronze-headed Cowbirds and Black-billed Cuckoos (Hughes 2015). The YBCUs breeding behavior seems to be modified by the abundance of food. They do not start breeding behavior unless there is an adequate food supply available, so the exact month in which they start breeding may vary. In years when food is very plentiful, the female YBCU may dump some of her "extra" eggs in another cuckoo's nest after her nest is completed or sometimes in the nest of another species of bird. Apparently, this only occurs if there an ample food supply readily available, which seems to stimulate extra egg production in the female.

Both female and male YBCUs participate in nest building, incubation, and feeding of their young. The nests are a rather flimsy open oblong cup design, loosely made from twigs, rootlets, dried leaves, and pine needles. Eggs are sometimes laid before the nest is completely finished, in which case the male continues to bring in nesting material to the female to finish the nest. One egg is laid per day and clutches usually contain two to four eggs.

There are conflicting reports whether YBCUs have only one brood or two broods per year, and where and how high the nest is placed. Some studies say nests are placed as low at 2 ft. off the ground or placed up to 20 ft. high or even higher at 90 ft. off the ground. Reports of such varied nest height placement may be due to habitat location or loss since they have nested across the U.S. in various habitats.

YBCU chicks mature very quickly. Incubation starts with the first egg laid, so the birds may hatch on different days. Hatch weight varies from 8.5–10 g. The naked birds can hold their heads up to be fed almost right after hatching and can open their eyes and stand usually the next day. Although born naked, they start to develop feather sheaths within 24 hours which will quickly grow long and burst into to fluffy feathers (all at once) in about 6–7 days. They quickly learn to perch on the edge of the nest, and between day 7 and 9 become "branchers" that can run along a limb to greet a parent for food and do not return to the nest. It will take about 3 weeks after hatching before the young birds can truly fly and be independent (Preble 1957; Potter 1980).

Nesting cuckoos are very sensitive to disturbances, especially during pairing or nest building. If an active nest has too many disturbances, reports of nest abandonment are common. Nothing is known on whether cuckoo chicks can be "re-nested" and the author would advise against trying. Other cuckoo chicks may be put at risk of abandonment by human presence while trying to find the nest or placing a bird back in the general area. Fledgling YBCUs move away from their nest location, so returning a "healthy fledgling" to the same location where it was found is probably not a good idea since they are not self-feeding and are dependent on their parents for food for several weeks after leaving the nest. The adults may have left the area with their other fast-growing fledges. It is not known if they are "good" parents and return to feed chicks that may be left behind, like some species do.

## Wild Diet

YBCUs feed heavily on caterpillars, including hairy caterpillars. They are known to eat insects, especially katydids, cicadas, dragonflies, moths, flies, beetles, grasshoppers, ants, and other bugs. YBCUs also have been seen eating small lizards, frogs, raspberries, mulberries, grapes and other berries, small fruits, and the eggs of other birds.

## Record Keeping

Because they are a species in great decline, it is very important to get as much information from the finder as to where the bird was found and the circumstances of why the bird was brought in for care. Knowing the exact location where the bird was found may help biologists learn more about these secretive birds and where they nest. You may want to check to see if any YBCU studies are being done in your state and contact the biologists regarding your young bird.

Weighing cuckoos daily is important. Young cuckoos have some peculiar eating habits so weighing the bird daily at the same time of day will help you to know that the bird is progressing well, eating enough food, and does not have an underlying medical problem. Keeping detailed progress notes on the birds' care may help improve future care and knowledge about these secretive birds.

## Initial Care and Stabilization

Upon intake, make sure the bird is gradually warmed up and hydrated. To hydrate the chick once it is warm, dribble tiny drops of warm fluid at the tip of bill and watch the bird swallow. If a bird is still in the stringy pinfeather stage and its skin visible, it definitely needs to be kept warm (Figure 29.1). If it comes in after the stringy pinfeather stage and has a fluffy-feathered look, feel the bird to check to see if it is chilled. The chick should always be warmer than a warm human hand. Remember, most birds will look fully feathered but may only be a few days old. If they have a very short tail less than ½ in. (1 cm) long, they may enjoy still being kept on low heat. With proper feeding, additional adult contour feathers will quickly fill in over more of their body and face as they get older. If they are active and perching on the side of the nest cup, they no longer need low heat.

When warmed and hydrated, a complete bird exam should be gently given (see Chapter 1). In most cases the bird was probably a "cute lost baby bird" that fell and was picked up by a person, or pilfered from a branch or nest by another bird or predator and escaped. Consequently, it should be carefully checked over for bruising and puncture wounds. Note that if a young bird is not thriving,

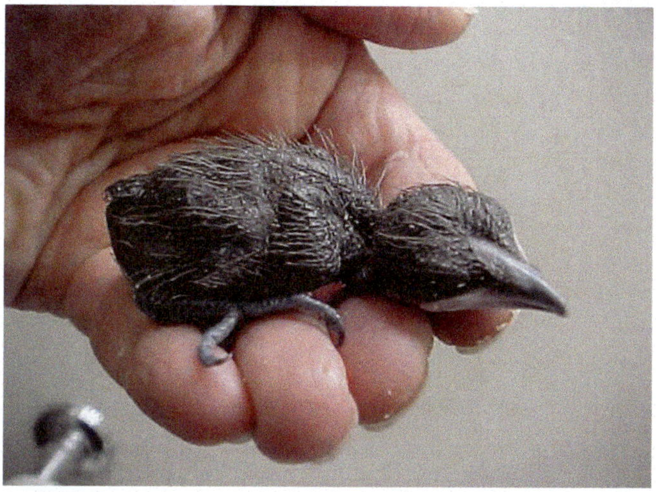

Figure 29.1 Yellow-billed Cuckoo (YBCU) hatchling.

a YBCUs parents will abandon them. Check for lack of plumpness on the bird's breast and any signs of starvation, like greenish tinged urates and no or scant stool.

## Diets and Feeding

When the chick is warm, has been hydrated, and has passed droppings, slowly introduce pulverized insects mixed with enough fluid to make an insect slurry. Another option is to slowly give about 1 cc of diluted Emeraid® IC Carnivore (Lafeber Company) with the insect slurry. YBCUs are used to being fed only insects; consequently, very wet fluids are hard for them to understand how to swallow. Be careful to not aspirate the bird with too much liquid food at once. The bird should be fed an insect diet as soon as it begins producing normal-looking droppings.

Sometimes lack of food or a high-stress situation will cause the bird to start to shut down and become stoic. If the bird does not willingly open its mouth after being warmed up and hydrated, it may be necessary to force-feed the bird for a few feedings. Use squished waxworms and water-soaked live mealworms or pupae in a bolus. Usually young fledges do not take more than 24 hours to understand that their new caregiver is the source of food and they should open their mouths willingly. If a stoic bird that will not eat is received, provide a calm and noise-free environment when force-feeding. If the bird does not normalize after 24 hours, try placing it with a buddy, which can be a soft fake bird or maybe a nice American Robin chick of similar size. Also try playing YBCU bird calls. The chick should be willing to eat when offered food by 36 hours. Because of their extremely fast growth rate, it is not a good idea to have to force-feed a young cuckoo for days on end.

Keep in mind that these birds need to grow up really fast, so feed, feed, feed! Day old nestlings are fed slightly pulverized food (mostly caterpillars) by their parents only for the first day or two. Thereafter, they are fed whole prey items, mostly live or slightly stunned caterpillars and other fairly large insects. In rehabilitation their diet should be mixed gut-loaded insects. The preferred diet would be waxworms, mealworms, mealworm larvae, blue bottle fly larvae, black soldier fly larvae, grasshoppers (with legs removed), and as many natural bugs as can be gathered. Drown live mealworms in water, dab once or twice on a paper towel to eliminate excess water, and feed to make sure the bird is getting enough fluids. Watch the birds' droppings to make sure the birds are properly hydrated and well fed. Weigh the birds daily.

YBCUs rely on an all insect diet to grow, but because feeder insects have certain nutritional deficiencies, additional supplements must be used to make sure the birds are getting the proper nutrition. See Chapters 43 and 44 for information regarding supplements necessary for feeding all-insect diets. Commercial diets of use include Harrison's Recovery Formula (Harrison's Bird Foods) or Wombaroo Insectivore Rearing Mix (Wombaroo Food Products); either formula powder should be mixed up like a thick pudding and can be syringed or have several insects dipped into it and then fed to the young cuckoos at several feedings. Dip the insects into the mixture for needed supplementation and then feed. Make sure any formula "dips" do not spoil and are made fresh every day. Do not use mixed formula as a primary food source. Use mixed formulas only as a supplement (see Figure 41.4).

### Feeding Schedule

Young YBCUs have an odd feeding schedule; they can eat a lot in one sitting and then, depending on what they were fed, may not be hungry for a period of time. This is unlike most songbird chicks that seem to be hungry every 15, 20, or 30 minutes like clockwork. The cuckoo's hunger seems to

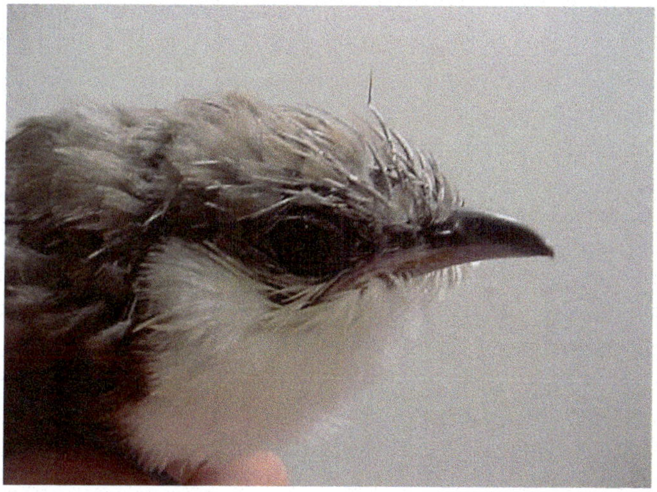

Figure 29.2 YBCU chick with unopened contour feather sheaths around its face, which is a sign of poor nutrition in chicks.

be related to what they were fed and how long it takes them to digest that food. Each cuckoo is different and needs its hunger/feeding rhythm worked out. Average weight gain should be about 2–3 g per day after their feathers burst open. One sign that a bird went through a period of not getting enough food is that stress bars will develop on their tail feathers. Also, lots of unopened pinfeathers may also start showing up, especially near the bird's face (Figure 29.2). These extra scrawny pinfeathers develop and do not open, but rather seem stuck. Ample food and consistent weight gain in a well-nourished chick help prevent this.

Sometimes the birds will get a bit picky as to what they want to eat; be aware they may be still hungry and want to eat, but might need a mealworm switched out for a waxworm or a small berry.

As the birds get older, with tails will be about 1.5–2 in. (3–5 cm) long, they should be presented with food in dishes. They may start picking at the food and eating some on their own, but will still need to be hand-fed as well. In the wild, the birds rely on their parents for food for many weeks after they have left the nest. Some observers say at least 2–3 weeks, others have reported birds still being fed by their parents up to 4 weeks after leaving the nest. In the author's experience, when the cuckoos' tails are nearly full grown, at about 4–5 in. (10–13 cm) long, then they completely stop accepting hand-fed food. Until then, count on a bird coming over to you for a hand out; make sure to continue to feed them.

Weigh chicks regularly even after they are fully self-feeding to ensure they are getting enough to eat. Premature weaning can lead to problems. If the initial flight feathers are of poor quality, they can molt bad tail or wing feathers in the fall, but be aware of migration dates in the area to ensure the bird will not miss migration.

## Housing

Young chicks may be housed in a knitted nest lined with often-changed tissue in a warm environment until perching, then can be housed in larger enclosures with appropriate size perches. Be aware that as their tails get longer, they can easily break or fray, so perch placement is very important. Place food and water cups where the birds can reach them from a perch so they do not have to go down to the ground for food (Figure 29.3). Use almost any kind of enclosure to house them as long as there are ample places for perches. Plastic bird carriers (making sure the birds can't get their bodies stuck between the bars) or large parrot cages with ½ or ¾ in. bar spacing are usually sufficient. Proper perch and food cup placement will keep them from damaging their tails between any vertical cage bars.

A light misting with water daily is recommended to encourage preening. Move birds to an outdoor aviary as soon as possible, but remember the bird may still need to be hand-fed. The aviary should have a good view of the stars at night and be open to the elements. Miller (2012) recommends a flight aviary of 16×8×8 ft. (4.9×2.4×2.4 m) for cuckoos >12 in. (30 cm) long. Natural leaves still on natural branches should be provided as the bird will spend many days under them after it is released.

YBCUs can be ornery birds as they get older and merit monitoring to make sure they get along with each other. Check frequently that none is picking on other birds or being picked on by cage mates.

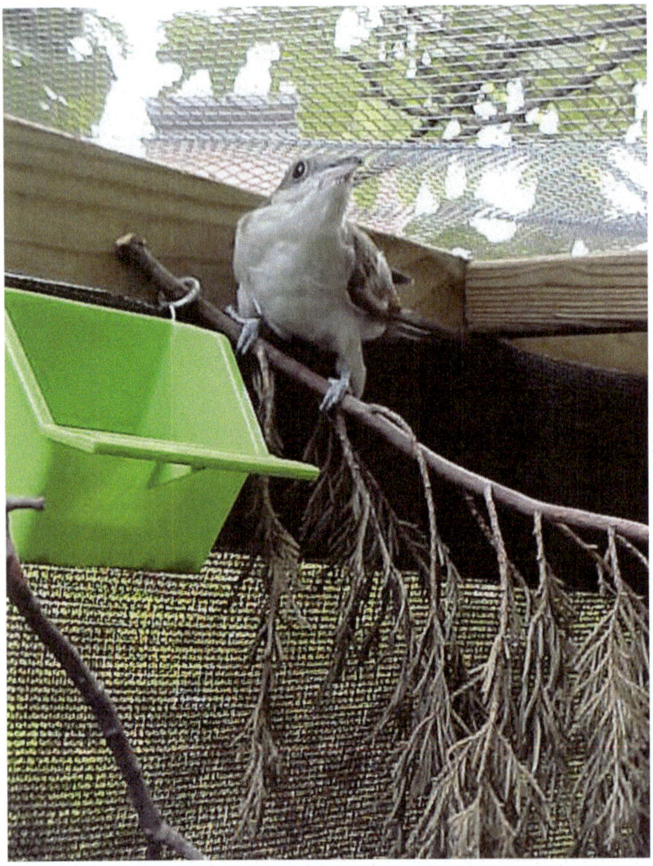

Figure 29.3 YBCU in an aviary with food dishes oriented such that the bird can eat from the perch. Note that feathers extend far down the legs.

### Foraging Ideas for the Aviary

Find webworms to put in the outdoor aviary for foraging and feeding the birds. Roll up mealworms in the mealworm bag and clip to a branch for the birds to eat them as they wiggle their way out (Figure 29.4). Add just-hatched mealworm beetles or live crickets to the diet and anything else that moves or can climb up a screen. Fruit/berries can be poked on branches or sprigs of berries attached to bigger branches. Add food cups attached to branches in various locations in the aviary to encourage flying as they get older.

## Release Criteria

YBCUs are long-distance migrants. Not much is known about their migration route other than it is thought that some birds go through Mexico and then further south, while eastern birds probably cross over the Gulf of Mexico, or island hop to Central America. Check eBird or other online birding sites for last migration dates for the area and to see if (or where) any YBCUs have been recently sighted; good release sites may be found that way. Make sure each bird's body condition and feathers are in good shape for migration (Figure 29.5). No wing feathers should be frayed or not nicely zipped. Their chest muscles should be filled out and they should be able to take short flights in the aviary. Cuckoos do not get as "flighty" as other species do when they "want out," so just flying from one branch to another is a good sign. The bird should be able to pull fruits off of sticks/vines and catch grasshoppers or other live prey.

When sprayed, the bird should be water resistant and water should bead up on the bird's feathers. Hopefully it will have had a few days in the aviary when it rained so the bird has learned what rain is. If not, trying using a water mister or sprinkler to see how the bird fares.

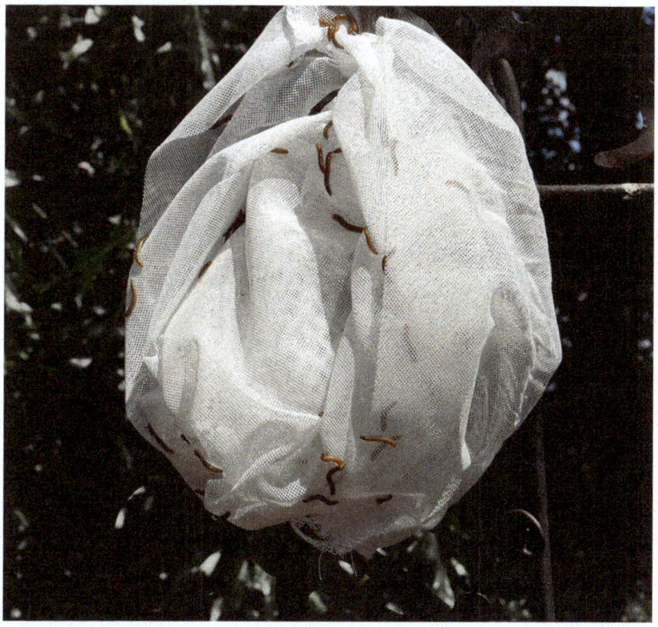

Figure 29.4 Mealworms escaping from a cloth bag to provide foraging opportunities in the aviary.

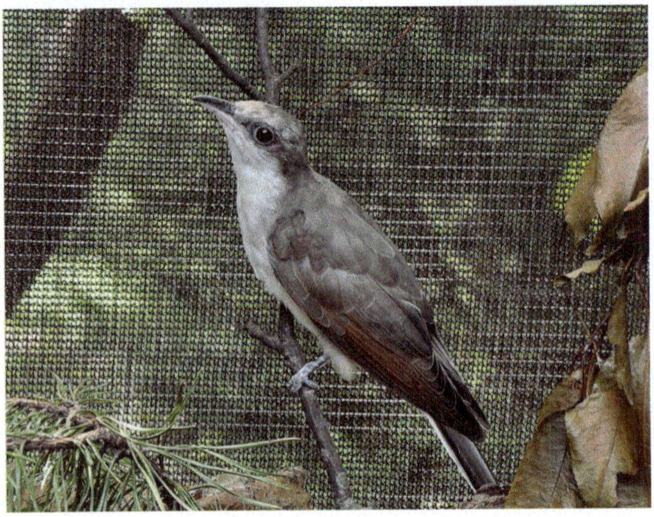

Figure 29.5 Fledgling in pre-release aviary basking in the sun, note the beautiful feathering.

Check the forecast for the timing of release, which should show at least 3 days of good weather and no future storms coming. Release in an area where there are still fruits and insects available for the bird to be able to find food. Usually that means someplace somewhat close to water.

Remember that a lot of time and effort went into getting the chick to the point of being able to be released; hence, make sure its release area will also provide what it needs.

## Conclusions

Because there is little information on the life habits of these species, there is conflicting and probable misinformation about YBCUs. But, from experience hand-rearing their chicks, we know that YBCUs need to eat a lot and need a variety of insects to thrive. They have odd feeding habits and need to be hand-fed much longer than most similar birds. Their tails can get damaged very easily if perches and food cups are not placed properly, or if they are malnourished. They don't always get along with other birds. They are declining species. We should do our best to try and keep YBCUs from becoming extinct, so when in doubt or having problems, ask for advice from another rehabilitator who has successfully raised cuckoos. When you have set one free, you may have helped save their species.

## Acknowledgments

Many thanks to Janine Perlman for always answering my nerdy questions about bird stuff, Jean Chamberlain for her unbiased input and for exchanging ideas, Jodi Swenson for her laughter and knowledge when I get stuck, and Suzie Gilbert for connecting me to other great rehabilitators on Facebook.

## Sources of Products Mentioned

Emeraid IC Carnivore: Lafeber Company, Cornell, IL 61319, (800) 842-6445, http://www.lafeber.com.

Harrisons Recovery Formula: Harrison's Bird Foods, 7108 Crossroads Blvd. Suite 325, Brentwood, TN 37027, (800) 346-0269, http://www.harrisonsbirdfoods.com.

Wombaroo Insectivore Rearing Mix Wombaroo Food Products, PO Box 151, Glen Osmond, South Australia 5064, www.wombaroo.com.au.

## References

American Bird Conservancy. (2019). Yellow-billed cuckoos. https://abcbirds.org/bird/yellow-billed-cuckoo (accessed 21 January 2019).

Hughes, J.M. (2015). Yellow-billed cuckoo (*Coccyzus americanus*), version 2.0. In: *The Birds of North America* (eds. A.F. Poole and F.B. Gill). Ithaca, NY, USA: Cornell Lab of Ornithology https://doi.org/10.2173/bna.418.

Miller, E.A. (ed.) (2012). *Minimum Standards for Wildlife Rehabilitation*, 4e. St. Cloud, MN: National Wildlife Rehabilitation Association.

Potter, E.F. (1980). Notes on nesting yellow-billed cuckoos. *Journal of Field Ornithology* 51 (1): 17–29.

Preble, N.A. (1957). Nesting habits of the yellow-billed cuckoo. *The American Midland Naturalist* 57 (2): 474–482.

# 30

# Roadrunners

*Elizabeth Penn (Penny) Elliston*

## Natural History

*Geococcyx californianus,* the Greater Roadrunner, is also known by many local names such as Chaparral Cock, Snake Killer, Lizard Bird, Churca, Paisano, and Correcamino. The only American cuckoo to take up permanent residence north of approximately 26° N latitude, this bird inhabits the arid environment of the American Southwest and north central Mexico. These cuckoos start nesting early and frequently choose thick evergreens or stationary farm equipment as a nesting site. They may have as many as three broods in a season. Both male and female are exemplary parents, and pairs may produce broods of up to six young in a clutch (Ohmart 1973). Parents start incubating as soon as the first egg is laid, for an incubation period of 17–20 days. Consequently, there may be a great variation in the age and development of chicks in a nest. Chicks may leave the nest at about 2 weeks of age, but are under the supervision of their parents for another 30–40 days (Whitson 1976) as they refine their foraging skills.

Upper parts of the adult bird are streaked brown and white with some iridescent shades of green, blue-black, and purple on the wing. Tail feathers have white "thumbprint" markings on the tips typical of cuckoos. The blue/black erectile crest on the head may be raised and lowered in displays, which may also expose brightly colored apteria, which are unfeathered post-orbital spaces colored bright blue close to the eye, fading and blending to bright orange distal to the eye. The eye, shaded by prominent protective lashes, has a pale yellow or gray to reddish-orange iris. The black decurved bill is about 5 cm in length. Legs are long and bluish terminating in a zygodactyl toe arrangement with toes number 2 and 3 pointing forward and 1 and 4 pointing backward. Normal adult body temperature has been reported by Calder (1968) as 104 °F (40 °C) and confirmed by the author. Adult weights range from 221 to 538 g (Dunning 1984).

Roadrunners are obligate faunivores. They hunt and eat any kind of small prey such as mice, lizards, snakes, small birds, insects, and snails. They may pick up and eat a variety of nonanimal material (chili peppers), which is usually cast out when the indigestible material builds up in the muscular stomach. Prey is prepared for swallowing whole by whacking it on a nearby rock or other hard surface.

*Hand-Rearing Birds*, Second Edition. Edited by Rebecca S. Duerr and Laurie J. Gage.

## Criteria for Intervention

Roadrunners may be brought into captivity as eggs from nests displaced from machinery, as hatchlings from similarly displaced nests, as fledglings that have been kidnapped or caught by dogs or cats, or as adults that have met with some accident. Roadrunners are very dedicated parents and seemingly uninjured fledglings should have a physical exam to rule out both subtle and obvious injuries. If the results are satisfactory, they should be reunited with their parents.

## Record Keeping

See Chapter 1 for record keeping suggestions.

## Initial Care and Stabilization

The main rule of initial baby bird care is to provide warmth, rehydration, and feeding, in that order. Warm chicks before giving fluids, and then hydrate them until they start passing droppings. Only then is it safe to commence feedings. Feeding a cold or dehydrated baby bird before it is warm and hydrated will probably kill it.

New patients should be allowed to rest for 15–20 minutes in a warm, dark, quiet container before examination. If the bird is not able to stand, it should be placed in a soft support structure such as a rolled cloth donut or paper nest. Do not allow the bird to lie on its side or other abnormal positions. Hatchlings and nestlings should be placed in a climate-controlled incubator if available. When the animal is warm and calm, it may be hydrated orally and/or subcutaneously (SQ). Warm sterile fluids such as 2.5% dextrose in 0.45% sodium chloride or lactated Ringer's solution may be administered SQ at 5% of body weight (50 ml/kg) once, although repeated administrations may be needed for extremely dehydrated birds. Gaping, active hatchlings or nestlings should be orally hydrated until they produce droppings. Give a few drops of warm oral fluids every 15–20 minutes with a small syringe or eyedropper and allow the bird to swallow completely before giving more. Once the amount the chick is able to swallow is understood, the amount may be raised to 2.5–5% of body weight in several mouthfuls. Human infant electrolyte fluids (unflavored) are excellent for oral rehydration of baby birds. Ensure that the bird is warm before administering fluids, and that the bird is both warm and well-hydrated before receiving food. Start the bird on a hand-feeding formula after it begins passing droppings.

If the bird is depressed or not swallowing well, oral rehydration must be performed very carefully, because there is a greater risk of aspiration of fluids into the respiratory system. It may be better in this circumstance to wait for the animal to absorb SQ fluids, rather than giving oral fluids too quickly. If SQ fluids are not an option, give tiny amounts of oral fluids deep into the mouth and ensure that the bird swallows everything before giving more.

## Common Medical Problems and Solutions

Young roadrunners usually present with injuries from animal bites, or as orphans from loss of parents. Injured birds may require splints for broken bones. Dense styrofoam makes a very nice supportive but lightweight splint. See Duerr and Purdin (2017) for more information on the management of orthopedic injuries in wild birds. For lacerations, the author prefers covering with a bio-occlusive dressing such as Op-site (Smith and Nephew, Inc.) or Tegaderm™ (3M) to sutures or any other closure. In the author's experience, these dressings are well tolerated by most birds and do not require a decision about closure or drainage because the material acts as a substitute skin. These dressings also serve to keep feathers out of wounds. Some brands of this type of product absorb exudate as well.

Subcutaneous emphysema (air under the skin) may occur as the result of a cat attack. This usually resolves without treatment. If the bubble is interfering with mobility or compromising breathing, it may be necessary to remove the pressure by puncturing the bubble with a sterile needle, avoiding any visible skin blood vessels. If the internal puncture into an air sac has not closed, the bubble will re-inflate. A slightly elastic pressure bandage may help resolve the emphysema, but is often hard to apply and may be stressful to the bird. Consult your avian veterinarian for medical advice regarding antibiotic treatment for puncture wounds.

## Diet Recipes

Roadrunners are obligate faunivores and do well on diets that are fed to raptors. See Chapter 20 for diet information. However, unlike raptors, roadrunners typically do not cast (regurgitate) bones, fur, teeth, or chitinous insect exoskeletons. In adults, the entire ingested animal is reduced to a thick, tarry, malodorous fecal dropping. In the healthy nestling, droppings are very large and encapsulated in a gelatinous envelope.

These rapidly developing youngsters evolved in the desert, and they need the proper calcium-to-phosphorus ratio (2 : 1 by weight) with adequate vitamin $D_3$ and sun from the earliest age. Characteristic of all cuckoos, roadrunners typically do not pick up and eat dead food unless they have learned to do so. In training young roadrunners for release, they are given an advantage if they are trained to pick up almost anything that could be food, live or dead, and examine it.

## Feeding Procedures

Roadrunner hatchlings, after being well-hydrated so that they produce large gelatinous droppings, can be fed pieces of food as large as they can swallow. The food should be lifted from a soak of fluid (water or 0.9% saline) to provide plenty of fluid and prevent dehydration. Hatchlings have bright red gapes with a fringed pattern in the mouth that includes both white spots and a black tip to the tongue. They gape vigorously and make a whining, growling sound when begging. They should be fed whenever they beg in response to stimulus. If even the slightest wrinkle appears on the abdomen, they are becoming dehydrated. This condition should be immediately corrected by hydration with isotonic fluid.

The amount of food needed each day can be calculated with the formula $(BW_{kg})^{0.75} \times 78 \times 1.5 = 24$ hour maintenance requirement. A young bird needs 1.5–3 times maintenance for healthy growth. A good way to measure the amount fed is to weigh the day's planned food at the beginning of the day and at the end of the day after feeding has ceased. The difference is, of course, the weight of the food consumed. Each prey species will vary in caloric density, but the author's rule of thumb is to estimate faunivore prey items at 1 kcal/g.

Self-feeding roadrunners coming in to rehabilitation may have a difficult time learning to eat nonmoving food. It is often important to give them foods that they do not have to kill, so that they receive sufficient calories and variety during the healing period. Encouraging them to self-feed is important because force-feeding these birds, even only twice a day, is very stressful to them. Sometimes presenting the food with a puppet will help, sometimes dressing a piece of meat up with spare feathers or fur will be enough to let the roadrunner know that this is food. Once they learn that this unlikely looking stuff is food, they will often begin to self-feed easily.

As with raptors, roadrunners imprint when their eyes have opened and cleared. As this process is occurring, it is important to provide chicks with a conspecific imprint model. This may be a foster parent, a slightly older sibling that responds to begging, or a puppet made from a roadrunner skin (Elliston 1998) (Figure 30.1). Puppets may be used with feeding implements such as long hemostats or a syringe with a long rubber tube attachment for feeding liquid diets. Also see Chapter 15 for more ideas to avoid imprinting and habituation in susceptible species.

### Hatchlings

Hatchlings, between 13 and 18 g, should be weighed every morning, hydrated, and fed 5 times/12–14-hour day or whenever they gape. Allow the birds to get plenty of sleep between feeds and at night. The internal temperature of hatchling roadrunners is about 105 °F (40.6 °C) (author, unpubl. data). They should feel hot to the touch and look like little black balloons with sparse white down on their feather tracts (Figure 30.2). If a bird refuses food, re-evaluate the temperature, hydration status, and physical condition.

### Nestlings and Fledglings

Fully and partially feathered birds should be fed two to three times a day when they call or beg (Figure 30.3). Roadrunners stop begging when they are full. In nature, their parents probably start to feed them when the day becomes warm and cease when they go to roost about 1 hour before dark. They can be fed by a surrogate parent (foster sibling or adult) or blunt forceps and a puppet surrogate.

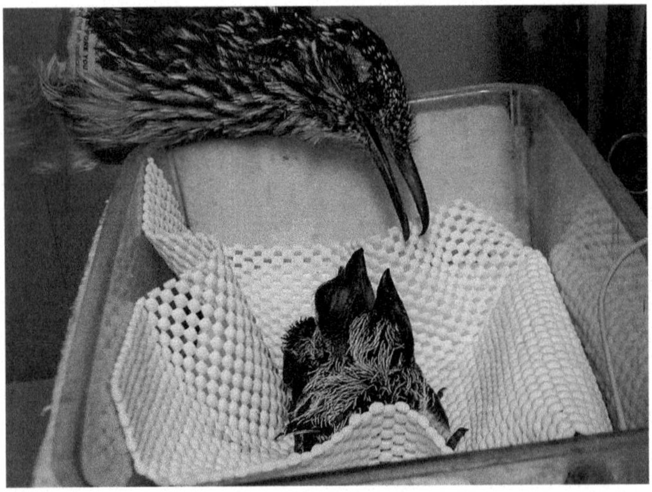

Figure 30.1 A puppet surrogate parent with very young chicks expectantly focusing on it for the next meal.

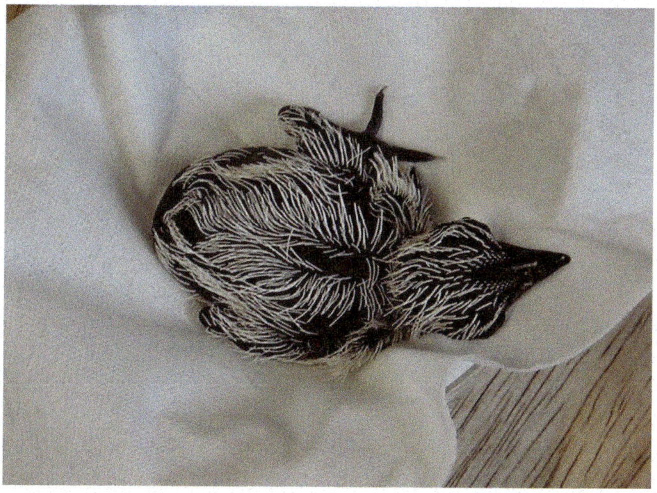

Figure 30.2 Hatchling roadrunner. Note the white down on black skin.

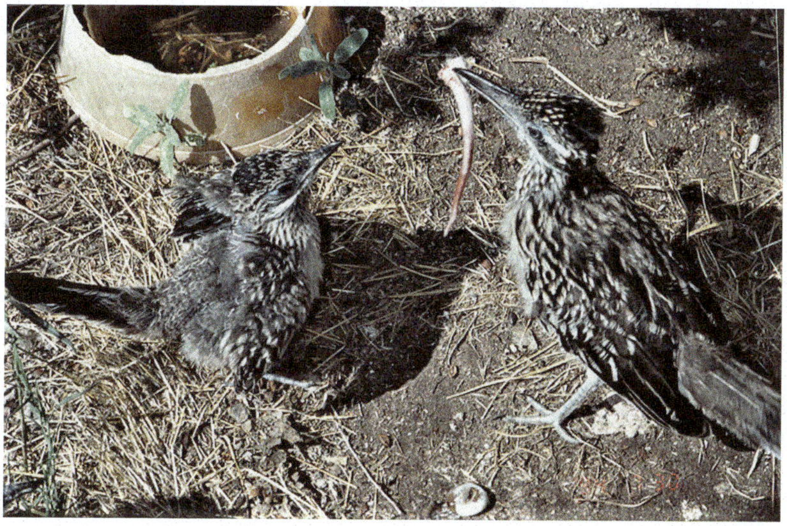

Figure 30.3 Two fledgling roadrunners in an aviary learning to pick up food.

## Expected Weight Gain

Unlike many other species, roadrunners do not gain their full adult weight before learning to forage. Their exact age may be determined by the length of the central rectrices, unless, of course, the bird has met with some mishap that has caused feathers to be lost or damaged (Figure 30.4).

## Housing

Hatchlings should be kept at around 99 °F (37 °C) and 40–50% humidity. A variety of materials may be used to create a replacement nest. A woven basket of the right dimensions makes a perfect

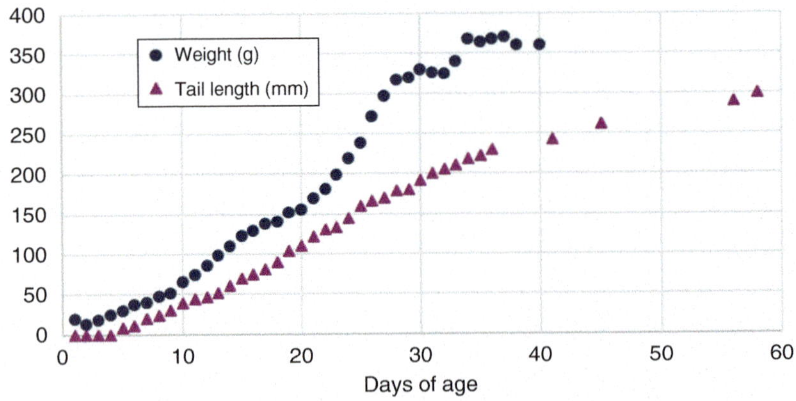


Figure 30.4 Mean weight and growth of central tail feathers in Greater Roadrunner chicks ($n$ = 10).

substitute nest for roadrunners. It can be lined with soft material when the birds are very young, and droppings can be removed with toilet paper. However, the sticks of the basket provide a perfect substrate for developing legs and feet. Young birds should sit in the nest with their legs folded underneath their heavy bodies. Legs allowed to splay may become deformed. A healthy nestling will deposit droppings over the rim of the nest, which makes maintaining cleanliness easy.

At 10–11 days, when they are fully feathered and beginning to move around, the nestlings can be placed outside where they can interact with their environment. The 16×8×8 ft. (4.9×2.4×2.4 m) enclosure for a maximum of six birds (Miller 2012) should contain plenty of room to sun- and dustbathe. Perches at various heights are important for exercise and night use. A pool of water is attractive, but not necessary for these desert birds. It is wise, however, to provide drinking water at all times.

As soon as the youngsters are able to manage their heavy bodies on their legs, they begin to exhibit typical roadrunner sunning behavior. Their bodies are extended, their wings spread, and their rumps exposed to the sun. In this way, since they don't need to generate their own heat, their daily caloric requirement for food may be reduced by 41–50% (Calder 1968; Ohmart 1971).

By 2 weeks of age, young birds pick up and play with objects but rarely swallow them. In the third and fourth weeks they begin to whack and eat their prey. At this time, they should be offered mealworms (*Tenebrio molitor*) and superworms (*Zoophorba moriom*) to stimulate foraging behavior. By the end of the fourth week, they may be picking up dead mice and whacking them, soon graduating to catching and killing live mice. Not surprisingly, birds raised by a conspecific surrogate (Figure 30.5) learn to hunt sooner than those raised by a puppet, and those that have had early experience opening snails are at an advantage after release. When they have left the nest, birds should be weighed less frequently than every day, to prevent too much habituation.

## Weaning

As soon as the birds begin jumping in and out of the nest and are old enough to begin exploring their environment, desert furnishings such as hunks of bark, cactus skeletons, and other similar objects should be provided. It is important to confine the live food of these animals so that it cannot escape, but it is equally important to stimulate foraging. Leaves and detritus, as well as game bird starter, chopped fruit, and potatoes, can be placed in large pans with Tenebrio or Zoophorba larvae,

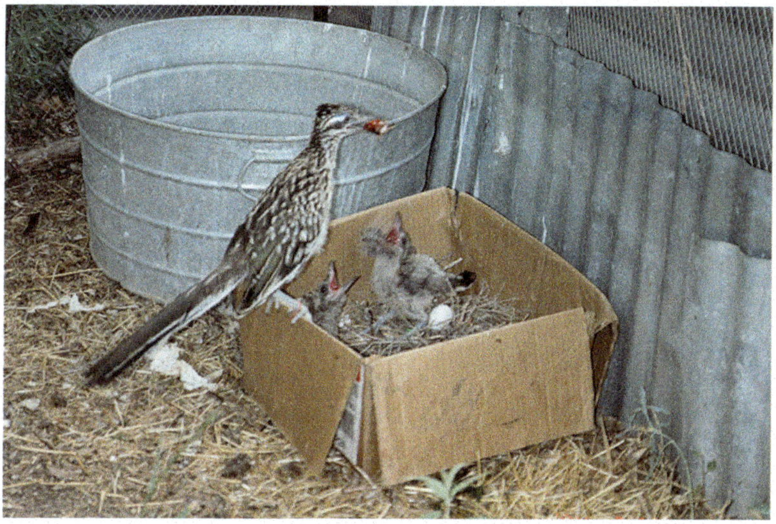

Figure 30.5 A fledgling roadrunner feeding younger chicks.

which may attract other "wild" insects into the hunting area. As the birds become competent killing large superworms, they can be introduced to live mice. It may be necessary to continue to feed some nonliving meat material (chicken neck pieces, ground turkey balls supplemented with calcium) to the youngsters because live prey is costly, and also to provide variety and good nutrition in the diet. However, learning to pick up and eat nonmoving food is clearly very advantageous to the young hunter in the wild because it allows the bird to scavenge while refining its hunting skills.

It is difficult to keep captive hand-reared roadrunners for long without having them become habituated to people. Making sure that they are exposed to only one caregiver helps keep them wild, as does only one or two approaches with food per day once the birds are weaned. If birds are heard calling, it may mean that they are not being provided with adequate foods stores in which to forage. If an individual ever appears lethargic or less active than usual, it should be removed and its condition assessed.

## Preparation for Wild Release

To avoid habituating young roadrunners to humans, restrict human contact to one person and only when food is being presented. It may be necessary to call other rehabilitation facilities to find conspecifics for placement of single orphans. Success at avoiding habituation should be seen by the time the birds are ready for release. They should be wary of humans rather than coming up to caretakers for food.

## Release

Roadrunners are not migratory and are quite territorial. It is important to release them at a time and in areas in which they can find plenty of prey and will not be harassed by domestic pets. In the season of plentiful range locusts and other prey, young birds are well tolerated by resident adults until natural dispersal occurs. Each chick should weigh at least 275 g on release and be exclusively foraging and sunning to fulfill its energy requirements. There should be no begging from the caregiver if food is present. A good way to catch up a young roadrunner for release is for the regular caregiver to approach them in the dark, pick them off their perch, and place them in a dark cardboard box. They can then be transported to the release site with as little stress as possible. The box should be opened on the ground and the birds allowed to exit at will.

## Acknowledgments

Thanks to Nancy Lee Olsen for sharing her extensive collection of literature and Janine Perlman for critical reading. Thanks to the Albuquerque office of the U.S. Fish and Wildlife Service and the New Mexico Department of Game and Fish (NMDGF) for permits and for bringing us displaced eggs and young of New Mexico's state bird. Thanks to the Share with Wildlife Program of the NMDGF for continued support of Wildlife Rescue Inc. of New Mexico (WRINM). Most of all, thanks to the supporters and members of WRINM who made the acquisition of this information possible through giving displaced nestling roadrunners their careful attention.

## Sources for Products Mentioned

Op-site Flexifix dressing: Smith & Nephew, Inc., 11775 Starkey Road, P.O. Box 1970, Largo, FL 33779-1970, (800) 876-1261, http://www.opsitepostop.com.

Tegaderm: 3M, 3M Center, St. Paul, MN 55144-1000, (800) 364-3577.

Invertebrate food supplier: Rainbow Mealworms, 126 E. Spruce St., Compton, CA 90220, (800) 777-9676, https://www. http://rainbowmealworms.net/home.asp.

Invertebrate food supplier: Fluker Farms, 1333 Plantation Ave., Port Allen, LA 70767-4087, (800) 735-8537, http://www.flukerfarms.com.

## References

Calder, W.A. (1968). There really is a roadrunner. *Natural History* 77 (4): 50–55.

Duerr, R.S. and Purdin, G.J. (eds.) (2017). *Topics in Wildlife Medicine, Vol. 4: Orthopedics*, 206 pp. St. Cloud, MN: National Wildlife Rehabilitators Association.

Dunning, J.B., Jr. (1984). Body weights of 686 species of North American Birds. *Western Bird Banding Association Monograph No. 1*. 39 pp.

Elliston, E.P. (1998). MOM—Made to Order Mother. International Wildlife Rehabilitation Council Conference Proceedings, p. 138.

Miller, E.A. (ed.) (2012). *Minimum Standards for Wildlife Rehabilitation*, 4e. St. Cloud, MN: National Wildlife Rehabilitation Association.

Ohmart, R.D. (1971). Roadrunners: energy conservation by hypothermia and absorption of sunlight. *Science* 172: 67–69.

Ohmart, R.D. (1973). Observations on the breeding adaptations of the roadrunner. *Condor* 75: 140–149.

Whitson, M.A. (1976). Courtship behavior of the greater roadrunner. *Living Bird* 14: 215–255.

# 31

# Owls

*Lisa (Elisa) Fosco*

## Natural History

Owls make up the order Strigiformes and are divided into two distinct families based on natural history as well as anatomical differences. Barn owl species make up the family Tytonidae, which includes about 14 species. The family Strigidae, also known as the "typical" owls, includes about 167 species worldwide and is further divided into two subfamilies: Striginae (long-eared and forest-adapted owls) and Buboninae (small-eared and visual hunting species.)

Owls are found on all continents except Antarctica. Most species are nocturnal and all are hunters that will scavenge only when necessary. They hunt by both sight and sound, and most species have feathers adapted for silent or noiseless flight. In general, owls are relatively sedentary, and typically only the smaller and more specialized species are migratory.

The reproductive period of owls tends to be prolonged compared to other raptor species. They have a long incubation period, and the pre-fledging period is also comparatively long. Cavity-nesting species usually remain securely hidden in their nest for most of their pre-fledging time where they are visually isolated from their surroundings. Unlike other owls, most of these species use no visual cues in any of their food-begging behaviors.

Tree-nesting species tend to grow and develop at a faster rate. They are more physically active and mobile, climbing up and around the nest as legs develop. This behavior often results in owlets of these species leaving the nest before they are flighted. Unlike most other avian and raptorial species, this is considered a natural or normal behavior and rarely impacts parental care. Also, unlike other raptors, juvenile owls of most species tend to remain with the parents for (comparably) longer periods of time after fledging while they are learning and refining their hunting skills.

## Criteria for Intervention

Whenever possible, healthy owlets should be returned to the nest site for familial recovery. Healthy owlets are well-fleshed, bright-eyed, and responsive to all stimuli. Feathered nestlings are usually accepted when placed safely off the ground in the vicinity of the nesting tree or structure. If the owlet repeatedly grounds itself, is in a structurally questionable nest, or is in an urban or visible location, protective measures may be helpful. Temporary barriers surrounding the tree base at a

*Hand-Rearing Birds*, Second Edition. Edited by Rebecca S. Duerr and Laurie J. Gage.

minimum distance of 8 ft. in radius may provide a protective barrier against domestic predators and human attention.

Unfortunately, owlets are commonly kidnapped due to their visibility on the ground and their proximity to people and domestic animals. Uninjured owlets should not be considered orphans unless the parent clearly and unquestionably rejects them. Captive-rearing of the highest standards still tends to have a permanent impact on their learned abilities and skills, as well as their general behavior. These factors are crucial for long-term survival.

Many species have been known to readily accept young that have been gone for several days and even extended periods. In 2001, the author rehabilitated a nestling Great Horned Owl with a fractured ulna for 22 days and then successfully reunited it with the family group where it fledged naturally.

Young owlets that are repeatedly forced from the nest, or those that have been actively ignored by parents, are often candidates for intervention. Those with large numbers of ectoparasites or those attracting flies are also candidates for rehabilitation, as this is a common indicator of parental absence.

If captive-rearing is the only option, owlets that are to be released into the wild should ***never*** be raised alone. Every effort should be made to house all sub-adult birds with conspecifics and ideally in view of the natural habitat. Regardless of the age or condition of the bird, human interaction and all contact with people or domestic pets should be minimized whenever possible.

## Record Keeping

All records should include detailed information on the location where the bird was found as well as the circumstances of the rescue. Regulating wildlife agencies should be consulted for specific requirements or for local, licensed wildlife rehabilitation options.

In addition to basic legal documentation, records should be kept on individual animals throughout their care. Birds should be weighed, aged as best as possible, and have a physical exam to identify or rule out any potential health concerns or injuries.

Proper development and general health status may be best assessed by closely monitoring and documenting body weight, feeding habits and behavior, digestive function, and feather condition, as compared to their wild counterparts. Physical development of most owl species has been observed, documented, and is accessible for reference with minimal research. This information is an essential resource when rearing any unfamiliar species. Special attention should be given to diet, nutritional needs, and feeding behaviors throughout development, because these factors impact bone growth and behavioral maturation.

## Initial Care and Stabilization

New patients that appear to be stable should be assessed for thermal needs and then should be left alone to settle down and de-stress. Covering the box or cage with a dark towel and moving it to a quiet room for a few minutes is often sufficient.

Once the animal is warm and calm, it should be weighed, rehydrated, and given an initial physical exam. Record its initial body weight in grams or in the smallest and most accurate unit available (Figure 31.1). Check the bird's keel and pectoral muscle to assess its overall state of health. The

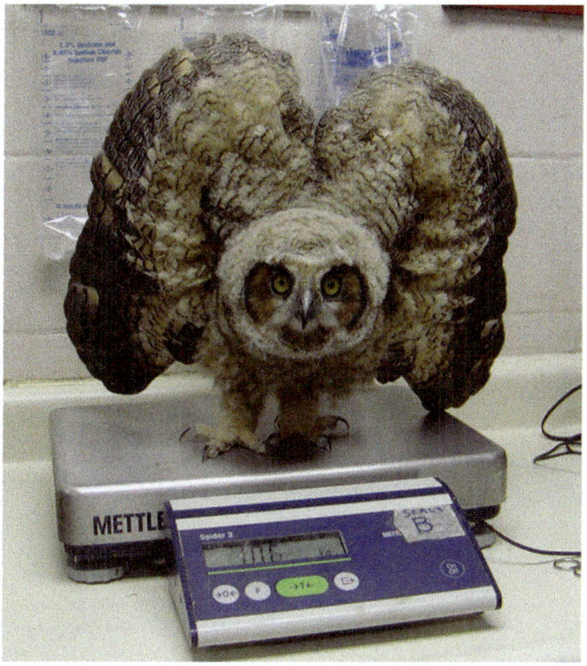


Figure 31.1 Great Horned Owl standing on scale.

keel should not be "sharp" or remarkably prominent in owlets of any age. It is normal for owls to have asymmetrically placed ears for sound localization of their prey. Severely malnourished or emaciated birds should be fed a few pieces of organ meat as soon as the bird is warm and hydrated. A little food goes a long way when stabilizing a weak or starving baby. For clinically emaciated birds, consult with experienced raptor rehabilitators for the best and most current nutritional recommendations for these critical animals. Birds in very poor body condition (BCS$\leq$2 on a 5-point scale) or those with a total protein less than 2.0 g/dl should be considered candidates for emaciation protocols. It is informative to collect a small amount of blood into microhematocrit tubes for a packed cell volume, total plasma protein, and a blood smear.

In general, owlets should be bright eyed and active before feeding and may sleep soundly after a satisfying meal. Weak, slow babies with dull eyes should be evaluated as quickly as possible. It should be noted that it is not uncommon for hatchling owls to have red, and sometimes swollen-looking eyelids (Figure 31.2). Hydration and adjustment of supplemental heat can often make a significant difference for weaker or lethargic owlets. Compromised individuals of any age should be fed small amounts often and should be given highly digestible and balanced foods until they are digesting and processing food correctly. Body weight, digestive function, and general behavior should be monitored throughout growth.

All new birds should be rehydrated. Rehydration volume should be based on the approximate level of dehydration. Healthy, non-, or mildly dehydrated birds should receive a bolus volume of 5% of their body weight in grams (50 ml/kg), those that are severely dehydrated (mucoid or tacky mouth, sunken eyes, wrinkled skin and eyelids) may require additional fluids. Consult or enlist an avian veterinarian if necessary. Warm, sterile, isotonic fluids such as lactated Ringer's solution or 0.9% sodium chloride should be administered subcutaneously or, in critical cases, intravenously. Large liquid volumes should not be given orally unless that is the only option. Owls are anatomically designed to eat and digest solid prey items only. They may easily aspirate liquids while swallowing or

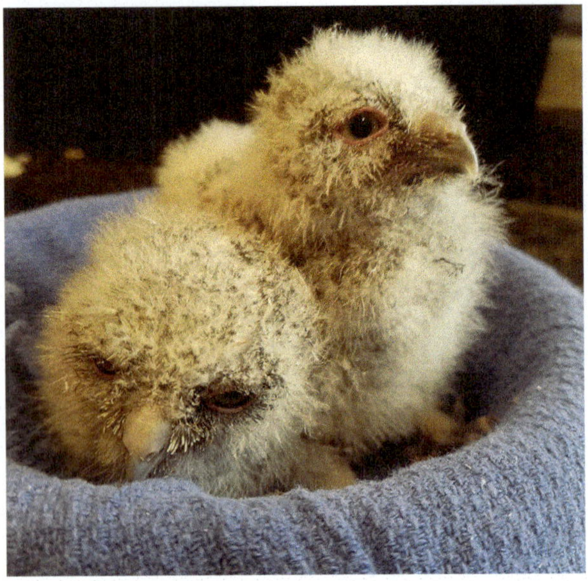

Figure 31.2 Young nestlings in a fabric-covered bowl nest.

in any body position where the head is not elevated above the body. Small volumes or sips of liquids can be given orally to those requiring additional gastrointestinal hydration or those not capable of processing whole foods.

Once the bird is warm and hydrated, a physical examination should be performed, and any injuries or remarkable conditions should be recorded and addressed. The approximate age should be established based on physical development and feeding initiated. Ideally, the bird should be fed relatively soon after being admitted. It is best to feed after handling because stress can increase the likelihood of regurgitation and therefore the risk of aspiration. For malnourished, very weak, or unstable birds, all handling should be as quick as possible. In these circumstances, check the weight, hydrate quickly, and, if warm enough, feed one or two pieces of organ meats. Then leave the bird alone on heat in a dark, quiet area. An hour or two later, the bird is likely to be at least a little stronger.

Well-fleshed, healthy owlets should be encouraged to reach for and take their own food as soon as they are capable of holding up their heads. Size and presentation of food items should be based on the digestive abilities of that stage of development. Never force-feed a young owl unless absolutely necessary. It is not unusual for a new chick to ravenously accept food on intake, and then, after a forcible and negative feeding experience, to avoid eating on its own or even to actively refuse food when offered. Carefully assess dietary needs and make a feeding plan before feeding a new patient.

It should be noted that well-fleshed animals with no apparent injuries should be kept in captivity only when there is no other option. It is after this initial exam that plans should be made to return any potential candidates to their family.

## Common Medical Problems and Solutions

### Traumatic Injuries

Traumatic injuries in owls should be treated as they would be in other avian species. Due to the anatomical absence of a protective brow bone, eye injuries are common in owls and, unfortunately, are rarely documented. A thorough eye exam should be performed in all owls with any suspicion

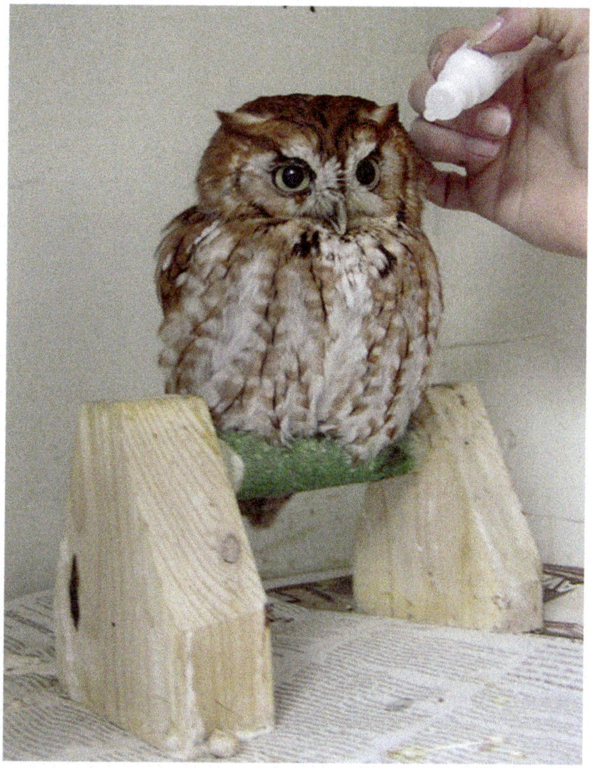

Figure 31.3 Administration of eye medication without restraint.

of trauma because these injuries may result in functional limitations that may affect flight, as well as hunting ability. All cases with a history of ocular trauma should be considered for release based on the proven ability to hunt live prey in optimal light conditions for that species.

Injuries to the cornea can be confirmed by the positive uptake of fluoroscein stain on the corneal surface. Treatment with nonsteroidal ophthalmic agents may be helpful. Do not use steroids if there is corneal damage (with positive fluorescein stain uptake). Corneal scars and opacities in the outer areas of the cornea may or may not affect visual function depending on their density and location. Visible blood in the anterior chamber (hyphema) may be a common result of traumatic injuries. Treatment with topical corticosteroids may be helpful, although blood is often reabsorbed without treatment. Age-related retinal degeneration in owls has been documented (Redig 1993).

Based on the natural behaviors of the larger-bodied owls, they can often be given topical eye medications without necessitating restraint. Often, if the protected hand holding the medication is brought in from the side of the bird, the owl will remain focused on the individual and not respond to the hand or the administration of the medication (Figure 31.3).

## Parasites

Wildlife species are common hosts to many species of parasites. Like other opportunistic pathogens, they may become a significant strain on compromised individuals and should be treated in compromised or recovering patients. Gastrointestinal parasites should be diagnosed by fecal analysis and treated accordingly.

### Blood Parasites

Several blood parasites are commonly identified in owl species, including *Plasmodium, Leucocytozoon,* and *Haemoproteus.* Routine bloodwork should include analysis of a blood smear in these species. *Plasmodium* species are the causative agent of malaria in birds as well as humans. Vectors include three genera of mosquitoes. The primary vector of *Leucocytozoon* is black flies in the genus *Simulium. Haemoproteus* species are commonly transmitted by hippoboscid or flat flies. Infections are often subclinical. Consult an avian veterinarian for treatment options.

### Ectoparasites

Feather mites, lice, and hippoboscids (flat flies) may be found all over the body. Due to the prevalence of vector-borne diseases, these parasites should be eliminated in clinical or group settings. Older juveniles or fully feathered birds can generally be safely de-parasitized with pyrethrins or permethrins, but for younger birds a light dusting of Sevin Dust™ (diethylcarbamazine, GardenTech™) works well. Lightly spray (or rub powder) through feather layers down to the skin. Avoid the facial area in those birds with respiratory concerns. One good treatment on intake will not only benefit the host, but will reduce the transfer of parasites to other patients or resident birds. It is prudent to wear gloves when applying pesticides to patients. See Chapter 1 for information regarding the use of pesticides.

Maggots and fly eggs should be manually removed as soon as possible. Sites that allow penetration or are easily penetrated, such as wounds and bodily orifices, should be cleared immediately. Although some species of flies target only compromised tissue, the larva of most common fly species are much less selective and are just as likely to feed on healthy structures. Once the eggs hatch, they can burrow through healthy tissues and often result in damage worse than the original trauma. Capstar™ (Nytenpyram, Novartis) is often administered orally to weaken and reduce the number of deeper and less-accessible active larvae. It is also dissolved in water and used to flush wounds, as a topical application. Birds should be closely monitored for continued hatching as well as for any resilient live maggots and treated twice daily until all larvae are eliminated.

## Diet

Owls are studied and even admired for their efficient breakdown of whole food. Only the most digestible and nutritious parts (organ meat, muscle, fat) are utilized, and the remaining less-digestible parts (bones, hair, feathers) are efficiently collected and formed into a pellet or casting that is ejected or spit out orally. Owl pellets are often used in educational programs.

As in other areas of captive wildlife management, the optimal and most healthy diet is one that most closely resembles the wild diet of that species. Although adult birds may tolerate modified diets, growing juveniles with developing bones may be permanently and irreversibly affected by incomplete or unbalanced diets. Ideally, owlets that are physically capable of digesting whole food should be fed a complete and fully balanced diet. Calcium, phosphorus, and fat content should be optimal in selected food sources. Whole adult prey items are always preferred. In captive environments, most birds are fed what is readily available, such as *adult* mice, rats, rabbits, and quail. Avian chicks (chickens or quail) are too young and not an ideal food source due to the deficient calcium levels.

In situations where food quality and availability are limited, care should be taken to supplement the necessary vitamins, minerals, and deficient components as needed for each meal. It must be emphasized that supplementation should be calculated carefully based on analysis of the food source as well as nutritional requirements for that species. As with other growing birds, calcium and phosphorus must be balanced at a 2 : 1 ratio by weight to avoid development of metabolic bone disease. Feeding whole adult prey animals avoids this problem. As a general rule, if whole adult prey items are not fed, calcium must be supplemented at a level that provides twice as many milligrams of elemental calcium as phosphorus in the deficient food. Powdered calcium carbonate is the calcium supplement of choice.

## Feeding Procedures

Frequency of feeding should be based on the digestion and clearance time of meals. Since owls lack a true crop, the gizzard is often used as an indicator. An empty, flaccid, or ill-defined lower abdomen represents a presumably empty gastrointestinal tract. When full, the gizzard is easily palpated as an obvious, dense, round mass in the lower abdomen. Body weight should be monitored daily and should begin to show a consistent daily increase within no more than 48 hours after intake. Stagnant weight curves would be a concern as growing birds must gain weight steadily for healthy growth and development.

Careful consideration should be used when formulating a feeding plan for growing owls. Hatchlings and young unfeathered nestlings do not have fully developed digestive systems. In most species, the male provides the food and the female stays with the young as a source of heat, protection, and feeding. She will tear food into edible pieces depending on the age of the chick. When cutting food into bite-size pieces, the size of the mouth and throat should be considered. The following sections on feeding considerations are based on the natural history and development of growing owls. Captive recommendations should ideally replicate general natural behaviors.

### Hatchlings

The digestive system of newly hatched owls may take as long as 36 hours to be functional in most species. Hatchlings may be hydrated orally with a few drops of water once vocalizations become persistent. Solid food should not be offered to most species for the first 24 hours; the chick's vocalizations at this age are believed to stimulate specific hormonal responses in the parents, not to actually acquire solid food yet. Digestive function in unfeathered hatchlings can be confirmed by the passage and elimination of droppings.

Young hatchlings of most owl species are usually fed every few hours, with four to five feedings daily (Figure 31.4). At this young age, food should be torn into small pieces of easily digestible parts, such as organ meat, muscle, and skin. These bite-size pieces are gently rubbed on the edge of the beak. Food should not be colder than room temperature and should be fresh. Although easily digested parts are preferred, parents do not debone or carefully eviscerate prey. Fragments of bone, skin, fur, and stomach contents are included in the natural diet at all ages. Using this as a reference, a small fragment of bone should be included in the diet of healthy owlets over 4 days of age, because they require calcium even at this young age. Be sure to remove any sharp edges that may irritate or injure their sensitive esophageal tissue. Tenderizing pieces by crushing or with a mortar and pestle may be helpful when necessary.

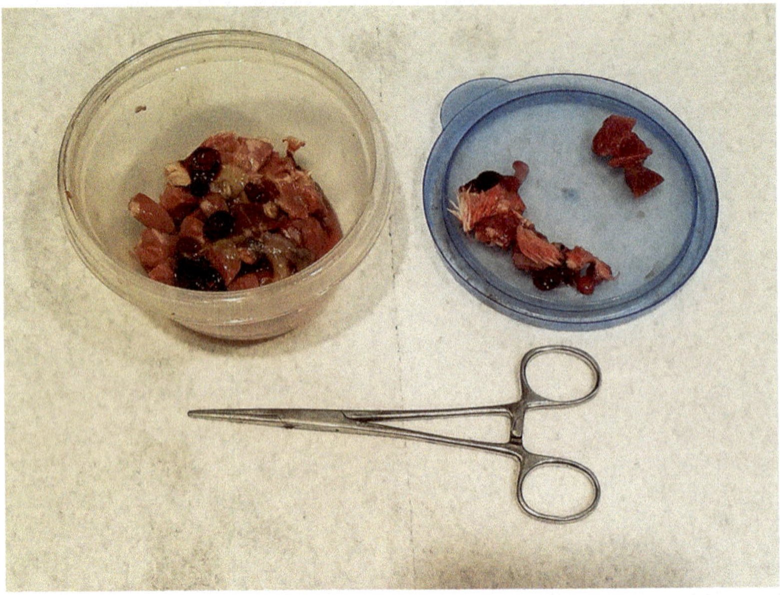

Figure 31.4 Small pieces of rodent prey to be offered with hemostats.

### Nestlings and Fledglings

Size and quality of food pieces should be increased as the baby grows and develops. Skin, fur, and feathers should be gradually added and pellet formation monitored and recorded. Digestibility of bones is also evident in pellet appearance. Healthy birds that are gaining weight, eating well, digesting food efficiently, and producing normal-looking pellets should be offered increasingly complete meals until food can be presented in its whole form. Healthy babies that are old enough to physically process whole food should never be offered anything less. Tree-nesting species learn to tear whole food at an early age. Exceptions should be made only when necessary in individual cases.

## Expected Weight Gain

Chicks should consistently gain weight up until fledging age. Some species may overshoot their adult weight during fledging. As an example, after hatching at around 50 g, Great Horned Owls should reach 800–1000 g by 25–29 days of age, then the rate of gain slows until they reach their adult weight several weeks later; adult weights vary fairly widely by region (Artuso et al. 2013). Barred Owls follow a similar pattern, reaching 50–75% of adult weight in the first 30 days (Mazur and James 2000). Barn Owls reach maximum weight at about 40 days of age (Marti et al. 2005). Eastern and Western Screech, Boreal, and Saw-whet Owls reach their maximum weight at about 20 days of age (Ritchison et al. 2017).

## Housing

### Hatchlings and Nestlings

At this young age, the mother's body provides a constant source of heat. Owlets will huddle against or burrow underneath her for warmth or may move or lean away to cool off. Incubators are ideal and are recommended, but heating pads can be used if an incubator is not available. The nest floor should be placed safely on a protected heating pad set on the lowest setting and should be positioned with up to 80% of the floor on heat to create a heat gradient. Owlets should seek or use heat as they would a warm-bodied parent. Any individual actively and continually moving off or away from heat should be watched closely because this is often the first observable behavior change of dying chicks. If noted, consult an avian veterinarian immediately.

Artificial nests should be designed with respect to each species' nesting style and should be placed in the back corner of the cage or incubator. Cavity-nesters should be offered a nest box large enough to allow movement, with solid walls for natural security as well as for a physical boundary. These species tend to huddle and lean in corners and will likely fall over the rim of conventional open nests. Tree-nesters should be offered bowl-shaped nests with a few small sticks in the middle. The edges should be high enough to crouch behind and lean against but low enough to reach heads out over the rim (Figure 31.2). Heavy crocks and dog bowls padded and covered with fabric can be used as a nest structure for larger bodied clutches and smaller heavy bowls may be ideal for smaller species. Many owl species will sleep with their neck limp and head hanging over the edge.

Whatever style of housing is used, the front of the cage should be adequately covered to provide the nest with a visual barrier to human activity but should also allow partial exposure to light. Thermoregulatory abilities develop as feathers grow, and supplemental heat can be gradually removed once the bird is adequately insulated.

Owlets may be housed in heavy, dark plastic kennels. The nest should be placed in a back corner with adjacent holes covered. Natural perches of the appropriate size for these birds should be provided to ease the first step out of the nest. The size of the kennel should be at least as wide as the length of the wingspan and should be enlarged as the birds grow.

As vision improves with age, the young nestlings become increasingly aware of their surroundings. It is presently believed that programmed identification and recognition behaviors develop during this period (McKeever 1987). Social development and permanent associations are consistently linked to this stage of cognitive development. Owlets that remain in their natural environment through this stage usually exhibit much wilder and more aggressive behaviors. They actively respond to human presence and seem to recognize natural threats. Those that were captive or in a modified environment during this stage may still recognize and avoid handling and human activity in general, but they are usually less aggressive and behave more passively in comparison.

It is imperative that growing owls are housed with conspecifics. Ideally, surrogate or foster owl parents should be present or at least visible at all times, and human presence should be reduced or, if possible, eliminated. As soon as each owlet is reliably self-feeding, growing, and able to maintain body temperature, the cage should be set up outside for increasing lengths of time until the bird is acclimated to ambient outdoor temperatures. If extreme weather and drastic temperature changes necessitate indoor shelter for these young babies, they should still be placed near a window for visual stimuli. Protected structures with open doors or windows (porches, garages, sheds) may help acclimation in questionable climates. If the temperature drops more than 15 °F (8 °C), a supplemental heat source should be offered as an option to all ages.

### Pre-fledglings and Older Juveniles

Owlets quickly become more physically active and mobile. They start to stand and will begin to branch or climb on and around the nest edge and beyond (Figure 31.5). In many tree-nesting species, family groups (including the mother bird as well as siblings of varying sizes) may be easily observed throughout the tree. As active and mature as these adolescents may appear, their flight feathers have a long way to go. Fledglings raised in captivity should be housed outdoors as early as possible. They spend much of their time watching their new world from the comfort of their perch.

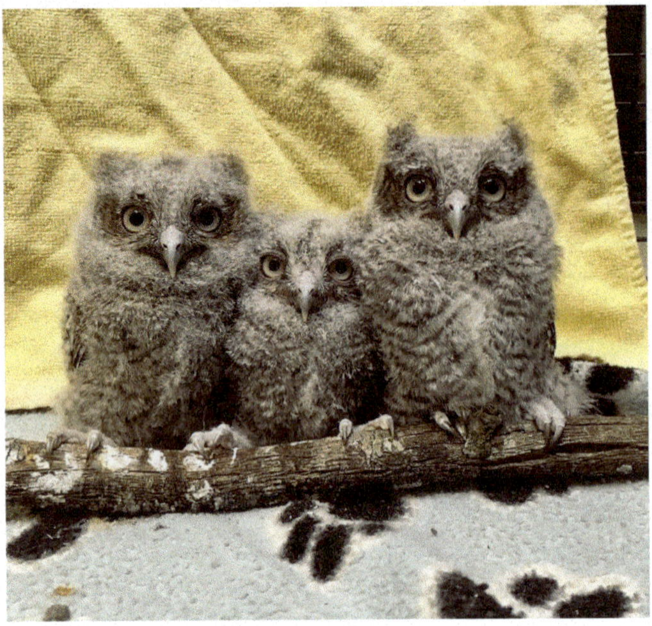

Figure 31.5 Three young Eastern Screech Owls branching, starting to grasp perches or nest edges.

Aviaries for small owls have a recommended minimum size of 8×8×8 ft. (2.4×2.4×2.4 m). Medium-sized species such as Barn Owls should have aviaries of at least 10×30×12 ft. (3×9×3.6 m). Large owls such as Great Horned Owls require large flight cages of minimum dimensions 10×50×12 ft. (3×15×3.6 m) (Miller 2012). Development of flight agility can be enhanced by designing the aviary in an L shape or by placing movable baffles extending from the side walls that birds must bank and turn to fly past. Live-prey arenas must be included for all species. These can be as simple as a large metal tub in which live rodents are placed, or an arena that may be set into the floor of the enclosure. Prevention of prey escape is an important factor. As birds become more adept at catching prey, the rodents should be allowed more hiding places within the arena.

## Release Considerations

Flighted juveniles of most owl species remain in the nesting territory for a considerably long period of time. Parents continue to provide food as owlets leisurely practice their flight and hunting skills. Owls seem to require more overall support during their training than other species of raptors. Young owls should be restricted to hunting of live prey for at least 3 weeks before release. Late-season captive-reared birds that were not exposed to what seems to be necessary training are less likely to survive their first winter. Many facilities overwinter fall owlets to allow extra time for practice and overall maturation. First-year owls that are released in the fall should be soft-released and provided with a feeding station. It is not uncommon for Great Horned Owls to return to a recognized feeding spot several times over the course of the winter. Nature would not provide this extra time and amount of assistance unless it was necessary for survival.

## Acknowledgments

I would like to gratefully acknowledge and dedicate this writing to Donald L. Burton DVM.

## Sources for Products Mentioned

Sevin Dust: GardenTech, PO Box 24830, Lexington, KY 40524-4830, (800) 969-7200. https://www.gardentech.com.
Capstar (Nitenpyram): Novartis Animal Health, (800) 637-0281.

## References

Artuso, C., Houston, C.S., Smith, D.G., and Rohner, C. (2013). Great horned owl (*Bubo virginianus*), version 2.0. In: *The Birds of North America* (eds. A. Poole and F. Gill). Ithaca, NY, USA: Cornell Lab of Ornithology https://doi.org/10.2173/bna.372.

Marti, C.D., Poole, A.F., and Bevier, L.R. (2005). Barn owl (*Tyto alba*), version 2.0. In: *The Birds of North America* (eds. A. Poole and F. Gill). Ithaca, NY, USA: Cornell Lab of Ornithology https://doi.org/10.2173/bna.1.

Mazur, K.M. and James, P.C. (2000). Barred owl (*Strix varia*), version 2.0. In: *The Birds of North America* (eds. A. Poole and F. Gill). Ithaca, NY, USA: Cornell Lab of Ornithology https://doi.org/10.2173/bna.508.

McKeever, K. (1987). *Care and Rehabilitation of Injured Owls*, 128 pp. Lincoln, Ontario, Canada: W.F. Rannie Publishing.

Miller, E.A. (ed.) (2012). *Minimum Standards for Wildlife Rehabilitation*, 4e. St. Cloud, MN: National Wildlife Rehabilitation Association.

Redig, P.T. (1993). *Medical Management of Birds of Prey*. St. Paul, MN: The Raptor Center at the University of Minnesota.

Ritchison, G., Gehlbach, F.R., Pyle, P., and Patten, M.A. (2017). Eastern Screech-Owl (*Megascops asio*), version 3.0. In: *The Birds of North America* (eds. A. Poole and F. Gill). Ithaca, NY, USA: Cornell Lab of Ornithology https://doi.org/10.2173/bna.easowl1.03.

## Further Reading

Bent, A.C. (1938). *Life Histories of North American Birds of Prey*. New York: Dover Publications.

Engelmann, M. and Marcum, P. (1993). *Raptor Rehabilitation*. Carolina Raptor Center.

Fosco, L. (1997). Great Horned Owls: Natural history and its role in wildlife rehabilitation. In: Proceedings of the International Wildlife Rehabilitation Council Annual Conference, Oct. 4, 1997, Concord, California, pp. 173–177.

Johnsgard, P.A. (1988). *North American Owls: Biology and Natural History*, 295 pp. Washington, D.C.: Smithsonian Institution Press.

Long, K. (1998). *Owls, A Wildlife Handbook*, 181 pp. Chicago: Johnson Publishing Company.

Macleod, A. and Perlman, J. (2003). *Wildlife Feeding and Nutrition*, 73 pp. International Wildlife Rehabilitation Council.

Tyler, H.A. and Phillips, D. (1978). *Owls by Day and Night*, 208 pp. Happy Camp, California: Naturegraph Publishers, Inc.

Walker, L.W. (1993). *The Book of Owls*, 255 pp. Austin: University of Texas Press.

# 32

# Goatsuckers

*Linda Hufford*

## Natural History

The goatsuckers are classified within the order Caprimulgiformes, which consists of five diverse but fascinating families with many unusual metabolic and lifestyle adaptations. The goatsuckers' family Caprimulgidae, nighthawks, and nightjars, will be discussed in this chapter in detail as representatives of their order.

Other Caprimulgids include the owlet-nightjars (Aegothelidae), sometimes referred to as *moth owls* in their native Australasia. These tiny long-tailed birds with an upright posture are capable of torpor during cold days. Also Australasian natives, the Frogmouths (Podargidae) are named quite descriptively for their wide cavernous mouths as well as their booming night sound. Prey consists of mostly insects, some of which are enticed within range by an odor exuded from the mouth of the bird. Frogmouths are kept in many zoological institutions because, unlike many birds in this order, they can adapt to eating out of dishes. Potoos (Nyctibiidae) are South American birds that have a unique feature of the eyelids: two small slits that allow the bird to see even with the eyes closed. Perched on a tree with their beaks upraised, these long-clawed birds look like broken branches. Among the most interesting and unique of all birds, the Oilbirds (Steatornithidae) of South America are so named because the young are fed rich, oily fruits until at about 30 days of age when they are 150% the weight of the adults. At one time, the chicks were rendered to make torch oil. These cave-dwelling frugivores are thought to be unique in that they use echolocation in near-total darkness.

The term *goatsucker* (family Caprimulgidae) is a common inclusive name that includes subfamilies of the New World nighthawks (Chordeilinae) and the typical nightjars (Caprimulginae). In North America, the birds known by the common names of Chuck Will's Widow, Common Pauraque, Whip-poor-will, Common Poorwill, and Buff-collared Nightjars are considered nightjars. Those known as Common Nighthawks, Antillean Nighthawks, and Lesser Nighthawks are usually referred to as nighthawks. Surprisingly few ornithological studies have been conducted on these birds.

Both subfamilies have common general physical traits. Their large flat heads blend into a rounded body to give the appearance of the birds' having no necks. A tiny bill with prominent nares (the nostrils of which are flexible tubes) conceals a cavernous mouth that is shockingly large when opened (Figure 32.1). Short, tiny, weak legs seem to disappear when the bird is perched. Caprimulgids have an anisodactyl toe arrangement with three toes forward and one toe back, and

*Hand-Rearing Birds*, Second Edition. Edited by Rebecca S. Duerr and Laurie J. Gage.

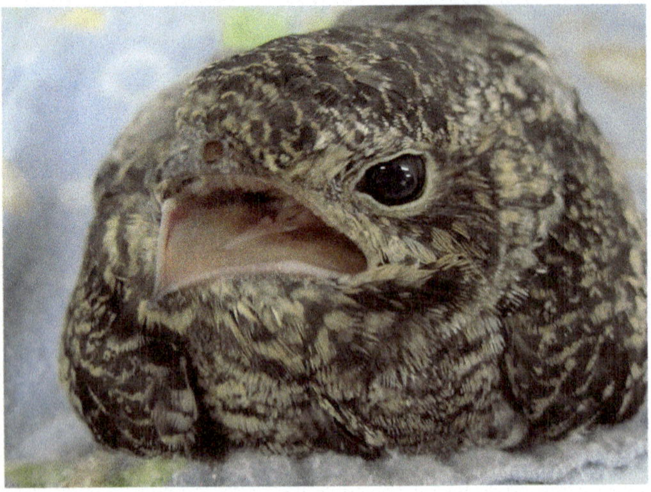

Figure 32.1 Common Nighthawk showing the petite bill with very large mouth typical of these species. *Source:* photo courtesy of Yvonne Wallace Blane, Fellow Mortals Wildlife Hospital.

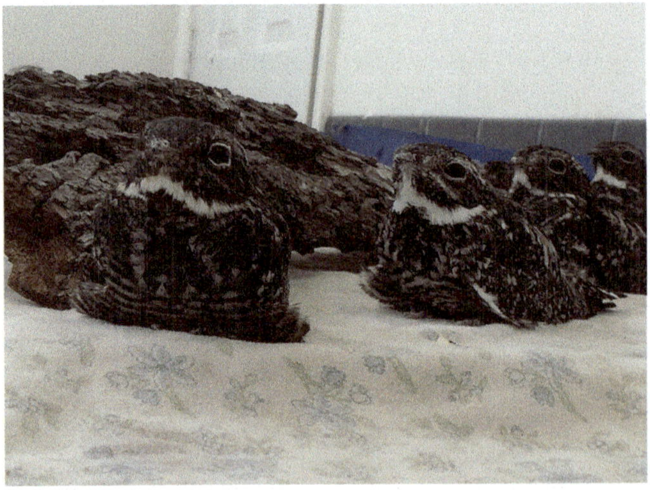

Figure 32.2 Four Common Nighthawk chicks showing cryptic coloration. *Source:* photo courtesy of Yvonne Wallace Blane, Fellow Mortals Wildlife Hospital.

there is partial webbing between the front-facing toes. Located on the inner claw of the middle toe of some species is a pectinated claw, also known as a *feathercomb*.

Virtually silent flight is accomplished with softened leading edges of the primaries, much like owls. Also owl-like is the lack of development of a true crop. Camouflage coloring, combined with a unique horizontal perching position, make these birds virtually disappear when resting on a branch or in leaf litter (Figure 32.2). The fragile, loose feathers are shaded brown, tan, gray, or rust and cryptically designed with penciling, blotching, and mottling. The variegated hues blend well with the natural background of their chosen environments; generally, the birds living in higher altitudes and those in desert areas are lighter in color than their forest- or field-dwelling relatives.

All species engage in dust-bathing to condition their delicate feathers. Adult birds may also indulge in aerial bathing when relaxed. Because the oil gland in goatsuckers is atrophied, preening consists of distributing fat from the feathers of the breast with the use of the bill and the pectinated claw. Some species are noted to have a strong, earthy smell.

Goatsucker wings are designed for maneuverability and swiftness to pursue the variety of insects that compose the majority of their diet (see Figure 32.3). The wings are proportionately long and powered by large pectoral muscles.

Even the eyes of the goatsuckers are designed for their crepuscular hunting habits; the large liquid-looking dark eyes have a tapetum that reflects unabsorbed light, resulting in a distinctive red or red-orange eye-shine. The eyes are situated laterally, offering a wide view during flight. One feature unique to goatsuckers is the ability to control their loose upper eyelids.

Generally, nightjars have rounded wings with no white feathering. They are nocturnal or crepuscular feeders and have obvious rictal feathering. The wingtips do not extend past the tail, and they have feathered tarsi. Nighthawks, on the other hand, have pointed wings with white covert feathers that are visible when they are sitting. There may be white patches on the wings, the specific markings of which vary by species. The adult wings cross over the back and extend beyond the tail. Rictal feathering is obscure or does not exist. The long, forked tail is also distinct.

Although most goatsucker chicks are raised in a similar manner, it becomes essential near release time to identify the proper release criteria and to recognize the signs of physical maturity of each species. The use of a good field guide may help identify specific species or subspecies of goatsuckers; weights and territorial ranges may also be helpful. In the northern parts of the U.S. and Canada, most species can be ruled out by location, although this is not always possible in the southern U.S. or northern Mexico during migration.

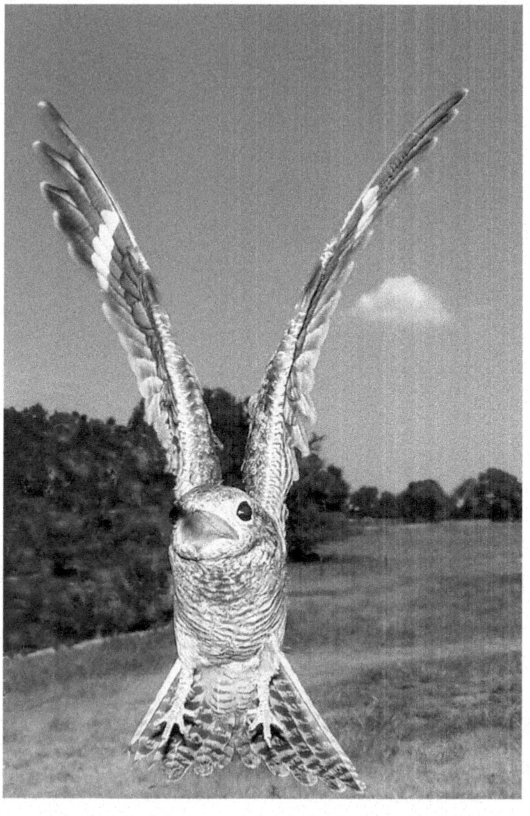

Figure 32.3 Goatsuckers are extremely agile fliers and must have full flight dexterity to qualify for release.

## Migration

Migration is achieved for some species in flocks during daylight hours. Nonmigratory species, primarily the Common Poorwill, may enter torpor, a state resulting in a lowered heart rate, breathing rate, and metabolism with reduced response to external stimulation during inclement weather or temperatures.

## Reproduction

After an aerial courtship, during which the male often "booms" and tail-flashes, the pair bond and breed. Generally, two eggs (very rarely up to four eggs have been found in a nest, possibly the eggs of a second female) are laid on consecutive days on the ground, on broken tree stumps, or on flat roofs. The nest has little or no nesting materials.

Incubation is 17–21 days, with either the male or the female being the primary daytime caregiver, species-specifically. Also species-dependent is whether the eggs hatch together or on consecutive days. When necessary, the adult is thought to move the eggs out of direct sunlight or dangerous circumstances by pushing the eggs with its feet or breast.

With weak feet and a tiny bill, goatsuckers are basically defenseless against predators; camouflage is one of the few defenses available. The nest site is on natural materials, the eggs are patterned to be obscure, and the still chicks' down blends well with the surrounding area. Adults on a nest use techniques to change their body profiles by flattening the upper feathers to the body, lowering the head to the ground, and changing the posture of the body to engulf the nest in an effort to be unseen. The bird then closes its eyes and maintains complete stillness. If this camouflage attempt does not work, the adult will aggressively defend the nest by flaring its feathers to appear larger and will launch an intimidating but harmless open-mouth attack while hissing.

If threats are not effective, attempts to lure and confuse may follow. The female may feign a broken wing in an attempt to lure the predator away from the nest or the male may circle and dive on the intruder while wing-clapping to create a distraction.

## Development of Chicks

The chicks begin peeping before hatching. The usual two eggs pip, and then open in perfect halves, generally within a day of each other. The semi-precocial chicks are capable of movement within the nest on the day of hatch. For species where hatch weights are published (Brigham et al. 2011; Cink et al. 2017), the chicks weigh 5–6 g and have a very sparse covering of soft down.

Pinfeathers emerge along the wing and scapular tracts and pterylae is visible on other parts of the body by day 10. When the nest is disturbed, chicks will rapidly scatter, with each chick going in a different direction away from the nest, apparently as an effort to confuse the predator. By day 16 for nightjars, and day 18 for nighthawks, the primaries are unsheathed and chicks respond to parental warning cries by hopping or flying short distances. Chicks become thermally independent between days 20–23, depending upon species. They are no longer brooded, but continue to be fed by the parents at this age. By day 30, the chicks of all species are feeding independently, flying well, and will leave their nest permanently. At about 32 days of age, chicks are capable of catching their own food, although parents may still furnish backup feedings. Migratory species will join a flock in preparation for a long journey at about 7 weeks of age.

## Criteria for Intervention

Chicks may come into care for a variety of reasons. They are often found when remodeling or repairing a flat roof, or recovered from construction sites where nests are accidentally disrupted or disturbed by cats or other predators, and have even been recovered from the backs of delivery trucks. Re-nesting recently discovered uninjured chicks is the best resolution, but if that is not possible chicks can be raised in captivity relatively easily.

## Initial Care and Stabilization

As with any young bird, warming first is essential. Place the bird in a padded container on a heating pad set on low for 15–20 minutes until it is relaxed and warm. Please see Chapter 1 for stabilization of newly admitted birds (Figure 32.4).

Goatsucker feathers are extremely delicate, and extreme measures must be taken to ensure that damage is not sustained in captivity. Use a silk or polyester material (such as a scarf) to protect the feathers during handling. If it is an emergency situation and such material cannot be located immediately, thoroughly wash and rinse the examination area and the examiner's hands with soap and water to remove any oils that might contaminate the feathers.

Be aware that even young chicks will probably hiss and gape in a very threatening manner; this is a harmless but startling tactic. Do not hold the bird by the legs. Many goatsuckers will remain still at approach, and then suddenly flush. To avoid injuries to the bird, one hand can be placed above the bird, while the second hand does a slow approach from the side. Uninjured chicks may be quite adept at evasive running maneuvers and may leap unexpectedly off the examination table.

The eyes should be clear and liquid-looking, and the eyelids rather loose-fitting. During daylight or under bright lights, the eyelids may appear to be half-opened; this is normal for these nocturnal birds. Hold the bird with the feathers laying in proper alignment and the wings folded against the body. To check wing alignment, hold an index and third finger on either side of the neck, pinning the bird down with the heel of the hand. A detailed palpation of the wings can be achieved by

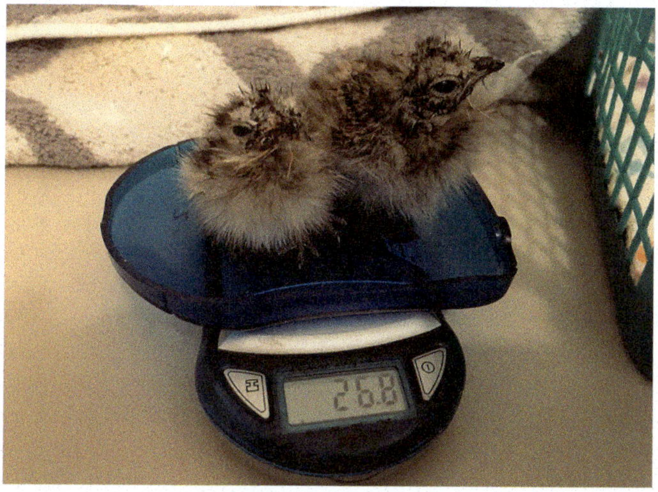


Figure 32.4 Two Common Nighthawk chicks being weighed. *Source:* photo courtesy of Yvonne Wallace Blane, Fellow Mortals Wildlife Hospital.

holding one folded wing against the body while examining the other. To check the mouth, brush gently or blow softly on the rictal feathering. This may trigger a snapping motion, so be prepared with a halved tongue depressor or a large paper clip to enter from the side of the mouth. Once in place, these devices can then be slowly turned sideways from the front of the mouth to open the mouth enough for viewing, without risking injury to the jaws. Examine the remainder of the body as you would any species of bird.

Common Poorwills found during cold weather should be evaluated for torpor. Torpid birds should be slowly warmed before examination in order to fully evaluate their condition. Torpor is an energy-conserving reduction of the heart, respiratory, and metabolic rates. Torpor can be induced by either a 20% weight loss or by cold weather; even young poorwill chicks have been found in torpor.

The torpor of a Common Poorwill studied in 1994 recorded body temperatures of less than 41 °F (5 °C), which constitutes the lowest body temperature ever recorded for any species of wild bird. One experiment kept a poorwill in torpor at 50 °F (10 °C) for 100 days, with a resulting weight loss of only 10 g of stored fat (Howell and Bartholomew 1959).

## Common Medical Problems

Little is known about the medical disorders of these species; goatsuckers are rarely brought into care from illnesses. Suspected poisonings may occasionally be brought in but generally are at very late stage to have allowed capture. Adult goatsuckers most commonly arrive with injuries from vehicles. The birds hunt insects, which are often attracted to car headlights. Many times, this collision results in a compound fracture or semi-amputated wing. Most rehabilitators consider goatsuckers with serious wing fractures to be candidates for euthanasia, due to the release criteria of nearly perfect flight maneuverability. Well-aligned, midshaft fractures of the radius, ulna, or metacarpal bones with minimal soft tissue damage may have a better prognosis, but should be evaluated on a case-by-case basis. All wing injuries must be considered extremely serious; a nighthawk or nightjar without viable flight is a nonreleasable bird. Goatsuckers occasionally present with skin lacerations from predator attacks. Keep any feather removals from wound cleaning to an absolute minimum, and any tape applied in the course of wing wraps or other bandaging must take the loose and delicate feathers into account. See Chapter 1 for more information.

## Feeding Procedures

In captivity, all goatsuckers must be hand-fed. There are no reported cases of a goatsucker self-feeding in captivity, aside from the apparently incidental ingestion of small moving prey. Chicks usually adapt easily to hand-feeding, and will come to the realization that food is imminent when the caretaker nears the cage. Caution should be used because the chicks will lunge toward the feeder with wings outspread and mouths wide open, often with a frantic-sounding peep. Chicks should be fed as much and often as demanded. A short rest during the feeding period, followed by an offer of additional food, works well.

The technique used while feeding is important. Perhaps because of the lateral eyes, goatsuckers appear not to recognize a still body as food. When hand-feeding, use a "zooming" motion with the food held in blunt forceps, hemostats, or by hand. Lightly brush or tickle the rictus feathers. Goatsuckers taken into captivity at an early age will usually become familiar with the routine.

At about 3 weeks of age, these youngsters will begin flying and may be enticed to come to familiar foods when the familiar motion is seen.

Adults, on the other hand, are notorious for being difficult to feed in captivity. The normal heavy feeding times of most species are during the 45-minute period just before dawn and again just after dusk. The birds will be more cooperative during this time period while in care. To reduce stress, first attempt to use the zooming motion mentioned in the general feeding section. Many adults will quickly adapt to this method. For the less cooperative, gently open the jaws and insert the food toward the back of the mouth. Hold the head up slightly with one fingertip beneath the jaw after the feeding as it is common for the adults to shake their heads in an effort to dislodge the food, or they may hold and dispose of food later without swallowing. Check the substrate several minutes after each feeding for signs of regurgitation.

If repeated feeding attempts during these times fail and the bird is in danger of starvation, force-feeding may be necessary. Hold the bird's body wrapped with a scarf in the left hand (for right-handed caregivers), and use the right hand to come beneath the body with the thumb and fourth finger on either side of the bird's temporal–mandibular joint (the intersection of the upper and lower jaws). Very gently pry open the joint with both sides receiving equal pressure. As soon as there is gape, insert a paper clip from the side of the mouth to the opposing side. Gently turn the distal end of the clip until the mouth is opened. Food can then be pushed to the back of the mouth, using care to place the food on top of the tongue.

In the wild, parents feed their chicks regurgitated insects in two or three feeding sessions around dusk and again near dawn. In captivity they are fed three or four times a day on a diet of primarily commercially available insects such as mealworms, waxworms, superworms, and crickets dipped in an insect-replacement formula (see Chapters 41, 43, and 44 regarding feeding 100% insect diets). As wide a variety of insects should be used as possible; insects most often found in stomach contents of smaller wild goatsuckers are beetles, moths, flies, mosquitoes, grasshoppers, plant lice, locusts, horseflies, winged ants, wasps, bees, chinch bugs, and caterpillars. The much larger Chuck Will's Widow has even been found to have consumed whole small birds and mice.

An insectivore hand-feeding formula (see Chapter 43, Diet section) can be used with a Catac ST1 nipple (Catac Products Limited) at the end of a syringe using the same approach. Goatsuckers are difficult to feed by gavage; great care must be taken when forcing the mouth open because the mandibles are very easily broken. However, if necessary, a 6 in. (15 cm) section of cut-off IV extension set or other narrow flexible tubing may be used to tube-feed. Burn the cut end of the tube to avoid sharp edges and attach the female fitting of the tubing to an appropriately sized syringe. Open the mouth as described previously while restraining the bird on a table, and then visualize the opening to the esophagus within the mouth. Spiral the tubing down this opening such that the tube curves around to follow the esophagus as deep as the end of the bird's ribcage. When inserting the tube it may feel as though the bird has a 90° bend in the esophagus from straight down toward the table and then abruptly curving to be parallel to the table. Adults have been successfully maintained for several weeks during care in captivity using this method. Again, beware of causing any damage to the delicate feathers during handling. Feed 5% of body weight in volume of hand-feeding formula (50 ml/kg) 4–6 times a day: for example, 2 ml formula 4–6 times a day for a 40 g bird (R. Duerr pers. comm.). Weigh the bird at the same time each day to track trends. Weight loss is a danger sign; the diet and frequency of feedings should be scrutinized.

After feeding, all birds should be wiped carefully with a damp cotton swab or cotton ball to remove any residual food or fluids from the rictal and facial feathers and nares. When old enough for flight, place the bird in a large flight cage and introduce into the cage flying insects such as dragonflies, beetles, moths, butterflies, and bees. Each bird should be weighed daily to assure no weight loss, and backup hand-feeding should be continued until the birds are released.

Some goatsuckers, primarily Chuck Will's Widows and Lesser Nighthawks, have been observed in the wild picking up small pieces of rocks and swallowing them. This may be due to a need for supplemental minerals, or it may be as an aid in digestion. While in care, crushed eggshells or oyster shell calcium can be made available by sprinkling on the substrate surface.

## Expected Weight Gain

Chicks usually gain weight daily and should reach or exceed adult weight by 4 weeks of age. See Table 32.1 for adult weights of several goatsucker species.

## Housing

Wire cages should be avoided at all times. Most rehabilitators use solid-sided caging for young birds or injured adults during recovery. Plastic port-a-kennels or airline kennels for dogs are a good choice if the front grates are covered with insect screening. A light stitching with heavy thread through the weave of the screening will hold it in place. Avoid using duct tape or any other type of adhesive that may come loose and cause feather damage. In an emergency, a draped cardboard box may be used. Some rehabilitators furnish these chicks with comfort objects similar to other species, such as mirrors and stuff animals for companionship or simulated parenting (Figure 32.5).

### Substrate

Clean sand is recommended as a substrate, and it provides the additional benefit of heating evenly. The sand can be sculptured to provide indentations and raised areas. An added benefit to sand is that the birds may use it for dust-bathing, which will help with feather conditioning.

Egg-crate foam, actual egg cartons, or clean gravel piled irregularly can be laid across the bottom of the cage to provide contoured flooring. This substrate can then be covered with fleece. Fleece is

Table 32.1 Characteristics of six species of North American goatsuckers.

| Common Name | Chick Down | Bill Color | Legs/Feet Color | Adult Weight |
|---|---|---|---|---|
| Common Nighthawk | Gray, buff w/mottled dark-brown upper parts | Dark blue-black | Drab brown | 58–91 g |
| Lesser Nighthawk | Buff with mottled brown upperparts | Black | Gray, brownish | 34–55 g |
| Chuck Will's Widow | Golden brown or yellowish ochre | Dusky, pinkish beige, black tip | Dull buff | 94–137 g |
| Whip-poor-will | Cinnamon, pale buff, brown, fades to yellow tan | Dark brown, black | Purple-gray or brown | 49–68 g |
| Common Poorwill | Pale buff, gray-buff, tinged purple | Brown or black | Pinkish-brown | 31–58 g |
| Common Pauraque | Brown, pinkish buff | Black | Gray | 43–66 g |

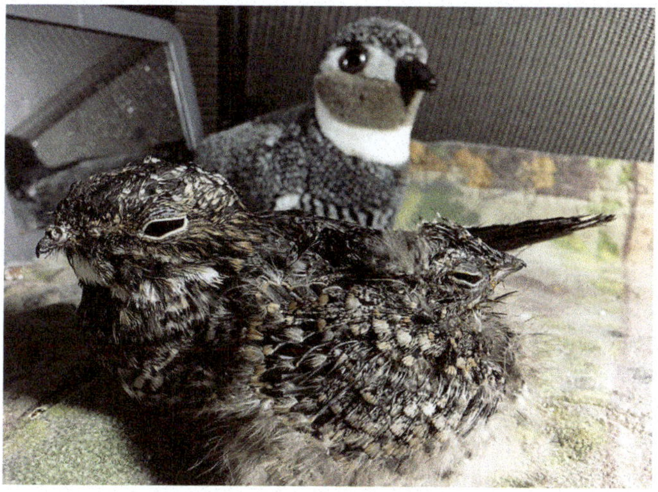

Figure 32.5 Common Nighthawk chick with a mirror and stuffed animal. *Source:* photo courtesy of Yvonne Wallace Blane, Fellow Mortals Wildlife Hospital.

washable, inexpensive, and has the additional benefit of being available in various patterns. If given a choice, choose a darker variegated pattern. Fleece will not catch the tiny toes of the bird, as will a looped towel, nor does it have feather-damaging oils, as newspapers do. Insecticide-free dry leaf litter may also be placed on the bottom of the cage in uneven piles if replaced regularly to avoid mold. Darker colors or camouflage patterns seem to provide comfort to the birds, even the youngest chicks will generally choose to sit or lie on the colors with which they best blend.

Cleanliness is of extreme importance, whatever substrate material is chosen. The substrate must be maintained meticulously to avoid feces or spilled formula from contacting and damaging the delicate feathers. Occasionally, a casting may be found, which will contain undigested insect parts; this should also be disposed of during cleaning.

### Perches

Typical songbird perches are not utilized by goatsuckers. They will perch either on the ground, or laterally and horizontally on a wide branch or rock. While in care, an elevated area may be provided through the use of a contoured substrate, a large branch or small log, or a large rock. Rocks and sand will retain heat better than woods, and both rocks and woods can be elevated enough to keep the delicate feathers away from feces.

### Water Availability

Some rehabilitators have noticed that the birds will defecate in water dishes, but none have reported goatsuckers actually drinking water while in care. In the wild, some goatsuckers have been observed drinking by skimming still water with their lower jaws while flying, or rarely while sitting at the edge of a still-water pond. Moisture is presumed to be primarily provided by the fluid content of insects, many of which are comprised of 70% fluids. As young chicks or injured adults may drown or become chilled, supplemental water should be made available only to healthy adults in pre-release housing.

### Supplemental Heating

There are two important considerations when artificially heating. Temperatures that are too cool may induce torpor in some species, too hot may induce gular fluttering. When chilled, the metabolism is slowed. Gular fluttering uses metabolic energy to cool the body. Neither of these conditions is conducive to the bird's wellbeing. Heat should be furnished for any chick less than 3 weeks of age, or for a traumatized adult. Heat can be provided in the form of a heating pad placed under the cage, through the use of an overhead heat lamp, or with reptile ceramic radiant heaters. Heaters have the advantage of raising the temperature without producing light, which is a consideration for nocturnal species. Full-spectrum lighting can be provided with the use of heat lamps. Generally, the ambient air should be approximately 90 °F (32.2 °C) for older chicks or injured adults, slightly higher for younger chicks. Whichever method is chosen, be certain the heat source is placed to avoid overheating the enclosure. Overhead heat lamps should be encased to prevent contact that may cause singed feathers or legs.

Observation is essential. Watch the movements of the bird; if it prefers to sit far away from the heat source, consider reducing the temperature. If sitting directly beneath or above the heat source, consider increasing temperatures by small increments and continue to observe. Although studies have shown that Common Poorwills efficiently tolerate the extreme heat of their desert and prairie environments by using gular fluttering to facilitate a heat exchange, this fluttering may be an important sign of overheating when you are using an artificial heat source. If you observe this behavior, immediately remove the heat source until the ambient air has cooled, and watch carefully as you slowly reintroduce a lesser heat.

## Weaning

Because goatsuckers will not self-feed from a dish, an approximation of weaning occurs when the bird proves that it is capable of feeding itself by catching free-flying insects. Once the flight feathers have fully emerged, move the chicks to an outdoor aviary. A lightbulb (enclosed in a wire basket to prevent close contact) placed in the cage and away from the birds should invite native flying insects at the appropriate feeding times. If necessary, insects can also be netted and put into the cage for testing purposes. Miller (2012) recommends an aviary size of 8 × 16 × 8 ft. (2.4 × 4.9 × 2.4 m) to contain a maximum of six birds.

Prior to release, a complete physical examination is important. Feathers should be checked carefully for any signs of distress that may hinder flight maneuverability, any previous fractures checked for alignment, and jaw and eyes examined. If there is no obvious reason not to release, the bird should be flight-tested and exercised in the largest flight cage available to build up muscle strength.

Maneuverability must be exceptional. A flight cage with obstructions, such as hanging branches or sheets of canvas, should be utilized for observations of banking and swerving capabilities. Keep in mind the hunting practices used by the individual species; these will range from sustained flight as in nighthawks, to short sallies by many other species. All birds must have the ability to corner, bank, dive, swerve, and gain altitude quickly.

## Release

If possible, sedentary birds should be released into the area where originally found; however, during migration, the bird may not have a local home territory, so release should be in an area that is safe, provides the proper foods, and allows the bird a high likelihood of survival. After a full feeding, release less than an hour after dusk or an hour before dawn. Choose a safe area away from traffic, raptors, and, if possible, where the recent use of insecticides is unlikely. This provides the birds with an opportunity to begin their freedom safely. Whenever possible, time releases according to weather and moon phases. A clear forecast and a full moon will enhance foraging.

Goatsuckers that are not physically capable of catching sufficient numbers of insects to sustain themselves should never be released. Almost no nonreleasable birds are placeable because few care facilities are willing to maintain a feeding regimen for the life of the bird.

## Acknowledgments

The author wishes to acknowledge and thank many fellow rehabilitators who generously contributed their experience and expertise, among these particularly Gloria Halesworth, Sigrid Ueblacker, Rebecca Duerr, Nancy Eilertsen, and Shirley Needham. The author also wishes to thank her husband of 43 years for being half of a rehab team.

## Sources for Products Mentioned

Catac nipples: Catac Products UK Ltd., 3 – 5 Chiltern Trading Estate, Earl Howe Road, Holmer Green, High Wycombe, Bucks, HP15 6QT, Tel: +44 (0) 1234 360116, www.catac.co.uk/xcart/home.php.

Catac nipples: Chris's Squirrels and More, LLC, P.O. Box 365, Somers CT 06071, (860) 749-1129, www.thesquirrelstore.com.

## References

Brigham, R.M., Ng, J., Poulin, R.G., and Grindal, S.D. (2011). Common nighthawk (*Chordeiles minor*), version 2.0. In: *The Birds of North America* (ed. A.F. Poole). Ithaca, NY, USA: Cornell Lab of Ornithology https://doi.org/10.2173/bna.213.

Cink, C.L., Pyle, P., and Patten, M.A. (2017). Eastern whip-poor-will (*Antrostomus vociferus*), version 3.0. In: *The Birds of North America*. (ed. P.G. Rodewald). Ithaca, NY, USA: Cornell Lab of Ornithology https://birdsna.org/Species-Account/bna/species/whip-p1.

Howell, T.R. and Bartholomew, G.A. (1959). Further experiments on torpidity in the poor-will. *Condor* 61 (3): 180–185.

Miller, E.A. (ed.) (2012). *Minimum Standards for Wildlife Rehabilitation*, 4e. St. Cloud, MN: National Wildlife Rehabilitation Association.

## Further Reading

Bent, A.C. (1962). *Life Histories of North American Cuckoos, Goatsuckers, Hummingbirds, and their Allies*, 506 pp. New York: Dover Press.

Cleere, N. (1998). *Nightjars: A Guide to Nightjars and Related Nightbirds*, 317 pp. New Haven, Connecticut: Yale University Press.

Forbush, E. and May, J. (1939). *Natural History of American Birds of Eastern and Central North America*, 553 pp. Boston: Houghton Mifflin Company.

Ligon, J.D. (1970). Still more responses of the poorwill to low temperatures. *Condor* 72 (4): 496–498.

Perrins, C. (1979). *Birds: Their Life, Their Ways Their World*, 411 pp. Pleasantville, New York: Reader's Digest Association.

Sibley, C.G. and Ahlquist, J.E. (1990). *Phylogeny and Classification of Birds: A Study in Molecular Evolution*, 976 pp. New Haven, Connecticut: Yale University Press.

Terres, J. (1991). *The Audubon Society Encyclopedia of North American Birds*, 1053 pp. New Jersey: Wings Books.

# 33

# Swifts

*Jayne Neville and Veronica Bowers*

## Natural History

There are 113 species of swifts and swiftlets in the family Apodidae worldwide (Gill and Donsker 2018), with four species occurring in North America: Chimney (*Chaetura pelagica*), Vaux's (*Chaetura vauxi*), White-throated (*Aeronautes saxatalis*), and Black (*Cypseloides niger*) Swifts. Superficially, these species resemble swallows, but taxonomically swifts are more closely related to hummingbirds. Swifts are historically common and widespread, though their numbers are dropping significantly, possibly due to a reduction in insect availability with the increased use of pesticides.

Swifts are aerial insectivores with long narrow wings, a short tail, and a wide mouth opening. In flight, they're described as "flying cigars," and hold their wings stiffly, alternating between short quick bat-like wing flaps and gliding. Swifts exclusively eat 100% flying insects on the wing, and never eat from dishes; hence, they require hand-feeding the entire time in captivity. Historically, swifts roosted and nested in hollow trees, caves, or shafts, but some species have adapted to use human-built structures such as chimneys as these artificial structures offer increased roosting and breeding sites. White-throated Swifts often nest in drain holes in bridges or other concrete structures. Vaux's Swift occupies chimney-like structures in the west during migration. Other swift species have been shown to touch land very rarely, remaining airborne for months at a time (Hedenstrom et al. 2016).

In rural areas, Chimney Swifts will nest in the large stone/brick chimneys of old farmhouses. In the city, smokestacks and chimneys in historic buildings (factories and mills) can be used. In most cases, Chimney Swifts are not able to utilize chimneys that have clay or stainless steel liners, or those that have been capped. However, the author has witnessed swifts nesting successfully in some types of lined chimneys as well as chimneys that have caps that are not fully enclosed.

North American swifts spend the entire day on the wing, only coming in to roost at night. They can fly up to 500 miles in one day searching for food and consume large numbers of small aerial insects with their wide mouth opening that allows them to snap up a single insect, or to fly through swarms, bill agape. They drink water by swooping low over bodies of water, scooping water into their bill as they fly above the surface. They also bathe on the wing by skimming the surface of the water with their breast.

Swifts are not capable of perching as passerines do; instead, they cling to vertical surfaces with specialized toes, bracing with woodpecker-like stiffened tail feathers. Their legs are very short, with four toes that are small but strong and give the foot a "hand" shape. The toes are anisodactyl

*Hand-Rearing Birds*, Second Edition. Edited by Rebecca S. Duerr and Laurie J. Gage.

and the nails are very long and sharp, allowing the birds a tenacious hold on anything they are clinging to. In some species, the hallux rotates forward to change the foot to appear as if all four toes face forward.

The four species that breed in the United States and Canada are present during the summer breeding season but spend the winter months in Central and South America. Chimney Swifts begin arriving along the Gulf of Mexico coast in March or April. The young spend the first 30 days of their lives in a chimney, and most will go on to breed and roost in them for the rest of their lives. Most Chimney Swifts fledge in July and August, and Vaux's Swifts largely fledge by mid-July. By September, most swifts begin feeding and roosting in large flocks, preparing to migrate to South America. White-throated Swifts migrate southward from northern parts of their range, but most populations in California are resident year-round.

## Criteria for Intervention

Swift nests are built of small twigs adhered together and to vertical walls with sticky saliva. Heavy rains or dirty chimneys can cause a nest to become unglued or not adhere properly and fall down. Asking the right questions is critical to knowing whether chicks need assistance or can be returned to the nest. Age is a large factor. Hatchlings and nestlings are at greatest risk, especially if the nest has fallen down (Figure 33.1). These birds will need to be rescued due to inability to re-attach the nest in the chimney. Time is also critical as to how long chicks have been separated from the adults: was it a few minutes, a few hours, all day long, or days? Where the birds are located is also very important, especially if they had been removed from the chimney. Did they have exposure to outside elements such as cold, rain, or sun? If yes, rehabilitation will be necessary.

Chimney Swift chicks may be able to be returned to the chimney if they are warm, fully feathered, bright eyed and alert, the wings appear even and are not damaged, the chick is not injured, and can cling with both feet. Always return the chick back to the fireplace it was found in. Place the bird as high as possible above the damper to the chimney wall, where it should be able to grab onto the wall and climb to where it needs to go.

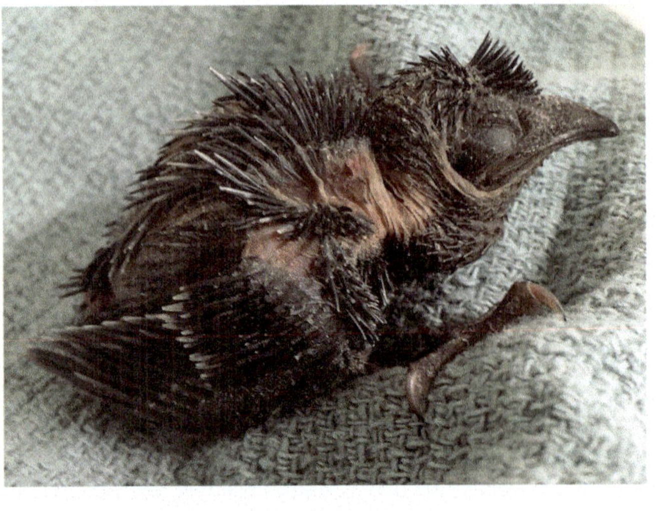

Figure 33.1 Vaux's Swift nestling.

Chimney Swifts are often evicted from chimneys for several reasons, such as the building owner having chimney work done and the birds being discovered during the repair, or the older nestlings' loud begging call being heard in the home or business and the owner being disturbed by it. Lastly, some people just will not tolerate birds in their chimney despite all efforts to convince them otherwise.

Dampers and stovepipes are also a hazard to swifts. Dampers left open in fireplaces can result in adults or young ending up trapped behind glass doors in or at the bottom of fireplaces, or flying around the home looking for a way out. Older homes and historic buildings, which are highly attractive to swifts as nest sites, do not have dampers. The author recommends purchasing foam rubber at a craft store and cutting it to the size of the fireplace opening and putting it in place whenever the fireplace is not in use. Stovepipes can cause a trapping hazard as birds fall down into stovepipes and are unable to get out. These birds can get covered in soot and become exhausted.

Take the time to educate the public each time you receive a call regarding a Chimney Swift. Explain that swifts are losing more and more of their nesting sites with old factories and mills being torn down and people lining and capping their chimneys, they eat tons of the pesky flying insects around their home or building, and that they came all the way from South America just to raise their young in your chimney; it's a genuine privilege to host them! Reassure the building owner the loud begging calls will diminish in 2 weeks and the swifts will be gone by October, when it will be safe to use the fireplace again. By allowing them to remain, they will be directly contributing to the conservation of a declining species – making a real difference.

Chicks that have become cold or dehydrated but are old enough to be placed back in the chimney can be brought into rehabilitation, stabilized, and returned later that day to be reunited with their parents. Follow up is very important. Ask the homeowner to monitor closely, as it is important to ascertain that the young are being cared for by the adults, lest they starve. Wing sounds of the adults flying in and out of the chimney can usually be heard by standing near the fireplace or adults can be observed entering from outside. Loud chattering calls of begging young following the observation of the adults entering the chimney is confirmation all is well. A flashlight can be used to check on the chicks. If the parents do not return, or the chicks do not appear to be being cared for, or if they fall again, they need rescue. This guidance applies to White-throated and Vaux's as well.

## Record Keeping

See Chapter 1 for record keeping suggestions.

## Initial Care and Stabilization

At arrival, swifts may still be clinging to the original nest that fell down (Figure 33.2). Care must be taken when removing a swift from something it is clinging to. Nails can be torn from the toes resulting in bleeding and permanent loss and damage of a toenail. Even though swifts typically come into rehabilitation during warm temperature months, if the bird's body temperature does not feel toasty warm it needs supplemental heat. The author uses a gooseneck lamp with a 60-W ceramic reptile heat emitter (LLL Reptile). Warmed lactated Ringer's solution can be given orally one drop at a time, as many drops as the bird will swallow on a closed bill every 15 minutes for 1 hour. Capillary action should pull the drops into the mouth where a swallowing motion can be observed. Liquid calories in the form of the Hatchling diet for Insectivores (see Chapter 43) can be used orally after 1 hour of

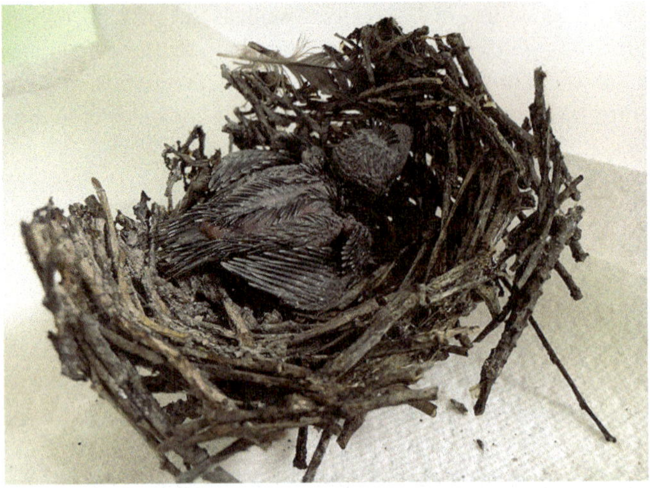

Figure 33.2 Vaux's Swift in natural nest.

hydration therapy if additional easily digestible calories are needed before insect introduction. It is very important to assess the bird's condition after fluid therapy. Is the bird more responsive? Are the eyes brighter, has its activity level increased? Has the bird defecated? Are the droppings normal? Do not introduce food until the bird has defecated. Normal droppings are wet, dark brown, semi-spiral "logs" with urates concentrated at one end. Droppings completely covered in urates reflect a fluid-depleted (dehydrated), and probably starving, bird. Birds with zero food in their system may produce pure white urate droppings. Most chicks will require more fluids in the form of water and drowned insects (in water) for the first 24–48 hours.

## Common Medical Problems and Solutions

Assume every swift received is dehydrated. Leg injuries can occur due to falls from the nest and can be easily splinted using a porous tape. See Duerr et al. (2017) for helpful information on managing orthopedic injuries in small birds. Bleeding toenails from improper handling by the finder are also a common injury. Nails can be torn from toes resulting in bleeding and loss of toenails. Bleeding can be stopped by applying a styptic powder or any clotting agent (corn starch, flour, baking soda) directly to the area and packing it gently.

Feather parasites are common in swifts but not all birds admitted are impacted by them. If a bird is in poor condition and is being overwhelmed, use a pet bird spray Ultracare® Mite & Lice Spray (8-in-1) on a tissue and wipe down the bird's body systematically, starting with the head and ending at the tail. Another option is to treat affected birds with ivermectin at usual avian doses (Hawkins et al. 2018).

## Diets

Swifts require a live insect diet, plus appropriate supplementation to compensate for deficiencies in the nutritional content of available feeder insects. See Chapter 44 for supplementation instructions and Chapter 41 for more information about insects as food. Supplements for hand-reared birds are given once a day on insects. These birds will do very poorly and fail to thrive when a blended formula is substituted. Feeder insects can be easily purchased in bulk; appropriate choices include small to medium mealworms, small to medium crickets, and waxworms. Insects need to be appropriately sized and also require proper care to remain healthy and nutritious. When buying or cultivating mealworms, do not use large or super-sized worms, as the skins are tough and difficult to digest. Mealworms should be made more nutritious by feeding them for at least 24 hours before feeding to chicks. The authors use a basic dry dog food plus carrots (JN) or poultry crumbles with carrots/yams (VB). Crickets are an excellent insect to feed. They also require proper care until used as food. Fluker Farms sells a cricket food and cricket gel for moisture that is nutritious and easy to offer, although some rehabilitators have concerns about the orange food coloring added to the gel; see Box 43.1 on keeping and feeding crickets within Chapter 43. Waxworms are another insect that can be offered; however, waxworms do not eat in this stage so cannot have their nutritional content improved by feeding. Waxworms should only be fed in conjunction with other insects and never fed solely as a diet.

## Feeding Procedures

Using hemostats, feed small or medium insects depending upon the size and age of the chick, killed before each feeding. Feed every 30–60 minutes, 12–14 hours a day. After every feeding, give as much water as the bird will take using a 1 cc syringe with a cannula tip on the end. Feathered swifts also enjoy being misted with a water bottle during hot temperatures, but this does not substitute for droplets from a syringe by mouth.

Saliva transfer is critical for the survival of hatchlings or any swift under 7 days old and will require saliva from a conspecific. Use a healthy older nestling, juvenile, or adult swift's saliva. Take an insect using a hemostat and swab the mouth of older swift with it, then remove it and feed it to the young bird. Swab at least once each feeding until feathers unfurl. Do NOT raise single swifts. Hatchlings that do not receive saliva transfer may be at higher risk for bacterial infections.

Chimney Swifts that are chattering and gaping can be a challenge to feed. In the wild, the parent flies down the chimney and feeds the young from below. The young hang their heads over the nest, chattering loudly, swinging their heads left or right. They do not open their mouth and keep it open; instead, they snap it open briefly and quickly between chatters.

In the rehabilitation setting, the birds will need to adjust to being fed from above. The younger the bird, the quicker the adjustment. Some adjust within just a few feedings. Fledgling/juvenile birds can take days or longer to make the adjustment. One method of easing the transition is to hold one hand over the bird with your thumb positioned near the bird's mouth. In your other hand, hold forceps with a balled up soaked (in water) waxworm (balled up waxworms or soaked cricket abdomens may simulate the ball of insects fed by the parents and are refused less often). When feeding crickets to very young swifts, kill the cricket, remove the wings and legs, and feed just the abdomen. Stick your thumb in its mouth when the bird snaps, holding it open long enough to give the food. Transition to soaked mealworms and then freshly killed mealworms, crickets, and waxworms. Feed every 30 minutes. Continue water droplets after every feeding. Hatchlings or any swift under 7 days old (unfeathered nestlings) require a small dab of nonfat plain yogurt on an insect at each feeding.

Assisted feeding may be necessary for birds who will not chatter or gape. Gently, being careful to avoid bill damage, use your fingernail to open the lower mandible and place the food. You may need to gently hold the bird's mouth closed until it swallows. Start with a drowned (in water) waxworm, torn open and balled up, then graduate to larger mouthfuls of waxworms in the same manner. Once eating these readily, try drowned mealworms, torn open mealworms, and then freshly killed mealworms and crickets (feed the abdomen only to nestlings), using a syringe afterwards to give water droplets. Feed at least 6–7, up to 10–12, mealworms, waxworms, or crickets at each feeding.

All immature swifts require time to adjust to being fed in captivity. Be patient, gentle, and understanding. Older fledglings and juveniles will arrive frightened and unwilling to accept food from hemostats. When chicks are reluctant gapers, make sure they are fully hydrated. If they are healthy, they can be placed with other healthy begging swifts. Waving a tissue above the birds to simulate the "wind" of the parent's wings can evoke a begging response. Sometimes a door closing or a similar noise will also work. Gently stroking a swift on the side or head can also result in gaping. Be ready and quick to get food in when they do gape. Adults need to be assist-fed until released.

Yeast infections can also be a cause of nongaping. Both Vaux's and White-throated Swifts are prone to yeast infections. Reluctance to gape, pale mouth color, and tacky/stringy saliva can be indications of a yeast infection. Diagnosis is by microscope examination of mouth and fecal swabs to look for budding oval organisms. Fluconazole (which seems more effective than nystatin) can be used to treat or can be administered prophylactically for the first week in care. See Hawkins et al. (2018) for dosing information.

Feeding techniques for Chimney Swifts are applicable to Vaux's Swifts too. However, White-throated Swifts can be a little tricky. In general, they are tactile and don't respond to feeding calls, whistles, or things waved in front of their face. They do respond to touch and vibration. To facilitate getting a reluctant White-throated to gape, place a thick hand towel with one end rolled or folded on a flat surface. Rest the swift's feet and upper body on the folded/rolled part of the towel, and place one hand over the bird's body so that four fingers are cupping one side of the body and the thumb tip is resting on the opposite side of the body at the commissure of the bill. With the other hand, secure an insect in a pair of hemostats. Most swifts mistake the thumb placed by its mouth for a parent swift approaching from the side to feed. When the young swift turns to put their mouth on the thumb, quickly stuff the insect on the hemostats into the swift's mouth. Eventually they get the idea and start accepting the food from the hemostats without having to be handled and removed from their basket/nest. If nongaping persists, gentle assist-feeding is required. Use extreme care when assist-feeding any bird, but especially a swift. The lower mandible is a thin, somewhat flexible rib of bone that is easily fractured when excess pressure or rough handling is applied.

Chimney Swifts are highly intelligent birds that will make direct eye contact with you. They are highly sensitive to your emotions. If you treat them with confidence, love, and gentle hands they will relax. If you become frustrated or angry, they will become equally stressed.

Once swifts are readily begging and eating, gradually increase the amount you feed on the forceps. Work up to six to seven mealworms at a time, or as much as you can hold in the forceps, and/or a couple of cricket abdomens and/or three to four waxworms. This makes feeding a quick and easy experience. Feed each bird as much as it will eat at each meal.

## Expected Weight Gain

Chimney and Vaux's Swifts hatch pink, blind, and naked, weighing 4.5–5.5 g. Shadows appear where pin feathers are to emerge. Pinfeathers are present by 7–8 days, when chicks weigh 12–13 g and nestlings still have their eyes closed. By 12–14 days old, chicks weigh 19–20 g and resemble a bristle brush or porcupine of quills, with eyes starting to open and feathers on the wings and back

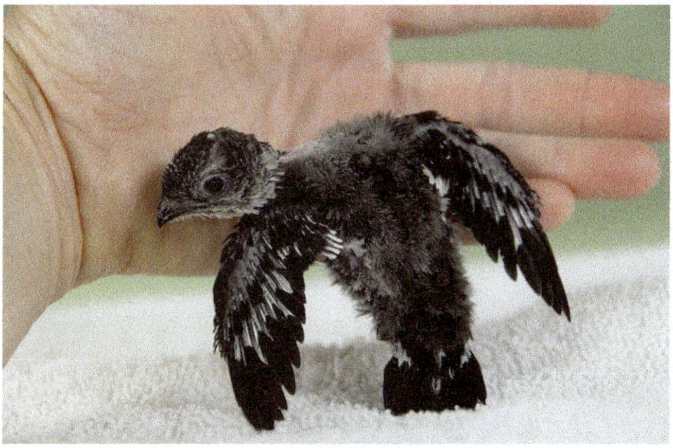

Figure 33.3 White-throated Swift nestling.

beginning to unfurl. At 18–20 days of age, chicks are fully feathered but those around the head are still in sheaths, eyes are fully open, and chicks weigh 24–25 g. White-throated Swifts mature similarly but are somewhat larger, with fledgling weights around 40 g (Figure 33.3).

## Housing

Hatchlings can be housed in a small, shallow bowl lined with soft cloth, placed in a small shoebox-sized container. Nestlings as they start to cling to more vertical surfaces can be housed in a small plastic rectangular set-up, with cloth secured at a gentle slope. Fledgling Chimney Swifts should be placed in an artificial chimney in an outdoor flight cage. Older juveniles or adults recovering from injury can be housed in reptariums, which can be used vertically while the birds are recovering, but watch for damage from tail feathers becoming abraded on the screening.

### Flight cage

**Chimney and Vaux's Swifts**

Swifts are the most aerial of all birds which means they are going to require a large flying space. They are only capable of clinging to vertical surfaces and will require suitable housing to cling to. Chimney use is important. Swifts in rehabilitation will require an artificial chimney to be raised in and to learn to navigate in and out of. Swifts need a large open space for flying, in order to be aerobically fit at release time. They require room to fly, turn on a dime, and maneuver honing their skills for fly-catching upon release. A flight cage of this size works well: 24 × 12 ft. (7.2 × 3.6 m), with height <8 ft. (2.4 m) lest you are unable to remove clinging birds at greater heights without a step ladder. Screen netting, and/or textured plywood (e.g. T1–11), is required on the interior for the birds to cling to vertically. They will also require an artificial/real chimney for roosting and feeding. When you transition fully feathered swifts outdoors, they should be placed, nest and all, in the bottom of the artificial chimney and allowed to climb up at will. Continue to feed every 30 minutes. An artificial chimney can be constructed using textured plywood. Make the structure about 20 in. (50 cm) square, and waist high. Use cinder blocks to adjust the height. Place in the center of the flight cage under solid roof. A brick and mortar chimney can also be constructed with the same

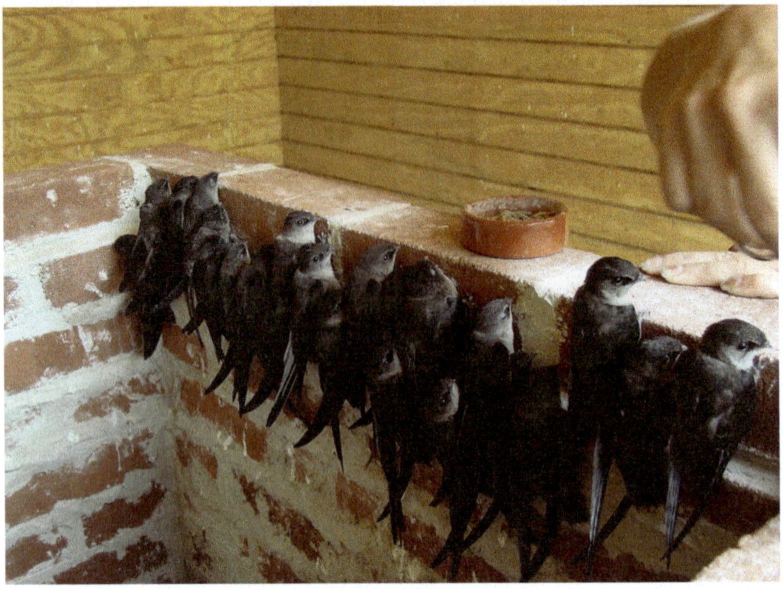

Figure 33.4 Chimney Swifts being fed in an artificial chimney within an aviary.

design; however, make a false bottom, with a drain that stands waist high (Figure 33.4). Place in the center of the flight cage under a solid roof.

Once outside, swifts begin to strengthen their wings by rearing back and practicing flapping. Their first flight usually takes them straight to the wall where they cling and look nervous, obviously overwhelmed at all the open space in relation to an enclosed and dark chimney.

Once swifts have begun flying out of the chimney, the birds will have to be collected off the walls and returned to the chimney for every feeding. This is going to encourage them to fly into the chimney to be fed when they see you and give them experience flying into and out of a chimney. Feedings are now every 60 minutes. In 1 week's time, swifts should begin flying into the chimney to be fed. All it takes is one bird and the others quickly learn. Now, they will gain practice and improve their ability flying into and out of the chimney. The fun begins! By week 2, swifts will be gaining confidence, strength, and ability, flying in and out of the chimney and chasing each other nonstop. Swifts will interact with you and you do not need to have any concerns regarding habituation or bonding. Always do a body check for clinging swifts before leaving the flight cage. Enjoy them! They are an amazing bird to have the privilege of having this up-close and getting personal interaction with.

#### White-throated Swifts

White-throateds appreciate a towel to hide under during nestling stage. They do not require an aviary for pre-release conditioning; however, access to an enclosed, large, safe space is required to confirm the bird can fly well before release. This species fledges the nest site fully flighted and capable of hunting alongside their parents on their first day of fledging.

At older nestling/pre-fledge stage, they will begin to wander from the nest and cling to vertical surfaces (Figure 33.5). They are not flight capable at this stage, but will soon begin to flap their wings and exercise. An extra-large laundry basket with interior sides lined with surgical towels, cotton or flannel sheet material, or other low-pile fabric is suitable at this point. However, as they

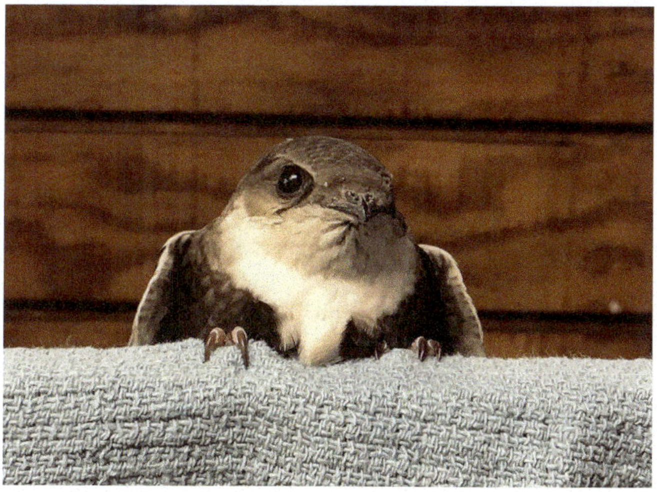

Figure 33.5 White-throated Swift perched on top of a cloth-covered caging wall.

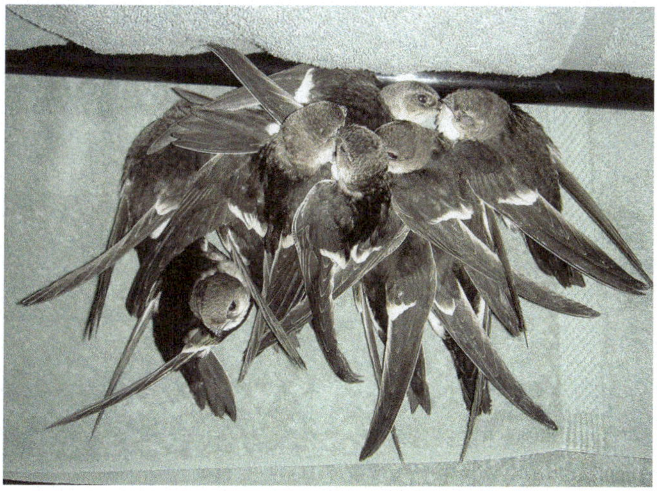

Figure 33.6 White-throated Swifts roosting together in a cloth-lined reptarium.

become more mobile, they will eventually require a slightly larger space, such as a 4 ft. (1.2 m) reptarium. Walls of the reptariums should be lined with fabric as previously described to prevent toenails from becoming caught on the reptarium mesh (Figure 33.6).

Alternatively, once fully feathered, they can be housed in an aviary as described above. In fact, White-throateds cohabitate very well with Vaux's and may be raised together. A word of caution: White-throateds are not flighted until they are almost 6 weeks old, so will likely climb out of the chimney and end up on the floor of the aviary, eventually making their way to a wall to climb up. Walk in the aviary carefully and take a mandatory headcount upon entering. They can somewhat utilize the space in a 24 ft. (7.2 m) aviary for flight, but it is awkward for them due to their large wingspan and unique takeoff and flight capabilities. But remember, it isn't really necessary to provide pre-release conditioning for this species.

## Release

### Chimney Swifts

Swifts need to be fully grown, meaning no visible feather sheaths on the underside of the wings. They must be waterproof, which means water will bead up on their feathers when misted. Swifts should be spending most of the day flying, able maneuver flawlessly, turn on a dime, and go in and out of the chimney. Swifts are a challenge to release; many factors must be met. Swifts cannot be soft released, but rather an active swift roost needs to be located where swifts are gathering socially and preparing to migrate prior to release. Check out potential sites the day before, about 1 hour or less before dark when they begin to gather in the area. The birds will require at least 3 days of clear weather. Birds will need to be transported to the release site, and should be released 1–3 hours before dusk. Never release at dusk! These birds have been confined to a flight cage for 2 weeks, flying with their tail spread to control their speed and unable to catch insects. Once released they are finally able to fly the way they are meant to and can catch diverse insects of their own choice. Give them plenty of time to adjust and enjoy their freedom. Releasing them when birds are circling to enter a roost at dusk is highly stressful and may result in failure. Even if there are not any swifts present at release, as long as you confirmed an active roost the day before, the juvenile swifts will stay close by and will soon be joined by others. When first released, swifts will flap hard, spiraling up in circles to get altitude, but soon will reach above the treetops and stretch out and fly the way they are meant to! Soon the jerky movements left and right will signal they are catching insects. I come back at dusk and count birds, otherwise stay until completely dark to be assured that all birds entered the chimney roost and count the roosting birds – which is great information to submit to the swift counts.

### Vaux's Swifts

In Western North America, massing and large roosts of Vaux's Swifts typically do not occur until late August/early September, which is well after orphans have fledged and their caregivers need to release them. A suitable release protocol for Vaux's is to release back to their natal site in the evening if parents are still present and utilizing the nest site as a roost, or release into a foraging flock of Vaux's Swifts during the day.

### White-throated Swifts

White-throated Swifts should be released late morning back to their natal site when other swifts are present, or into a foraging group of conspecifics located in the geographic area of the natal site.

## Acknowledgments

Our sincere gratitude to the amazing passerines whose beauty and song grace this earth each day.

## Sources of Products Mentioned

Crickets: Fluker Farms, P.O. Box 530, Port Allen, LA 70767–4087, (225) 343–7035, https://flukerfarms.com/.

Ultracare Mite and Lice Bird Spray: 8 in 1 Pet Products, Hauppauge, NY, (800) 645-5154.
LLLReptile and Supply Company Inc., 609 Mission Ave, Oceanside, CA 92054, (760) 439-8492, www.lllreptile.com.

## References


Duerr, R.S., Purdin, G.J., and Bowers, V. (2017). Small-bodied birds: Passerines, doves, woodpeckers, others. In: *Topics in Wildlife Medicine, Vol. 4: Orthopedics* (eds. R.S. Duerr and G.J. Purdin), 53–74. St. Cloud, MN: National Wildlife Rehabilitators Association.

Gill, F. and Donsker, D. (eds.). (2018). IOC World Bird List (v8.1). doi: https://doi.org/10.14344/IOC.ML.8.1.

Hawkins, M.G., Barron, H.W., Speer, B.L. et al. (2018). Birds. In: *Exotic Animal Formulary*, 5e (eds. J.W. Carpenter and C.J. Marion), 167–375. St. Louis, MO: Elsevier.

Hedenstrom, A., Norevik, G., Warfvinge, K. et al. (2016). Annual 10-month aerial life phase in the Common Swift *Apus apus*. *Current Biology* 26: 3066–3070.

# 34

# Hummingbirds

*Elizabeth Penn (Penny) Elliston*

## Natural History

American ornithologist Robert Ridgeway captured the uniqueness of hummingbirds when he wrote, "Of all the numerous groups into which the birds are divided there is none other so numerous in species, so varied in form, so brilliant in plumage, and so different from all others in their mode of life" (Johnsgard 1983). There are over 300 species in the family Trochilidae, all of which are found in the Western hemisphere. Most occur in South America (although several of the southern species occasionally stray north into the U.S.), and at least 23 species in five genera occur regularly in North America, from the southern states to Alaska (Johnsgard 1983).

Hummingbirds are perching birds in the order Apodiformes. They typically fly anywhere they desire to go, using their feet only for perching. Wing use is unique to the family Trochilidae in that the shoulder structure allows a rotational, or sculling, motion of the wings. This enables the bird to hover for long periods and even fly backward, an ability possessed by no other type of bird.

Hummingbirds eat nectar found in a wide variety of flowers and feeders provided by humans. For over a century, it has been known that they also consume large numbers of tiny insects and spiders (Bendire 1895; Bent 1940; Scheithauer 1967; Camfield et al. 2013; Healy and Calder 2006; Baltosser and Scott 1996; Weidensaul et al. 2019; Baltosser and Russell 2000). A bird may perch to gather nectar or hover while feeding.

It has long been believed that hummingbirds draw nectar by capillary action up into the tongue and squeeze it into the crop, but new studies and techniques have produced new hypotheses. Alejandro Rico-Guevara's (Rico-Guevara and Rubega 2011; Rico-Guevara 2017) intricate examination of the hummingbird bill and tongue suggest that the tongue is "a fluid trap, not a capillary tube." The trap is formed by forces including "surface tension, Laplace pressure, and the elastic properties of the keratinous materials making up the tongue tip" and the perfect way the tongue fits the surrounding bill. This produces a much more rapid and efficient means of drinking. However, Rico Guevara also concluded that much additional research is needed to completely understand how the birds ultimately ingest nectar.

Insects are obtained by hawking, and reportedly also by gleaning. Scheithauer (1967) described some captive hummingbirds as using a "hazing" behavior, in which the bird flushes the insect into the air before catching it. Gleaning appears uncommon at best (the author has observed it only rarely in captive Black-chinned hummingbirds), and caregivers should not assume that the species they are housing will glean enough unflighted insects to fulfill dietary requirements.

*Hand-Rearing Birds*, Second Edition. Edited by Rebecca S. Duerr and Laurie J. Gage.

These birds typically nest in feltlike cups that are made of plant fibers, down, fur, and cotton and are lined on the outside with lichen, bark, paint chips, or similar materials. Females lay two eggs about a day apart but begin incubating immediately, which results in an asynchronous hatch. Incubation can last from 12 to 19 days (14 days is the most common), and its length is probably influenced by the weather. The young are altricial, with closed eyes and naked black skin decorated by a few filamentous white or yellowish feathers on the head and along the back-feather tracts. They typically fledge at about 21 days but remain dependent on their mother for as long as 14 days after leaving the nest. Males do not participate in family life beyond copulation.

## Criteria for Intervention

Hummingbirds brought into captivity fall into three major categories. The first of these comprises adults with wing or other injuries (from a collision with a window, an interaction with a cat, or some other trauma) that has rendered them nonflighted. These mishaps commonly occur during summer months in North America; hummingbirds injured this way may or may not recover flight with little treatment other than a safe place to rest, remain still, and recuperate.

The second category consists of uninjured orphaned fledglings. These are birds that have left the nest but have not yet become independent. Overzealous people concerned about the fledglings' wellbeing may kidnap them, or the birds may be true orphans whose mothers have met with some mishap. These birds are typically capable of flight, but their bills have not grown to full length. In addition, they may be making the high frequency "peep" call used so their mothers can locate them (Elliston and Baltosser 1995). Birds in this category can easily be brought to release stage with proper nutritional support and foraging practice.

Populating the third group are nestlings, which have come to the attention of people and been brought into care. These birds are rarely "kidnapped," because people tend to attentively watch the nest and remove the young only when it is apparent that something has gone wrong. Indications of imminent nest failure are the nonreturn of the mother to feed the young every hour or so, her failure to cover the naked birds at night, and the young calling from the nest. Not infrequently, the young are found on the ground, calling and seemingly unable to fly, usually because they have fallen from the nest, likely because of agitation arising from food deprivation (Elliston 1995).

## Record Keeping

Detailed information on the date and where the bird was found should be recorded. A record of location serves as a guide to suitable habitat for release and also for placing the bird back where its genetic pool already occurs. The date will be of interest if the bird becomes a museum specimen or for species breeding records.

Pertinent data should be recorded as they are observed so that details for each bird will be preserved. For unflighted juvenile hummingbirds, this may include daily body weights, length of bill (exposed culmen) in millimeters, progress of treatments, record of food given, and notes on behavior.

Wildlife regulatory agencies have minimum record-keeping standards mandating that individual animals be tracked while undergoing rehabilitation, so check with your regulating agencies for pertinent information. At a minimum, the following information should be kept: date and location found, species (when known), age (when determined), reason brought into captivity, initial condition assessment, final disposition, and release location. There is often confusion between reason for acquisition and initial condition. *Reasons* can include such things as apparently abandoned (in hummingbirds, calling from nest or parent not seen for ~12 hours), found on ground, rescued from predator, or "kidnapped." *Condition* includes such things as dehydration, out of nest, cold, starving, etc. Every attempt should be made to keep these categories distinct.

A detailed medical record should be kept on each animal, with results of the initial examination recorded and any updates added as they happen. When large numbers of diverse species are being raised en masse with different caregivers, it is useful to have a "feeding instructions" sheet that tells the next caregiver what to feed and any tips for food delivery. A chart for recording the actual time of each feeding and how much was fed is invaluable.

## Initial Care and Stabilization

As is true for all types of baby birds, the main goals of initial care are warmth, rehydration, and feeding, in that order. Hummingbirds that are in pinfeathers (~14 days of age), feathered, or perching and too old to display gaping behavior, are probably able to regulate their own temperature and thus need only temporary warming until their behavior indicates that they are normothermic. Then they must be persuaded to drink an isotonic rehydrating solution before hypertonic nutrition is offered. For the initial stages of rehydration, 5% dextrose will suffice and will provide a tiny bit of nutrition. This isotonic fluid tastes acceptable to the bird (if a fluid does not taste good to the bird, it will refuse to drink). Gavage for hummingbirds is possible, but it is highly undesirable, so persuasion is the best route. Once the bird passes some fluid droppings, feedings can commence.

For hummingbirds that are naked or in early pinfeathers, adequate heat is extremely important. Newly hatched hummingbirds can weigh as little as 250 mg, so heat loss is rapid. Also, because of the birds' tiny size, hot and cool spots in incubators dictate how much heat they are actually receiving. Measuring heat with an indoor–outdoor wire probe-style thermometer (available at many home and garden stores) in the nest and under the birds is an effective way of monitoring the birds' temperatures. Placing nestlings in a natural nest in an incubator at 100 °F (37.7 °C) and covering with a small piece of flannel may provide adequate heat for all but the tiniest of chicks. If a bird heated to that temperature fails to gape, the heat can be increased to register as high as 104 °F on the probe under the bird. At that temperature, the nestling usually kicks off the covering blanket. Under all these conditions of high heat, it is important to also monitor humidity in the chamber. A wide-mouth jar containing water and a cotton wick should keep the air adequately moist. Warm hydrating fluid can be introduced into the gaping bird with any tiny plastic catheter placed on the end of a 1 ml syringe. The response of a healthy vigorous nestling will be to "climb" the catheter with the pulsing pumping motion observable in parent-fed birds. Depending on the size of the bird, amounts of fluid from 0.05–0.5 ml can be given at each feeding. Observation of the crop, easily visible around the neck, can aid in determining what volume to give (Figure 34.1). Though hummingbirds manage their liquid food very well, it is better to underfill than overfill a tiny crop. Because these birds are gaping and won't taste the food, they can immediately be given a hydrating solution containing electrolytes, such as lactated Ringer's solution (LRS) or a mixture of LRS and 5% dextrose. When they look plump and start passing wet droppings, they can be fed insects and a nutritious fluid diet.

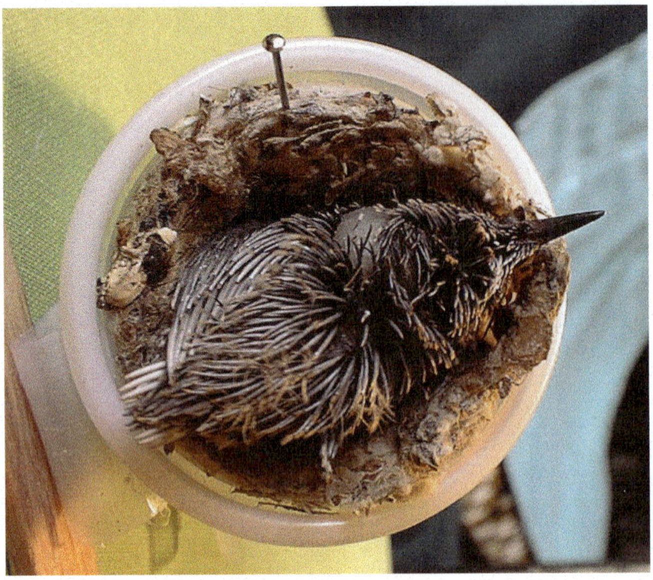

Figure 34.1 Black-chinned Hummingbird nestling. Note the full crop visible at the neck, plus many feathers still in quills. Hummingbirds do well when kept in their original nest inside another container.

## Common Medical Problems and Solutions

A common problem for orphaned or injured hummingbirds coming into care is that they are covered with sugar water from finders' attempts to feed them. Nestlings may often be stuck to the nest, which can interfere with their movement or even excretory functions. It is important to free the young birds with warm water as soon as they have been stabilized, and to clean their feathers and vents. Then, be aware that each bird's vent must be kept clean until the caregiver is confident that the bird is regularly lifting its behind and defecating out of the nest.

Young hummingbirds rarely present with medical conditions. There have been occasional anecdotal reports of cases of trichomonas in flighted birds and outbreaks of microsporidia in nestlings in care. These can be treated with one of the nitroimidazoles, when detected (Diane Waters, pers. comm.). Fungal spores and *Escherichia coli* are not uncommon in examinations of fecal smears, but unless some symptoms are evident, the best treatment is usually good nutrition and supportive care. If a self-feeding bird is holding its tongue out continually or shows signs of growth on the tongue, a drop of miconazole lotion (Butler Schein) in 3 cc liquid food may be used to address the condition (Trish Mazolini DVM, pers. comm.). Oral nystatin is also used for yeast infections (Hawkins et al. 2018).

Feather mites, which usually appear late in the season, are a common parasite in hummingbird nests. They can be treated by removing the nestlings from the nest, treating the nest with a miticide such as Kelthane (Dow Agrosciences), and returning the birds to the nest. Residual mite poison in the nest usually takes care of any mites remaining on the birds, and this poison, which is very specific to mites, is unlikely to harm the birds. If the parasites seem to be excessive on a feathered bird, one remedy is to gently wipe a cotton-tipped swab dampened in miticide over the outer feathers, especially at the top of the head.

Another mite, Ascidae, is sometimes found on nestling hummingbirds. This type was first described by Baker and Yunker in 1964, and now has grown to 60 described species. These little mites can be seen clustered around the nares, running to the tip of the bill when the bird opens its mouth, and running back to the top of the bill when the bird closes its mouth. They are often yellow, pink, or brownish, and are flower mites – they eat the nectar and pollen of particular flowers and hitch a ride from flower to flower on visiting hummingbirds (Baker and Yunker 1964). Once these mites get off onto a nestling bird, where there are no flowers, they live only a few days. Thus, the birds need no treatment other than time or perhaps a damp cotton swab to remove the mites.

## Diet Recipes

The first priority of a newly hatched bird is to build its skeleton and organs and, concurrently, to develop the feathers that will cover and insulate its body and provide the tools needed for flight. Poor quality feathers in a hummingbird are a life-threatening condition; if the bird cannot fly, it cannot catch the flying insects required, nor can it travel to gather the nectar needed to fuel its engines. As early as 1890, Ridgway observed that the mother hummingbird almost exclusively fed small arthropods to hatchlings (Johnsgard 1983). Inadequate plumage has been the most apparent problem for rehabilitators raising very small hatchlings.

Development of an optimal diet for the youngest of hummingbirds is an ongoing effort. Although a number of details on the components of suggested diets are clear, there have always been problems collecting adequate growth data to rank the recipes. Either people keep meticulous data but get too few birds to compare results, or people get numerous birds but are too busy raising them to collect the necessary data, or people have data but do not make them available to others. In any case, the work goes on, and the hope is that those raising baby hummingbirds will make every effort to communicate with others regarding new findings.

Regrettably, by 2018, Abbott labs had stopped making Vital HN, which was a heavily used, highly palatable ingredient in hummingbird diets when the first edition of this book was written. Abbott now produces a canned liquid diet that contains whey (Vital HP) and therefore more protein. One might hope that the addition of whey protein to what is purported to be a diet similar to the powdered diet and producing it as a liquid would save rehabilitators time in diet preparation. However, the birds appear to find the Vital HP diet noticeably less palatable based on personal experience and communications with other rehabilitators. They will drink the fluid, mixed in varying concentrations and with varying amounts of sugar, if it is the only food they are offered. However, given a choice of these preparations and plain 1:4 sucrose in water, they invariably prefer the sugar water. [Editor's note: Vital HP also contains cellulose gel and gum, which may cause intestinal passage problems in hummingbirds (Kirk Klasing, pers. comm.). Vital HN did not include these ingredients. Several rehabilitators have reported abdominal bloating in young chicks fed Vital HP.]

An alternative diet can be made by simply replacing the no longer available Vital HN with Vivonex® Plus (Nestle), which comes in both unflavored and powdered forms. After one season of trial, Vivonex Plus seems to be an adequate replacement. Juvenile and older birds accept it readily, and the nutritional contents are very similar to the formerly used Vital HN (Table 34.1).

It is important to remember that any human elemental powder (such as Vivonex Plus) is used only to ensure that sufficient calories are being delivered to a *very* small bird, and that the major food component for hummingbirds should always be invertebrates (insects, other tiny arthropods) in the greatest achievable quantities. Protein is what enables the bird to grow its essential strong feathers. A hummingbird without strong feathers will not survive in the wild.

Table 34.1 Vivonex® Plus/whey/sugar recipe for fledglings and unflighted adults.

| Ingredient | Amount |
|---|---|
| Water | 75 ml |
| Vivonex Plus powder | 4 g |
| Granulated table sugar | 25 g |
| Whey, powdered 100% concentrate | 1.8 g |
| *Mix the above and freeze as ice cubes* | |
| *Thaw enough for each day and add per 10 ml:* | |
| Yogurt, plain live-culture[a] | 0.5 ml (~10 drops) |
| 5 : 1 cod liver oil, vitamin E oil, mixed | 1 drop |
| B complex plus C tablet, crushed | Small pinch, to turn solution light lemon-yellow color |
| *Add the following to the diet of any growing or skeletal-injury bird:* | |
| Calcium glubionate (23 mg/ml) | 0.25 ml |

[a] Though some feel that the addition of a probiotic such as Lactobacillus acidophilus and its yogurt-producing relatives is beneficial, this author feels that adding a live bacillus to a rich medium is asking for contamination issues.

Caregivers may find the task of sticking "bites" of insects into a hummingbird's throat via forceps to be daunting. Blending or grinding the insect component in the liquid component may be a better route. However, one must then remember that very small birds need lots of hydration in order to avoid the risk of dehydration. The way to rectify this issue is to add more water. The most reliable way to determine whether a hummingbird is adequately hydrated is to pay close attention to its naked skin, making sure there are no wrinkles, and to its feeding behavior, which should be vigorous.

## Hatchlings and Nestlings

If one is starting with a 250 mg chick, it is unlikely that human implements can introduce many of even the smallest of insects into the crop. It would be difficult to deliver the 0.77 kcal per day in insects necessary to provide adequate nutrition to this growing bird. Three versions of a liquid food can be fed with the use of a tiny intravenous catheter that acts as a substitute for the mother's bill, including a recipe based on Liquid Vivonex Plus (Table 34.2), one based on Nektar Plus with whey (Table 34.3), or a mix containing Vivonex Plus, Nektar-Plus (Nekton Products), and whey (Table 34.4). These liquid foods, containing only the carbohydrates present in the commercial preparations (no extra sugar), alternated with insect slurry, can be introduced into the crop and will suffice to get the bird started. Since at this age the bird is receiving gavage, palatability is not an issue. The recipe shown in Table 34.3, when alternated with feedings of insect slurry, has proven successful at Wildlife Rescue of NM for very tiny birds until they stop gaping (Christy Brant, pers. comm.).

These liquid diets can pass through the very tiniest of catheters. As the bird grows, and larger catheters can be used, tiny insects that may have a greater particulate component than ground

Table 34.2 Hatchling Recipe Option 1: Vivonex® Plus.

| Ingredient | Amount |
|---|---|
| Water | 33 ml |
| Vivonex Plus powder | 8 g |
| B complex plus C tablet, crushed | 1/20 tablet, to turn solution light lemon-yellow color |
| Supplemented oil (see Table 34.6) | 0.025 ml |
| Yogurt, plain live culture[a] | 0.05 ml per ml diet fed |

[a] Though some feel that the addition of a probiotic such as Lactobacillus acidophilus and its yogurt-producing relatives is beneficial, this author feels that adding a live bacillus to a rich medium is asking for contamination issues.

Table 34.3 Hatchling Recipe Option 2: Nektar Plus with whey.

| Ingredient | Amount |
|---|---|
| Water | 30 ml |
| Nektar Plus | 1 tsp |
| Nekton I vitamins | 1/8 tsp |
| Whey powder | 1/16 tsp |

Table 34.4 Hatchling Recipe Option 3: Vivonex® Plus, Nekar Plus, and whey.

| Ingredient | Amount |
|---|---|
| Water | 50 ml |
| Nektar Plus | 6.5 g |
| Vivonex Plus | 1.5 g |
| Whey protein isolate | 2 g |

insect larvae can be added to the slurry or to the fluid mix. As with all baby birds, diverse foods are always beneficial. "White" mosquito larvae, fruit flies, and dried versions of these – all are good foods. Frozen tropical fish dealers have a variety of such foods to choose from. Cricket powder can also be obtained commercially and is a very finely ground insect material. The innards of mealworms are not recommended because they seem to make the birds logy and unresponsive. It is beneficial to add some recently live insects to the mixture to provide certain enzymes and microbes that may not be present in the dried or preserved foods.

Tiny arthropods such as fruit flies, midges, leaf hoppers, or even brine shrimp can be fed whole with forceps to gaping birds. The chitinous coverings of any of these little animals all break down into tiny plates that can be digested without problems by baby hummingbirds.

"Bloodworms," which are actually midge larvae (blood, red, or black), may be either live or frozen, and should be drained on a paper towel before weighing. Crush the worms with a mortar and pestle. Grind ingredients together, mixing well, and draw into a 1 ml syringe. Freeze stock and keep amount in use very cold. A very small container in an ice-filled thermos is an excellent way to keep this food very cold between feedings.

Any form of calcium supplementation may be used that can be measured precisely enough to add the elemental calcium required. Calcium glubionate comes in a convenient pediatric suspension that provides 23 mg/ml.

Various other diets have been reported as successfully used for raising young hummingbirds. It is the author's opinion, however, that successful feather development cannot be achieved unless the foods contain large amounts of animal protein with the amino acid profile required for a growing insectivore (MacLeod and Perlman 2001). Indeed, personal communications with numerous rehabilitators have revealed poor outcomes using commercial diets based on soy protein for both hummingbirds and passerines (Elliston and Perlman 2002). The author strongly recommends against using any commercial hummingbird diets that contain significant amounts of soy protein. These diets have been known to cause gastrointestinal stasis in young hummingbirds and do not provide adequate types or quantities of protein for growing birds (Elliston and Perlman 2002). Although these products may be more convenient to make, the younger the bird in question is started on these inadequate diets the higher the probability that they will grow substandard feathering or suffer greater mortality rates. Nektar-Plus is meant only for adult birds and is inappropriate for growing chicks without the additional supplemental animal-based slurries suggested. Because hummingbirds have evolved eating insects, there is little reason to believe they can utilize the vegetable protein provided by soybeans.

### Fledglings and Adults

If fledgling and adult food contains 20 mg/ml of protein, eating 5 ml/day will provide the approximate amount needed to sustain an adult's protein requirements. It has been observed that the older the bird is, the more personal the preference may be for sweetness. Adjustments for taste may be needed with small additions of sugar to coax the bird into readily drinking presently available diets.

## Feeding Procedures

The best way to approach meeting the nutritional needs of hummingbird chicks may be to just do what the mother hummingbird does: stuff the little crops with insects at every opportunity. Begin each day with fresh diet. Refrigerate all liquid diets between feedings, or keep the day's food in a thermos filled with ice. Whey is available in several consistencies, and individual measuring spoons may vary considerably. It is important to weigh powders until the relationship of volume to weight has been established for each individual's equipment.

Some rehabilitators have adopted the technique of putting insects in the fluid to deliver by syringe (Van Epps 1999). Because some birds may regurgitate when fed insects mixed into their liquid diet, the author prefers to use catheters that are too small to pass whole insects (except daphnia, the water flea) and to feed whole insects with forceps (Figure 34.2). Accurate assessment of a bird's tolerance for solids in the crop, and maintenance of hydration, is possible by feeding solids and fluid separately. However, another option is to create a slurry by grinding insects and adding an appropriate amount of calcium to balance the phosphorus content of the insects (0.03 ml 23 mg/ml calcium glubionate per 100 mg insects fed) (Table 34.5). There may be fewer problems if the slurry and Vivonex Plus mix are fed alternately as the crop empties.

As the caregiver and bird become accustomed to the feeding techniques, feeding becomes easier to accomplish. Packing the crop first with insect and arthropod slurry until the bird ceases to gape, and adding vitamin-enriched liquid elemental protein mix, if the bird will accept it, every

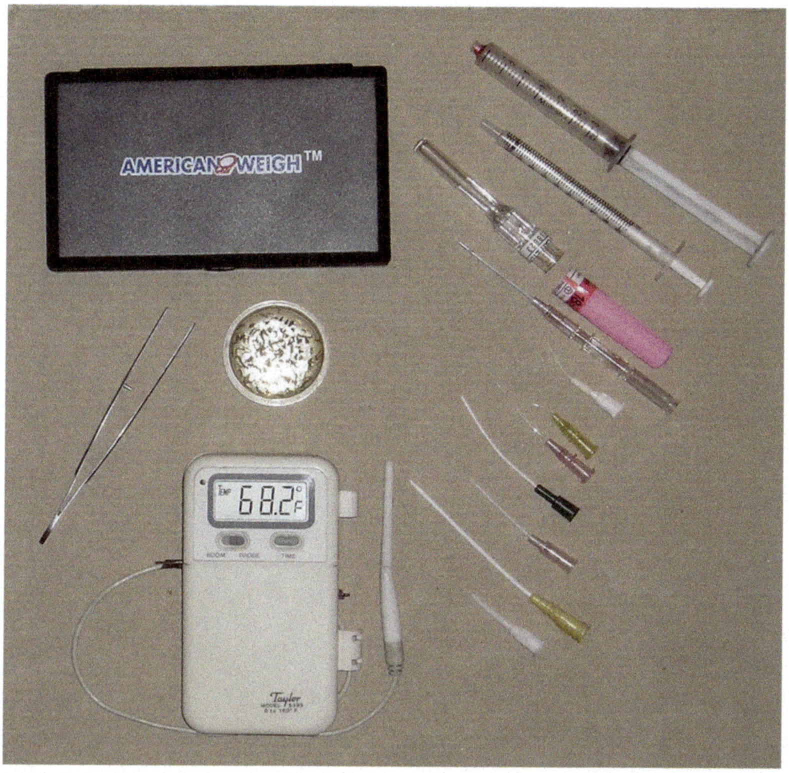


Figure 34.2 Clockwise from top left: American Weigh scale, 3 cc syringe with tip shortened and colored with red nail polish, 1 cc O-ring syringe, a variety of intravenous catheters to be used as feeding implements (shown are 18–24 gauge), white plastic irrigation cannula, digital thermometer with probe, feeding forceps with a small dish of tiny insects.

Table 34.5 Hatchling and nestling recipe: Insect slurry.

| Ingredient | Amount |
|---|---|
| "Bloodworms" and mosquito larvae | 2 g |
| Supplemented calcium glubionate (see Table 34.7) | 0.60 ml |
| Yogurt, plain live culture[a] | Toothpick-tip-sized amount per ml fed |

[a] Though some feel that the addition of a probiotic such as Lactobacillus acidophilus and its yogurt-producing relatives is beneficial, this author feels that adding a live bacillus to a rich medium is asking for contamination issues.

30–60 minutes or as the crop empties, becomes an easy routine. Insects and slurry are digested more slowly than fluid nutrients. As the day progresses, the bird may accept less insect material and more liquid protein mix at a feed. If the crop slows and fails to empty, feed water and liquid protein mix until the crop is moving well again (Figure 34.3).

Liquid food can be offered in 3 ml syringes. Any food mix containing protein and other nutrients is more susceptible to bacterial and fungal growth than is water or sugar alone, and it should be monitored carefully for signs of spoilage. Dripping is a sign of gas formation and fermentation. The birds will not eat something that tastes at all sour. They will starve first.

Table 34.6 Supplemented oil.

| Ingredient | Amount |
|---|---|
| Fish body oil (omega 3) | 7 drops |
| Cod liver oil | 2 drops |
| Vitamin E | 1 drop |

Table 34.7 Supplemented calcium glubionate.

| Ingredient | Amount |
|---|---|
| Calcium glubionate (23 mg/ml) | 10 ml |
| B complex plus C tablet, crushed | 1/20 tablet, to turn solution light lemon-yellow color |
| Supplemented oil | 1 tiniest drop |

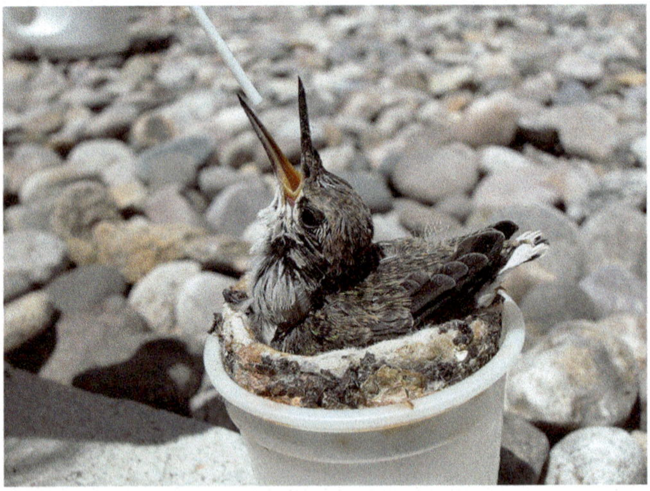

Figure 34.3 A Black-chinned Hummingbird chick gaping for a meal. Note the size of the feeding catheter in relation to the chick's bill. *Source:* photo courtesy of Mark Gruber.

Mother hummingbirds regurgitate the contents of their crop into their young. Healthy young hummingbirds can be observed to open their bills at the approach of their mother and make vigorous "pumping" movements in accepting their mother's bills. As with many baby birds, the key to getting them to gape is to find the appropriate stimulus. Blowing on them prior to feeding seems to do the trick. As the mother hummingbird approaches, the movement of her wings agitates the filoplumes on the smallest of birds, which stimulates gaping. When the bird is gaping and reaching up, a "pinch" of insects in the tip of a pair of blunt-eye forceps can be plunged down the throat into the crop. Slightly release the grip on the insects and allow the motion of the feeding bird to dislodge them from the forceps. Remove the forceps and repeat the feeding procedure until the bird ceases to gape. The author has found that the best posture for this kind of feeding is to brace the forearm on a flat surface adjacent to the bird in its nest such that the arm can act as a lever over the bird.

Holding the forceps or syringe directly over the bird, bring it down ready to plunge into the gape. Then blow on the bird. A syringe tipped with a catheter of appropriate size can be used in the same way and is, initially, easier to manipulate.

## Hatchlings

Hatchlings should be fed every 20–30 minutes for 12–14 hours a day, whenever they gape. Chicks should never be overstimulated or forced. A 1 ml syringe with an IV catheter tip of 18 gauge or smaller makes an excellent feeding implement for fluid food or slurry. Attach the tip securely to avoid the possibility of it disconnecting and making a mess on the bird. Administer the food in a controlled manner while the bird is actively accepting the food. Watch the crop increase in size, and stop delivery before it becomes too full. Occasionally, fluid may well up into the mouth and be swallowed again. This is not a matter of concern because healthy young hummingbirds can control fluid intake very successfully. It is better to give both solid and fluid food in small increments until the bird refuses to gape than to overfill in one application, which may cause some distress or, worse, aspiration.

If a bird with an empty crop refuses food, reevaluate the temperature, hydration status, and physical condition. Check the vent to ensure that it is clean and not stuck to the nest.

## Nestlings and Fledglings

Fully and partially feathered birds should be fed every hour or when they gape for 12–14 hours a day. When the bird is large enough, bite sizes of about five fruit flies stuck together with water can be delivered with blunt-tipped eye dressing forceps. Care must be taken to get the tip of the forceps far down past the glottis, because the tongue rarely helps in swallowing insects. If the solid material is not placed far enough into the crop, the tongue will bring the particle out and wipe it off. Birds with open eyes will learn to distinguish between the forceps with solid food and the catheter with fluid food. Typically, they will open their mouths for insects until they have received enough, but will gape again when offered fluid food. The fluid food can be used to fill up the crop when insects or slurry are rejected. When whole insects are fed, calcium, in the levels noted above, should also be included in the liquid component of the daily diet (0.03 ml of 23 mg/ml calcium glubionate for every 100 mg insects).

If young hummingbirds are received fully feathered and perching, they are unlikely to gape for anyone but their mother. It is here that palatability becomes an issue. They can quickly be taught to self-feed with the presentation of a 3 ml syringe containing a food, if they like the taste. Though they will readily accept a proven food source, it may be helpful to initially present the tip of the syringe with some kind of color. The tip of the syringe can be painted red, a bright piece of yarn can be tied around the tip, or a bright piece of cellophane can be stuck on the syringe. Since young birds have fairly short fat bills, slicing the tip of a luer syringe to about 1/4 its length, or boring out the hole in the syringe, provides better access to the food. Another syringe containing plain water should also be placed within reach.

Hummingbirds have very wet droppings that they typically eject over the edge of the nest. Fecal boli should appear very black and bulky with a spot of white urates on top. The bolus is ejected in copious amounts of urine. Try to keep the nest and surroundings clean and dry.

A culture of flying fruit flies should be made available to flighted birds so that they will learn through practice how to catch small insects. As they become proficient at foraging and consume more flies, intake of the protein-rich liquid food will diminish, and plain nectar or water consumption may rise.

## Expected Weight Gain

Because hummingbirds may start life outside the egg at a weight of well under 1 g, a triple beam or "gram scale" balance will not be accurate enough to measure growth reliably. An electronic balance that weighs a maximum capacity of 200 g in gradations of 0.01 g can be obtained from American Weigh™, among other places, for a price in the neighborhood of $50.00 (as of early 2019). A standard analytic pan balance can also be used. Because a bird may grow in increments of 100–900 mg a day, depending on age, this will provide an appropriate level of accuracy.

Weights must be taken before the first feeding in the morning because the crop can contain a significant proportion of the bird's weight. Defecation in a bird of this size can also reduce its weight by as much as 30–50%. Hummingbirds should gain weight daily and reach or exceed the adult weight for the species at about 14 days of age. This may be as little as 3 g for smaller species and up to about 5 g for Anna's Hummingbirds. By 10–12 days of age, the young will be covered with pinfeathers and, in nature, the parent ceases to sit on them at night. By 14 days of age, the weight reaches a plateau. If a bird is not gaining weight or is calling from the nest persistently, there is something seriously wrong and the feeding and housing regimen should be evaluated.

## Housing

Hatchlings should be kept at 90–95 °F (32.2–35 °C) or somewhat higher (see "Initial Care and Stabilization," above) and at 40–50% humidity. Nestling hummingbirds are very intimately associated with their nests, and hummingbirds may be the only species for which keeping them in or replacing them into a natural nest is desirable (Figure 34.4). If the nest is infested with ectoparasites, the birds can be removed (peeled out), the nest treated as mentioned in "Common Medical Problems," above, and the birds returned. When daily weights are taken, it is preferable to allow the birds to remain in the nest, weighing the whole thing. After the birds fledge, a tare weight can be obtained. Using these two methods of weighing may result in a slight variance in the actual

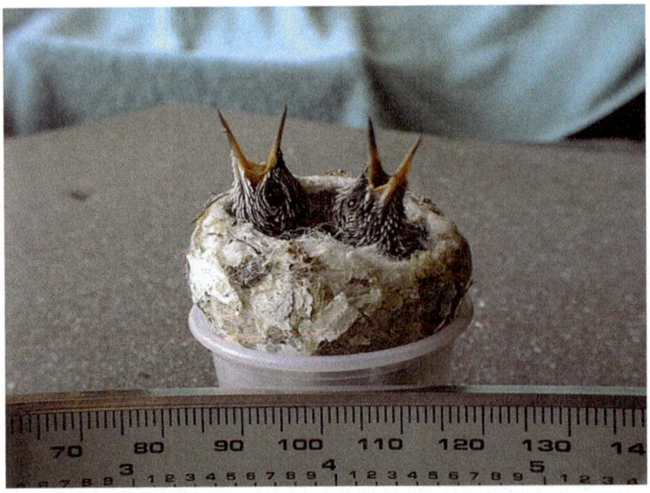


Figure 34.4 A very young Black-chinned Hummingbird chick with a chick nearing weaning age.

growth record, but it is unlikely to be more than a few milligrams – and a good visual assessment of growth can be obtained during the nestling phase.

An alternative method for weighing nestlings relies on the use of a scrap of single-ply toilet paper to line the nest. The bird is lifted from the nest in its liner "hammock," the liner with the bird in it is weighed, and the bird is rolled out of its hammock back into the nest, where a new, clean replacement liner has been placed. This method tends to result in more accuracy of weight for a very small bird (250–1500 mg) because an accurate tare weight can be obtained each time.

Hummingbirds become able to control their body temperature at 10–14 days of age. At this point, the mother stops covering them at night in the wild, so they can be removed from an incubator in care. Safety is still a major concern for these tiny young and thus should be considered. For example, rodents patrolling the care facilities at night can easily eat them.

At 19–20 days of age, the birds in their nests should be placed in a secure enclosure so that they will be safely confined when they fledge. When a nestling hummingbird takes its first flight, it starts by buzzing its wings while hanging onto the edge of the nest. At some point, it lets go of the nest and shoots off in an uncontrolled direction. If it is unconfined while in care, there is no telling where it will land – behind the refrigerator or filing cabinet, or in the toilet. In the wild, it will vanish. It may sit where it has landed for several days, or it may experiment again within hours. But it has little control of its flight and is completely dependent on its mother for food. It is at this stage of increased mobility that, under optimal circumstances in nature, the bird begins to "peep" to call its mother. In care, it is important that during these first few days out of the nest, the bird's food be placed where it is easy to reach. As a bird becomes more competent in managing its flight capabilities, food can be placed where the bird must hover to reach it (Figure 34.5). In addition, a flying fruit fly culture should be introduced.

The enclosure can start at a relatively small size and be increased as the birds acquire flight proficiency. Unlimited activity aviaries should be at least 2×4×6 ft. (0.6×1.2×1.8 m) or provide an equivalent flight volume (Miller 2012). Over the next 14 days, the birds will learn to be proficient

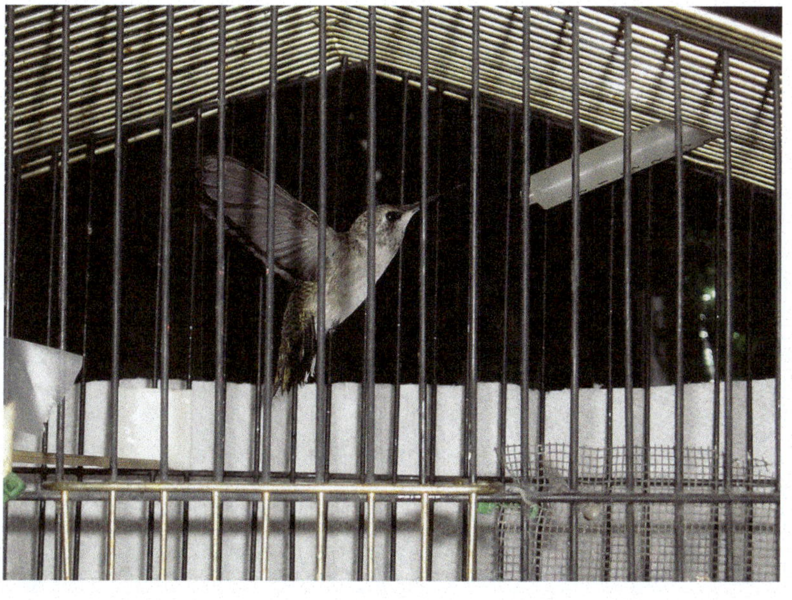

Figure 34.5 Fledgling hovering to eat from a syringe.

flyers, to hover as they feed, to feed from a variety of sources, and to catch insects. Their housing should be enlarged as they learn and become skilled, resulting in release from a final large outdoor aviary.

If two or more fledglings are housed together, they will sit shoulder to shoulder at night. As they age, become more successful at foraging, and experience their hormones beginning to flow, males may become more antagonistic toward other residents of the enclosure. Sufficient syringes of food should be placed to ensure adequate intake by all birds.

## Weaning

At about 19–20 days, the birds can be trained to self-feed. In order to persuade them to drink the food, sugar must be added. At this stage, the birds can be offered the Vivonex Plus/sugar formula or whatever has been found to be palatable to the birds. Since it will only be a few days before the birds will be catching flies, supplying adequate protein may not be a critical factor to their health.

Hummingbirds are not as difficult to wean to self-feeding as many other species. They will, in fact, self-feed from the nest. However, they need to be given adequate time to learn to catch insects efficiently, and to bathe and perform other independent behaviors. Acquiring these skills comes readily and is rarely a concern for caregivers.

When the birds are in an outdoor aviary, presentation of an adequate number of insects to forage can be challenging. The most reliable technique is to contain a healthy fruit fly culture in a jar, with the mouth of the jar covered with fiberglass netting. This will allow the flies to move in and out of the jar without risking the bird falling in. A collection of decaying fruit covered with hardware cloth can also be placed in the enclosure to attract other insects, such that the birds can approach and perch on dry, nonsticky surfaces and haze the flies attracted to the food into the air. One option is to use a handful of raffia sticking out of the fruit fly culture for the flies to sit on and be hazed from (Christy Brant, pers. comm.). It is important to anticipate and prevent ways that the birds can get into trouble by getting caught in crevices or cobwebs, or covered with sugar water or fruit juice. A small, very shallow pan of water or a small fountain of cascading water over rocks should be made available for bathing. Misting may be time consuming but useful. Water for drinking should also be available in hanging tubes or feeders. The pre-release enclosure of the author is made predator-proof with 0.5 × 0.5 in. (1 × 1 cm) hardware cloth through which a 3 ml syringe hangs very nicely. This makes it easy to place syringes of water and Vivonex Plus/sugar solution in a variety of changing locations from which the birds will feed ad lib. It is wise to place some Vivonex Plus/sugar solution within reach of a perch so that birds which, for any reason, have difficulty hovering can reach nutritious food. The skill of the birds can be assessed by whether these tubes empty more rapidly than those that require hovering or whether one hears calls (peeps) from the birds.

Nectar-containing (one part sugar to four parts water) feeders of various designs, such as those that the birds reach down into (satellite) and those that offer a tubelike delivery, should be offered to optimize the birds' chances for success after release.

If the birds make any "peep" calls, check to see that all the food is available and fresh and that the bathwater is clean. Any bird that peeps is not ready for release, and the reason for its distress should be addressed. Flighted birds should not be frequently weighed, as this causes them stress. Their health and condition can be assessed by their flying and feeding behavior. If birds are found in torpor during the day or having difficulty awakening in the morning, they should be removed to a smaller, more intensive care enclosure, with food and water available to them as they perch, and monitored carefully.

## Preparation for Release to the Wild

Approximately 14 days after fledging, the birds are ready to be assessed for release. Black-chinned Hummingbirds have a bill length of 13 mm when they fledge at 21 days. Their bills reach adult length 14 days later (Elliston and Baltosser 1995).

A characteristic of hummingbirds is that they are fearless. Their lack of apparent fear at the approach of people may be interpreted as habituation. However, after a certain age, with only a modicum of isolation in pre-release life, it is unlikely that a newly released hummingbird could be walked up to and captured. This is not to suggest that simply offering some attractive nutrient cannot lure a purely wild hummingbird. Lack of fear, coupled with plentiful curiosity, can be a real hazard to a hummingbird's wellbeing.

## Release

Birds should spend a couple of weeks in the aviary prior to release, with feeders hung within view outside the housing. They can observe the behavior of wild birds at those feeders, listen to the ambient sounds, and locate possible sources of nectar. Release is accomplished by opening the door of the aviary and allowing the birds to leave when they are ready. If no "peep" calls are heard after release, the process should be considered successful.

Hummingbirds are migratory in most of America north of Mexico. However, some vagrants remain in warmer climates after the others have left. If they are normally migratory within the release area, they should be released within the normal migration time, or overwintered. Young hummingbirds leave the natal area after the departure of adults, so the release window is relatively flexible. If there is doubt about late-season release, local birding organizations and 10-day weather forecasts can be consulted.

## Acknowledgments

Many thanks to Christy Brant for communicating her experience raising most of Wildlife Rescue Inc.'s hummingbirds in 2018 and 2019, and to Jennifer Opean for her diligent work on hatchling and nestling diets. Thanks to the Albuquerque office of the U.S. Fish and Wildlife Service (USFWS) and the New Mexico Department of Game and Fish (NMDGF) for permits. Thanks to the Share with Wildlife Program of the NMDGF for continued support of Wildlife Rescue Inc. of New Mexico (WRINM). Thanks to the New Mexico Department of Parks and the Rio Grande Nature State Park for providing a central clinic location (RGNCSP). Most of all, thanks to the supporters and members of WRINM who made the acquisition of this information possible through giving displaced nestling hummingbirds their careful attention.

## Sources for Products Mentioned

Cricket powder, Thailand Unique, https://www.thailandunique.com/cricket-flour-protein-powder, obtainable from Amazon.

Kelthane miticide: Dow AgroSciences LLC, 9330 Zionsville Rd, Indianapolis, IN 46268, (317) 337-3000.

Miconazole Nitrate lotion 1%: Butler Schein, Dublin H 43017 Vet supplies.

Nektar Plus: Nekton-S: Nekton USA, 600 F Street, Arcata, CA 95521, (707) 822-2417, www.nekton.net.

Scale: American Weigh Scales Inc., 1836 Ashley River Rd, Suite 320, Charleston, SC 29407, (866) 643-3444. Look in the category 1/100th Gram.

Vivonex Plus: Nestle HealthCare Nutrition, Inc., 1041 US Highway 202, Bridgewater, NJ 08807, https://www.nestlehealthscience.us/brands/vivonex/vivonex-plus-hcp.

## References


Baker, E.W. and Yunker, C.E. (1964). New Blattisociid mites (Acarina: Mesostigmata) recovered from neotropical flowers and hummingbirds' nares. *Annals of the Entomological Society of America* 57: 103–126.

Baltosser, W.H. and Russell, S.M. (2000). Blackchinned Hummingbird (*Archilochus alexandri*) version 2.0. In: *The Birds of North America* (eds. A. Poole and F. Gill). Ithaca, NY, USA: Cornell Lab of Ornithology https://doi.org/10.2173/bna.495.

Baltosser, W.H. and Scott, P.E. (1996). Costa's Hummingbird (*Calypte costae*). In: *The Birds of North America* (eds. A. Poole and F. Gill). Ithaca, NY, USA: Cornell Lab of Ornithology https://doi.org/10.2173/bna.251.

Bendire, C.E. (1895). Life Histories of North American Birds. *United States National Museum, Special Bulletin 3.*

Bent, A.C. (1940). Life Histories of North American Cuckoos, Goatsuckers, Hummingbirds and Their Allies, Part II. *Bulletin of the United States National Museum* i–viii, 1–506, 73 pls. https://doi.org/10.5479/si.03629236.176.

Camfield, A.F., Calder, W.A., and Calder, L.L. (2013). Broad-tailed Hummingbird version 2.0. In: *The Birds of North America, No. 16* (ed. A.F. Poole). Ithaca, NY, USA: Cornell Lab of Ornithology https://doi.org/10.2173/bna.16.

Elliston, E.P. (1995). Security behavior in Blackchinned hummingbird mothers and nestlings. *Journal of Wildlife Rehabilitation* 18 (2): 3–4.

Elliston, E.P. and Baltosser, W.H. (1995). Sex ratios and bill growth in nesting Black-chinned hummingbirds. *Western Birds* 26: 76–81.

Elliston, E.P. and Perlman, J. (2002). Meeting the protein requirements of adult hummingbirds in captivity. *Journal of Wildlife Rehabilitation* 25 (2): 14–19.

Hawkins, M.G., Barron, H.W., Speer, B.L. et al. (2018). Birds. In: *Exotic Animal Formulary*, 4e (eds. J.W. Carpenter and C.J. Marion), 167–375. St. Louis, MO: Elsevier.

Healy, S. and Calder, W.A. (2006). Rufous Hummingbird (*Selasphorus rufus*) version 2.0. In: *The Birds of North America* (ed. A.F. Poole). Ithaca, NY, USA: Cornell Lab of Ornithology https://doi.org/10.2173/bna.53s.

Johnsgard, P.A. (1983). *The Hummingbirds of North America*, 11. Washington D.C.: Smithsonian Institution Press, 24.

MacLeod, A. and Perlman, J. (2001). Food for thought. *Journal of Wildlife Rehabilitation* 24 (2): 30–31.

Miller, E.A. (ed.) (2012). *Minimum Standards for Wildlife Rehabilitation*, 4e. St. Cloud, MN: National Wildlife Rehabilitation Association.

Rico-Guevara, A. (2017). Relating form to function in the hummingbird feeding apparatus. *PeerJ* 5: e3449. https://doi.org/10.7717/peerj.3449.

Rico-Guevara, A. and Rubega, M.A. (2011). The hummingbird tongue is a fluid trap, not a capillary tube. *Proceedings of the National Academy of Sciences (PNAS)* 108 (23): 9356–9360.

Scheithauer, W. (1967). *Hummingbirds*, 48. New York: Thomas Y. Corwell.

Van Epps, L. (1999). Care and feeding of the newborn hummingbird. International Wildlife Rehabilitation Council, 22nd Annual Conference Proceedings, Tucson, AZ, p. 72.

Weidensaul, S., Robinson, T.R., Sargent, R.R. et al. (2019). Ruby-throated Hummingbird (*Archilochus colubris*), version 2.1. In: *The Birds of North America*. (ed. P.G. Rodewald). Ithaca, NY, USA: Cornell Lab of Ornithology https://doi.org/10.2173/bna.rthhum.02.1.

# 35

# Mousebirds

*Kateri J. Davis*

## Natural History

Mousebirds, or colies as they are also known, are small, gregarious birds, so named because their scampering movements through bushes combined with their gray coloring and long, skinny tails are quite mouselike. They can be found throughout most of Africa except for the northern and far western regions, inhabiting trees and bushes of dry scrubland forests and savannas as well as cultivated zones. They avoid desert and rainforest areas. They are mainly herbivores, eating ripe and unripe fruit as well as leaves, buds, and flowers. Insects, such as grubs, are taken on occasion.

Truly unique birds, there are six closely related mousebird species within two genera comprising the entire order of Coliiformes. Coliiformes is the only modern avian order to be entirely endemic to the continent of Africa. Mousebirds have no close relatives, although they share some characteristics with turacos and parrots.

Mousebirds have unusual thermal physiology and are some of the very few avian species that employ torpor. They also employ sunning, clustering, and sociability techniques to help ensure their survival in an environment where food is relatively low in energy and often unpredictable in availability.

Mousebirds do not perch in typical avian fashion but rather rest their bellies on the perch. Their legs are widely spaced and appear splay-legged to the mousebird novice. Mousebirds also hang with their feet above their heads with their tails pointing down, even sleeping in this position.

Mousebirds are all sexually monomorphic. They are generally monogamous and live in small flocks breeding cooperatively. They help each other build loosely formed open-cup nests out of small twigs, leaves, and similar material. The young are fed by regurgitation.

All mousebird species have similar anatomy, habits, and voice, thus sharing the same avicultural care and housing requirements. Speckled, Blue-naped, Red-faced, White-head, and White-backed are the species that have been seen in aviculture (Figure 35.1).

## Criteria for Intervention

In the United States and Europe, mousebirds of all species are highly sought after as pet birds; thus hand-rearing is important. Although parent-raised or adult imported birds can be tamed, generally

*Hand-Rearing Birds*, Second Edition. Edited by Rebecca S. Duerr and Laurie J. Gage.

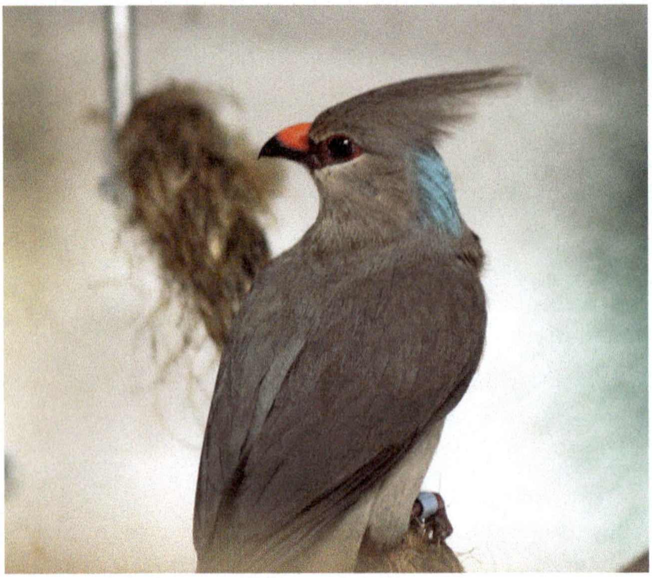

Figure 35.1 Adult Blue-naped Mousebird.

hand-reared birds make the best human companions. A hand-raised mousebird can rival any species of hand-raised parrot in terms of suitability as a pet bird in a human home.

Despite making excellent pet birds, mousebirds continue to be quite rare in aviculture, mostly because of the lack of interest in consistently breeding them. All the mousebird species have a hard time garnering and keeping breeders. However, without breeders, there are no pet birds.

The pet market cannot be ignored as pet birds increase the interest in a species, but with so few actual individual birds available, a mousebird taken out of the breeding equation to become a pet bird can be devastating to the future of the birds in aviculture. With each hatched chick, mousebird breeders should weigh carefully whether or not their breeding program can survive taking that bird out to make a pet. This is a tough choice, especially since breeder birds do not sell as well and sell for less than a pet-quality bird. There is a great need to encourage people to get into the joy of breeding birds.

If all mousebirds raised go into the pet trade, then the species heads toward extinction in aviculture rather quickly. Breeding mousebirds can be difficult because of their messy habits and short lifespans. A mousebird is at peak breeding condition between 2 and 5 years of age. Generally, breeding success diminishes after 6 years. The average life span in captivity is between 7 and 10 years, with a maximum age recorded as 15 years.

Hand-raising mousebirds for the pet trade is not difficult, and mousebirds are probably the easiest of the softbill chicks with which to work. Mousebird chicks that are to be hand-raised for pet quality are best removed from the nest at 6–9 days of age. Aviculturists often use the term *pulled* for this. At this time, the chick is mostly feathered, although flightless, and very alert. It can grip well with its extra-large feet, and can hang and climb within days.

In their native African environment and in some avicultural settings, young and adult mousebirds sometime need rescuing, especially in stormy weather when the birds may become drenched. Rehabilitation, including hand-feeding, is sometimes needed.

## Record Keeping

At this time, no U.S. federal permits are required to keep and raise mousebirds. However, state laws vary and should be checked before attaining mousebirds.

Record keeping varies with each aviculturist, but should include the basics, such as date hatched, parents and bloodline, sexing information, and any medical issues. Leg bands or microchipping is recommended to identify and track individuals. Traditionally in aviculture, the gender of sexed birds can be visually marked by bands placed on the right leg for a male and left for a female. Tattoos are used on the appropriately sided wingweb.

## Incubation of Eggs

There is little reason to incubate mousebird eggs artificially, and successfully raising a mousebird chick from hatch is extremely difficult. In avicultural settings, mousebirds are usually very prolific reproductively, so it is not a necessity to save every egg. Dealing with a rare species or a special case of emergency rescue would be the only instances where artificial incubation would be needed.

Mousebird eggs can be incubated at a temperature of 99–100 °F (37.2–37.8 °C) and 45% humidity in a standard incubator unit. They should be turned 180° in opposite directions every 1–5 hours. Evidence of fertility can be seen by candling methods around day 5 to 7. Incubation usually lasts 12 days. Once the chick pips, it will generally hatch within the day. It is quite noisy, making short calls throughout the process.

## Initial Care and Stabilization

Heat must be given immediately to young, sick, or otherwise compromised mousebirds. Heat, from 90 to 100 °F (32.2–37.8 °C), can be provided by heat lamps, heating pads, or incubator/brooder set-ups (Figure 35.2). When a mousebird becomes chilled, especially a youngster, whether due to environmental conditions or health problems, it can cause the bird to go into a torpid state in which the bird's bodily functions slow down, and the bird may even appear dead. Chicks and young birds can become torpid at lower temperatures, even room temperatures. Compromised mousebirds have a difficult time successfully coming out of a torpid state.

Torpidity should be avoided in aviculture. Keep birds well fed, in good feather condition, and healthy. Unfortunately, mousebirds are not fastidious in their grooming, but cleanliness is very important in maintaining body heat. Pairs or groups of mousebirds can handle lower temperatures than a single bird, because multiples will hang and cluster together belly to belly to conserve body heat.

If a cold mousebird is found that is not responding to physical stimuli, it is recommended to provide the bird with heat before pronouncing it dead; torpid mousebirds often resemble dead birds. There are cases of "dead" mousebirds reviving once warmed.

## Common Medical Problems and Solutions

Mousebirds are relatively hardy creatures and typically have few health problems. Chilling and intraspecies aggression are the number one killers of mousebirds in aviculture. Housing needs to

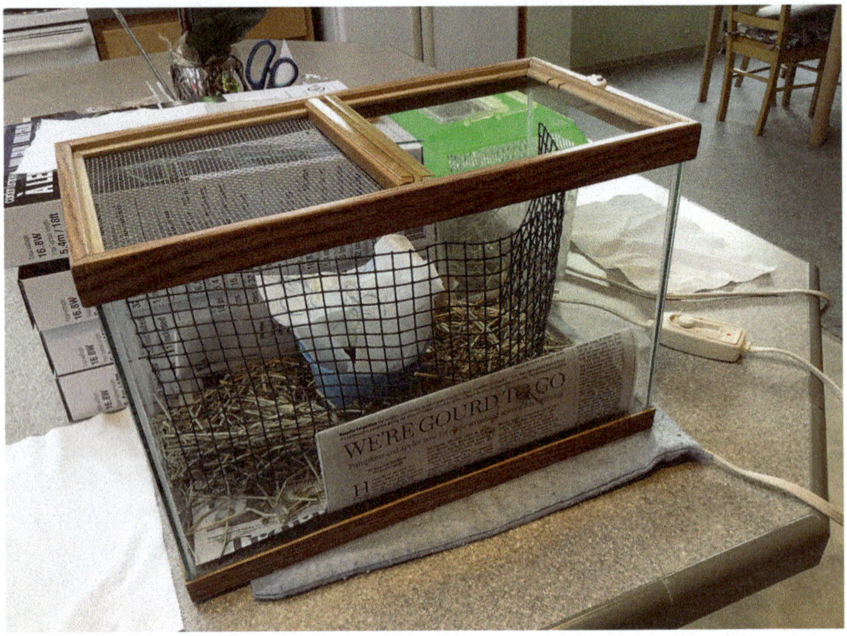

Figure 35.2 A brooder set-up for a fledged mousebird chick. Note the heating pad, the small bowl "nest" with paper towels. The hay substrate and wire screen for hanging both reduce damage to the tail and help keep the chick away from his own feces.

be carefully planned to avoid both. Iron storage disease, which is common in some softbilled birds, is not documented in mousebirds.

Because of the soft nature and copious quantity of a chick's feces, the brooder and cage environments need to be religiously cleaned. If not, mold and bacteria will quickly grow, putting the chick's health at risk for aspergillosis and other infections.

Recently emptied or half-emptied food bowls attract mousebirds as resting places, which can make breast feathers soiled. Unfortunately, juvenile and adult mousebirds are poor self-groomers, are oblivious of contact with their feces and food, and will soil their plumage even to the point where it impacts the feathers' ability to insulate the bird properly, which leads to chilling.

Mousebird tail plumage is easily damaged and soiled, yet the tail provides much needed balance for the often clumsy birds. Birds that lose their tails completely do not fly or maneuver well and are at risk. Unlike what is sometimes done with other bird species to encourage new feather growth, it is not recommended to purposely pull damaged mousebird tail feathers unless the feathers are broken short. Although slow, it is best to allow the natural molting process. When hand-feeding, chicks' tails need to be kept clean and can be washed under gentle streams of warm water when dirtied. Place perches and other things the bird can hang from with a focus on allowing the tail to hang clear of obstructions.

Fecal impacting can occur and can be life threatening if not remedied in time. Impactions most frequently happen with chicks from day 2–10. It is important to gently stimulate the chicks to defecate at feeding times and frequently throughout the day. Once a mousebird is defecating on its own, continue to monitor the output until it is totally weaned.

## Hand-feeding Diet

### Days 1–6

Mix together with warm water:

- 2 parts commercial hand-feeding formula for parrots, such as Kaytee Exact® brand Hand Feeding Formula (Kaytee)
- 1 part strained fruit human baby food, such as Gerber's pear, apple, papaya, or banana

Formula should be fed warm but not hot, and should be made fresh. As the chick develops, the formula should be made with less water for a thicker pancake-batter consistency. Mashed water-soaked softbill pellets can be substituted for the hand-feeding formula in emergencies.

Probiotics can be used but are not necessary; indeed, they are premixed into some commercial diets such as Kaytee Exact. Some aviculturists mix a small amount of the parents' fecal matter into the first few days' formula to promote beneficial bacteria and antibodies in the chick, but there is the possibility of introducing pathogenic bacteria and parasites.

### Day 6 to Weaning

- Very small chunks of soft fruit, such as apples, melons, pears, papaya, and others. Avoid citrus fruits and tomatoes because of their high acid content.
- Small softbill pellets, soaked in water.
- Large pellets, such as Mazuri Softbill, can be water-soaked and then broken into small pieces.
- Water should be offered in a shallow dish.

A variety of fruits should be fed, not only to ensure nutritional variety but also to keep the bird from becoming a picky eater as an adult. Formula can be used to supplement feedings at this age, but the mixture should be made thicker every day and the majority of the diet should be the fruit mix.

## Feeding Procedures

### Hatchlings

Hatchlings do not have to be fed for the first 20–24 hours, getting their nutrition from the absorption of the yolk sac. The first feedings should be every 15–30 minutes, starting with only a drop or two of formula. The feeding schedule should start at about 6:00 a.m. to 11:00 p.m., with a few extra nighttime feedings for the first few days.

Mousebirds do not have crops. Their esophagus expands when fed, so a bulge can be seen on the right side of the chick's neck as he feeds. Clean the beak area after each feeding with a clean, damp swab to reduce the chance of spoiled food causing a health problem.

As the chick ages, feeding frequency can be expanded to every 1–2 hours, and amounts of formula can be gradually increased. By day 6, the chick can take 1–1.5 cc of formula per feeding.

Once the chick realizes the feeding procedure, he will readily gape at the feeder. Chicks will signal their hunger by buzzing sounds, half-opened wings, and spastic-type movements. Speckled Mousebirds have especially pronounced movements that resemble seizures when begging.

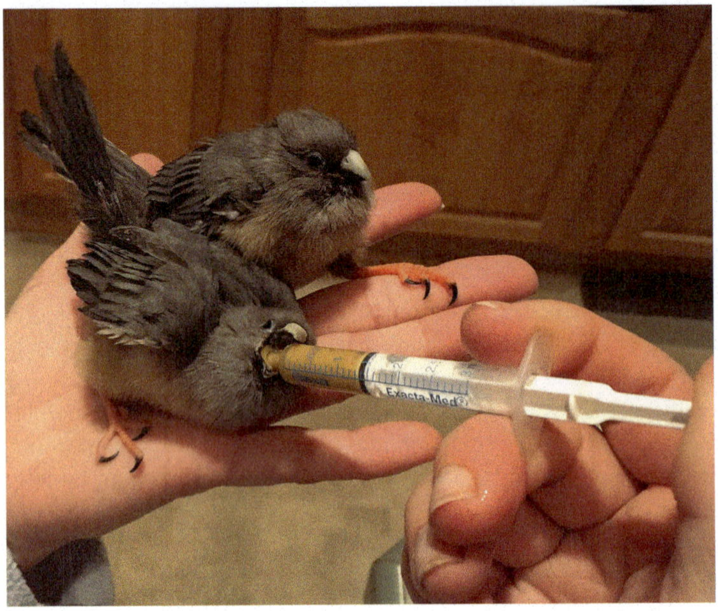


Figure 35.3 Two White-back Mousebirds chicks getting their formula. Note the posturing on the one being fed.

Mousebird chicks will make pumping motions while being fed and may continue to beg, even when full, and food can be visualized in the esophagus from the mouth (Figure 35.3). Beware of overfeeding, which may lead to aspiration. Smaller, more frequent meals are better than larger, less frequent meals.

Mousebird chicks will need to be stimulated to defecate after each feeding. Use a soft tissue touched to or gently rubbed on the vent. Feces are not in a fecal sac and are quite voluminous and soft. As the chick ages, it will defecate more and more on its own, but it is recommended that the caregiver stimulate defecation at every feeding to help keep the brooder clean.

Unfortunately, the method of hand-feeding a mousebird chick from day 1 to day 6 has still not been perfected. Obviously, there is more avicultural work to be done in this area. Although there have been some success stories, chicks this young often start to gape less, weaken, and die by day 5 of the hand-feeding. The chick that makes it to day 6 will usually continue to thrive. Pulling chicks from the nest is not recommended until day 6 because of this difficulty of raising the younger ones by hand.

## Nestlings

Young mousebirds aged 6 days and older should be kept well fed with feedings every 1–2 hours from approximately 6:00 a.m. to 11:00 p.m. An extra feeding or two during the night is recommended the first night or two of pulling a chick.

Recently pulled mousebird chicks, especially if after day 7, can be difficult to hand-feed in the beginning, and some are downright stubborn. Chicks tend to tuck their heads down and refuse to gape at the hand-feeder initially. The edge of a fingernail can be used to very gently wedge the beak open to insert the food item or syringe tip. The food should be placed just inside the beak. Care must be taken that the bird does not aspirate the food, especially with formula, and that the handler does not damage the young beak. Once the food is in the chick's mouth, it should swallow on its own. Usually the chick will start to gape after a day or two of force-feeding.

Table 35.1 Adult mousebird weights.

| Species | Weight (g) |
|---|---|
| Blue-naped | 50–60 |
| Red-faced | 65–75 |
| Speckled | 50–80 |
| Red-backed | 50–75 |
| White-backed | 50–55 |
| White-headed | 35–45 |

### Expected Weight Gain

Mousebird chicks grow very quickly and should gain weight every day. Healthy chicks should not have a sharp keel, and, although they are generally thinner than adults, there should be muscle mass on both sides of the breast. Mousebirds do not achieve their adult weight until approximately 3 months of age. Speckled Mousebirds are the heaviest of the species at between 50 and 80 g. See Table 35.1 for adult weights of mousebird species.

## Housing

For the first day, hatchlings can be kept in the incubator in a small plastic bowl with a terry cloth liner. Make a small depression in the lining to simulate a nest. The substrate enables the chick to grip with its feet as it grows. A lightweight cloth or tissue is draped loosely over the bowl so that the chick feels like it is being brooded by parents.

After the chick and its replacement nest is moved to a brooder enclosure, the temperature can be gradually lowered to 90 °F (32.2 °C) during the next few days. Crumpled tissues can be used over the cloth substrate for ease of cleaning, but make sure that the nest material is able to be gripped by the chick or leg problems may occur. Mousebird chicks are very messy. Do not allow them to become soiled or damp.

By day 6, the chick will be hanging on the edge of the bowl and may hop out at feeding time. The bowl substrate can be switched to crumpled paper towels to aid in clean up.

By day 8–10, the chick is out of the nest more of the time, and it is time to provide perches and/or toys for him to start hanging on. He will soon want to hang at night instead of using the nest, and he may be moved to a more typical cage situation at this time as long as supplemental heat, such as a heat lamp, is given. The temperature may be gradually lowered every day until it is at room temperature by about day 14. Watch temperature and behavior closely because the chick may become torpid if the temperature goes down too quickly. If multiple chicks are being raised together, watch for aggression such as feather plucking.

Chicks that are being raised for pet quality can be placed in separate enclosures around day 10 to ensure that they will bond closely with humans, and they must be handled daily to become successfully socialized. Mousebirds are so social that keeping a mousebird of any age by itself with no human or bird contact is cruel. If a pet-quality bird is the goal, typically isolating the chick from other mousebirds for several months with only human contact is recommended.

If a breeding bird is the ultimate goal, the act of hand-raising a chick is not usually a deterrent. Mousebird chicks revert to wild behavior quickly if not handled daily, if pulled from the nest too late, or if allowed to mix with other mousebirds. However, if a long-term pet bird is put into a breeding situation years later, or if the aviculturist tries to keep handling a hand-raised bird while with a mate, breeding success declines compared with similarly aged wild birds.

## Weaning

Mousebirds wean quickly and easily. By day 11, a shallow bowl of small soft fruit chunks (75%) and soaked pellets (25%) can be placed in the enclosure for the chick to start investigating on its own. This proportion may be continued into adulthood. At each feeding, place the bowl in front of the begging chick and move the pieces around with a finger (Figure 35.4). This will encourage the chick to put its beak in the bowl while gaping, thus touching the food. Feed him at an angle as close to the bowl as possible. Some birds will catch on in one day, but others may take a week more. Blue-naped Mousebirds tend to take longer weaning than Speckled or White-backed.

Do not discontinue the hand-feeding until the bird is about 16 days old and eating everything completely on its own. Monitor weight gain and keel muscle mass carefully. A mousebird chick is not ready for an aviary or new home release until he is a month old, eating well, and has not had supplemental heat for at least 2 weeks. At this time, he should also be able to fly, although not expertly. Mature birds should be fed a variety of fruits and some vegetables with dry and/or soaked pelleted softbill diets.

Make sure that young mousebirds, generally up to 3 months of age, have food available to them at all times. They have tremendous appetites and, if they are allowed to go hungry too often, they lose weight very quickly and may go torpid.

A well-raised, hand-fed mousebird is a cuddly and loving bird that requires no extra training before entering a pet home. Because most pet bird owners are used to only parrot species, the new owner must be thoroughly educated on the unique attributes and different diet of mousebirds so that proper care will be given.

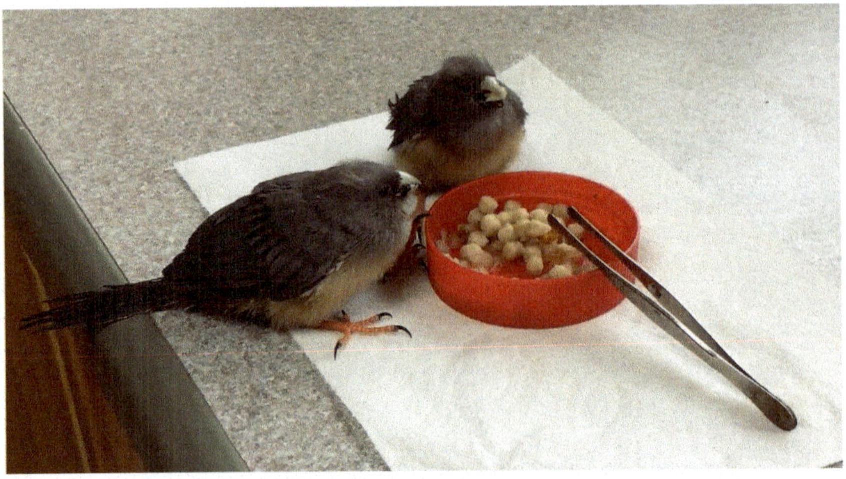

Figure 35.4 Two White-back Mousebird chicks learn to eat on their own. Forceps make it easy for the hand-feeder to handle the small food pieces.

## Introduction to Captive Flock

Care must be taken when introducing mousebirds to each other, especially to established individuals or flocks. Intraspecific aggression is common and often fatal. Chicks can even be aggressive with each other once fledged. Typically, juveniles are accepted into flocks faster than adults. Mixing mousebird species is not recommended for novices because it can be even trickier to establish harmony. Speckled Mousebirds are typically a more aggressive species.

The best method is to release all the mousebirds into a new environment at the same time. If any of the established birds are breeding at the time, it is riskier to introduce new birds. Use a "howdy cage" technique, in which either the new bird or the established birds are placed in a smaller cage inside the enclosure. Because mousebirds hang on the wire, a cage within a cage in the enclosure is even better; otherwise, the birds will bite each other's toes and feet. This "howdy cage" arrangement allows the newcomer a chance to introduce himself to the other birds safely.

Once released, continue to monitor closely for signs of aggression, which include bloody toes, face, and rump area. Loss of head and tail feathers or a bird hiding on the ground signals problems.

## Author's Note

Previously, little has been documented about this fascinating order of birds in captivity or in the wild. After years of working with mousebirds herself, and compiling experiences and studies from zoological institutes and other aviculturists, the author wrote *Mousebirds in Aviculture,* the only book written on the subject. The book covers mousebirds' natural history and all aspects of the care, diet, housing, and breeding of all species of mousebirds. See https://sites.google.com/site/birdhousepub for information on ordering a copy.

The author owns Davis Lund Aviaries, which specializes in softbilled birds, and more pictures and information about mousebirds and other softbill birds can be found on the author's website, https://dlaviaries.wordpress.com. She has bred and raised all species of mousebirds except for the Red-back Mousebird which has never been in U.S. aviculture. Currently, she has the largest flock of White-back Mousebirds in the country. She would like to make contact with other people that are working with mousebirds and can be reached at (541) 895–5149 or DLAviaries@aol.com.

## Acknowledgments

Thank you to all the softbill aviculturists who have shared their experiences throughout the years.

## Source for Products Mentioned

Kaytee products: 521 Clay St, PO Box 230, Chilton, WI 53014, (800) KAYTEE-1, https://www.kaytee.com.

Mazuri, PMI Nutrition International, LLC, PO Box 66812, St. Louis, MO 63166, www.mazuri.com.

## Reference

Davis, K.J. (2001). *Mousebirds in Aviculture*, 140 pp. Creswell, Oregon: Birdhouse Publications.

# 36

# Hornbills, Kingfishers, Hoopoes, and Bee-eaters

*Patricia Witman and Nicole LaGreco*

## Introduction

Both facilities of San Diego Zoo Global, the San Diego Zoo and the San Diego Zoo's Safari Park, have a long history of caring for and breeding a variety of members of the orders Bucerotiformes and Coraciiformes. Eleven species have been reared from the three families of Bucerotiformes: Upupidae (hoopoes), Phoeniculidae (woodhoopoes), and Bucerotidae (hornbills). Ten species have been hand-reared from three of the six families of Coraciiformes: Alcedinidae (kingfishers), Meropidae (bee-eaters), and Coracidae (rollers).

## Natural History

There are 62 species of hornbills in the family Bucerotidae, with 31 species found in tropical Africa and 31 species found in Asia to the Solomon Islands. The eight species of woodhoopoe in the family Phoeniculidae are found in sub-Saharan Africa, and the two species of hoopoe in the family Upupidae are found in the Palearctic, Afrotropical, and Oriental regions.

There are 120 species of kingfishers in the family Alcedinidae with a worldwide distribution. The 31 species of bee-eaters in the family Meropidae and the 13 species of rollers in the family Coracidae are all found in the Old World (Table 36.1).

Members of the orders Bucerotiformes and Coraciiformes are typically described as large-headed, short-necked, and short-legged. Most have large or long bills and have short toes on relatively weak feet, with the third and fourth toes fused at the base pointing forward. Plumage may be iridescent or with green and blue pigment colors, although hornbills are black and white with some gray, brown, and cream. All are hole-nesters, whether in tree cavities, termite mounds, mud holes in banks, or some in excavated rock outcroppings. Most unusual are the hornbill species that "mud up" the nest cavity opening with mud, food, or feces, thus sealing the female and subsequent chicks inside. The female and chicks are then solely dependent on the male or helpers for food. All have white eggs that hatch into altricial chicks (Fry et al. 1992; Kemp 1995; del Hoyo 2001).

Some species nest cooperatively, but most pair up monogamously. There is a wide range in size of different species, from the pygmy kingfishers to the largest hornbills. Likewise, there is a wide range of incubation periods, clutch sizes, and nestling periods (Table 36.2).

*Hand-Rearing Birds*, Second Edition. Edited by Rebecca S. Duerr and Laurie J. Gage.

Table 36.1 Family distribution of orders Bucerotiformes and Coraciiformes.

| Family | Common Name | # Species | Distribution |
|---|---|---|---|
| Bucerotidae | Hornbills | 62 | Afrotropical and Oriental; marginal in Australasian |
| Upupidae | Hoopoes | 2 | Palearctic, Afrotropical, and Oriental |
| Phoeniculidae | Woodhoopoes | 8 | Sub-saharan Africa |
| Meropidae | Bee-eaters | 31 | Old World |
| Coraciidae | Rollers | 13 | Old World |
| Brachypteraciidae | Ground rollers | 5 | Madagascar |
| Todidae | Todies | 5 | Greater Antilles |
| Momotidae | Motmots | 14 | Neotropical |
| Alcedinidae | Kingfishers | 120 | Worldwide |

Table 36.2 Incubation period, clutch size, and nestling period.[a]

| Species | Incubation Period (Days) | Clutch Size | Nestling Period (Days)[a] |
|---|---|---|---|
| Southern Laughing Kookaburra (*Dacelo novaeguineae*) | 21–26 | 3 | 32–44 |
| Guam Kingfisher (*Todiramphus cinnamominous*) | 20–23 | 1–3 | ? |
| White-breasted Kingfisher (*Halcyon smyrnensis*) | 18–25 | 4–7 | 26–27 |
| Collared Kingfisher (*Todiramphus c. chloris*) | ~22 | 2–5 | 29–30 |
| Carmine Bee-eater (*Merops nubicus*) | 19–22 | 2–5 | ~30 |
| White-throated Bee-eater (*Merops albicollis*) | 19–20 | 4–7 | ~30 |
| White-fronted Bee-eater (*Merops bullockoides*) | 19–20 | 2–5 | ~30 |
| Blue-bellied Roller (*Coracias cyanogaster*) | 18–21 | 2–4 | 25–30 |
| Purple Roller (*Coracias naevius*) | 17–23 | 2–4 | 25–30 |
| Oriental Dollarbird (*Eurystomus orientalis orientalis*) | 18–22 | 3–5 | ~23 |
| Common Hoopoe (*Upupa epops*) | 16–18 | 5–8 | 24–28 |
| Green Woodhoopoe (*Phoeniculus purpureus*) | 17–18 | 2–5 | 28–30 |
| Abyssinian Ground Hornbill (*Bucorvus abyssinicus*) | 37–41 | 2 | 80–90 |
| Southern Ground Hornbill (*Bucorvus leadbeateri*) | 37–43 | 1–3 | 86 |
| Black Hornbill (*Anthracoceros malayanus*) | 30 | 2–3 | 50 |
| Great Hornbill (*Buceros bicornis*) | 33–40 | 1–4 | 72–96 |
| Sulawesi Hornbill (*Rhabdotorrhinus exarhatus*) | 28–30 | 2–4 | 50–60 |
| Trumpeter Hornbill (*Bycanistes bucinator*) | 28 | 2–4 | 50–60 |
| Knobbed Hornbill (*Rhyticeros cassidix*) | 32–35 | 2–3 | ~100 |
| Wrinkled Hornbill (*Rhabdotorrhinus corrugatus*) | 29 | 2–3 | 65–73 |
| Writhed Hornbill (*Aceros leucocephalus*) | 29 | 2 | ? |

[a] del Hoyo (2001), merged with SDZG data.

A wide variety of insects, other invertebrates, small mammals, small reptiles, amphibians, bird eggs, and nestlings make up the bulk of the diets of the kingfishers, bee-eaters, rollers, woodhoopoes, hoopoes, and ground hornbills. Kingfishers prefer beating their prey items against a branch prior to eating. Bee-eaters mostly hunt in flight, eating bees, wasps, and related stinging species, manipulating the items until the stingers fall out. Most rollers go to the ground to feed, except the Dollarbirds that mainly take their prey in flight. Hoopoes probe for food in the ground with their long narrow bills. Although most other insectivorous birds cast a pellet made up of the indigestible chitin of the exoskeletons, hoopoes excrete it in their feces. The woodhoopoes use their long narrow beaks to probe behind bark eating, among other things, lots of caterpillars.

Although most hornbills are omnivorous, there are species that are mainly carnivorous or mainly frugivorous. When the frugivorous species are breeding, there are often many animal prey items included in the diet. The carnivorous species tend to live in the savanna and are semi-terrestrial. Most of the frugivorous species live in the forest and are arboreal. Most hornbills do not drink water and rely on food as a source of hydration.

## Criteria for Intervention

Although parent-reared birds are preferred at both facilities, chicks may be brought in for hand-rearing as a result of parental neglect or a history of failures due to a variety of causes. Most chicks that are hand-reared are hatched using artificial incubation. This eliminates, for the most part, any chance of exposing them to parasites or infectious diseases. Chicks removed from parental care are isolated from others until the veterinary staff can evaluate their health via fecal gram stains and culture results. If parent-hatched chicks are healthy and well-hydrated (Figure 36.1), they may be relatively easy to hand-rear when removed from the nest prior to fledging. However, it may be extremely time consuming to successfully hand-rear a chick whose health has been compromised by less-than-adequate parental care.

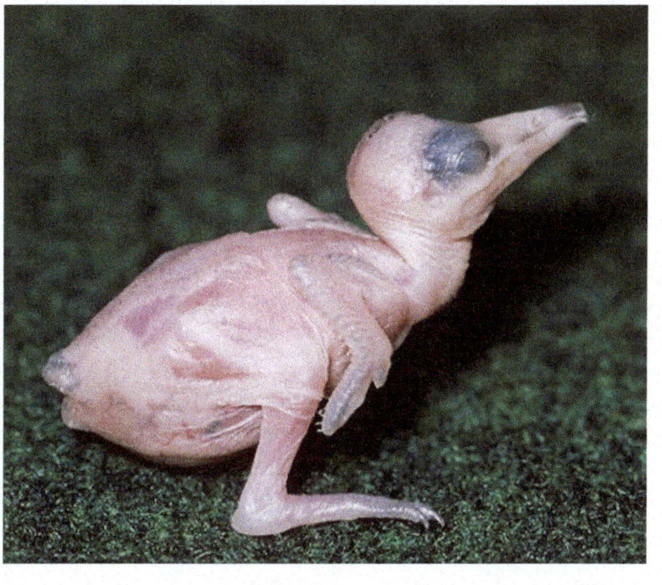

Figure 36.1 Well-hydrated White-fronted Bee-eater during first week. *Source:* photo © Zoological Society of San Diego.

## Record Keeping

Detailed hand-rearing records are kept to ensure the ability to repeat successes, share data, or track changes that lead to success. Specific information about their location, parents' identification, age, reason for removal, and condition of chick at time of removal is recorded. Care is taken to either place a band on, or mark with nontoxic colored felt pens, all chicks for identification purposes. Detailed feed and weight records should be kept. Target amounts to feed are entered along with the frequency of feedings, which are determined from past successes. The actual amounts fed are recorded, tallied, and compared to the target. Chicks are weighed every morning before their first feeding. Decisions related to target amounts to feed are based on whether weight gains or losses are in the normal range.

## Incubation of Eggs

Artificial incubation is used if the parents have a history of failure to hatch eggs or if there are conditions within their enclosures that would make it difficult to rear young. Incubation parameters have been determined based on past successes of closely related species. Incubation periods have been difficult to establish in cavity-nesters, as it disturbs the parents to have someone investigate the nest, and there are very few that have been set up with cameras for monitoring.

All of the successfully reared hornbill species and the Kookaburra were artificially incubated at 99.0 °F (37.2 °C) at 56–62% relative humidity (RH). The smaller eggs of the other kingfisher species, all the rollers, and bee-eaters were incubated at 99.5 °F (37.5 °C) at 50–66% RH. These RH settings are the starting point for incubation, but the percentage of egg weight loss is monitored for most eggs and the humidity adjusted accordingly. If eggs are not losing enough weight, the humidity is lowered, and conversely if they are losing too much weight, the humidity is raised. The earlier these changes are made, the more effective they will be. Several small adjustments early in incubation are safer to the developing embryo than one drastic change later in incubation. Decreasing or increasing the surface area of water within the incubator will change the humidity. For example, if an egg loses only 9%, water pans with a smaller surface area would replace the original pans in an attempt to lower the RH by 6–7%. RH should not be raised or lowered drastically; aim for less than 10% each week.

Eggs are weighed twice a week during incubation. One method used to calculate egg weight loss is the following formula:

$$\left\{ \frac{\left[ \left( \frac{S-E}{D} \times I \right) \right]}{S} \right\}$$

where $S$ = set weight, $E$ = end weight, $D$ = # days incubated since set weight, and $I$ = incubation period. *Set weight* is the weight of the egg when it is pulled from the nest. *End weight* is the weight of the egg on any given day of artificial incubation. This formula allows the egg weight loss to be calculated even if the fresh egg weight was not obtained, and may be used at any point during incubation to determine the trend of the egg weight loss. For example: if an egg is removed from

Table 36.3 Guam Kingfisher (GKF) egg weight loss sample.

| Egg # | Actual I | Date of 1st Wt. | Date of 2nd Wt. | D | S | E | I1 | I2 | GKF @20 Day I % Wt. Loss | GKF @23 Day I % Wt. Loss |
|---|---|---|---|---|---|---|---|---|---|---|
| 5 | 20 | 27-Jun-95 | 16-Jul-95 | 19 | 7.89 | 7.00 | 20 | 23 | 12% | 14% |
| 6 | 21 | 20-Dec-97 | 6-Jan-98 | 17 | 7.98 | 7.23 | 20 | 23 | 11% | 13% |
| 231 | 21 | 9-Apr-98 | 17-Apr-98 | 8 | 7.58 | 7.25 | 20 | 23 | 11% | 13% |
| 197 | 21 | 28-Apr-99 | 30-Apr-99 | 2 | 7.10 | 7.03 | 20 | 23 | 10% | 11% |
| 222 | 21 | 24-Apr-00 | 30-Apr-00 | 6 | 6.08 | 5.88 | 20 | 23 | 11% | 13% |
| 209 | 23 | 19-Mar-04 | 5-Apr-04 | 17 | 7.81 | 7.14 | 20 | 23 | 10% | 12% |

$S$ = set weight; $E$ = current or end weight; $D$ = # days artificially incubated; $I$ = incubation period, I1 = low incubation period; I2 = high incubation period.

the parents after 5 days of parental incubation, the egg weighs 26 g, the incubation period is 30 days, and after 7 days of artificial incubation the egg weighs 25 g, the formula would look like this:

$$\left\{\frac{\left(\frac{26-25}{7}\times 30\right)}{26}\right\} = 16.5\%$$

and the egg weight loss would be 16.5%. This would be within normal limits if this were a chicken egg. However, if this is a species such as the White-fronted Bee-eater, and all of the successfully hand-reared chicks had hatched artificially from eggs with weight losses averaging 11.2%, the decision would be made to increase the humidity in the incubator in an attempt to slow the rate of weight loss of the egg (Table 36.3).

Another method is to use the following formula:

$$\left\{\frac{F-P}{F}\right\}\times 100$$

where $F$ = fresh weight and $P$ = pip weight. This can be used at any time during incubation, even if the fresh weight was not obtained and prior to pip, if these values are extrapolated mathematically. The actual egg weights can be plotted on a graph along with these extrapolated values. It is then possible to determine whether the weights are in the expected range (Figure 36.2).

The percent weight loss is 10–14% in the kingfisher's, bee-eater's, roller's, and hornbill's eggs that have been artificially incubated. Some of these eggs were collected as freshly laid and artificially incubated for the entire incubation period; others were collected after varying amounts of parental incubation. Eggs were transferred to hatchers approximately 3 days prior to hatching, where the temperatures were lowered by 0.5–1 °F and the humidity settings were raised to 63–73% RH.

There are routine sanitation protocols that apply to incubators and hatchers to help ensure that chicks hatch with minimum exposure to bacterial or viral contamination. Once a year, the incubation and hatching rooms are disinfected with a liquid disinfectant (Sani-cide 94 Maintex) from floor to ceiling, including all incubators, hatchers, and related equipment. On a weekly basis, the outside of all machines is wiped down with a liquid disinfectant and a UV sterilizer (Hanovia Inc.) is used

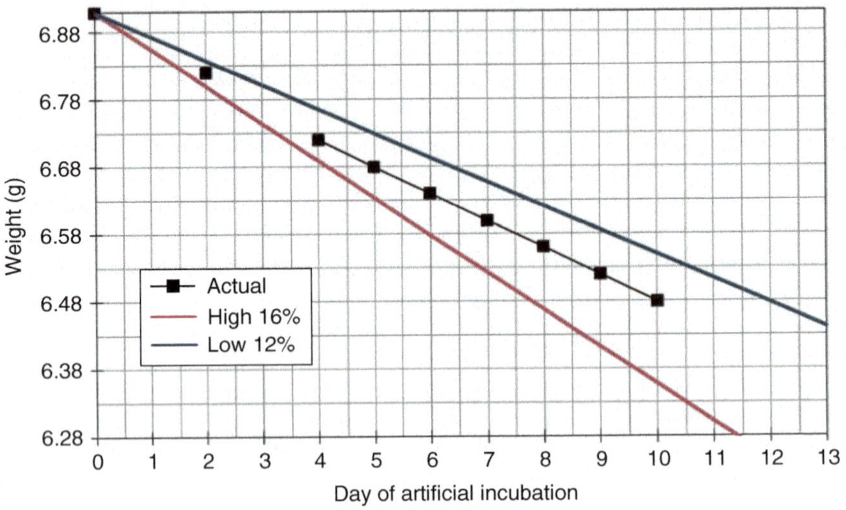


Figure 36.2 Guam Kingfisher egg weight loss graph.

within both rooms, covering windows to protect both humans and eggs. Egg trays within all machines are disinfected between clutches. Floors are disinfected at least twice weekly, with foot baths at the entrance. Traffic within the facility is limited. An ozone generator has been used routinely in the incubators historically as another means of maintaining a clean environment for eggs. The water source for humidity within all machines comes from a reverse osmosis system with a UV sterilization component. Hands are washed with soap before and after handling eggs. Employees wear clean uniforms daily and are expected to arrive with clean hair that is short or tied back.

## Initial Care and Stabilization

Most neonates come to the facility via the hatchery where they've been artificially incubated. Once the chick has dried off in the hatcher, it is brought into the brooder room. The temperature of the appropriate brooder is adjusted and stable prior to the expected hatch date. Avian neonates are fed at the first sign of feeding response or within 24 hours of hatching. All food items are dipped in bottled drinking water to moisten and provide fluids.

If a chick has been removed after hatching with the parents, its condition is evaluated and recorded. If it is determined by "tented" skin, sunken eyes, and lack of feeding response that a chick is dehydrated, it receives 5–10% of its body weight in subcutaneous fluids (2.5% dextrose and 0.45% NaCl Injection USP). If a chick has injuries, it receives treatment by a staff veterinarian. A latex glove filled with warm water is sometimes used to warm up a small cold neonate by placing it among the fingers of the glove, taking care to frequently check the temperature of the glove to ensure it has not cooled off.

## Common Medical Problems

As with many species of avian neonate, bacterial infections are the most common problem encountered. A well-nourished chick reared in sanitary conditions is the least susceptible to infections.

Observations about feeding responses, feces, skin, and feather condition are recorded as changes occur. Any changes that are outside the normal range are addressed as either developmental or medical abnormalities. Developmental abnormalities can occur as a result of improper nutrition, improper quantities fed, or improper feeding techniques.

All of the species discussed in this chapter have been observed casting a pellet of indigestible materials (insect chitin or rodent fur) with the exceptions of the Common Hoopoe, which excretes this material, and the frugivorous hornbills that are not fed as many of the prey items as the more insectivorous or carnivorous species. In the mid-1980s, when not many of this group of birds had been hand-reared, there were occasions when a chick's lack of feeding response may have been misdiagnosed as a medical issue as opposed to the normal pause some chicks need prior to casting a pellet.

Intestinal impactions associated with feeding too much chitin or fur were problems with the ground hornbills when first reared in the mid-1980s. As ground hornbills also became impacted on sand, it was determined that their rearing enclosures had to be free of foreign objects that were small enough to swallow. In general, it is safer to rear chicks in relatively bare enclosures until they are old enough to be moved in with cohorts that may distract them from picking at everything around them or until they are big enough for some foreign objects to pass harmlessly through their digestive systems.

White-fronted Bee-eaters' first primaries were shorter than normal, but they grew in normal length after their first molt. At least one parent-reared chick was also observed to have abnormal tail feathers. Speculation centered around a possible nutritional imbalance, but no cause was determined.

Star-gazing was observed in one Northern Ground Hornbill and one Guam Kingfisher at day 11 and day 8, respectively. Both birds received injections of B-complex vitamins, and the hornbill's condition improved within 5 days. The kingfisher did not improve for 30 days with repeated injections. It was not until the chick was placed in a plastic cup with a screen lid shut, holding the head in the normal position, that it did improve; and it was completely normal 5 days later.

## Diet Recipes

Most of the species discussed are insectivorous or carnivorous species, with the exception of some of the hornbills that tend to be more frugivorous. Regardless of the adult requirements, all chicks need protein to grow and develop normally. The most readily available commercial sources of protein are mice, insects, soaked cat or dog pet food, and supplemented meat products. Well-hydrated, plump, and juicy naked neonate mice are a source of protein that is efficient to use for many of these species. Many insects have considerable amounts of indigestible chitin that can cause impactions in the digestive tracts of avian neonates. By using 3-week-old crickets, white molted mealworms, and waxworms during the first 7–10 days impactions may be avoided. Ground meat products supplemented with vitamins and minerals are available as another source of protein.

Converting an avian neonate from an easily digestible diet to an adult diet is done with a series of transitions. For species such as the ground hornbills and kookaburras, which have adult mice in their adult diets, juvenile mice from approximately 7–10 days provide a small amount of fur for these gradual changes. Removing the head, legs, and wings of crickets may be used as a transitional step from the soft-bodied 3-week-old crickets prior to adding adult crickets with chitin to the diet.

Some food items that are found in the captive adult diet may not be needed for hand-rearing, but adding them prior to weaning may increase the likelihood that the bird will consume a well-balanced diet as an adult. It is far easier to introduce new items to a dependent chick that is being hand-fed versus one that is already weaned. Soaked dry dog or cat food and processed meat products are two such items. Anoles are added to the diet of Guam Kingfishers because they are an item that is usually available, and the male uses them in courtship when feeding the female.

Because none of these adult diets have a significant amount of a commercial avian pellet as a nutritionally balanced component, all of the diets used for hand-rearing are supplemented with calcium carbonate (1% of the amount of food fed the previous day) and a liquid B-complex high potency vitamin (Nature's Answer Hi potency liquid dietary supplement for humans). This product contains 3.3 mg Vitamin $B_1$ (thiamine), 3.3 mg $B_6$ (pyridoxine), and 6.6 mcg $B_{12}$ (cyanocobalamin) dosing 1 ml/50 g of the amount of food fed the previous day. For instance, if 50 g of food was fed the previous day, the calcium supplement would be 0.5 g of calcium carbonate and the vitamin supplement would be 1.0 ml of the liquid vitamin B for the following day. Crickets and mealworms are gut-loaded with a commercial calcium-based feed for 3 days prior to being fed.

The frugivorous hornbill neonates are fed approximately 70% high-protein items (neonate mice and insects) with 30% fruit for the first 10 days. The proportions gradually shift to 75% fruit and 25% protein items by approximately day 28. Papaya has traditionally been used in this facility as a source of hydration in some high-protein hand-rearing diets. By 30 days of age there is a change to a fruit mix composed of melon, apple, and other fruits as seasonally available.

The carnivorous ground hornbill chicks are fed 100% protein items. A ground meat product is introduced gradually at about 2 weeks, as is fur from adult mice (Table 36.4).

Determining when to make these changes was initially by trial and error. Once success was achieved, that became the starting point for other closely related species. This underscores the importance of keeping careful records. Actual intake may vary from the target as the response of the chick and the rate of growth are taken into consideration (Figure 36.3).

## Feeding Procedures

There are three basic concerns to be addressed when hand-feeding chicks: when to feed (frequency), how much to feed (quantity), and how to feed (technique). Each of these factors changes during the rearing of a chick. These transitions are what make hand-feeding such a dynamic process.

Changes in frequency of feedings occur related to each species' capacity for larger quantities of food and the greater periods of time they can go without food. As greater quantities are fed, chicks will stop eating and make it clear that it is time to reduce the frequency again. Healthy chicks are never fed by force. Keepers learn to "read" a chick's behavior and modify what they are doing to get a strong feeding response. The small bee-eaters were started at 13 times a day (every hour); all the others were started at 7 times a day (every 2 hours). Feedings occur between 6:30 a.m. and 6:30 p.m.

Forceps or curved spoons are used to feed chopped fruit or prey items (Figure 36.4). Diet items are cut into small bite-sized pieces and are gradually cut larger as chicks grow and can easily swallow larger bites. Using blunt-tipped forceps, the food is dipped in bottled drinking water and placed far back into the mouth. By feeding in this manner, chicks are less apt to spit the food item back out. Chicks may regurgitate all or part of a feeding if they are fed too much, too fast, or if either they or the food items are too cold. Curved spoons have been used for hornbill chicks as they get older, and a teaspoon that was modified with the sides bent up was more efficient for delivering larger quantities.

The quantity fed has been determined differently over the years. At times, chicks have been fed to satiation or ad lib, but more often a percentage of the body weight has been used to determine

Table 36.4 San Diego Zoo's Avian Propagation Center hand-rearing protocol.

**Common Name: Northern Ground Hornbill**
**Species Name: *Bucorvis abyssinicus***

| Day | Brooder/temp. | Freq. | Diet (by weight) | Intake (as % BW) | Misc. |
|---|---|---|---|---|---|
| 1 | AICU/95 °F, drop 1°/day. Nest cup lined with paper towel/tissue. | | Wait 12–24 hrs posthatch to feed. | | |
| 2 | | 2 hr (7×) | 100% chopped pinkies dipped in bottled drinking water. | 20% | Supplement w/calcium carbonate and liquid vitamin B. |
| 3 | | 2 hr (7×) | | 25% | Begin sunning. |
| 4 | | 3 hr (5×) | Change to whole pinkies. | 30% | |
| 5 | | 3 hr (5×) | | 35% | |
| 8 | Add Nomad mat to nest. | 4 hr (4×) | | 35% | May increase intake to 45% to get 15–20% wt gains. |
| 12 | | 5 hr (3×) | Change to fuzzies. | 35% | Change from $CaCO_3$ to dicalcium phosphate. |
| 13 | | 5 hr (3×) | Add 25% carnivore meat (75% fuzzie). | 35% | |
| 14 | | 5 hr (3×) | 50% carnivore meat, 50% fuzzie. | 35% | |
| 15 | | 5 hr (3×) | Gradually change to mouse torso with no fur. | 35% | Eyes open. |
| 17 | | 5 hr (3×) | Add small amount of fur (1 in. square) and gradually increase. | 35% | Pin feathers. |
| 21 | | 6 hr (2×) | | 35% | May cast pellet. |
| 24 | Move to 1/2 floor with heat, in a tub. | 6 hr (2×) | | 35% | |
| 30 | | 6 hr (2×) | | Ad lib | |
| 33 | No heat inside. | 6 hr (2×) | | Ad lib | ~Day 40, self-feeding begins; leave dish between feedings. |
| 52 | Outside at night with heat. | 6 hr (2×) | | Ad lib | |
| 53 | | 6 hr (2×) | | Ad lib | May be out of tub. |
| 56 | Outside w/out heat. | 6 hr (2×) | | Ad lib | May be able to fly. |
| 63 | | 1 × | | Ad lib | Weaned. |

Weight gains should be maintained at 15–20% per day.
Hornbill chicks will impact on fur, feathers, dirt, sand, and rocks.

the amount to be fed. This amount typically starts off at 20% of body weight and gradually increases to 35–50% in the hornbill species and 50–75% in the other smaller species during the first week. It may be held at that highest level until the chick starts regulating the amount eaten or it may be reduced gradually. The goal is to wean the chick at the same age as a parent-reared chick.

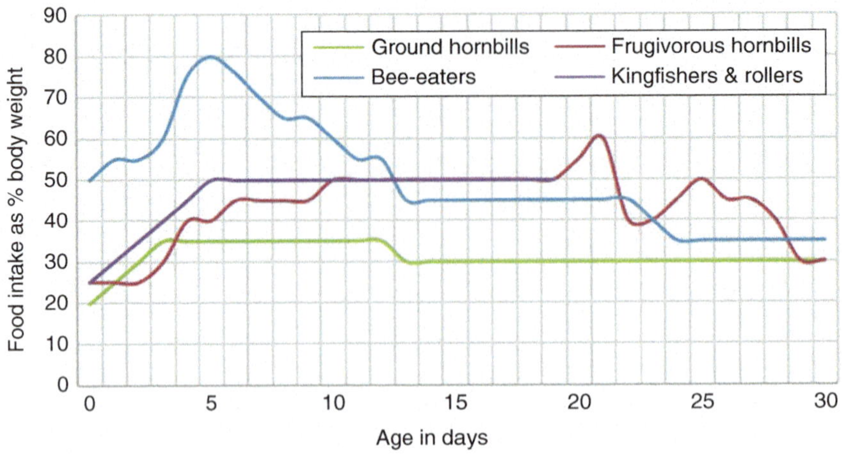


Figure 36.3 Intake targets for hornbills, bee-eaters, kingfishers, and rollers.

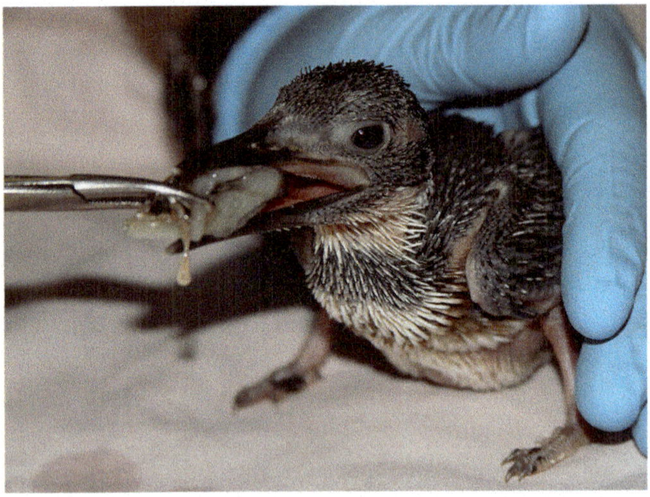

Figure 36.4 Belted Kingfisher at 2 weeks being fed with hemostats. *Source:* photo courtesy of International Bird Rescue.

Hatchlings, nestlings, and fledglings respond to feeding in different ways. Avian hatchlings' neck muscles are relatively weak and may cause their heads to sway as they reach up with beaks open for feeding. Care and attention are needed to avoid injuring the mouth with the feeding forceps. Missing the target may result in a dirty chick. Cleaning the chick with a warm damp cloth may prevent bacterial infections in the eyes and keep the feather follicles free of debris that could hinder normal feather development. Nestlings are stronger and may fall out of a nest cup in their enthusiasm to feed. It is important to ensure the safety of the nestling by never leaving it unattended while outside the brooder and to use nest cups that are deep enough to prevent a nestling from falling out. Nestlings that are close to fledgling, on the other hand, must be in a cup that they can get out of as they become more mobile.

The goal is to allow the chick to fledge at the same age as a parent-reared chick (Table 36.2). Feeding responses often decrease near fledging. It is a difficult decision to make between allowing the chick to refuse feedings and getting enough food into it to meet its energy requirements. Using a growth curve of normal surviving chicks as a guide may make those decisions easier (Figure 36.5a–d).

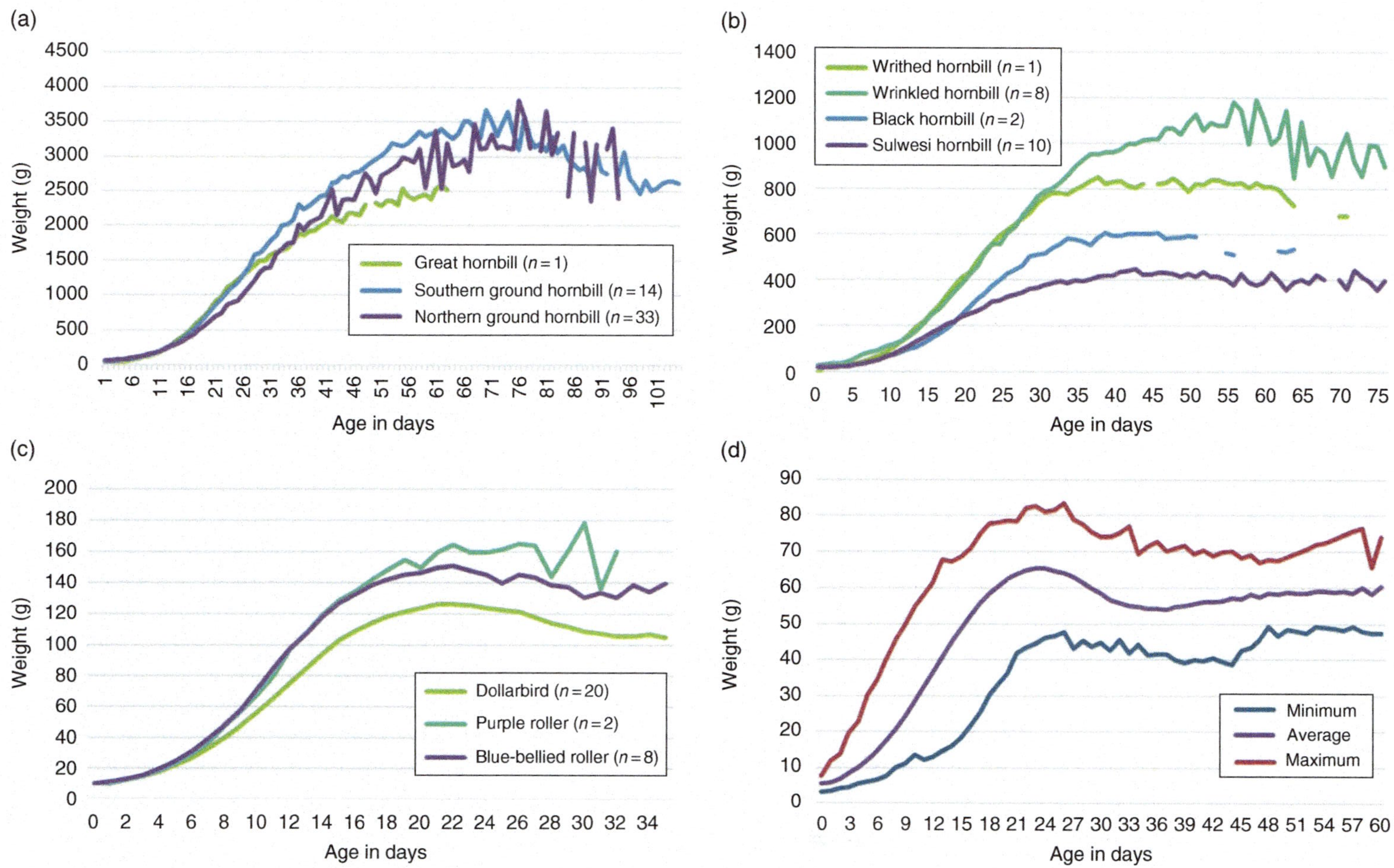


**Figures 36.5** (a) Average chick growth curve for three species of hornbills; (b) average chick growth curve for four species of hornbills; (c) roller chick growth curve; (d) Guam Kingfisher chick growth curve.

Nowhere is it more important to have good sanitation habits than in the area of food preparation. Food is prepared indoors on stainless steel counters using separate cutting boards and knives for fruit and meat items to minimize bacterial contamination. Keepers wash their hands regularly during the preparations. All perishable food items are kept refrigerated and are not allowed to sit out in the sun after being delivered. Live forage items – such as crickets, mealworms, anoles, and mice – are housed for 3–4 days prior to being fed to chicks. The housing, food, and water containers for these items are cleaned regularly. The sources where prey items are obtained are inspected to ensure that the product is high quality.

## Expected Weight Gain

Chicks are weighed daily prior to feeding until fledged and less frequently thereafter. Weights are recorded and added to a growth curve to be compared with weights of previously reared normal chicks (Figure 36.5a–d). Amounts of food fed are recorded, along with a rating of feeding response and the presence of feces. Feed charts are computer spreadsheets with formulas to calculate percent weight changes in chicks and to tally amounts fed of solids and fluids. On a daily basis, keepers enter the chick weight; intake target, based on a percent of body weight; and frequency of feedings, as prompted from a protocol. The target amount to be fed for the day and for each feeding is automatically calculated on the spreadsheet. For instance, if a chick weighs 10 g, the desired intake is 35% and the frequency of feedings is 7 times a day; then one multiplies 10 times 0.35 and divides by 7 to determine that the chick will be fed 0.5 g per feeding. Comparisons are then easily made between the goals for the day and what was actually ingested. Quantities of supplements given are also calculated based on the amount fed the previous day.

Observations of growth and development milestones, such as eyes opening and fledging, are documented during the rearing process (Figure 36.6). If chicks survive and have developed at the same rate as parent-reared chicks, one wants to use those same milestones as a measure for the next chicks reared (Table 36.5).

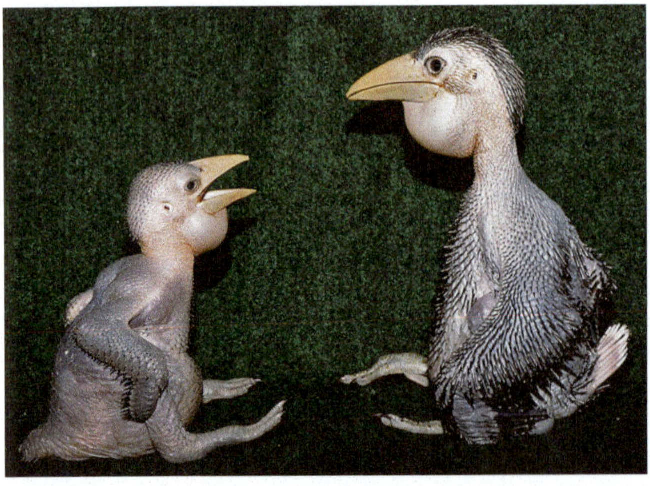

Figure 36.6 Wrinkled Hornbill chicks at day 23 and 28. *Source:* photo © Zoological Society of San Diego.

Table 36.5 Developmental milestones.

| Developmental milestones (approx. in days) | Kingfishers | Bee-eaters | Rollers | Woodhoopoe | Sulawesi Hornbill | Wrinkled Hornbill | Ground Hornbill | Great Hornbill |
|---|---|---|---|---|---|---|---|---|
| Casting pellet | 6 | 11 | 20 | – | 10 | | 20 | – |
| Eyes open | 12 | 12 | 12 | – | 12 | 15 | 15 | – |
| Mobile/active | 14 | 14 | 14 | 14 | 30 | 30 | 50 | 55 |
| Fed ad lib | 20 | 30 | 20 | 30 | 30 | 30 | 30 | 30 |
| Self-feeding begins | 20 | 17 | 30 | 26 | 30 | 40 | 40 | 40 |
| Weaned | 25 | 30 | 35 | 35 | 50 | 60 | 60 | 65 |
| Flying | 30 | 30 | 30 | 30 | 40 | 65 | >55 | 75 |

## Housing

Neonates are housed in electronic metal brooders with a starting temperature of 94.0–96.0 °F (34.4–35.6 °C). The temperature is reduced by approximately 0.5–1 °F (0.3–0.6 °C) each day, depending on the chick's reaction. Observations are made of the chick's behavior, noting whether there is shivering, panting, legs and wings splayed out, moving away from clutchmates, or huddling together. Feeding responses and fecal output may both decrease if the temperature and humidity are not optimal. For the first 10 days, water pans, which are disinfected every other day, are placed in the brooders to provide humidity, starting at approximately 50–59% RH. This may prevent dehydration and reduce flaking skin. Brooders are covered to simulate nest cavities and to reduce contact with keepers. Brooders are disinfected between clutches or more frequently as needed.

Chicks are placed in plastic bowls lined with paper towels and tissue paper. Looped vinyl matting (Nomad matting) is used in the bottom of the bowls to keep the chicks from sitting in their feces and to give their toes something to grip. Paper is changed after each feeding, and bowls and matting are disinfected daily.

When pinfeathers open, chicks are moved into heated box brooders, wire cages, or rubber tubs on the floor (Figure 36.7). When chicks are fully feathered and perching, they are allowed access to an outside run with perches and access to a heat lamp. After a few transition days, birds are left outside day and night. Heat lamps are removed within approximately 3 days or when the ambient temperature does not drop below 50 °F (10 °C).

## Weaning

Weaning begins when a chick can physically pick up food unaided and continues until the chick refuses to be hand-fed. Food is left with the chick between feedings when it becomes mobile and the eyes are open. The first feeding will be omitted shortly after the chick is observed picking up food on its own. Prompting occurs at feeding time until the chick refuses all attempts to hand-feed and growth is determined to be normal.

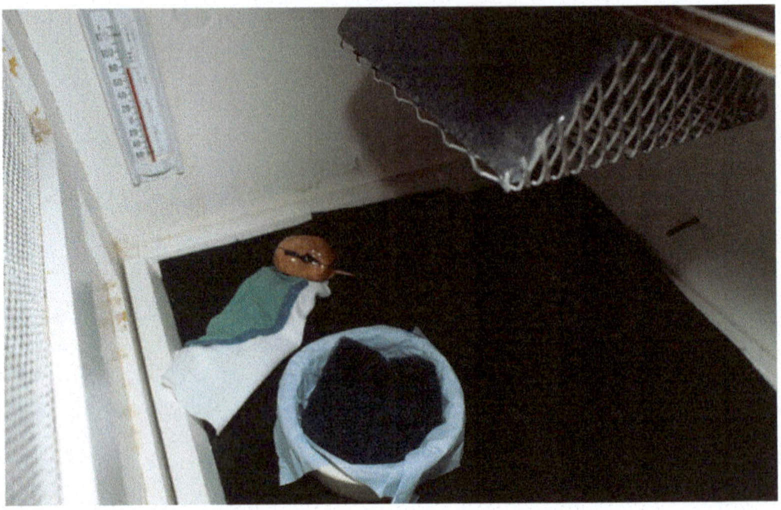

Figure 36.7 Guam Kingfisher puppet in a box brooder. *Source:* photo © Zoological Society of San Diego.

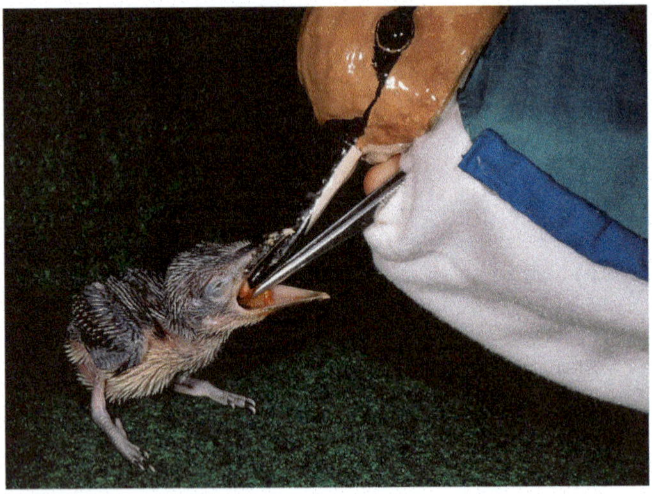

Figure 36.8 Guam Kingfisher at -30 days being hand-fed by a puppet. *Source:* photo © Zoological Society of San Diego.

## Preparation for Introduction to Captive Flock

If there is more than one chick in a clutch, they are raised in the same brooder, but in a separate nest cup to avoid siblicide. They are permitted to fledge together and continue to be housed together after that. Chicks that hatch without siblings may be housed either next door to older chicks of the same species or a closely related species if available.

A hand puppet has been used to rear the Guam Kingfisher as a precaution against imprinting on humans (Figure 36.8). "Ghost-rearing" may be used in the absence of a puppet, where the keepers cover their body with a sheet and wear a sock over their hand while feeding. These species have not seemed to be especially susceptible to maladjusted behaviors associated with imprinting.

Table 36.6 Results of hand-rearing.

| Species | # Hand-reared | # Survived (30 days) | % Survivability |
|---|---|---|---|
| Laughing Kookaburra | 8 | 8 | 100% |
| Guam Kingfisher | 56 | 50 | 89% |
| Sulawesi Collared Kingfisher | 1 | 1 | 100% |
| White-breasted Kingfisher | 9 | 9 | 100% |
| Carmine Bee-eater | 2 | 1 | 50% |
| White-throated Bee-eater | 2 | 2 | 100% |
| White-fronted Bee-eater | 21 | 12 | 57% |
| Blue-bellied Roller | 6 | 6 | 100% |
| Purple Roller | 2 | 2 | 100% |
| Dollarbird | 21 | 19 | 90% |
| Common Hoopoe | 1 | 1 | 100% |
| Green Woodhoopoe | 1 | 1 | 100% |
| Northern Ground Hornbill | 42 | 34 | 81% |
| Southern Ground Hornbill | 2 | 2 | 100% |
| Black Hornbill | 2 | 1 | 50% |
| Great Hornbill | 1 | 1 | 100% |
| Sulawesi Hornbill | 11 | 10 | 90% |
| Trumpeter Hornbill | 1 | 1 | 100% |
| Knobbed Hornbill | 4 | 3 | 75% |
| Wrinkled Hornbill | 10 | 8 | 80% |
| Writhed Hornbill | 2 | 1 | 50% |
| Totals: | 205 | 175 | 85% |

## Results

Hand-rearing protocols evolve over time as challenges are overcome and success is achieved. Changes occur related to housing, feeding frequency, diet items, and quantities to feed. Learning from past observations is the key to making changes that result in greater successes (Table 36.6).

## Acknowledgments

The authors would like to acknowledge the tremendous efforts of all the bird keepers at the San Diego Zoo's Avian Propagation Center, Bird Department, and San Diego Zoo's Safari Park. Their care of eggs and chicks, and collecting data during artificial incubation and hand-rearing, have made this possible. Thanks to the curators – David Rimlinger, Andrew Stehly, and Michael Mace – for their continued support in these endeavors.

## Sources for Products Mentioned

Animal Intensive Care Unit, Grumbach Hatcher, and Hi-intensity candler: Lyon Technologies, Inc., 1690, Brandywine Avenue, Chula Vista, CA. 91911, (619) 216-3400, https://lyonvet.com.

Commercial avian pellet: Marion Jungle Pellets, manufactured by Marion Zoological, 14149 21st Ave N, Plymouth, MN 55447, (800) 327-7974, www.marionzoological.com. Outside the United States: (763) 559-3305.

Disinfectant: Sani-cide 94, manufactured by Maintex, 13300 E. Nelson Avenue City of Industry, CA 91746 (800) 446-1888 www.maintex.com.

Dog food: Iams Less Active For Dogs, manufactured by Iams Company, (800) 675-3849, www.iams.com.

Forced air hatcher: AB Newlife Hatcher, manufactured by A.B. Incubator Ltd., PO Box 215, Moline, IL 61265.

Forced air incubator: Humidaire Model 20, manufactured by Humidaire Incubator Co., 217 W. Wayne St., PO Box 9, New Madison, OH 45346 (out of business).

Forced air incubator: Petersime Model 1 Incubator: Petersime Incubator Company, 300 North Bridge Street, Gettysburg, OH 45328 (out of business).

Insect calcium feed: High Calcium Cricket Diet manufactured by Marion Zoological, 14149 21st Ave N, Plymouth, MN 55447, (800) 327-7974, www.marionzoological.com. Outside the United States (763) 559-3305.

Liquid B-complex vitamin: Nature's Answer Liquid Vitamin B-complex, high potency formula, manufactured by Nature's Answer, 85 Commerce Dr., Hauppauge, NY 11788, www.naturesanswer.com.

Looped vinyl matting: Nomad Matting, manufactured by 3M Product Information Center, 3M Center, Building 042-6E-37, St. Paul, MN 55144-1000, (866) 364-3577, http://solutions.3m.com/en_US.

Meat products used until 1999: Nebraska Bird of Prey Diet, manufactured by Central Nebraska Packing, Inc., PO Box 550, North Platte, NE 69103-0550, (308) 532-1250, (877)900-3003, (800)445-2881, fax (308)532-2744, http://www. nebraskabrand.com, info@nebraskabrand.com.

Meat products used between 2000 and 2015: Natural Balance® Meat-eating Bird Diet, processed by Dick Van Patten's Natural Balance Pet Foods, Inc., 12924 Pierce Street, Pacoima, CA 91331, (800) 829-4493, www.naturalbalanceinc.com (discontinued).

Meat products used since 2015: Nebraska Feline Premium Horsemeat Diet, manufactured by Central Nebraska Packing, Inc., PO Box 550, North Platte, NE 69103-0550, (308) 532-1250, (877)900-3003, (800)445-2881, fax (308)532-2744, http://www. nebraskabrand.com, info@nebraskabrand.com.

Pedialyte®: Abbott Laboratories, Columbus, OH 43215-1724, www.abbott.com.

Scale: Ohaus scale, manufactured by Ohaus Corporation, 7 Campus Dr., Suite 310, Parsippany, NJ 07054, www.us.ohaus.com

UV sterilizer: Hanovia Inc./Hanovia Lamp Division, 6 Evans St., Fairfield, NJ 07004, (973) 651-5529.

## References

Fry, C.H., Fry, K., and Harris, A. (1992). *Kingfishers, Bee-eaters & Rollers*. Princeton, New Jersey: Princeton University Press.

del Hoyo, J. (2001). *Handbook of the Birds of the World, Vol 6. Mousebirds to Hornbills* (eds. A. Elliott and J. Saragatal). Barcelona: Lynx Edicions.

Kemp, A. (1995). *The Hornbills*. New York: Oxford University Press Inc.

## Further Reading

Woodall, P.F. and Kirwan, G.M. (2019). Guam kingfisher (Todiramphus cinnamominus). In: *Handbook of the Birds of the World Alive* (eds. J. del Hoyo, A. Elliott, J. Sargatal, et al.). Barcelona: Lynx Edicions https://www.hbw.com/node/55769. Accessed June 16, 2019.

# 37

# Toucans

*Martin Vince*

## Introduction

The Toucan family, Ramphastidae, comprises a total of 35 species of toucans, toucanets, and aracaris. *Ramphastids,* as they are generally known, are in the Order Piciformes along with their close relatives the woodpeckers and barbets. Toucans nest in tree cavities that are either abandoned parrot nests or cavities excavated by the birds themselves within the trunks and boughs of rotting trees. Aracaris and toucanets are the smallest members of the family; their nest cavities are approximately 7 in. (17 cm) in diameter and extend to 12 in. (30 cm) below the entrance hole. The large toucans, genus *Ramphastos,* require cavities of approximately 9 in. (22 cm) in diameter that extend to 16 in. (38 cm) or more below the entrance hole. The ideal nest site may be a semi-rotten palm log approximating these dimensions that can be modified by the birds themselves. Toucans have fairly strong beaks and are capable of excavating a nest chamber in soft wood. In captivity, nest boxes may also be used. However, they are poorly accepted by members of the genus *Ramphastos,* which are generally much harder to breed than the aracaris and toucanets.

Toucans have a lightweight, honeycomb-structured bill. For the chick, however, the structure becomes increasingly unwieldy; and the only way the bird can remain upright is to sit in a backward-leaning position with feet up in the air (Figure 37.1). Young toucans have a patch of boney ridges on the back of each leg that acts as a shoe while the feet themselves are elevated for the first couple of weeks. The boney "shoes" disappear at fledging as they are no longer needed. This apparently comical situation is important for the caregiver to understand because older chicks will fall forward if left unaided on a countertop.

All toucans are omnivores, using their serrated bills to eat small animals, as well as an array of vegetation and fruits. The sexes are alike in nearly all species. Two to four plain white eggs are laid directly on the floor of the nest chamber, with no materials added. Both sexes incubate the eggs. Aracaris and toucanets incubate for about 16 days; the large toucans incubate for about 18 days. Chicks fledge at 6–7 weeks of age, and can feed themselves reliably at 10–12 weeks of age.

## Criteria for Intervention

Most toucans are hand-reared by design, either from incubator-hatched eggs, or as older chicks taken from the nest for taming. Some, however, will be found abandoned on the aviary floor or may be retrieved from a nest because they are sick or abandoned or the parents are incapable of rearing

*Hand-Rearing Birds*, Second Edition. Edited by Rebecca S. Duerr and Laurie J. Gage.

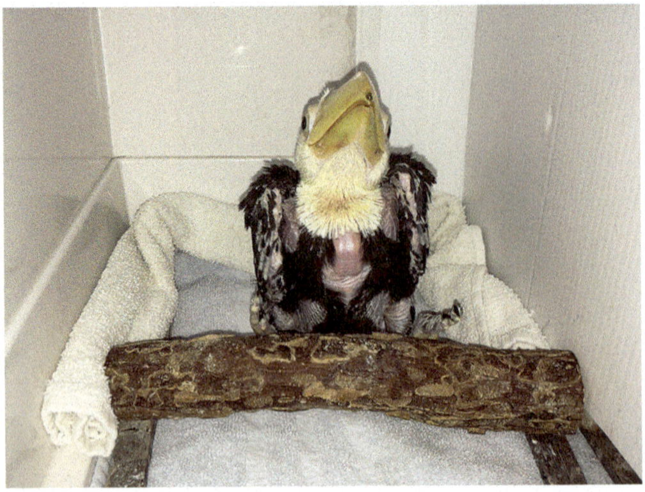

Figure 37.1 Toucan chick resting on the boney ridges on the back of each leg.

them. All require immediate care, and the proactive aviculturist will be prepared with an incubator or brooder that has been operating at the correct temperature for some days.

## Record Keeping

Although hand-rearing a chick is a memorable experience, inevitably memories fade, making detailed record keeping essential if successes are to be repeated and failures avoided. The ability to hand-rear toucanets and aracaris is a rare skill, and the ability to hand-rear large species of the genus *Ramphastos* is even more uncommon. It is important, therefore, that all hand-rearing information is carefully recorded to ensure the probability of future successes with these species.

Computerized records are strongly favored over paper ones. Hand-feeding notes may be recorded in a table, which eliminates illegible handwriting, makes email consultations simple, and facilitates graphing and other statistical operations. Miniature photographs of the chick are also easily inserted into a table, providing perfect benchmarks for future chicks.

## Initial Care and Stabilization

A chick found on the aviary floor will usually be hypothermic and should be cupped in warm hands and carried to an incubator or brooder. If the chick is uninjured, vigorous movement will usually be detected as its body temperature begins to rise. Toucan chicks are robust and, depending on age and injuries, have moderately good prospects of surviving such an event.

## Common Medical Problems

### Misaligned Beak

Toucans have extremely malleable beaks until about 3 weeks of age. The tip of a toucan's bill (1/8 in./3 mm) may become misaligned for various reasons, including syringe pressure during feeding. The defect is relatively easy to rectify by applying gentle pressure to the tip of the bill in the direction that opposes the curvature. Gently bend the tip of the mandible 20–30° beyond center, repeating the procedure three or four times per day, or as often as recommended by your veterinarian.

### *Candida* Overgrowth

Some aviculturists use the antifungal drug Nystatin (Bristol Myers Squibb) orally as a prophylaxis treatment in the hand-rearing of toucans. The use of Nystatin for the first 2–3 weeks seems to do no harm and should help reduce the risk of *Candida*. There is enough anecdotal information to suggest that the use of Nystatin is helpful. However, it is also the case that toucans may be successfully hand-reared without using Nystatin. Ultimately, the decision is made by the aviculturist and the avian veterinarian.

### Impaction from Organic Material

When young chicks are taken from the nest, be aware that they may have been fed inappropriate items such as wood chips, sticks, cable ties, or other small nonfood items by their parents. The chick itself may also have eaten bark and soil from the cavity floor. Watch for poor weight gains or the appearance of soil in feces for clues as to whether the chick could be impacted. A chick may be given a small amount of mineral oil (between 0.1 and 0.2 ml depending on the size of the chick) as a laxative after being removed from the nest. However, the chick will normally defecate or cough up nonfood items by itself in the first 24 hours.

## Diet Recipes

When fed by their parents, toucans receive a high-protein diet for the first several days, beginning with large insects and progressing to small animals such as baby birds, mice, and small reptiles. Even though fruit is the mainstay of the adult diet, it is only when the chicks are 4–7 days old, depending on the species, that they receive fruit from their parents. This seemingly unusual initial diet is normal for fruit-eating birds and should be taken into account when hand-rearing their chicks.

Toucan chicks may be successfully reared using a small amount of pureed fruit (apple or papaya, for example), "pinkie" (newborn) mice, and a proprietary hand-rearing formula developed for parrots, such as Kaytee® Exact® Hand Feeding Formula (Kaytee). The precise recipe is probably not critical, but an approximate mix by weight of 20% pureed apple and/or papaya and 80% Kaytee Exact made to the appropriate ratio of water : Kaytee Exact powder (Table 37.1) seems to be satisfactory. In addition to this mixture, and in keeping with the natural feeding pattern, the author recommends dribbling the innards of pinkie mice into the chick's mouth or pureeing pinkies for syringe feeding. It is recommended that a calcium supplement (calcium carbonate) be used daily until fledging. Chicks are fed approximately 0.5 g of pharmaceutical grade calcium carbonate per day from 1 to 10 days of age, gradually increasing to 1.5 g per day for chicks 10 days and older.

The abovementioned foods produce very satisfactory results. It must be said, however, that the ingredients are intended to cover all the nutritional "bases" because the rearing of toucans is still a rare event, which lacks scientific study. The success of this diet disguises the fact that it still needs improvement. The fruit component is arguably questionable at a life stage that does not receive fruit in nature (i.e. during the period 1–7 days of age). Future work may explore the benefits of

Table 37.1 Feeding chart for young toucan chicks.

| Age | Water | Kaytee ® exact ® Hand Feeding Formula (powder) |
|---|---|---|
| Day 1 | 6 parts | 1 part |
| Day 2 | 5 parts | 1 part |
| Day 3 | 4 parts | 1 part |
| Day 4 | 3 parts | 1 part |
| Day 5 | 3 parts | 1 part |
| Day 6 | 3 parts | 1 part with the introduction of small pieces of pellets and fruit |

reducing or eliminating the fruit component from diets fed to chicks aged 1–7 days old. The feeding of pinkie mice may also cause concern due to the well-known risk of iron storage disease. However, in the initial days of life, a chick has an especially high nutritional requirement and the heme-iron of meat is not likely to give rise to iron storage disease. Withholding small amounts of pinkie mice, at least during the first several days, is more problematic than not, producing sluggish or negative weight gains. In any case, the threat of iron storage disease to modern toucan collections is now practically nonexistent thanks to good nutrition, health care, and successful captive-breeding.

## Feeding Procedures

As with many species, toucan chicks may be hard to rouse in the morning. Gently tapping on the countertop may be needed to stimulate activity because the vibration and sound equate to an adult landing on the tree trunk; making whistling or chirping sounds may also be helpful, as well as creating a shadow as if the parent had just arrived at the nest hole.

A toucan chick has poor control of its head, which tends to flail about during feeding. One's fingers can be ringed around the head, to control it without actually holding it or fear of damaging the delicate beak.

Toucans lack a crop, and they may become temporarily full after receiving only a small part of the diet. Once the portion of food has been swallowed, however, the chick will again appear hungry and demand more. Once a chick reaches 10 days of age, it is normal for a feeding to take at least 15 minutes, as the bird goes through multiple full–empty cycles. Finally, however, the head flops completely backward as the bird truly becomes full. Feeding a toucan chick properly, therefore, takes considerably longer than other species the reader may be familiar with, such as parrots. An expert may feed a parrot chick in less than a minute, but no amount of practice can speed the feeding of a toucan.

After each feed, the author recommends cleaning food residue from inside and outside the chick's mouth using a moistened cloth or cotton-tipped swab.

### Days 1–6

To promote yolk sac absorption, wait several hours before giving the first feed. The initial feed should be mostly liquid, such as distilled water or an oral electrolyte such as Pedialyte® (Abbott Labs), with only a minimal amount of Kaytee Exact. For subsequent feeds, the Kaytee formula should be progressively thickened according to the approximate schedule in Table 37.1.

Hatchlings should be fed every 60–90 minutes for 14 hours. Initial feeds on day 1 should be approximately 2–3% of body weight (e.g. 2% of a 9 g bird: $0.02 \times 9 = 0.18$ ml per feed), increasing to 3–4% of bodyweight by the afternoon of day 1. It is a good idea to deliver the food in amounts as small as 0.05 ml until greater confidence is achieved, rather than giving a single food delivery as one might with a parrot, for example.

For at least the first 4 days, the chick should be fed using a 1 ml syringe. Depending on personal preference, the syringe may be fitted with a feeding tip, such as a plastic teat infusion cannula tip (see Figure 1.4). A plain 1 ml syringe may be equally preferred, especially in the case of large species (genus *Ramphastos*). Accidental food aspiration is a significant cause of mortality in hatchlings at this stage. Within the first week, consideration should be given to transitioning the chick onto small food pieces. This approach creates a more natural presentation for the chick and carries a lower risk of aspiration than syringe-feeding. From 6 days of age, the toucan chick is able to eat small pieces of pellet that are thoroughly soaked in water. The caregiver should use the same brand of pellet that is intended for the bird's adult diet. Low iron pellets are recommended, such as those manufactured by Kaytee, Mazuri, and ZuPreem.

### Day 7 Onward

At approximately 7 days of age, it is relatively easy to feed pieces of the adult diet either from forceps or one's fingers. This may be possible as early as 4 or 5 days of age in the case of large chicks. Delivering food directly into the mouth tends to be easier with a pair of forceps, but fingers are safer for older chicks because they are far more active. At 7 days of age, feeding frequency may be reduced to 6 or 7 times per day over 12 hours. At 2 weeks of age, 5 feeds per day are sufficient, and by 5 weeks of age 3–4 feeds per day are sufficient.

At about 3 weeks of age, toucans become fussy eaters and routinely spit out their food. One's index finger may be used to push food into the bird's mouth to encourage swallowing. Otherwise, food will sit unnoticed in the mouth and may create a choking hazard when the bird slouches.

Toucans are very light-sensitive at this age, perhaps instinctively knowing that a change in lighting signals the arrival of a parent at the nest hole. Be careful not to cast a shadow over the brooder when checking the chick unless you plan to feed it at that moment. Even before the eyes are open, the bird will know you are there; and certainly do not turn the room light on or off unless you are prepared to disturb the chick. This is most awkward at the end of the day when the room lights have to be turned off. In the case of incandescent bulbs, a dimmer switch will greatly alleviate the problem because the lights may be gradually dimmed.

## Expected Weight Gain

Weigh the chick at the same time every 24 hours. Digital scales are ideal since they are quick and easy to read, minimizing the disturbance to the chick. An acceptable daily weight gain can fall within a range as wide as 5–15%, although the average (mean) daily weight gain should be about 10%. If the weight gain is outside the range of 5–15%, either adjust the amount per feed or the time interval between feeds.

### Poor Weight Gains

*Example:* if a chick is fed every 75 minutes but only experiences a 2% weight gain, the feeding frequency may be increased to every 60 minutes. Changes should be gradual. Normally, either the feeding frequency *or* the amount per feed will need to be changed to achieve the desired weight increase. Weigh the chick after 12 hours to help predict the 24-hour weight. If the 12-hour weight suggests that action is needed before waiting until tomorrow, one has the option of giving additional late feeds to better support the chick through the night. It is easiest to preempt tomorrow morning's poor weight by taking action tonight. If the weight does not improve the following day, consider these possibilities:

- Dehydration may be the problem, especially if the chick has recently suffered parental neglect. Provide liquid feeds of approximately half the amount of a normal feed two to four times during the day.
- The brooder temperature may be too low. Consider a 1–2° increase, and look for changes in feeding response/attitude.
- Add pinkie mice to fortify the diet for chicks aged 1–7 days, as described in the section on "Diet Recipes, earlier in this chapter.
- Weight gains will fall to near zero at 4 weeks of age because nutrition is used for feather production – not physical growth.

In general, the caregiver must carefully calculate daily weight changes using an array of tools to correct the course according to the individual chick's performance. If extraordinary weight gains are achieved (such as 40–50% in 24 hours), check for a mathematical error or fluid retention, both of which are possible. Do not panic if one day produces a low or negative weight gain, especially if the previous days saw large increases. Add pinkie mice if weight gains are sluggish; monitor the chick and look for panting or lethargy that may be suggestive of overheating or being cold, respectively. Overall, the chick should be as comfortable and as unstressed as possible to maximize weight gains and promote wellbeing.

## Housing

If more than one chick is being hand-reared, experience has shown that chicks are best kept together for the first couple of days. The long neck of each bird drapes over a sibling, with the arrangement appearing to be comfortable and self-supporting; perhaps the touch is even stress-reducing.

Likewise, a single chick appears to be more restful when supported by a suitable surface, such as a cloth-covered golf ball. Chicks may be contained in a small bowl lined with a towel. The towel provides important traction for the bird's feet, as well as a soft rim over which the chicks will drape their heads (Figure 37.2). After only a few days they will prefer the edge of the bowl for neck support. By this time their flailing heads will have become a hazard to each other, and separating the birds into individual bowls is recommended.

Thus, at about 3 weeks of age, it is advisable to separate the chicks into their own brooders, or at a minimum they should be protected from each other by cardboard barriers. Providing a perch in the brooder at about 34 days of age allows the feet to develop normally, avoiding the risk of foot injuries caused by staying in a bowl for too long. The perch also encourages a healthy standing posture which prevents the hind claws from cutting into the legs. The perch can be made portable and stable by screwing wooden "feet" beneath each end (Figure 37.3). Feeding two or three toucans in a single container may be hectic, and the birds' faces will get whacked by wildly competitive siblings if each is not protected from the others. At about this age, the chicks are large enough to be removed from the bowls. Toweling on the floor of the brooder is the ideal substrate, providing traction and cushioning, as well as being removable for easy cleaning. A lot of work is created by using towels because they have to be changed at every feed, but they are excellent for the purpose.

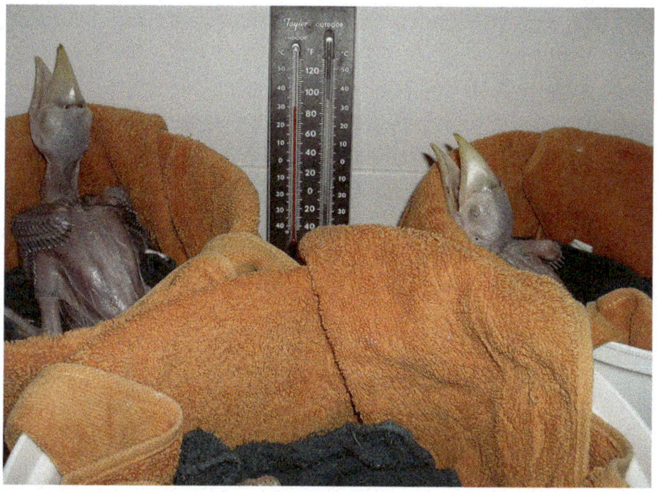

Figure 37.2 Thick, heavy towels provide traction that is important for foot health for these 18-day old toucan chicks.

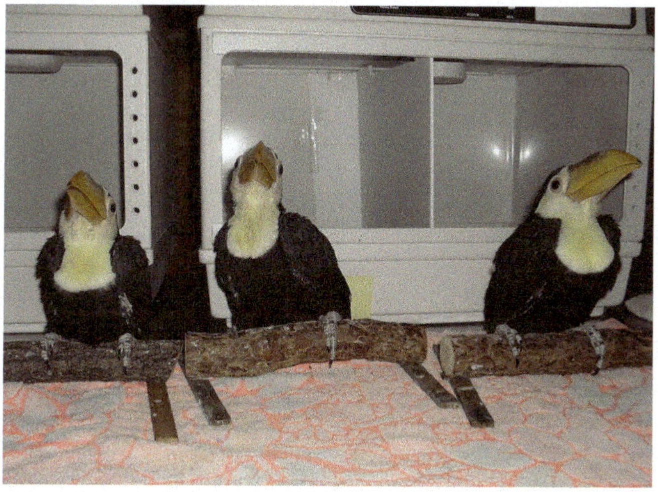

Figure 37.3 Perching is essential for foot health: 34-day old chicks.

## Fledging

At about 6 weeks of age, the most precarious part of the rearing process begins. Parrots may be content to languish in the brooder for a prolonged period of time, calm and tame after having been hand-reared. Toucans, on the other hand, have a powerful urge to fledge and will bounce and crash about in their brooder if that urge is forestalled. Fledging will happen, whether one is ready or not. Watch for signs of fledging, such as a readiness to fly from the brooder. When the time is right, move the brooder into a small aviary or enclosure. If the bird is tame, it can be carried on a perch to the aviary. The bird may fly immediately into the new surroundings, or more likely will observe them cautiously for a few more days before "fledging" at its leisure.

Do not clutter the aviary with too many perches. Select straight tree branches of about 2 in. (4.8 cm) in diameter with rough bark that the birds can use to clean their bills. Fledgling toucans can fly only about 4 ft. (1.2 m). However, after just a few days, young birds will fly greater distances and will need perching to accommodate that growing ability. Three perches, spaced 4 ft. (1.2 m) apart, are ideal because they provide both a short distance and longer distance of 8 ft. (2.4 m) for when the bird is ready. If possible, provide at least one high perch for roosting, with the main perches being about 5 ft. (1.5 m) above the ground. Also, provide a perch that reaches the ground so the bird can recover when it falls.

Toucans are inquisitive. They are constantly exploring their environment and thus have a frightening capacity to locate and swallow loose nails, screws, and the like if given the opportunity. Constantly check the fledgling's environment for dangerous foreign objects.

Expect the birds to begin feeding themselves at about 8 weeks of age, becoming completely self-feeding at 9–10 weeks of age. If possible, attach the food pan at perch level to make feeding easier for them.

## Acknowledgments

Thanks to all of the staff of the Riverbanks Zoo Bird Department, especially Bob Seibels, Curator of Birds Emeritus, for their great passion and dedication. Without such professionalism and countless hours of dedication, the knowledge described in this text would never have been developed.

## Sources for Products Mentioned

Calcium Carbonate USP Precipitated Light, manufactured by PCCA, 9901 S Wilcrest, Houston TX 77099, (800) 331-2498, www.pccarx.com, Item# 30-1944-500.

Kaytee exact® Hand Feeding Formula and Kaytee exact Rainbow® pellets: Kaytee Products Inc., 521 Clay St, Chilton, WI 53014, (800) Kaytee-1 or (920) 849-2321, www.kaytee.com.

Mazuri® ZuLiFe® Soft-Bill Diet: Mazuri, PMI Nutrition International, LLC, PO Box 66812, St. Louis, MO 63166, www.mazuri.com.

Nystatin: Bristol Myers Squibb, 345 Park Avenue, New York, NY 10154-0037, (212) 546-4000, www.bms.com.

Pedialyte: Abbott Laboratories, Columbus, OH 43215, www.abbott.com.

Zupreem® low iron softbill diet: Zupreem PO Box 9024, Mission, KS 66202, (800) 345-4767, www.zupreem.com.

# 38

# Woodpeckers

*Nancy Barbachano and Rebecca S. Duerr*

## Natural History

Woodpeckers are one of the oldest groups of birds, perhaps going back as far as 24–50 million years (Backhouse 2005). There are approximately 236 species of woodpeckers found throughout the world, including wrynecks and picolets (Gill and Donsker 2019); 22 species breed in North America (Rodewald 2015) including seven genera: *Picoides, Melanerpes, Sphyrapicus, Colaptes, Piculus, Dryobates,* and *Campephilus*. Many woodpeckers are local residents, although some such as Northern Flickers move to lower latitudes or elevations in winter (Wiebe and Moore 2017). One of the more important roles played by woodpeckers is that of "keystone species" in that they provide an important ecological role in maintaining healthy forests and woodlands (Aubry and Raley 2002). They excavate cavities (making homes for many other species), control insects, facilitate decay, and provide food for other species (sapsuckers).

All species in this order nest in holes and cavities and hatch altricial, blind, naked, and helpless young. The pink skin of hatchlings is very thin and translucent, so organs and blood vessels are visible; they are bald with no down at all (Figure 38.1). Their necks are longer than those of passerine chicks and they can be observed flinging their heads around in an uncontrolled manner or draping their necks over each other in the nest.

Woodpeckers nest in cavities, hence chicks are not exposed to direct light until they are mobile. Woodpeckers have a short incubation period of 10–14 days with both parents performing incubation duties. It is usually the male that does the incubation at night. Only the Acorn Woodpecker and the Red-Cockaded Woodpecker are cooperative breeders (Jackson 1994; Koenig et al. 1995).

Most woodpeckers have a zygodactyl (also called ectropodactyl) toe arrangement with two toes pointing forward and two pointing backward, and this assists in differentiating very young woodpeckers from similar-appearing passerine hatchlings. A few species, such as the Three-toed and Black-backed Woodpeckers, have only three toes: two forward, one back.

Woodpeckers have several unique physical features that make them unusual, including an elaborate hyoid apparatus that extends the tongue to impressive distances and retracts it to reside inside the mouth at rest. The bones of the hyoid curve around both sides of the back of the head between the mandibles and skull, then travel across the crown to insert at the right nare or continue to wrap around the right orbit (Bock 1999; Lovette and Fitzpatrick 2016). The tip of a woodpecker tongue is not only highly sensitive to touch, but its shape also varies depending upon the way it feeds. The various types of tongues are smooth (wrynecks), brush-like (Acorn

*Hand-Rearing Birds*, Second Edition. Edited by Rebecca S. Duerr and Laurie J. Gage.

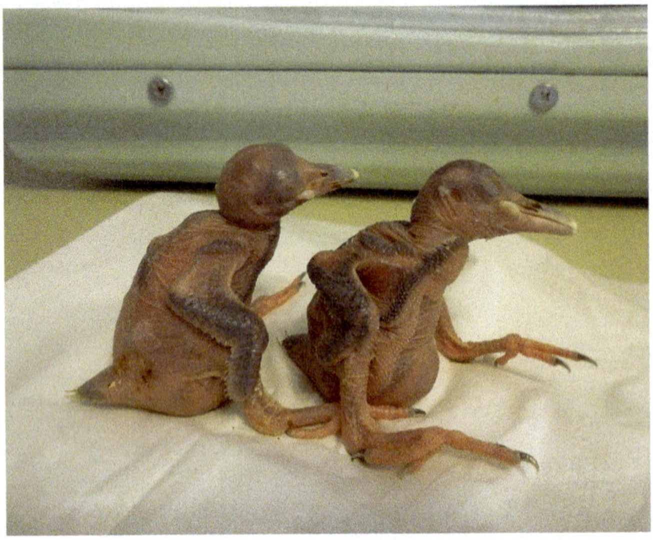

Figure 38.1 Hatchling Acorn Woodpeckers.

Woodpecker, Yellow-bellied Sapsucker), 1–3 barbs (Green-barred Woodpecker), 1–6 barbs (Lineated Woodpecker), and grouped barbs of different sizes (Pale-Billed and Golden-Fronted Woodpecker), in accord with the species' feeding style. It is imperative in any type of housing being used that the woodpecker tongue cannot get caught or stuck.

All woodpeckers, to some extent, are insectivores. They eat insect eggs, larvae, pupae, other invertebrates, and especially spiders. The most common insects eaten are ants, in all of their stages, and larval and adult beetles. Depending on the species, woodpeckers may eat fruit, nuts, seeds, berries, sap, flower nectar, cambium, and flower buds. Some woodpeckers are even fly catchers. Adult woodpeckers will change their diet seasonally and many species cache food for winter consumption. The majority of adult woodpeckers bring food to their young by the beakful; only a few species feed by regurgitation (Shunk 2016). Woodpeckers (e.g. Northern Flicker) may have a distensible esophagus that acts as a crop (Wiebe and Moore 2017).

Caregivers should make every effort to become informed about the natural history and behavioral specializations of the species in their care, since the social structures of some species such as Acorn Woodpeckers complicate the release of captive-reared young. Raising a single woodpecker and releasing it back into the wild guarantees a dead bird; every effort should be made to find a conspecific companion for singletons. It may be necessary to call other facilities to match up single birds. It is not recommended that woodpeckers be mixed with passerines or other species of similar-sized woodpeckers. Woodpeckers are naturally aggressive toward their nest and housemates; only place nestlings and/or fledglings with conspecifics of the same size. To avoid habituating the birds to humans, interact with them only at mealtime and avoid raising solitary birds. Usually, woodpeckers that are admitted as older nestlings or fledglings do not readily habituate to humans.

## Criteria for Intervention

Most woodpeckers brought into captivity as hatchlings or nestlings are the result of untimely tree removal, or if a tree with a nest falls. Because nests are located inside cavities, they are usually not discovered until the tree (or cactus) has been removed and someone has noticed the young vocalizing from inside a log. By this time, it is typically too late for the nest to be left undisturbed or replaced.

Young and adult woodpeckers are often brought into captivity after encounters with domestic pets or other mishaps, such as collisions with windows or cars, or due to being shot. As Northern Flickers feed primarily on the ground, they are occasionally caught by hawks. Fledglings found on the ground often have problems that require medical attention, but they may occasionally be captured by overzealous rescuers. Any seemingly uninjured fledgling that is a candidate for reunion with its parents should have a physical exam and flight test to rule out both subtle and obvious injuries. It is critical if a fledgling is returned to where it came from that careful observation in maintained to ensure a parent is still in the vicinity or, in the case of an Acorn Woodpecker, it is not rejected by the colony.

## Record Keeping

Orphaned and/or injured woodpeckers should be cared for only by those licensed and permitted to undertake their care. In the United States, woodpeckers are protected under the Migratory Bird Treaty Act and possession is regulated by the U.S. Fish and Wildlife Service and state natural resources departments. Basic information regarding the species, location found, date found, final disposition, and disposition date must be recorded. A medical record for each bird to track progress toward recovery is very useful. Record each bird's weight at admission and re-weigh frequently during care to ensure the bird is growing properly. Most larger organizations have their own intake forms, and many have moved to using online electronic records in recent years. See Appendix A for an example of a paper record, and Chapter 1 for more information regarding record keeping and electronic records.

## Initial Care and Stabilization

The main rule of initial baby bird care is warmth, rehydration, and feeding, in that order. Cold or unfeathered woodpeckers should be immediately placed into an incubator (aka brooder) at 90–95 °F (32.2–35 °C) and 40–50% humidity. Hatchlings have no ability to thermoregulate, so it is imperative they be placed into an incubator immediately upon intake. Do not feed chicks until they have begun to pass droppings. Feeding a cold or dehydrated baby bird before it is warm and hydrated will probably kill it.

When the bird is warm and calm, it may be hydrated orally or subcutaneously (SQ). Gaping, active hatchlings or nestlings should be orally hydrated until they produce droppings. Human infant electrolyte fluids (unflavored) are excellent for oral rehydration of baby birds. Give a few drops of warm oral fluids every 15–20 minutes with a small syringe or eye dropper and allow the bird to swallow completely before giving more. Keep a close watch on the bird's crop so that it does not become overly full. Once comfortable with the amount the chick is able to swallow, the amount may be raised to 2.5–5% of body weight in several mouthfuls. Never use a cannula tip when hydrating or feeding a woodpecker, lest the chick pull the tip off and swallow it in their enthusiasm to eat. Warm sterile fluids, such as 2.5% dextrose in 0.45% sodium chloride or lactated Ringer's solution, may be administered SQ at 5% of body weight (50 ml/kg) once, although repeated administrations may be needed for extremely dehydrated birds.

If the bird is depressed or not swallowing well, oral rehydration must be done very carefully because there is a greater risk of aspiration of fluids into the respiratory system. It may be better in this circumstance to wait for the animal to absorb SQ fluids, rather than giving oral fluids too quickly. If SQ fluids are not an option, give tiny amounts of oral fluids deep into the mouth and ensure that the bird swallows everything before giving more.

If an altricial bird does not begin passing droppings within 1 hour of giving the fluids, begin feeding the appropriate diet. Feed mini or very small mealworms, one at a time. They can also be squished for easier consumption.

## Common Medical Problems and Solutions

Woodpeckers may become stressed and/or depressed if they are restrained by either wraps or splints; older woodpeckers may peck at the wrap or splint and ultimately remove it. They can even remove a pin from a wing that has been stabilized. See Duerr et al. (2017) for information on management of orthopedic injuries in wild birds.

Lacerations can be closed with either sutures or tissue glue. Woodpecker chicks that have been caught by cats are typically treated with a broad-spectrum antibiotic such as Clavamox (amoxicillin with clavulanic acid) at 125 mg/kg orally twice daily (Hawkins et al. 2018) until wounds have completely healed. For more information regarding physical examination and wound care, see Chapter 1.

Different woodpecker species have their own unique smell. It can be informative to be able to distinguish the normal smell of a woodpecker from a smell that would indicate a disease or injury. It is uncommon for woodpeckers to present with pathologic parasitic infestations, but performing routine fecal smears and flotation is recommended. Possible parasites include coccidia, intestinal worms, mites, and feather lice.

Woodpecker vocalizations are primarily innate; from hatchlings to fledglings, they are constantly vocalizing. If they are not, further examination may be warranted to determine if there is a problem. A quiet chick is abnormal.

## Diet Recipes

Woodpeckers should be fed a mixed species, all-insect diet during growth, then other natural food items that are part of the species' adult diet added as chicks reach maturity. However, commercially available feeder insects are deficient in several nutrients that must be compensated for with supplements. See both supplementation guidelines for all-insect diets in Chapter 44, and Chapter 41 which discusses the use of insects as food.

## Feeding Procedures

Woodpeckers make a vigorous pecking motion that makes it a challenge to get food into their mouth rather than all over their body. It is normal woodpecker behavior for them to peck at each other, especially at feeding time. It is not necessary to separate them as this would not be possible in the wild. Rather, feed the most vocal one first until it is full, then move on to the next one being sure each one has been fed. Blunt forceps or hemostats may be used to feed insects.

As with many altricial young birds, woodpeckers may eat approximately 5% of their body weight per meal in volume (e.g. 1.5 ml for a 30 g bird). Watch the crop as well as the droppings to gauge how much should be fed. Droppings should be moist and well-formed. A lack of droppings often indicates dehydration. Each bird should produce roughly the same amount of droppings in volume as the amount of food being fed. Any bird that has stopped producing droppings should be orally hydrated until the food currently in the digestive tract has passed. At that point, restart feedings with smaller quantities of moister food to alleviate further dehydration, such as by dipping insects in water prior to feeding or by offering a small amount of water with a syringe after each meal. Woodpeckers grow very quickly and feeding amounts may need to be adjusted daily.

Feather condition is extremely important, especially tail feathers on species that will need to use their tail as a stiff support when climbing trees. Do not allow any stray food or droppings to dry on growing feathers. If this occurs, feather loss and skin or eye infections are a possible consequence.

## Hatchlings

Woodpecker hatchlings are exceedingly strong and within a day they are able to extend their long necks to be fed; they usually double their weight within 1–2 days of hatching. Hatchlings should be fed every 20–30 minutes for 12–14 hours a day. Hatchlings can be fed small- to medium-sized worms depending on their weights. Even at this age, woodpeckers will fling their heads around and fight with each other for food. This makes it difficult to feed them, but it is their natural behavior and should not be discouraged.

Woodpeckers, especially Northern Flickers, have extremely large gape flanges that bulge out at the corners of the mouth. If a woodpecker is not gaping, touching the ends of these flanges will help to stimulate them to eat (Figure 38.2).

New birds that will not take offered food may need to have their beaks gently opened and a small amount of food placed at the back of the mouth to stimulate swallowing. Be careful not to bend the bird's beak to one side when opening the mouth, or the growing beak or jaw may be damaged. If a bird refuses food, reevaluate the temperature, hydration status, and its physical condition, and correct any problems found.

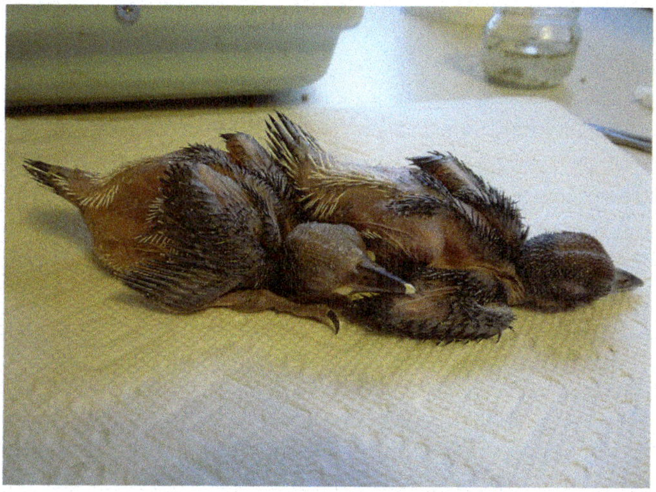

Figure 38.2 Nestling Acorn Woodpeckers, with feather tracts just emerging.

### Nestlings and Fledglings

Nestlings should be fed every 30 minutes from sunrise to sunset. Once they have climbed out of their nest and can cling to the side, the feeding time can be extended to every 45 minutes. The nestling that puts its head up first is fed and, once full, goes back into the nest and the next one pops up to be fed. Woodpeckers truly epitomize the saying "pecking order." The young birds will typically remain in the nest until about 4 weeks of age.

## Weaning

As soon as the birds begin to climb out of their nest, it is necessary to provide them with the appropriate enrichments, such as logs, pieces of bark with suet in the cracks, and routered logs (see below) with suet and worms stuffed into the holes. Hanging plastic baskets on the side with worms and water can also be provided. Woodpeckers love to take baths so a dish, appropriate for their size, should be provided. Acorn Woodpeckers should have whole acorns and crushed acorns provided. Sapsuckers and Northern Flickers can be given fruit juice, such as orange or mango, in a hanging plastic dish. Presentation of food items to encourage self-feeding should begin at this time. Ideally, the birds should be weaned onto the identical natural food items they will be eating when they are released, although substitution for easily available items is often necessary.

Exposing the birds to the types of food items (i.e. live insects, nuts, sap, berries, etc.) they will be eating when released is essential. Woodpeckers forage using a variety of techniques, such as subsurface excavation, flaking, bark removal/scaling, probing with bill and tongue, gleaning, and aerial pursuit. Providing them with as many of these types of foraging opportunities as possible will facilitate their adaptation to feeding in the wild. Creativity in developing ways of presenting food to the birds, to both wean them off of hand-feeding and also to teach them food-finding skills, is required. Examples of food presentation that have been found to be effective are as follows.

#### Worm Pillow

Cut out a 1 ft. (30.5 cm) square or circle of gauze cloth. Place a handful of mealworms in the center and lay a few slices of apple on top. Bundle up the four corners and snug the worms up into a twisted-off pillow of worms. Secure the pillow with tape or string. Cut several small slits in the fabric to help catch the birds' attention, but don't make them large enough to allow the worms to escape. The apple serves to keep the worms hydrated and less interested in escape. Suspend the pillow(s) in an obvious spot. Evidence of the birds pecking at the pillow will be seen when the holes become frayed and stained with worm juices. Replace or refill as necessary. The worm pillow is also useful for nuthatches and other passerine species that glean insects from the bark of trees. Pay careful attention that the woodpecker's tongue and claws do not become stuck in the pillow.

#### Routered Log

Drill numerous holes and depressions in various sized stumps and logs that fit in the caging. Fill the depressions with nuts, acorns, killed fresh or thawed frozen crickets, mealworms, or other insects. Woodpeckers love suet and this can also be placed in the holes. When using sticky food items, be careful not to create a feather-contamination hazard.

### Stump-Mounted Dishes

Standard plastic wall-mounted pet bird dishes may be adapted to hang on the side of a vertical stump or attached to the side of the caging. Insert appropriately sized eye screws into the wood to allow the wire-hook variety of dish to be attached. This type of dish may also be hung at the top of a stump by wedging the wire hangers between the bark and wood. Also remember that woodpeckers may peck at and destroy plastic dishes, so be sure to replace them as needed. Woodpeckers will use various types of commercial woodpecker feeders. Their preference for food is suet, shelled peanuts, and hulled sunflower seeds.

When the birds are consistently at or above adult weight, have fully grown-out feathers, and are showing an interest in the food choices offered, it is time to begin weaning them. Continue to use forceps or hemostats to feed the birds meals of more adult food items. Clean and stock the cage in the morning with a fresh assortment of food choices.

There are many possible regimens for reducing and then eliminating the birds' dependence on human caregivers for meals. Some rehabilitators cut back on the morning feeds first in order to encourage hungry interest; others make the intervals between feedings longer. The authors prefer to extend the length of time between feedings.

From the former feeding interval of 45 minutes, extend it first to 1 hour for 2–3 days, and then 2 hours for 2–3 days. If the birds are holding their weight at 2-hour feeds and their droppings have ample solids, continue cutting back feeds to 3-hour intervals for a few days and finally discontinue feedings entirely. Once a woodpecker begins to reject food, discontinue feeding but monitor its weight to verify it is indeed self-feeding. If the birds were above adult weight when weaning began, it is normal for them to drop up to 10% of their body weight while weaning. If uncertain about the bird's weight status or unable to weigh birds daily, monitor the plumpness of the breast muscling closely. If any bird has dropped significant amounts of weight during the process, lost breast muscle mass, or has sparse lime-green or urates-only droppings, return the bird to 45-minute feeds and reexamine for any medical problems. Try again after the bird has fattened up and reevaluate food presentation.

## Expected Weight Gain

In order to determine that chicks are gaining weight, each one should be weighed individually using a gram scale. Within 24–48 hours after hatching, their body weight will typically double. After a day of rehydration and adjustment to their new diet, woodpeckers should gain weight daily and quickly reach or exceed the adult weight for the species (Figure 38.3). If a bird is not gaining weight, the feeding regime should be critically evaluated. Older nestlings and fledglings may be difficult to feed, especially by novices, and the bird may not be getting enough calories per day. The chick should be examined again for any potential medical problems. Weight gain in sick or injured birds may be delayed while healing occurs. Birds should be at or above adult weight before beginning the weaning process.

Caregivers may be able to judge a body weight to be normal even if it varies from published accounts. It is important to chart weights over time to determine optimal body weights for each species in a region. The Cornell Lab of Ornithology's Birds of North America Online is a valuable resource (available by subscription) not only for typical bird weights, but also for detailed descriptions of everything ranging from natural history to breeding to vocalizations.

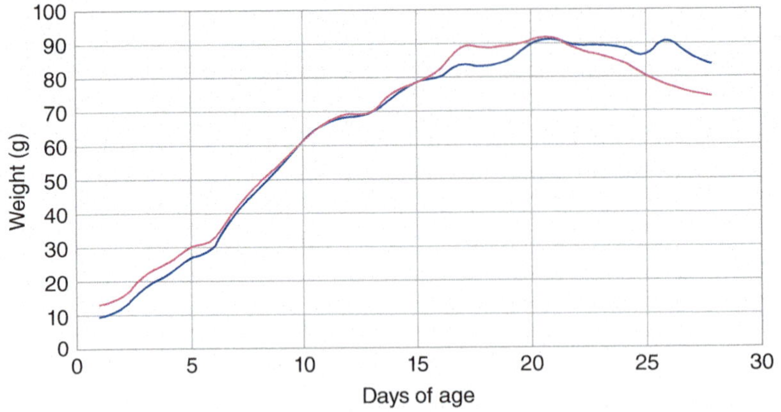


Figure 38.3 Growth of two Acorn Woodpeckers.

## Housing

Dim lighting is fine for hatchlings and nestlings because they would be in a dark cavity in the wild. However, once birds are feathered, use light-colored sheeting as a visual barrier to block views of human activity without blocking the light. Hatchlings should be housed in an incubator (aka brooder) at 90–95 °F (32.2–35 °C) and 40–50% humidity, with the temperature reduced as chicks become feathered. Different materials may be used to create a replacement nest: berry baskets, rolled newspaper, and plastic or ceramic dishes have been used. Knit nests are another option used by some rehabilitators. Line the nest with tissue or paper toweling, which will allow for easy cleaning throughout the day. Change the tissues as necessary, and do not allow the chicks' feathers or skin to become soiled. Young birds should sit in the nest with their legs folded underneath their bodies. Do not allow the legs to splay out to the sides or malformed legs or hips may result.

When the birds are feathered and begin to climb out of their nest, place it into a large container such as a laundry basket (Figure 38.4). Do not use reptariums, cardboard boxes, or fish tanks. Woodpeckers need to be able to cling to the side of whatever enclosure they are in. Their tongues can get caught in reptarium walls, they will easily destroy a reptarium or cardboard box, and they are unable to cling in a fish tank. The container needs to be lined with heavy duty pet screening (Stanek Netting Co., Inc.). Place the nest box directly adjacent to the side of the basket so the woodpecker can venture out and begin to cling to the side. Once they are clinging to the side, they become much easier to feed. Place a hanging dish for water and a hanging dish for mealworms on the side of the basket. Also put in a log that has been drilled with holes and secured to a plywood base. Fill the holes in the log with suet, mealworms, etc. If a log with a natural hole is available, this can also be placed in the basket, but it is preferable to wait until the bird is moved to a larger enclosure before doing this.

Once the bird is fully feathered and beginning to show signs of self-feeding, graduate it into a larger wire cage that is fully screened. Feather damage can occur if the caging is not properly screened. Depending on the size of the woodpecker, small or large parrot type cages are good to use. They have small doors that can be opened to facilitate hand-feeding and some may even have tops that lift off. It is ideal if the top lifts off as the birds can climb to the top of the cage to be fed, they then take their turn and go back down again (Figure 38.5). A parrot cage that is 24 × 24 × 30 in. (61 × 61 × 76 cm) is good for smaller woodpeckers. Caging that is 28 × 26 × 36 in. (71 × 66 × 91 cm)

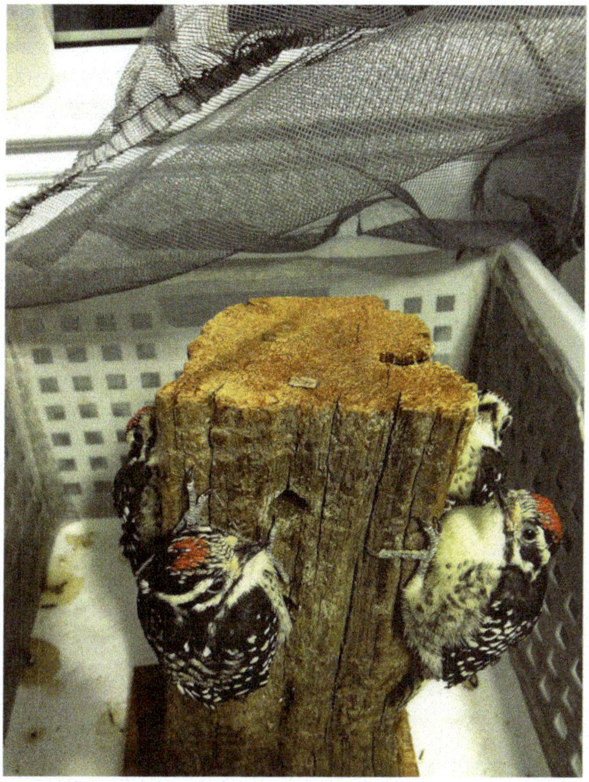

Figure 38.4 Four Nuttall's Woodpeckers in laundry basket housing; note the screened sides and top with a small stump to begin to learn climbing and foraging skills.

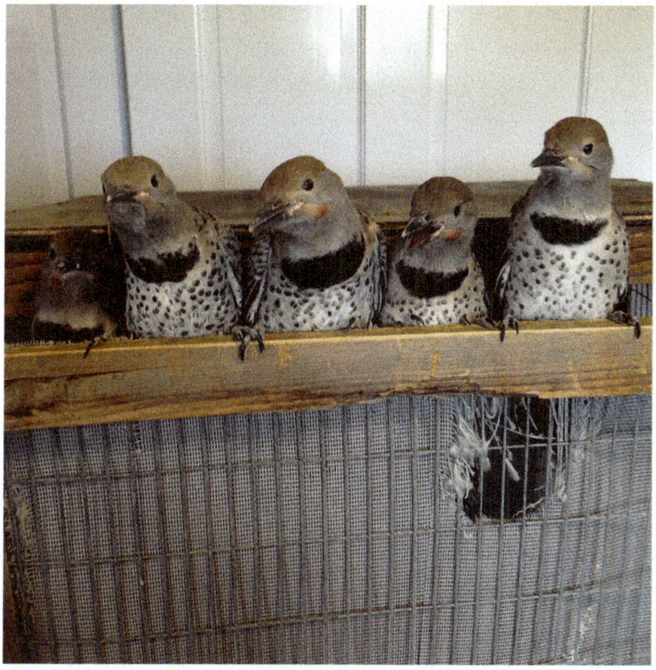

Figure 38.5 Northern Flicker chicks coming to the removable top of their cage at feeding time. Note the typical damage all woodpeckers quickly do to caging.

high with a removable top is good for medium-sized woodpeckers; 32×32×58 in. (81×81×147 cm) with a removable top is good for larger woodpeckers. Caging with removable tops works exceedingly well for woodpeckers as the top can be slid backwards just enough for the woodpecker to climb to the top, be fed, and then climb back down again. Any type of caging used for woodpeckers should be lined with heavy duty pet screening. This is imperative in that woodpeckers use their tails as props and thus their tails must be maintained in perfect condition. Any screening will need to be periodically repaired as woodpeckers will peck at and through it. Caging should be properly cleaned on a daily basis to maintain a hygienic environment. While this scenario is not always available to larger centers, woodpeckers should definitely be placed into housing that allows them to climb.

Once the birds are eating consistently in their small cage and maintaining weight without any supplemental hand-feedings, they are ready for an aviary. If the outdoor climate is significantly different from indoor temperature, the birds should be acclimated by gradual exposure over the course of 24–48 hours before being put in the aviary. Acclimation may be accomplished at the same time as the final stages of weaning. If acclimation is skipped, birds may die if they are suddenly subject to extremely hot or cold temperatures.

Aviaries should be at least 6×12×8 ft. (1.8×3.6×2.5 m) for small bodied woodpeckers and 8×16×8 ft. (2.5×5×2.5 m) for large-bodied woodpeckers (Miller 2012). The aviary the author prefers for smaller woodpeckers is larger than the 4×8×8 ft. (1.2×2.5×2.5 m) size listed by Miller (2012). There are different ways to construct an aviary. They can be constructed with heavy duty pet screening over a metal frame, or built with a wood frame with ½ in. (1.25 cm) mesh metal screening on the outside aspect and polypropylene netting on the inside. Ample logs and stumps should be placed at various locations throughout the aviary (Figure 38.6). Water should be provided for both drinking and bathing. Avoid areas of bare wire mesh because it can damage the birds' tail feathers. At least half the aviary should be shaded for protection from the elements, and the log furnishings should provide a wide variety of climbing opportunities. Food should be presented as described in the "Weaning" section above. Never place the aviary in proximity to caging for raptors or mammals.

## Preparation for Wild Release

Success at avoiding habituation should be seen by the time the birds are in the aviary. They should be wary of humans rather than coming up to caretakers for food. Commercial woodpecker feeders used within the aviary can be helpful during preparation for release, and for providing supplemental food after release. Placing these feeders outside the release cage provides them with an option for additional food as they become adjusted to their new environment. A water source outside the aviary is also useful.

## Release

When woodpeckers fledge in the wild, their wing flight feathers and their tail feathers are not fully grown; parental care continues while the chicks are learning to forage and navigate their world. This period can range from 3 weeks up until 5 months. Therefore, it is important that woodpeckers are given a soft release with supplemental food being made available. Birds should spend 7–14 days gaining flight experience in the aviary prior to release, and should be capable of short-duration

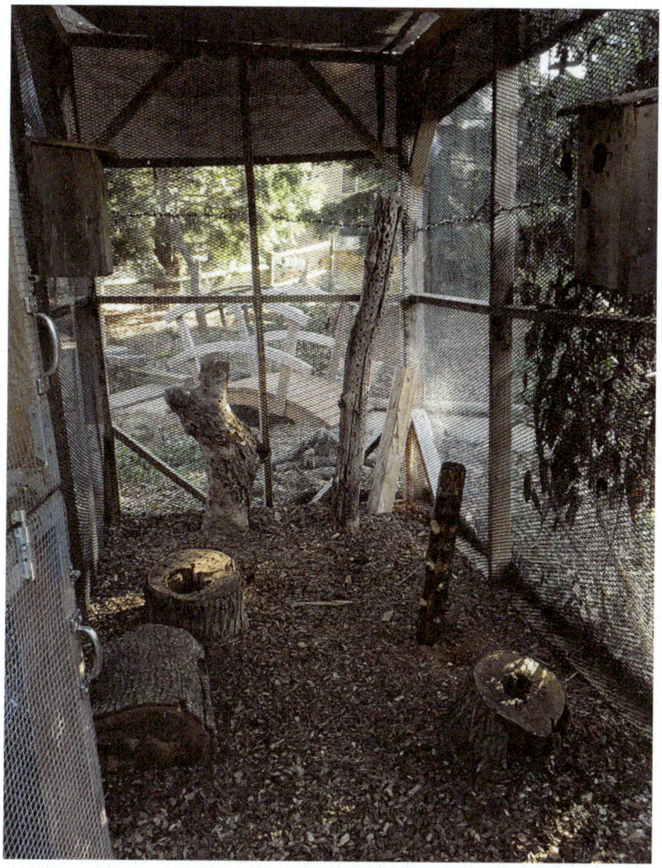

Figure 38.6 Aviary for small- to medium-sized woodpeckers. Note the ample logs and stumps to provide foraging and climbing opportunities, plus boxes for roosting.

flights lasting for 5–10 minutes of continuous flight at ambient temperatures without panting. Birds should shed water when misted and should weigh as much as a normal adult. Whenever possible, release birds in their home neighborhood. Choose the release day to avoid weather extremes. Release in the morning, because woodpeckers are diurnal.

If it is late in the year when the bird is ready for release, consideration should be given as to whether or not the bird should be overwintered. This is especially true of late babies as some woodpeckers will have a brood into the early fall.

Some species, such as Acorn Woodpeckers, will not accept unfamiliar fledglings into an established territory, although the family should recognize missing members if they are returned within a few weeks. It is preferable for Acorn Woodpeckers to minimize aviary time in order to get the bird back to its home territory quickly.

The author has had success in consolidating hatchling, nestling, and fledgling Acorn Woodpeckers from different groups to form a new social colony. As each colony has its own language, it is important that a group be kept together for 1 to 2 months before release so they can communicate with each other or learn the language of a group that may be in the area they are going to be released. A soft release is recommended. As Acorn Woodpeckers are colony birds, it is unfair to place them alone in a captive environment.

## Acknowledgments

Thanks to Dr. Walt Koenig, for allowing me (NB) to research and study Acorn Woodpeckers under his guidance. We would also like to thank the wildlife rehabilitation centers of northern California that admit these wonderful birds and go to such great lengths to ensure each one has the best care.

## Sources for Products Mentioned

Polypropylene Netting: Stanek Netting Co., Inc., 111 Orange Street, Bloomfield, NJ 07003, (973) 680-1616, https://www.staneknetting.com.

## References

Aubry, K.B and Raley, C.M. (2002). The Pileated Woodpecker as a keystone habitat modifier in the Pacific Northwest. *USDA Forest Service Gen. Tech. Rep. PSW-GTR-181*, pp. 257–274.

Backhouse, F. (2005). *Woodpeckers of North America*, 232 pp. Firefly Books, Ltd.

Bock, W.J. (1999). Functional and evolutionary morphology of woodpeckers. *Ostrich* 70 (1): 23–31.

Duerr, R.S., Purdin, G.J., and Bowers, V. (2017). Small-bodied birds: passerines, doves, woodpeckers, others. In: *Topics in Wildlife Medicine, Vol. 4: Orthopedics* (eds. R.S. Duerr and G.J. Purdin), 53–74. St. Cloud, MN: National Wildlife Rehabilitators Association.

Gill, F. and Donsker, D. (eds.). (2019). IOC World Bird List (v9.1). https://doi.org/10.14344/IOC.ML.9.1.

Hawkins, M.G., Barron, H.W., Speer, B.L. et al. (2018). Birds. In: *Exotic Animal Formulary*, 5e (eds. J.W. Carpenter and C.J. Marion), 167–375. St. Louis, MO: Elsevier.

Jackson, J.A. (1994). Red-cockaded woodpecker (*Dryobates borealis*), version 2.0. In: *The Birds of North America* (eds. A.F. Poole and F.B. Gill). Ithaca, NY, USA: Cornell Lab of Ornithology. https://doi.org/10.2173/bna.85.

Koenig, W.D., Stacey, P.B., Stanback, M.T., and Mumme, R.L. (1995). Acorn woodpecker (*Melanerpes formicivorus*), version 2.0. In: *The Birds of North America* (eds. A.F. Poole and F.B. Gill). Ithaca, NY, USA: Cornell Lab of Ornithology. https://doi.org/10.2173/bna.194.

Lovette, I.J. and Fitzpatrick, J.W. (2016). *The Cornell Lab of Ornithology's Handbook of Bird Biology*, 3e, 173. UK: Wiley Blackwell.

Miller, E.A. (ed.) (2012). *Minimum Standards for Wildlife Rehabilitation*, 4e. St. Cloud, MN: National Wildlife Rehabilitation Association.

Rodewald, P. (ed.) (2015). *The Birds of North America*: https://birdsna.org. Ithaca, NY: Cornell Laboratory of Ornithology.

Shunk, S.A. (2016). *Peterson Reference Guide to Woodpeckers of North America*, vol. 28, 258–259. Houghton Mifflin Harcourt Publishing Company.

Wiebe, K.L. and Moore, W.S. (2017). Northern flicker (*Colaptes auratus*), version 2.1. In: *The Birds of North America* (ed. P.G. Rodewald). Ithaca, NY, USA: Cornell Lab of Ornithology. https://doi.org/10.2173/bna.norfli.02.1.

# 39

# Wild Parrots

*Nikki Buxton and Sophie Hebert Saulnier*

## Natural History

The parrots or Psittacine order contains roughly 398 species in four families: Psittacidae (African and New World parrots), the Cacatuidae (cockatoos), Psittaculidae (Old World parrots), and the Strigopidae (New Zealand parrots) (Gill and Donsker 2019). They are very popular in the pet trade the world over. The only parrot naturally found in the continental U.S., the Carolina Parakeet (*Conuropsis carolinensis*), is now extinct. Many feral populations of escaped pets are gradually becoming established, including in the U.S. and elsewhere in the world. About a third of all parrot species are listed as near-threatened to endangered, making them one of the most imperiled groups of birds.

Theoretically, parrots mate for life, although many birds do re-mate if something happens to their partner, especially if they are still of breeding age. Mating season in Belize begins in late January to early February and there are mid-air battles over mates and nesting sites. Pairs start copulating as soon as a cavity has been identified, and eggs begin to appear in March. The season lasts until August, during which time birds with failed clutches have the opportunity to re-nest and second-clutch.

Most species of parrots are cavity-nesters, with some exceptions, such as Quaker Parrots (*Myiopsitta monachus*), which are communal nest-builders. Some prefer open-space pine savanna, some deep forest, some nest in trees or power poles in the city. Parrot nests have also been documented in termite nests. Most have deep, slim cavities: having once tried to extract two pre-fledges from a power pole (to circumvent malicious poachers), the author knows how hard it is to extract a biting chick from a nest hole once your hand is balled into a fist. Often poachers will chop down the tree or cut a new entrance hole at the base of the cavity with a machete, which has the double devastation of destroying the nest site as well as removing the chicks and potentially injuring the birds.

A typical parrot clutch is 2–4 eggs depending on the species, and incubation periods are usually 16–30 days. Parrots begin to incubate eggs as soon as they are laid, and clutches thus contain chicks of different ages. The young are altricial and as such are born blind, naked, and totally dependent on their parents. The oldest chicks usually have a better chance of survival, since younger chicks often struggle with their larger siblings to be fed. It is rare for more than two chicks to reach fledgling age due to restricted cavity space. Old nests are often lined with the bones and feathers of dead

*Hand-Rearing Birds*, Second Edition. Edited by Rebecca S. Duerr and Laurie J. Gage.

Table 39.1 Duration of life stage events for White-fronted and Yellow-headed Amazon Parrots.

| Key stages | Average duration |
|---|---|
| Egg incubation to hatching | 26–32 days |
| Eyes opening | 14 days |
| Fledgling (move to outdoor enclosure) | 10 weeks |
| Weaning | 8–24 weeks |
| Flight aviary | 16 weeks |
| Initial release periods | 18–24 months |
| Breeding age | 4 years |
| Life span | 45–60 years |

siblings. Chicks fledge at 6–12 weeks (depending on the species) and do not return to the nest cavity once fledged. Generally, fledglings stay with the parents until the next clutch and all young will be integrated into the flock and develop a place within its complex social structure. A chick forages alongside his parents for about 12 months in order to learn the territory and the location and season of each food source. As the chick matures, it remains within the flock, reinforcing familiarity with the territory and forging bonds with other members of the flock. These early flock bonds often result in a life-pair bond.

Flock language is complex and extensive. Studies show that birds have their own names given to them by their parents in the nest (Berg et al. 2012). They use the name to identify themselves during flight and landing in foraging and roost trees. Communication among the flock includes location of food and water, when and likely where to gather for pre-roost and roosting, and, of course, predator awareness. Amazons share a common roost site and usually gather at a pre-roost, appearing from every direction in pairs and small groups. At dusk, they fly as one to the night roost. There are no noises from the flock arriving at the roost or throughout the night, unless disturbed by a predator. Most parrots do not defecate during the night as this would alert a predator to the presence of parrots in the canopy above. Many parrot owners can attest to this "morning poop." Parrots do not see well at night and silence is one of their best defenses against being localized by a predator during sleep. Sleeping in groups is most likely a good defense against predators as their large number, up to a few hundred, will increase the survival of more birds. See Table 39.1 for timing of life stages and rehabilitation milestones.

## Criteria for Intervention

Belize Bird Rescue (BBR) has been rehabilitating and releasing locally endemic parrots since 2004. The majority of BBR's intakes are confiscated chicks brought in by local authorities or those surrendered by pet owners. In many cases these chicks are sick, have nutritional deficiencies, or both. Clipping the flight feathers is a very common practice, often with long-term detrimental effects. Occasionally, injured wild birds will be brought in, but this is rare.

Some at-risk wild chicks, especially those of endangered or threatened species, may be removed from their nests by permitted organizations or authorities and brought in for hand-rearing. Reasons for intervention in wild nests include avoidance of poaching, prevention of siblicide associated with overcrowding, pest or parasite infestation, predation, parental abandonment, or threat from natural disasters such as flooding or fires. Optimum at-risk chick removal for a planned intervention is at about 3 weeks of age.

Re-nesting is a consideration but a risky one. Foster parents may fail to feed the introduced chick or abandon the nest completely. They and the original nestmates may also attack the newcomer. However, nest manipulation has been successful with Scarlet Macaws. More studies are needed on the subject. If re-nesting is attempted, an introduced chick must closely match the ages of potential nestmates and be closely monitored.

Birds that have been habituated during captivity in the pet trade can be rehabilitated and re-socialized for successful wild release, but the process is time consuming and may require a prolonged period of care. If time and resources are limiting, do not try to rehabilitate ex-captive or hand-reared wild parrots. This is a seriously long-term investment for a long-lived and intelligent species. You cannot cut corners or accelerate the process.

## Record Keeping

Daily weight records are important along with periodic biometrics during chick development (Figure 39.1). It is the best way to detect the beginning of many problems early. Records should include the diet being fed, quantity, frequency of feeding, weight gain, and notes on droppings and crop emptying if needed. Compare weights to other chicks of the same age, or to species-specific weight charts, if available.

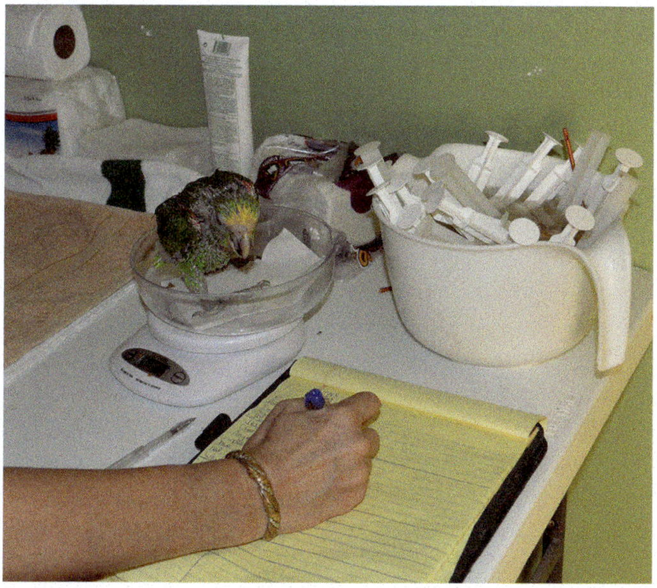

Figure 39.1 Chick being weighed.

Use colored plastic bands on young chicks and change those out for numbered stainless steel open bands as they fledge. BBR uses a stainless steel open leg band which remains post-release. Microchips inserted into the pectoral muscle can also be safely used, but for visual identification of a rehabilitated bird in the wild, the leg bands are more practical. (Editor's note: Local governmental agencies may have regulations regarding banding or marking animals released to the wild.)

## Initial Care and Stabilization

Initially, perform a brief examination to identify any life-threatening issues and address them accordingly. See Chapter 1 for physical examination and basic medical care information. Hydration is paramount, especially in young chicks. The majority of new arrivals are dehydrated, particularly in Mesoamerica because the height of the breeding season falls in the dry season. Most of the cavities chosen by parrots have been shown to maintain the optimum temperature range, but it is not always the case and some artificial nest boxes can be warmer than natural cavities.

If the chick is warm, active, and swallowing or head bobbing, it can be hydrated orally. Hydrate each chick using a pediatric electrolyte solution such as Pedialyte® orally. In very dehydrated babies, subcutaneous (SQ) fluids may be needed. If the bird is lethargic or not swallowing normally, SQ fluids will be safer: 50 ml/kg of lactated Ringer's solution (LRS) is used in mildly dehydrated babies. Repeat if still dehydrated after complete absorption. If nonsteroidal anti-inflammatory drugs (NSAIDs) are to be used to treat injuries, they should only be started after optimal hydration is reached to limit the risk of kidney damage.

New intakes have usually been though considerable stress during capture, handling, and transport. Following any urgent rehydration and a simple weight check, a recuperation period should be observed. A dog crate with toweling substrate and a solid perch is preferred: cover the door with another towel to minimize stimulation and keep them in a warm, calm environment. A temperature of 85–90 °F (29–32 °C) is optimal.

If a chick already has food in the crop, it is important to wait for this to empty and the bird to pass regular droppings before attempting feeding. Continue oral or SQ rehydration if necessary. Sometimes, a crop flush might be needed, especially if the baby was fed inappropriate food (bread, corn flour) or if the digestive system is severely affected, producing "sour crop" or slow crop clearance (see "Crop Motility" section).

Once the baby is well hydrated, is passing droppings, and the crop is fairly empty, it is safe to start feeding. Assessing age, development, and behavior will help determine whether or not a bird is already weaned. Any parrot chick with incomplete feather development will always require hand-feeding. Fully feathered birds that still requiring feeding will react to stimulation of the pads next to the commissures of the beak. Head bobbing and a gentle (or urgent) begging sound will indicate an unweaned chick. If in doubt, offer recognizable natural solid foods, provide a secure and quiet environment, and observe. Never force a chick to take hand-feeding formula unless every other approach has been exhausted; however, don't wait too long before starting to hand-feed a chick that is not self-feeding, as they weaken quickly if not self-feeding adequately.

Once the chick is settled and over the initial stress, assess for any other issues that may require intervention: parasites; fungi (including yeast); bacteria; splayed legs; ear, nose, throat, or eye infections; poor stool quality; or dirty feathers, feet, or vent. See "Common Medical Problems" section ahead.

Do not under any circumstances mix species: inappropriate pair-bonding happens very easily at young ages, and it will unquestionably preclude release of both birds. It is incredibly rare for there to be any aggression within chick groups.

### Quarantine

Textbook quarantine periods are not always possible, as birds may arrive in large groups or there may simply be too many intakes to house individually. Try to keep individuals or groups isolated as much as possible. Ideally, a strict quarantine of 30–45 days should be respected before introducing any bird or group of birds into an already established group. Whatever the initial circumstances, it is always recommended to perform a fecal test on intake, repeated after 14 days or at the end of the quarantine period before introducing to *any* other birds. If resources permit, a gram stain for mouth, respiratory, and GI microbes of at least one bird per group is ideal. Periodic random testing is useful once the birds are outside in the rehab enclosures.

It is always preferred to quarantine new birds in case of infection, disease, or parasites. However, if presented with a single bird and others of its species are in care, it may be better for the chick's psychological development to fast-track the quarantine, or introduce that baby and continue the quarantine as a group starting at the newest introduction. This decision should be made on a case-by-case basis, taken in conjunction with all reasonable precautions of fecal and crop/fecal swab tests.

## Common Medical Problems and Solutions

See Table 39.2 for a list of common problems and potential treatment options.

### Parasite Control

Ectoparasites are common (feather lice, mites, and beef worms/bot flies) and can be treated using topical or oral ivermectin; only use in otherwise healthy birds of good weight and hydration. Infestations in downed and debilitated birds should be treated with diatomaceous earth applied carefully to the feathers, avoiding the head. Once the bird is stronger, ivermectin can be used safely. Periodic dosing of rehabilitated birds is recommended, such as every 4 months or during a significant husbandry move or introduction, especially when the birds would be handled anyway.

It is ideal to always perform a fecal analysis and identify the parasites present in the patient. A fecal flotation is best for eggs, but a direct smear is also very useful to identify protozoa. Ivermectin treats many gastrointestinal parasites and systemically works on ectoparasites, and may be used as a routine all-round preventative and to treat roundworms, which are the most common internal parasites encountered.

### Crop Motility and Impaction Problems

Crop motility might be affected by different factors such as stress, lack of warmth, inadequate diet, or infection. The crop may be noticed to not be emptying normally between meals, especially when the chick is new. Impactions are usually caused by the ingestion of nonedible material (wood chips, pebbles) or inappropriate food (bread, flour) that is unable to exit the crop. Maldigestion could be caused by an infection or sickness. To be sure that the maldigestion is not simply stress-related, it is advisable to tube a small amount of oral fluids, bring the bird to optimum temperature, and leave overnight in dark, calm conditions.

To address severe crop stasis, the first step should be to use a feeding tube and empty syringe to empty as much of the crop contents as possible. To ease the process, inject a few ccs of warm fluids,

Table 39.2 Common medical problems of wild parrot chicks. See Hawkins et al. (2018) for drug dosing information.

| Issue | Treatment(s) | Notes |
|---|---|---|
| Roundworms (Ascaris) and ectoparasites | Ivermectin (oral or injectable) | Don't treat severely debilitated birds until they are stable. |
| Capillaria | Fenbendazole | |
| Tapeworms | Praziquantel | Bird might exhibit neurological symptoms, especially head incoordination when attempting to eat. Many dewormers with praziquantel contain ivermectin, so take care not to overdose. |
| Bacterial infections (GI) | Antibiotic | In young chicks, use in conjunction with nystatin against secondary yeast infections. |
| Fungal infections (GI) | Antifungal | Usually nystatin for yeast infection, use a systemic antifungal, such as fluconazole or terbinafine, if systemic infection is suspected. |
| Fungal infections (external or mouth) | Antifungal | Avoid creams or ointments as these can seriously damage the feathers. Gentian violet can safely be used for mild infections (Maley and Arbiser 2013). |
| Crop stasis | Flush and give clay water. Analyze flush for microbial or parasitic issues | New intakes (diet changes, stress) may need 24–36 hours to adjust. Give oral fluids, massage crop, and wait for changes. Treat with antibiotics or antifungal if needed according to lab results. Prokinetics can be added also in advanced cases. Restart feeding with very diluted food and small amounts but multiple meals a day, making sure the crop is mostly empty between meals. |
| Splayed legs | Toggle (hobble) legs with tape at mid-tarsometatarsus for 2–3 weeks, change regularly according to growth | Caused by smooth substrate in nest or poor care. Usually not reversible in adults. Can cause foot deformities and difficulties with egg incubation. |
| Broken blood feather | Grip the base of the bleeding feather with hemostats and, holding the wing firmly where the feather is attached, pull the feather straight out of its follicle and apply pressure until the bleeding stops | Make sure the whole root of the feather is removed otherwise the bleeding might restart later and can promote infection in the affected follicle. Do under anesthesia in nervous birds. Consider using pain medication after the procedure as some flight feathers are anchored in the bone. |
| Respiratory infections | Antibiotics and/or antifungal | Identify quickly as it can be deadly in birds. Enrofloxacin or amoxicillin/clavulanic acid are usually good choices. In case of older birds with suboptimal diet or hygiene, consider adding antifungal drugs (terbinafine, itraconazole) and supplement in vitamin A. Vitamin A deficiency is often an underlying cause. |
| Pododermatitis (bumblefoot) | Depends on the severity | Mild: improve perches (use natural branches of various sizes, around 40–60% of the perch circumference should be covered by the parrot's feet) and supplement with vitamin A.<br>Advanced: bandaging, pain medication, antibiotics, and wound care might be needed. In very severe cases, surgery might be needed. |

and massage gently if the material is solid. Repeat the flushing procedure until the crop is completely empty and the liquid coming out is relatively clear. Beware of aspiration during the procedure. Make sure the tube is really in the crop before injecting. Stop immediately if the chick is coughing or sneezing. Keep some of that withdrawn liquid to perform a gram stain and a direct smear looking for any bacterial, parasitic, yeast, or other fungal causes.

Once the crop is empty, begin with hydration. Use lactated Ringer's solution and/or clay water (water taken from a settled solution of Bentonite clay) in small amounts and monitor that the solution is absorbed in about 1–2 hours. Once well hydrated, the crop should empty of liquid fairly quickly. Then, restart feeding with formula diluted with fluids (about 1 : 2) in small amounts. If digestion appears normal, gradually increase the number of feedings and quantity of food throughout the day and decrease the dilution until it reaches normal consistency. As digestion improves, reduce the frequency of meals but increase the amount. If the emptying is still slow or if you are dealing with an infection, start with injectable (usually SQ) fluids and injectable antibiotics (if needed) as the medication may not be absorbed orally. Injectable prokinetic drugs (e.g. metoclopramide) can also be used up to three times a day in severe cases only. Look for an underlying cause, such as infection, heavy metal intoxication, or other medical problem.

### Clipped Wings and Feather Condition

Most parrots confiscated from Belizean homes have clipped wings and poor feather condition due to vitamin deficiencies. Stress bars are common; even chicks that are brought in quickly can develop serious stress bars. Natural causes are diet deficiencies, dehydration, nest overcrowding, or predator presence. In severe cases, the feathers break at the stress point on fledging. This is not a factor limiting the ultimate releasability of a bird as long as there are no injuries to the wing or follicle deformities. The normal molting process is long, but birds will learn to fly normally once completed. The bird's plumage condition is a crucial factor to evaluate when judging if a bird is ready for release or not. Release is not even considered for less-than-optimally hand-reared chick until the bird has had a complete annual molt under optimum diet and husbandry conditions, which translates as an absolute minimum rehabilitation period of 18 months.

## Imprinting and Habituation

Avoiding habituation or imprinting of hand-reared chicks is absolutely impossible. Chicks are naturally curious, intelligent, and rapidly develop an affinity with their human caregiver: this trait is exactly why they are sought after as pets. Many of these birds have already been exposed to humans when admitted. Unless the bird was removed from the nest very close to fledging, or has experienced serious pain and distress at the hands of humans, they are unlikely to be afraid or even wary of us. Thankfully, habituation can be largely reversed. From the start, interactions should be kept to a minimum, which includes avoiding unnecessary talking when birds are present. Feeding time should be efficient and limited. Limit exposure and proximity to human activity during weaning, and as soon as the chicks are weaned they should be moved to a suitable outside location which reduces and restricts interactions with humans. As their contact with humans decreases and they experience healthy flock interaction with other birds of their species, they will gradually lose their unhealthy interest in humans. Even habituated ex-pets develop healthy intraspecific behaviors, lose their human vocalizations, and revert back to natural sounds given sufficient time and circumstance. However, expect that a hand-raised baby parrot will not lose their interest in humans until they approach 12 months of age and even beyond.

## Length of Rehabilitation

Most rehabilitators are amazed at the time invested in getting a former captive parrot or even a hand-raised chick ready for release. Any chick that has spent time with a member of the public will be imprinted, habituated, likely vocalizing human sounds, and have poor feather condition. Hopefully there will be no permanent metabolic, physiological, or deformity issues. Adding together the multiple issues of habituation, dependency on the parents and the flock, a seasonal and extensive wild foraging range, poor feather condition, lack of communication and social skills, and poor developmental diet, chicks are never ready to release under 12 months of age. Under optimum hand-rearing conditions, 14 months in care would be the minimum, and for hand-reared ex-captives with clipped wings, be prepared to invest 20–24 months or more. Birds under 14 months old are not released unless there are special circumstances (e.g. the youngster has been adopted by a releasable adult). The worst cases are the species most renowned for mimicry that have been long-term captives with poor diet and husbandry. So far, our longest rehab that has resulted in release was for a flock of 26 Yellow-headed Amazons, many of which had spent 9 years in the program before being released successfully.

## Fostering

Fostering chicks to unrelated adults is always tricky. Although inherently altruistic, some species and some individuals can be aggressive toward the unrelated offspring, and a parrot attack on a chick can be rapid and devastating and often come without warning. In a captive situation, a gradual introduction is best, with the chicks protected by double mesh initially. Watch carefully for any signs of aggressive behavior. Typical signs are eye-pinning, tail splaying, growling, lunging, and stereotypical head movements. Some species have a gentler and more maternal temperament than others, making some introductions easier and others riskier. It is recommended to gather information on previous experience with the species under consideration for fostering. Fostering into wild nests is the riskiest situation, as it is almost impossible to monitor continually or intervene should aggression be recognized. It takes only a few moments for an aggressive adult to permanently maim or even kill a chick. The risks have to be carefully weighed up against the benefits and the success potential of other less risky alternatives.

### Introducing Chicks to Adult Flocks

Over the years BBR has accumulated nonreleasable birds that are receptive to new birds. These older birds live in larger aviaries and adjacent or connecting aviaries are used to acclimatize babies to their new adult flockmates. The connecting aviaries allow for the smoothest introductions, as once the connecting hatch is opened, each group remains in their familiar space until they are ready to explore. Because eating is an important part of the social structure of parrots, feeding platforms in the hatch area make for faster integration of groups. In the early stages, watch for any immediate signs of aggression or any subtle and prolonged bullying that may prevent a bird from eating well or drive them to exhaustion. Introductions are not advisable during breeding season as adult birds become much more aggressive and territorial. By the same token, be aware of dynamic shifts and aggression in existing groups as breeding season approaches.

Some ex-captive adult birds may be poor role models for fledglings and should not be used to model wild normal social behaviors due to aberrant vocalizations or behaviors. This is a problem seen with Yellow-headed Amazons at BBR.

## Hand-feeding Formulas

There are some excellent commercial hand-feeding formulas on the market specifically for Psittacines, including Tropican (Hagen Inc.), Nutri-Start Baby Bird Formula (Lafeber Company), and Kaytee Exact Hand Feeding Formula (Kaytee, Inc.). With macaw chicks, a higher amount of fat will be required; use a high-energy hand-feeding formula formulated for macaws. The availability of these diets may vary by region. The author's facility supplements these diets with an (off label) formula made of Mazuri® Parrot Maintenance commercial pellet (Mazuri) plus Prime (Hagen Aviculture Research Institute, HARI®) (or other avian) multivitamin, papaya, and apple juice. The authors have found that banana is not very palatable in the mash, and some blended fruits and juiced vegetables, like cucumber and mango, can go rancid very quickly. Papaya seems to be the most stable fresh ingredient and it gives the food a fluid quality that makes tubing and syringe-feeding easier.

### Recipe

- 450 g Mazuri Parrot Maintenance pellets (or other available parrot pellets)
- 2 cups (473 ml) hot apple juice
- 1¼ cups (296 ml) water
- 300 g papaya
- 2 teaspoons Prime avian vitamins (Hagen)
- 1 teaspoon calcium carbonate powder

Combine the parrot pellets, apple juice, and water in a bowl and soak for at least 1 hour. Add the rest of the ingredients and blend in a food processor until smooth (2+ minutes).

When ready to feed, mix two tablespoons of commercial hand-feeding formula to a smooth paste with warm water and add to 200 g of Mazuri mix. Additional water may be added to the mixture if necessary. The consistency should be similar to a thick soup or apple puree. If it is too thin, the chicks will not gain enough weight, but if it is too thick, it could slow emptying of the crop and promote dehydration. It must be blended well or it won't go through the feeding tube easily, and that's frustrating for all and very messy. Supplement or thicken this formula with any amount of commercial hand-feeding formula.

### Heating Formula

Temperature is critical as crop motility can be slowed if the food is not warm enough. Colder food in a slow crop promotes bacterial growth. When syringe-feeding, many chicks will refuse the food if it is not warm enough. On the other hand, food that is too warm can severely burn the crop, causing major injuries and possibly death. Ideally, warm the water to the correct temperature and mix it quickly when using powdered diets. Food should be fed between 103–105 °F (40–41 °C) and can be kept warm by placing the syringe in a container of water heated to the target temperature. Microwave ovens should be used with extreme care. The uneven heating of microwaves commonly causes crop burns when gavage feeding and, if used, caregivers must ensure there are no hot spots whatsoever in the warmed formula. Stir extensively to homogenize the mix. Check and then check again, stirring multiple times with your finger along the sides and bottom of the bowl to minimize the risk of feeding overheated formula, or use a thermometer to check the temperature.

As with most feeding techniques, hygiene is very important, especially between clutches of birds. Use a different set of equipment for each group. Wash hands, syringes, and tubes between groups. Flush and at least cold-sanitize the tube; seemingly healthy birds may harbor yeast and bacterial infections that can be easily transmitted.

## Feeding Procedures

### Tubing vs Syringe-feeding

The author uses 6–8 in. (15.2–20.3 cm) metal gavage "feeding needles" (aka tubes) attached to a syringe for chicks. A curved #12 is ideal, although a #10 or #14 can be used depending on age and species. Most chicks get accustomed quickly to swallowing the tube without fear of injury or distress after a few feedings. Stimulate the feeding response by gently pushing on the oral commissures. The chick will usually answer by head bobbing and simultaneously closing the glottis (opening of the trachea), reducing the risk of aspiration. Warming your fingers in hot water beforehand can increase the feeding response. Insert the tube gently from the left side of the beak toward the cranial esophagus located on the right side of the throat. Be sure to feel the tube in the crop (palpate the trachea and the tube next to it in the esophagus) before ejecting food to be sure the tube is not in the trachea. Hold the syringe lightly between thumb and forefinger, allowing the bird to swallow the tube. There is no need to handle the beak during gavage but do support the head and neck as the bobbing movement during insertion of the tube can damage the oropharynx.

Hatchlings require three to four feedings a day, decreasing to two feeds in pre-fledglings, and one evening feed for the fledglings as they are being weaned (at about 2–6 months, depending on species). Very young hatchlings might need more frequent meals, but usually after 48 hours old, 4 meals will be sufficient as the crop stretches and can contain more food. The food during the initial days of life should be more dilute and gradually thickened to reach the optimal consistency. The crop doesn't need to be completely empty before the next feeding but should be mostly empty. Fill the crop until the food begins to just barely fill the cranial esophagus. Overfeeding results in regurgitation and possible aspiration of food.

Syringe-only feeding, without the tube, is clearly more fun for everyone, but is not recommended for wild parrots. The reasons not to syringe-feed include: (i) food-association and pleasurable feeding encourages habituation, which should be avoided in releasable birds; (ii) it is messy and therefore risks damaging feathers; (iii) it is wasteful, which makes it almost impossible to know exactly how much has been ingested; and (iv) it takes a lot longer to complete. The disadvantages of using a crop needle to feed are the risk of damage to the esophagus, potential for harm with crop burns, risk of spreading infection, and risk of overfeeding as the rapid filling encourages the baby to beg for more even after it's full. All these risks can be easily managed with good hygiene, good technique, and experience.

Groups of birds routinely mimic parent feeding behavior with one another, especially before and directly after feeds. This is totally normal, although they are not technically feeding one another. If a bird is regurgitating, it is likely he has been tubed too much food.

### Weaning

Soft food is usually introduced around 6–8 weeks of age depending on the species. Weaning is a gradual process where the babies will start refusing feeding and their crop will shrink gradually as they start to eat on their own. Provide a plate of varied food items and they will begin to pick up pieces. Do not expect it to happen before the chick is 16–20 weeks, or even longer in some

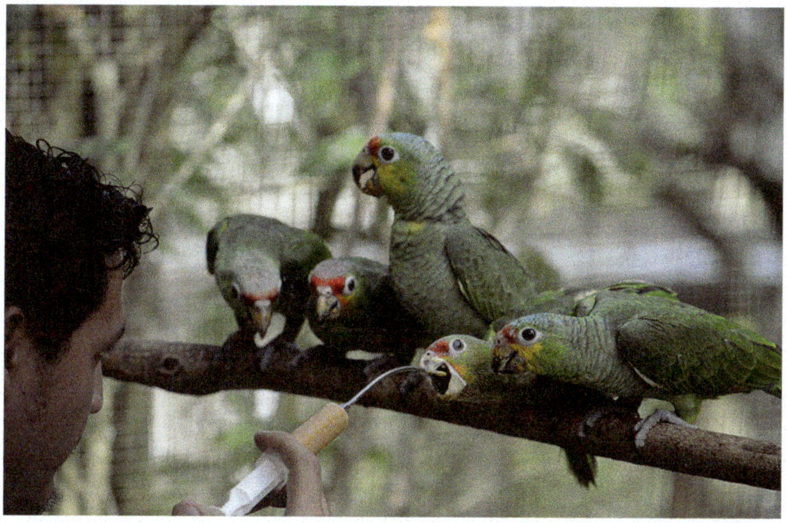

Figure 39.2 Feeding with a steel feeding needle while chicks perch. Note that no handling is needed.

cases: usually the larger the bird, the later the weaning. At this stage, the birds will have been outside for several weeks. For the benefit of the feeder, it is advisable to train the birds to line up along a single perch for feeding (Figure 39.2). At first it is a free-for-all, but they soon get the hang of it. Stay strong and don't be tempted to deviate from the feeding protocol otherwise you will always have a battle and feeding will be unpleasant for everyone. Chicks that have been tubed will feed better with the tube attached to the syringe: even if you don't actually put the tube into the esophagus, the birds will lean into it. This method is less messy and forms less of an attachment than getting closer with the syringe tip, as that usually involves more contact to control the head. Weaning depends on the temperament of the bird(s), and the species and the number of birds in the flock.

As our young flocks acquire more members throughout the year, we have as many as 40 chicks with an age spread of ~4 months difference. Because of the way we build the flocks and the importance placed on this process of socialization, once chicks are old enough to leave the nursery, we don't separate the weaned from the unweaned birds. The only segregation would be for a few weeks maximum at fledgling age, and even then we would try our best not to leave a single chick by itself if it was last to fledge.

Provide ample solid foods throughout the aviary and supplement with two hand-feeds a day, morning and afternoon, and gradually make each feed later and later until the evening feed is eliminated entirely, and the morning feed becomes an early afternoon feed. There is a point when it is clear that the birds are "playing" and no longer require the nutritional benefit of the food, even if they still continue the begging noises and behavior. Bring feeds down to alternate days for about a week, making sure to increase the amount of solid food available throughout this process to allow for the natural weaning process to take place. The weaning process is usually accompanied by a weight drop of about 10–15%. Take a final weight a week after weaning and, providing there has been no dramatic losses, consider them weaned.

## Self-feeding Diet

Because of their vast territory and distances traveled in 1 day, it is impossible for anyone to say exactly what the natural diet of a wild parrot consists of. Their foraging territory is huge and the blooming and fruiting of each tree is seasonal and usually brief. We do have an understanding of their nutritional needs, however, and this is what most captive parrot diet recommendations are based on.

Unlike the aviculture sector, parrot rehabilitators have other considerations to take into consideration. Is the food we are presenting grown as people food? If a bird learns to recognize a commercial crop such as corn, apples, citrus, or bananas as food, then you could put them at risk of lethal deterrents should they encounter one of these crops post-release. The fat content and caloric value of foods should be higher for a wild bird than a pet bird, as their energetic requirements are higher. These are not perch-potatoes. They should be active in their large enclosures, flying (hopefully), but if they were clipped as babies and are awaiting a full molt, then they should be interacting with their flock, working with foraging foods and enrichment that promotes active behavior, such as climbing on swings, ropes, and hanging branches of berries and fruits.

BBR's foundation diet is limited due to cost and seasonal availabilities. The staples at BBR are cooked corn and beans, including kidney or pinto beans that are soaked overnight, washed, and cooked. Ideally, we would use garbanzo beans (chickpeas) but they are prohibitively expensive. We avoid peanuts because of the risk of aflatoxins; almonds would be perfect, but these and any other nut is again prohibitively expensive. However, we grow coconuts and the birds get fresh coconut meat every day. We use oranges as we have them for free, but these are a commercial crop and too much vitamin C can cause issues with iron in some species – all tropical birds have a propensity to store excessive iron, toucans especially, but is not usually an issue with most Psittacines. We have access to a commercial pellet (Mazuri Parrot Maintenance) which the birds simply won't eat easily, so we use it as a base for "Birdy Bread."

**Birdy Bread Recipe**

- Warm 3 cups of apple juice
- Add 3 cups of any commercial parrot pellets

Soak for 20+ minutes until soft (add more liquid if required). Mix the pellets to a paste, then add:

- 2 tbsp (30 ml) peanut butter
- 3 eggs
- 1 cup (237 ml) coconut oil
- 1 cup (237 ml) wholewheat flour
- 2 cups (474 ml) yellow cornmeal
- 1 cup (237 ml) oats
- 2 cups (474 ml) grated (unsweetened) coconut
- 1/4 cup (60 ml) crushed red pepper
- 1 large grated carrot

Mix thoroughly to dough consistency. Add more liquid or more dry ingredients if required. Spread to about 1 in. (2.5 cm) thickness in a shallow baking tin greased with coconut oil. Push down firmly with your hands to limit cracking during cooking. Slow bake at 170 °C/325 °F for 1 hour. Cool completely before cutting into small cubes. Give three to six pieces per bird per day. This recipe makes a large cake which can be frozen after cutting and will last one bird several weeks. Scale down the ingredients to make a smaller cake if desired. Keep frozen or refrigerated. Variation: add grated pumpkin or other veggies, banana, apples, ground nuts, and dried fruits.

Birdy quiche is simply a dozen beaten eggs. Mix in six of the shells, left-over spaghetti or rice, chopped spinach, chili peppers, or anything yummy, pour into a greased deep dish and bake in a moderate oven until cooked through.

We give sunflower seeds daily, unless we can get pumpkin seeds (seasonal and rare). Other foods offered include any vegetable (apart from onion), papaya, banana, any fruit other than pineapple (which they don't like) and avocado (that can be toxic), occasional eggs with rice or pasta (beaten eggs mixed with whole-grains rice or pasta and leafy-greens, then baked). A variety of fruits and ideally vegetables is recommended, with an emphasis on dark green and dark orange vegetables, such as leafy-greens, carrots, peppers, pumpkins, squash, and sweet potatoes. A multivitamin supplement is also added to the food at least twice a week.

### Feeding in the Aviaries

High feeders are at the top of ladders at least 15 ft. (4.6 m) in the air. Use hatches for changing out the baskets of food once each day at the top of these ladders. Hatches in the walls are a great way to minimize human interaction and involvement with the birds. Hoisted swinging platforms are excellent, and mimic wild feeding behavior really well; however, caregivers do need to enter the enclosure to deal with them.

## Expected Weight Gain

Hatchlings and nestlings should gain steadily every day and reach their adult weight by 6–8 weeks. A weight loss or even absence of weight gain during more than 2 consecutive days should arise concerns. Be attentive of general condition, especially crop emptying time and stool amount and consistency, as it could show signs of malabsorption or maldigestion. A fecal analysis for parasites, and a gram stain of the crop contents and stool, should be a first step in assessing a chick that is not gaining weight adequately.

In general, expect a daily weight gain of 10% until all feathers are present and out of the pin-feather stage. The birds will plateau and then drop slightly (around 10% from maximum) just before fledging.

Weight checks should be carried out daily throughout hand-feeding, at least every other day for the first week in their outdoor enclosure, twice weekly during the initial weaning phase, and weights should be stable once the birds are weaned and in their final flight enclosure.

## Housing

### Chicks

All parrots in Belize, and the majority of Psittacine species everywhere, are cavity-nesters. Knowing this, sympathetic housing is paramount: try to mimic the womb-like confine of a cavity, including a minimal patch of light to mimic the cavity entrance. Allow ventilation without drafts. Cavities are efficient thermoregulators, so be aware of day and night temperature fluctuations and adjust your efforts accordingly. In the early weeks, most chicks require access to a heat pad; even with older chicks it is advisable to give them the choice of extra heat. Full strength artificial light should be used only when necessary for feeding and cleaning. Use dimmed lights or draped windows otherwise, as they would not be exposed to sunlight and stimulation before fledging from the cavity.

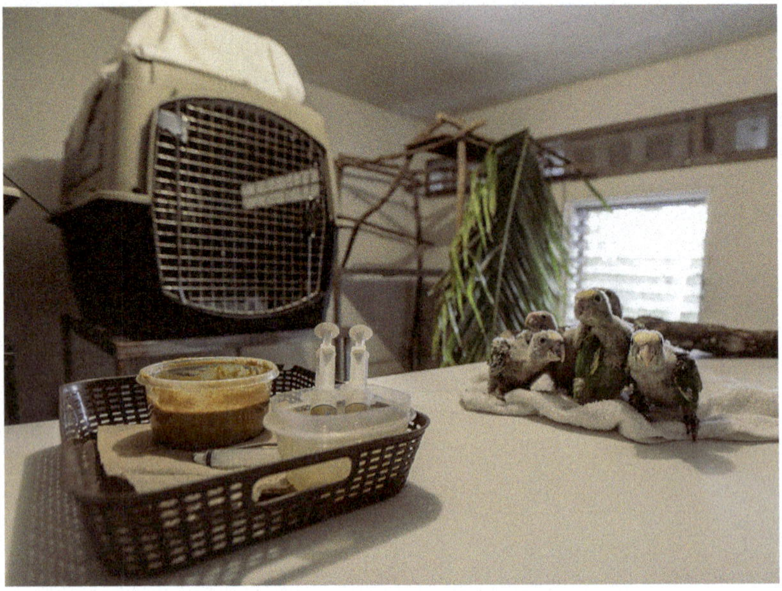

Figure 39.3 Chicks removed from crate for a feeding, which is a good time to clean the crate.

The choice of housing depends entirely on the available resources and space at the facility and the developmental stage of the birds. Very young hatchlings can be kept in a knitted nest or suitable container lined with paper towel. Hatchlings and nestlings can be kept in open containers, such as laundry baskets or vegetable crates, but covering these proves challenging. Dog crates are our preference, although the disadvantage here is that each chick needs to be removed for every feeding as there is no access to them from above. However, parrots are incredibly messy birds and don't eject poop from the nest like songbirds, so are likely to need cleaning after every feed (Figure 39.3). Many wild chicks are encountered with balls of rock-solid feces adhered to every toe. Sometimes the nailbed or even the toe is damaged, which may explain why we see so many otherwise-healthy wild chicks with missing nails and digits. Increase the size of the crate to accommodate age differences and clutch sizes, upgrading to larger crates as the birds start to become more mobile.

## Crate Substrate

Fabric without loops, such as rough drapes or old t-shirts, or towels with a close weave and smallest loops possible, are preferred as housing substrate. Cover the towels with a wrinkled, absorbent nonshiny paper towel to cut down on laundry. Natural substrates such as wood shavings are not recommended because oils can cause breathing issues (especially soft woods as cedar or pine), and they don't absorb feces any better than towels. Additionally, loose substrates such as wood shavings, corn cob, or rice hulls run the risk of ingestion. Because they cannot be digested, these may cause impaction or obstruction. Any substrate that does not provide a good grip for the chick's feet is not recommended either, as even a slight amount of slide can cause feet to turn or legs to splay at varying degrees. Create a large donut shape of fabric at the back of the crate, as babies tend to huddle together away from the door.

The towels need to be changed at least daily if not several times a day depending on the numbers of chicks in the group. The crate should be changed and disinfected regularly. With larger groups, remove a chick, check its weight, feed, then transfer to a clean crate at every meal. This minimizes handling and stress and makes it easier to keep track of who has been fed. Group size in one large dog crate may be up to 12 birds.

Low-level perching is made available at around 6 weeks of age. Use movable, very low t-stands and position them at the front near the door of the crate. Most young nestlings huddle to the back if they are not ready for perching or solid food, so the perch will not distress the younger birds of the group. Increase the height and variety of perches as they are utilized by more birds.

## Fledging

Fledging for most Amazons usually happens between 8 and 12 weeks in the wild (6–16 weeks across all parrot species). In our captive-rearing situation, pre-fledge chicks are mobile, extra-curious, perch well, and are proficient at eating solid fruits. They are much more difficult to hand-feed as they won't remain in the feeding basket and they flap and explore once outside the crate. The biggest indicator of a fledged parrot, however, is that they actually fly! Good protocol practice has any doors closed at all times during feeding.

At this stage, start taking the fledglings to a close-by outdoor enclosure so they can get used to using their new wings. Solid foods are offered at multiple feeding stations throughout the enclosure. Endure adequate climbing access for clumsy babies. Put a well-perched, large dog crate on a trolley or shelf as a safety retreat. The majority of birds will use these at some stage during the day. Offer food and water in the crate in case they remain inside all day. If intending to leave the chicks out at night, then the crate will provide security for sleeping initially. Enclosures must be 100% rat-, snake-, and other predator proof. In the wild, chicks would never return to the cavity after fledging, but this is not a natural situation for these birds. Wild parrots have incredibly strong parent–chick bonds and the transferred knowledge and confidence of the parents is paramount to survival during this treacherous fledging stage. As compensation for the lack of parental protection and guidance, a crate provides a safe-haven for less confident chicks. With wild parrots, do not push chicks to advance a developmental stage before they are ready. They all have different personalities and we must allow for these idiosyncrasies throughout their rehabilitation.

As chicks mature, try not to leave a single younger bird alone in the feeding room. A pre-fledge age chick will be fine in the crate outside with his "siblings." If concerned about falls from perches or crates, then cushion the ground; use palm leaves or similar leafy branches. Otherwise, hold back a couple of the less-advanced birds for a few days to keep the youngest one company.

The first couple of nights the birds will cling to the wire as it gets dark. Either bring them in overnight if concerned for their safety, or just keep putting them into the crate until it is too dark for them to climb out. They will soon settle down.

## Food and Water Tips

Once the birds are weaned, they are fed a large tray of food at the start of the day and then have no contact with humans. When feeding outdoors, the food plate needs to be low enough that stepping on the side doesn't cause it to tip over. It needs to have holes to drain any water. It needs to be chew resistant, or cheap enough to replace once chewing commences, and needs to be easily cleaned. A double plate can be very useful: the bottom one is fixed in place and the top plate is placed (full of food) onto the fixed plate (Figure 39.4). Offer full stainless steel bowls of water (for easy cleaning). Parrots are heavy and they will climb on the water bowl and play with it and overturn it. If it is full of water, destruction becomes more difficult.

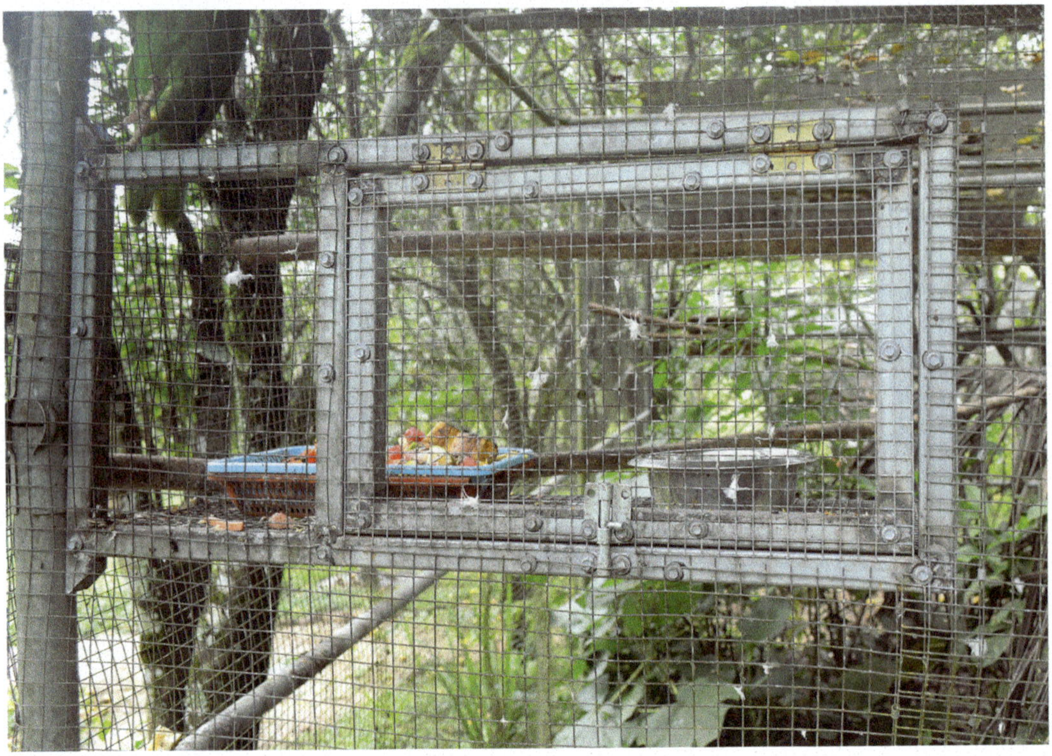

Figure 39.4 Double plate system for food trays and a stout water bowl, with a wall hatch that allows food delivery without direct interaction with the birds.

## Enrichment

Enrichment is as important for wild birds that will eventually be released as it is for long-term captive birds. Choice of enrichment depend upon the species, the number of birds in the enclosure, and whether or not they are able to be released into the wild.

The optimum enrichment for a flock of healthy wild releasable birds should be natural foraging branches of berries, fruits, flowers, etc. Avoid the use of manufactured toys and artificial items such as beads. If you are making toys, use natural wood or branches cut into slices and strung up, or use food itself as the enrichment: corn cobs impaled on dowelling attached to branches, whole papaya hung in nets or simple wire baskets, or a stand of bananas. The more closely related to natural food, the better training it is for these birds awaiting release. Natural food items available to them after release should be introduced to them prior to release to facilitate their adaptation later on. As with the entire diet during rehabilitation, beware of teaching wild parrots to eat farmed crop foods, turning them into targets for lethal deterrents or exposing them to pesticides and herbicides.

## Aviary Furnishing

Perches should be natural branches, not manufactured dowel, metal, or PVC perches which are too smooth. The bird's nails should stop ¾ of the way around the perch if it is adequately sized. Connect perches with screws and washers through the wire and with cable tie connections to other

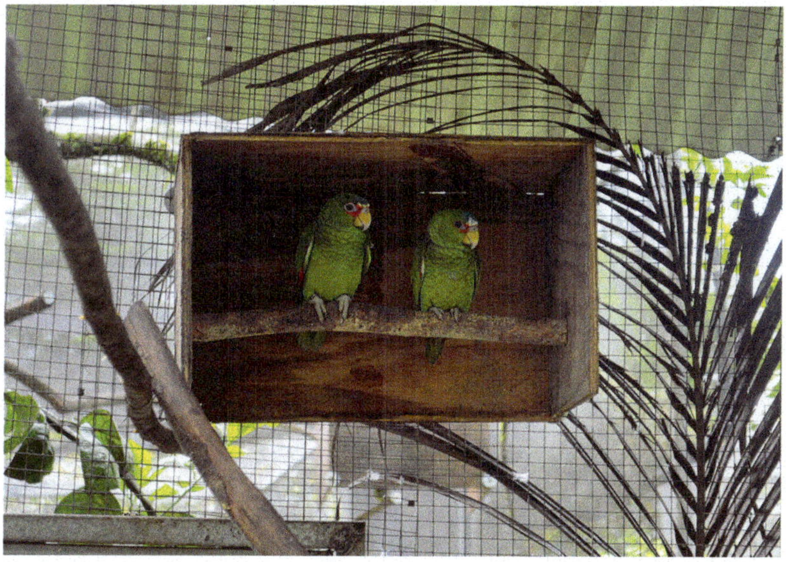

Figure 39.5 Roost boxes allow birds to feel secure and have their own space within the social environment of an aviary.

perches. If a bird has foot deformities, wrap the branches with cohesive bandage material or sisal rope. Always give several different thicknesses and various angles. Knowing that parrots gravitate toward the highest point, install perches as high as possible or they will use the metal rafters of the enclosure. Use chains instead of rope to build swinging perches. Cover the roof of the flight cages with large palm leaves to provide shelter, shade, and a feeling of security. Roost boxes are essential: basically, a long, four-sided, wooden box with a perch inside, which provides roof, sides, and rear protection and shelter (Figure 39.5). Roost boxes are attached high up on the side of the enclosure, giving single or multiple birds their own territory within this artificial and unnaturally small environment.

A double door "airlock" is great for preventing escapes. They don't need to be as secure as the main cage door, so are cheaper to construct: hardware cloth or even well-secured shade cloth could be used. In the absence of a double door, have the doors open outward and use a shade-cloth curtain to prevent escape during entry. Feeding hatches also help minimize opportunities for escape. When designing entrances, be sure to allow access for large dog crates, extremely long perches, and large branches of browse. For door closers: rubber bungees work, but the parrots like to chew on them. If a screen-door closer is used, slide a piece of PVC pipe over it first: the spring can pinch their feet if birds land on it while it is closing. Use latches that allow for a clip or padlock, especially if security is an issue.

## Preparation for Wild Release

Birds should be transferred into a large aviary as their flight abilities progress. Human contact should be increasingly limited. This last step is a large pre-release aviary located in an isolated area away from all human sounds or view (except briefly for food once a day). Avoid talking and try not to make eye contact with the birds. Use high platform feeders accessed via ladders or on hoisted platforms to encourage natural elevated feeding positions. Diverse natural foods should be introduced seasonally, more often than in previous steps, but supplemental (unnatural) foods should continue to be given in sufficient quantities and locations for all birds in the enclosure.

## Flight Aviaries

These aviaries are where the fledged and weaned flock will spend their last 8–24 months of rehabilitation preparing for life in the wild, so they need to be spacious and robust (Figure 39.6). Ultimately, aim for enclosures as large as resources permit: 50 ft. (15.2 m) in length and 30 ft. (9.2) in height is a good size for up to 45 small or 35 larger birds. See Appendix 39.1 at the end of this chapter for more information on aviary construction and perches. These birds fly great distances

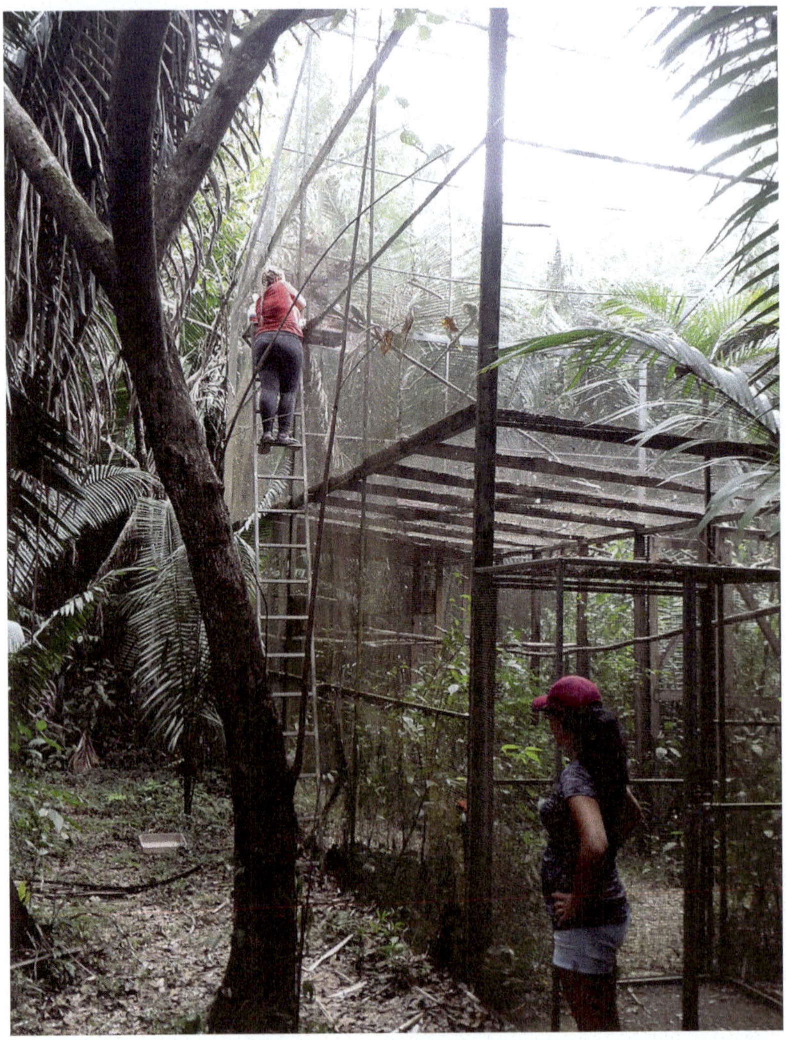

Figure 39.6 A large footprint, tall aviary is needed for pre-release activity and social interaction. Note the hatch that allows feeding at elevation.

and they need space to become athletically fit. Height is very important during the pre-release stage. Parrots will naturally gravitate to the highest point, so make sure there is adequate perching up high for all of the birds to prevent squabbles. Swinging perches attached to chains secured to the rafters have proven the easiest to install and the longest-lasting. Swinging motions mimic tree movement and reinforce core strength and balance skills. Be aware of positioning and be sympathetic to natural behaviors. Ensure adequate foliage cover above the high perches. Don't leave roosting birds exposed to the night sky; it is unnatural and not instinctive, and if birds get accustomed to being exposed yet safe, it could prove fatal upon release. Take care also not to position perches above food dishes for obvious reasons.

### Indications of Release Readiness

As the birds progress toward release, they should be evaluated for release suitability. A complete physical exam is necessary to assess the condition of joints, wings, and feathers, and observation of the bird in flight will shed light on abnormalities or deficiencies. Social behavior is continually assessed throughout the process. The birds should be cooperating and coexisting within the integrated social group and be familiar to some extent with the appearance of natural food sources. The aim is to release the group at the same time; being part of a social group greatly increases everyone's chance of survival.

Any injuries that significantly reduce a bird's ability to survive should be assessed early in the rehabilitation process so that the birds can be rehabilitated or given long-term care with sympathetic husbandry. Examples include permanently impaired flight, multiple complete toe amputations that reduce gripping ability, conditions leading to chronic pain or arthritis, joint issues, or beak or bone deformities that preclude normal mobility or foraging. The aim is to avoid any inappropriate pair bonding between a releasable and a nonreleasable bird.

### Catching and Relocating for Release

To catch birds for offsite release, we have constructed catch-enclosures within the aviaries. In these, although food is provided throughout care, we find that the birds become increasingly reluctant to enter the area as the months go on. They become ever-more suspicious of us, and leave the area rapidly on our approach. As a result, catching the birds for relocation and release is incredibly stressful for all parties. We have not yet found a perfect method of capturing birds from a large aviary. The best we have come up with is to chase them to exhaustion with our long-reach nets. Ultimately, they don't like us very much, which is, of course, the goal. Since offsite release often involves a journey, catch the birds from the large aviaries 1–2 days before. Then, allow them to destress in a smaller, more controlled enclosure where recapture can be swift and stress-free. A last dose of ivermectin before transfer is prudent.

### Release Site and Timing

The location of an adequate release site can be an issue. The ideal site is located away from human communities and activity as much as possible. The release location must have the correct habitat for the birds, a current or historical population of wild conspecifics in the area with breeding habitat close by, and the local human population must be sympathetic to the efforts and not set out to recapture released parrots. A wild flock of conspecifics will greatly help the new birds to integrate, learn natural behaviour, and locate food sources. Accessibility of the release site is also an issue here in Belize; flooding precludes access to many nesting grounds where common species are known to congregate.

Timing of the release is gauged on flock behavior and attitude, diminished or ceased vocalization, and perfect physical condition including feathers and flight. Weather patterns and seasonal hazards such as fires, floods, or hurricanes are additional considerations.

## Release

Never hard-release hand-raised chicks or ex-captives. It is ideal to soft-release the birds at the chosen release site. This necessitates building a suitably sized, predator-proof, soft-release cage at the location with a trusted person close by who can monitor the release process and keep providing food for the birds in the cage; field staff can also attend to the birds (Figure 39.7). The birds are transported to the enclosure and will remain inside for a minimum of 14–21 days.

A drop-down hatch doubles as the release opening and also a secure place to return for supplemental feeding until all birds have exited the enclosure and no longer return. Enclosures with "normal" human doors are a nightmare for release; hence the hatch. If the opening does not go right to highest point, then the birds may have serious trouble finding the exit. For the first few nights, some birds may come back, in which case the hatch should be closed at night to avoid predation. Once they no longer return to the aviary (usually a couple of days), discontinue the hatch and start supplemental feeding on alternate platforms nearby. Position platforms to give the security of foliage while giving clear view of approaching predators and a fast escape route. Suspended

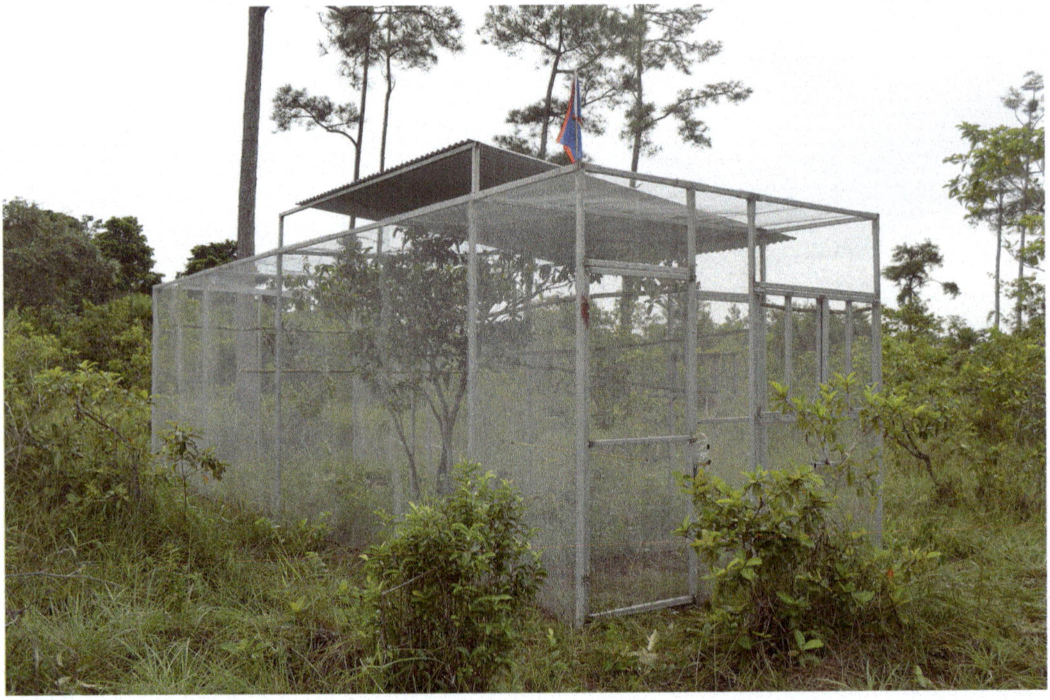

Figure 39.7 Smaller, modular aviary to allow birds to become accustomed to the release site prior to soft release when the hatch is finally left open.

platforms are a more natural method of feeding. Food continues to be supplied for as long as required, up to 6 months or longer. Purists argue that the unnatural foods increase dependency and "wild weaning" time. This may be true, but in our experiences, the birds that have stayed around the longest are without doubt the most ecologically successful birds. In our experience, a soft-release gives these birds the time, space, and resources to figure things out for themselves while remaining safe and fed.

### Sources of Products Mentioned

Kaytee products: 521 Clay St, PO Box 230, Chilton, WI 53014, (800) KAYTEE-1, https://www.kaytee.com.
Lafeber products: Lafeber Company, Cornell, IL 61319, (800) 842–6445, www.lafeber.com.
Tropican: Hagen Avicultural Research Institute (HARI), https://hari.ca.

## Appendix 39.1 Outdoor Enclosures for Parrots

### A.1 General Information

Ideally, parrots need to have a series of enclosures with increasing heights, perching availability, and space. This allows gradually increasing group size while permitting them to adapt physically to an expanding environment and to flock social dynamics. Include multiple feeding platforms to alleviate territorial aggression. Provide plenty of perching pathways leading both to and from feeding platforms for access and escape. If wing-clipped birds are included in a flight aviary (perfectly acceptable provided they have some flight/controlled fall ability), then provide a floor substrate that will cushion a fall and extra perching for them to move around with ease. It is advisable to introduce young birds to one another as soon as possible. As they get older, they become less inclined to accept new birds into the flock and bullying begins.

BBR uses two sizes of outdoor quarantine/acclimatization cages: 6 × 6 ft. (1.8 × 1.8 m) with a 7 ft. (2.1 m) height for one or two larger birds, and 6 × 10 × 7 ft. (1.8 × 3 × 2.1 m) high for multiple pre-fledge chicks, especially of the smaller species. These cages are moveable steel-framed boxes with wire floors. They rest on thick gravel beds and have large handles welded onto the sides so they can be moved periodically for cleaning and flexibility of introduction and isolation. For larger groups of just-fledged birds, a predator-proof enclosure 15 × 10 × 7 ft. (4.6 × 3 × 2.1 m) high is used, having a cement floor with a row of cement blocks connecting the floor to metal mesh/hardware cloth walls.

First-stage fledgling enclosures are 20 × 10 × 10 ft. (6.1 × 3 × 3 m) for a maximum of 12 birds. Pre-flights are 20 × 20 × 10 ft. (6.1 × 6.1 × 3 m). At this stage, BBR doesn't worry about wire or cement floors as the enclosures are close to the facility and in areas of low plant density. However, if the enclosures are in the bush, they need secure floors and the whole structure needs to have double-layered wire walls to protect birds at night.

Field pre-release cages are 15 × 10 × 10 ft. (4.6 × 3 × 3 m), constructed in sections with a steel box-frame, double-wire walls, home-made steel connectors, and a wire floor (Figure 39.7). Transported flat-packed on a trailer, they can be easily relocated and assembled onsite using self-tapping metal screws (roofing screws with rubber washers). The release door is a dropdown hatch that doubles as a temporary food platform. Make sure the hatch starts at the roof: the birds are slow to figure out regular doors as they always gravitate to the highest point.

## A.2 Construction

Wooden frames have been used, and the author has never experienced issues with the birds chewing them. However, the wood rotted close to the ground, the door frames warped becoming hard to shut, and bolts became misaligned in damp weather. Frames are now almost exclusively steel; which doesn't warp, shrink, or settle, but is more expensive and more labor intensive to work with. Do not paint anything as parrots will likely pick at it and ingest paint flecks.

The load-bearing of the enclosure is important: the higher the structure and longer the span, the stronger the gauge of tubing and the more corner braces are necessary. Use square tubing throughout as it makes it easier to build doors that fit snugly. Round fence-pipe with commercially produced connectors was not as durable, rusting badly at joints and welds; nor were all necessary connectors available. For the majority of the smaller enclosure sizes, 1¼ in. (3.1 cm) galvanized steel square tubing is adequate. Use 1½ in. (3.8 cm) tubing to create the sleeve connectors: these are much stronger than welding a joint. For flight enclosures, use 2 in. (5 cm) square tubing throughout with possible 2×4 box steel for the rafters if the enclosure is more than 30 ft. (9.1 m) wide (Figure 39.8).

If possible, every enclosure should have double-layered wire walls throughout to prevent predator attack and toe-chewing through the wire by previously released parrots or those in adjacent caging. Do not use chicken wire, it is too flexible and the holes are too wide to exclude predators. Use of ½ in. (1.3 cm) hardware cloth wire is preferred, doubled if possible. With anything larger, small snakes and rodents can get through while opossums and raccoon will reach their paws in. There have been cases where captive birds have literally been pulled apart by predators reaching into caging with wide mesh walls. This sort of attack doesn't happen in the large flight aviaries when there's plenty of foliage inside for parrots to climb and all of the birds are well-flighted.

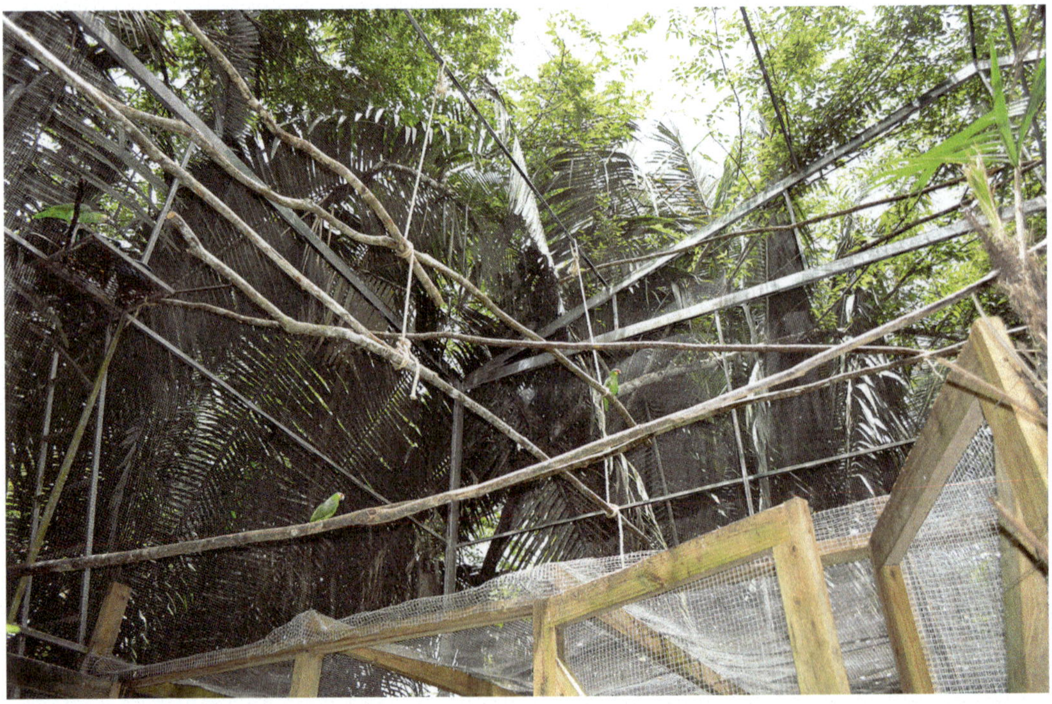

Figure 39.8 Box steel 2 ×4 primary supports in a very large aviary, with a variety of ropes and perches.

Quarter-inch wire mesh tends to be made of a thinner and weaker gauge metal than the ½ in. (1.3 cm), and is therefore less durable to the elements and the parrots. It also makes it difficult to secure perching using a screw and washer method and the cage clips don't fit. If ½ in. (1.3 cm) is used, alternative methods of joining the wire would be needed. The wire is screwed onto the frame at 2 in. (5.1 cm) intervals using the self-tapping rubber-washer metal-screws.

The 100 ft. (30.5 m) lengths of ½ in. (1.3 cm) hardware cloth (in Belize) have a 4 ft. (1.2 m) width maximum. To work with this size material, lay out three entire rolls side-by-side and use commercial stainless steel cage clips to clip them together, creating a 100 ft. (30.5 m) roll of 12 ft. (3.7 m) width. Wind it back onto a steel pipe and use ropes to haul it to the top of the enclosure lengthways, secure the pipe to the frame and pull down the wire needed for one half the roof and the side, then let the remaining wire roll down the other side. Use galvanized wire or it will rust; post-welded galvanized is recommended. No problems have been seen with birds chewing on galvanized steel and acquiring problems with zinc toxicosis. Avoid "deals" and other cheap options: experience has shown they rust and degrade very quickly.

BBR uses a flat roof on the smaller enclosures as it is much cheaper and easy to clear off leaves if necessary (fallen leaves actually make a nice visual barrier). On the large flights, use a pitched roof for extra height. The rafters in an A-frame make for great perching braces too. All BBR's aviaries and enclosures have a ¾ in. (1.9 cm) PVC pipe watering system along the roof. The pipes have a shut-off valve for each enclosure and the roof length is drilled with small holes a few inches apart, creating a simple shower. Wiring the bottom securely in an enclosure 10×10 ft. (3×3 m) or less is strongly recommended since rats and other predators burrow through dirt floors at night. Use shade-cloth screening between adjoining aviaries: this creates a visual barrier as well as a physical one to avoid toe-chewing. Wherever practical, cover up to half of the roof with tin, especially over the feeding platforms.

## A.3 Methods of Securing the Wire at Ground Level

- At least 2 ft. (>0.6 m) deep trench with wire buried either into or secured onto cement or wedged in place with rocks. Note: wire in the ground rusts easily, so the lower areas will need periodic replacement.
- Cement floor with one or more layers of block wall: use the wall to attach the wire. Be aware this is a permanent hard floor, so drainage has to be good
- Wire floor with gravel. This is 100% foolproof as there is a secure wire floor and any breaches are instantly visible. Only practical for smaller enclosures.

## A.4 Drainage

Over the years, the authors have tried several methods of providing drainage, each having its own pros and cons. When deciding, consider if there is need to vent the drains into a septic system or soakaway pit.

- PVC pipe in cement floor: plan very carefully to get everything in place before the cement is poured. Don't ever use 90° bends, instead use two 45°s or it blocks up constantly. Anything smaller than 2 in. (5.1 cm) diameter pipe blocks up easily. A way to close off the pipe when not in use is needed, lest snakes and rodents take up residence in the aviary.
- V-ditch and/or pipe vent at ground level: this has the same predator proofing issues as the in-floor drain but some other advantages, like needing less pipe. It can also be installed after the enclosure is built to target a natural low spot. It rarely blocks up.

- Floor-door: great for the larger acclimatization enclosures. Create a cat-flap sized hole at floor level and cover it with a metal "door" on runners. Pull the door up and pin in place through the wire when sweeping, then let it drop back down and securely lock it closed after cleaning.
- Wire floor on gravel: difficult to rake clean, but provides great drainage and plants can still grow through it.
- Natural dirt floor, no structured drainage: the sensible option for bigger enclosures. It's natural, plants grow in it, it's relatively soft for landing, plus it's "free" and practical. As parrots don't often go to the ground, the crawlies (at least in Belize) will take care of much of the food spillages, so raking is only needed once a week or so. Don't use sand on the floors as parrots can ingest this.
- Laid slabs or bricks: cheaper than cement and provides drainage, but very little advantage otherwise. A determined predator could excavate though, given time.

## References

Berg, K.S., Delgado, S., Cortopassi1, K.A. et al. (2012). Vertical transmission of learned signatures in a wild parrot. *Proceedings of the Royal Society B* 279: 585–591. https://doi.org/10.1098/rspb.2011.0932.

Gill, F. and Donsker, D. (eds). (2019). IOC World Bird List (v9.1). https://doi.org/10.14344/IOC.ML.9.1.

Hawkins, M.G., Barron, H.W., Speer, B.L. et al. (2018). Birds. In: *Exotic Animal Formulary*, 5e (eds. J.W. Carpenter and C.J. Marion), 167–375. St. Louis, MO: Elsevier.

Maley, A.M. and Arbiser, J.L. (2013). Gentian violet: a 19th century drug re-emerges in the 21st century. *Experimental Dermatology* 22 (12): 775–780. https://doi.org/10.1111/exd.12257.

# 40

# Lorikeets

*Carol Stanley*

## Natural History

Lorikeets are generally active, strikingly colored birds of small to medium size. With 53 species, Loriinae is a subfamily of Psittacine birds and are part of the family Psittaculidae that also includes budgerigars and fig parrots. Lories and lorikeets are widely distributed in the Southeast Asian islands and Australia. Their habitats include subtropical, tropical rainforest, woodland, coastal bush, and mountainous areas. Care should be taken for those from cooler, mountainous elevations as they have a difficult time with higher temperatures.

The name "Lory" is generally attributable to those birds with shorter, blunt tails. Lorikeet refers to those with long tails but is used to describe both tail types. Both names are used for all lories. A lack of sexual dimorphism in most lorikeets makes sexing reliant on DNA from blood, feather, or eggshell samples, or surgical sexing.

The structure of their brush-tipped tongues makes them and their diet unique among parrots. The tongue consists of *papillae,* hair-like projections that are used to eat soft fruit, pollen, and nectar in the wild. Their method of eating makes them natural pollinators. The occasional insect or two may also be consumed. Lacking a gizzard, lorikeets require a soft diet.

Lories in captivity are ready breeders when appropriate diet, housing, a clean nest box, and breeding age have been achieved. Lories will nest in a cockatiel box, but a 24-in. tall × 8 × 10 in. (61 × 20.3 × 25.4 cm) grandfather nest box works well (Figure 40.1). Substrate can be dust-free aspen or pine shavings, or equine bedding pellets. Unlike some parrots that only use the nest box during breeding season, lories will use a nest box as sleeping quarters throughout the year. Check the nest box periodically and keep the substrate changed and clean.

Altricial lory babies are totally dependent on their parents for food and warmth. Parents feed by regurgitating what they have eaten into the chick's mouth. Parents keep the food mixture off the feathers by cleaning the chick with their tongues. As the chicks get older, they will clean each other and keep their feathers in good condition.

Incubation of the 1–3 eggs is started when the first egg is laid and lasts 22–27 days, depending on species. Eggs are laid every other day. Candling of the egg in a dark area can show signs of fertility at approximately 5 days (see Chapter 3). Both males and females incubate the eggs in some species.

*Hand-Rearing Birds*, Second Edition. Edited by Rebecca S. Duerr and Laurie J. Gage.

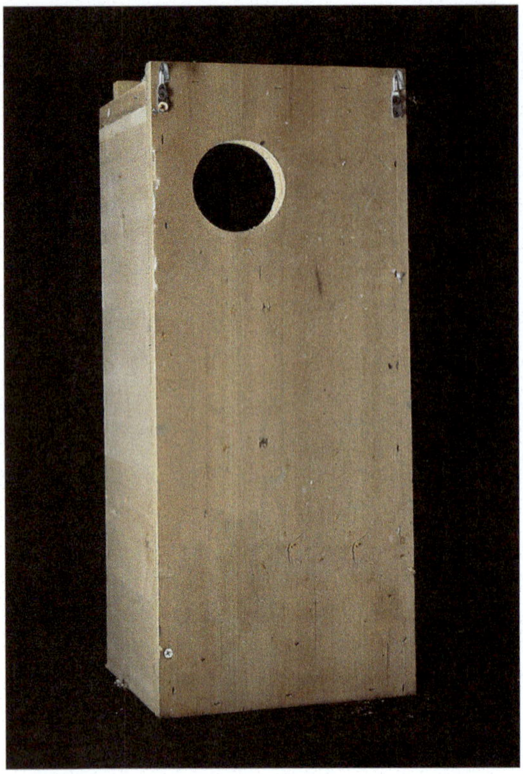

Figure 40.1 Grandfather nest box. *Source:* photo by Carol Stanley.

## Criteria for Intervention

Some lories will breed year-round. When this occurs during the hottest weather, overheating may cause high chick mortality. Countermeasures against overheating include strategically placed misters and fans. Alternatively, pulling the chicks for hand-rearing may be the wisest choice. Cold-weather hatching sometimes requires intervention if the parents are not diligent about keeping their young warm, or if it is just too cold for them to do so. Heat lamps with 250-W red bulbs placed in the vicinity of the nest box, but not too close, will help. When all else fails, pulling and hand-feeding may be the only alternative.

Installation of a nest box camera will provide valuable information on how the chicks are being cared for by the parents. Wireless cameras may be used for this purpose and require only electricity to send video to a smartphone or computer. Viewing the nest in real-time may alleviate the need for physically disturbing the chicks and parents, which may put both at risk. Novice parents should be monitored more closely and evaluated for the level of care given to their chicks. Abandoned nests or chicks thrown out of the nest can be seen immediately through a nest box camera, making intervention timely and lifesaving.

If the camera shows a chick that is lethargic and not begging its parents for food, the chick should be pulled for veterinary evaluation. If a chick appears to have died in the nest, it should be pulled immediately, and a necropsy performed to determine the cause of death. If the remaining clutch is pulled for hand-feeding, they should be kept in isolation and away from other clutches being hand-fed. Utensils and feeding instruments used for a potentially ill clutch should not be used for any other clutch. Disposable gloves should be worn and replaced before servicing the next clutch.

When pulling chicks from the nest box, care should be taken to keep them warm, especially those under 14 days. A warm, portable brooder or a bowl with paper towels and a towel for covering will work for quick removal and placement in a brooder.

Chicks should be pulled if either parent shows signs of illness, with the sick bird receiving veterinary attention immediately, and determination of whether the illness is potentially communicable to the chicks. Never start medicating without consulting your veterinarian.

If rearing chicks to be pets or to be in an interactive display, pulling the chicks may be done at any time but pulling before the eyes open, at about 10–14 days, makes transitioning to hand-feeding more easily accepted. Chicks at this age will generally accept feedings without fuss.

## Record Keeping

Keeping records of the dates eggs were laid will help determine the approximate hatch date. For example, Rainbow Lories will lay from 1 to 3 eggs and will incubate for 25 days before hatching. If the parents started incubation with the first egg, a newly hatched chick should be seen on or about 25 days after the egg was laid. Any additional chicks will hatch out according to the date the egg was laid. In the case of 3 fertile eggs, the oldest chick would be 4–5 days old when the third egg hatches. Lories are generally good parents and can handle the difference in chick size without a problem, and a nest box camera will allow you to monitor the condition of the chicks as they grow.

Banding chicks (L&M bird leg bands) is highly recommended for identification purposes and for record keeping for the life of the bird. Bands should be ordered well in advance of chick season. At approximately 10 days of age, the band may be applied. Placing a drop of olive oil on the band and foot area will make band application much easier. Apply the band by gently holding the four toes together and inserting them into the band. Gently slide the band up and over the joint. Note the leg band that was applied and all band information in records for that chick.

Once chicks are pulled from parents, their weights should be documented. If it is too early to band, marking them with a permanent fabric marker will make it easier to tell them apart. Marvy Uchida DecoFabric Paint Markers come in a variety of colors, are nontoxic, and are readily available at craft stores. Apply the color onto the "fuzz" down of the chick and note in the chart.

Records should be kept so that anyone working with the chick can easily see when the last feeding was, how much was fed, the behavior, environmental information such as humidity and temperature in the brooder, and what chicks, if any, are being kept together. Note the consistency and amount of fecal matter and note any changes or things out of the ordinary, and document those in the daily record.

## Hatching

See Chapter 3 for information regarding incubation and hatching of birds. Once draw down and internal pip is determined to have occurred, the egg may be moved to a hatcher/brooder set at 97 °F (36.1 °C). Humidity should be at 75%. To prevent waterborne disease, a few drops of grapefruit seed extract (GSE) or salt should be mixed into the water to deter the growth of bacteria. The egg should be place in a shallow bowl lined with a large nonstick pad, such as Band-Aid® Large Non-Stick Pads (Johnson & Johnson). This prevents the membrane sticking to the substrate during the hatching process. The external pip happens 24–48 hours after the internal pip and hatching usually

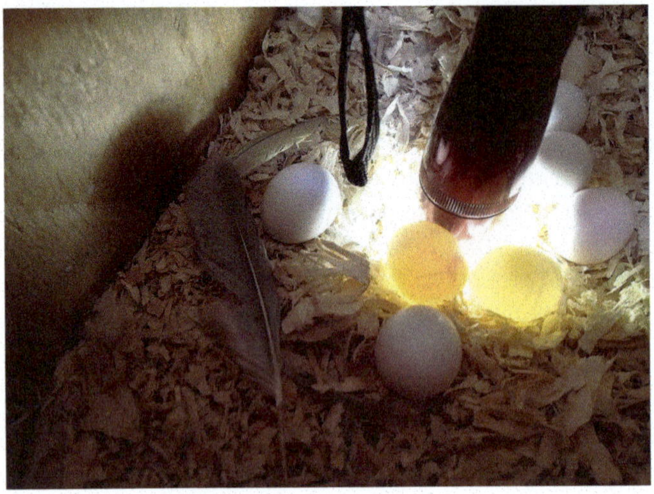

Figure 40.2 Candling lorikeet eggs. *Source:* photo by Gregory Sercel.

occurs within 24 hours after that. Lory eggs are sometimes almost round and the chick may move in every direction during the hatching process. Watch its progress by occasionally checking with a candler (Figure 40.2). Newer candlers utilize LED bulbs which emit very little heat. Initially, there will be many visible red veins lining the egg wall when candling the egg. The blood in these is slowly being absorbed, as is the yolk, by the chick. Be patient! Interference could cause the chick to bleed out or the yolk to not be absorbed completely. The chick will exhibit spurts of energy and then rest quietly, preparing for the next spurt. Eventually, the star-shaped crack in the egg made by the external pip will expand around the egg until the chick is able to use its feet and hatching neck muscle to push out of the egg.

Once hatched, a drop or two of lactated Ringers solution may be given orally for hydration but food should not be offered for 24 hours. During this time, the yolk sack is internally processed. The yolk can usually be seen through the skin of the abdominal wall of a newly hatched chick and will disappear after about 24 hours.

## Initial Care

See Chapter 1 for information about management of cold, dehydrated, injured, or ill chicks, including initial care. If pulling very young chicks, a brooder should be set up in the nursery a few days beforehand, if possible, to regulate its temperature. Brooder temperature should be set according to the age of the chicks being brooded (Table 40.1). The nursery room itself should ideally have a stable temperature 78–82 °F (25.5–27.7 °C) (Hagen Avian Research Institute, HARI).

Chicks pulled from the nest after their eyes have opened and pinfeathering has begun will be frightened and may resist being fed with a syringe. This is stressful for the chick, as well as the hand-feeder. Do not force it to eat. Offer drops of formula on the beak. The chick will start licking. If it resists, try again in a couple of hours. Eventually, especially when time for the morning feeding, the chick will be more accepting of hand-feeding efforts. Thereafter, they will eat from the syringe.

Table 40.1 Approximate brooder temperature (HARI).

| Age | Temperature °C | Temperature °F |
|---|---|---|
| Hatch to day 2–3 | 35.0–36.5 | 96–98 |
| Day 3 to day 14–21 | 31.1–34.0 | 88–94 |
| 3 weeks to weaning | 25.0–30.0 | 76–86 |

## Common Medical Problems

Bacterial infections are common in lories. Lories will use their brush tongues to lick everything, even if they have defecated on the object. Bacterial growth is compounded in hot weather. Therefore, it is important to keep surfaces clean and disinfected. Enclosures should periodically be wiped down and disinfected with veterinary disinfectant. Larger aviaries can be hosed down, scrubbed, and then, utilizing an electric mister, disinfected with a solution of F10SC Veterinary Disinfectant mixed as directed with water. Food and water bowls must be cleaned, and new food and water replenished throughout the day to avoid bacterial contamination.

When keeping lories outside, rodents may be a problem. Mice can get through ½ in. (1.25 cm) mesh hardware cloth while ¼ in. (0.75 cm) mesh hardware cloth stops them, but they have been known to chew through that. Watch for telltale signs in the aviary. Even a few droppings may be a sign of an infestation. A professional exterminator will be helpful but other trapping methods are also available. Mice and rats deposit their urine and feces throughout the aviary and feeding dishes which may cause bacterial infections in the birds if the rodents are not eliminated.

Overheating in the nest box is possible during hot days. Chicks should be pulled to the nursery and appropriate brooding temperatures and methods should be administered.

Cold temperatures bring the possibility of hypothermia. Pull chicks and place in brooder or appropriate housing at an appropriate temperature. Do not feed cold chicks; return hypothermic chicks to normal body temperature prior to feeding.

Care should always be taken not to press on the just-filled crop when handling birds during feeding. Formula may come up the esophagus and be aspirated down the trachea in an instant, which may result in death. If you think a chick has aspirated formula, seek veterinary advice.

## Diets and Tools

Commercial psittacine hand-feeding formulas, such as HARI Hand-feeding Formula, work well for lories. Follow mixing and temperature directions on the packaging. Always save the original container or packaging with the lot numbers, as they may be needed in case of a recall notice. Mix formula with heated water in a measuring cup using a small whisk.

The following is a recommended list of supplies to keep on hand:

- Psittacine baby bird feeding formula (Hagen)
- nectar powder
- feeding charts
- Gram Scale
- bedding (linens and/or equine bedding pellets)

- 1 ml syringe
- 10 ml syringe
- small (shallow) feed dish or bowl
- small mixing whisk
- 2 C (500 ml) glass measuring cup
- F10SC Veterinary Disinfectant
- lactated Ringer's solution
- small bottle brush for cleaning 10 cc syringes
- pipe cleaners for cleaning 1 cc syringes.

## Feeding Procedures

Wear gloves if feeding birds from different clutches. This will minimize crosscontamination and help prevent disease transmission. Change gloves for each group being fed. Thoroughly clean and then sterilize syringes and utensils by submerging in F10SC Veterinary Disinfectant, or a similar product, until the next feeding. Rinse before use.

### Hatchlings

Hatchlings that are 1–5 days old should be fed formula mixed as directed on the packaging, except substitute lactated Ringer's solution for water when mixing to assist with hydration. The temperature of the formula should be 100–105 °F (38–40.5 °C) to ensure the chicks will accept it. Cold formula can chill a newly hatched chick. Formula the first few days is thin and watery for hydration. Using a 1 ml syringe, feed approximately 0.5–1 ml (Figure 40.3). Feed chicks every 2 hours, making sure the crop is emptied before the next feed. Watch the crop fullness to determine the amount to feed; overfeeding may result in aspiration. As the chicks grow, increase the amount and slowly increase the thickness of the formula each day. After 5 days, use the formula manufacturer's recommended mixing ratios. Water may then be used for mixing formula and the lactated Ringer's

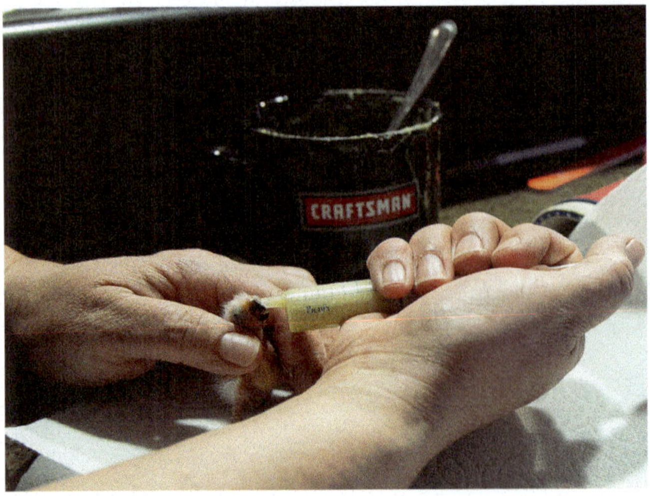


Figure 40.3 Feeding a 2-day old hatchling lory. *Source:* photo by Carol Stanley.

discontinued. Record all feedings and observations for each chick's record. Some caregivers take a 6-hour rest from hand-feeding hatchlings overnight, resuming the 2-hour schedule the next morning. A range of 55–70% humidity produces quieter, fatter chicks with a greater growth rate than those kept at levels of 15–35% (Clipsham 1991).

Lorikeet chicks will consume between 5 and 20 ml of formula depending on age and species. Mix formula fresh for each feeding. Ensure the formula is at a safe temperature for feeding by squirting a tiny amount on your wrist. It should feel very warm but not hot or cold. See package directions on the formula for recommended temperatures. When feeding multiple chicks, syringes of food may be immersed in a glass of very warm water to keep the formula warm. Do not feed cold formula or crop stasis may occur.

When feeding, remove the chick from the container and feed on a paper towel on a flat surface. Chicks will defecate shortly after feeding. A heat lamp may be necessary to ensure the chick does not get chilled during feeding. When chicks are housed in small containers, change the substrate (paper towels) when chicks are removed for feeding.

### Older Chicks

As chicks approach 3 weeks of age, feedings can be gradually reduced to 4 times a day. An example schedule would be 8:00 a.m., 12:00 p.m., 4:00 p.m., and 8:00 p.m. Weigh chicks before the first feeding of the day and compare to previous weights to measure progress. If there is no weight gain two days in a row, or the weight drops in a pre-fledging hatchling, seek veterinary advice. Observe the chick for lethargy, abnormal skin tone, or abnormal behavior.

Clean feathers after feeding. Dried formula may damage feathers. Once the chicks are older, they will begin cleaning each other. Once the chicks are moved to a weaning cage, a shallow bowl of prepared commercial lory nectar will encourage them to learn to feed themselves. Feeding by syringe should continue until they are clearly filling their crops with nectar on their own. Once eating nectar on their own, start introducing blueberries, papaya, apple, and other fruit.

## Expected Weight Gain

A growth chart for the species being raised can be used as a guideline for the development of the chicks you are feeding. Weights can vary or be erratic and the chick still be normal. Observation is your best tool for minimizing problems.

Stoddard (1988) monitors the health and development of young chicks by the:

A) Plumpness of the toes, wings and rump.
B) Skin color – should be beige-pink.
C) Skin texture – should be translucent and soft.
D) Anatomical symmetry – malnourished chicks often have thin feet, toes, and wings as well as a disproportionately large head.

The expected weight gains of three species of lorikeets are shown in Figure 40.4.

## Housing

Brooders are available from several sources. Lyon Technologies offers animal intensive care units that may be used for brooding. Addition companies offer portable brooders that will plug into a wall outlet and a car cigarette lighter. Water brooders, such as described by HARI, are heated with

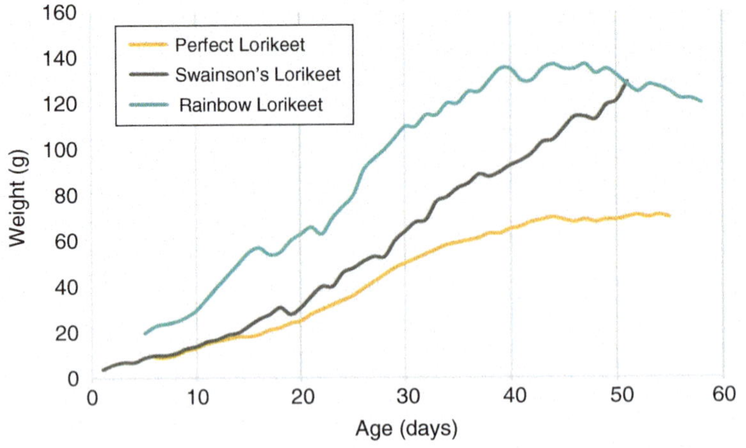


**Figure 40.4** Perfect, Rainbow, and Swainson's Lorikeet weight gain graph.

submersible aquarium heaters and utilize an aquarium inside an aquarium. Whatever the brooder, monitoring the comfort of the chicks is paramount.

Humidity can be increased in brooders by placing covered plastic bowls with holes in the lids to prevent a chick from accidentally falling in and drowning. The temperature of the water will affect the brooder temperature. Use warmer water to achieve a warmer brooder temperature relatively quickly. As before, use GSE or salt in the water to prevent bacterial growth. Change the water and clean the container every other day and keep the brooder clean using F10SC Veterinary Disinfectant.

Raising chicks with siblings or other chicks is preferable to raising a lone chick, unless there are medical problems. Chicks will clean each other after eating and huddle for security. A shredders piñata or feather duster may be attached and hung on the lid of the tub in a back corner. The chicks will stay in the corner under it. Ensure the toy or feather duster is not touching the substrate. Clean periodically to remove any fecal matter. Clean and sanitize toys periodically with F10SC Veterinary Disinfectant to remove any fecal matter. Lory chicks are very vocal, even after being fed, and this is normal.

## Hatchlings

Place hatchlings in plastic containers lined with paper towels or tissues, making sure the wall of the container is taller than the chick. Do not use material that is frayed or snags, such as terrycloth. Day-old chicks, if alone, should be kept in a brooder at 97° F (26 °C) and temperatures lowered by one degree every day. If raising multiple chicks of varying ages, this may be too warm. Check for signs of overheating. Older chicks will help keep younger chicks warm. When chicks are comfortable, they huddle loosely together. When too warm, they will pant, extend their wings, and sometimes lay prone. When chicks are chilled, they huddle tightly together and may shiver. Either way, adjustments to brooder temperatures should be made immediately. Overheating is much more harmful than being chilled. If overheated, turn the temperature down a couple degrees and open the brooder lid or door to allow fresh, cooling air in until chicks are comfortable. Keep a vigilant watch until the temperature has stabilized and the chicks are resting comfortably. Ensure the brooder settings are adjusted. To warm chilled chicks, adjust the brooder settings a couple of degrees at a time and wait for the new temperature to be achieved. Repeat if necessary. Adjusting brooder temperatures too quickly can cause erratic temperature swings and careful monitoring is warranted until the desired temperature is stabilized. External room temperatures have great influence on the brooder temperature and care should be taken to stabilize both.

Brooder temperatures are guidelines. Visual inspection of the condition of the chicks is crucial. Watch for signs of overheating and stress: panting, unrest, hyperactivity, and dry, reddened skin. Cold temperatures may result in death, poor gut motility, crop stasis or other digestive disorders, failure to feed or beg, inactivity, or shivering (Clubb and Clubb 1986). Never feed a cold chick. They will not be able to process food and may develop crop stasis.

Continue adjusting temperatures downward slowly until room temperature is reached. At that point, the chicks will have pinfeathers and be better able to thermoregulate and can be moved into plastic tubs without external heat, as long as the ambient room temperature does not fall below 78 °F (25.5 °C).

## Older Chicks

At 3 weeks of age, chicks are ready to be moved from the brooder to a tub where temperature control is not as crucial. At this age, chicks start climbing out of the small containers in the brooder and have developed pinfeathers (Figure 40.5).

Tub preparation: Sterilite 20-quart plastic tubs, or similar plastic tubs are acceptable. With the lid on the tub, drill 3/4 in. (1.8 cm) holes, approximately 1 in. (2.5 cm) apart in a series of rows and columns (Figure 40.6). These holes provide adequate ventilation and are the appropriate size to hold the sanitized 10 cc syringe to be used only for the chicks in that tub. Line the tub with a scent-free tall kitchen plastic garbage bag (13 gal/42 l) and place newspaper on the very bottom for absorbency. Place approximately 2 in. (5.1 cm) of equine bedding pellets in the tub on top of the newspaper. Equine bedding pellets eliminate odors and disintegrate when wet, preventing the crop impaction that is sometimes experienced with pine shavings. Change the bedding pellets every other day or as needed. These pellets work very well to keep chicks dry.

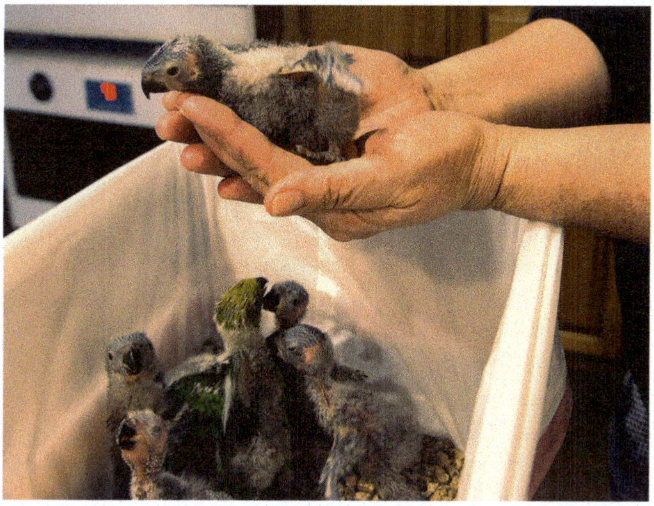

Figure 40.5 Swainson's Lorikeet chicks at 4–5 weeks old. *Source:* photo by Carol Stanley.

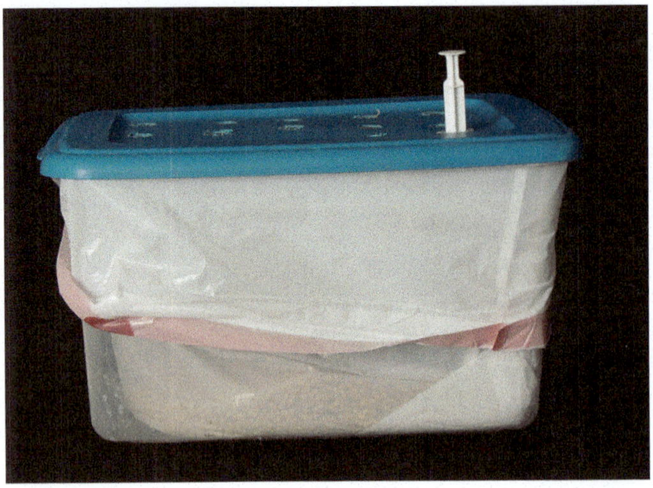

Figure 40.6 Lorikeet brooder tub. *Source:* photo by Carol Stanley.

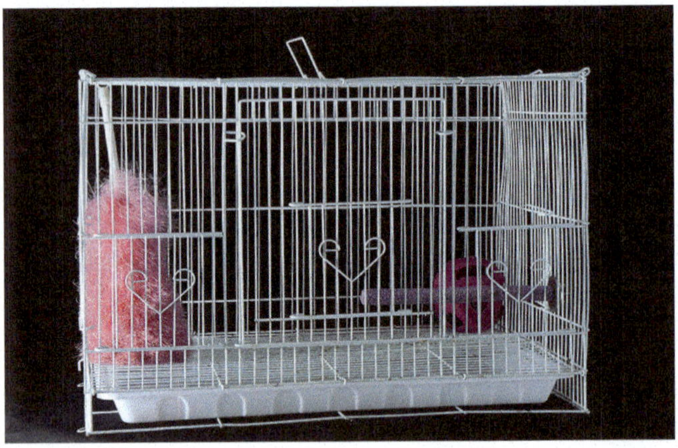

Figure 40.7 Weaning cage and feather duster. *Source:* photo by Carol Stanley.

## Weaning

As chicks continue to grow and become more active, they will need more room and can be moved to a weaning cage. The weaning cage should be small enough to prevent any errant flight attempts that might cause harm from the gaining of speed or altitude (Figure 40.7). Continue hand-feeding, but add a shallow dish of nectar in the bottom of the cage. Follow the package directions for mixing. Dip their beaks a few times into the nectar until they begin eating from the nectar dish. Hand-feeding may be discontinued when they are actively eating the nectar and filling their crops. During this period the chicks will huddle in a corner. Clean the dish and replenish nectar regularly (every four hours) throughout the day to prevent bacterial infections. Perches should be placed far enough away from the food dish to prevent the chicks from soiling their food.

As the chicks develop further in the weaning cage, they will begin to climb the walls. At this stage they will perch and are starting to explore more. If the chicks are to be raised as pets, hand-feeding should be started again and chicks encouraged to step up onto your hand or finger to eat. At first, there may be hesitation, but soon they will be eager to get on your hand to eat. Requiring chicks to step up to eat establishes a positive experience for the birds with hands and prevents hand fear in most species of parrots.

## Fledging

When chicks become more active, climbing cage sides and practicing short flight attempts, it's time for them to move into a fledging aviary. If the fledging aviary is outdoors, the addition of 250-W portable heat lamps should be used initially if the temperature is below 60 °F (15.5 °C). Arrange perching so they have a choice of what distance from the heat lamp is comfortable for them. They will tend to stay close together for warmth and not use the lamp. Leave the lamp available for potential colder nights.

This is a good time to introduce bird-safe toys, branches, and various perches for good foot exercise. Avoid toys with long cords or chains that could wrap around the neck or body. Cotton perches should be monitored for fraying and repaired or replaced promptly. Tiny cotton fibers may be dangerous and can wrap around a toe and cut off circulation. Shower curtains, bed linens, plastic tablecloths, or plastic sheeting may be use on walls behind cages and washed periodically to stay clean. Finely chopped fruits may be added to the diet at this time.

Flying comes naturally to most birds. It is a time when they develop into graceful flying machines. Fledging aviaries need not be very large. A 6 × 6 ft. (1.8 × 1.8 m) aviary with a safety door to prevent escape works very nicely for these relatively small birds. Aviaries may be outdoors if protected from the elements and predators.

## Preparation for Aviary Release

After the birds have had some time to practice flying, they may be taken to an introductory aviary, which is a small aviary large enough for them to fly in, and may house calm, nonaggressive birds, or other fledged chicks. This allows them to socialize with other birds. Allow them to spend 2–3 hours per day in this aviary for a few days, gradually increasing the time. This requires close supervision to ensure that the other birds are acting appropriately and that the young birds are eating. If no other birds are available for the introductory aviary, housing the young birds in an aviary adjacent to the main aviary is the next best option for socialization. Weigh the chicks daily until they have maintained their weight for at least 2 weeks. The young birds are now ready to be introduced to their final aviary housing.

## Acknowledgments

Thanks to Steve Duncan with Avian Resources, Gregory Sercel at Gregory's Aviary, Alycia Antheunisse at Cedar Hill Birds, and Jordan Daniels at Nurilory Aviary.

## Sources for Products Mentioned

Bird Sexing Solutions: Bird Sexing Solutions, 1348 LadyFern St., Plumas Lake, CA 95961, (530) 923-2974, https://www.birdsexingsolutions.com.

Leg Bands: L&M Bird Leg Bands, Inc., PO Box 2636, San Bernardino, CA 92406 USA, (909) 882-4649, http://www.lmbirdlegbands.com.

Lory Nectar: http://LoryNectar.com, PO Box 1751, Dawsonville, GA 30534, www.lorynectar.com.

Nekton-S: Nekton USA, 600 F St., Arcata, CA 95521, (707) 822-2417, www.nekton.net.

Tropican: Hagen Avicultural Research Institute (HARI®), (800) 225-2700, https://hari.ca.

Wingz Store: 9565 Pathway St., Santee, CA 92071, USA, (800) 447-CAGE, (800) 447-2243, www.wingzstore.com.

## References

Clipsham, R. (1991). Preventative medical management of aviary diseases. Proceedings of the Parrot Management Seminar, Concord, NH, pp. 23–56.

Clubb, S.L. and Clubb, K.J. (1986). Psittacine pediatrics. Proceedings of the Association of Avian Veterinarians, pp. 317–332.

Stoddard, H.L. (1988). Avian pediatric seminar. Avian Pediatric Seminar Proceedings (Supplement), pp 1–19.

## Further Reading

Hagen, M. (n.d.). Psittacine Pediatrics: Housing and Feeding of Baby Parrots. Hagen Avicultural Research Institute. https://hari.ca/hari/research-facility/hari-research-papers/psittacine-pediatrics-housing-feeding-baby-parrots (accessed 18 June 2019).

Low, R. (1998). *Encyclopedia of the Lories*. Blaine, Washington: Hancock House Publishers.

# 41

## Insects and Other Arthropods as Food

*Mark Finke, Liz Koutsos, and Diane Winn*

### Introduction: Definitions and Taxonomy

It is estimated that 61% of North American birds are primarily insectivorous, with an additional 28% partially insectivorous (Capinera 2010). Tremendous variability is shown in the types of insects consumed by different avian species. Additionally, there may be seasonal changes in feeding behavior, as is the case for some birds during breeding season, presumably to enhance their nutrient intake for egg production and delivery of optimal nutrition to growing young. The purpose of this chapter is to provide a nutritional primer for wildlife professionals raising nestlings of species that, in the wild, would be fed predominantly insects or other arthropods (Figures 41.1 and 41.2).

Arthropods are the largest group of animals on earth. While insects are the most well-known of the arthropods, other groups include, spiders, ticks, mites and scorpions (Arachnida); woodlice/pillbugs, crabs, crayfish and shrimp (Crustacea); millipedes (Diplopoda); and centipedes (Chilopoda). The arthropods familiar to most people are insects, which have a body with three distinct regions (head, thorax, and abdomen) and three pairs of legs. Although many animals are termed insectivores, most of them prey on a variety of invertebrates, some of which are likely an important source of select nutrients that may not be obtained in sufficient quantities from most insect species.

Generally, insects fall into two fairly distinct groups: those with simple metamorphosis (hemimetabolous) and those with complete metamorphosis (holometabolous). The young of hemimetabolous insects are called nymphs, and in most cases they resemble adults, sharing similar habitats and food. Examples of hemimetabolous insects include crickets, grasshoppers, and roaches. In contrast, the young of holometabolous insects are called larvae and are distinct from the adults both in appearance and food habits. The larvae are essentially specialized to accumulate nutrients, while adult holometabolous insects are specialized for dispersion and reproduction. Examples of holometabolous insects include beetles, butterflies and moths, flies, and ants.

More than 1 000 000 species of insects have been named, and there are an estimated 5.5 million species worldwide grouped into 31 orders (Wheeler et al. 2001; Stork 2018). While an in-depth review of insect taxonomy is not required, some of the major orders of insects likely used as food by those who gather wild insects include beetles (Coleoptera), bees and ants (Hymenoptera), flies (Diptera), true bugs and cicadas (Hemiptera), grasshoppers and crickets (Orthoptera), butterflies and moths and their larvae (Lepidoptera), and cockroaches (Blattodea). In addition to insects,

*Hand-Rearing Birds*, Second Edition. Edited by Rebecca S. Duerr and Laurie J. Gage.

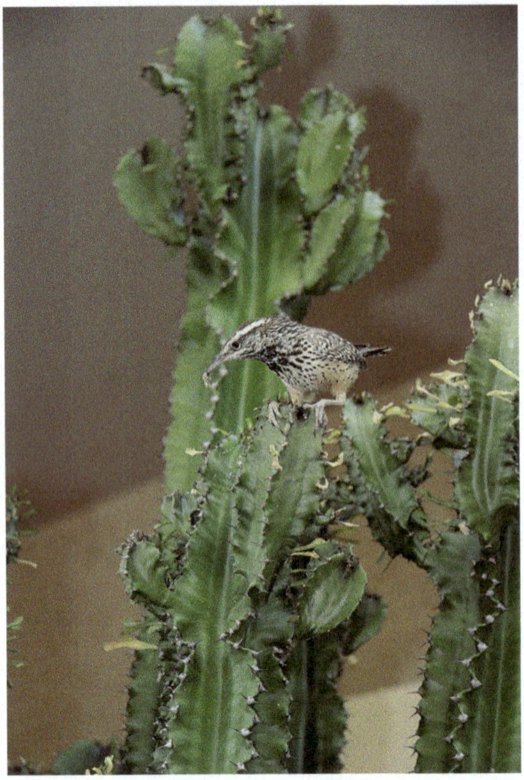

**Figure 41.1** Cactus Wren with food for nestlings. *Source:* photo courtesy of Mark Finke.

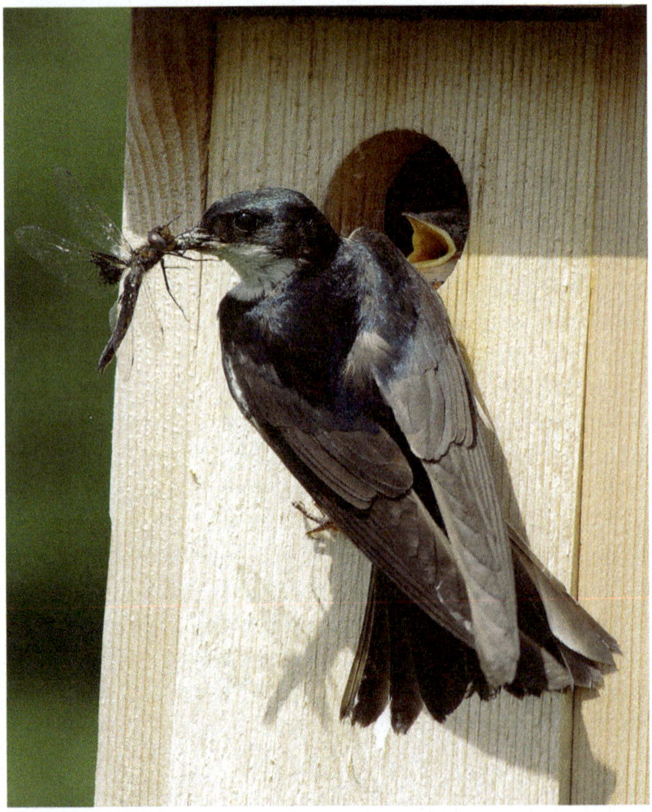

**Figure 41.2** Tree Swallow with food for nestlings. *Source:* photo courtesy of Kshanti Greene.

other arthropods that might be used in a feeding program include spiders, woodlice/pillbugs, and millipedes. Although earthworms (*Lumbricus terresstris*) are not arthropods (they are annelids), they are included here because of their use by many rehabilitators.

## Nutritional Composition of Insects

The insect species most commonly cultured for food include house crickets (*Acheta domesticus*), waxworms (larvae of the wax moth: *Galleria mellonella*), mealworms and superworms (larvae from two species of beetles: *Tenebrio molitor* and *Zophobas mori*), soldier flies (larvae of the black soldier fly: *Hermetia illucens*), fruit flies (*Drosophila melanogaster* and *Drosophila hydeii*) and several species of roaches. Nutritional information for these species and other feeder invertebrates is summarized in Tables 41.1–41.2 (original sources are Finke 2002, 2013; Oonincx and Dierenfeld 2012). To facilitate comparisons between different papers, these data have been recalculated from the original data to express the information on an as-fed basis, because most insects are fed live, with the moisture they naturally contain. More comprehensive reviews of the nutrient content of a wider range of insects are available (Bukkens 1997; Finke and Winn 2004; Finke and Oonincx 2017).

### Moisture, Protein, Fat, and Other Macronutrients

The moisture, protein, fat, ash, and fiber content of selected invertebrates are shown in Table 41.1. Whole invertebrates generally contain 55–85% moisture. After water, the nutrient in highest concentration is usually protein, which is not surprising given the protein-rich exoskeleton of insects. The protein content of whole invertebrates shown in Table 41.1 ranges from a low of 9.3% for silkworms to 26.3% for six-spotted roaches. In addition to protein, fat is a major component of most invertebrates, with the fat content of whole invertebrates ranging from a low of 1.4% for silkworms to a high of 29.4% for butterworms. Generally, there is a negative relationship between insect moisture content and insect fat content, with high-fat insects having less moisture than low-fat insects. In several instances, insects contain more fat than protein. Generally, female insects contain more fat than males, and commercially-raised insects usually contain more fat than wild-caught insects (Finke and Oonincx 2017). Most invertebrates contain only small amounts of ash (which represents minerals) because they lack the internal calcified skeleton found in vertebrates. The exceptions are soldier fly larvae and woodlice/pillbugs, both which have a mineralized exoskeleton (Oonincx and Dierenfeld 2012; Finke 2013).

Protein is composed of amino acids, and there are a number of published reports on the amino acid composition of insects that show them to be a good source of protein that provides sufficient quantities of most of the essential amino acids (Finke 2002, 2013; Finke and Oonincx 2017).

There are multiple reports on the fatty acid composition of most commercially-raised insect species (Finke 2002, 2013, 2015b). Importantly, all the insects tested contained significant amounts of the essential fatty acids linoleic acid (18 : 2) and linolenic acid (18 : 3). Commercially-raised insects generally contain higher levels of omega-6 fatty acids and lower levels of omega-3 fatty acids than wild-caught insects. Long chain omega-3 fatty acids eicosapentaenoic acid (EPA) and docosahexaenoic acid (DHA) are typically only found in any significant amounts in aquatic insects (Ghioni et al. 1996; Fontaneto et al. 2011). However, the fatty acid content of insects can be modified by diet, so there may be significant variation between insects of the same species from various suppliers (Finke 2015b; Starčevića et al. 2017). Soft-bodied insects like silkworms usually contain less

Table 41.1 Moisture, protein, fat, fiber, and ash content of selected invertebrates.

| Species – Life stage | Moisture (%) | Crude Protein (%)[a] | Crude Fat (%) | Acid Detergent Fiber (%) | Ash (%) | Energy (kcal/g) |
|---|---|---|---|---|---|---|
| Waxworms (*Galleria mellonella*) – larvae | 58.5 | 14.1 | 24.9 | 3.4 | 0.6 | 2.75 |
| Mealworms (*Tenebrio molitor*) – larvae | 61.9 | 18.7 | 13.4 | 2.5 | 0.9 | 2.05 |
| Superworms (*Zophbas morio*) – larvae | 57.9 | 19.7 | 17.7 | 2.7 | 1.0 | 2.42 |
| Silkworms (*Bombyx mori*) – larvae | 82.7 | 9.3 | 1.4 | 1.1 | 1.1 | 0.67 |
| Butterworms (*Chilecomadia moorei*) – larvae | 60.2 | 15.5 | 29.4 | 1.4 | 0.8 | 2.98 |
| Soldier flies (*Hermetia illucens*) – larvae | 61.2 | 17.5 | 14.0 | 3.0 | 3.5 | 1.99 |
| Crickets (*Acheta domesticus*) – adults | 69.2 | 20.5 | 6.8 | 3.2 | 1.1 | 1.40 |
| Crickets (*A. domesticus*) – nymphs | 77.1 | 15.4 | 3.3 | 2.2 | 1.1 | 0.95 |
| Rusty red roaches (*Blatta lateralis*) – nymphs | 69.1 | 19.0 | 10.0 | 2.2 | 1.2 | 1.60 |
| Six-spotted roaches (*Eublaberus distanti*) – adults | 56.6 | 26.3 | 13.6 | ND | 1.65 | 2.27 |
| Fruit flies (*Drosophila melanogaster*) – adults | 69.1 | 21.0 | 5.9 | 3.1 | 2.2 | 1.37 |
| Woodlice/pillbugs (*Porcellio scaber*) – adults | 67.8 | 13.3 | 3.7 | 1.6 | 10.5 | 0.83 |
| Earthworms (*Lumbricus terresstris*) | 83.6 | 10.5 | 1.6 | 0.1 | 0.6 | 0.71 |

ND = Not determined.
[a] Crude protein measured as nitrogen ×6.25.

fiber than those with a hard exoskeleton like beetles (Finke 2007). The "hard" body parts of some insects (i.e. the wing covers of beetles or the legs and wings of grasshoppers and other insects) is largely a result of sclerotized proteins, not chitin. These proteins are hardened via a cross-linking or tanning process. That is the reason newly-molted insects like mealworms are soft and white in color. The cross-linking process occurs after molting and results in a darkening and hardening of the insect cuticle. Insects that are high in fiber are often mistakenly thought of as being high in chitin, but quantitative data suggest that chitin is only a minor component of most insect species (Kaspari 1991; Kramer et al. 1995; Finke 2007). While chitin is sometimes thought to be unique to insects, it is much more widely distributed, being found in fungi, mollusks, fish scales, and most species of arthropods.

## Minerals and Vitamins

Mineral analyses of invertebrates are shown in Table 41.2. As expected, most insects contain little calcium and high levels of phosphorus, resulting in a calcium : phosphorus ratio of <1. Some arthropods, including a few species of insects such as black soldier fly larvae, which have a mineralized exoskeleton, are exceptions to this rule. Soldier fly larvae can contain up to 6.6% calcium on a dry-matter basis depending on diet, while millipedes and isopods contain from 7 to 20% calcium

Table 41.2 Mineral content of selected invertebrates.

| Species – Life stage | Calcium (%) | Phosphorus (%) | Magnesium (%) | Iron (mg/kg) | Zinc (mg/kg) | Copper (mg/kg) | Manganese (mg/kg) |
|---|---|---|---|---|---|---|---|
| Waxworms (*Galleria mellonella*) – larvae | 0.024 | 0.19 | 0.03 | 20.9 | 25.4 | 3.8 | 1.3 |
| Mealworms (*Tenebrio molitor*) – larvae | 0.017 | 0.28 | 0.08 | 20.6 | 52.0 | 6.1 | 5.2 |
| Superworms (*Zophobas morio*) – larvae | 0.018 | 0.24 | 0.05 | 16.5 | 30.7 | 3.6 | 4.3 |
| Silkworms (*Bombyx mori*) – larvae | 0.070 | 0.17 | 0.06 | 9.0 | 15.2 | 2.2 | 1.9 |
| Butterworms (*Chilecomadia moorei*) – larvae | 0.012 | 0.23 | 0.03 | 14.0 | 35.7 | 3.0 | 0.7 |
| Soldier flies (*Hermetia illucens*) – larvae | 0.934 | 0.36 | 0.17 | 66.6 | 56.2 | 4.0 | 61.8 |
| Crickets (*Acheta domesticus*) – adults | 0.041 | 0.30 | 0.03 | 19.3 | 67.1 | 6.2 | 11.5 |
| Crickets (*A. domesticus*) – nymphs | 0.027 | 0.25 | 0.02 | 21.2 | 68.0 | 5.1 | 8.9 |
| Rusty red roaches (*Blatta lateralis*) – nymphs | 0.038 | 0.18 | 0.02 | 14.8 | 32.7 | 7.9 | 2.6 |
| Six-spotted roaches (*Eublaberus distanti*) – adults | 0.043 | 0.24 | 0.04 | 48.2 | 93.6 | 11.1 | 2.4 |
| Fruit flies (*Drosophila melanogaster*) – adults | 0.052 | 0.41 | 0.05 | 123.9 | 69.0 | 5.0 | 5.1 |
| Woodlice/pillbugs(*Porcellio scaber*) – adults | 4.621 | 0.39 | 0.15 | 139.7 | 54.7 | 41.5 | 27.3 |
| Earthworms (*Lumbricus terresstris*) | 0.044 | 0.16 | 0.01 | 50.4 | 17.7 | 1.5 | 1.3 |

on a dry-weight basis (Reichle et al. 1969; Gist and Crossley 1975; Graveland and van Gijzen 1994; Oonincx and Dierenfeld 2012; Spranghers et al. 2017). Earthworms from soil in chalky areas contain significant amounts of calcium for nestling common blackbirds (*Turdus merula*) and song thrushes (*Turdus philomelos*) (Bilby and Widdowson 1971).

While calculations suggest that insects contain insufficient calcium for most insectivores, in the wild, insectivorous animals seek out either prey unusually rich in calcium or other sources of calcium, especially while breeding. For example, Collared and Pied Flycatchers (*Ficedula albicollis* and *F. hypoleuca*) preferentially feed on calcium-rich isopods during reproduction (Bureš and Weidinger 2003). Isopods were also found by to be unusually prominent in the diet of nestling European Starlings (*Sturnus vulgaris*) (Moore 1986). Birds may also obtain extra calcium via the ingestion of eggshells, snail and clam shells, calcareous grit, bones, crawfish exoskeletons, limestone gravel, or mortar (St. Louis and Breebaart 1991; Graveland and van Gijzen 1994; Graveland 1996; Dhondt and Hochachka 2001).

Most insects and other invertebrates appear to be good sources of magnesium, sodium, and potassium, as well as the trace minerals iron, zinc, copper, and manganese. Invertebrates with a mineralized exoskeleton have higher amounts of magnesium and manganese, while flies appear to be a rich source of iron (Oonincx and Dierenfeld 2012; Finke 2013). Mineral composition in general probably largely reflects the food sources of the insect, both that present in the gastrointestinal tract and that incorporated into the insect's body because of the food it consumed. Studies of wild insects show seasonal variation as well as variations between different populations of the same species living in the same general area (Reichle et al. 1969; Studier and Sevick 1992; Graveland and van Gijzen 1994).

Vitamin A is provided by a group of compounds composed of both retinol (preformed vitamin A) and various carotenoids, such as β-carotene, α-carotene, and β-cryptoxanthin. Like most vertebrates, insects obtain retinoids via the cleavage of these carotenoids (Von Lintig 2012). However, unlike vertebrates in which cleavage takes place largely in the intestine, insects convert carotenoids to retinoids only in the compound eye (Von Lintig 2012). This explains why adult insects contain very low levels of vitamin A/retinoids and why holometabolous insect larvae, which lack compound eyes, do not contain retinoids (Pennino et al. 1991; Barker et al. 1998; Giovannucci and Stephenson 1999; Finke 2002, 2013; Oonincx and Dierenfeld 2012).

The conversion of carotenoids to vitamin A (retinol) varies widely among animal species, but conversion takes place in several species of birds, including chickens, turkeys, quail, and geese (Olson 1989). High levels of carotenoids, including those that can be converted to vitamin A, are found in various wild insect species, whereas commercially-produced insects contain far lower quantities (Finke 2002, 2013, 2015b; Isaksson and Andersson 2007; Eeva et al. 2010). While most commercially-produced insects contain few carotenoids, insect carotenoid levels can be enhanced by feeding them a carotenoid-enriched diet (Finke 2015b).

Data on vitamin D in insects are limited. Most commercial insects contain low levels of vitamin D (typically <400 IU/kg dry matter) (Finke 2002, 2013; Oonincx et al. 2010). More data is needed to better understand the vitamin D content of wild insects and its application to feeding insectivores.

The vitamin E content of commercial feeder insects varies widely (Pennino et al. 1991; Barker et al. 1998; Finke 2002, 2015b; Hatt et al. 2003). This variation is likely due to diet resulting in different amounts of vitamin E being incorporated in the insect's tissues as well as from food remaining in the insect's gut. In contrast, the limited information available suggests that wild insects contain higher levels of vitamin E than those typically found in commercially-raised insects (Pennino et al. 1991; Barker et al. 1998; Cerda et al. 2001; Finke 2015a).

While there are only limited data on the B-vitamin content of wild insects, there is a significant amount of information for commercially-raised insects (Finke 2002, 2013, 2015a, 2015b). These data suggest that, in general, insects are good sources of most B-vitamins. Some species such as crickets are moderately low in thiamine, but a diet of mixed species of insects should provide adequate amounts of all the B-vitamins.

### Other Nutrients

In addition to the known nutrients, insects contain a variety of other compounds that may be utilized by insectivores. These include inositol, cholesterol, taurine, and other compounds (Cerda et al. 2001; Ramsay and Houston 2003; Finke 2015b). While some of these compounds are required by other species (i.e. taurine for cats and inositol for some species of fish), there currently are no data to suggest they might be required by insectivores, including birds. Taurine, an amino sulfonic acid, is of particular interest. It is found in a wide variety of animal tissues, including some species of invertebrates. Crickets, grasshoppers, flies, moths, and spiders are rich sources of taurine, while most species of insect larvae contain little if any taurine (Bodnaryk 1981; Massie et al. 1989; Finke 2002, 2013, 2015a; Ramsay and Houston 2003). Ramsay and Houston speculated that the preference of blue tits (*Parus caeruleus*) for spiders during their nesting season may be due to their high levels of taurine.

## Feeding Captive Insectivorous Nestlings

As the primary food for many wild nestlings, insects in general should supply adequate levels of protein, amino acids, fatty acids, plus most minerals and vitamins. As noted in the previous section, during the breeding season, adult wild birds of many species provide additional calcium to their nestlings in the form of either calcium-rich invertebrates or calcium supplements to support skeletal mineralization (Reynolds et al. 2004; Reynolds and Perrins 2010). Assuming an adequate supply of foodstuffs, wild birds are presumably able to select a variety of arthropods that, in the proper proportions, provides nestlings a diet that is sufficient for growth. Because nestlings in captivity are often fed only a few species of cultured insects (typically, crickets, mealworms, and waxworms), several nutrients are of special concern. Rehabilitators feeding insects to growing birds should be primarily attentive to calcium, vitamin A, and, if adequate sunlight or full-spectrum lighting is unavailable, vitamin D. The importance of additional nutrients such as omega-3 fatty acids (and overall fatty acid profile) and taurine may be significant, although more work in this area is warranted.

### Insect-based Diets

Cultured insects presumably offer a close approximation to the natural diet of insectivorous nestlings; however, they are expensive, and supplementing them with appropriate amounts of selected nutrients can be challenging. Supplementation of insects is typically done in one of several ways.

The most common practice used in zoos is gut-loading, which involves feeding insects diets that augment their nutrient profiles via food retained in their gastrointestinal tracts. The calcium content of waxworms, house crickets, mealworms, and silkworms can all be increased 5 to 20-fold by feeding a high calcium diet (e.g. Strzelewicz et al. 1985; Klasing et al. 2000; Hunt et al. 2001; Finke 2003). Other nutrients such as vitamin A can also be added using this method (e.g. Finke 2003;

Ogilvy et al. 2012). However, the results can be inconsistent, due to a variety of factors that impact how much of the diet and the supplemental nutrient in question is actually consumed by the insect (Finke 2003; Livingston et al. 2014). This inconsistency was demonstrated by the fact that only one of seven commercially-available gut-loading products sold in pet stores significantly increased cricket calcium content above that of the control group (Finke et al. 2004, 2005). Further, gut-loading foods are not suitable maintenance diets and may negatively impact viability when used for more than a few days (e.g. Klasing et al. 2000). This means that a rehabilitation facility would have to keep two colonies of each insect species used, one on a maintenance diet and another on the gut-loading diet. A comprehensive review of these issues may be found in Livingston et al. (2014), and although this article focused on crickets, the issues are similar regarding other species of insects. In summary, care is required in selecting and implementing gut-loading diets, especially those that are not supported by published research.

Dusting is another method used to supplement feeder insects (Figure 41.3). This approach involves using a fine powder, typically calcium carbonate with or without other nutrients, and applying it to the insect just prior to offering it as food. Dusting can be an effective means of supplementation, but the amount that adheres to the insect depends on factors that include the characteristics of the powder, the species and age/size of the insect, and the ability of that insect to remove the powder by grooming over time since the dust was applied (Winn et al. 2003; Michaels et al. 2014). The previously-mentioned review by Livingston et al. (2014) also contains a discussion and summary of research on dusting crickets. While dusting can be effective, care must be taken, as the results can be inconsistent.

Another strategy is delivering supplements in oily pastes that can be applied to insects in greater quantities than would be possible with powders. For nestling and fledgling passerines raised on 100% insects, Perlman (2016) suggested creating a package of human supplements comprising calcium, vitamins A, C, D, and E, plus taurine and omega-3 marine oil. The supplement mix is either applied daily to a feeder insect or fed directly in small amounts that vary according to the size of the bird. Because the supplements are packaged for human consumption, users must estimate small fractions of a total mixture volume, which may affect accuracy. Also, without

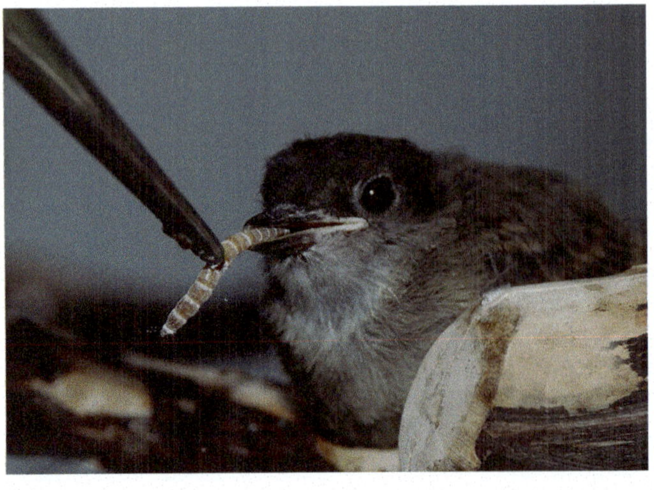

Figure 41.3 Eastern Phoebe fed calcium-dusted mealworm. *Source:* photo courtesy of Diane Winn/Avian Haven.

specifying the types and amounts of insects that are fed, it is not possible to accurately calculate the nutritional composition of the resulting diet. See Chapters 43 and 44, for more information on feeding supplemented all-insect diets.

## Insect-substitute Diets

As an alternative to insect-based diets, blends of commercially-available ingredients may be utilized to prepare insect-substitute diets. These formulas are designed with the nutrient composition of insects in mind, as well as ease of preparation and access to components. Over the years, several formulas have been published or described, and subsequently modified as new knowledge and/or changes in commercial ingredients occurred. Tables 41.3 and 41.4 provide the diet ingredients and nutrient composition of several formulas currently in use. There are many other formulas used in rehabilitation settings, but due to lack of complete information (and thus the inability to accurately estimate nutrient levels in the finished product), such formulas are not evaluated in this text.

One incredibly important consideration with insect-substitute diets is that they are formulated around the inclusion of specific components. Therefore, substitution of those components (e.g. replacement of one cat food product with another brand) is ill-advised, as the nutrient composition of the finished formula will change and may no longer be suitable. As our knowledge of the composition of insects evolves, more modifications to these formulae will be possible. Essential nutrients for which our knowledge is still limited, such as fatty acids, trace minerals, and vitamins, may be further optimized in the future, and this progress is already evident in revisions of commonly fed formulas (e.g. Winn 2002; Winn and Finke 2004, 2017).

As noted in several of the insect-substitute diets, insects may be a component of a total diet. For example, the BuNS© formula incorporates dried crickets, mealworms, and soldier fly larvae, plus calcium and vitamin supplements, with all components in specified amounts. After the combination has been processed, water is added to the ground mixture to achieve a consistency appropriate for forceps-feeding (Winn and Finke 2017). A suitable feeding program for any given organization or individual should be available to meet economic needs, animal needs, and provider comfort level.

There have been only a few efforts to compare diets such as these in actual practice. The challenge in such attempts is controlling extraneous variables that could provide alternative explanations for results seeming to favor one diet or another.

Seage et al. 2010 reported results of a feeding trial comparing FoNS© and Mazuri® Nestling Meal (MNM). On admission, healthy clutchmates from various species were randomly assigned to the two dietary treatments but were housed together. Staff caregivers were experienced in syringe-feeding and followed standard facility protocols for nestling birds (Figure 41.4). Gains in weight and feather development were similar in the two groups, with the two diets judged equivalent in ability to support healthy growth. Birds in the MNM group had more vivid yellow mouth color, likely due to the marigold extract in that diet. Fusté et al. (2013) reported a comparison of several hand-rearing diets, including a formula somewhat similar to FoNS© (but using a different base product) compared to cricket- or mealworm-based diets (with supplementation). Lower fledging weights were observed in the formula group relative to the insect groups, but, unfortunately, this project did not use split-clutch assignment to dietary treatments, and thus initial body weights and ages were quite variable between treatments. Additionally, several factors other than the primary food varied among conditions, including various unquantified vitamin and mineral supplements in the insect groups, and total feed intake level (and thus total energy and nutrient allocation to birds). Further research evaluating optimal feeding programs for a given avian species is needed but is very challenging to undertake in a controlled manner.

Table 41.3 Ingredient composition of various insect-substitute diets.

| Gut-loaded mealworms[a] | Gut-loaded crickets[b,c] | BuNS 2019[d] | FoNS 2018 Wellness[e] | Mazuri Nestling Meal[f] | Robyn's Songbird Diet[g] | Basic Nestling Diet[h] |
|---|---|---|---|---|---|---|
| Mealworms | Crickets | 15 g dried crickets | 135 g (1 cup) Wellness Core Kitten Formula soaked in 360 ml (1.5 cups) water | Primary Ingredients – Soy protein concentrate, dried egg, dried chicken, fishmeal | 187 g Wellness Complete Health Kitten Diet | 122 g (1 cup) Purina ProPlan Kitten Chicken and Rice dry diet |
| Gut-loaded with high calcium gut loading diet w/ 14.4% Calcium | Gut-loaded with 83% Timberline Cricket Power Food and 17% T-Rex 2.0 Calcium/ No Phosphorus Supplement | 5 g dried mealworms | 18 g (3 tbsp) dried egg white | Water varies by desired consistency | 70 g Science Diet Adult Light Feline | 300–360 ml (1.25-1.5 cups) water |
| | | 2 g dried soldier fly larvae | 5 g (1/2 tsp active culture plain yogurt | | 142 g Gerber 2[nd] Food, chicken and gravy | 12 g (2 tbsp) dried powdered egg white |
| | | 0.8 g $CaCO_3$ (powder) | 4.6 g (1 tsp) corn, canola or sunflower oil | | 130 g hardboiled egg (no shell) | 1.85 g $CaCO_3$ (powder) |
| | | 0.4 g (4 scoops) Avi-Era vitamins (Lafeber) | 2.0 g $CaCO_3$ (powder) | | 6 g $CaCO_3$ (powder) | 1 g (1/4 tsp) Avi-Era vitamins (Lafeber) |
| | | 0.05 g active culture plain yogurt per 1.0 g dry mix | 1 g (1/4 tsp) Avi-Era vitamins (Lafeber) | | 3 tsp Avian Formula LA 200 (Fox Valley Animal Nutrition) | |
| | | 2.5 g water per 1.0 g dry mix | | | 1 g (1/4 tsp) Avi-Era vitamins (Lafeber) | |
| | | | | | 1 tablet Simply Right B-complex + C | |
| | | | | | 720 g water | |
| | | | | | Supplemental Insects or ½ cup dried insects | |

For all blended diets: Add dry ingredients to water to soften prior to mixing (e.g. BuNS) or blending (e.g. Basic Nestling Diet). BuNS is intended to be fed as moist clumps by forceps; other blended diets should be smooth enough to feed by syringe.

[a] Bernard and Allen 1997.
[b] Finke 2002.
[c] Finke et al. 2005.
[d] Modified by the authors from Winn and Finke 2017.
[e] Winn and Finke 2017.
[f] http://www.mazuri.com/product_pdfs/5S90.pdf
[g] Grabowski. 2014.
[h] Duerr 2007.

Table 41.4 Nutrient composition of various insect-substitute diets (DMB = dry matter basis).

| | Gut-loaded mealworms[a] | Gut-loaded crickets[b,c] | BuNS 2019[d] | FoNS 2018 Wellness[e] | Mazuri Nestling Meal[f] | Robyn's Songbird Diet[g] | Basic Nestling Diet[h] |
|---|---|---|---|---|---|---|---|
| Moisture (%) | 57.8 | 70–73 | 73 | 71 | 65–85 | 76 | 68–72 |
| Crude Protein (%, DMB) | 38.9 | 66.6 | 57.2 | 51.2 | 50.0 | 42.0 | 45.0 |
| Crude Fat (% DMB) | 45.4 | 22.2 | 24.9 | 20.0 | 24.0 | 24.0 | 19.5 |
| Fiber (% DMB) | 7.7*** | 10.2 | 8.6 | 2.8 | 3.3 | 2.6 | ND* |
| Carbohydrate (% DMB) | 4.4 | 3.6 | 1.7 | 17.5 | 5.4 | 24.0 | ND* |
| Energy (kcal/g DMB) | 5.8 | 4.7 | 4.5 | 4.5 | 3.1 | 4.5 | 4.7** |
| Ash (% DMB) | 3.5 | 3.6 | 3.6 | 7.4 | 7.3 | 7.4 | ND* |
| Calcium (% DMB) | 0.69 | 1.16 | 1.73 | 2.05 | 1.40 | 1.79 | 1.66 |
| Phosphorus (% DMB) | 0.57 | 0.96 | 0.86 | 1.18 | 1.10 | 0.87 | 1.07 |
| Ca:P | 1.21:1 | 1.21:1 | 2.01:1 | 1.73:1 | 1.27:1 | 2.06:1 | 1.55:1 |
| Iron mg/kg DMB | 58 | 63 | 88 | 230 | 215 | ND* | ND* |
| Zinc mg/kg DMB | 86 | 218 | 182 | 180 | 72 | ND* | ND* |
| Vitamin A (IU/kg DMB) | ND* | 3630 | 18 000 | 29 200 | 4550 | ND* | ND* |
| Vitamin D (IU/kg DMB) | ND* | 313 | 2,253 | 2,463 | 2,294 | ND* | ND* |

[a] Bernard and Allen 1997.
[b] Finke 2002.
[c] Finke et al. 2005.
[d] Modified by the authors from Winn and Finke 2017.
[e] Winn and Finke 2017.
[f] http://www.mazuri.com/product_pdfs/5S90.pdf
[g] Grabowski. 2014.
[h] Duerr 2007.
* Not determined
** Determined from published values on individual product composition, where provided, or using Atwaters factors of 4 kcal/g protein, 9 kcal/g fat, 4 kcal/g carbohydrate
*** Acid detergent fiber, not crude fiber.

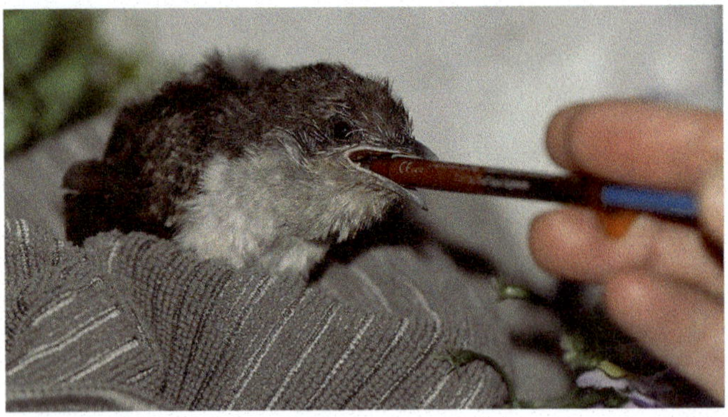

Figure 41.4 Syringe-feeding a Black-billed Cuckoo nestling. *Source:* photo courtesy of Diane Winn/Avian Haven.

## Comparative Analyses and Evaluation

As previously noted, primary nutrients of concern in a rehabilitation setting should be calcium, vitamin A, and, if adequate sunlight or full-spectrum lighting is unavailable, vitamin D. In addition, moisture levels of diets can be a critical component for success of nestling chicks, and other nutrients, including fatty acids, fiber, and carotenoids are worthy of consideration in nestling diets.

Moisture content of the insect-substitute diets, and insects themselves, ranges from 55 to 85% moisture. Water is a critical component of the diets of hatchling and nestling birds, as evaporative losses in small birds can be very high. Very small birds (e.g. less than 50 g) can lose up to 25% of body weight as water per day (Bartholomew and Cade 1963), and Psittacine hatchlings (*Nymphicus hollandicus*) have been shown to require ~ 80% moisture for the first few days of life for optimal survival and fledging (Roudybush and Grau 1986). The hydration level of the chick is often apparent in a smooth, "plump" appearance of skin versus the wrinkled, "tight" appearance of the skin of a poorly hydrated chick.

The calcium content of insects is generally low, as previously noted, but can be modified by supplementation (e.g. gut-loading, dusting), resulting in insect-based diets containing close to 1% calcium (dry matter basis). Insect-substitute diets are generally higher in calcium, resulting in ~1.4–2.1% dietary calcium (dry matter basis, Table 41.4). Unfortunately, almost nothing is known about the daily calcium requirement for most species of nestling wild passerines. In very occasional reports of the accretion of body calcium with age as the skeleton mineralizes, less than 30 mg calcium per day has been estimated, depending on age and species (e.g. Common Blackbird (*T. merula*), Bilby and Widdowson 1971; Eastern Bluebird (*Sialia sialis*) Hungerford et al. 1993). Using the blackbird as an example, and based on predicted basal metabolic rate (Aschoff and Pohl 1970), consequential daily energy intake, and relative bioavailability of calcium at 68% (based on work in domesticated poultry using a variety of sources) (Soares 1995), the reported deposition of calcium into body tissues during growth would require ~ 1.08% dietary calcium. Obviously, this is merely a calculation and should be considered as such, but it does correspond well to the recommendations made for nestling passerines (i.e. 1.5–2.0% calcium; Duerr 2007), and with formulated levels of calcium in various insect-substitute diets. However, users of daily supplements should remain mindful that excessive calcium intake can cause several problems, including visceral gout, kidney nephrosis, and secondary deficiencies of several other minerals (see Klasing 1998).

Dietary fatty acids, while not defined in each of the insect-substitute diets, are critical not only to chick development via energy provisioning, but also to immune function. The recent focus on omega-3 : omega-6 fatty acid levels in diets has demonstrated that insects, both commercially-available and wild, are a source of omega-3 fatty acids (Thompson 1973; Finke 2002, 2013). However, commercially-available insects may be more enriched with omega-6 fatty acids than their wild counterparts due to the fatty acid profile of diets fed to these insects during commercial rearing (Finke 2015b). Omega-3 fatty acids, and particularly longer chain omega-3 fatty acids, are known to impact immune responses, and generally drive more anti-inflammatory responses as compared to omega-6 fatty acids (Fritsche 2006). Therefore, inclusion of omega-3 fatty acids in the diets of nestling birds is likely appropriate.

There are several forms of omega-3 fatty acids that may be useful in these diets. Alpha-linolenic acid (ALA, 18:2n3) is a commonly offered omega-3 fatty acid and is found in flaxseed oil, for example. In some species, ALA can be converted to longer chain omega-3 fatty acids, such as EPA and DHA. Recent work has demonstrated that insectivorous Tree Swallow chicks (*Tachycineta bicolorswift*) were capable of converting ALA to EPA and DHA (Twining et al. 2018). These data would support the thought that provisioning of ALA in diets of insectivorous chicks would be sufficient to meet their needs for longer chain omega-3 fatty acids (EPA and DHA). However, other species of birds may not have this capacity, and the level of ALA in the diet would need to be high enough to allow for bioconversion. For this reason, enrichment with longer chain omega-3 fatty acids such as EPA and DHA may support improved growth and fledging success, as demonstrated in Tree Swallows (Twining et al. 2016). Further research is needed in this area to examine species differences in this response. Also, it should be noted that supplementation with omega-3 fatty acids does increase the need for antioxidant levels (e.g. vitamin E) in the diet for the bird consuming it. Thus, this type of supplementation should be carefully considered before implementing broad-scale diet changes.

As previously mentioned, the "fiber" content of insects is generally related to the proteinaceous and chitinous components of their exoskeletons. The crude fiber content of insects tends to be a bit higher than that of insect-substitute diets (Table 41.4). Fiber is generally thought of as beneficial for animals due to its effects on gastrointestinal bacterial profiles and on development of gastrointestinal musculature. However, in large amounts, it may adversely affect the growth of young animals due to negative impacts on overall nutrient digestibility and energy intake. For all other insectivorous animals, there is no evidence that mixtures of a variety of insect species, including those containing high amounts of fiber, are harmful. In order to replicate fiber and chitinous components in insect-substitute diets, the use of insects or commercially-available alternatives such as shrimp or crab shell meal (with concerns about deposition of heavy metals), purified chitin (very expensive), or cellulose (which chemically is similar to chitin, but without nitrogenous components) would be required. Cellulose may be adequate for birds that cannot digest chitin (i.e. that lack chitinase enzyme), and for which chitin likely serves as a prebiotic and/or fiber source. Unfortunately, there are no data available to determine whether chitinase activity is present in nestling birds. Further research into the needs and/or digestibility of various type of fibers, including chitin by nestling birds, would be very valuable to our understanding of the need for chitin and/or fiber in the diets of hand-reared insectivores.

Additional dietary components that are likely of value to birds are carotenoids, as previously mentioned as a source of pro-vitamin A activity (e.g. β-carotene), in order to enhance immune function (e.g. Koutsos et al. 2006, 2007), and for signaling to parents and prospective mates. For the latter reason, it may be especially important to ensure that birds to be released have appropriate pigmentation, if only to allow for integration back into wild environments with maximum chance of social success. However, different birds use different carotenoid pigments for coloration, and many avian species will transform a dietary carotenoid into the preferred substrate for coloration

(McGraw 2004). Thus, there are still many questions remaining about the optimal level and type of carotenoid that should be provided to chicks. Sources of dietary carotenoids include insects (naturally enriched, or enriched via their feeding and/or gut-loading; Ogilvy et al. 2012; Finke 2015b), produce items, or commercial supplemental forms (e.g. marigold extract, a source of the yellow pigments lutein and zeaxanthin or canthaxanthin, a source of red pigmentation). Again, further research is needed to characterize the optimal level of these pigments in avian diets, but the risk of toxicity from these compounds is low.

As mentioned previously, it has also been suggested that the preference of Blue Tits (*P. caeruleus*) for spiders during their nesting season may be due to their high levels of taurine (Ramsay and Houston 2003). Supplementing the diet of wild Blue Tit nestlings from 2 to 12 days of age with taurine resulted in juveniles that took significantly greater risks when investigating novel objects and were more successful at a spatial learning task than controls (Arnold et al. 2007). Adult insects and commercial cat/kitten foods are rich sources of taurine, while insect larvae and vegetable protein-based commercial products (unless supplemented) would typically contain little taurine.

## Conclusions

It is crucial to note that animals require nutrients and appropriate substrates to deliver those nutrients, as opposed to specific diet ingredients. Thus, it is completely reasonable that insect-substitute diets may serve as a complete diet item in a facility. Alternatively, commercially-available insects with appropriate supplementation may be more appropriate for a particular situation. There are several options for feeding insectivorous nestling birds in rehabilitation settings. Each comes with pros and cons, and institutions should determine what feeding program(s) best meet their needs with regard to chick success, resource allocation (human and monetary), and availability of food items. It is likely that more than one option is optimal within an institution. Care should be taken to document feeding programs, such that educated decisions about modifications can be made for future improvements to protocols. Additionally, when utilizing recipes for insect supplementation or for insect-substitute diets, it is critical to follow recipes precisely or the intended nutritional profile may not be achieved. Ideally, nutrients are provided to chicks in a way that is appropriate to their digestive physiology, nutrient needs for development of robust immunity, skeleto-muscular systems, and neurological functions to provide optimal chances of success post-fledging and release.

## References

Arnold, K.E., Ramsay, S.L., Donaldson, C., and Adam, A. (2007). Parental prey selection affects risk-taking behaviour and spatial learning in avian offspring. *Proceedings of the Biological Society B* 274: 2563–2569.

Aschoff, J. and Pohl, H. (1970). Rhythmic variations in energy metabolism. *Federation Proceedings* 29 (4): 1541–1552.

Barker, D., Fitzpatrick, M.P., and Dierenfeld, E.S. (1998). Nutrient composition of selected whole invertebrates. *Zoo Biology* 17: 123–134.

Bartholomew, G.A. and Cade, T.J. (1963). The water economy of land birds. *The Auk* 80 (4): 504–539.

Bernard J.B. and Allen M.E. (1997). Feeding captive insectivorous animals: nutritional aspects of insects as food. https://nagonline.net/wp-content/uploads/2014/01/NAG-FS003-97-Insects-JONI-FEB-24-2002-MODIFIED.pdf.

Bilby, L. and Widdowson, E. (1971). Chemical composition of growth in nestling blackbirds and thrushes. *British Journal of Nutrition* 25: 127–134.

Bodnaryk, R.P. (1981). The biosynthesis, function and fate of taurine during the metamorphosis of the noctuid moth *Mamestra configurata* Wlk. *Insect Biochemistry* 11: 199–205.

Bukkens, S.G.F. (1997). The nutritional value of edible insects. *Ecology of Food and Nutrition* 36: 287–319.

Bureš, S. and Weidinger, K. (2003). Sources and timing of calcium intake during reproduction in flycatchers. *Oecologia* 137 (4): 634–641. https://doi.org/10.1007/s00442-003-1380-7.

Capinera, J. (2010). Insects and Wildlife: Arthropods and their Relationships with Wild Vertebrate Animals. Hoboken, NJ: Wiley-Blackwell.

Cerda, H., Martinez, R., Briceno, N. et al. (2001). Palm worm: (*Rhynchophorus palmarum*) traditional food in Amazonas, Venezuela – nutritional composition, small scale production and tourist palatability. *Ecology of Food and Nutrition* 40: 13–32.

Dhondt, A.A. and Hochachka, W.M. (2001). Variations in calcium use by birds during the breeding season. *The Condor* 103 (3): 592–598.

Duerr, R. (2007). Passerines: hand-feeding diets. In: Hand-Rearing Birds (eds. L. Gage and R. Duerr), 377–380. Ames, IA: Blackwell Publishing.

Eeva, T., Helle, S., Salmine, J.P., and Hakkarainen, H. (2010). Carotenoid composition of invertebrates consumed by two insectivorous bird species. *Journal of Chemical Ecology* 36: 608–613.

Finke, M.D. (2002). Complete nutrient composition of commercially raised invertebrates used as food for insectivores. *Zoo Biology* 21 (3): 269–285.

Finke, M.D. (2003). Gut loading to enhance the nutrient content of insects as food for reptiles: a mathematical approach. *Zoo Biology* 22: 147–162.

Finke, M.D. (2007). Estimate of chitin in raw whole insects. *Zoo Biology* 26: 105–115.

Finke, M.D. (2013). Complete nutrient content of four species of feeder insects. *Zoo Biology* 32: 27–36.

Finke, M.D. (2015a). Complete nutrient content of three species of wild caught insects, pallid-winged grasshopper, rhinoceros beetles and white-lined sphinx moth. *Journal of Insects as Food and Feed* 1: 281–292.

Finke, M.D. (2015b). Complete nutrient content of four species of commercially available feeder insects fed enhanced diets during growth. *Zoo Biology* 34: 554–564.

Finke, M.D. and Oonincx, D.G.A.B. (2017). Nutrient content of insects. In: Insects as Food and Feed from Production to Consumption (eds. A. Van Huis and J.K. Tomberlin), 290–316. Wageningen: Wageningen Academic Publishers.

Finke, M. and Winn, D. (2004). Insects and related arthropods: a nutritional primer for rehabilitators. *Journal of Wildlife Rehabilitation* 27: 14–27.

Finke, M., Dunham, S., and Cole, J. (2004). Evaluation of various calcium-fortified high moisture commercial products for improving the calcium content of crickets, *Acheta domesticus*. *Journal of Herpetological Medicine and Surgery* 14: 6–9.

Finke, M., Dunham, S., and Kwabi, C. (2005). Evaluation of four dry commercial gut loading products for improving the calcium content of crickets, *Acheta domesticus*. *Journal of Herpetological Medicine and Surgery* 15: 7–12.

Fontaneto, D., Tommaseo-Ponzetta, M., Galli, C. et al. (2011). Differences in fatty acid composition between aquatic and terrestrial insects used as food in human nutrition. *Ecology of Food and Nutrition* 50: 351–367.

Fritsche, K. (2006). Fatty acids as modulators of the immune response. *Annual Review of Nutrition* 26: 45–73.

Fusté, E., Obon, E., and Olid, L. (2013). Hand-reared common swifts (*Apus apus*) in a wildlife rehabilitation centre: assessment of growth rates using different diets. *Journal of Zoo and Aquarium Research* 1 (2): 61–68.

Ghioni, C., Bell, J.G., and Sargent, J.R. (1996). Polyunsaturated fatty acids in neutral lipids and phospholipids of some freshwater insects. *Comparative Biochemistry and Physiology B* 114: 161–170.

Giovannucci, D.R. and Stephenson, R.S. (1999). Identification and distribution of dietary precursors of the Drosophila visual pigment chromophore: analysis of carotenoids in wild type and ninaD mutants by HPLC. *Vision Research* 39: 219–222.

Gist, C.S. and Crossley, D.A. Jr. (1975). The litter arthropod community in a southern Appalachian hardwood forest: numbers, biomass and mineral element content. *American Midland Naturalist* 93: 107–122.

Grabowski, R. (2014). Robyn's baby bird diets. *Wildlife Rehabilitation Bulletin* 32: 5–7.

Graveland, J. (1996). Avian eggshell formation in calcium-rich and calcium-poor habitats: importance of snail shells and anthropogenic calcium sources. *Canadian Journal of Zoology* 74 (6): 1035–1044.

Graveland, J. and van Gijzen, T. (1994). Arthropods and seeds are not sufficient as calcium sources for shell formation and skeletal growth in passerines. *Ardea* 82: 299–314.

Hatt, J.M., Hung, E., and Wanner, M. (2003). The influence of diet on the body composition of the house cricket (*Acheta domesticus*) and consequences for their use in zoo animal nutrition. *Der Zoologische Garten* 73: 238–244.

Hungerford, B., Studier, E., Szuch, E. et al. (1993). Aspects of caloric, nitrogen and mineral nutrition during growth in nestling eastern bluebirds, *Sialia sialis*. *Comparative Biochemistry and Physiology* 106A: 385–389.

Hunt, A., Ward, A., and Ferguson, G. (2001). Effects of a high calcium diet on gut loading in varying ages of crickets (*Acheta domestica*) and mealworms (*Tenebrio molitor*). In: Proceedings of the 4th Conference on Zoo and Wildlife Nutrition (eds. M. Edwards, K. Lisi, M. Schlegel and R. Bray), 94–99. AZA Nutrition Advisory Group.

Isaksson, C. and Andersson, S. (2007). Carotenoid diet and nestling provisioning in urban and rural great tits *Parus major*. *Journal of Avian Biology* 38: 564–572.

Kaspari, M. (1991). Prey preparation as a way that grasshopper sparrows (*Ammodramus savannarum*) increase the nutrient concentration of their prey. *Behavioral Ecology* 2: 234–241.

Klasing, K. (1998). Comparative Avian Nutrition. New York: CAB International.

Klasing, K., Thacker, P., Lopez, M., and Calvert, C. (2000). Increasing the calcium content of mealworms (*Tenebrio molitor*) to improve their nutritional value for bone mineralization of growing chicks. *Journal of Zoo Animal Medicine* 31: 512–517.

Koutsos, E.A., Garcia Lopez, J.C., and Klasing, K. (2006). Carotenoids from in ovo or dietary sources blunt systemic indices of the inflammatory response in growing chicks (*Gallus gallus domesticus*). *Journal of Nutrition* 136: 1027–1031.

Koutsos, E.A., Garcia Lopez, J.C., and Klasing, K. (2007). Maternal and dietary carotenoids interactively affect cutaneous basophil responses in growing chickens (*Gallus gallus domesticus*). *Comparative Biochemistry and Physiology B* 147: 87–92.

Kramer, K.J., Hopkins, T.L., and Schaefer, J. (1995). Applications of solids NMR to the analysis of insect sclerotized structures. *Insect Biochemistry and Molecular Biology* 25: 1067–1080.

Livingston, S., Lavin, S., Sullivan, K. et al. (2014). Challenges with effective nutrient supplementation for amphibians: a review of cricket studies. *Zoo Biology* 33: 565–576.

Massie, H.R., Williams, T.R., and DeWolfe, L.K. (1989). Changes in taurine in aging fruit flies and mice. *Experimental Gerontology* 24: 57–65.

McGraw, K.J. (2004). Colorful songbirds metabolize carotenoids at the integument. *Journal of Avian Biology* 35: 471–476.

Michaels, C.J., Antwis, R.E., and Preziosi, R.F. (2014). Manipulation of the calcium content of insectivore diets through supplementary dusting. *Journal of Zoo and Aquarium Research* 2 (3): 77–81.

Moore, J. (1986). Dietary variation among nestling starlings. *The Condor* 88 (2): 181–189.

Ogilvy, V., Fidgett, A., and Preziosi, R. (2012). Differences in carotenoid accumulation among three feeder-cricket species: implications for carotenoid delivery to captive insectivores. *Zoo Biology* 31: 470–478.

Olson, J.A. (1989). Provitamin A function of carotenoids: the conversion of beta-carotene into vitamin A. *Journal of Nutrition* 119: 105–108.

Oonincx, D.G.A.B. and Dierenfeld, E.S. (2012). An investigation into the chemical composition of alternative invertebrate prey. *Zoo Biology* 31: 40–54.

Oonincx, D.G.A.B., Stevens, Y., van den Borne, J.J. et al. (2010). Effects of vitamin D3 supplementation and UVb exposure on the growth and plasma concentration of vitamin D3 metabolites in juvenile bearded dragons (*Pogona vitticeps*). *Comparative Biochemistry and Physiology B* 156: 122–128.

Pennino, M., Dierenfeld, E.S., and Behler, J.L. (1991). Retinol, alpha-tocopherol, and proximate nutrient composition of invertebrates used as feed. *International Zoo Yearbook* 30: 143–149.

Perlman, J. (2016). Supplements for nestling and fledgling passerines hand-reared on an 100% insect diet. In: Passerine Fundamentals: Native Songbird Care & Conservation (ed. V. Bowers), 45–46. Sebastapol, CA: IWRC.

Ramsay, S.L. and Houston, D.D. (2003). Amino acid composition of some woodland arthropods and its implications for breeding tits and other passerines. *Ibis* 145: 227–232.

Reichle, D.E., Shanks, M.H., and Crossley, D.A. (1969). Calcium, potassium, and sodium content of forest floor arthropods. *Annals of the Entomological Society of America* 62: 57–62.

Reynolds, S. and Perrins, C. (2010). Dietary calcium availability and reproduction in birds. *Current Ornithology* 17: 31–74.

Reynolds, S., Mänd, R., and Tilgar, V. (2004). Calcium supplementation of breeding birds: directions for future research. *Ibis* 146: 601–614.

Roudybush, T.E. and Grau, C.R. (1986). Food and water interrelations and the protein requirement for growth of an altricial bird, the cockatiel (*Nymphicus hollandicus*). *Journal of Nutrition* 116: 552–559.

Seage, E., Miller, E., and Koutos, L. (2010). Feeding trial evaluating Mazuri® Nestling Meal compared to FoNS® as a diet for nestling and fledgling passerines in a rehabilitation setting. Abstract, National Wildlife Rehabilitators Association, Annual Symposium, Bellevue, WA.

Soares, J.H. (1995). Calcium bioavailability. In: Bioavailability of Nutrients for Animals (eds. C. Ammerman, D. Baker and A. Lewis), 95–118. New York: Academic Press.

Spranghers, T., Ottoboni, M., Klootwijk, C. et al. (2017). Nutritional composition of black soldier fly (*Hermetia illucens*) prepupae reared on different organic waste substrates. *Journal of the Science of Food and Agriculture* 97: 2594–2600.

St. Louis, V.L. and Breebaart, L. (1991). Calcium supplements in the diet of nestling tree swallows near acid sensitive lakes. *The Condor* 93 (2): 286–294.

Starčević, K., Gavrilović, A., Gottstein, Z., and Mašek, T. (2017). Influence of substitution of sunflower oil by different oils on the growth, survival rate and fatty acid composition of Jamaican field cricket (*Gryllus assimilis*). *Animal Feed Science and Technology* 228: 66–71.

Stork, N.E. (2018). How many species of insects and other terrestrial arthropods are there on earth? *Annual Review of Entomology* 63: 31–45.

Strzelewicz, M., Ullrey, D., Schafer, S., and Bacon, J. (1985). Feeding insectivores: increasing the calcium content of wax moth (*Galleria mellonella*) larvae. *Journal of Zoo Animal Medicine* 16: 25–27.

Studier, E.H. and Sevick, S.H. (1992). Live mass, water content, nitrogen and mineral levels in some insects from south-central lower Michigan. *Comparative Biochemistry and Physiology A* 103: 579–595.

Thompson, S.N. (1973). A review and comparative characterization of the fatty acid compositions of seven insect orders. *Comparative Biochemistry and Physiology Part B* 45 (2): 467–482.

Twining, C.W., Brenna, J.T., Lawrence, P. et al. (2016). Omega-3 long-chain polyunsaturated fatty acids support aerial insectivore performance more than food quantity. *Proceedings of the National Academy of Sciences* 113 (39): 10920–10925.

Twining, C.W., Lawrence, P., Winkler, D.W. et al. (2018). Conversion efficiency of α-linolenic acid to omega-3 highly unsaturated fatty acids in aerial insectivore chicks. *Journal of Experimental Biology* 221 (3): jeb165373.

Von Lintig, J. (2012). Metabolism of carotenoids and retinoids related to vision. *Journal of Biological Chemistry* 287: 1627–1634.

Wheeler, W.C., Whiting, M., Wheeler, Q.D., and Carpenter, J.M. (2001). The phylogeny of the extant hexapod orders. *Cladistics* 17: 113–169.

Winn, D. (2002). Formula for nestling songbirds: down payment on fitness and survival. *Journal of Wildlife Rehabilitation* 25 (3): 13–18.

Winn, D. and Finke, M. (2004). Formula for nestling songbirds (FoNS): updates for 2006. *Journal of Wildlife Rehabilitation* 27 (3–4): 28.

Winn, D. and Finke, M. (2017). Formula for nestling songbirds (FoNS): update and options for 2018. *Wildlife Rehabilitation Bulletin* 35 (2): 37–39.

Winn, D., Dunham, S., and Mikulski, S. (2003). Food for insects and insects as food: viable strategies for achieving adequate calcium. *Journal of Wildlife Rehabilitation* 26: 4–13.

# 42

# Corvids

*Elaine Friedman*

## Introduction

Corvids are highly intelligent birds with well-developed social skills. They show anger, fear, jealousy, and the ability to deceive, which allows them to mask a physical problem. They are excellent observers and quick to notice any difference from the norm. They exhibit food preferences and have a wide range of personality traits. In order to successfully raise or rehabilitate corvid species, one must be a good observer and make judgment calls based on the history, body language, behavior, and physical condition of each individual bird. The caregiver must be able to adapt a set of instructions to each bird's particular needs. For example, too much food gavaged or force-fed to a weakened bird will be regurgitated and possibly aspirated.

These birds operate not only on instinct but also by the learned experiences they have had in their life. If they have never experienced red berries or a white mouse in their diet, putting this in their food bowl might cause them not to eat at all. And if as a juvenile they never see natural foods in their diet, they might starve, once released, before locating food. These are birds that express thoughts and intentions in their vocalizations, feather position, and body language, Plan to research corvid natural history in more detail than presented here. This chapter provides guidelines and insight to help you make educated decisions on how to proceed in raising an injured or orphaned corvid.

## Natural History

The family Corvidae are members of the order Passeriformes, and include the largest of the songbirds, which are perching birds with three toes in front and one long toe behind. These birds are ruled less by instinct and more by their superior mental capabilities than other bird species. There are 20 species of corvids grouped in 8 genera, including ravens, crows, magpies, jays, and Clark's Nutcracker, within the borders of the United States, with approximately 134 species worldwide (Gill and Donsker 2019). Protected by the United States federal government, corvids are included in the laws pertaining to migratory birds even though many members of the various corvid species do not migrate but may simply relocate to follow ample food supplies. It is illegal to keep a corvid as a pet.

*Hand-Rearing Birds*, Second Edition. Edited by Rebecca S. Duerr and Laurie J. Gage.

These are social birds, often found in small to very large groups numbering thousands of birds. Some species, including the American Crow and Florida Scrub Jay are cooperative breeders. The birds as a group are omnivorous, with some species being heavily dependent on certain food items including insects, nuts, cone seeds, and carrion. The focus of their diet fluctuates with the changing seasons and the natural foods available. Uneaten food is cached, a skill that should develop as a juvenile matures.

The nest for this family is a bulky cup of sticks in a tree or other convenient tall structure. At times some species will nest in a bush. Magpies add a roof when structurally possible and some ravens nest on ledges and manmade structures.

Each species in the Corvidae family has specific behaviors relating to conspecifics and these behaviors may complicate release possibilities, especially if birds are not raised with siblings, similarly aged juveniles, or adults of the same species. Adult ravens, for example, may be intolerant of older juveniles, forcing the juveniles to form a group to defend food finds from the resident adults. Raven nestlings vocalize loudly back and forth to one another after feeding, which is not typical of the other species. Ravens have a different natural history compared to crows and the two species should not be combined during the rehabilitation process. American Crows are cooperative breeders and may live their entire lives within an extended family group. When unrelated crows need to be combined, there will be a small amount of determination of the birds' positions in the pecking order, but generally a new addition will be accepted. Combining ravens requires care because older juveniles could prove to be highly aggressive to a newcomer. Ravens move their young on within a few months after hatching and live their lives paired, as single birds foraging or roosting in groups of unmated individuals, or in a group consisting of a mated pair plus a third bird. Once past the fledgling stage, ravens can be aggressive to a new group member and there is a risk of injury to a newly introduced bird. The situation must be carefully monitored in a rehabilitation setting; but beware, these highly intelligent birds may temper their aggressive behavior until they determine that you are not present. Magpies are also extremely aggressive to an inferior or poorly socialized member of the species.

American Crows (*Corvus brachyrhynchos*) are common across most of America and can also be found in Canada. Their diet is highly varied, including small animals, their young, and eggs; insects; plant material such as seeds, grains, nuts, fruits, berries; plus carrion and garbage. The Fish Crow (*Corvus ossifragus*) is found in flocks by marshes and lowland rivers of the eastern United States, but in recent years has moved much farther inland following large river systems. They feed primarily on animals, especially amphibians, crab, shrimp, small live fish, dead fish, plus the eggs and chicks of other species in their habitat. They may flock with American Crows, The Northwestern Crow (*Corvus caurinus*) is distinguished from other crow species by its limited range in the coastal Pacific Northwest, intermixing with the American Crow in the most southern parts of the range. This bird is omnivorous with a focus on marine environment items such as crabs, shellfish, carrion, stranded fish, and the eggs of seabirds.

The Common Raven (*Corvus corax*), a species proven to be capable of stepwise thought, is an omnivore with a focus on carrion. They will also prey on nestling birds, eggs, and vulnerable species including mammals, amphibians, and reptiles. The Chihuahuan Raven (*Corvus cryptoleucos*) is omnivorous with an emphasis on carrion.

The United States is home to two close-related species of magpie, the Black-billed Magpie (*Pica hudsonia*) found in the northwestern part of North America and the Yellow-billed Magpie (*Pica nuttalli*) found in central and southern California and nowhere else in the world. The Yellow-billed Magpie favors more acorns in the diet than the Black-billed Magpie and tends to require the milder climate found in sheltered valleys of California. They are highly social, so release of this species requires definite knowledge of magpie appropriate territories.

Jay species vary significantly from one another. A caregiver must correctly identify the jay species in order to supply the proper diet, accurate care prior to release, and proper release site. The natural history of the Gray Jay (*Perisoreus Canadensis*) is an excellent example of the special needs of some species. Gray Jays do best in areas of coniferous trees, especially black spruce. In the United States, these birds breed mostly in northern and mountain coniferous forests.

Blue Jays (*Cyanocitta cristata*) are found in the central and eastern areas of the United States. They are omnivores with a fondness for acorns. These crested members of the jay family are capable of hybridizing with the Steller's Jay. Steller's Jays (*Cyanocitta stelleri*) also have a crest and are found in the western part of the United States with preferred habitat being evergreen forests. This omnivorous species is also well known for stealing food from picnic tables, sorting through garbage, and frequenting feeders. The Green Jay (*Cyanocorax yncas*) can be found in southern Texas. They can be found in mainly sedentary small flocks heavily dependent on an insect diet. Brown Jays (*Cyanocorax morio*) are also found in southern Texas, frequently visit feeding stations, and travel in flocks of 5 to 10 birds. The California Scrub Jay (*Aphelocoma californica*) can be found in California, Oregon, and southwest Washington. The Woodhouse's Scrub Jay (*Aphelocoma woodhouseii*) is found in Nevada east to Texas. Florida Scrub Jays (*Aphelocoma coerulescens*) may live their entire lives within ½ mile of their hatch site and are found only in Florida. The Island Scrub Jay (*Aphelocoma insularis*) is found only on Santa Cruz Island in the Channel Islands south of Santa Barbara, California. The Pinyon Jay (*Gymnorhinus cyanocephalus*) is dependent on the seeds of the Pinyon Pine. The Mexican Jays (*Aphelocoma ultramarina*) are common residents of pine and oak canyons of southwestern mountains.

Clark's Nutcrackers (*Nucifraga columbiana*) are found in the west. The birds' pointed bill is adapted to opening cones and extracting seeds. Most of their eggs are laid by March or early April, enabled by their ability to store thousands of pine cone seeds.

Individuals must become familiar with the natural history of each species of corvid they hand-rear to prevent unintentional injury, taming, or imprinting of the bird being raised. Release criteria must be based on the needs of each species, especially the natural habitat and the expected interaction with wild conspecifics.

The natural diet of corvids consists of insects and other invertebrates, grains, seeds, especially those gathered from cones, fruits including berries, vegetables, nuts including acorns, small mammals, carrion, eggs and young birds, frogs, lizards, salamanders, worms, garbage, and just about any other natural food source found in the wild.

When raising corvids in captivity, particular problems appear that are related to the natural history of these birds. Crows and ravens are unusually large songbirds. Their size may cause caregivers to not recognize they are still a juvenile and might not be self-feeding or might still be a nestling requiring a nest rather than a perch. Due to the social nature of the various corvid species, fledglings usually leave the nest well before becoming self-feeding, with the adults giving weeks or months of supportive care and training. The caregiver for a juvenile corvid must supply more training than would be expected with other songbirds. Corvids are sensitive to changes in spatial relationships, an important component to a caching bird with a highly developed hippocampus portion of the brain. When in captivity, changes in housing may greatly affect corvids, which at times may cause them to stop eating. Corvid family nestlings appear more susceptible to overheating and dehydration than many other bird species, at times quickly becoming dehydrated after initial hydration even when housed in an incubator. Dehydration may cause the birds to become unresponsive to the stimuli that usually cause them to gape. If they are forcefully given food at this point, they lack the ability to successfully swallow or digest it. The bird may rapidly

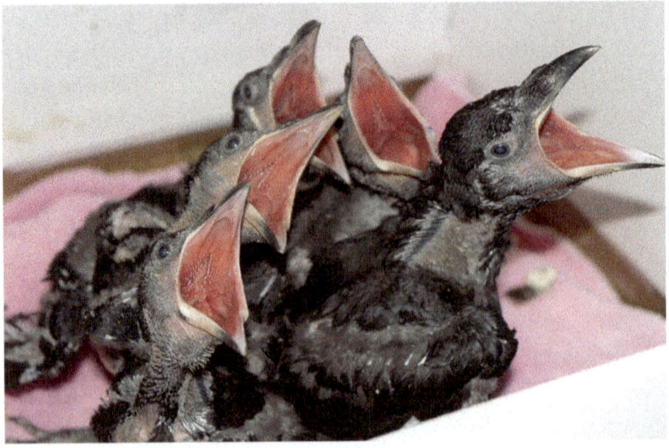

Figure 42.1 Healthy raven nestlings have a vivid pink mouth.

become critically ill unless the caregiver recognizes the cause of the problem and rehydrates the bird. A healthy juvenile usually exhibits a vivid pink mouth lining (Figure 42.1).

## Criteria for Intervention

Corvids may be brought into captivity for a variety of reasons. Hatchlings, nest and all, may be blown out of a tree during wind storms. Badly timed tree trimming or tree removal also accounts for many disruptions to nests. If nestlings are relocated to a neighboring tree, or even put back into the same tree but not in an identical nest, the adults may not continue to support the birds. Older nestlings move about in the nest, stretching and flapping, possibly causing younger siblings or even themselves to fall out of the nest. Predators may injure a nestling or cause it to fall out of the nest.

During periods of low humidity and high temperatures, fledglings may become dehydrated and disoriented. If the area where the fledgling has landed appears unsafe for adult birds to support or assist the juvenile, the adults may vocalize to the younger bird but not give it supportive care. Because most fledglings must spend some time on the ground before they master flight, even a healthy fledgling may become frail from lack of food and hydration if parents are unwilling to risk their own safety to support the bird. Fledglings must not only learn to fly but also to eat on their own by following the example set by older birds and by trial-and-error pecking and exploring; hence they are vulnerable to injury by predators, including domestic pets.

Fledglings may be docile, especially if they are stunned or injured from a collision with a window or other object, and many times they are picked up by humans. A physical examination must be performed before reuniting a juvenile with its family, because a large percentage of corvids found by humans have injuries to the skeletal or nervous system or are fatigued by a lack of food and hydration. See Chapter 1 for information on performing a physical exam. If a corvid is simply observed on the ground and adult birds are present, this may not be enough to ensure its safety. Observe from a distance far enough away that adults are willing to approach the juvenile. If adults are repeatedly feeding the juvenile, no predators are present, and the juvenile appears alert and agile, it can be left undisturbed. But if adults are not actively feeding the juvenile or prodding it to a safe area or branch, the bird should be captured and evaluated. Returning the juvenile to the nest bears careful consideration. If other juvenile corvids are present in the nest and not quite ready to fledge, they might prematurely jump out of the nest when the sibling is returned. If the juveniles are not fully feathered and therefore more docile, returning a sibling to the nest is generally more successful for all of the birds. Some corvid nests, including those of ravens, are located on cliffs or in tall trees and would require an experienced climber or special equipment to reach the nest. If an attempt is made to re-nest a corvid nestling in a substitute nest, the situation must be observed until the adults are seen directly feeding the young.

## Record Keeping

Corvids living in the United States are covered under the Migratory Bird Treaty Act and any time spent in captivity is, by law, regulated by the United States Fish and Wildlife Service and by individual state agencies. Injured or orphaned corvids should be cared for only by individuals or organizations permitted by both the state and the federal governments. Outside of the United States, the laws regarding wild birds vary. Beware that an inexperienced caregiver raising a single bird is almost guaranteed to produce an imprinted or tame bird, and caregivers need guidelines to successfully rehabilitate corvid species. Some rehabilitation centers do not accept corvids. Search state and federal organization websites to locate a rehabilitator willing to care for the species.

Basic information including species, age, location found, finder's contact information, reason for bringing the bird into captivity, behavior of the bird when found, medical problems found on initial exam, final disposition, and release location must be included in a record for each bird. A detailed medical record should include initial exam and updates, such as body weights, response to treatments, medications, daily types and amounts of food consumed, behavioral notes, and results of laboratory tests.

Recording the location the bird was found is critically important. Corvids are social birds, with family members congregated in a specific area. Returning a bird to a support network upon release will enhance its chance of survival. Detailed records about the habitat in the location the bird was found will allow a caregiver to pinpoint areas with habitat beneficial to a particular species of corvid. This will aid in the successful release of birds unable to be returned to their home territory. Because much of a corvid's behavior depends on its familiarity with its environment and learned skills, it is critical to release a "city bird" in the city and a "country bird" in a more rural area.

Multiple caregivers may result in inconsistent and inappropriate care; therefore, feeding and housing instructions including amounts to feed and feeding methods for each stage of the bird's growth or recovery should be available.

Finally, corvids require the company of conspecifics to decrease stress and to develop social ties. They may carry illnesses or parasites that are infectious to other birds. Records should detail interactions or contact between birds in captivity to enable caregivers to keep social groups together through release and to track and locate transmission of contamination or illness. Corvids should be raised in stable groups to prevent the spread of disease to the entire rehabilitation collection of corvids.

## Initial Care and Stabilization

A newly admitted corvid should be allowed to stabilize in a warm, quiet, and dark enclosure for at least 15 minutes before having an initial exam unless immediate care is indicated. The initial exam should consist of a systematic search for lesions, fractures, or other abnormalities. If indicated, further diagnostics may be conducted once the bird has stabilized. Corvids, as a result of their diet, are susceptible to trichomoniasis. An oral swab viewed under a microscope, even if lesions are not present, can prevent future problems and potential contamination of other birds. A fecal analysis prior to introducing the bird to others is also recommended since many corvids carry parasites such as capillaria, coccidia, and tapeworm. Examine the body for pox lesions and ectoparasites. Weigh the bird on a gram scale. This will aid in determining the quantity of fluids to offer initially. Hydration is of paramount importance. Without proper hydration, the bird cannot be fed or treated successfully. The safest method for rehydration is the administration of subcutaneous fluids. Give 2–3% of the body weight in fluids if the bird appears dehydrated. If hydration must be done orally, give initial fluids with a 1 ml syringe. For magpies and jays a narrow-tipped 1 ml syringe or a teat cannula (syringe extender) is useful (Figure 1.4). The bird must be warm before it can swallow and process fluids. A small portion, less than 0.1 ml, of warm oral solution (lactated Ringer's solution or equivalent), should be placed past the glottis down the bird's right side of the throat to ensure that it is capable of swallowing the liquid. Tissues become compressed and sticky when a bird is dehydrated, rendering it incapable of swallowing the liquid. In this case, administer subcutaneous fluids for the initial rehydration. Once the bird can gape and swallow, administer orally whatever portion of the calculated rehydration amount remains, divided over the next 2–3 hours.

For example: for a 200 g corvid fledgling, 2% of its body weight in fluids is $200\,g \times 0.02 = 4\,ml$. This amount would then be divided and given to the bird orally over the next 2–3 hours. The size of the portion depends on the responsiveness of the bird. Weaker 200 g birds may be able to handle only 0.5–1 ml at a time.

Administer only what the bird can manage at a given time, regardless of the amounts quoted in the literature. It may have health problems preventing normal processing of fluids and could die if handled too aggressively. Once it begins to defecate, the focus may switch to the feeding regimen.

Housing during stabilization should be stress-free. Place hatchlings in an incubator if available, or use a heating pad set on the lowest heat setting, placed under the container the bird is housed in. When using a heating pad, insulation from the pad may be required to prevent overheating. Nestlings and hatchlings require a nest. Larger corvids such as crows and ravens might require a rolled towel placed in a donut shape as a nest to support their weight. Smaller birds may be placed in a plastic margarine-type container lined with multiple layers of toilet paper. Use a plastic container suitable in size for the species of hatchlings. Pile the paper high enough to allow nestlings to defecate over the side of the nest; a hatchling should rest in an indentation in the toilet paper. The toilet paper should be crumpled enough to provide support for the birds to prevent splayed legs. If the heat supplied to a hypothermic bird in a nest is from a heating pad under the container, increase the layers of toilet paper as the bird warms to prevent overheating. A pre-warmed nest would be optimal. A sheet or two of toilet paper placed over the bird also helps maintain warmth in the nest, especially for single hatchlings. Stabilization of older birds may be done in a heated cardboard cat carrier or similar device that provides quiet isolation. Newspaper lining is nonabsorbent and not recommended due to profuse defecation. A pillow case or tightly looped towel with rolled towel nest or perch is best.

Corvids tend to harbor pathogens that may be infectious to other birds. Do not combine a newly admitted bird with those already being hand-reared. Corvids are especially susceptible to West Nile virus (WNV). Newly admitted corvids should be isolated if WNV is prevalent in the area; however, the social needs of a new bird must be balanced with the stress of being isolated. If the single chick or fledgling appears healthy upon admission, it may be isolated for just for 2–3 days, even with the presence of WNV in the area. Then place the chick with only one or two others the first week and monitor closely. A sign of a healthy chick is one that preens after the completion of hand-feeding (Figure 42.2).

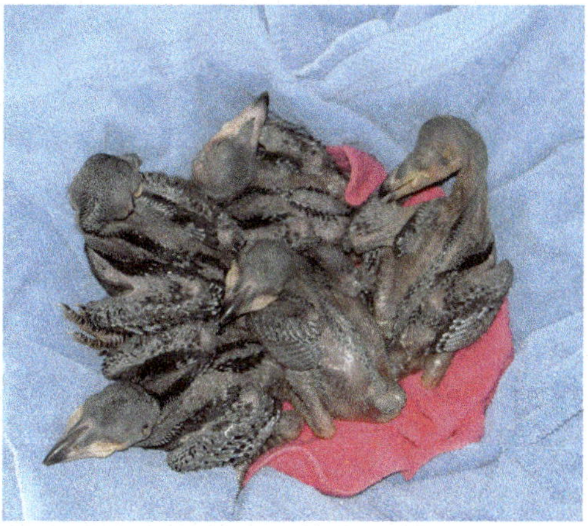

Figure 42.2 Pinfeather ravens preen after hand-feeding.

## Common Medical Problems and Special Care Problems

Juveniles have a weaker immune system than adults. When introduced to an aviary, corvids at times develop bacterial infections or might have a rise in previously undetected parasites. If a bird appears quiet, is perched inappropriately (i.e. in the sun when other birds are in the shade), is being picked on by the other birds, is perching much of the time with nictitating membranes or eyes shut, has a weak cry, is fluffed, or does not appear to be eating, remove the bird from the aviary and examine and weigh it. Bacterial infections may come from many sources in the aviary, especially during hot weather. Consult a veterinarian regarding administering antibiotics. Observe for sprains, strains, or breaks that may develop as birds learn to fly. Periodic fecal analysis of samples in the aviary should prevent recurring problems with parasites.

Corvids often accept Clavamox but may refuse Baytril. They may form a pellet after being medicated and expel the medication. Medication may be injected into waxworms or pinky mice or into a food that the bird will take and swallow without tearing the food item apart.

### Behavioral Issues

#### Activity at Dusk

Corvids naturally move to a roosting area at dusk, and this urge ignites in older juveniles with a frenzy. If juveniles are still housed indoors, place them in a room that may be darkened completely before dusk or cover the enclosure with a light-blocking cloth. Failure to do so may cause feather damage from the birds flying into the sides of the enclosure.

#### Aggression by Conspecifics

Be cautious when adding a new bird to an established group of juveniles. Even removing a bird for an extended medical procedure and returning it to the group might lead to aggression from the group to the newcomer. If the newcomer is compromised or ignorant of social skills it might not be able to avoid aggression from members of the group. Injury or death may result. When introducing a new bird, observe the interactions from a distance. It might be necessary to remove all of the resident birds from the housing, allowing the newcomer to acclimate. Then, one by one add the conspecifics. The new bird could also be housed with just one other resident bird. If it has a health problem, it may need to fully recover before introduction to other birds. An imprinted bird might never achieve acceptance. The most aggressive of the corvids appear to be ravens and magpies when it comes to introduction of any new bird, especially those ignorant of accepted social rules.

#### Fear

Corvids survive by being fearful of new things. This can cause major problems in the rehabilitation process. Keep housing as consistent as possible including food bowls. Don't use highly patterned or colored towels or wear overly bright or patterned clothing. Birds may be fearful of pictures on a shirt including images of other birds. California Scrub Jays may move away from bright blue shirts, while the color black seems to evoke instinctual reactions such as panic or sexual curiosity in crows and ravens. Most significant is the fear of going to the ground or bottom of a new enclosure. Provide food and water at perch level to prevent weight loss or starvation until the bird is observed eating at floor level.

#### Stress and Boredom

Wild birds in captivity will show signs of stress, such as panic flight, open-mouthed breathing, repetitive movements, and feather picking. Corvids need natural types of stimulation in captivity to reduce negative behaviors. Introduce natural items such as rocks, pine cones, acorns, twigs, small branches with leaves, dried sunflowers, bark, and containers of soil to dig and cache in. Aviaries should have a substrate on the floor for foraging, digging, and caching. Add small trees or bushes in pots, impale fruit on branches, or hang suet baskets (Arcata Pet Supplies) with fruit, suet, mice, or other food inside. Indoor birds should be allowed to see outside and hear natural bird sounds. Avoid capturing the birds for occasional medication or examinations at the same time that they are being cleaned or fed. Otherwise, the birds will fear being caught every time the cleaning routine begins.

#### Imprinting

Imprinting occurs when a hatchling is exposed to humans and not their own species. A bird that recognizes its own identity can be either tame or habituated. An imprinted corvid will not seek a relationship with its own kind and is not a good candidate for release. A tame or habituated bird needs to be placed with members of its own species for an elongated period of time to allow it to make the choice between humans and a social relationship with another corvid. Becoming a member of the corvid group the bird has been paired with might allow the bird to be returned to the wild as long as the bird does not continue to seek the companionship of humans (Figure 42.3).

### Feather Problems

#### Bald Head

This is normal in corvids if it occurs during the spring–summer-early fall molt period (Figure 42.6). Even the juveniles go through a body molt after flight feathers have established themselves. Magpies especially lose head feathers all at once. If a bird has experienced a traumatic health episode or has been in captivity for a period of time, it may be more prone to a balding-head molt.

#### Feather Damage

Wing flight feathers should never be pulled from magpies, crows, or ravens for any reason. Only a veterinarian should remove these feathers from jays and must take steps to keep the feather follicle open until a new feather emerges. Pulling flight feathers usually results in impacted feather follicles which prevents the formation of healthy, normal feathers. If wing and tail feathers are broken on a juvenile, the feathers will not be replaced until a molt the following spring and summer. Tail

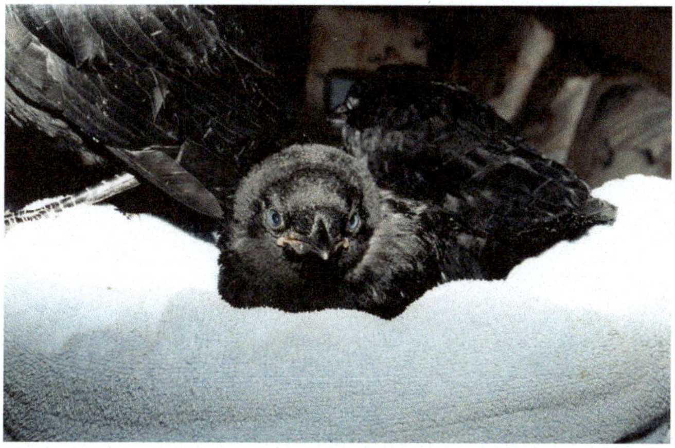

Figure 42.3 A young crow sporting blue eyes that will soon turn brown demonstrates his distaste for human presence with raised feathers.

feathers may be successfully pulled under a veterinarian's care to stimulate early replacement of the feathers. A better way to replenish damaged wing feathers is to house the bird in an aviary lined with a fine screen material (Pet Screen, Phifer Co.), fiberglass screening, shade cloth, or aviary netting. Provide step-like perching and do not have branches so close to perches that they brush against and break growing blood feathers. Supply a flutter climbing pole, which is a sturdy pole, such as a closet pole or straight tree branch, covered with AstroTurf and long enough to rest against a horizontal perch at about a 45° angle to the ground. This allows a bird having difficulty with flight to sidestep up to a perch. It may naturally flap its wings as it climbs up the pole. Permitting a feather-damaged bird to get off the ground prevents further feather damage caused by failed attempts to jump from the ground to a perch. If a juvenile repeatedly develops impacted feather follicles, suspect and check for staph infection of the follicles.

## Respiratory Distress

Corvids will demonstrate open-mouthed breathing when stressed or overheated; however, if this type of breathing is present when the bird is calm and at the proper temperature, it could be signs of a respiratory infection (bacterial or fungal) or signs of aspiration of food or liquids. Do not ignore the symptoms as this is a definite sign of a seriously ill bird. A high pitched "hick" sound indicates respiratory distress if uttered repetitively.

## Dehydration

Corvids become dehydrated easily in captive care. They become sluggish and may cease gaping even within hours after rehydration. Rehydrate the bird, ensure the food contains ample moisture, and ensure the housing is not too warm. In intensely warm climates cooling packs may be placed around the nest of older nestlings to prevent overheating.

## Emaciation

Emaciated birds have a sharp keel. Evaluate total protein and packed cell volume to develop a course of action including the probability of survival, and whether a liquid diet or baby songbird food recipe diet (BSFR) should be provided. A corvid will regurgitate and possibly aspirate any food

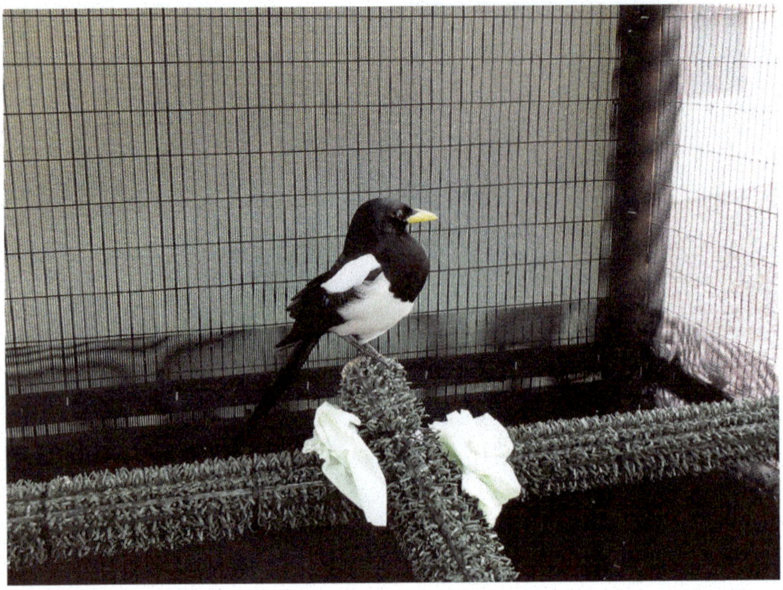

Figure 42.4 A Yellow-billed Magpie afflicted with juvenile cataracts perches on bumblefoot preventive Daisy Doormat.

that its body cannot tolerate. Begin the feeding process more slowly than the feeding chart might suggest. As the bird gains strength, feeding amounts may be increased.

## Eye Problems

Examine the eyes for discharge, swelling, or discoloration. Common causes of eye lesions may be injury, pox, bacterial infection, trichomoniasis, or mycoplasma. If the bird does not respond to visual stimuli correctly or exhibits a tracking-type of behavior with the head, suspect visual problems or impairment. Juvenile corvids may have cataracts or corneal ulcers which may be easily visible or may require staining the eye and use of a scope (Figure 42.4). Juvenile birds that continue to gape while others of similar age are self-feeding, or that gape but not necessarily in the direction of the food source, may have vision problems.

## Foot Abnormalities

### Abnormal Perching

Observe how the juvenile perches or sits in the nest. If the bird repeatedly places the hallux forward together with the other toes, a wrap or cardboard or plastic "shoe" may be required to reposition the hallux. If left unattended, the hallux will continually fold under and prevent grasping of a perch. Allow for growth while a wrap or shoe is being used. A wrap applied too tightly may result in permanent damage to the foot. A wrap or shoe might only be required for a few days on young birds.

### Bumblefoot

Bumblefoot is an unusual finding in a corvid fledgling, so problems that resemble bumblefoot may have another etiology. Overweight birds are prone to bumblefoot especially if a secondary problem restricts movement. Damage to a joint in the foot may result in leakage of joint fluid that causes swelling of the area around the joint. Pox lesions may also form on the foot and should not be misdiagnosed as bumblefoot.

## Head Injury

Many juvenile corvids fall from the nest or have unsuccessful initial flights, which may result in a head injury. A weak cry, labored breathing, eye problems, balance problems, or an abnormally quiet bird may be indications of a head injury. Keep the bird warm and quiet and seek veterinary assistance. Provide a rolled towel nest if support is needed to keep the bird upright and use caution in giving hydration and food because the ability to swallow might be compromised. Familiarize yourself with the avian tongue structure. A wound to the top of the head might reveal the movement of the "appendages" to the tongue.

## Metabolic Bone Disease

Juvenile corvids often exhibit signs of metabolic bone disease, which include lameness and reluctance to move due to painful degenerative changes in the bones. This problem is often seen if the bird was the runt of the clutch, kept as a pet, or raised by inexperienced parents or a member of the public. The BSFR diet will help in supplying necessary calcium to the bird, but extra supplementation of calcium may be necessary. Supply a balanced diet. Offer corvids portions of hard-boiled egg with the shell. Seek veterinary assistance concerning calcium supplements for birds showing signs of metabolic bone disease.

## Infectious Diseases

### Avian Pox

Avian pox is common in young corvids. To mitigate the potential spread of the virus, house corvids in stable groups that will go through the raise and release process together. Spray newly admitted birds for ectoparasites and periodically check for possible infestation. Ensure feeding utensils are not shared between groups. Examine the legs, feet, face, abdomen, vent, mouth, or other exposed areas for raised areas or sores. Pox is contagious to similar species by direct contact or an insect vector. Isolate all exposed birds for a minimum of 2 weeks. Birds exhibiting signs of the disease should be kept in a screened, insect-free area until lesions are healed and scabs, which may contain the virus, are shed. Disinfect all surfaces after use and discard contaminated cardboard crates or carriers. Pox virus may be transmitted on clothing. Treatment involves supportive care to prevent secondary infections and promote healing. If lesions become grossly large or do not heal, the veterinarian should rule out bacterial or fungal infection or mite infestation. Wash your hands or change gloves before handling a new bird or nest of birds. Unwashed hands are frequently responsible for the spread of pox virus!

### Beak Deformities

There are many reasons for beak deformities, among them diet and injury. There is also new research indicating a newly discovered Poecivirus may be responsible for a number of beak abnormalities initially recognized in birds, including crows from Alaska (Zylberberg et al. 2016). Juvenile corvids with metabolic bone disease may exhibit "bendable" beaks. Time and proper diet usually mitigates the problem.

#### West Nile Virus

Corvids are sensitive to WNV, and the mortality of infected birds is high. The best treatment is prevention. If WNV is in your area, isolate newly admitted corvids for a few days in case they are carrying the virus but are not yet symptomatic. Placing new birds together in small groups exposes fewer birds if one bird develops WNV. Keep mosquitoes and other biting insects out of enclosures. Spray newly admitted birds for ectoparasites. Direct contact between birds may spread the illness. Check with your veterinarian for current treatment protocol if you suspect WNV.

### Antibiotic Sensitivities

Trimethoprim sulfamethoxazole may cause corvids to regurgitate after dosing. Birds sensitive to this drug may suffer from dehydration combined with a lack of medication. Use only if necessary and monitor for problems.

### Parasitic Diseases

#### Ectoparasites

Mites will appear as grayish patches on featherless areas, such as the legs and feet. A skin scraping and microscopic examination will help determine if burrowing mites are present which if left untreated, may cause gross distortions that may appear as grayish protrusions with holes in the center. Treatment with ivermectin and the application of an avian lice and mite spray will usually eradicate the parasites. Length of treatment depends on severity of the infestation. Any visible infestation of external parasites should immediately be treated with an avian lice and mite spray.

#### Endoparasites

Common parasites in corvids are capillaria, coccidia, and tapeworm. Examine feces soon after the bird is acquired, and treat promptly to prevent infection of other birds. Praziquantel (Droncit) is effective for tapeworm, fenbendazole (Panacur) or ivermectin for capillaria, and sulfadimethoxine (Albon) for coccidia. Baycox and Ponazuril have been used to treat coccidia with varying success. Check with your veterinarian. Do not administer Albon and Panacur simultaneously. Some corvids lose their appetite, become depressed, or develop a weakened immune system after being dosed with this combination, or with Panacur alone, so monitor food intake and behavior after dosing.

#### Trichomoniasis

Trichomoniasis infections are caused by flagellated protozoan parasites and may be present but visually undetectable. A wet mount of a mouth and throat swab should be examined under the microscope for the telltale "Pac Man"-like swimming organisms. Carnidazole administered orally is routinely used to treat this condition. Check with your veterinarian for the correct dosage.

## Diet Recipes

Table 42.1 lists the ingredients for the BSFR. Mash kibble with a fork after water has been absorbed. Puree egg and banana in a blender. Mix all the ingredients using a food processor. Freeze in small containers. Thaw only enough diet for 1 day. Warm the mixture by placing the container in warm

Table 42.1 Baby songbird food recipe (BSFR).

| |
|---|
| 1 C (100 g) Science Diet Canine Growth (Puppy) soaked in 1 C (240 ml) cold water |
| 1–4 oz jar (112 g) banana baby food or 4 oz (112 g) ripe banana |
| 1 peeled hard-boiled egg |
| 1/2 tsp. (2.5 ml) bird vitamin (Avi-Era, Lafeber or equivalent) |
| 1 tsp. (5 g) ground calcium carbonate (approximately 1800 mg calcium) |

Table 42.2 Adult bird kibble mix.

| |
|---|
| 4 C (400 g) Science Diet Canine Growth (Puppy) soaked in 2 C (474 ml) water |
| 1/2 tsp. (2.5 g) bird vitamin (Nekton S, Arcata Pet Supply, or equivalent) |
| 1/2 hard-boiled egg |
| 1/6 C (~40 ml) fruit, such as apples, pears |
| 1/6 C (~40 ml) green vegetables, such as zucchini, cucumber |
| 1/6 C (~40 ml) yellow or orange vegetable, such as carrots, squash |

water or on a warming plate set on low. In warmer climates the diet should be discarded midday and fresh diet supplied to finish the day.

If the BSFR appears too stiff to feed via syringe, add a small amount of water and mix until the consistency is moist enough to easily syringe-feed but not too moist as to possibly cause aspiration of the food.

Table 42.2 lists the ingredients for the adult bird kibble mix. Ensure the selection of fruits and vegetables will not spoil easily or be so watery as to make the kibble mushy. Pulse-chop eggs and fruit/vegetables in a food processor until coarsely chopped. Do not over-process. Mix all the ingredients. Store in a refrigerator for up to 2 days. Adult bird kibble mix can be tweezer-fed to juveniles with the addition of chopped whole meats such as mice, rats, smelt, or day-old chicks. Tweezer-feeding does not supply the same hydration as syringe-feeding BSFR, so supplementary hydration may be required.

## Diet Supplements

Offer a variety of nutrients and textures in addition to the kibble mix. Study the natural history of each species you plan to rehabilitate. Recognize that not all species within the corvid family have the same diet. This is especially true of the various jay species. For instance, the Pinyon Jay is uniquely dependent on the seeds of the Pinyon Pine. Green Jays are heavily dependent on insects in their diet. It is imperative that species that remove seeds from cones be given the opportunity to do this as a fledgling. Species frequenting oak habitats should be exposed to acorns. The Gray Jay caches food among the branches of trees. It is therefore logical to supply branches with crevices for the birds to explore prior to release. Do not overfeed any one of the supplements as it may create an unbalanced diet. Supplement additions are based on the caregiver observing the current status of the bird. A young bird just learning to eat will require mostly kibble plus a small amount of supplements to taste and move about. As the bird learns to manipulate food, more supplements may be given. Nuts must be cracked open at first and later may be supplied whole once the bird learns what to do with the nut.

Add any of the following to the kibble mix diet:

- Chick (1 day old).
- Mouse, starting with pinkies or cut mice initially, and working up to whole mice as the bird learns to grip and tear the food.
- Hard-boiled egg, with shell on.
- Unsalted nuts of all kinds, especially those found wild in the bird's native area (i.e. acorns).
- Insects (including mealworms, waxworms, crickets, and those found naturally).
- Vegetable chunks.
- Vegetable bits, i.e. frozen corn kernels, chopped string beans, broccoli bits, peas.
- Fruit chunks and whole fruits, especially those found in the bird's natural habitat.
- Fruit tidbits for pecking exploration stage – raisins, raisin-sized bits of strawberries, grapes, cantaloupe, and watermelon.
- Cooked sweet potato as a good source for vitamin A.
- Colored kibble bits, for example: Kit and Kaboodle cat food (Purina).
- Peanuts, unsalted, in the shell, cracked, and out of shell.
- Cones that are found in the habitat of the species being cared for.
- Berries, especially those found in the bird's native habitat.
- Carrion/roadkill.
- Jays should be exposed to bird seed, especially seed containing dried corn and nuts. Even crows show an interest in this. Species that depend on a particular seed should be given the particular seed that they require.

When ravens become self-feeding, their diet is largely whole meats or carrion. Even in the final stages of hand-feeding they will reject the BSFR and gape only for cut-up meats like rats, chicks, or mice. Older juvenile crows also develop a taste for whole meats. A varied diet should continue to be offered to these species for self-feeding in preparation for a successful release.

## Feeding Procedures

Warm and hydrate all birds before introducing food. Once this is accomplished, if the young bird is actively gaping, begin syringe-feeding with the BSFR. If the young corvid is warm and hydrated but refuses to gape, it may be force-fed. During force-feeding or when feeding a corvid hatchling, support the head and extend the neck using gentle finger pressure. Place an appropriately sized syringe (Table 42.3) containing the BSFR down the right side of the bird's throat, positioning the tip past the glottis when force-feeding or when feeding a hatchling. For older, vigorous birds, the syringe may be placed in the back of the mouth and the bird will swallow as the food is pushed in via the syringe. Use a 1 ml syringe with a stainless steel feeding tube or teat cannula syringe extender if necessary for a tiny (25 g) or weak bird, and 0.5 ml or less of the BSFR for the initial portion for any corvid. Begin with small amounts of food and ensure that the bird does not expel the food or gag. Refer to Table 42.3 for approximate feeding amounts for the following categories: hatchlings (nakeds), nestlings (pinfeather birds and pre-fledglings), and fledglings.

## Expected Weight Gain

Corvids vary greatly in size between and within a species. Charting the daily weight in grams versus feather growth for members of the common species in your area will be useful for future reference. The birds increase rapidly in size and weight, and tend to level off as pinfeathers develop and

Table 42.3 Feeding regimen.

| Corvid | Age | Amount | Syringe | Frequency |
|---|---|---|---|---|
| Crow | Naked | 1 ml or less | 1 ml | Every 30–45 min |
| | Older naked | 3–6 ml | 1–3 ml | Every 30–45 min |
| | Pinfeathers | Up to 6 ml | 1–3 ml | Every 30–60 min |
| | Pre-fledgling | 6–12 ml | 3 ml | Every 1–2 hour |
| | Fledgling | 9 or more ml | 3 ml | Every 1–3 hour |
| Jays*<br>*Jay species vary quite a bit in size. Try to coordinate food amounts with active gaping.<br>The Brown Jay can be equivalent in size to a large magpie. For this jay follow the magpie feeding regimen. | Naked (1–6 days old) | 0.1–1 ml or more | 1 ml with teat cannula | Every 20 min from 7:00 a.m.–10:00 p.m. |
| | Naked (more than 6 days old) | Variable: 1–2 ml | 1 ml; use teat cannula if not a strong gaper | Every 20–30 min from 7:00 a.m.– 9:00 p.m. |
| | Pins (with pinfeathers) | Variable: 1–3 ml | 1 ml | Every 30–60 min from 8:00 a.m.–9:00 p.m. |
| | Pre-fledgling | Variable: 1–3 ml or more | 1 or 3 ml<br>For older pre-fledge (cut-off syringes) | Every 1–2 hours from 8:00 a.m.–8:00 p.m. |
| | Fledgling | Variable: 3 ml or more | 3 ml (cut-off syringe) | Every 1–3 hours from 8:00 a.m.–7:00 p.m. |
| Magpies, Black and Yellow-billed | Naked | 0.1–2 ml or more if bird is still gaping | 1 ml; use teat cannula for recently hatched or weak birds | Every 30 min from 7:00 a.m.–9:00 p.m. |
| | Pins (with pinfeathers) | Variable: 1–3 ml | 1 ml | Every 30–60 min from 8:00 a.m.–8:00 p.m. |
| | Pre-fledgling to fledgling | Variable: 1–6 ml | 1 or 3 ml syringe (cut-off syringe); larger syringe for older, stronger birds | Every 45 min for younger birds up to every 120 min for older fledglings |

(*Continued*)

Table 42.3 (Continued)

| Corvid | Age | Amount | Syringe | Frequency |
|---|---|---|---|---|
| Ravens | Naked to pin | Same as for crows, but increase amounts as bird gapes for more | For youngest raven, begin with 1 ml syringe and increase to 3 ml as soon as bird can tolerate it; use cut off syringe | Every 30–60 min |
| | Pre-fledgling to fledgling | Ravens grow rapidly and vary greatly in size. Older birds may take 20–30 ml. Allow bird to determine food amounts through gaping. Many ravens will refuse BSFR and need whole meats, such as cut-up mice | 3 ml syringe or larger, (cut-off syringe); use forceps to feed cut-up meat | Every hour for pre-fledglings up to every 3 hours for oldest fledglings |

Table 42.4 Developmental milestones in the American Crow.

| Age/ days | Weight/ Grams | Integument | Eyes | Reaction to observer | Notes |
|---|---|---|---|---|---|
| 1–3 | 15–30 | Pink | Closed | Gaping | Brooding by parent; yolk sac persists |
| 3–5 | 30–45 | Smoky | Closed | Gaping | Brooding by parent; yolk sac persists |
| 5–10 | 45–110 | Black | Closed/ then slit | Gaping | Brooding by parent/tapers off; yolk sac persists |
| 10–15 | 110–210 | Growth of pins | Slit/then opening | Gaping | Brooding tapers off, then ends traces of yolk sac, then gone |
| 15–18 | 210–255 | Growth of feathers | Dull | Gaping | Voice changes to lower pitch |
| 18–25 | 255–300 | Growth of feathers | Clear gray-violet | Gaping, then crouching | Projection of middle primaries beyond sheaths is 2 in. or less |
| 25–30 | approx. 300 | Growth of feathers | Clear gray-blue | Crouching, then escape | Projection of middle primaries beyond sheaths is greater than 2 in. |

change into feathers. Some birds bulk-up in the aviary prior to release, significantly increasing their body weight (Table 42.4).

An optimal method of weight evaluation is to palpate the amount of muscle on either side of the keel. A bird with small breast muscle mass is not ready to be released. If this evaluation is done after the bird has been in captivity for a number of weeks and the muscle mass is low, a reevaluation of the health status of the bird should be done, checking for infection or parasites. If the diet varies from the ones listed in this chapter, a review of the nutrition supplied should be done. As the weight levels off, usually around the pre-fledgling stage, note the hydration of the bird, because its food intake typically decreases. It may be necessary to supplement the syringed diet with oral fluids. First-year corvids tend to develop fat supplies to aid in getting them through their first winter. This has the potential of making them heavier than adult birds of similar dimensions in wingspan and body length.

## Housing

### Jays and Magpies

Hatchlings should be placed in an incubator or in a heated, windowed cardboard pet carrier (Portapet); nestlings may go directly into a pet carrier or other suitable enclosure. An optimal pet carrier is constructed of cardboard with a 7×9 in. (18×23 cm) hole cut in one side and covered by a piece of flexible, clear plastic taped in place with clear packaging tape, creating a window. The pet carrier is lined on the bottom with a towel covered by a folded pillowcase.

A small towel rolled into a donut shape is provided in the carrier or incubator to be used as a nest or to hold in place a margarine container nest (lined with sheets of toilet paper) used for hatchlings. Hatchlings may require only a very light towel under the nest plus another towel wrapped around the nest to promote enough warmth from a heating pad. Heat is supplied by placing a heating pad set on the lowest heat setting partially under the carrier for nestlings and fully under the carrier for hatchlings. Loss of heat may be adjusted by partially covering the top of the carrier with a pillowcase and by placing a layer of toilet paper over the nest. This carrier may be adapted for juvenile jays just leaving the nest by adding a sisal rope (natural fiber rope) perch. Two holes are made at perch level on the largest sides of the carrier. The sisal rope is strung through and held in place by knots tied on the outside of the carrier. Ensure the rope placement leaves room for the bird to stand and also have ample room so the tail is not pushed against the carrier side. The window side of the carrier should be placed near a window to provide stress relief for the bird or birds inside. Nestlings may also be housed in plastic baskets lined with fiberglass screening, with a layer of screening held in place by clothespins on top or in a small soft sided basket or reptarium (a netted enclosure sold for reptiles).

Once the birds are able to perch and sample food, they should be moved to a pre-flight cage. If the cage is not already soft sided, line it with fiberglass screening to protect the feathers. If a kennel is used at this stage, line any openings or metal grates with fiberglass screening to prevent feather damage. A pre-flight cage may be set up indoors, permitting birds to be hand-fed as they are learning to eat on their own. Perches in the cage should be arranged to allow the birds to hop back and forth easily without their long tails touching the sides of the caging. Consider using soft sided playpens covered with fiberglass mesh for perching magpies. Place food bowls away from areas where the birds defecate. Jays should be completely self-feeding before moving to a larger enclosure or aviary. Even friendly juvenile jays become nervous about a radical housing change and may refuse to accept hand-fed food. The final step prior to release is for the bird to spend at least 3 weeks in an outdoor aviary.

Due to probing corvid beaks, most enclosures will sustain some damage, especially to lining materials. Pet Screen (Phifer) seems more resilient than other products.

Cages and aviaries should have a variety of perches. Avoid using smooth branches. Corvid feet are prone to developing bumblefoot with the use of improper perching. Perches covered with a plastic turf material (AstroTurf) are recommended for areas where the birds perch for extended periods. Perching alternatives include rough branches such as oak, live trees and plants, and sisal rope, which is a natural fiber rope that is rough enough to support healthy bird feet.

Optimal incubator temperatures will vary among corvid hatchlings. Some songbird hatchlings are kept at temperatures as high as 90–95 °F (32.2–35 °C) and 40–50% humidity, but this is generally too hot for a corvid and could easily cause dehydration, especially if the incubator is not maintaining steady high humidity. Many rehabilitation centers keep a number of incubators warm with 5 °F (2.8 °C) differences between them. After placing a hatchling in an incubator, observe breathing and feeding patterns. Open-mouthed breathing in a healthy hatchling indicates the temperature is too warm and that the bird should be moved to a slightly cooler incubator. The number of hatchlings placed together also makes a difference with corvids, because they have large bodies as compared to other songbirds. Single birds have a large unfeathered surface area from which to lose moisture; four to six birds grouped together supply a fairly resilient reservoir of warmth.

### Larger Corvids (Ravens and Crows)

Larger corvid juveniles are usually started in a windowed pet carrier or a small kennel equipped with a rolled towel nest or plastic turf (Astroturf) perch, unless they are recently hatched. Openings or grates on the kennel should be lined with fiberglass screening. A soft-sided reptarium or a soft-sided playpen can also be used for larger corvid nestlings. The playpen can be covered with fiberglass screening held on top by plastic clips. If the birds attempt to cling to the top cover, replace with a light-colored sheet. The soft-sided enclosures can be equipped with rolled towel nests or floor perches and the bottom of the enclosures can be covered with large string-free towels or sheets. Follow the protocol under jays and magpies for recently hatched birds. If the bird's ability to eat or

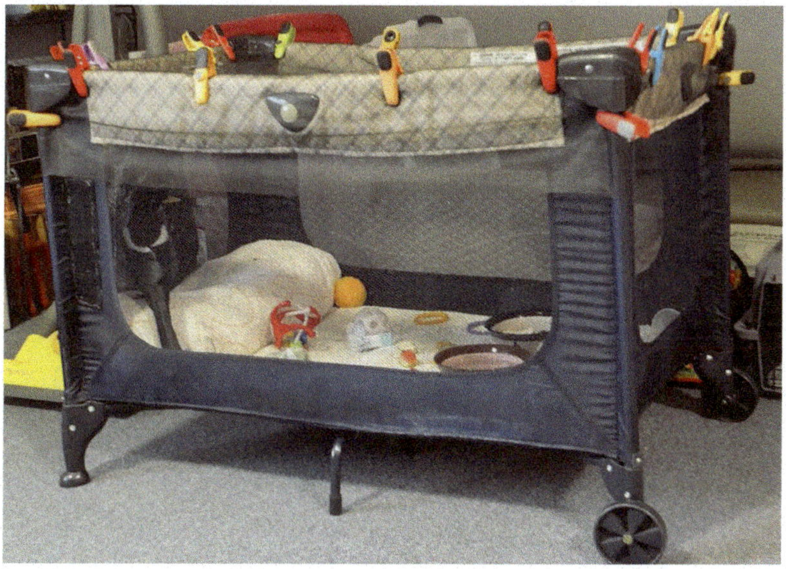

Figure 42.5 A soft sided playpen is feather-friendly housing for corvids.

defecate normally is unclear, the bird should be kept in the carrier overnight for observation. Nestlings that are first placed in the windowed carrier or equivalent on a heat source must be moved when they begin to perch or become too large for the unit. They are then moved to a larger enclosure (kennel, reptarium, playpen) equipped first with a rolled towel nest, and then a perch. If the birds thrive in the new enclosure add one or two perches fitted with Astroturf that is cable-tied around a closet pole cut to fit the kennel width or designed to be placed on the floor. If a kennel is used the perch is wedged into the kennel using folded paper toweling at both ends. The birds should be allowed to stretch and flap their wings during the cage cleaning periods, either by placing them on top of the kennel, on the floor (if they cannot yet fly), or in a mesh playpen covered with a sheet (Figure 42.5). The opportunity to build wing strength ensures a stronger bird upon placement in an aviary. The final housing before release is an outdoor aviary. If a small 6×6×6 ft. (1.8×1.8×1.8 m) aviary is available, the birds may be placed outside while still gaping. The small aviary allows hand-feeding of the still-gaping birds. Once the birds become self-feeding and comfortably go to the ground to eat rather than just from hanging bowls, they are moved to the large aviary.

## Social Groupings

Form small groups of juveniles upon admission and allow the birds to remain with this social group throughout the rehabilitation period. Release the birds as a group. Corvid social bonds are strong, and disrupting the bonds will cause stress. Do not mix or switch the birds as new birds are admitted. Following this policy also prevents the spread of viruses and parasitic infections.

## Aviary

Check with your state Fish and Wildlife agency for their specifications for aviary sizes for corvids. Another good source is Miller (2012). A 10×10×7 ft. (3×3×2 m) aviary would suffice for magpies and jays and 20×10×7 ft. (6×3×2 m) is enough for the larger corvids, such as ravens and crows.

An aviary must be constructed to withstand weather conditions at your location. Long periods of freezing conditions or temperatures above 100 ° F (38 ° C), high or low humidity, large amounts of rain or drought, or whether the aviary is located underneath trees or not shielded at all, are conditions that must be addressed when designing and outfitting an aviary. Basic aviaries can be constructed with wood, metal, powder-coated metal, or netting or a combination of these items. All aviaries should have at least a partial roof and a blind area where the bird can perch undisturbed by outside forces. Line the aviary with insect screening to prevent feather damage and to protect from mosquito-borne illness. Pet Screen (Phifer) is stronger than regular fiberglass insect screening and appears to sustain less damage from corvids. Most damage occurs to the aviary sides where the ends of perches contact the netting. These areas may be further lined with plastic 1/2 in. hardware cloth over the screening to act as a buffer to deter probing beaks.

A variety of perching must be supplied both for prevention of bumblefoot and to familiarize the birds with perching possibilities in the wild. The highest perch should be placed in a protected area of the aviary and it is recommended that this perch be covered with plastic turf material (Astroturf, Clean Machine, or Daisy Doormat) (Figure 42.4). This is where the birds will spend much of their time. Sisal rope, rough natural branches, and live plants are good alternatives. Most corvids are hesitant to go to the ground to eat or drink when first placed in an aviary. This behavior may last for a number of days. To prevent dehydration and starvation, hang bowls containing water and basic foods near the most frequently used perch for the first few days of aviary usage. Feeding platforms placed near heavily used perching are an alternative to the hanging bowls. Place favorite foods at ground level to inspire exploration. The bowls used to hold food and water at ground level should be sturdy nontip crocks. Always have climbing poles, fitted with plastic turf material reaching from the ground up to a perch in the aviary, to allow nonflighted birds to climb to a perch where they will feel safe. The perch should not be so high that they might fall and be injured. A climbing pole aids in stress relief and encourages healthy feather growth. Nonflighted birds left on the ground often injure themselves trying to gain height. Be aware that simple changes made to the aviary, such as putting in a larger water bowl, may cause the birds to stop eating for a period of time. Corvids are highly spatially oriented and notice the slightest change in environment. The aviary must be partially covered for protection from the elements and have a substrate on the floor to inspire digging and caching. Bark and 0.75–1.5 in. (2 × 3.8 cm) smooth light pebbles (Lodi rock) are good choices. An alternative to inspire caching would be to have dig boxes filled with dirt, leaves, or shredded bark on the aviary floor. The aviary should have a safety enclosure at the entry door to prevent escapes. An internal water system can be installed in this area and outfitted with a "quick connect" hose connection through a small hole in the side wall in order to permit a safe, escape-proof water supply. The aviary roof should be sloped to prevent water accumulation. If screening is used on part of the roof, it should be the upper layer to facilitate easy removal of leaf debris. Frigid climates will require a heat source whereas overly hot temperatures could benefit from misters.

## Weaning

In the wild, corvids may spend many months learning from their parents and relatives. Corvids fledge well before they are self-feeding and may be supported and protected out of the nest by an extended family group. They must be able to locate food, water, and shelter and be aware of what to fear. They may not have the benefit of the family support group, so to improve survival, birds must be educated before release. Because of their high sensitivity to spatial relationships, corvids fear unknown areas and might be too afraid to seek food in a new area. Juveniles benefit greatly by being housed in an outdoor environment replicating the release area as much as possible. Housing the young bird with a surrogate or other adult corvid of the same species so it can learn from the more experienced bird is optimal.

Weaning should include the bird being placed in enclosures with live plants, tree branches, and substrates such as dirt, bark, and rocks to dig and cache in, and logs to pound on and use for cracking nuts. Additionally, it should be able to hear other wild bird sounds, especially those of the species involved, so it can learn which vocalizations are connected with dangers located outside of the enclosure. Present the natural foods that will be in season when the bird is released for recognition purposes. Expose the bird to seed feeders, suet baskets, fruit and nuts hung on branches of bushes, nuts wedged in pine cones, food wedged in the cracks of logs, and anything else you can devise to educate the birds on finding food. In some areas, crows frequent fast food restaurants, so they are taught to tear apart a paper bag to obtain the enclosed food item.

The weaning process also involves allowing the bird to test natural food items while learning to eat on its own. As soon as a bird begins to leave the nest it should be given food items to explore. Certain species, especially among the jays, survive on a limited diet or specialized habitat and those needs must be addressed while the bird is in captivity. When the bird begins to hold some food in its mouth rather than swallow during syringe-feeding, it means that it is eating some food on its own but probably not enough to sustain itself. When gaping becomes intermittent, make feeding intervals longer, maintaining at least four feedings a day. As the bird becomes more proficient at eating on its own, reduce the number of feedings per day to three, then two, then one, and finally cease hand-feeding support while keeping weight records. Most caregivers give fresh food in the morning and allow the bird to eat and explore the fresh food, and then offer support later in the day until it is no longer gaping and is maintaining its weight. Evidence that the bird is eating is also present in profuse defecation and normal activity levels. In the weaning period, offer feeding support if the bird stops eating due to a change in the enclosure, and continue the support until it is evident that the bird has resumed eating on its own. This process may be aided by supplying food and water in hanging bowls at perch level in a kennel and especially in an aviary. During the weaning period, offer a variety of food. Fledglings need to explore, taste, and move about natural food items as they learn to take in enough food to support themselves. Sprinkling a few wiggly worms on fruits, kibble, and other food items will encourage exploration. Bright colors like corn kernels also inspire probing beaks. Colored items such as egg yolks, persimmon, watermelon tidbits, and blood-red mouse parts will often elicit at least a taste. Allow the bird to practice its eating prowess, to learn to crack nuts, and to pull apart a whole mouse before placing it in a large enclosure where progress is not easily monitored. Before a bird is moved outside, it must be acclimated to more adverse conditions than that of a temperature-controlled environment. A bird should be gradually exposed to more extreme temperatures during the weaning process.

## Preparation for Wild Release

Preparation for wild release of the bird should begin upon entry of the bird into your care. Never treat a wild bird as a pet. Corvids are social birds and should never be raised alone. A bird devoid of the social rules of its species will be shunned or possibly injured by birds that would ordinarily socialize with it. Find another caregiver with a bird similar in age to the one in your possession or arrange to pair the bird with an injured adult or permanently injured captive adult. During the time you are waiting to combine birds, supply the singlet in your care with a mirror at eye level, a

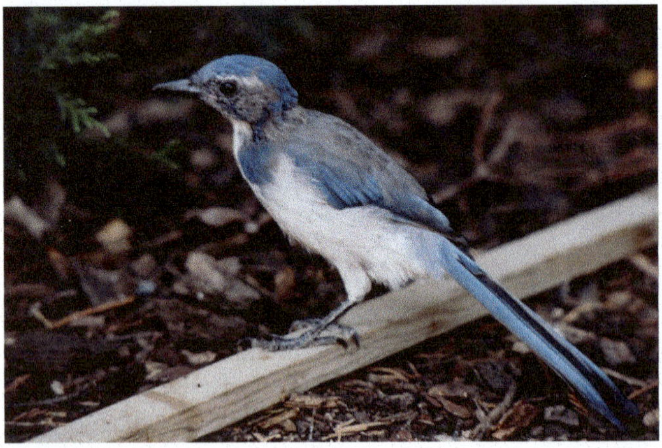

Figure 42.6 California Scrub Jays molt their gray head feathers prior to the end of their first summer.

species-specific stuffed toy, or an actual mount to view up-close. If the stuffed toy is the size of the actual bird, place it in the nest with the bird so the "companion" can be leaned on and pushed against. Face an indoor enclosure up against a window so that the bird views the outdoors rather than human activity. Interact with the bird only when necessary and then not in a way you would with a pet.

Once in the aviary, the birds will demonstrate distrust of humans if they have been successfully reared. A wild-raised fledgling is usually already fearful of humans and therefore does not require as much concern over taming or imprinting. Recognize that all corvids, even juveniles, go through a body feather molt during the summer months and that it is normal to occasionally have bald areas on the body during this molt. If so, delay release for the short period that it takes for feathers to grow in (Figure 42.6).

## Release

To be considered for release, a corvid should be parasite free, well-fleshed, difficult to catch in the aviary, and fully feathered with the feathers having a water-repellent quality called *weathered*. The fledgling should be adapted to varying temperatures and able to fly easily to the top of a tree, eat on its own, identify and locate natural foods, successfully interact with others of its species, and be fearful of people and predators, before being considered a candidate for release. A minimum of 3 weeks in an outdoor aviary with other birds of the same species is necessary to acclimate a corvid and maximize its survivability in the wild. Realize that for the first week in the aviary the bird might not come down to the floor and that the bird must be comfortable foraging on the ground in order to survive.

Release a corvid in an area where there are others of its own kind. Optimally return any bird to its family territory. If this is not possible, find an area where multiple groups gather so that the new bird will have a better chance of acceptance. Release groups of corvids raised together in the same location so they continue to interact with and support one another. Be aware of the special requirements of a specific species. For instance, it is especially important with Common Ravens to release a juvenile in an area with other juveniles if the original parents cannot be found. Juvenile ravens support one another and lead each other to food, while adults might chase an unknown juvenile.

Because these birds are diurnal, release them early in the day in good weather. Preview the release area to discover the movements and locations at the proposed release time of flocks, pairs, or families.

### Sources for Products Mentioned

AstroTurf, www.astroturfmats.com., www.grassworxllc.com.
Kit and Kaboodle cat food, Purina Mills, Nestlé Purina PetCare Company, Checkerboard Square, St. Louis, MO 63164, (314) 982-1000, www.http://purina.com.
Pet Screen, Phifer Inc., P O Box 1700, Tuscaloosa, AL 35403-1700, (205) 345-2120, www.phifer.com.
Portapet-Cardboard Pet Carrier, www.amazon.com, www.petsmart.com, optimum size is 24 in. × 12 in. × 18 in.
Sisal Rope (natural fiber rope): LeHigh, 2834 Schoeneck Road, Macungie, PA 18062, (610) 966-9702, www.lehighgroup.com.
Suet Baskets, Item #1472: Arcata Pet Supplies, (800) 822-9085, www.arcatapet.com.
Teat Cannula (Cannula): www.squirrelstore.com.
Trimethoprim-sulfamethoxazole (Septra), www.pfizer.com.

## References

Gill, F. and Donsker D. (eds.). (2019). IOC World Bird List (v9.1). https://doi.org/10.14344/IOC.ML.9.1.
Miller, E.A. (ed.) (2012). *Minimum Standards for Wildlife Rehabilitation*, 4e. St. Cloud, MN: National Wildlife Rehabilitation Association.
Zylberberg, M., Van Hemert, C., Dumbacher, J.P. et al. Novel picornavirus associated with avian keratin disorder in Alaskan birds. *mBio* 7 (4): e00874–e00816. https://doi.org/10.1128/mBio.00874-16.

## Further Reading

Alderfer, J. (2006). *National Geographic Complete Birds of North America*. Washington, DC: National Geographic.
Angell, T. (1978). *Ravens, Crows, Magpies, and Jays*. Seattle, Washington: University of Washington Press.
Caffrey, C. (2003). Determining impacts of West Nile Virus on crows and other birds. In: American Birds, Summary of the 103rd Christmas Bird Count. National Audubon Society, pp. 12–13. https://www.audubon.org/sites/default/files/103_c-wnvintro.pdf.
Ehrlich, P.R., Dobkin, D.S., and Wheye, D. (1988). *The Birder's Handbook*, 406–421. New York: Simon and Schuster Inc.
Elston, C.F. (1991). *Ravensong*. Flagstaff, Arizona: Northland Publishing Co.
Emlen, J.T. Jr. (1936). Age determination in the American Crow. *The Condor* 38 (3): 99–102.
Emlen, J.T. Jr. (1942). Notes on nesting colony of Western Crows. *Bird Banding* 13: 143–154.
Friedman, E. (2004). Magpie rehabilitation. In: Selected Papers from the 22$^{nd}$ annual National Wildlife Rehabilitation Association symposium, Orlando, FL, March 2–6, 2004.
Friedman, E. and Petersen, S. (2001). Care for the Western Scrub Jay and Steller's Jay. In: Selected Papers from the 19$^{th}$ annual National Wildlife Rehabilitation Association symposium, Lake Tahoe, NV, March 13–17, 2001.

Goodwin, D. (1976). *Crows of the World*, 173–183. New York: Cornell University Press.
Heinrich, B. (1999). *Mind of the Raven*. New York: HarperCollins Publishers, Inc.
Kilham, L. (1989). *The American Crow and the Common Raven*. College Station, Texas: A&M University Press.
Madge, S. and Burn, H. (1994). *Crows and Jays: A Guide to the Crows, Jays and Magpies of the World*. New York: Houghton Mifflin Company.
Marzluff, J. and Angell, T. (2012). *Gifts of the Crow: How Perception, Emotion, and Thought Allow Smart Birds to Behave like Humans*. New York: Atria Paperback.
Marzluff, J. and Balda, R. (1992). *The Pinyon Jay: Behavioral Ecology of a Colonial and Cooperative Corvid*. London: T&AD Poyser.
Savage, C. (1997). *Bird Brains – The Intelligence of Crows, Ravens, Magpies, and Jays. Sierra Club*. San Francisco.
Save Those Eggshells (1998). *Birder's World*. Waukesha, Wisconsin: Kalmbach Publishing Co.
Sibley, D.A. (2001). *The Sibley Guide to Bird Life and Behavior*, 408–415. New York: Alfred A. Knopf.
Sibley, D.A. (2001). *The Sibley Guide to Birds*, 350–361. New York: Alfred A. Knopf.
Terres, J.K. (1991). *The Audubon Society Encyclopedia of North American Birds. Wings Books*, 124–144. Avenal: New Jersey.

# 43

# Small Insectivores

*Veronica Bowers*

## Natural History

### Bushtits

Bushtits are one of the smallest North American passerines. Their range extends throughout western North America. Adults are approximately 4 in. (10 cm) in length and weigh only 6 g. Their bodies are gray with light brown on the head, long slender tails, dark pointed bill, and dark long legs. They are strictly insectivorous. At one time, Bushtits were grouped by ornithologists with the chickadees and titmice in the family Paridae. Recent research has shown that they are most closely related to the Old-World group known as long-tailed tits.

Bushtits are highly social birds. During the nonbreeding season, large flocks of up to 40 or more birds can be seen foraging together. The flocks are usually comprised of several family groups. While foraging, they remain in constant contact with each other, using light, high-pitched call notes. They roost communally in dense cover and huddle closely together for warmth. They are very active foragers, spending the majority of daylight hours searching for food. As foliage gleaners, Bushtits pick insects and spiders from leaf and twig surfaces, hanging upside down to reach prey items on the underside of leaves. Bushtits are often seen foraging in mixed species groups, such as with chickadees, kinglets, and titmice.

During the breeding season, birds pair off and become somewhat territorial. They construct a fully enclosed pendulous nest suspended from a group of small twigs in a tree. The foundation of the nest is bound together with spider webs, and then a variety of plant material such as moss and small leaves is used to camouflage the exterior. The interior is lined with feathers and animal hair; dryer lint is also a common nest material. The average clutch size is five to seven, with one to two broods per season. Most Bushtits typically complete their breeding cycle by late June. The male and female build the nest, incubate the eggs, and brood and feed the young. Some pairs have helpers. Helpers are usually unmated male Bushtits or adults whose own nest has failed. In exchange for helping raise their young, helpers are allowed to roost in the nest at night.

### Wrens

There are 76 species of wrens worldwide, 7 of which occur in North America. Wrens are small, brown birds that are very active and vocal. They dwell in scrubby habitat and dense undergrowth, from marshes and forests to deserts. They are strictly insectivorous and use their slender pointy

*Hand-Rearing Birds*, Second Edition. Edited by Rebecca S. Duerr and Laurie J. Gage.

bills to glean their food from the ground, plant surfaces, and cracks and crevices of rocks and trees. Some wrens, like the Carolina and Bewick's, are known to consume tiny amounts of berries and seeds during the winter. Some species of wrens in North America are migratory; others are not.

Wrens are well known for their complex and loud song and can develop large repertoires of song. Young wrens learn their paternal song between 30 and 60 days of age. Wrens use their song to defend territory and attract a mate. Wrens are extremely territorial during the breeding season, and nonmigratory species defend their territory all year.

All wrens nest in some form of enclosed space, including rock crevices, tree hollows, nest boxes and even abandoned automobiles. Both the male and female participate in nest building and raising the young. Clutch sizes range from 3 to 10 eggs. Young fledge the nest at 10–23 days of age depending on the species. The distinctive up-pointed tail posture of wrens can be discerned on nestlings as soon as the tail feathers begin to emerge, aiding in identification.

### Warblers

There are over 100 species of New World warblers, typically referred to as wood-warblers. Members of this family consist of some of the smallest, ranging from 6 to 20 g, and most colorful passerines in the Americas. They belong to the family Parulidae and are not related to Old World warblers or the Australian warblers.

Most warbler species are obligate insectivores; however, some species may consume fruits, seeds, and even nectar during fall and winter. Warblers are migratory and, more specifically, are nocturnal migrants. Like wrens, all warbler species belong to the suborder Oscines of passerine birds and as nestlings and fledglings must learn their song from a paternal tutor.

Due to the diversity of this family of birds, the nesting habitat and location ranges from ground nesting to nesting 10–40 ft. (3–12 m) off the ground in trees and shrubs. The nest structure also varies with open cup style as the most common type; however, species such as Lucy's and Prothonotary nest in cavities. The average clutch size is four to five eggs. Nestling growth and development is rapid as they gain approximately 0.5–1 g per day between 1 and 7 days of age. Young of most warbler species fledge the nest between 9 and 13 days of age and become fully independent 25–28 days post-fledge.

Most species belonging to this family are highly arboreal and occupy the forest canopy, gleaning insects from twigs and leaves. Warblers may opportunistically flycatch prey from the air, but hover and glean is their standard form of food procurement. There are several species that occupy other foraging niches such as mid-story shrubs, bark crevices on tree trunks, and a few species that forage for insects on the ground. Due to the wide range of behavior and habitat among warbler species, it is incumbent upon the caregiver to correctly identify the species and research the natural history thoroughly to establish an appropriate care plan.

### Vireos

Vireos are another small, insectivorous passerine found in the New World as well as Southeast Asia. Thirteen species occur in North America and Bermuda. North American species of this family have subtle plumage color ranging from grayish to greenish. They occupy a wide range of habitats including mixed forests, deciduous woodlands, riparian areas, and mangrove. All but the Hutton's Vireo are migratory species. The average clutch size is three to four eggs. Young fledge the nest at approximately 2 weeks of age and are mostly flighted at time of fledging. Young are dependent upon parental care for approximately three weeks post-fledge. Vireos belong to the suborder Oscines and therefore the young must learn their song from a paternal tutor.

Members of Vireonidae have small, strong bills with a tiny hook at the tip that aid in the capture and dismemberment of their prey. Their foraging behavior is similar to warblers, as they tend to be very active foragers, constantly moving from branch to branch as they search leaves, twigs, and flowers for insect prey. Some employ flycatching behavior to capture flighted insect prey. Vireos species are known to consume varying amounts of fruit opportunistically or seasonally; however, the majority of their diet consists of insects. Other species of small insectivorous passerines typically have similar needs to the species covered in this chapter; see Box 43.2 "Kinglets" for an example.

## Criteria for Intervention

### Bushtits

Bushtit nests are extremely well camouflaged and are commonly cut down during springtime tree trimming. If the nest is undamaged and the nestlings are uninjured, the nest should be reattached to the tree. If the nest is still attached to the branch that was cut, the entire branch should be reattached using wire to secure it to another branch in the tree. The nest should be placed no more than 1 ft. (30 cm) from its original location and should not be accessible or visible to predators. Do not attempt to put the nest in another tree. The nest should be observed for at least 1 hour from a distance of 30 ft. (9 m) or more to be certain the parents find the nest and continue to care for the young.

Domestic cats, jays, and squirrels are common predators of Bushtit nests. If a nest has been disturbed or destroyed by a jay or squirrel and there are surviving nestlings, attempts should not be made to re-nest the youngsters because the predators will return and predate the nest again. If a domestic cat has attacked a nest of Bushtits, all survivors should be brought to a wildlife rehabilitator for care because cats carry bacteria in their mouths and claws that can be lethal to birds.

### Wrens

Wrens may choose inappropriate nest sites. Nest relocation is rarely successful because wrens are shy species and very wary of change in their surroundings. Chicks are also often admitted after being caught by cats.

### Warblers and Vireos

Cats also frequently capture these species and cause often-lethal injuries. Warblers and vireos are also common victims of humans kidnapping, particularly when a newly fledged youngster is found on a trail out in the middle of nowhere by hikers, who mistakenly assume the chick is orphaned. Unfortunately, these chicks are typically transported long distances away from the area, with no hope of ever being returned to his/her parents.

## Record Keeping

See Chapter 1.

## Initial Care and Stabilization

Gaping, active hatchlings, nestlings, and fledglings can easily be rehydrated orally with a rehydration fluid appropriate for the condition of the bird (Figures 43.1 and 43.2). More severely dehydrated birds may require fluids to be administered subcutaneously. It is not uncommon to keep a dehydrated bird on fluid therapy for several days after intake. The oral rehydration solution listed in Perlman (2016) works exceptionally well as part of initial care. Always supply supplemental heat on

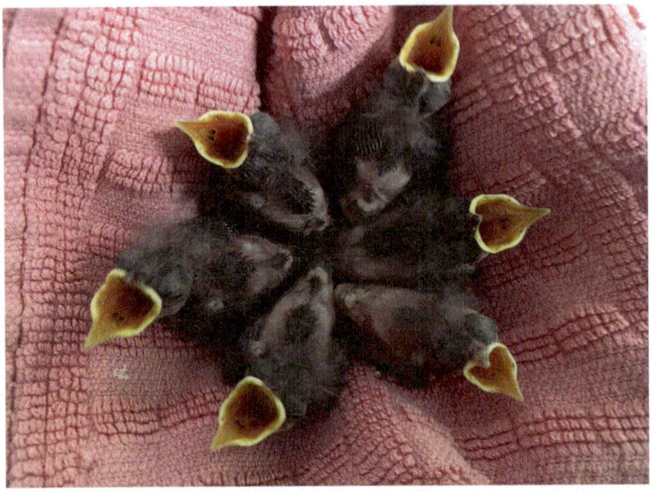

Figure 43.1 Bewick's Wren nestlings. Note the two spots at the back of the tongue.

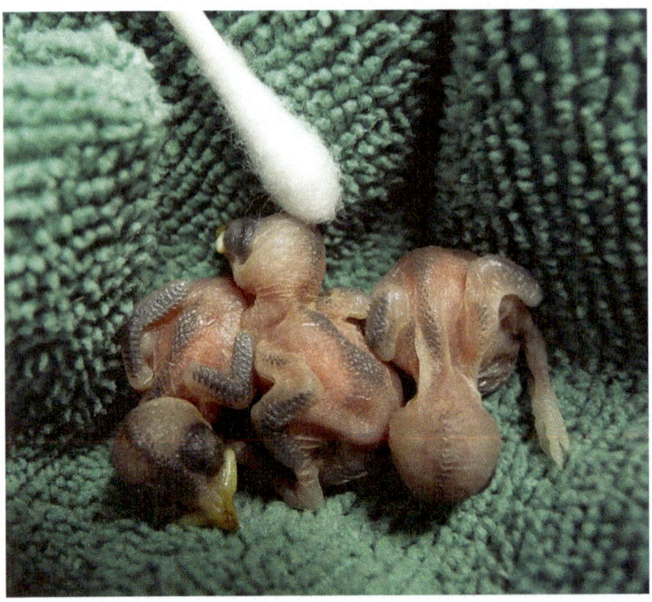

Figure 43.2 Hatchling Bushtits, note their tiny size and lack of down.

intake for these species. Depending on the age and condition of the bird, the ambient heat of an incubator set between 85 and 92 °F (29.4–33.3 °C) will be required to keep the bird comfortable.

These species are very prone to stress in captivity. Consequently, oral administration of fluids is much preferred over subcutaneous injection in order to minimize handling. See Chapter 1 for more information on physical examination and wound management.

## Common Medical Problems and Solutions

### Caught by Cat

Cat-caught birds should immediately begin a course of an antibiotic such as Clavamox (Hawkins et al. 2018). Small wounds should be cleaned with warm water or sterile saline. Bushtits and wrens are very small birds, which may make it difficult to palpate fractures or locate puncture wounds. Using a damp cotton swab can be helpful to brush back feathers when looking for puncture wounds. A tiny amount of silvadene cream, or other water-soluble ointment, can be applied if necessary.

### Fractures

Fractured wings must be carefully evaluated. Full recovery of flight and agility is essential to qualify for release. Bushtits are intensive foragers, spending the day in constant search of food with their flockmates. They must be able to keep up with the flock at all times and require full use of their legs and feet to dangle from tips of branches while gleaning insects from the underside of leaves. Although wrens are not intensely aerial, a few species are migratory and therefore must have full recovery and perfect flight upon release. Warblers and vireos must have full recovery from wing injuries, as all species in these families are intensive foragers, some employ flycatching to capture prey, and most species are obligate long-distance migrants.

Leg fractures are common among nestling Bushtits whose nest has been displaced through unseasonal tree trimming, or attacked by free-roaming cats or jays. Although Bushtit legs are tiny, they are long relative to their body size and fairly easy to splint. Material such as vet wrap is rigid enough to stabilize a leg fracture of a nestling Bushtit. The splint should be removed and the fracture site checked after 3 days. More rigid splinting materials can be used for older mobile birds. See Duerr et al. (2017) for more information on managing fractures in small birds.

### Parasites

Ectoparasites, such as mites and lice, occur among these species and are easily treated with a pyrethrin spray such as Ultracare Mite and Lice Bird Spray (8-in-1). Mist the spray onto a cotton ball or swab and gently swab the affected areas of the bird. Change the bedding and caging frequently until parasites are no longer present. Quarantine infested birds until all parasites are gone. These species rarely present with internal parasites, but it is always good practice to conduct a fecal smear or float.

### Sticky Traps

Fledgling wrens and Bushtits are often victims of sticky rodent and fly traps. Birds should be carefully removed from traps using the protocol described in Appendix C. Conduct a thorough physical examination once the bird is removed from the trap and is stable enough for handling. A course of antibiotics is recommended if the skin is injured or abraded. Glue removal, decontamination, and washing the feathers should only be conducted after the bird has been stabilized, which could be a day or two after intake. Provide fluids, correct diet, and housing appropriate for the condition of the bird. A small hospital basket placed in an incubator set at 90 °F (32.2 °C) provides a supportive environment until the bird has been decontaminated, washed, and feather condition has been restored.

### Stress

Stress in captivity can be detrimental to any wild bird, but these species are especially susceptible to stress. When hand-raising these species, they are best cared for under the supervision of one caregiver and must be provided with a quiet and calm environment.

## Diets

Insectivorous species must be hand-raised using an all insect diet. These species are obligate faunivores; more specifically, they are insectivores. This means they must eat insect protein. Depending on the age of the bird, insects for hand-feeding can include domestically cultivated mealworms, waxworms, crickets, dubia roaches, fly larvae, flightless stingless wasps, and fruit flies. Feed hatchlings the slurry recipe described below. Nestlings and fledglings should be fed whole insects supplemented as described in Chapter 44, Box 44.1: "Supplementation.". Micronutrient supplements are essential to a complete and nutritious all-insect hand-feeding diet because commercially cultivated feeder insects are deficient in several important nutrients. Make sure that birds being hand-fed using an all-insect diet receive their supplements every day until they are self-feeding.

### Diet for Hatchling Passerines, 0–3 Days of Age

Combine:

- 80 g "wet weight" of insects: 30 g of small mealworms, 20 g defrosted bloodworms, 30 g cricket bodies
- 500 mg elemental calcium (from 1250 mg calcium carbonate powder)

Place ingredients in electric mini spice grinder and puree to a consistency that is easily drawn up into a 1 cc syringe. Diet may be frozen: portion out 8.5–9.5 g increments into 10 mini containers with lids. Label and freeze (Figure 43.3).

To serve to birds:

Defrost one container and add:

- 1 cc live-culture yogurt (plain, low-fat)
- a sesame seed-sized bit of Taurine
- a sesame seed-sized bit of Thiamine
- a sesame seed-sized bit of vitamin C

  0.05 cc of the following mix:
  - 4 cc omega-3 marine oil
  - vitamin D3, 4000 IU
  - vitamin A, 4000 IU
  - vitamin E, 400 IU

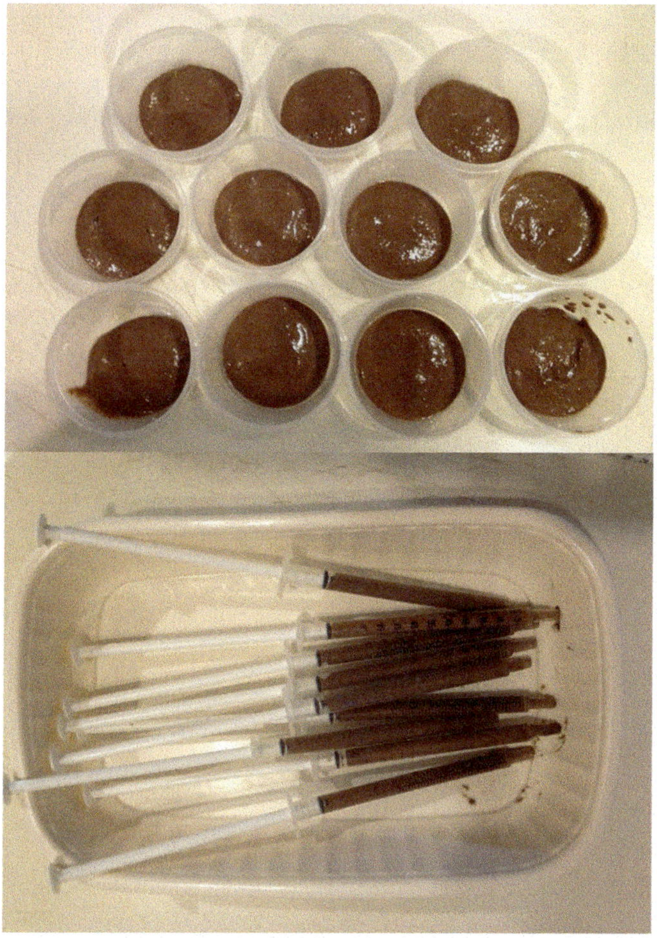

Figure 43.3 Hatchling diet portioned into small freezer containers for storage, and into syringes when thawed.

Mix well. Draw the slurry up into 1 cc syringes and store in the fridge. Warm each syringe of food in a warm-water bath before feeding. Discard unused food at the end of the day. Attach a cannula tip to a 1 cc syringe, especially when feeding tiny hatchlings, such as of wrens and Bushtits.

Possible additions to the slurry:

- A dab of Pancrezyme®: Pancrezyme provides pancreatic enzymes to pre-digest the food and may be beneficial for hatchlings of species who are fed regurgitant, such as woodpeckers and possible others – do your research. Pancrezyme could also be added when using this diet for emaciated birds.
- A speck of feces from a *healthy* adult conspecific for the *first feeding of the day only*. This may help establish good gut flora. Do this ONLY for hatchling birds who may not have received a food/saliva transfer from their parents and may have arrived with a sterile GI tract.

## Nestling, Fledgling, and Adult Diet

When purchasing cultivated insects for small insectivores, order small and mini sized mealworms, not to exceed ½ in. (1.25 cm) in length for fledglings, and ¼ (0.6 cm) for nestlings. Pinhead crickets are best for nestlings and 2-week-old crickets work well for fledglings. The smallest size of Dubia roaches is ¼ in. (0.6 cm) which is easy for most fledglings and nestlings to ingest; however, the roach should be squeezed in the middle for smaller nestlings such as warblers and Bushtits. Waxworms can be added for variety, but it can be difficult to find them in a small enough size for these species. Waxworms provide hydration in the diet, but are not very nutritious and should only comprise a small amount of the daily insect intake, approximately 5%.

Live, cultivated insects, such as mealworms, crickets and Dubia roaches, should be fed a nutritious diet before being used as a food source for avian patients. The author prefers to feed mealworms and Dubia roaches a diet of bran, nonmedicated poultry starter crumbles, and vegetables that are high in carotenoids, such as carrot and yam. Care and feeding of crickets can be found in the Box 43.1: "Cricket and Dubia Roach Care" below. For ease of hand-feeding, crickets and Dubia roaches can be pre-killed.

### Box 43.1 Cricket and Dubia Roach Care

#### Preparation for Hand-feeding

Crickets and Dubia roaches must be fed a nutritious diet before using them for hand-feeding or as live food in aviaries. The author feeds crickets and roaches a mixture of dry dog kibble, yam, and apple for 24–48 hours before feeding the insects to the birds.

*Storage and Preparation of Frozen Crickets and Roaches*

Keep the insects in the container they arrived in from the supplier and add food as described above. After the insects have eaten for 24–48 hours, place the sealed container in the freezer. The insects should be completely frozen within 24 hours.

For crickets, remove the box from the freezer and shake the box vigorously to break off legs and wings. Open the box and empty crickets into a strainer or colander with large enough holes to separate and sift out broken legs and wings. Working quickly, portion the frozen cricket bodies into smaller freezer-safe containers, place the lids on the containers, label and store the containers in freezer. Use as needed. Frozen cricket bodies keep well for up to 2 months in the freezer.

For Dubia roaches, remove the container from the freezer and separate the roaches from any leftover food. Place the frozen roaches in small freezer-safe containers, place the lids on the containers, label and store the containers in the freezer. Frozen roaches keep well for up to 2 months in the freezer.

*Hand-feeding Fresh Frozen Crickets and Roaches*

If the weather is mild, per each group of birds, portion out enough frozen crickets for 1 to 2 hours' worth of feedings. Putting each portion in a small dish with a little water keeps them moist. Don't feed the crickets to the birds until they have defrosted; it usually takes approximately 5 minutes for crickets to defrost at room temperature. Do not defrost crickets in microwave.

Left at room temperature, defrosted fresh frozen insects will begin to spoil after 2 hours. They will turn black and develop a sour smell. This means they have spoiled and should be discarded. Do not feed spoiled food to the birds. During extremely hot weather, it is best to portion out what can be used in 1 hour or less.

**Preparation for Use as Live Prey and Foraging Enrichment**

Live crickets and Dubia roaches that will be for foraging enrichment are provided the same diet of dry dog kibble, yam, and apple, but the insects are not put in the freezer. Instead, the insects, food items, cardboard egg crate, and empty paper towel rolls are placed in a 56 qt. plastic Sterilite® bin. Use separate bins for crickets and roaches. A mesh cover is placed over the top of the bin to prevent crickets from escaping. The insects will hide in the paper towel rolls and under the sections of paper egg crate. To distribute live insects to birds in aviaries, place an insect-filled paper towel roll or section of egg crate in an appropriate area of the aviary. The author prefers to hide the insect-filled paper rolls on a tray of dirt placed on the ground topped with a pile of leafy branches or grass, depending on the species of birds in the aviary.

## Feeding Procedures

These species require small, frequent feedings every 10–20 minutes for 14 hours a day to ensure healthy weight gain and development. Extreme care must be used to keep their feathers, face and body parts free of food and fecal matter at all times. Perfect feather condition is essential to a bird's survival upon release. Food accumulated in the nares and around the eyes can cause infection. Food left on the bill or bill commissure of hatchlings and nestlings can result in bacterial infection and bill deformity. Contaminants on skin can cause hypothermia; when on feather tracts, can inhibit healthy growth and emergence of feathers. It is imperative that birds are kept clean at all stages of development. Immediately remove any contaminants from the bird using a cotton swab or soft cloth dampened with warm water.

Hatchlings, 0–3 days of age with eyes still closed or barely cracked open, are fed the Diet for Hatchling Passerines every 10–15 minutes, 14 hours a day. Use a cannula tip attached to a 1 ml syringe to deliver the diet. Nestlings, 4 days of age and older, should be transitioned to a diet of small whole pre-killed insects and the Supplements for Hand-rearing Birds. Supplements are administered to all chicks once daily.

Due to the tiny mouth and huge appetite of nestling Bushtits and warblers, the author finds it more efficient to feed nestlings these species the Diet for Hatchlings Passerines until they are 5 to 6 days old. By 6 days of age, the author transitions nestling Bushtits and warblers to the whole insect diet and supplementation protocol (see Chapter 44 for supplementation protocol).

Heads of mealworms should be crushed and bodies of the mealworms should be squeezed once in the middle by pinching with forceps. Avoid tenderizing the entire body of the mealworm. Doing so can result in expelling most of the nutritious viscera from the exoskeleton of the larvae, which makes this food source less nutritious for the bird. It is wise to get into the habit of feeding the mealworms to the bird head first. Bushtits in particular, will often eject mealworms that are not fed head first. The author assumes this may have something to do with the direction in which the scales lay on the exoskeleton of the mealworm. Crickets and Dubia roaches may require the same preparation. Again, take care not to squeeze out the nutritious viscera of the insect and do not feed any insect that is too large for the age and species of bird.

At nestling stage, feed each individual as much as they would like during each feeding interval of every 15–20 from sunrise to sunset. Intervals more frequent than every 15–20 minutes may be indicated. Use the bird's behavior as a guide and make appropriate adjustments to the feeding schedule. There is no risk of overfeeding healthy gaping nestling insectivores.

Keep the nest and nestlings clean. Even the tiniest amount of food or feces left on the bird can damage feathers, or if near the face, it can cause infection. While in the nest, Bushtits raise their rear ends almost over their heads to defecate toward the center of the nest. This is normal behavior and usually perfectly timed during their scheduled feeding. Fecal sacs can easily be removed from the nest with forceps at this time.

Nestling and fledgling wrens are especially fearful when they are brought into captivity. Be patient. A small wiggling worm held at the tip of forceps is likely to pique the interest of a shy but hungry wren. Learn to make their food call, be patient and set up their housing to ensure they are comfortable in their environment (see "Housing" section).

Newly admitted fledgling warblers and vireos tend to be very vocal. Persistent food calls can be a sign of stress and hunger. The food call of most warblers is a rhythmic rapid chip note. Vireos produce a nasally whine. Ensure proper housing, enrichment, and companionship is provided to reduce stress. Feed at more frequent intervals of every 10 minutes until the bird settles into the new surroundings. If the bird was orphaned for any length of time, more frequent than usual feedings may be required for a couple of days to make up for a nutritional deficit.

As the fledglings get older, continue feeding insects and supplements on a frequent feeding schedule every 20–30 minutes for 14 hours per day. At fledgling stage, it is no longer necessary to pre-kill mealworms for wrens and vireos; however, Bushtits and warblers may find it easier to ingest pre-killed mealworms when being hand-fed. As birds continue to pick up more food on their own, gradually reduce the frequency of their feedings by increments of 15 minutes over the course of 2–3 weeks until they're proficiently self-feeding. Patience is essential as these species can be slow to become independent. Careful observation of self-feeding is critical. Although birds may be observed picking up insects and killing them on their own, they may not be ingesting enough to sustain themselves. As soon as the birds are no longer begging for food and have been self-feeding proficiently for at least 3 days, they can be moved to an aviary for pre-release conditioning.

**Box 43.2 Kinglets**

Golden-crowned and Ruby-crowned Kinglets can be hand-reared in the same manner as the warblers and vireos described in this chapter. During the breeding season, kinglets are found in conifer forests. They spend most of their foraging time high in the canopy and feed exclusively on insects. Hunting methods include hovering, gleaning, and hawking prey from the tips of branches or the underside of leaves and between tufts of conifer needles, and probing underneath the bark of conifer branches and tree trunks. Some populations of each species are more migratory than others. Caregivers of these species should research the migratory behavior for the species in their geographic area.

Kinglets fledge the nest at 16–19 days of age and are mostly flighted at time of fledging (Figure 43.4). They reach independence approximately 17 days after fledging the nest. A post-fledging behavior shared with Bushtits is that young kinglets commonly perch and huddle together throughout the day and at night to roost.

It is noteworthy that the mouth color of nestling Golden-crowned Kinglets is distinctly bright pink, a departure from the yellow to orange mouth color associated with most insectivorous passerines. This is a common cause for misidentification and can be a detriment to the survival of the kinglet nestling if it is treated as a finch or sparrow species. The mouth color of Ruby-crowned Kinglets is pinkish-orange.

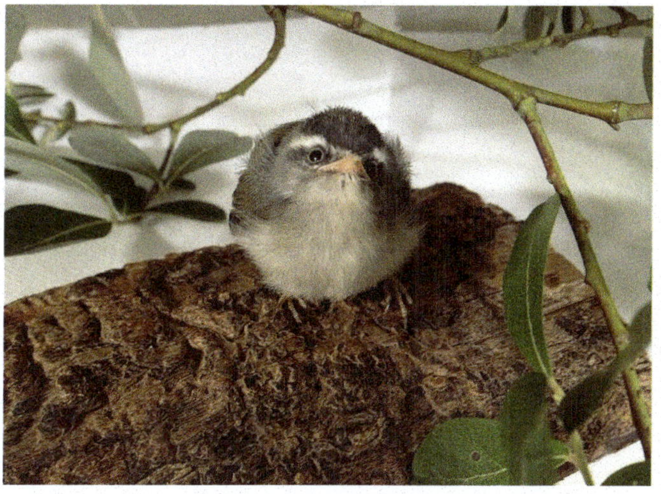

Figure 43.4 Golden-crowned Kinglet fledgling.

## Expected Weight Gain

All species gain approximately 0.5–1 g of weight each day between 0 and 7 days of age and reach their maximum weight by 7 days of age.

## Song Development

Young wrens, warblers, and vireos must be exposed to the song of their species. Song development in most species of young passerines is critical to their success as breeding adults. Raw unprocessed geographically appropriate recordings of bird songs are available from Cornell's Lab of Ornithology Macaulay Library of sound (see resources). Research the available materials for the species in question. Download the sound file to a computer or smart phone and play the recording at dawn and dusk. It is also possible to make a recording of the song by visiting the location where the orphaned bird was found and recording the dawn song at that location. Birds in care should have access to their song from nestling through fledgling stage. Providing song at hatchling stage may be impractical as it is unlikely to be heard over the din of the incubator.

## Housing

### Hatchlings and Nestlings

Hatchlings should be kept in an incubator set at 92–95 °F (33.3–35 °C) with 50% humidity. An artificial nest can be created using a small, round plastic container lined with a face cloth or similar fabric for insulation and softness. Fill the center of the nest with tightly crumpled tissue or a square soft felt fabric to form the shape and shallow cup of a natural nest. Proper texture of the lining and shape of the nest interior provide important support for the body of a developing young bird. Choose a size of container that will comfortably accommodate the number of hatchlings/nestlings to inhabit the nest.

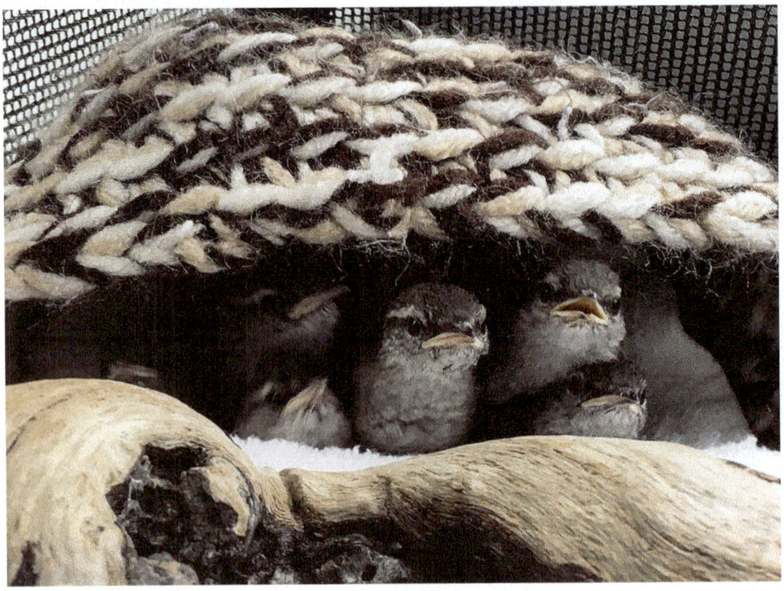

Figure 43.5 Young fledgling Bewick's Wrens in nest that provides warmth and security.

Lay a piece of soft felt or a folded tissue over hatchlings to simulate a brooding parent and provide warmth and security (Figure 43.5). The addition of a folded face cloth folded over the top of the nest to create a dome will help nestlings feel more secure and minimize stress. Placing the nest in a small nest box is also a comfortable option for certain nestling wren species, such as Bewick's, House, and Carolina Wrens. The nest box must have a lid that opens for ease of hand-feeding the birds. Depending on their condition and amount of emerging feathers, young nestling (5–6 day old) wrens, warblers, and vireos are comfortable in an incubator set at 85–89 °F (29.4–31.7 °C) with at least 50% humidity. Bushtits of similar age may be kept slightly warmer at 89–90 (32 °C). As feathers emerge and nestlings are able to thermoregulate, they should be transitioned out of the incubator and into regular hospital housing.

As long as nestlings are healthy, thermoregulating, and have two or more nestmates, the author removes nestlings of these species from the incubator at 6 days of age. Remaining in their nest, nestlings can be housed in a soft-sided 38-gal. reptarium or similar housing as long as they're healthy, able to thermoregulate, and pinfeathers have emerged. If needed, offer supplemental heat for a few additional days until nestlings are at least 50% feathered. Supplemental heat can be provided using a heating pad on the lowest setting or a gooseneck lamp with a ceramic heat bulb. At this stage of development, nestlings' eyes will be open. Keep in mind Bushtits, wrens, and certain warbler species nest in cavity-like structures and their eyes are not fully exposed to daylight until they fledge at approximately 12–14 days of age. Therefore, maintaining a cavity-type nest structure in captivity is appropriate and may be important to eye health.

In anticipation of fledging, an appropriate environment must be created in the nestling enclosure. On fledge day, Bushtits and wrens tend to scatter frantically out of the nest rather than cautiously exit. However, most of the frantic scattering can be avoided if the enclosure containing the nest has been furnished with an abundance of leafy branches at all levels to support a more natural environment and less scary process of fledging the nest. Warblers and vireos also require a properly furnished environment, but usually have a more graceful exit from the nest as they have typically prepared themselves by perching on the edge of the nest and exercising their wings a couple of days prior to fledging.

Never raise or release a single baby bird. Conspecifics or compatible species are necessary to provide warmth, physical support, interaction, and companionship in the nest. As fledglings, conspecifics or compatible species also inspire competition, which fosters healthy behavioral and physical development. Conspecifics are obviously the ideal companions during rehabilitation; however, when that is not an option there are compatible species that can be considered. Bushtits, vireos, warblers, and kinglets are all mutually compatible. Chickadees are compatible with the aforementioned species. Small Empidonax flycatchers are compatible with vireos and warblers, but at fledgling stage can become aggressive toward Bushtits. Bewick's Wrens can be safely co-housed with the previously mentioned species; however, at fledgling stage wrens in general can act aggressively toward other species and may require a separate aviary.

In the wild, House Wrens are known to invade and take over the nests of other cavity-nesting species. The risk of desensitization toward a natural enemy should be considered when contemplating co-housing House Wrens with other wren species and cavity-nesting species. The author frequently has young House and Bewick's Wrens in care during the breeding season. Every effort is made to house the species separately; however, on occasion a single House Wren may be housed with a group of Bewick's Wrens, but never vice versa.

Bushtits are highly social species and require the companionship of a minimum of two other Bushtits. This is especially important during fledgling stage to allow time to form a small flock during pre-release conditioning in the aviary and upon release.

## Fledglings

Nests must remain in the enclosure for Bushtits and wrens until fledglings are no longer returning to the nest for naps and to roost at night. A day or two after fledging, the housing size should be increased to a 175-gal. reptarium (4×3×3 ft./1.2×0.9×0.9 m) or similar housing to provide more room for flight and behavioral development. This size enclosure is adequate to house eight Bushtits or six wrens during their first week post-fledge. At the second week post-fledge, it is optimal to graduate them to a larger enclosure or an aviary as described below.

On the day they fledge, vireos and warblers should be moved to a 175-gal. reptarium (4×3×3 ft. /1.2×0.9×0.9 m) or similar housing for flight and behavioral development. If practical and safe for the birds, it is strongly recommended that these species be moved outdoors to an aviary where they will continue to receive frequent hand-feedings. When they are fledglings, it is the author's experience that these species, as well as wrens, thrive when moved to aviaries for the duration of the hand-rearing process. A more natural environment, access to natural sunlight, exposure to the night sky, and elimination of stressors from a busy clinic benefit the wellbeing of these shy and stress-prone species.

Whether housed indoors or in an aviary, furnish the enclosure with perches at different heights and natural branches complete with leaves to encourage foraging. Hang dishes of small mealworms, Dubia roaches, fly larvae, and freeze-dried domestic flies at varying heights in the cage. For wrens, also include dishes of small mealworms on the floor of the enclosure hidden behind logs and pieces of bark (Figure 43.6).

Scatter leaf litter and grass on the bottom of the enclosure. Include a shallow dish of water for drinking and bathing. Make sure the dish is large enough to accommodate at least two birds from head to tail. A 6 in. (15.2 cm) plastic plant saucer works well in an indoor enclosure. It is very

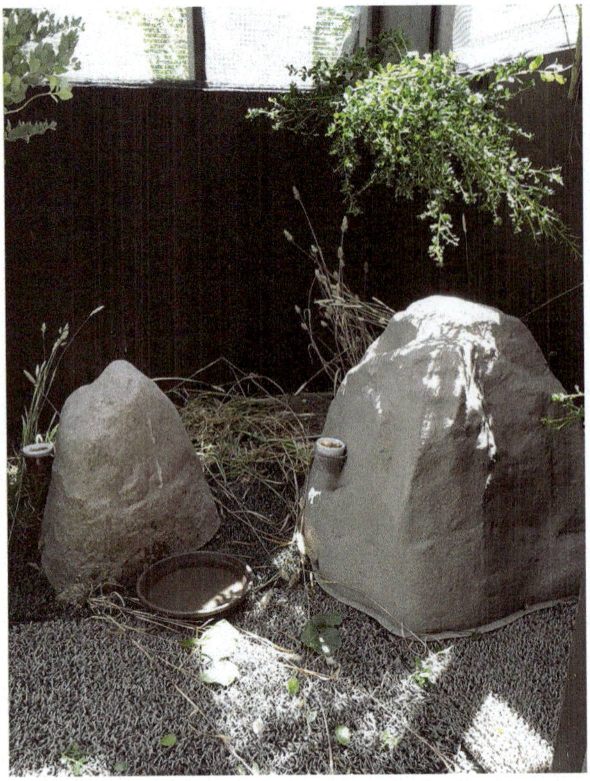

Figure 43.6 Dish arrangement in an aviary set up for Rock Wrens.

important to offer a shallow dish of clean dirt – birds must have access to dirt, but wrens in particular require it for dust baths. A source of free-choice calcium, such as ground cuttlebone or crushed sterilized eggshell, should be provided in a small dish.

In the fledgling cage, most wren species will roost at night in a cavity of some sort. Young wrens enjoy roosting in enclosed domestic finch nests, small nest boxes, or other similarly enclosed structures that are safe, hygienic, and have an opening. Do not use facial tissue boxes as they are not safe or hygienic. The size of the roosting nest will depend on the number of wrens in the enclosure. It may be necessary to offer two roosting options. Tightly crumpled tissue or a folded face cloth can be placed in the nest and changed regularly. Fledgling wrens will often retreat to the nest during the day for short naps.

Vireo fledglings may exhibit anxious behavior as they prepare to go to roost in the evening. They may be observed flying around the enclosure frantically searching through branches and vocalizing incessantly just after sunset. In the author's experience, this behavior is consistently observed with all species of vireo regularly in her care and has been witnessed among vireos in the wild. The birds finally settle into their roost once they have identified the perfect leaf under which to roost for the night. When setting up enclosures for vireos, it is essential to provide branches with leaves that are at least 3 in. (7.6 cm) wide and 4–5 in. (10.2–12.7 cm) in length (Figure 43.7). Arrange branches with leaves approximately 3 in. (7.6 cm) above perching branches. These branches should be placed in the upper elevation of the enclosure to facilitate the ideal roosting area for a vireo.

A note of caution: once flight-capable, each of these species is quick to escape their enclosure if given the opportunity. In certain environments, such as overcrowded busy nurseries, reptariums may not be a suitable or safe form of housing for these species. Alternatively, a screen-lined wire

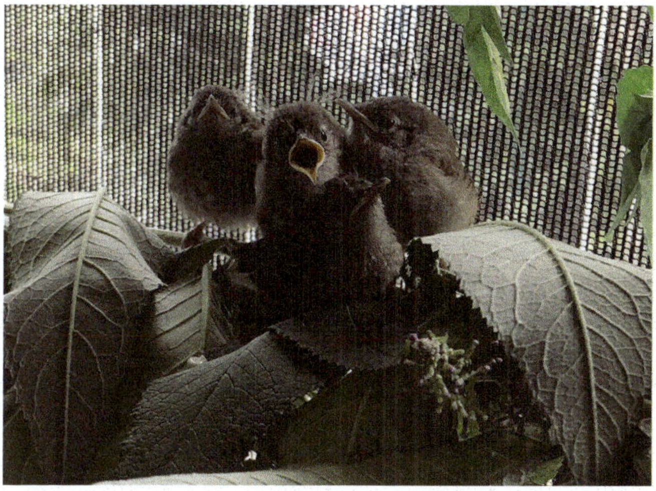

Figure 43.7 House Wren fledglings clustering together around greenery in an aviary.

cage approximately 4×3×3 ft. (1.2×0.9×0.9 m) with a small entrance can be used. A small square of window screen secured at the top of the entrance with safety pins or clothespins between the cage and the door of the cage to cover the entrance can prevent unwanted escapes when the cage door is opened for feeding and cleaning.

From 5 to 7 days after fledging, it is the author's preference to move Bushtits and wrens outdoors to an aviary while completing the hand-rearing process. Warblers and vireos are moved outdoors to an aviary approximately 2 to 3 days after fledging. Initially, birds are housed in a small 6×4×8 ft. (1.8×1.2×2.4 m) or 10×6×8 ft. (3×1.8×2.4 m) aviary that is furnished with appropriate enrichment and food presentation. The birds will remain on frequent hand-feeding in the outdoor enclosure and graduate to a larger pre-release conditioning aviary as soon as they are self-feeding. Hand-feeding small, highly active, stress-prone songbirds loose in an aviary may not be sensible or safe for the birds at a high-volume wildlife hospital with multiple caregivers.

When combining fledgling Bushtit groups or introducing a single Bushtit into an established group in an enclosure, be observant and watch for squabbles. A dominant bird in the flock may attack other members. Use extreme caution and watch for aggression when introducing a single fledgling to an established group.

Due to the variety of wren species in North America, enrichment and food presentation will vary. Previously described enclosure set up and care protocols are appropriate for Bewick's, House and Carolina Wrens. Cactus, Rock, Marsh Wren, and other less common wren species whose natural history and habitat criteria are unique will require research. Guidance for enclosure design, enrichment, and food presentation can be formulated based on the natural history unique to the species. A good place to start is the Birds of North America Online by the Cornell Lab of Ornithology, a comprehensive web-based resource that provides detailed species accounts of all North American birds.

## Create a Comfortable and Stress-Free Environment

Never house corvids, starlings, or grackles with or near other passerine species; these birds are aggressive and/or predatory species that most passerines seek to avoid in the wild. Do not house passerines within sight or sound of other predatory species such as mammals, birds of prey, and domestic pets.

## Pre-release Conditioning

An 8×8×8 ft. (2.4×2.4×2.4 m) aviary lined with fiberglass window screen to prevent feather damage and injury works well for up to 6 wrens, vireos or warblers; or 8 Bushtits; a 12×8×8 ft. (3.6×2.4×2.4 m) enclosure works well for up to 8 wrens or 15 Bushtits. One third to one fourth of the aviary should include a covered roof and solid walls to protect against weather and provide a secure place to roost and flee from the visual range of predators. The outside of the aviary should be lined with hardware cloth for protection against predators. A double-door system at the aviary entrance is strongly recommended to prevent premature and accidental escapes.

The aviary should be enriched with ample vegetation to simulate an appropriate habitat for the species. Suspend freshly cut leafy branches from the ceiling to create a forest canopy and introduce wild insects. Potted living shrubs and trees as well as logs with rough bark are also excellent enrichments to add in the enclosure. Create mid-story cover by affixing leafy branches to the walls of the enclosure. Vegetation should be dense at each end of the aviary for foraging and roosting, but some space in the middle should be left open for areas to fly without obstructions.

Using small metal binder clips or clothespins, fasten small, hanging domestic bird dishes of mini and small mealworms to branches. Bushtits, warblers, and vireos do not feed on or the ground, so their food sources should be elevated to mid-story and canopy level in the aviary. Wrens forage at all levels, but focus mostly at the mid-story and very low to the ground. Change branches frequently to introduce fresh wild insects. Shallow water dishes for bathing and drinking should be provided, as well as a shallow pan of fresh, clean dirt for dust baths on the floor of the aviary. A source of free-choice calcium, such as ground cuttlebone or crushed sterilized eggshell, should be provided in a small dish.

Brush piles are essential because wrens spend a great deal of time foraging low to the ground. Create brush piles using cut branches from trees, live potted shrubs and trees, or sections of artificial Christmas trees. Dishes of mealworms and fly pupae should be hidden in the piles of brush. A roost box or nest box should be secured high in the enclosure for roosting at night.

It is important to provide a variety of insects and foraging opportunities. Cultivated tiny stingless wasps can be purchased in pupae form and hatched in the aviary. Place the pupae in small domestic bird seed dishes and secure the dishes to branches. The wasps will hatch and disperse among the leafy branches to create insect gleaning opportunities. A compost bucket of rotting fruit to cultivate fruit flies is an inexpensive and effective means of providing additional foraging opportunities. When using a compost bucket in the aviary, cover the bucket with small gauge aviary wire to prevent accidents. For wrens, the bucket can be camouflaged with leafy branches. The insects will climb out of the bucket onto the leaves of the brush providing a natural environment for foraging. Warblers and vireos will take advantage of flycatching opportunities if the bucket is elevated on a milk crate or suspended a few feet from the ceiling.

Live 1- and 2-week old crickets are another excellent option to add variety to the diet and foraging in the aviary. Use the protocol described in Box 43.1 to care for and house live crickets. Secure a cricket-filled paper towel or toilet paper role into a dense leafy branch in the aviary with the ends folded in to create just one or two small holes where the crickets can crawl out one at a time, or place two cricket-filled toilet paper rolls in a suet cake basket hung in a cluster of leafy branches. One and two-week old crickets can be provided to wrens by dispensing the crickets into a brush pile in the aviary or containing the crickets in a cricket feeding rock found at reptile suppliers.

Self-feeding Bushtits should spend at least a full week in the aviary for pre-release conditioning. The pre-release conditioning enclosure should be located where local Bushtit flocks are present. To facilitate acceptance into the local flock, orphaned Bushtits raised from hatchling and nestling stage must learn the local language and develop a rapport with the local flock before release. The same process is required if releasing Bushtits back to their natal site. Hard releases into unknown territory will likely result in hostile attacks from the local Bushtit flock. Self-feeding wrens, warblers, and vireos should spend 10–14 days in the aviary for pre-release conditioning.

## Release

Birds ready for release should be aerobically fit, at adult weight, waterproof, have excellent feather condition, be totally self-feeding, recognize their natural diet, be able to forage for their natural diet successfully in the manner appropriate for the species, be free of disease and parasites, have fully recovered from injuries, and demonstrate a healthy fear of and appropriate response to all predators, including humans.

Bushtits must be released in a group in the appropriate habitat where there are other Bushtits present. Every effort should be made to release wrens, warblers, and vireos back to their natal territory. However, if that is not possible, select a location with appropriate habitat where the species is present. Releases should occur in the mid to late morning upon a forecast of 3 days of clear weather.

## Acknowledgments

Gifts of knowledge, advice, opportunity, humor, and experience have been bestowed upon me by many wonderful humans and birds. In numerous ways, they have supported me and helped me grow in my work as a wildlife rehabilitator. I am especially grateful to the late Rich Stallcup, Janine Perlman, PhD, Jayne Neville of Mount Vernon Songbird Sanctuary, my husband Lance Groody, Dr. Rebecca Duerr, DVM, Dr. Dan Famini, DVM, Dr. Shannon Riggs, DVM, and the amazing volunteers at Native Songbird Care & Conservation. And finally, my deepest gratitude to all of the magnificent passerines that grace this earth each day with their beauty and song.

## Sources for Products Mentioned

Cannula tip for feeding (aka teat infusion cannula): Jorgensen Labs, 1450 Van Buren Ave, Loveland, Colorado 80538, (800) 525-5614, https://www.jorvet.com/.

Flightless stingless wasps and freeze-dried insects: Arbico Organics, 10831 N. Mavinee Drive, Ste. 185, Oro Valley, AZ 85737-9531, (800) 847-2847, www.arbico-organics.com.

Mealworms, waxworms, Dubia roaches, fly larvae, fruit flies, and crickets: Rainbow Mealworms, 126 E. Spruce St, Compton, CA 90220, (800) 777-9676. https://www.rainbowmealworms.net/.

Mesh butterfly enclosures: Amazon.com.

Mesh reptariums, logs and bark, Cricket Rock feeder: LLLReptile and Supply Company Inc., 609 Mission Ave, Oceanside, CA 92054, (760) 439-8492, www.lllreptile.com.

Pancrezyme: Virbac Corporation, Fort Worth, TX, (844) 484-7222, https://us.virbac.com/products/digestive/pancrezyme-powder-and-tablets.

Recordings of song: Macaulay Library, Cornell Lab of Ornithology, 159 Sapsucker Woods Road, Ithaca, New York USA 14850 (607) 254-2404 www.macaulaylibrary.org.

Ultracare Mite and Lice Bird Spray: 8 in 1 Pet Products, Hauppauge, NY, (800) 645-5154.

## References

Duerr, R.S., Purdin, G.J., and Bowers, V. (2017). Small-bodied birds: passerines, doves, woodpeckers, others. In: *Topics in Wildlife Medicine, Vol. 4: Orthopedics* (eds. R.S. Duerr and G.J. Purdin), 53–74. St. Cloud, MN: National Wildlife Rehabilitators Association.

Hawkins, M.G., Barron, H.W., Speer, B.L. et al. (2018). Birds. In: *Exotic Animal Formulary*, 4e (eds. J.W. Carpenter and C.J. Marion), 167–375. St. Louis, MO: Elsevier.

Perlman, J. (2016). *Wildlife Rehabilitation: A Comprehensive Approach*, 120. International Wildlife Rehabilitation Council.

## Further Reading

Bowers, V. (2018). *Passerine Fundamentals*, 199 pp. Sebastopol, CA: Native Songbird Care and Conservation.

Elphick, C., Dunning, J.B., and Sibley, D.A. (2001). *The Sibley Guide to Bird Life and Behavior*, vol. 588. New York: Alfred A. Knopf, Inc.

International Wildlife Rehabilitation Council (2003). *Wildlife Nutrition and Feeding*, 73 pp. Eugene, OR: International Wildlife Rehabilitation Council.

MacLeod, A. and Perlman, J. (2001). Adventures in avian nutrition: dietary considerations for the hatchling and nestling passerine. *Journal of Wildlife Rehabilitation* 24 (1): 10–15.

Rodewald, P. (ed.). (2019). The Birds of North America: https://birdsna.org. Cornell Laboratory of Ornithology, Ithaca, NY.

# 44

# North American Swallows

*Veronica Bowers*

## Natural History

There are approximately 90 species of swallows found worldwide, except in Antarctica, and the greatest number of species is found in Africa. Eight of the 90 species occur in North America. All North American swallows are migratory, spending the breeding season in the U.S. and migrating as far as South America during the winter.

Swallows have long pointed wings, short bills, short legs, small delicate feet, and an anisodactyl toe arrangement with three toes forward and one toe back. Swallows are more aerial than other passerines and are graceful while in flight, much like swifts. All swallows are aerial insectivores, frequenting open areas for foraging, often near bodies of water. Swallows feed almost exclusively on flying insects. Tree Swallows are the only North American swallows known to occasionally consume certain types of berries during the winter.

Some species, such as Tree and Violet-green Swallows, nest in dispersed territories. Others, such as Barn Swallows, nest in aggregated groups. Cliff and Bank Swallows nest in colonies. Nest sites range from burrows to holes in trees, banks, and cliffs, to nest boxes or cup or gourd-shaped nests made of mud.

All species hatch altricial, naked, blind, and helpless young. Incubation ranges from 13 to 18 days. Both parents care for the young in all swallow species. Young swallows fledge the nest at approximately 3 weeks of age.

## Criteria for Intervention

The mud nests of Barn and Cliff Swallows are frequently knocked down by humans. Nests can also legitimately fall from structures on their own if an old nest was reused or there is a prolonged spell of extreme weather such as intense rain or a heatwave.

If a Barn Swallow nest has fallen, the nest remained mostly intact, and the young in the nest are uninjured, a nest replacement should be considered. To replace the nest, construct a cup-shaped basket out of 0.25 in. (0.5 cm) chicken wire and affix the basket in the exact location of the original nest. Make sure the basket is free of sharp edges or protruding pieces of wire that could cause injury to parent birds arriving at the nest or young in the nest. Insert the original nest with the

*Hand-Rearing Birds*, Second Edition. Edited by Rebecca S. Duerr and Laurie J. Gage.

chicks in the wire basket. Observe the nest from a distance until there is confirmation that the parents are tending to their young.

Nest replacement for Cliff Swallows is often not practical due to the physical structure of their fully enclosed gourd-shaped mud nests and the nature of their colonial nesting habits. When a human knocks a Cliff Swallow nest down, they usually remove a significant portion of or the entire colony, which may lead to dozens or a hundred or more nestlings requiring care simultaneously. Fostering some of the uninjured orphaned nestlings into nests of other Cliff Swallow families is possible, but must be done with extreme care. To evaluate potential foster families for an orphaned swallow, consider the following: age of young in the recipient nest, number of chicks in the recipient nest, and health of the orphaned swallow. The ages of the foster family and orphan must be the same and not older than 12 days old, the number of chicks in the nest should not exceed 5, and the orphaned swallow must be in good health without injuries, illness, or parasites. The recipient nest must also be accessible by a human. Due to the structural nature of Cliff Swallow nests, it can be very difficult to make these observations, especially if the young in the potential recipient nest are less than 10 days old. Never stick hands into Cliff Swallow nests because there is a high risk of damaging nests. There is also high risk of premature fledging for any swallow species if they are disturbed in the nest at 12 days of age or older. Fostering an orphaned Barn Swallow into another Barn Swallow family is slightly less challenging because their nest style and young are visually accessible, making them easy to evaluate without getting too close to the nest. Fostering opportunities for Northern Rough-winged Swallows are rare due to the often-obscure location (drainpipes, bridge weep holes, etc.) of their nest.

Always observe from a distance first to determine approximate age of the foster family's nestlings. Nestlings 12 days and older are very vocal and often poke their heads out the nest entrance. Their faces will be well feathered and have a few tufts of natal down may still be intact on top of the head. Observe the behavior of the parents after they deliver a meal to the nestlings. Typically, swallow parents cease removing fecal sacs from the nest when their young reach 8–12 days of age (Purple Martins continue removing fecal sacs from the nest through fledging). Never attempt to stick anything into or closely approach a nest containing this age group of swallows as doing so may cause the inhabitants to fledge prematurely.

If the initial assessment appears to be a promising candidate for a foster family and the nest is accessible, proceed with closer inspection of the nestlings. A small dental mirror and penlight can be used to gain more direct visual access to assess foster potential of Cliff, Tree and Violet-green Swallow nests as well as Purple Martin. A more effective and less invasive means to inspecting a cavity-type nest is the use of a wireless endoscope. These devices are relatively inexpensive (around $50 on amazon.com), can be used with a smartphone, and require fewer implements and maneuvering to view the inside of a nest with minimal disturbance. Make sure the operator of the scope has very steady hands and practice using the device before attempting to evaluate a nest.

Tree and Violet-green Swallows are cavity-nesters. They will nest in tree hollows as well as nest boxes. If an active nest is destroyed by tree removal, healthy vocal nestlings can easily be re-nested in a nest box mounted on a pole in the same location where the tree was. Remove the nest and nestlings from the cavity of the tree and place in the nest box. Observe the nest box from a distance and watch for the parents to respond to the food cries of the young. Do not leave the young alone in the nest box until parents have been observed entering the nest box and have been confirmed as feeding the young. As described above, fostering healthy orphans of Tree and Violet-green swallows into active nests of same species is also an option. Foster nests should not be disturbed if the young in the nest are 12 days or older. Young of these species at this age can prematurely launch from the nest and will likely continue to launch themselves from the nest even after attempts to re-nest.

Fledgling swallows are often brought into rehabilitation centers for care after they have collided with a structure or car or have had an unfortunate encounter with a domestic cat. Rarely are they victims of kidnapping. Swallows are flight capable when they first fledge the nest. During the first day out of the nest they may not be strong enough to sustain flight for extended periods of time, so it is common to observe vulnerable-looking youngsters resting on a fence, rooftop or less typically on the ground. When approached, a healthy fledgling should fly away; if it does not, it is likely in need of rescue.

## Record Keeping

See Chapter 1.

## Initial Care and Stabilization

Follow the basic steps for Intake and Initial Care described in Chapter 1. As is good practice for all species' chicks, warm chicks to normal body temperatures, then provide fluids as per each chick's hydration status, then commence feedings once chicks start producing droppings. Depending on the age and condition of the bird, the ambient heat of an incubator set between 85 and 92 °F (29.4–33.3 °C) will be required to keep the bird comfortable. Emaciated or chilled birds will require more thermal support, up to 95 °F (35 °C).

Gaping active hatchling, nestling and fledgling swallows can easily be rehydrated orally with a rehydration solution appropriate for the condition of the bird. Oral fluids can safely be administered by inserting a 1 ml syringe into the mouth, make sure the hub of the syringe has passed the glottis before carefully administering 0.05 ml of fluids at a time. Remove the syringe from the mouth after each administration of fluid and allow the bird to swallow before offering more fluids. It is important to remember that severely dehydrated birds may require fluid therapy for up to 72 hours. Of course, this does not mean that food is withheld until they are fully rehydrated. Once the bird is stable, continue to carefully administer fluids orally in tandem with their hand-feeding diet at scheduled intervals appropriate for their age until they are fully rehydrated. During initial care, soaking cricket bodies in the Oral Rehydration Solution found in Perlman (2016) is an effective means to provide important nutrients and hydration to dehydrated nestlings and fledglings that are stable enough to receive whole food. Always monitor droppings to ensure there are no issues with digestion and assimilation of food during initial care.

Swallows are obligate faunivores and should be fed a diet consisting exclusively of insects and micronutrient supplements. Nestling and fledgling swallows should receive a hand-feeding diet of assorted whole insects (mealworms, crickets, Dubia roaches, waxworms) supplemented with vitamins and calcium using the Supplements for Hand-rearing Passerines (see Box 44.1 in this chapter). Hatchling swallows, 0–3 days old, should be fed the Diet for Hatchling Passerines in Chapter 43.

Commercially prepared or homemade hand-feeding formulas are inappropriate diets for swallows and other obligate insectivores. These diets do not provide optimal nutrients to support rapid growth and development of passerines. In addition to problems such as soiled feathers and accidental aspiration, formula-based hand-feeding diets also seem to be less palatable to swallow species and other obligate insectivores.

## Box 44.1 Supplements for Birds Hand-reared on an Insects-only Diet

*©Janine Perlman, PhD, 2019*
*Used with permission*

*Introduction*

All nestlings whose parents feed them insects in nature should be reared on an all-insects diet (Fusté et al. 2013; Perlman 2016). Use supplements made for humans. Products made for animals are often poorly formulated and have inadequate quality control. Each chick fed an insect-only diet must be supplemented daily with EACH of the TWO nutrient mixes described below to avoid deficiencies.

*Calcium/Taurine/Thiamine/Vitamin C Mix*

Open and squeeze the contents of one capsule of 600 mg elemental calcium (as $CaCO_3$) in oil containing 500 IU vitamin D (Puritan's Pride) out on a flat surface.

Separately, mix 500 mg taurine powder with 500 mg vitamin C powder and 50 mg thiamine. Mix 1/5 of this taurine/thiamine/vitamin C mixture with the contents of one capsule of the calcium/vit D paste. Mix to make a uniform paste. This results in a mixture containing 100 mg of taurine, 10 mg thiamine, 100 mg vitamin C, 600 mg elemental Ca, and 500 IU vitamin D. Feed by daubing onto one (or more, if needed) insects.

Feed 1/10 (one-tenth = 60 mg elemental Ca) of the mixture for each 10 g of live (wet weight) insects fed. This is the most accurate method of supplementation.

A less precise (and less preferable) dosing method: For nestlings under 20 g, give 1/10 of the total (60 mg elemental Ca) daily; over 20 g, give 1/5 of the total (120 mg elemental Ca) daily.

*Oil-Vitamin Mix*

- 5 cc omega-3 marine (fish) oil
- 10 000 IU vitamin A
- 400 IU vitamin E
- If vitamin D3 is not present in the Calcium/Taurine/Vitamin C mix supplement, 5000 IU vitamin D3 should be added to the Oil-Vitamin mix

Squeeze out contents of gel caps and mix thoroughly, minimizing oxygenation; store refrigerated, in the absence of air, for up to 2weeks.

Give 0.05 cc per day per 25 kcal, on food. Less precisely, give 0.05 cc to birds under 20 g; 0.1 cc per day to larger nestlings/fledglings. (Editor's note: See Table 41.1 for caloric value of typical feeder insects.)

This supplies approximately 4 IU of vitamin A, 2 IU of vitamin D and 0.2 IU vitamin E, per kcal consumed.

Each vitamin can be bought as an oil-based solution in gel caps from manufacturers such as NOW® Foods or Puritan's Pride™.

### Sources of Products Mentioned

600 mg calcium/500 IU Vit D capsules: Puritan's Pride, 1233 Montauk Highway, PO Box 9001, Oakdale, NY 11769-9001, (800) 645-1030, http://www.puritan.com/calcium-supplements-001/absorbable-calcium-1200-mg-with-vitamin-d-1000-iu-006272.
500 mg taurine: NOW Foods, 244 Knollwood Drive, Bloomingdale, IL 60108, (888) 669-3663, https://www.nowfoods.com/supplements/taurine-500-mg-capsules.

### References


Fusté, E., Obon, E., and Olid, L. (2013). Hand-reared common swifts (*Apus apus*) in a wildlife rehabilitation centre: assessment of growth rates using different diets. *J. Zoo Aquarium Res.* 1 (2): 61–68.

Perlman, J. 2016. Nutrition and nutritional management. In: *Avian Medicine* 3. J. Samour (ed.), Elsevier, St. Louis, MO, pp. 25–32.

## Common Medical Problems

### Parasites

Ectoparasites, such as mites and lice, are common among swallows and easily treated with a pyrethrin spray such as Ultracare Mite and Lice Spray (8 in 1). Mist the spray onto a cottonball or gauze pad and gently swab the mite-affected areas of the bird. Avoid the eyes, nares and mouth, and never spray directly onto the bird. Change the bedding and housing frequently until parasites are no longer present. Quarantine infested birds until all parasites are gone. Administer an oral dose of ivermectin at 0.2 mg/kg once (Hawkins et al. 2018).

Other ectoparasites such as blowfly larvae are also common, especially among Cliff Swallows. Birds infested with blowfly should be treated with an oral dose of ivermectin and an antibiotic. Remove larvae and eggs from the bird's body and feathers, and flush the affected area with warm saline, if needed. See www.birdblowfly.com for fascinating information about this parasite.

Swallows can present with internal parasites, so it is good practice to conduct a fecal smear or float, and sometimes a direct smear of the mouth and throat as well. In 2006, the author experienced an outbreak of oral trichomoniasis among several dozen young swallows and found that a course of ronidazole was an effective treatment; carnidazole was ineffective on that occasion. Consult your avian veterinarian for medications to treat internal parasite infection.

### Stress

Stress in captivity can be detrimental to any wild bird, swallows are especially susceptible to stress. When hand-raising these species, they are best cared for under the supervision of one caregiver and must be provided a quiet and calm environment dedicated to the unique needs of the species.

### Caught by Cat

Cat-caught birds should immediately be started on an antibiotic such as Clavamox (Hawkins et al. 2018). Small wounds should be cleaned with warm water or sterile saline. A tiny amount of sulfa silvadene, or other water-soluble antibiotic cream can be applied if necessary. Administer pain medication, such as meloxicam. See Chapter 1 for more information on wound care.

### Fractures

Wing fractures must be carefully evaluated. Swallows are migratory aerial feeding birds and therefore must have 100% recovery from a wing fracture. A fractured humerus typically has a poor prognosis. Keel fractures are not uncommon, especially for nestlings that fell from the nest or were victims of nest destruction. Less than perfect recovery from a keel fracture will impact ability for perfect flight. Confirmation of full recovery from any fracture affecting a bird's ability to fly should be evaluated post-healing when the bird is at the age it should be flying. The assessment should be conducted in an aviary no less than 24 ft. (7.3 m) in length and 12 ft. (3.7 m) in width. Anything less than those dimensions will not provide adequate space for evaluation, as the bird will not be able to gain reasonable speed nor bank and turn in flight.

Leg fractures are common in nestlings and have a higher success rate for recovery due to the feeding behavior and perching preferences of swallows. However, full functionality of legs and feet are required for release back to the wild, especially for species such as Cliff and Barn Swallows that cling to vertical surfaces during nest construction. See Duerr et al. (2017) for more information regarding management of orthopedic problems in small birds.

## Dehydration and Emaciation

A large percentage of young swallows delivered to rehabilitators will present with some degree of dehydration or emaciation or both. It is not uncommon to maintain a severely dehydrated swallow on a fluid therapy regimen for a few days after initial intake. More severely dehydrated birds may require fluids to be administered subcutaneously.

In addition to dehydration, orphaned swallows can present with varying levels of emaciation. For emaciated swallows, determine the cause and follow the appropriate protocol. The oral rehydration solution by Perlman (2016) works exceptionally well as part of the initial care of emaciated and dehydrated swallows. Emaciated fledglings should receive supplemental heat in an incubator set at 85–90 °F (29.4–32.2 °C), nestlings 90–95 °F (32.2–35 °C).

## Feather Damage

Fledgling and nestling swallows, Cliff Swallows in particular, occasionally present with damaged feathers. Blowflies, swallow bugs and deer mice are known to predate Cliff Swallow nests and, less frequently, other swallow species. These nest parasites cause damage to nestlings and their feathers by feeding on the blood-engorged developing feathers. Blowfly larvae will also burrow into the skin, nares, and ears of hatchlings and nestlings. Adult flies will puncture the skin and deposit their eggs under the skin of hatchling and nestling birds.

Feather damage as well as serious physical injury can be inflicted upon nestling Cliff and Barn Swallows when cruel humans remove active nests by power washing or scraping with rakes and poles.

Poor feather condition can also result from improper housing (too small, or not lined with soft screen material), confinement indoors too long, poor husbandry, and incorrect diet while in captivity. Broken and damaged feathers can be pulled to allow regrowth of healthy new feathers before it is time for the birds to depart on their fall migration. However, keep in mind that the process of pulling and regrowth can take 4–8 weeks depending on the number of damaged feathers. Due to time constraints and migratory departure dates, it may be necessary to overwinter a bird with damaged feathers and allow it to go through a natural molt.

Never pull damaged feathers that are still in blood and growing, only pull damaged feathers when they are fully grown with a mature shaft (rachis). Pulling feathers is painful for the bird and should only be done using proper technique and under the supervision of a veterinarian. Naturally, removal of feathers for regrowth of healthy feathers should not be pursued unless proper housing, diet, and other essentials of good husbandry can be provided. If the rehabilitator is unable to meet the needs of this species, the birds should be transferred to a facility specializing in swallows.

The number of damaged feathers and whether they are secondaries or primaries will dictate how many and in what order to pull at a given interval. Never pull all damage feathers at once, only pull every other feather. Wait for the pulled feathers to fully regrow, and then pull the next set of every other feather. If all the primaries are damaged and require replacement, the best practice is to begin with odd feathers first, P1, 3, 5, 7, and 9; then P2, 4, 6; and finally, P8 and P10. It is important to save P8 and P10 for last as they require the protection and stability provided by the other feathers.

## Diet

Swallows must be hand-raised using an all-insect diet. Swallows are obligate faunivores, more specifically, they are insectivores. This means they must eat insect protein. Depending on the age of the bird, insects for hand-feeding can include domestically cultivated mealworms, waxworms, crickets, dubia roaches, fly larvae, house flies and fruit flies. Nestlings and fledglings should be fed whole insects supplemented as described in the Supplementation instructions within this chapter. Supplements are essential to a complete and nutritious all-insect hand-feeding diet because available feeder insects are typically deficient in several important nutrients needed by growing birds. Hatchling birds should be fed the Diet for Hatchling Passerines shown in Chapter 43. Make sure that birds hand-fed with an all-insect diet receive their supplements every day until they are self-feeding.

Live cultivated insects, such as mealworms, crickets, and Dubia roaches, should be fed a nutritious diet before being used as a food source for avian patients. The author prefers to feed mealworms and Dubia roaches a diet of bran, nonmedicated poultry starter crumbles and vegetables that are high in carotenoids, such as carrot and yam. Care, feeding, and preparation for use as food for crickets and Dubia roaches can be found in Chapter 43.

When purchasing cultivated insects for swallows, order small (not to exceed ½ in. or 1.25 cm in length) mealworms, crickets, and Dubia roaches. As young birds begin to learn to self-feed, medium and large sized insects are difficult for swallows to pick up on their own and ingest, and are an inappropriate size of "prey" for birds their size. Waxworms can be added for variety, but should only comprise a small amount of the daily insect intake, approximately 5%. Waxworms offer hydration, but are not as nutritious as other available cultivated insects. Commercially available freeze-dried flies are also a good addition to the diet of self-feeding swallows when sprinkled over a dish of live mealworms (Arbico).

## Feeding Procedures

Swallows do not possess a true crop, such as a finch or dove, instead they have the ability to slightly expand their proventriculus to accommodate varying amounts of food delivered by their parents. Take care when a health condition requires assist-feeding (force-feeding) a swallow, as overfeeding can cause food to back up into the throat and aspirate the bird or even rupture the proventriculus.

To achieve optimum growth and healthy weight, young swallows should be hand fed for 14–16 hours a day, every 20–30 minutes, from sunrise to sunset, until they are self-feeding (Figure 44.1). If the bird is in good health, feed them as much as they wish to eat at each feeding interval. If the bird is in poor health with a suppressed appetite, you will need to calculate the kcals needed to support the growth and health condition of a young swallow. Feeding amounts for each feeding interval can be determined based on the kcal calculations and amounts shown in Appendix B. Table 41.1 shows the caloric value of typical feeder insects.

Extreme care must be used to keep their feathers, face, and body parts free of food and fecal matter at all times. Perfect feather condition is essential to any bird's survival upon release and it is a matter of life or death for a migratory aerial insectivore. Food accumulated in the nares, around the eyes, or on the bill or bill commissure of hatchlings and nestlings can result in bacterial infections and bill deformities. Contaminants on skin can cause hypothermia. Contaminants on feather tracts can inhibit healthy growth and emergence of feathers. It is imperative that birds are kept clean at all stages of development! Immediately remove any contaminants from the bird using a cotton swab or soft cloth dampened with warm water.

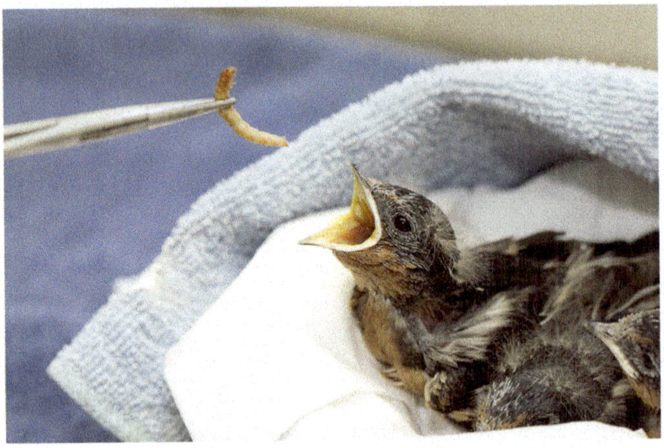

Figure 44.1 Hemostat feeding nestlings.

Observe the droppings at each feeding. Loose, runny feces can be the result of illness or incorrect diet. A lack of droppings can be a sign of dehydration or underfeeding. Droppings with an orange color can be a sign of underfeeding or bacterial infection. If whole undigested insects are present in feces, use smaller pieces of insect and tenderize the insect bodies first before feeding them to the birds. Healthy droppings should be well-formed, moist, and in a fecal sac.

It is advisable to establish a food call when hand-feeding swallows; a short double whistle is usually effective. This is helpful in stimulating a gape response and can be used later during the weaning process once the birds are in the aviary for pre-release conditioning.

Healthy young birds will readily gape when they are hungry. If a young swallow is not gaping, it may be dehydrated, cold, receiving an inappropriate diet, housed incorrectly, ill, or have a painful physical condition that needs to be addressed. It is common for older nestling and fledgling swallows to be fearful of humans and reluctant to gape when they are first delivered to a rehabilitator. If they are in good health, they should be housed with another swallow of similar age who is also in good health and gaping well. This will teach the reluctant gaper his new means of receiving food. If a nestmate is unavailable, a mirror placed next to the nest may be helpful in stimulating a gape response. This should be used as a temporary solution. Swallows should never be raised singly. If necessary, contact another rehabilitator to locate a swallow nestmate of similar age.

## Hatchlings (0–3 Days of Age)

Administer small amounts of the Diet for Hatchling Passerines (see Chapter 43 for recipe), 0.01 cc at a time, using a 1 cc syringe with a cannula tip (Jorgensen). Tiny pieces of white mealworms (mealworms that have recently shed their exoskeleton), or mini crickets (usually crickets 1 week of age) can be fed using a pair of blunt-end forceps or hemostats. Hemostats are preferred because forceps and tweezers can accidentally spring open in the mouth. Feedings should be small and frequent, every 10–15 minutes for at least 14 hours a day; 16 hours a day is optimal.

## Nestlings (4–9 Days of Age)

Nestling swallows are fed the supplemented all-insect diet every 20–30 minutes, 14–16 hours a day. Insects with tough exoskeletons, such as mealworms and crickets, may require tenderizing. To tenderize, pinch the body and head of mealworms with hemostats and remove the legs and crush the head and thorax of crickets. Tip: to prevent dehydration, mealworms can be drowned in a dish of water before hand-feeding to nestlings. To prevent aspiration, be sure to shake off excess water before feeding the worm to the bird.

### Older Nestlings (10–21 Days of Age)

Continue to feed older nestlings the supplemented all-insect diet every 30 minutes. Older nestlings can easily consume and digest live mealworms, so there is no need to pre-kill them. Pre-killing crickets and Dubia roaches as described in Chapter 43 is recommended for convenience and ease of hand-feeding. Insects with tough exoskeletons, such as mealworms, may still require tenderizing by squeezing the body with hemostats, crickets can be tenderized by crushing the head and thorax, and removing wings and legs. Dubia roaches have a fairly tender exoskeleton and should not require crushing if they are a small size appropriate for the age of the bird.

### Fledglings (21–23 Days and Older)

Feed fledgling swallows every 30 minutes, 14–16 hours a day. When they begin to pick up food on their own, slowly transition to every 45 minutes, 14–16 hours a day, until they are proficiently self-feeding. Continue to feed the all-insect diet with supplements. Discontinue supplements as soon as the birds are self-feeding.

At a certain point during the fledgling stage, swallows may resist accepting an insect dipped in the calcium paste component of the supplement. At this point, if more calcium is getting on the bird than in the bird, switch to powdered calcium carbonate sprinkled on the insects in a dish prepared exclusively for hand-feeding. IMPORTANT: calculate the amount of calcium carbonate powder needed based on the amount of worms fed. Remember to mix/shake the worms in the dish *before each feeding* to redistribute the calcium powder. Once secured in the hemostats, swirl the worm around the bottom of the dish to pick up additional calcium before administering to the bird. This technique is only for older fledglings. DO NOT use it for nestlings.

If the calcium paste component of the vitamin supplement protocol is discontinued and calcium carbonate powder is used, it is still necessary to administer the vitamin oil component of the supplement protocol once a day until the bird is self-feeding. Please note, if not already included in the vitamin oil preparation, vitamin D will need to be added.

### Transitioning to Self-feeding

Older fledgling swallows should remain on a 45-minute hand-feeding schedule until proficient self-feeding is confirmed. Reduce hand-feeding intervals to 1 hour when consistent signs of self-feeding are observed and the birds show less interest in receiving hand-feedings. There will always be a few individuals in a group that take longer to self-feed. Do not rush them. Continue with frequent and regular feeding intervals for as long as the need is indicated. Swallows will fail to thrive if rushed during this phase of their development. It is advisable to conduct a thorough physical exam and fecal analysis for individuals who have not shown interest in self-feeding.

### Expected Weight Gain

Hatchling swallow weights range from 5 to 8 g for birds 3–5 days old depending on the species. Nestling swallow weights vary widely, depending on the species. The greatest rate of growth and development occurs between days 5 and 10 for all swallow species, with an average weight gain of 2 g per day. Fledgling swallows will typically exceed adult weights by 2–3 g. It is important to chart weights over time to determine optimal body weights for each species in that region.

## Housing

### Hatchlings

Hatchlings are birds aged 0–3 days old. Their eyes are closed, they are naked with a small amount of natal down, and they cannot thermoregulate. Hatchling swallows should be kept in an incubator set at 92–95 °F (33.3–35 °C) with 50% humidity. An artificial nest can be created using a small round plastic container lined with a face cloth or similar fabric for insulation and softness. Fill the center of the nest with tightly crumpled tissue or a square, soft felt fabric to form the shape and shallow cup of a natural nest. Proper texture of the lining and shape of the nest interior provide important support for the body of a developing young bird. Choose a size of container that will comfortably accommodate the number of hatchlings/nestlings to inhabit the nest. Lay another piece of soft felt or a folded tissue over the hatchlings to simulate a brooding parent and provide warmth and security.

Never house more than five swallows in a nest as overcrowding and soiling each other with fecal matter will become an issue. To minimize handling of birds and reduce the number of times nest substrate is changed throughout the day, fecal sacs can be manually removed from the nest by using a pair of hemostats to carefully extract the sac. Take extreme care to avoid pinching a limb or other body part of the hatchlings.

### Nestlings

At 4 days of age, their eyes begin to open. At this point, a nest that simulates a more natural style of nest should be provided. Nestling swallows of all species are most comfortable in a slightly enclosed nest; even Barn Swallows who are not cavity-nesting species prefer this style of nest. Create an enclosed nest by forming a “cave” using a thick terry cloth hand towel folded in half and placed in a way that creates a dome over two-thirds of the nest (Figure 44.2). The opening of the towel cave should be large enough to allow the caregiver to administer food without moving the towel and disturbing the nestlings. The opening should also allow enough space for the nestlings to comfortably defecate out the entrance of the nest. It is essential to keep enclosures and nests clean. Towels and tissues must be changed as soon as they become soiled.

Nestlings that are 4–5 days old may also benefit from the ambient heat and humidity of an incubator at approximately 88–90 °F (31.1–32.2 °C). A group of nestlings 5 days and older, in good health with pinfeathers, are typically able to thermoregulate, and do not require housing in an incubator if the nursery has a mild ambient temperature. It is the author’s preference to house nestling swallows approximately 5–6 days old in the following manner: remaining in their nest with a towel cave, nestlings can safely be moved from the incubator and into a soft-sided 38-gal (144 l) reptarium or similar housing, as long as they are healthy, able to thermoregulate, and pinfeathers have emerged. If needed, offer supplemental heat for a few additional days until nestlings are partially feathered. Supplemental heat can be provided using a heating pad on the lowest setting or a gooseneck lamp with a ceramic heat bulb.

By 7–8 days of age, swallows begin defecating out the entrance of the nest. It is important that the nest is set up correctly with a towel cave to create a nest entrance. A layer of paper towels can

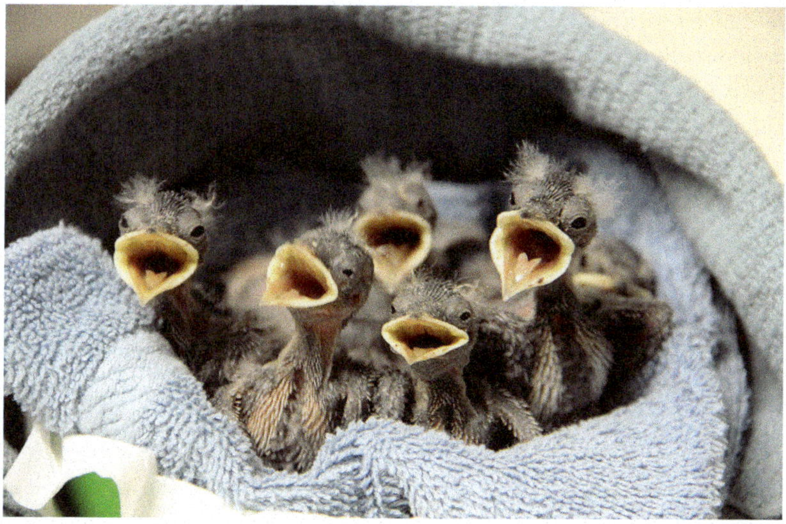

Figure 44.2 Cliff Swallow nestlings in a dome nest.

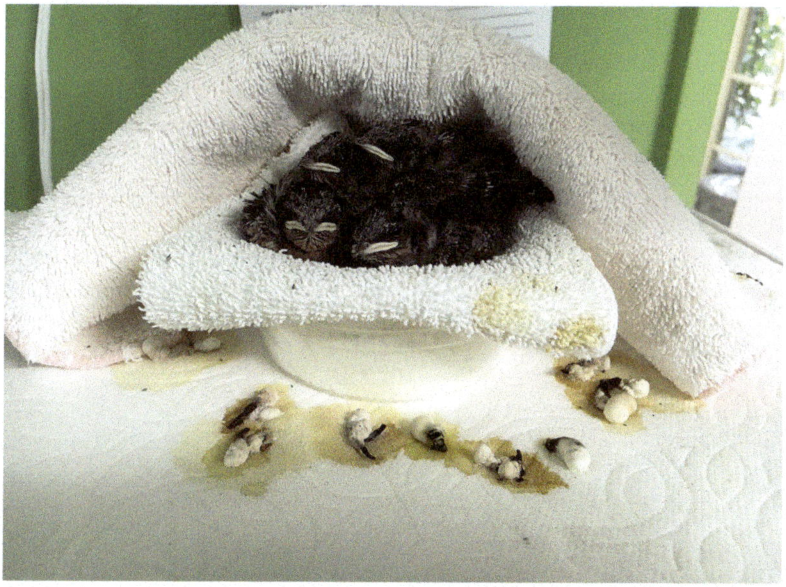

Figure 44.3 Nestling swallows with proper nest set up in a reptarium. The cave towel and nest opening supports natural defecation behavior so nestlings can easily defecate over the edge of the nest. Multiple layers of paper towels under nest facilitate easy clean-up throughout the day.

be placed on the substrate in front of the nest to catch the droppings and facilitate easy clean up (Figure 44.3).

By 18 days of age, swallows begin perching on the edge or entrance of their nests and exercising their wings. In preparation for "Fledge Day," the nest and/or towel cave should be moved to a larger reptarium, such as a 175-gal (4 × 3 × 3 ft./1.2 × 0.9 × 0.9 m) mesh reptarium or similar housing, so the birds have room to fledge from the nest naturally and enjoy a space to use their wings.

At fledgling stage, no more than six to eight birds should be housed in this size of reptarium. See "Fledgling" housing in the next section for setup criteria.

Once thermoregulating and partially feathered, nestling Purple Martins can be comfortably housed in nest boxes. This form of housing will provide a more typical nesting environment for the species and support their natural fledging process. Large wooden nest boxes used for breeding domestic exotic birds work well for young martins. Form a shallow cup-shaped nest inside the box using a non-terry towel. This style of nest box opens from the top, making access for hand-feeding easy, and the entry holes are usually a larger 3 in. (7.6 cm) opening. It is highly recommended that a wash cloth or small piece of fabric is folded over one side of the top of the box. This will keep the box lid slightly ajar, which eliminates a potentially disruptive noise when opening the box and prevents the lid from accidentally slamming closed. Once fledged, Purple Martins will return to their nest box for naps and to roost at night. The next box can also be placed in the aviary for fledglings.

Unlike many other passerine species, swallows have a long nesting period of approximately 3 weeks. If you are uncertain whether an orphaned swallow is a nestling or a fledgling, assume it is a nestling and provide a nest. Even if it is a fledgling, it will most likely appreciate the option of having the security of a nest as long as this is constructed properly.

## Fledglings

Depending on the species, swallows fledge the nest between days 20 and 23 (Figure 44.4). Purple Martins fledge at approximately day 28. At this time, a bungee cord or rope perch, a natural perch such as a willow branch with leaves, and a log should be provided in the 175-gal reptarium (4×3 ×3 ft./1.2×0.9×0.9 m) or similar size soft-sided screen-lined enclosure. The nest style should be changed for fledgling Cliff, Barn, and Northern Rough-winged Swallows and remain in the enclosure until the birds are no longer returning to sleep in it. When it is time to go to roost, newly fledged swallows will become anxious and active as they search for a place to roost. At this time, they are looking for their nest to retreat to. The nest should be securely attached in an upper corner

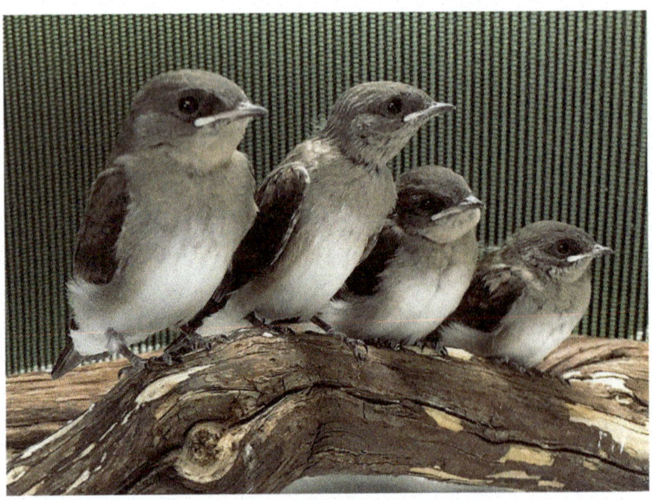

Figure 44.4 Four newly-fledged Northern Rough-winged Swallows perching on a log inside a reptarium.

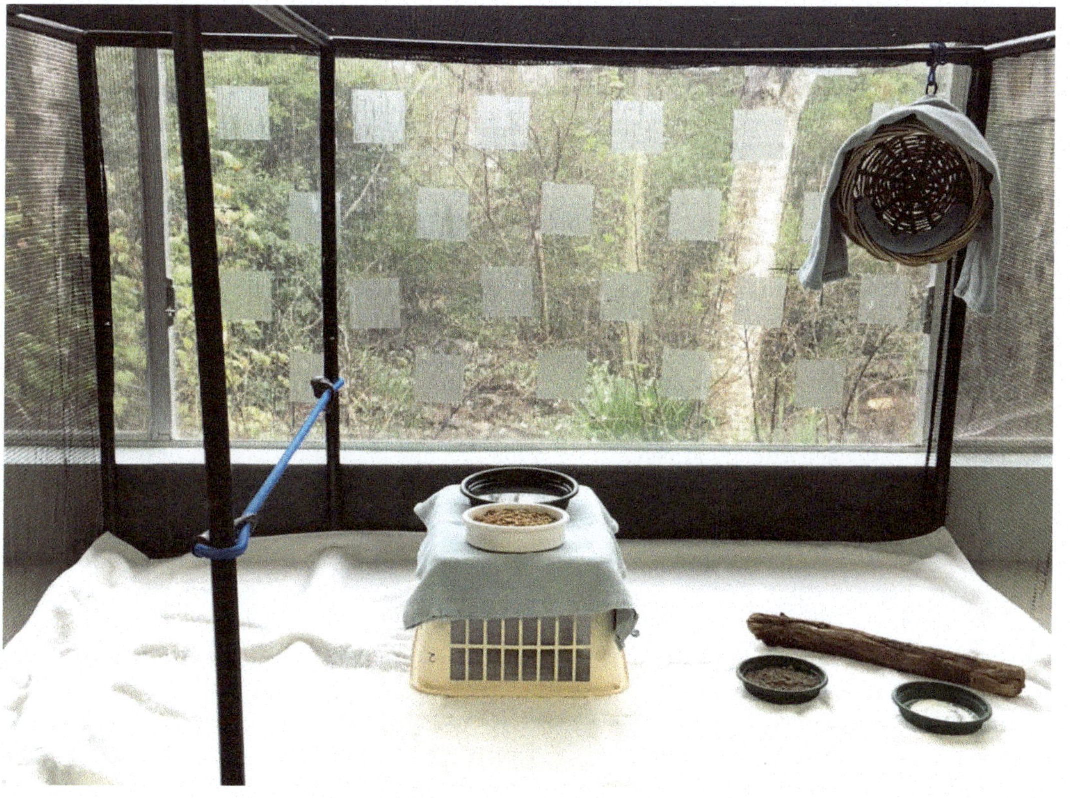

Figure 44.5 Inside housing in a reptarium. Note the elevated nest mounted in a corner of the reptarium for fledglings to rest and roost in overnight.

of the reptarium (Figure 44.5), or if in an aviary, in an upper corner of the sheltered end of the aviary. These species will continue to take naps during the day and sleep at night in the nest up to 1 to 2 weeks after fledgling. Purple Martins also tend to roost in their nest box at night, sometimes all the way up to release day. Violet-green and Tree Swallows generally do not return to their nest once they have fledged, so it is not necessary to provide a nest for fledglings of these species. However, if either of these species is housed with Barn Swallows, it is likely they will attempt to roost in the nest with Barn Swallows.

The new nest style will depend on the species. Fledgling Cliff and Northern Rough-winged Swallows require an enclosed nest. This can easily be achieved using a bowl-shaped small wicker basket and hanging it in one corner of the reptarium. Line the interior with a folded non-terry cloth towel. It is also a good idea to cover the top of the basket with a similar material as swallows can and will sit and defecate on the top of the basket. Barn Swallows prefer a simulated cup-shaped nest at fledgling age. Wicker baskets designed to hang on walls can emulate this shape and are easily found in craft and floral supply stores.

After fledging the nest, it is the author's preference to move fledgling swallows outside to aviaries as doing so supports their natural behavior and developmental process. At this stage, they are fully flighted and active. In the wild, their parents will feed them while perched in the open on fences and telephone wires, as well as provide mid-air food transfers when the young are in flight. Continuing the hand-feeding process in an aviary will foster development of strong flight and agility and support the behavior of obtaining food while in flight.

If fledglings are housed indoors, much of their natural behavior and development will be suppressed, so extra care must be taken to encourage food exploration and self-feeding as soon as the birds fledge the nest. Indoor enclosures for fledgling swallows should contain low-sided clear dishes of mealworms, waxworms, and freeze-dried insects presented at perch level. Perches should be elevated to approximately 10–12 in. (25–30.5 cm) from the floor of the enclosure. A "table" of some sort can be used to elevate the dishes to perch level (Figure 44.5). Provide a wide, shallow dish of water for drinking and bathing, a small saucer of clean dirt and a small saucer of free-choice calcium can be offered in a clearing on the floor of the indoor enclosure.

Although less optimal, food can be presented in hanging dishes used for pet birds and attached to the wall of the enclosure placed at perch level. Alternatively, the same type of dish can be attached directly to the perch if the type of perch is a rigid wooden branch rather than a bungee cord. Hanging pet food dishes present some difficulties. For example, if they are hung through the mesh wall of a reptarium, the dish often tips forward just enough to allow some mealworms to escape. Dishes attached directly to perches are often perched on and pooped in. Because of these issues, elevate food to perch level using an inverted plastic hospital basket, or similar item with a stable base and wide enough surface to accommodate the dishes for food and water.

On the day of fledging or shortly thereafter, move fledgling swallows outside to a 6 × 10 ft. (1.8 × 3 m) aviary. Here they will continue to be hand-fed at regular 30-minute intervals, 14–16 hours a day. As soon as they initiate self-feeding, they are moved to a 12 × 30 ft. (3.6 × 9.1 m) aviary where they remain on a hand-feeding schedule until they are completely self-feeding and refuse hand-feedings. Once self-feeding, they will remain in the same aviary for 10–14 days of pre-release conditioning.

When hand-feeding swallows in an aviary, birds should be encouraged to take their food on the wing. This can be done easily by holding an insect in the forceps up in the air several feet away from the birds while they are perched. Giving a food call to the birds and bobbing the forceps up and down a few inches will attract the swallow's attention. When the bird approaches the forceps to snap up the food, it is important to remember to release the food so the bird may take it (Figure 44.6). They should be encouraged to do this at least once at the beginning of each feeding. This technique encourages natural foraging skills as well as flight conditioning. The remainder of each feeding can be administered while the birds are perched and should be continued until the

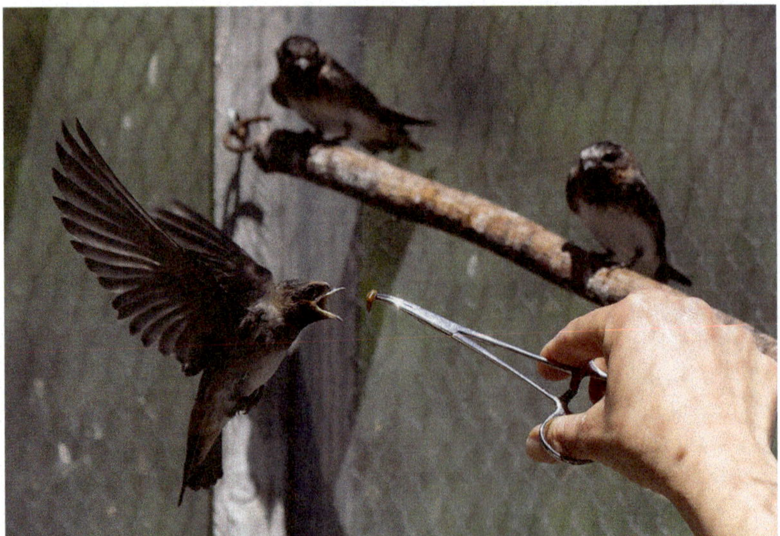

Figure 44.6 Hemostat feeding a Cliff Swallow fledgling in the aviary.

birds are no longer begging for food. The behavior and weight of the birds must be closely monitored using this hand-rearing technique and it should not be done with more than 10 birds in an aviary. It may become difficult to feed and monitor the condition of individual birds if there are too many birds in the aviary. Using plastic, temporary, colored leg bands (Red Bird Products) can be very useful in identifying individuals in a group.

Miller (2012) indicates that 8×16×8 ft. (2.4×4.8×2.4 m) is the minimum aviary dimension for swallows. This size is adequate for supporting the needs of very young fledging swallows or swallows recently recovered from an injury. However, an enclosure of this small size is not large enough to support the level of physical activity required for pre-release conditioning and successful preparation for release back to the wild. An aviary of this size severely inhibits a healthy swallow's ability to bank, turn, and gain speed in flight, and it does not provide sufficient space to fully assess a patient that has recovered from a wing injury. Minimum dimensions of a pre-release condition aviary for swallows should be 24×12×8 ft. (7.3×3.7×2.4 m).

Aviaries should be of wood frame construction with an exterior of protective wire, such as ½ in. (1.25 cm) hardware cloth to keep birds safe from predators, and the interior should be fully lined with light gray fiberglass window screen to prevent injury and damage to feathers. One-quarter to one-third of the aviary should be fully enclosed on the sides, back, and top with plywood to provide shade, privacy, and a safe place to roost and escape from the sight of predators. The substrate of the aviary can be composed of pea gravel for easy cleaning (Figure 44.7).

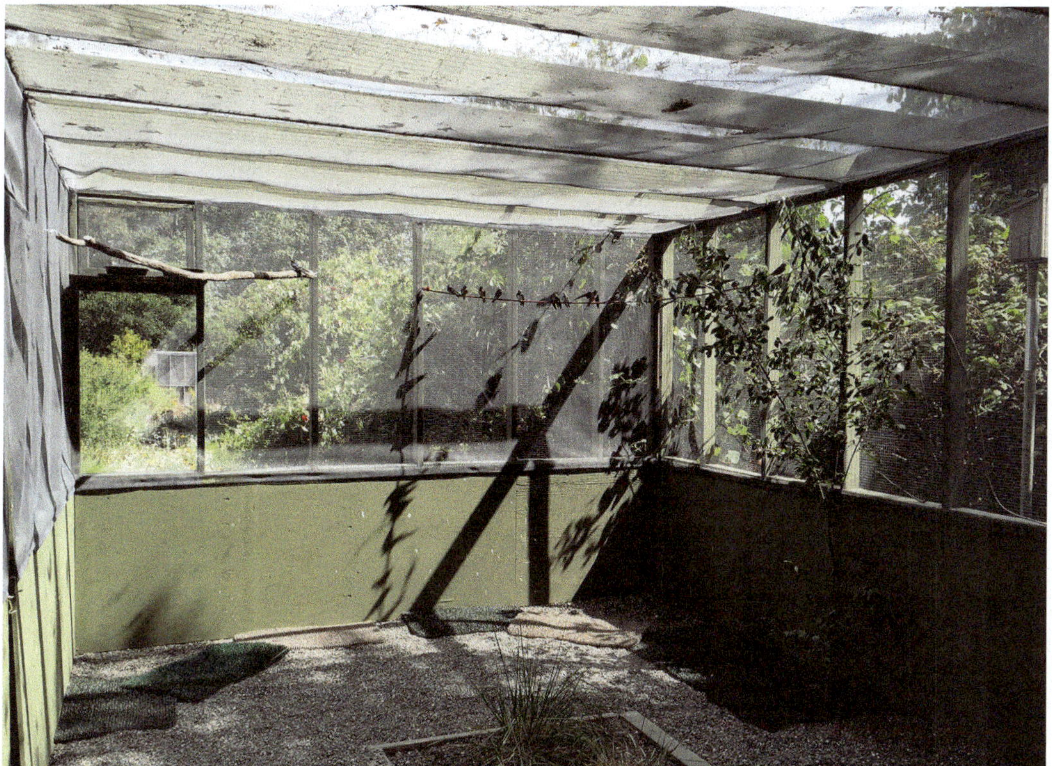

Figure 44.7 Swallow aviary: large open space in the middle to support unobstructed flight path and room to maneuver, perching options at the end include rope and natural branches, elevated shelf to hold water and food dishes, AstroTurf mats are placed directly under perching areas to facility easy clean-up of feces.

The aviary should be furnished with a variety of perches. A line of rope or a long bungee cord should be provided at each end of the aviary in addition to a couple of natural branches with leaves and a shallow shelf lined with Astroturf. Keep all perching areas at the ends of the aviary and do not obstruct the flight path. A roosting nook should be placed high in a corner at the sheltered end of the aviary.

### Food Presentation in the Aviary

Provide low-sided dishes of mealworms, waxworms, fresh-frozen cricket bodies, and freeze-dried insects at perch level in the aviary, but do not place dishes on the ground. Crème brulee dishes work exceptionally well for swallow food dishes. Clear glass ashtrays work well for fresh frozen crickets and waxworms. Dishes can be placed on small shelves affixed at perch height to the walls of the aviary. If shelves are not available, a large shallow dish, such as a cake pan or similar sized plastic plant saucer, can be placed in a hanging plant holder and suspended from the ceiling of the aviary. Food dishes can be placed within the cake pan or plant saucer. Similarly, a high standing platform-style bird feeding tray placed in the middle of the aviary can also be used to hold food dishes. Using shelves affixed to the wall to display food dishes is ideal as they don't obstruct flight paths.

Remember to offer a shallow dish of clean dirt and another shallow dish of free-choice calcium. The author provides sandy loam soil from her garden, which is free of pesticides and chemical fertilizers. Free-choice calcium is best offered in the form of ground up cuttlebone or finely crushed sterilized eggshells. Hand-reared songbirds of all species should always be offered calcium and dirt as free-choice items so that individuals who need it can partake. The author has observed over numerous years working with the species that fledgling Barn Swallows and Purple Martins, in particular, seem to partake in consuming a small amount of dirt and free-choice calcium each day, presumably for grit and minerals. The author has also observed Purple Martins select small bits of clam shell from the pea gravel substrate of the aviaries. A biologist who studies Purple Martins has observed wild conspecifics exhibiting this same behavior along the banks of the American River in Northern California.

Wide, shallow dishes of water should be provided for bathing and drinking. Dishes should be large enough to accommodate at least three swallows from head to tail. Water should also be elevated. Typically, swallows do not feel secure enough to go down to the ground for bathing and eating in a captive setting. Although it is not uncommon to observe Barn Swallows and Purple Martins waddling around on the floor of the enclosure exploring and picking up gravel, feathers, and runaway mealworms, swallows should not be forced to go to the ground to find food and water. They're aerial feeders, so keep their food elevated.

An abundance of flighted insects must be provided in the aviary to encourage natural foraging. The behavior of capturing prey in the air is innate for swallows; however, it takes practice for a young bird to become proficient in this skill. It is incumbent upon the rehabilitator to provide adequate space and appropriate food sources during pre-release conditioning for swallows to hone aerial maneuvers and hunting ability. It is cruel and unethical to release a hand-reared swallow that has not demonstrated proficiency of these skills.

Dishes of mealworms will provide the majority of daily nutrition for a self-feeding bird, but a variety of other insects must be offered, including flighted insects. Flighted insects can be provided by introducing wild caught moths, flies, and damselflies into the aviary and by stocking the aviary with commercially available live fly pupae that will hatch into houseflies. Large buckets of rotting fruit can be established to attract and cultivate fruit flies (Figure 44.8). As a precaution, buckets should be covered with ½ in. (1.25 cm) aviary wire before placing in the aviary.

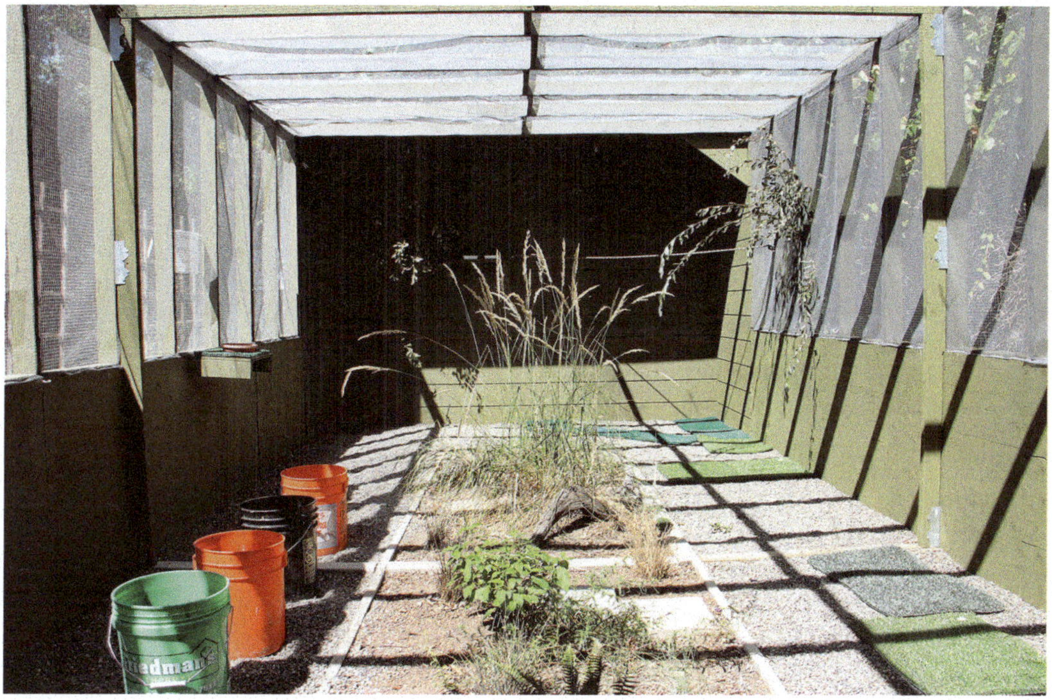

Figure 44.8 Several compost buckets provide ready access to clouds of live fruit flies. The aviary is lined with soft fiberglass window screen to protect feathers, three-quarters of the roof is unshaded to allow ample access to full sun; the substrate includes pea gravel and soil.

### Release

Once the swallows have been self-feeding in the aviary for 10–14 days, they should be evaluated for release back to the wild. Swallows are long-distance migrants and have stringent requirements for survival in the wild. A swallow ready for release should be able to sustain continuous flight for at least 5 minutes with ease, demonstrate the ability to catch flighted insects on the wing, be a healthy weight for the species, show an appropriate fear response to humans and predators, have impeccable feather condition, and be waterproof.

Swallows should be released back to their natal territory if their colony or family is still present. If their family has dispersed, then select another release site with suitable habitat for the species and where other swallows are present upon release. Release day should take place upon a clear forecast of at least 3 days of good weather. Avoid releases on days of high winds and temperature extremes. Before setting the swallows free from their transport carrier, check for aerial predators. An aerial predator is likely in the area if swallows are high above, swirling in a dense group, and making alarm calls. If there are swallows calmly feeding and flying about in the sky above, that is a good indication that the area is free of predators. Swallows should be released in the mid-morning to allow for exploration and adjustment to the new environment before it is time to find a roost for the night.

## Overwintering

Overwintering may be a consideration when a swallow is not ready for release in time for their fall migration. Well-managed, long-term care will be required to maintain good health throughout the winter. Exposure to natural sunlight and full-spectrum UV light must be provided as well as meticulously maintained hygienic conditions and a balanced diet. Their nails and bill will require grooming approximately every 30 days. Their weight should be monitored. Feathers should be carefully examined and checked frequently for ectoparasites and cleanliness. Feet should be checked regularly as swallows are prone to bumblefoot (pododermatitis) if they are sedentary. They must also be housed with another swallow. Swallows kept singly become depressed, which can lead to deterioration of their general health.

### Overwintering Flighted Swallows

Continue to provide all aspects of food presentation, perches, and enrichment as described earlier in this chapter for pre-release conditioning of swallows. If birds are flighted and housed in an aviary, provide domestic flies hatched from pupae, moths, and a compost bucket of fruit flies as long as weather and temperatures permit. Flighted insects are for the purposes of enrichment and physical activity, not a primary source of nutrition. As the winter weather becomes cool, flighted insects may become difficult to provide until warmer temperatures return in spring.

Flighted birds should only be housed outside for as long as the weather permits. Move birds indoors when nighttime temperatures drop to 45 °F (7.2 °C) and below. In captivity, swallows don't do well in the cold, they tend to become less active and drop weight easily. Large reptariums work well for indoor housing; however, they don't offer enough room for full flight. If nights are cold, but daytime temperatures are mild, put the birds in the outdoor flight during the day and move them indoors at night. If daytime temps are too cold, allow birds to have access to free flight in a safe indoor area.

The author, who lives in the mild climate of coastal Northern California, houses overwintering swallows outdoors in an insulated aviary with a heat source and full-spectrum lighting.

### Care of Feet

Swallows are highly aerial and not meant to remain sedentary for prolonged periods of time. They can easily develop pressure sores on their feet. Provide a variety of perching substrates to maintain healthy feet. For additional comfort and foot relief, straight perches can be wrapped in vet wrap or draped with a non-terry towel. Be sure to change the vet wrap on the perch each week or sooner if it becomes soiled.

If pressure sores develop, clean the bottom of the foot with dilute chlorhexidine and rub a small dab of silver sulfadiazine on the affected area. To protect the foot while it heals, a foot wrap can be fashioned using a thin strip of vet wrap. The sore usually disappears in less than a week. A topical preparation of enrofloxacin can also be effective in treating pressure sores. Consult with your vet for use and preparation of topical enrofloxacin.

### Diet for Overwintering Swallows

Feed overwintering birds mealworms and other insects prepared and presented as mentioned previously for self-feeding birds in aviary. To prevent fat soluble vitamin deficiencies during long term care, give 0.05 ml per 25 kcal insects (~12g mealworms) of the following mix: 5cc omega-3 marine oil (from fish body, not liver), 10 000 IU vitamin D3, 10 000 IU vitamin A, and 500 IU vitamin E. Administer daily to each swallow housed indoors; outdoor birds can receive the supplement added directly to their food.

For additional protein and variety, offer a dish of freeze-dried flies and ground up freeze-dried crickets. Waxworms and fresh frozen crickets with wings and legs removed can also be offered.

Waxworms should be offered in small amounts, one to two per bird per day, as they're not very nutritious. Fresh frozen crickets should be offered in small amounts because they're highly perishable.

### Swallows Are Social Creatures

NEVER overwinter a single swallow. It is cruel. Find another swallow from another rehabilitator, or prepare to transfer the bird to another rehabilitator. When temporarily housing a single swallow, position a vertical mirror directly next to their favored perch. Most swallows hunt for food communally, so place a dish of mealworms adjacent to the mirror and the perch.

Swallows seem to be prone to depression when kept in captivity too long, especially Cliff Swallows. The larger the group of birds, the more content they seem to be. Again, if you have a single swallow staying for the winter, please do the right thing and find another overwintering swallow buddy or two.

### Weekly and Monthly Health Check

Birds should be thoroughly examined and weighed every week. Watch feet carefully for pressure sores. Make sure their nares are clear and mouth color is normal. Monitor their respiratory condition. Bills and nails can overgrow. To maintain a healthy bill length, carefully file the tip of the bill with an emery board as needed. Observe their self-maintenance. Are feathers clean? Are birds preening and bathing regularly? Check for mites and lice. It's also good practice to perform a fecal exam once a month, or sooner if a problem with internal parasites is suspected.

### Lighting and Regulating the Photoperiod

Provide full-spectrum lighting. Do not use lighting designed for reptiles, it is not appropriate or healthy for birds. Full-spectrum lights, such as Phillips Natural Light bulbs, work very well for birds. These bulbs have a CRI of 92 and color temperature of 5000 k. The 18 in. (46 cm) bulb can be used in an aquarium light fixture and placed on top of a reptarium or cage. The bulbs can also be installed in an under-counter style fixture and mounted on the underside of a shelf directly above the cage. It is very important to leave half the perching area free of direct light so the birds have the option to bask under the light or not.

Manipulating the photoperiod during the winter to mimic the photoperiod on the swallows' wintering grounds helps retain their natural molt cycle and length of foraging time during the day while in captivity. Remember, most swallow species spend the winter very near or south of the equator. As the days grow shorter in our hemisphere, you can lengthen the day artificially so that the swallows receive approximately 12 hours of "daylight" each day.

Manipulating the photoperiod is easily done by setting a regular light and their full-spectrum light on staggered timers to create "sunrise" and "sunset." If housed indoors, set one light (any light will do – floor lamp, gooseneck lamp, etc.) away from their reptarium to turn on at 5:30 a.m., and the full-spectrum light directly over one section of their housing to turn on at 6:15–6:25 a.m. Do the reverse for "sunset" in the evening. Make adjustments to the lighting schedule as the length of daylight changes through the winter. Make sure the full-spectrum lighting is placed directly over their housing and approximately 18 in. (46 cm) above one of the perches. Make sure that the bird can perch comfortably in another area of the enclosure away from the full-spectrum light source.

### Overwintering Temporarily Nonflighted But Otherwise Releasable Swallows

Most swallow species received late in the breeding season or during fall migration that present with damaged or missing feathers should molt in late winter or early spring. Resist the temptation to pull damaged feathers to initiate regrowth, as doing so will disrupt their natural molt cycle, cause unnecessary discomfort, and prematurely expose fresh new feathers to inevitable wear and tear in captivity.

### Housing Temporarily Nonflighted Swallows

Follow all other aspects of care and diet for flighted swallows. Make food and water easily accessible to nonflighted birds by placing all food dishes and water at perch level next to the perch. Nonflighted swallows can be set up in a reptarium with perches placed 1.5 in. (3.8 cm) from the floor of the enclosure.

### Releasing Overwintered Swallows

Observe all standard criteria for release (fitness, behavior, good weather, etc.) and release overwintered swallows only when their species has returned for the breeding season.

## Acknowledgments

My sincere gratitude to the amazing passerines whose beauty and song grace this earth each day.

## Sources of Products Mentioned

Butterfly enclosures, wireless endoscope: http://Amazon.com.

Mesh reptariums, logs and bark, lighting: LLLReptile and Supply Company Inc., 609 Mission Ave, Oceanside, CA 92054, (760) 439-8492, www.http://lllreptile.com.

Mealworms, waxworms, Dubia roaches, fly larvae, fruit flies and crickets: Rainbow Mealworms, 126 E. Spruce St, Compton, CA 90220, (800) 777-9676. https://www.rainbowmealworms.net.

Flightless stingless wasps and freeze dried insects: Arbico Organics, 10 831 N. Mavinee Drive, Ste. 185, Oro Valley, AZ 85737-9531, (800) 847-2847, http://www.arbico-organics.com.

Leg bands: Red bird Products, Inc., P. O. Box 376, Mount Aukum, CA 95656-0376, (530) 620-7440, http://www.redbirdproducts.com.

Cannula tip for feeding (aka teat infusion cannula): Jorgensen Labs, 1450 Van Buren Ave, Loveland, Colorado 80 538, (800) 525-5614, https://www.jorvet.com.

## References

Duerr, R.S., Purdin, G.J., and Bowers, V. (2017). Small-bodied birds: passerines, doves, woodpeckers, others. In: *Topics in Wildlife Medicine, Vol. 4: Orthopedics* (eds. R.S. Duerr and G.J. Purdin), 53–74. St. Cloud, MN: National Wildlife Rehabilitators Association.

Hawkins, M.G., Barron, H.W., Speer, B.L. et al. (2018). Birds. In: *Exotic Animal Formulary*, 5e (eds. J.W. Carpenter and C.J. Marion), 167–375. St. Louis, MO: Elsevier.

Miller, E.A. (ed.) (2012). *Minimum Standards for Wildlife Rehabilitation*, 4e. St. Cloud, MN: National Wildlife Rehabilitation Association.

Perlman, J. (2016). *Wildlife Rehabilitation: A Comprehensive Approach*, 120. International Wildlife Rehabilitation Council.

## Further Reading

Birds of North America website: http://bna.birds.cornell.edu/BNA.

Bowers, V. (2018). *Passerine Fundamentals*, 119 pp. Sebastopol, CA: Native Songbird Care and Conservation.

Brown, C.R. and Brown, M.B. (1998). *Swallow Summer*. University of Nebraska Press.

# 45

# Thrushes, Mimids, and Thrush Relatives

*Linda M. Tuttle-Adams*

## Natural History

There are about 330 species of thrushes (family Turdidae) worldwide, with 18 species in North America. There are also five families whose diets, vocal capabilities, and other characteristics are similar enough to those of thrushes to place them in close taxonomic relationship within the passerine order of birds. These five families of birds, referred to as thrush relatives, are mockingbirds and thrashers (family Mimidae), with about 34 species in the world, all in the Americas; starlings and mynas (family Sturnidae), with about 113 species worldwide; waxwings (family Bombycillidae), with three species in the northern temperate zone; silky-flycatchers (family Ptilogonatidae), with four species; and babblers (family Sylviidae), with 270 species in the world.

The complex vocal organ, the syrinx, of thrushes and mimids enables them to produce some of the most melodious songs of any birds in the world. Mimids and sturnids are capable of imitating numerous birds' songs and other sounds, such as frog calls, barking dogs, and human words. The Brown Thrasher (*Toxostoma rufrum*) has perhaps the largest repertoire of any bird, with over 2000 song types and other sounds. The bills of thrushes and relatives are specifically adapted to dig into soil, catch insects, peck at fruit, or pick berries. In autumn and winter, when fruits are available, these birds switch from eating invertebrates to eating more fruits and seeds. The diet of waxwings and silky-flycatchers is primarily frugivorous. Waxwings are highly social, and known for their berry sharing. Both parents care for and feed young thrushes and thrush relatives. Foods fed to the young consist of a wide variety of invertebrates (mainly insects and other arthropods, as well as annelid worms); for the more omnivorous species, parents introduce fruits at species-specific stages. Nests are open cup and arboreal except in the case of starlings and some thrushes that prefer cavities. Thrashers nest on the ground or low in dense vegetation; thrushes nest in tree holes, rock crevices, cup- or dome-shaped nests, on the ground, and in burrows.

The American Robin (*Turdus migratorius*) is the most abundant and broadly distributed thrush in North America, as well as one of the most commonly admitted species in the rehabilitation setting. For the most part, the following care guidelines for the thrush relatives are based on years of experience with the young of American Robins. Since not all species have the same requirements, complete natural histories should be consulted for each species cared for in captivity. The European Robin (*Erithacus rubecula*) is not a thrush but rather an Old World flycatcher.

*Hand-Rearing Birds*, Second Edition. Edited by Rebecca S. Duerr and Laurie J. Gage.

## Criteria for Intervention

Because fledglings are not yet adept at flying, they are one of the most common age groups brought into care. Since young birds that are raised in open-cup nests are more exposed to potential predators, leaving before their wings and tails have finished growing is safer than staying. Well-meaning people find fledglings on the ground and assume they have "fallen" out of their nest. Fledglings are also susceptible to injuries from car strikes, dogs, and cats. Young birds that are injured, sick, or in immediate danger from domestic pets must be brought into care. Most uninjured fledglings can be reunited with their parents if the area is safe. All chicks should have an exam before nest replacement is attempted, as one or more may have been injured in the fall or may have been attacked by a predator before rescue. Healthy nestlings can be re-nested or placed with a foster family, but only after many criteria are met. Older nestlings may jump prematurely if their nest has been disturbed.

## Record Keeping

The care of each individual bird should be tracked. Plastic leg bands for identification can be used on all birds except tiny hatchlings; they must be of a diameter that will not impede leg growth (Red Bird Products). In addition to an intake form noting the circumstances of rescue, a detailed medical record noting diet, feedings, medications, and observations should be kept. Chicks should be weighed regularly to monitor health and to calculate medications and the amount of food required. A detailed record of the location where the bird was found is imperative for a re-nest or reunite possibility, and for eventual release.

## Initial Care and Stabilization

Before removing chicks from the transport container, note their posture and behavior and check for evidence of blood, ectoparasites, and fecal droppings. Newly admitted chicks should be treated only for urgent issues – the first goal is to allow de-stress time (15–20 minutes) in a pre-warmed, quiet, darkened area. Nestlings should be placed inside a nest (see "Housing," section) in an incubator or room warmed to 90–95 °F if the chicks are sparsely feathered, or 85 °F if feathered. Humidity should be 40–60%. Once the chicks are warmed, rehydration can begin. Resist the urge to feed chicks until they are warmed, hydrated, and consistently passing droppings. Normal droppings consist of clear watery urine, white (urates), and dark, formed feces.

Warm fluids should be given very slowly, starting with tiny amounts given deep into the throat past the glottis (tracheal opening), which is located at the base of the tongue. If using a syringe, ensure the plunger does not stick when depressed. The "crop," which is simply an expandable pouch of the esophagus and can easily be overfilled, runs down the *right* side of the bird's neck (alongside the trachea), into the stomach. Make sure the bird swallows before giving more fluid. A young nestling that is not gaping or not holding its head upright may be showing signs of shock or another serious condition. Administration of warm sterile isotonic fluids subcutaneously (SQ) at 5% of body weight (50 ml/kg) may be necessary. If SQ fluid is not an option, fluids may be given by applying small amounts along the beak side opening where capillary action draws the fluid inside the mouth (stay clear of the nares); this should elicit a visible swallowing action. Repeat this frequently until the chick strengthens. Once the chick is well hydrated and passing droppings, small amounts of age-appropriate food may be given. If the bird is starving or emaciated or has diarrhea (very loose, watery), give dilute (to start) formula or dilute Emeraid Intensive Care Carnivore (Lafeber) (absorbable high protein for critically ill) until droppings are normal. Digestive organs need to be fully functioning before regular foods are started.

Correct identification is essential (see Chapter 2). American Robins and Northern Mockingbirds are often mistaken for each other, but a rule of thumb is that a robin will always weigh more than a mockingbird at every stage of life. Starlings are sometimes mistaken for woodpeckers because they both nest in cavities, or mockingbirds due to both species' large yellow mouths when gaping (Figure 45.1). Bluebirds have a thinner whiter gape flange (Figure 45.2). The best way to avoid mistaken identities is to pay attention to bird's location, type of habitat, foot type, weight and age, interior mouth color, presence or absence of down, and details of the beak and gape flanges.

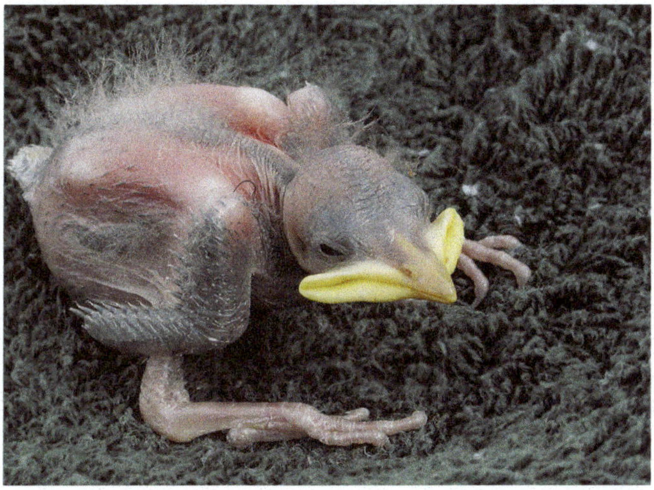

Figure 45.1 European Starling nestling with eyes just opening. Note enlarged lower bill, bright yellow mouth, sparse gray down on head shading to whitish on rump. *Source:* photo courtesy of Jackie Wollner.

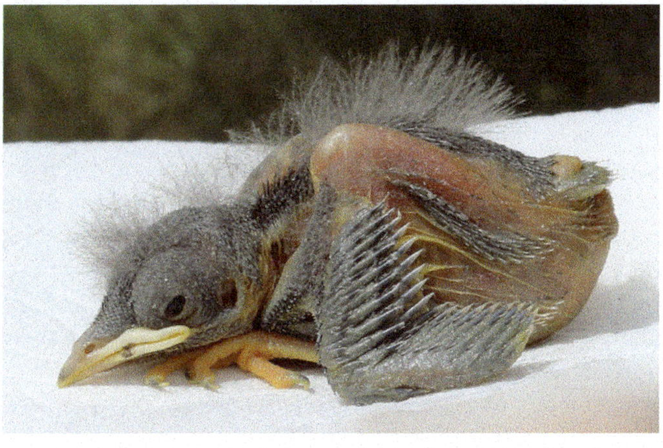

Figure 45.2 Western Bluebird nestling. Note whitish, thin gape flanges.

## Common Medical Problems and Solutions

### Caught by Cat

Victims of cat (or dog) attack often have punctures, lacerations, fractures, internal bleeding from crushing bites, and respiratory issues, including ruptured air sacs. Antibiotics must be given for 7–10 days depending on the severity of the injuries. Amoxicillin, cephalexin, enrofloxacin, and ciprofloxacin are the preferable drugs. Avoid trimethoprim sulfamethoxazone since some species are sensitive to it. For birds with severe injuries, wound treatment is needed (this is covered in Chapter 1). Ruptured air sacs should be left to resolve on their own unless they are causing the bird great discomfort and/or an inability to maintain balance or eat.

### Metabolic Bone Disease

Well-meaning rescuers create more complications by feeding birds inappropriate foods. Robins and mockingbirds are very susceptible to metabolic bone disease (MBD), which is typically caused by a diet deficient in calcium. Older nestlings or fledglings that demonstrate difficulty in standing or have drooping wings may have weak or broken bones. Supplementation with oral calcium glubionate or calcium carbonate (150 mg/kg SID or BID), a balanced diet, light supportive splints, and padded surfaces may help. If the disease is advanced (i.e. there are joint or limb abnormalities), euthanasia should be considered. See Duerr et al. (2017) for information regarding management of orthopedic injuries in small birds.

### Pesticides

Birds that feed on lawns and cultivated berries may be inadvertently passing on pesticides to their young. If this issue is suspected, the only treatment available is activated charcoal.

### Viruses

Avian pox and West Nile virus (WNV) may be more problematic in some areas or regions as outbreaks occur. Pox is a very contagious disease, transmitted through insect bites or direct contact, whereas WNV is transmitted by mosquito vector. Pox treatment can be labor intensive, and the risk of infecting other birds in care must be considered.

### Parasites

Some thrushes and thrush relatives present with infections from more than one parasite. Typical parasites for American Robins are coccidia, gapeworm, capillaria, and occasionally tapeworm and roundworm. The protozoan *Trichomonas gallinae* may occur in these species and may be diagnosed by a throat swab. Starlings carry many of these infections and may also present with giardiasis, caused by an intestinal protozoan. Routine fecal exams are recommended, especially for nestlings that have (smelly) diarrhea and are underweight for their developmental age. Many rehabilitation centers have protocols in place for prophylactic treatment. Remember, one fecal sample is just a point in time in a parasite's lifecycle, so even if an initial sample is negative, results can change over time in the captive setting. Prophylactic medications such as ponazuril (3 days) and ivermectin (one dose) may be given to fledglings and nestlings that are fully feathered and thermoregulating, if needed. Doses can be found in Hawkins et al. (2018). Newly arriving chicks should be kept separate from others already in care until they have a clear fecal or prophylactic treatment. Follow-up tests should be done 7–10 days following the bird's last dose.

Earthworms, land snails, and many insects are intermediate hosts to many parasites, such as protozoa, nematodes, and the gapeworm parasite, *Syngamus trachea*. Once gapeworm larvae migrate to the trachea, the bird will exhibit head shaking, or a soft coughing sound; in advanced cases, it will have difficulty swallowing and breathing. Treatment is a single dose of ivermectin.

Antiparasitic drugs commonly used to treat parasites in these species include carnidazole, ronidazole, fenbendazole, metronidazole, praziquantel, ponazuril, toltrazuril, and ivermectin. Medications and dosages should be prescribed by your avian veterinarian upon diagnosis. Probiotics help replenish gut flora whenever any medication is given, particularly antibiotics.

External parasites (lice, flies, ticks, mites) can be treated with over-the-counter mite/lice powder or spray and/or ivermectin. "Scaly leg," a thickening of scales on the feet that is often confused with dry pox, is caused by a mite. If untreated, it can lead to loss of digits or an entire foot.

Stringent disinfection and quarantine protocols should be in place at all times in any facility to prevent diseases from spreading. Aviaries should be treated to kill any eggs or larvae that may have been shed into the substrate if any birds had a parasitic infection while in the enclosure. Giardia and coccidia may be particularly difficult to eradicate from aviaries; steam cleaning can a helpful addition to routine cleaning and disinfection.

## Diet

Wild nestlings are fed regurgitated soft-bodied invertebrates for the first 4 to 5 days (only 1 to 2 days for waxwings). In general, these species feed hatchlings an all-arthropod diet for at least the first few days of life, then some species add in increasing amounts of other foods while others continue feeding all arthropods. Table 45.1 lists the wild diets fed to chicks of selected species of thrushes and thrush relatives, and the ages at which other foods are added. Older nestlings and fledglings receive a large variety of whole insects, worms, and soft fleshy fruit pieces, according to species.

Regardless of what hand-rearing diet is chosen, it must be of optimal quality and high in digestible protein. A captive diet of a variety of invertebrates, plant foods, and calcium-vitamin supplements, according to species for thrushes and thrush relatives, is ideal because it most closely simulates their wild diet. Some caregivers choose to use hand-feeding formula, but thrushes and relatives need a variety of animal and plant foods as a portion of their diet (Table 45.2, also see Tables 41.3 and 41.4 for formula options). Ideally, newly admitted nestlings should be started on insects before gradually introducing formula. If a "combo" diet (insects + formula + supplemental foods) is chosen, follow the percentages of arthropods and plants in the wild diet of the species, as listed in Table 45.1. For example, an acceptable ratio for an American Robin nestling is one-third formula, one-third live "insects," and one-third supplemental foods. Keep in mind that some pet foods may contain toxins, pesticides, and herbicides (especially glyphosate), particularly if they are not certified organic and grain-based. As nestlings are weaned from formula, they should be graduated to foods that resemble what they will receive in the wild. Chicks fed whole insects require supplements to compensate for deficiencies in the nutritional content of feeder insects. See Chapter 44, Box 44.1: "Supplements for Birds Hand-reared on an Insects-only Diet" for what is needed per amount of insects fed.

Table 45.1 Wild foods fed to nestlings of thrushes and thrush relatives.

| SPECIES | WILD FOODS |
|---|---|
| | **Note:** Foods listed are examples. % and type vary by location and availability. Arthropods include insects, spiders, moths, caterpillars, bugs, beetles, etc. Annelids are segmented worms such as earthworms. d = days of age. |
| Wrentit | All arthropods. Mostly butterfly and moth larvae at first. Coastal California: inchworm moth larvae and other caterpillars, some spiders, true bugs, and beetles. No mention of fruit for nestlings. Juveniles consume fruits and seeds late summer through winter. |
| Eastern Bluebird | All arthropods, few annelids, and small vertebrates. d 0–5: butterfly and moth larvae (41.6%) and spiders (31%). d 6–10: grasshoppers and crickets, are gradually added. d 11–18: more beetles and 5.2% earthworms. Small fruits uncommon in the diet during nestling stage. If berries available, a very small % when nestlings are completely endothermic (Pinkowski 1978) and just prior to fledgling. Newly fledged and juveniles consume more fruit in fall/winter. |
| Western Bluebird | Mostly arthropods, some annelids, and small vertebrates. Grasshoppers, caterpillars, and other soft-bodied invertebrates. No information if nestlings are given fruit. Small fruits consumed by juveniles and adults in fall/winter. |
| Hermit Thrush | All arthropods. Small larvae (minced at first); then insects, grasshoppers, moths, beetles, spiders. Older young fed whole arthropods. Berries not normally fed. |
| Wood Thrush | Soft-bodied invertebrates (ants, spiders, cantharid beetles, earthworms, millipedes) and pre-softened fruits (e.g. cherry, grape, elderberry). |
| American Robin | Regurgitated arthropods (d 1–4). Then pieces of soft invertebrates (beetle grubs, parts of earthworms). With growth, pieces of fruits (30%) added (of a very wide variety). |
| Gray Catbird | Mainly small invertebrates, insects (caterpillars, grasshoppers), and spiders; about 5% fruit, more added with growth (e.g. blackberry, elderberry, cherry, grape, blueberry, huckleberry, strawberry). |
| Brown Thrasher | Almost entirely earthworms and arthropods (the type varying geographically) and some berries (e.g. cherry, mulberry, strawberry, blackberry, grape). |
| Northern Mockingbird | Arthropods (82%) and fruit (18%). More fruit (25–30%) added with growth (e.g., blackberry, wild grape, buckthorn, cedar, elderberry). Arthropods: bees, beetles, wasps, cicadas, grasshoppers. Occasionally small lizards and flowers. |
| Starling | Small soft-bodied insects at first, then larger insects. Animal: beetles, grasshoppers, moths, millipedes, caterpillars, spiders, snails, earthworms. Plant: cherry, mulberry, elderberry, apple. Also, nectar. |
| Mynas | Young nestlings: small insects and larvae; older nestlings: larger insects (butterflies, dragonflies) and earthworms. Plant food: not before 10 d. |
| Cedar Waxwing | Mostly insects (d 1–2), then fruit added gradually. Animal: beetles, ants, flies, caterpillars, grasshoppers, crickets. Fruits: cherry, dogwood, blackberry, cherry, grape, strawberry, and many others. *Able to digest sucrose.* |
| Phainopepla | Mostly insects (d 1–4), ants, spiders, beetles. Fruit (small berries) added with growth. Fruits: mistletoe, elderberry, grape, buckthorn, mulberry, cherry. *Able to digest sucrose.* |

The young of species that receive earthworms in their natural diet should receive a limited number of earthworms (for American Robins, for example, up to six or seven per day). In the wild, the immune systems of these species are adapted to combat the gapeworm parasite; but the stress these birds experience in captivity or from being injured requires that they are healthy before

Table 45.2 Foods and supplements for thrushes and thrush relatives in captivity.

| | |
|---|---|
| Animal foods, cultured or wild-caught | Mealworms, crickets (live or frozen), waxworms, fly larvae (live or dried), fruit flies, moths, a limited number of earthworms. NEVER feed earthworms intended for bait, use home-raised earthworms or collect them in pesticide-free garden loam. |
| Plant foods, cultivated or wild-picked | Berries (blackberries, blueberries, mulberries, elderberries), grapes, cherries, plums, figs, apples, pears (minced, chopped, or whole, according to mouth size). DO NOT use fermented berries or those from the nonnative shrub Heavenly bamboo (*Nandina domestica*). Avoid fruit collected from any area suspected of herbicide or pesticide use, especially glyphosate. |
| Supplemental foods | Chopped hard-boiled egg, soaked currants, nutmeats (sunflower seeds, etc.), suet bits, dried flies in peanut butter crumble. |
| Vitamin and mineral supplements, per amount insects fed | For insect diets. See Chapter 44, Box 44.1, "Supplements for Birds Hand-reared on an Insects-only Diet." |

earthworms are added to their diet. Earthworms are necessary for these chicks, since the many benefits provided outweigh the risk of potential infection and better prepare birds for the real world.

Cedar Waxwing hatchlings, age 1–2 days, should be fed insects drowned in blueberry juice from thawed berries, plus vitamin and calcium supplements and digestive enzymes (e.g. Pancrezyme® powder), every 20 minutes. Starting on day 3, stop the enzymes and introduce fruits. Then gradually increase fruits by 5% each day, until at 14 days the birds are receiving 60% fruit + 40% insects every 30 minutes. By weaning, they should be up to 85% fruit. Waxwings could also be given formula in addition to insects, keeping the insect/fruit percentages as described.

## Feeding Procedures

Feed hatchlings every 20–30 minutes (more often for the smallest chicks); nestlings every 30 minutes; fledglings every 45–60 minutes, all for 12–14 hours/day. Wild baby American Robins receive >35 feedings/day, sometimes receiving food past dusk.

Solid food can be fed with blunt-end forceps. Use 1 ml (cc) syringes for feeding formula to young nestlings and 3 ml for larger nestlings (see Figure 1.4). The gaping response is stimulated by touch or movement on/at the nest. Nestlings whose eyes are still closed can be stimulated to gape by jiggling the nest. Newly admitted older nestlings and fledglings may be made to gape by *gently* tapping their beaks or holding a wiggling insect in front of them. Syringe-feeding must be done carefully. To prevent aspiration, feed in small bites and do not overfill the mouth; wait until the chick swallows before giving more. Also, some chicks gape even with food in their throats, so be careful to not overfeed. A bird's stomach capacity is approximately 5% of its body weight, so the amount of food for each meal should be calculated accordingly. For example, a 20 g bird should receive 1 ml or 1 g of food per feeding, starting with small doses to see what the bird can handle. Poorly formed droppings resembling undigested food or regurgitation may indicate overfeeding. Berry-eating birds have droppings similar in color to the fruits they consume, but those droppings should still be well formed.

Fledglings are very curious and active, and they may be more interested in exploring their surroundings than in being fed when they first leave their nest. This is normal behavior, and their appetite should resume in a day or two. If several fledglings are being housed together, it is important to monitor individual weight and behavior as the birds become self-feeding.

Self-feeding is stimulated by the movement of live insects. Attract the bird's attention by holding wiggling food in forceps, away from the beak so as to make the bird reach, and then over the food dish or to the ground. Be patient, and *never* withhold food. Many of the thrush relatives are helpers at the nest with successive broods of their parents. Slightly older birds make good "mentors," as some species learn by imitating their parents. Older robins and waxwings may even feed younger cagemates or encourage them to forage. It is very important for these family social types to be housed with members of their own species.

## Expected Weight Gain

The period of rapid growth begins about day 4 post-hatch; it then reaches a peak and levels off as birds reach adult size. Before the chicks become fledglings, parents will taper off feedings to encourage their chicks to leave the nest. It is normal for wild chicks to show a slight drop in weight just before fledging, to about 60–70% of their adult weight (see tables in Chapter 2). Captive-raised birds may not exhibit this normal weight loss, as feedings should *never* be cut back. Captive birds are already at a disadvantage from not being in the wild with their parents, so they should gain weight until they reach adult mass within 2 to 4 weeks after they fledge.

## Housing

The ambient temperature should be 90–95 °F (32.2–35 °C) for hatchlings and 85–90 °F (29.4–32.3 °C) for feathered chicks, with a humidity of 40–60%. An Animal Intensive Care Unit (Lyon Technologies) is ideal for young chicks in nests (Figure 45.3). Temperature and humidity are more difficult to control when heating pads are used. Two or more chicks combine body heat, and as their feathers unsheathe, the temperature inside the nest can rise. A probe thermometer placed under tissue layers beneath the birds helps monitor the temperature *inside* the nest. This way, if ambient temperatures fluctuate or as feathers unsheathe, the nest temperature can be adjusted or the heat source possibly removed as birds thermoregulate.

Consider the natural history of the species when preparing housing. A nest can be created using a small bowl or a knitted nest lined with crumpled tissue so the birds have something to grip. To ensure proper limb development, the cup-shaped nest should be formed so that the bird's legs remain underneath it and are not allowed to splay. Several nestlings should fit snuggly together. A piece of fleece can be placed on top to simulate a brooding parent. Species that in the wild are raised in a cavity or dome-type nest should be provided with an arched "cover" over the nest (see Figure 44.2). Fecal material should be removed immediately to avoid soiled feathers. It may be necessary to change the nest material after each feeding to keep the birds clean.

Fully feathered nestlings can be kept in a screen-lined laundry basket. When they begin perching on the nest rim, they are ready for a soft-sided pre-flight cage, one that allows light in but does not allow insects to escape. Other types of cages that have been used include wire cages lined with window screening (Figure 45.4), "reptarium" type enclosures, large butterfly cages, and toddler playpens with clipped-on screening for the ceiling. Birds should receive natural sunlight or full-spectrum lighting, and indoor daylight hours should match the outdoor photoperiod. The enclosure should be "outfitted" with various-sized perches that can be adjusted as the birds grow. Gently

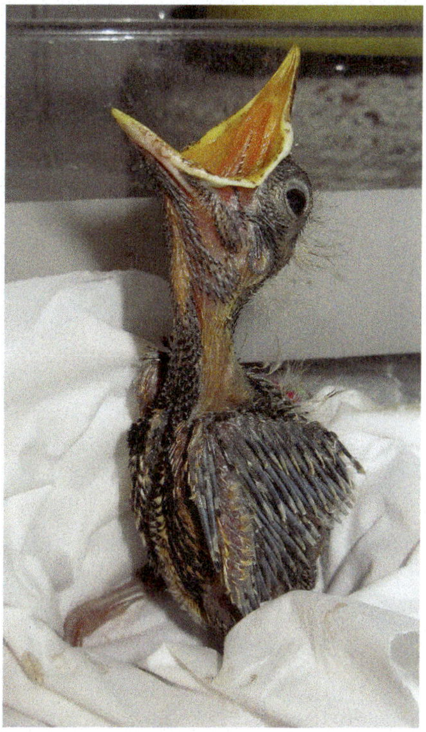

Figure 45.3 Newly admitted American Robin nestling in a replacement nest. *Source:* photo courtesy of Connie Black.

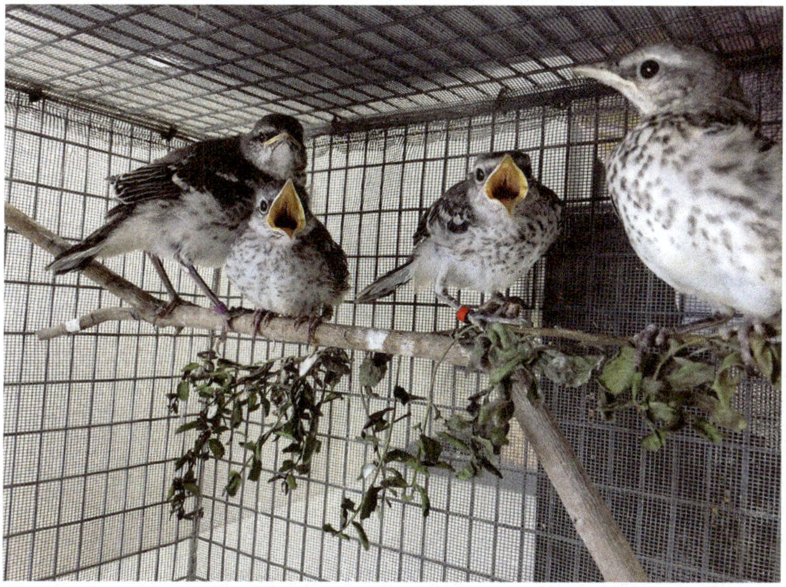

Figure 45.4 Northern Mockingbird fledglings in a window screen-lined wire cage. *Source:* photo courtesy of Linnaea Furlong.

swinging perches exercise legs and help birds learn landing skills on a moving target. Potted evergreens and full branches with leaves offer hiding places. Bluebirds and starlings need a sheltered area in their cage in order to mimic their wild behavior of returning to their nest cavity to huddle together at night. Keeping the cage clean is challenging during this stage of development. Fledglings tend to be messy as they explore the enclosure and develop their foraging skills. Supply water in nontipping containers to encourage drinking, since birds who are drinking are on their way to becoming self-feeding. At this stage, birds should also be offered mealworms, grubs, etc. in clean loam, and earthworms in dampened loam.

Behavioral enrichment helps relieve stress and encourages learning experiences. Offer hiding places and foraging opportunities, and play natural sounds, including the species' song. Always attempt to find a conspecific buddy for a chick, as these species are susceptible to habituation and imprinting – covered in Chapter 15 and others. If none is available, use a mirror and/or house the bird near a conspecific adult or juvenile, and attempt to find the bird an appropriate companion by networking with other rehabilitators.

## Weaning

The weaning process can begin when birds are self-feeding but should never be rushed. Many thrush relatives naturally begin refusing feedings as their feeding skills improve. They are stimulated to forage by the movement of earthworms in soil or in a mixture of mealworms with crumbled suet cake, dried flies, and pieces of nutmeats in a shallow container. Even if self-feeding is occurring, birds need to be regularly weighed to monitor weight gain. It is normal for fledglings to lose a little weight during the night, but their weight should remain stable or increase each day during the weaning period. When birds are regularly eating on their own, hand-feedings should be reduced. If any bird is not gaining weight, hand-feedings should be resumed, and a fecal sample may be warranted.

## Preparation for Wild Release

Before moving birds to an outdoor aviary, acclimate them by moving their enclosure near an open window or outdoors for increasing periods. Outdoor aviaries should be a minimum of 4×8×8 ft. (1.2×2.4×2.4 m) for most species, and 8×8×16 ft. (2.4×2.4×4.8 m) for larger-bodied species or groups of birds (Figure 45.5). Most thrush relatives tolerate being in mixed-species groups if they are in the larger-sized aviary and the total number of birds does not exceed 8–10. However, some species are highly territorial (e.g. mockingbirds) as fledglings and thus may not be the best cagemates in mixed-species enclosures. Territoriality may be shown by birds posturing about, displaying their white wing patches. Always monitor behavior in the aviary to make sure everyone is getting along.

Enclosure enrichment should include natural features, such as small trees, bushes, small logs, bark pieces, and grassy areas. Make a leaf pile where the birds can hunt for hiding insects. A *variety* of food promotes health, holds birds' interest, helps develop foraging skills, and helps them recognize wild foods. Bathing for some species is an essential, innately driven behavior. For these birds, shallow saucers 12 in. (30 cm) in diameter work well (Figure 45.6). The water in these baths should be changed daily, and separate shallow containers for drinking should be provided. Misting stimulates preening and bathing. As birds become adept at catching live prey, food can be scattered

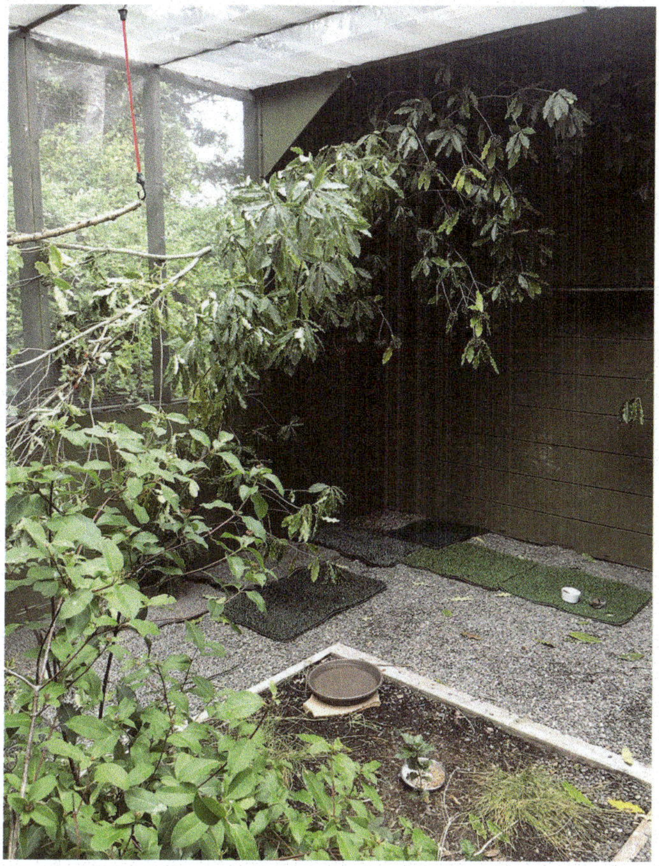

Figure 45.5 Aviary set up with diverse opportunities for perching, foraging, and flying. *Source:* photo courtesy of Veronica Bowers.

around the cage bottom and hidden among leaves or logs to encourage natural foraging. Branches of berries can be hung. A dish of bird grit (e.g. crushed cuttlebone or crushed boiled eggshells) should be included.

Once in the pre-release aviary, birds should see and interact with caregivers only briefly. NEVER allow birds to land on you! Observations are best from behind a "blind" to ensure each individual is eating and behaving normally and that no bird is being bullied. You should notice that the birds' behavior toward you changes as they "wild up" before release.

## Release

Most thrushes and thrush relatives need a minimum of 10–14 days in the pre-release aviary. Those birds that in the wild depend on parental support for longer periods than other birds may need more time. Before release, the birds should look more like juveniles with longer wings and tails than fledglings as flight feathers finish coming in. They should demonstrate a strong flight capability and an ability to find food and shelter, and their plumage should repel water. Ideally, the release site should be the bird's natal area, but keeping together birds that have been raised as a "family" unit is more important, since these family members will help each other find food and alert each

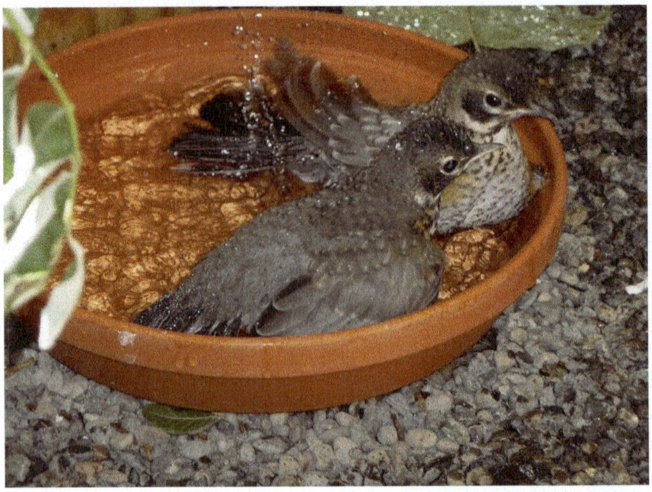

Figure 45.6 American Robins bathing in an aviary. *Source:* photo courtesy of Veronica Bowers.

other to predators. Soft-release is preferable – that is, providing food and shelter until the birds find their own food and gradually move on. Cedar Waxwings must be released into a flock, which can be located using online sources such as eBird. Weather should be mild the day or two following release so that the birds have the time and opportunity to find food and shelter and to develop a home territory.

## Acknowledgments

My sincerest appreciation to Connie Black for her procedures on Cedar Waxwing care, to Connie Anderson for her advice on American Robins, particularly regarding parasite protocols and housing enrichment, and to Janine Perlman for direction on nutrition and diets.

## Sources of Products Mentioned

Animal Intensive Care Unit: Lyon Technologies, Inc., 1690 Brandywine Avenue, Chula Vista, CA. 91911, https://lyonvet.com.

Flightless stingless wasps and freeze-dried insects: Arbico Organics, 10831 N. Mavinee Drive, Ste. 185, Oro Valley, AZ 85737-9531, (800) 847-2847, www.arbico-organics.com.

Leg bands: Red bird Products, Inc., P. O. Box 376, Mount Aukum, CA 95656-0376, (530) 620-7440, http://www.redbirdproducts.com.

Mealworms, waxworms, Dubia roaches, fly larvae, fruit flies and crickets: Rainbow Mealworms, 126 E. Spruce St, Compton, CA 90220, (800) 777-9676. https://www.rainbowmealworms.net.

## References

Duerr, R.S., Purdin, G.J., and Bowers, V. (2017). Small-bodied birds: passerines, doves, woodpeckers, others. In: *Topics in Wildlife Medicine, Vol. 4: Orthopedics* (eds. R.S. Duerr and G.J. Purdin), 53–74. St. Cloud, MN: National Wildlife Rehabilitators Association.

Hawkins, M.G., Barron, H.W., Speer, B.L. et al. (2018). Birds. In: *Exotic Anmal Formulary*, 5e (eds. J.W. Carpenter and C.J. Marion), 167–375. St. Louis, MO: Elsevier.

## Further Reading

Beaver, P., Brain, K., Schimmel, L., and Biyal, M. (1985). Effects of diet on the ontogeny of food preference and foraging in robins. NWRA Proceedings Vol. 4, pp. 98–104.

Cabe, P.R. (1993). European starling (*Sturnus vulgaris*), version 2.0. In: *The Birds of North America* (ed. A.F. Poole). Ithaca, NY, USA: Cornell Lab of Ornithology. https://doi.org/10.2173/bna.48.

Cavitt, J.F. and Haas, C.A. (2014). Brown thrasher (*Toxostoma rufum*), version 2.0. In: *The Birds of North America* (ed. A.F. Poole). Ithaca, NY, USA: Cornell Lab of Ornithology. https://doi.org/10.2173/bna.557.

Chu, M. and Walsberg, G. (1999). Phainopepla (*Phainopepla nitens*), version 2.0. In: *The Birds of North America* (eds. A.F. Poole and F.B. Gill). Ithaca, NY, USA: Cornell Lab of Ornithology. https://doi.org/10.2173/bna.415.

Dellinger, R., Wood, P.B., Jones, P.W., and Donovan, T.M. (2012). Hermit thrush (*Catharus guttatus*), version 2.0. In: *The Birds of North America* (ed. A.F. Poole). Ithaca, NY, USA: Cornell Lab of Ornithology. https://doi.org/10.2173/bna.261.

Evans, M., Gow, E., Roth, R.R. et al. (2011). Wood thrush (*Hylocichla mustelina*), version 2.0. In: *The Birds of North America* (ed. A.F. Poole). Ithaca, NY, USA: Cornell Lab of Ornithology. https://doi.org/10.2173/bna.246.

Farnsworth, G., Londono, G.A., Martin, J.U. et al. (2011). Northern mockingbird (*Mimus polyglottos*), version 2.0. In: *The Birds of North America* (ed. A.F. Poole). Ithaca, NY, USA: Cornell Lab of Ornithology. https://doi.org/10.2173/bna.7.

Gage, L.J. and Duerr, R.S. (eds.) (2007). *Hand-Rearing Birds*, 441 pp. Ames, Iowa: Blackwell Publishing.

Geupel, G.R. and Ballard, G. (2017). Wrentit (*Chamaea fasciata*), version 2.1. In: *The Birds of North America* (ed. P.G. Rodewald). Ithaca, NY, USA: Cornell Lab of Ornithology. https://doi.org/10.2173/bna.wrenti.02.1.

Gowaty, P.A. and Plissner, J.H. (2015). Eastern bluebird (*Sialia sialis*), version 2.0. In: *The Birds of North America* (ed. A.F. Poole). Ithaca, NY, USA: Cornell Lab of Ornithology. 10.2173/bna.381.

Guinan, J.A., Gowaty, P.A., and Eltzroth, E.K. (2008). Western bluebird (*Sialia mexicana*), version 2.0. In: *The Birds of North America* (ed. A.F. Poole). Ithaca, NY, USA: Cornell Lab of Ornithology. 10.2173/bna.510.

Kessel, B. (1957). A study of the breeding biology of the European starling (*Sturnus vulgaris L.*) in North America. *The American Midland Naturalist* 58 (2): 257–331.

Martin, A.C., Zim, H.S., and Nelson, A.L. (1951). *American Wildlife & Plants: A Guide to Wildlife Food Habits*, 500pp. New York: McGrawHill.

Miller, E.A. (ed.) (2012). *Minimum Standards for Wildlife Rehabilitation*, 4e. St. Cloud, MN: National Wildlife Rehabilitation Association.

Orendorff, B. (2003). The growth and development of a wild-reared eastern bluebird. *National Wildlife Rehabilitators Association Quarterly Journal* 21: 20–23.

Pinkowski, B.C. (1978). Feeding of nestling and fledgling eastern bluebirds. *The Wilson Bulletin* 90 (1): 84–98.

Sibley, D.A. (2001). *The Sibley Guide to Bird Life & Behavior*, 608 pp. New York: Alfred A. Knopf.

Smith, R.J., Hatch, M.I., Cimprich, D.A. et al. (2011). Gray catbird (*Dumetella carolinensis*), version 2.0. In: *The Birds of North America* (ed. A.F. Poole). Ithaca, NY, USA: Cornell Lab of Ornithology. https://doi.org/10.2173/bna.167.

Vanderhoff, N., Pyle, P., Patten, M.A. et al. (2016). American Robin (*Turdus migratorius*), version 2.0. In: *The Birds of North America* (ed. P.G. Rodewald). Ithaca, NY, USA: Cornell Lab of Ornithology. https://doi.org/10.2173/bna.462.

Wheelright, N.T. (1986). Diet of American Robins. *The Auk* 103: 710–725.

Witmer, M.C., Mountjoy, D.J., and Elliot, L. (2014). Cedar waxwing (*Bombycilla cedrorum*), version 2.0. In: *The Birds of North America* (ed. A.F. Poole). Ithaca, NY, USA: Cornell Lab of Ornithology. https://doi.org/10.2173/bna.309.

# 46

# Towhees

*Ashton Kluttz and Dana A. Glei*

## Natural History

Towhees belong to the Passerellidae family, which also includes New World Sparrows and Juncos. Towhees fall into two groups: the rufous-sided complex (*Pipilo* spp.) and the brown towhee complex (*Melozone* spp.). This chapter focuses on two species encountered in coastal Northern California: California Towhees (*Melozone crissalis*) and Spotted Towhees (*Pipilo maculatus*). Other species of towhees found in the Western U.S. include Canyon Towhees (*Melozone fusca*), Abert's Towhee (*Melozone aberti*), and the Green-Tailed Towhee (*Pipilo chlorurus*). Eastern Towhees (*Pipilo erthrophthalmus*) are found east of the Rockies and two species are endemic to Mexico: the White-Throated Towhee (*Melozone albicollis*) and the Collared Towhee (*Pipilo ocai*). The now extinct Bermuda Towhee (*Pipilo naufragus*) was endemic to Bermuda and closely related to the Eastern Towhee.

California and Spotted Towhees build a cup nest, often near the ground. Clutch size is typically two to three eggs for California (Benedict et al. 2011) and three to five eggs for Spotted Towhees (Bartos Smith and Greenlaw 2015). They may raise more than one brood per year. California Towhees feed their hatchlings solely animal food, mostly grasshoppers and caterpillars, but when the nestlings are 10 days old, parents begin introducing a small amount (<10%) of vegetable matter, mostly fiber with little fruit; at 2 weeks, the diet is still up to 95% animal-based – mostly beetles, wasps, and ants with fewer grasshoppers, caterpillars, and spiders (Benedict et al. 2011). Less is known regarding the diet fed to Spotted Towhee chicks, but it includes moths, caterpillars, grasshoppers, insect larvae, along with some seeds (Bartos Smith and Greenlaw 2015). As adults, California Towhees eat primarily seeds/grains (~80%) with ~15% insects (especially beetles and grasshoppers) and ~5% fruit (Benedict et al. 2011), whereas Spotted Towhees' diet differs between the breeding season (primarily insects) and nonbreeding period (mostly plant-based: seeds and fruit) (Bartos Smith and Greenlaw 2015).

### Why Are Towhees So Troublesome for Rehabilitators?

California Towhees are wary, furtive birds and easily stressed in captivity (Kasper 1998). Young towhees notoriously are troublesome for rehabilitators because of their reluctance or outright refusal to gape, which is exacerbated by trauma, pain, and captivity-induced stress. The rare Spotted Towhee may be less problematic than the ubiquitous California Towhee, but towhees may starve themselves to death before they will gape.

*Hand-Rearing Birds*, Second Edition. Edited by Rebecca S. Duerr and Laurie J. Gage.

Much of the care described here for towhees can be extended to the rest of their family (New World sparrows and juncos), which are generally much easier to rehabilitate. Anyone who can successfully raise and release towhees back to the wild is likely to have little difficulty raising sparrows and juncos.

## Criteria for Intervention

As ground birds, towhees are easy prey for outdoor cats; fledglings without fully-developed flight capability are particularly vulnerable. Over the past 3 years, nearly two-thirds of all towhees admitted to our rehabilitation center were preyed upon by a cat. Towhees comprise nearly 25% of our cat attack patients. Among towhees, kidnapping is the second most common cause of admission to our facility.

Although injured and predator-caught birds should be admitted to a rehabilitation facility, we have successfully reduced kidnappings by educating finders. Most finders are well-intentioned, but ill-informed regarding normal fledgling behavior, being unaware that most wild bird species spend at least a week on the ground with limited flight capability while the parents continue to feed and care for them. In questionable cases that lack a known predator interaction, noticeable weakness, or injury, we ask callers to send a photograph of the bird. If it appears to be a healthy fledgling, our phone personnel explain the fledging process and ask the finder to monitor the situation and confirm that a parent is caring for the fledgling. This request is typically well-received, and through such efforts we have prevented hundreds of healthy birds from entering our center.

If there is any evidence of predation, we ask the finder to bring the bird in for examination, but inform him/her that if we find no evidence of injury or illness, they will need to reunite the fledgling with its parents. It cannot be overstated that young birds are better off with their parents; no matter how thoughtful, captive care is a poor substitute. See Chapter 1 for more information about determining whether a chick requires rescue.

## Record Keeping

Small, colorful plastic leg bands can be used to identify individual birds (e.g. Red Bird Products). Identification is important for monitoring injury progress, tracking weight gain, administering treatments, and determining eating patterns.

## Initial Care and Stabilization

As with any chick entering care, warming chicks to normal body temperature followed by fluid therapy to ensure the GI tract is functioning is necessary before offering chicks food. See Chapter 1 for more information on stabilization of new birds.

## Common Medical Problems and Solutions

### Caught by Cat

For predator-caught birds, see Chapters 1 and 48 for protocols including treatments for immediate injuries and related complications. An oxygen concentrator and oxygen chamber have been very helpful in caring for new towhees. Given that towhees are easily stressed, they are placed in the warmed chamber upon arrival for the 15–20 minute rest period prior to examination. This protocol has significantly aided recovery for towhees and other stressed/injured birds. The bird must be stable and hydrated prior to injections, medications, or feeding.

Any predator-caught bird (e.g. cat attack victims) requires a full course of antibiotics and pain medication. Once the bird has been stabilized, our center, being a high-volume facility, provides prophylactic treatments to any bird suspected of cat contact due to the high prevalence of cat attack in these species in our area. See Chapter 1 for information on wound care and antibiotics for cat injured birds. Considering that towhees are notoriously difficult to get to eat in captivity, injectable antibiotics may be helpful in preventing a bird from associating an unpalatable medication with feedings, especially during initial care when birds are becoming accustomed to hand-feeding. Oral medications are better tolerated after this period has passed.

### Foot Problems

Compared with other species, we have encountered more foot dysfunction in towhees, especially California Towhees. A typical case exhibits normal blood supply to the foot with no fractures, but the bird shows a flaccid foot with an inability to position toes normally. We have successfully treated such cases with foot splints, utilizing corn pads, cardboard foot splints, or toe wraps, depending on the severity of the condition and activity level of the bird. The splint is visually evaluated daily to ensure appropriate fit with no edema. The splint should be temporarily removed to assess foot function after 3, 5, and 7 days as young birds develop and heal quickly. If function appears normal, we remove the splint for 24 hours to fully evaluate function before re-splinting if necessary. Typically, the splint needs to remain in place for approximately 1 week to recover proper foot function. See Duerr et al. (2017) for information on treatment of orthopedic problems in small birds.

## Diet

See Table 46.1 for what to feed by stage of development, which is based on the NWRA diet for Eastern Towhees (Scott 2013), our own observations of their feeding patterns while in captivity, and food source availability. Many rehabilitators would recommend against using formula because towhee parents would not feed chicks via regurgitation. Ideally, the diet for young towhees would be similar in composition and variety to the insect-based diet provided by towhee parents in the wild. Yet, most rehabilitation facilities, including ours, operate with limited resources and must be practical. We use primarily mealworms because they are readily available for purchase. At nestling and later stages, we generally try mealworms first, but offer everything available and developmentally appropriate. We find that some towhees prefer FoNS (see Table 41.3 for the recipe). Whenever possible, we prefer towhees to eat willingly. If a towhee wants blackberries, dusted with hard-boiled egg yolk, encrusted with seeds and chopped mealworms, and followed by a FoNS chaser, we will provide it. Insect diets must be supplemented to compensate for nutrients lacking in feeder insects. See Chapter 44, Box 44.1 for supplementation instructions based on the amount of insects eaten.

Food presentation for towhees differs from most other species. Towhees are essentially ground-feeders, known for their characteristic "double-scratch" method of foraging among the leaf litter. Therefore, we use towhee-specific dishes (Figure 46.1) in which mealworms are mixed in among seed. In larger reptariums/aviaries, the mealworm/seed dish is placed in a

Table 46.1 Example diet for young towhees by stage of development.

| Stage | Diet and Feeding Intervals | Notes[a] |
|---|---|---|
| Hatchling (day 1–4) | Hand-feed bloodworm hatchling diet[b] every 30 minutes for at least 12 hours a day | **At hatching (naked)**: Weight 9–11g[c]<br>**Day 2**: Downy<br>**Day 2–3**: Raises head and gapes in response to nest vibration.<br>**Day 3–4**: Pinfeathers only; no tail growth. Should produce well-formed fecal sacs. |
| Nestling (day 5–10) | Hand-feed mealworms[d] and FoNS every 30 minutes for 12+ hours a day | **Day 5**: Eyes begin to open; mean weight 17 g ± 5.5 SD.[e]<br>**Day 6–8**: Feathers begin to emerge from pins.<br>**Day 7**: Mean weight 29 g ± 3.3 SD.[e]<br>**Day 8**: Cowers rather than begs when approached; will jump from nest if disturbed.<br>**Day 8–10**: Begins hopping. |
| Pre-Fledge (day 10–13) | Hand-feed mostly mealworms[f] and FoNS; offer seed mixture, fruit, and hard-boiled egg. Feeding intervals progress from 30 to 45 minutes (still spanning 12+ hours a day) | **"Tail starter" phase** (2 cm long); often become reluctant gapers at this stage; very active; needs space, greenery, places to perch, leaf litter, and dirt tray. |
| Fledgling (day 14 to 2 months) | Diet same as for pre-fledge. Hand-feeding intervals gradually progress from 45 minutes to 1 hour to 2 hours (for 12+ hours a day) until weaning | Weight 35–45 g; tail growth average of 5 mm/day;<br>At beginning of this stage, should gain 2–3 g per day;<br>**Weaning** may begin once they attain a weight of 40 g+ and tail length of 5–6 cm[c]; in the wild, young begin foraging for themselves at 3–4 weeks.<br>**Pre-release conditioning** may begin by 4–6 weeks of age; should weigh around 50 g at release with a fully-grown tail 10.5–11.5 cm; for Spotted Towhee: 40 g with tail 9–10.5 cm.[c] |

[a] Refers to a development of a California Towhee unless otherwise noted; information for Spotted Towhees is more limited.
[b] Bowers, V. See Chapters 43 and 44 for hatchling diet and insect supplementation instructions.
[c] Kasper (1998).
[d] Cutting the worms in half is often helpful for towhees.
[e] Benedict et al. (2011).
[f] It may be helpful to dip a mealworm (or half a mealworm) in water and then in seed or egg before offering it to the towhee.

broad dirt tray with leaf litter. As they get older, mealworms are scattered among the dirt and leaf litter to encourage practice of the "towhee two-step." When placing their food, think about where towhees in the wild would find seed and insects (most likely on the ground) and fruit (NOT on the ground).

## Feeding Procedures

### Patience is Needed

California Towhees are generally good gapers until pre-fledge stage. At 2 to 3 days old, hatchlings will raise their heads and gape in response to nest vibrations or even changes in lighting over the nest, such as when a parent returns to the nest.

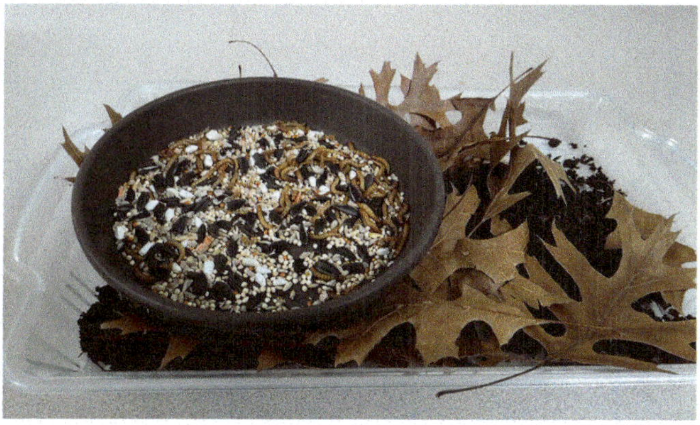

Figure 46.1 Towhee-specific dish (earth tones, shallow with low edges) in dirt tray with leaf litter. *Source:* photo by Dana A. Glei.

Anyone hand-feeding young towhees must be extremely patient. They cannot be rushed, which is why towhees are so demanding of rehabilitators (Kasper 1998). Bowers (2013 pers. comm.) explained that they must go through their ritual of hopping around, acting distracted, and ignoring you before they may finally be ready to gape. It may seem to take forever, and you might be certain this towhee will never gape, and then, seemingly magically, they do. Once a towhee begins gaping, they will usually keep gaping easily for the rest of that feeding. Yet by the next feeding, perhaps only 30 minutes later, that same towhee will have forgotten they ever gaped for the feeder. Unlike House Finches, overfeeding is rarely a problem. If you can get them to gape, keep feeding them as long as they gape. In our experience, it is a rare towhee who will continue to eat even after its crop becomes notably enlarged. If the crop becomes substantially enlarged, stop feeding until the next scheduled feeding.

Towhees must eat – or they will starve to death – but force-feeding induces further stress and thus may exacerbate the problem. Feeding towhees requires experienced volunteers who are willing to take the time and have the proper training to coax them to eat. Tips for encouraging gaping follow.

## Give the Towhee a Buddy (Preferably a Good Gaper)

No baby bird should be raised in isolation. It helps to pair difficult eaters with a good gaper to serve as a model. The pre-fledge stage is when towhees are most likely to become reluctant gapers. Adding a younger, gaping nestling may encourage a pre-fledge to gape, but can backfire if the good gaper also becomes reluctant to gape. We typically house the rarely admitted Spotted Towhee with California Towhees in a cohort, but towhees can also be grouped with other compatible species. A Brown-Headed Cowbird, generally eager to gape, can be a great nursemaid to towhees. Although cowbirds often parasitize towhee nests and can be responsible for evicting a nestling towhee that eventually ends up at a rehabilitation facility (Kasper 1998), we have not witnessed competition between cowbirds and towhees. Nonetheless, one should monitor carefully the interactions after introducing any new bird into an existing cohort. Other possible inter-species buddies include American Robins and Northern Mockingbirds – adult mockingbirds can be bullies, but when young, are compatible with towhees.

## "Time to Eat" Vocalization

Another trick recommended by Kasper (1998) and Bowers (2013 pers. comm.) is to mimic a "chipping song," which can help calm nervous birds and may trigger gaping when applied consistently. This vocalization is created by pressing air through your teeth while moving your lips to modulate a faint hissing-whistling sound (Kasper 1998). Fortunately, fledglings can become accustomed to a wide variety of feeding calls and are very forgiving if your attempt is not perfect. Bowers (2013 pers. comm.) warns that overusing it may further stress the bird; use it only once at the beginning of each feeding. We do not know whether the "chipping song" described here is suitable for other species of towhees, but we have used it with Spotted as well as California Towhees.

## Other Tricks

A bobbing motion with a worm-filled hemostat can help switch towhees into eating mode. While the towhee hops around the enclosure ignoring you or cowers in a corner with her beak firmly closed in a typical towhee frown (Figure 46.2), patiently follow the towhee offering up the food in front of the bird with the bobbing motion.

One towhee within a cohort will often gape first, upon which you should start feeding that individual but maintain watch on the others to note when another one begins gaping. Then, alternate between feeding the two (or more) towhees that are gaping. Continue feeding all gapers, and the others may catch on eventually. Take care to ensure that the towhees are, in fact, eating the worms they take; some troublesome towhees will spit them out when you look away to the fetch the next worm.

Offer mealworms first – cut in half and dipped in water to provide additional hydration – but switch to FoNS if the towhee displays no interest in worms. At the pre-fledgling stage, offer a variety of foods (see Table 46.1) and let each towhee decide what they want to eat. When many volunteers cover different shifts, it helps to leave notes for the next feeder detailing the feeding idiosyncrasies of each towhee. Colored leg bands help feeders track individuals to ensure that all towhees in a cohort are fed at every scheduled feeding. Towhees are finicky and their preferences change quickly; even with careful notes, "towhee whisperers" must be able to improvise and adapt as feeding behavior changes.

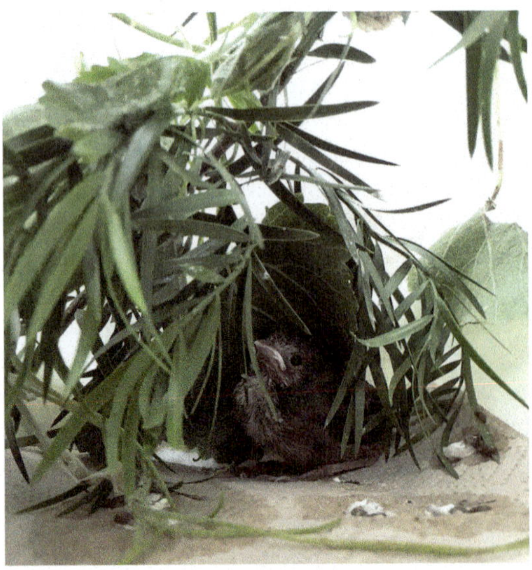

Figure 46.2 Towhee, with typical towhee frown, seeking shelter in the fresh greenery. *Source:* photo by Lucy Stevenot.

### How Long Should I Wait Patiently?

Given the importance of patience, volunteers often ask: How long should I wait? If the gaping behavior of a given towhee remains unknown, we counsel greater persistence (e.g. wait at least 1 minute). A full minute seems like an eternity when there is a room full of birds to be fed and you fear being unable to finish one feeding before the next begins. If multiple people have already patiently tried every trick, but failed to induce gaping, then you might wait only 30 seconds on the first attempt. If you also fail to elicit gaping, then it is reasonable to give up more quickly on subsequent feedings of that bird, unless seeing some indication of potential gaping behavior. If you manage to induce gaping behavior once, then be very patient and persistent with that towhee on all subsequent feedings. As Kasper (1998) warns, do not betray the trust a towhee displays by gaping; if you rush them or feed them too much in one mouthful, they will become even more difficult to feed.

### Last Resort: Assisted-feeding

Assisted-feeding should be a last resort, after exhausting all other means of inducing voluntary gaping. Never skip a feeding unless self-feeding has been confirmed, and the bird is demonstrating adequate weight gain. For an assisted-feeding (see also Chapter 32), it can be helpful to "burrito" the towhee in a small washcloth, making it easier to hold a squirmy bird without squeezing too tightly. Once in hand, the towhee may begin gaping on its own or gape more easily. If not, gently open its mouth and insert food using a hemostat. Allow the bird to swallow before administering additional food. Baby towhees eat a surprising amount of food for their size. Gauge the quantity of food you provide based on the consumption of similar-aged towhees who gape voluntarily, but remain alert to signals that the towhee has had enough for that feeding; stop if the bird begins regurgitating.

## Weaning

Kasper (1998) suggests that weaning can begin when tail length reaches 5–6 cm and their weight is at least 40 g. Do not cease hand-feeding until you visually verify that the towhee is self-feeding. Once it is confirmed that every individual in a cohort is self-feeding, fresh diets are offered every morning with replenishment as needed throughout the day. Continue weighing birds twice daily for 5 more days until they are moved into an aviary. After transfer to an aviary, they are weighed once daily for the first 3 days. Every few days after that, weigh or simply catch and assess the pectoral muscle mass at their keel, which should be plump. Release weights for California Towhees are between 50 and 60 g, and birds progress through our program from admission to release in about 30 days.

## Expected Weight Gain

Developmental stages are described briefly in Table 46.1. Young towhees should be weighed daily – particularly during the most difficult pre-fledgling and early fledgling stages – to ensure they are achieving adequate weight gain. If not, there may be a gap in feeding that needs to be addressed. Alert feeders to devote special attention to feeding those problem towhees. Birds in our care have gained about a 1 g per day throughout days 5–13 (Figure 46.3).

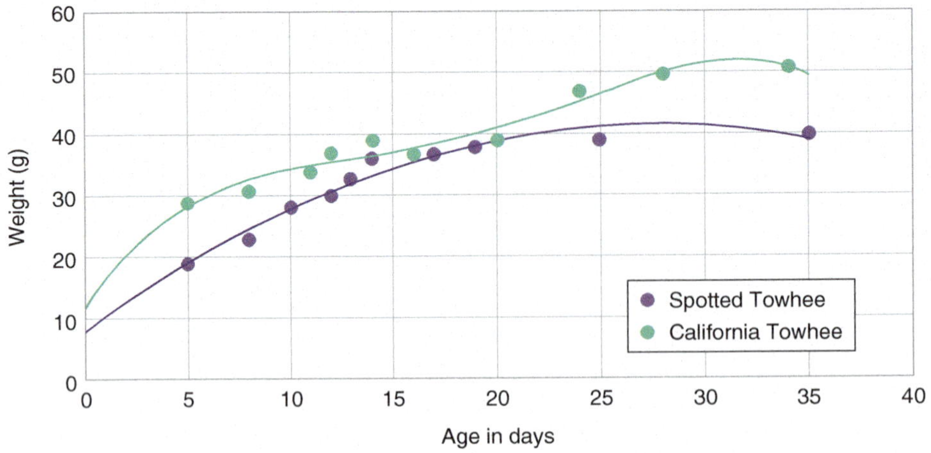


Figure 46.3 Towhee weight progression. Typical towhee weight progression, please note that weights younger than Day 5 are extrapolated but correspond well with known hatch towhee weights.

## Housing

Place hatchlings in an incubator (at 90–95 °F/32.2–35 °C with 50–60% humidity). Hatchlings and nestlings should produce well-formed fecal sacs. It is imperative for feather development, general health, and minimizing stress that nests and living areas be kept as clean as possible. The nestling stage begins on day 5, at which time their eyes begin to open. Feathers begin to emerge between days 6–8. We keep towhees in an incubator during the nonmobile portion of the nestling stage. When they begin to explore between days 8–10, we transition them from the incubator into our brooder area (ambient temperature ~90 °F/32.2 °C). At 8 days, California Towhees will cower rather than beg when approached and may jump from their nest if disturbed (Benedict et al. 2011); at this point, jiggling the nest to induce gaping is ill-advised. In the wild, they would stay with parents up to 6 weeks, unless their parents re-nest, in which case they may drive the fledges away at 4 weeks.

In late nestling and early pre-fledge stages, birds cannot fly yet, but are very capable runners that will try to escape any housing enclosure. We typically move them to our ICU (ambient temperature ~80–85 °F/26.7–29.4 °C) during days 10–13 when their tail is about 2 cm long and birds are about 25–35 g. A precocious nestling that begins hopping at a slightly younger age than normal may require additional heat sources (e.g. heating pad) longer than the typical mobile nestling. As they become more active, they will require more space, natural greenery, perches, leaf and dirt tray, and often become reluctant gapers. If so, weigh each bird first thing in the morning and again at midday, so as to gauge who may be starting to self-feed and who may need special attention. This protocol allows individual towhees to progress at their own pace within our larger facility.

The data shown in Figure 46.3 suggest that a transition stage occurs around day 16 in our center while we determine the towhee's eating preferences. If you can successfully manage these difficult few days, they typically start self-feeding during days 20–22. If there is steady weight gain, good feather development, and progressive healing of injuries, we begin gradually lengthening the feeding intervals (Table 46.1), but continue weighing them twice a day and monitor their feeding behavior.

## Emulate their Natural Environment

The housing suggestions provided in Chapter 48 also work well for towhees. To the extent possible within a rehabilitation setting, try to emulate towhees' natural environment. Wild towhees spend most of their time close to the ground and often hide in dense bushes; foraging in leaf litter is a favorite pastime; and they absolutely love bathing. Beginning at pre-fledgling stage, it is important to provide a dirt tray with leaf litter to encourage their "double-scratch" method of foraging for food. Do not neglect to provide a place for them to hide (Figure 46.2). Isolating towhees from predatory species will reduce their stress levels. Keep towhees, finches, juncos, sparrows, doves, and quail in a room separate from corvids whenever possible. Human caretakers should minimize their own noise and try to maintain a calm, quiet composure in the presence of the birds. Never talk to the birds and avoid unnecessary "peeking" in their enclosures. Once they are thermoregulating but not yet self-feeding, reptariums enriched with generous fresh greenery work well for towhees (Figure 46.4). Move towhees to an aviary as soon as possible; at the latest, once they are self-feeding.

## Keeping Them Clean

Cleaning is vital. Having dirty feathers/feet/face/bill or soiled housing can exacerbate stress levels and unwillingness to gape. During the nestling stage, parents remove fecal sacs, keeping the nest clean until fledging (Benedict et al. 2011). Tweezers are useful for removing fecal sacs from their housing/nest without unduly disturbing the nestling. As they become more active, keeping the birds and their enclosure clean is increasingly difficult. You may change the liners, add fresh greenery, replace soiled food with fresh diets, and provide clean water only to have the towhees excrete in the new food dishes or on each other before you have even left the room. It is important to provide young towhees with a bird bath. Even in small enclosures, a small, shallow plant saucer with a little water provides them the opportunity to bathe.

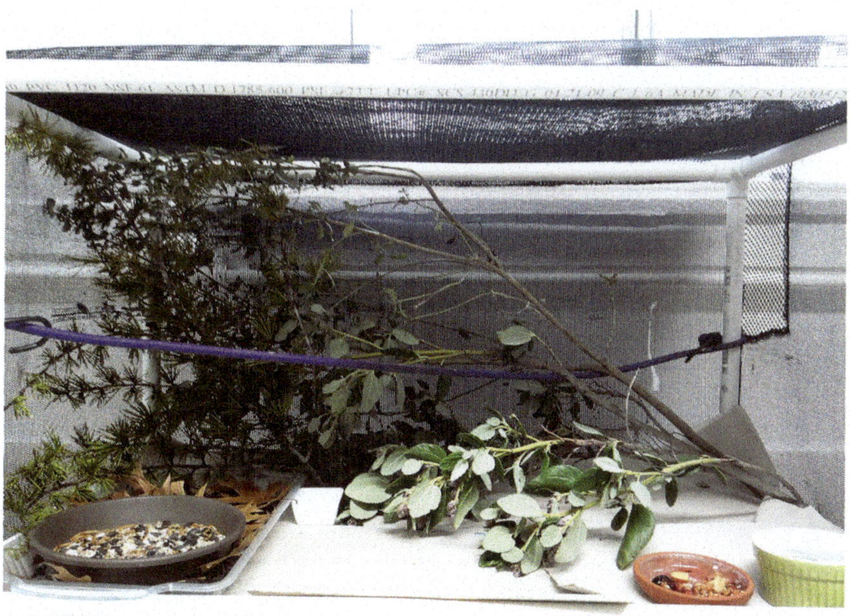

Figure 46.4 Model set up of reptarium for towhees. *Source:* photo by Dana A. Glei.

## Release

Unless towhees can be reunited with their parents, returning them to the wild too early could be a death sentence. Towhees mature slowly and must learn many survival skills before they can thrive on their own. For the best chance of survival, towhees should be grouped in a cohort of three to six birds that progress through rehabilitation together and are eventually released as a group.

Pre-release conditioning may begin by 4 to 6 weeks of age. Prior to release, towhees need at least 1 to 2 weeks in an aviary to socialize with the other towhees in their release cohort and to practice survival skills. For towhees, we recommend a minimum aviary size of 10×8×8 ft. (3×2.4×2.4 m) for three to four towhees. The bigger the aviary the better, but each facility must balance their limited resources to serve all the birds/wildlife in their care. During this phase, it is crucial to provide enrichment that approximates their natural environment. Minimize human intrusion to allow them to "wild up." Towhees learn by example, copying the behavior of older towhees; housing them with older towhees may speed the learning process.

When raised in the wild, California Towhees do not disperse far from their natal home. Yet, if we return each towhee raised in captivity to its natal home, it is less likely to survive on its own. Releasing a cohort of towhees at one of the original rescue sites is generally not a good option either because most towhees admitted for care are victims of a roaming domestic cat and/or the finder may not have the commitment to provide necessary support during the transition period from captivity to independence.

We rely on our volunteers and staff with towhee-appropriate habitat for soft-release sites. To better suit towhees, we developed a special soft-release enclosure: The Towhee Trailer (Figure 46.5). Its defining features include double walls with plastic fencing on the outside of the 2×2 in. (3.1×3.1 cm) wood frame coupled with fiberglass screen on the inside and a large door on the end

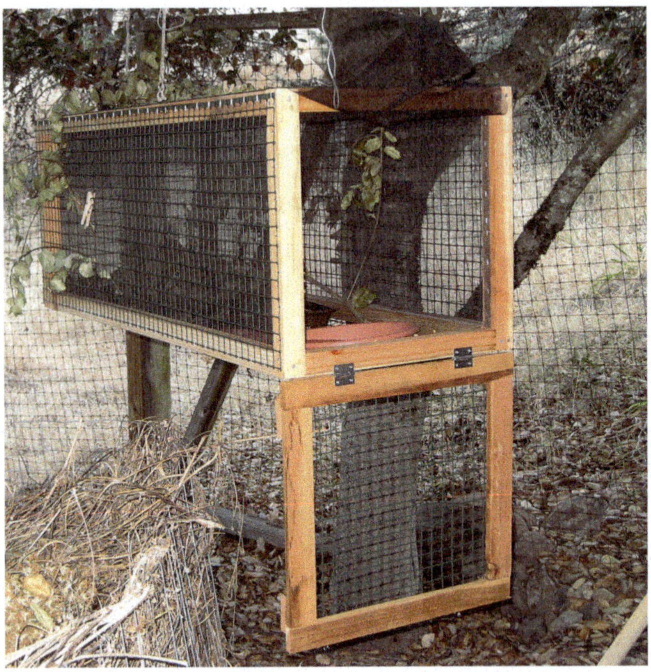

Figure 46.5 Towhee-specific soft-release enclosure ("Towhee Trailer"). *Source:* photo by Dana A. Glei.

that opens like a mailbox so that towhees might be more willing to return to the cage for food/water/shelter as needed.

After transporting a cohort in the Towhee Trailer to the release site and hanging it in a tree (day 1), the host allows a 3-day acclimation period during which the cage is kept closed and the host disturbs them only 2–3 times a day to replenish food and water, otherwise observing from afar. It is helpful to set up a ground-feeding station nearby as soon as the Towhee Trailer is installed in the new setting. Doing so encourages resident towhees to visit and perhaps make friends with the newly-introduced towhee cohort.

First thing in the morning on day 3, the host replenishes their food and water. A few hours later, the release hatch is opened completely, and the towhees are allowed to emerge when they are ready. Most towhees leave immediately, but some are more hesitant. In some cases, it may take many hours before the last towhee will have the courage to embark, during which time they are left alone, but may be monitored from afar.

After release, the host continues to replenish food and water inside the trailer for at least a few more days and maintains the nearby ground-feeding station and water bath for at least several weeks. After a few days, food and water are removed from the trailer. Over time, seed is dispersed on the ground more widely to encourage foraging and, eventually, food dishes are removed, although it is helpful to continue spreading food around the area for several more weeks.

## Acknowledgments

Many thanks to Veronica Bowers (NSCC) who shared her insights regarding the care of towhees with us. We are also grateful to the crucial groundwork laid by Kasper (1998) and colleagues at the Lindsay Wildlife Museum whose research and development of a towhee-specific protocol provided a crucial foundation for our own protocol. Most importantly, special thanks to the 125+ volunteers at The Bird Rescue Center and, in particular, the army of "towhee whisperers" who help coax young towhees to eat.

## Sources for Products Mentioned

Feeder insects: Rainbow Mealworms, 126 E. Spruce St, Compton, CA 90220, (800) 777-9676. https://www.rainbowmealworms.net.

Leg bands: Red bird Products, Inc., P. O. Box 376, Mount Aukum, CA 95656-0376, (530) 620-7440, http://www.redbirdproducts.com.

## References

Bartos Smith, S. and Greenlaw, J.S. (2015). Spotted towhee (*Pipilo maculatus*), version 2.0. In: *The Birds of North America* (ed. P.G. Rodewald). Ithaca, New York, USA: Cornell Lab of Ornithology. https://doi.org/10.2173/bna.263.

Benedict, L., Kunzmann, M.R., Ellison, K. et al. (2011). California towhee (*Melozone crissalis*), version 2.0. In: *The Birds of North America* (ed. P.G. Rodewald). Ithaca, New York, USA: Cornell Lab of Ornithology https://doi.org/10.2173/bna.632.

Duerr, R.S., Purdin, G.J., and Bowers, V. (2017). Small-bodied birds: passerines, doves, woodpeckers, others. In: *Topics in Wildlife Medicine, Vol. 4: Orthopedics* (eds. R.S. Duerr and G.J. Purdin), 53–74. St. Cloud, MN: National Wildlife Rehabilitators Association.

Kasper, A. (1998). *Natural History, Rehabilitation, and Medicine of the California Towhee (Pipilo [Melazone] Crissalis)*. Glendale, AZ: Wildlife Publications.

Scott, M. (2013). *Songbird Diet Index: A Guide to the Natural Food Habits of Ohio Songbirds and Substitute Diets for Use in Wildlife Rehabilitation Facilities*, 2e. National Wildlife Rehabilitators Association.

## Further Reading

Bowers, V. (2016). *Passerine Fundamentals*, 100 pp. Sebastopol, CA: Native Songbird Care & Conservation.

# 47

# Grackles, Blackbirds, and Other Icterids

*Maureen Eiger and Guthrum Purdin*

## Natural History

Icteridae is a New World family of birds including 109 species (Gill and Donsker 2019). Neonates are frequently presented for care at wildlife facilities in North America, among which Brewer's and Red-winged Blackbirds as well as grackles, orioles, and cowbirds are common. The Eurasian species, the Common Blackbird (*Turdus merula*), is not an icterid, but rather is in the Thrush family, see Chapter 45.

An unusual feature of the icterids is the ability of the jaw muscles to open the bill with great force against resistance, a technique known as "gaping." Whereas most birds with powerful jaws have muscles evolved to close their mouths to apprehend, tear, or crush food, icterids use their gaping ability as a method of exposing hidden food items like insects.

As a representative member of Family Icteridae, this chapter will largely focus on the Common Grackle (*Quiscalus quiscula*). These birds are found in flocks east of the Rocky Mountains, where they are considered resident or short-distance migrants. All adults have yellow eyes, with feathering considered black, though different subspecies can show varied iridescent colors on their feathers in sunlight; from bronze to purple to greenish coloring depending on the region. The corner flange of the bird's mouth is light colored and curves downward (like a frown) toward the throat. Adults have a distinctive long wedge-shaped tail, easily identified in flight. Females are smaller and duller-colored than males. Chicks have long gray down, especially on their head, and the inside of the mouth is red. Baby grackles have been described as looking like "tiny vultures" since the feathers around the birds' eyes come in last; this characteristic is also common in other icterids (Figure 47.1). Young and fledgling grackles are browner in coloring than adults and have brown eyes changing to yellow in the fall. They are one of the few birds that completely molt all of their feathers in the fall. Grackles are found in suburban backyards, city parks, farmlands, and swamps, and are not generally found in unbroken forests. They roost together in huge mixed flocks at night.

### Nesting

Common Grackles begin nesting at most locations in late March to early April (Peer and Bollinger 1997). Eggs are laid from March to June, with an average incubation period of 14 days, with 1–2 broods per year. Common Grackles nest in colonies or as a single family in a variety of locations,

*Hand-Rearing Birds*, Second Edition. Edited by Rebecca S. Duerr and Laurie J. Gage.

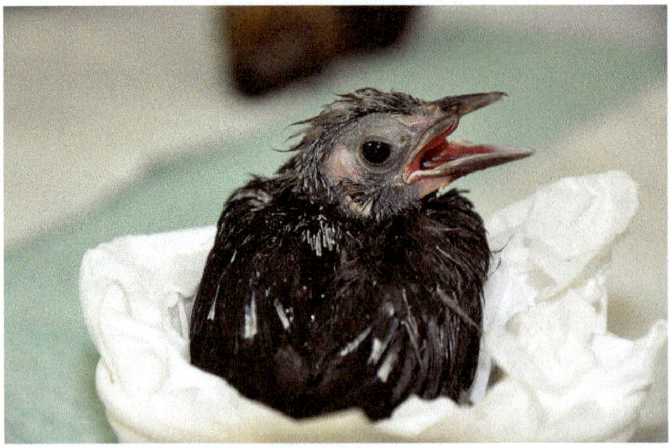

Figure 47.1 Common Grackle nestling displaying a typical icterid face where the feathers around the eyes come in relatively late during growth.

from evergreens or hardwoods to bushes or sometimes on buildings. Usually nests are built very high up or are well hidden, so it is difficult to re-nest fallen nestlings.

### Wild Diet

Adult grackles eat a variety of animal and plant foods, including grubs, grasshoppers, earthworms, boll weevils, army worms, caterpillars, ants, flies, cocoons, cicadas, crayfish, minnows, goldfish, small mice, small snakes and lizards, eggs of birds, baby birds, small birds (especially house sparrows), bats, acorns, chestnuts, weed seeds, all kinds of grain (especially corn), and wild and cultivated fruit. The adult diet is typically 70–75% plant matter, mostly seeds and fruits, and 25–30% animal matter (Peer and Bollinger 1997).

## Criteria for Intervention

Chicks may fall from their nests, especially in high winds. High temperatures may make nestlings restless and thus more likely to tumble to the ground. These individuals are usually dehydrated and may be overheated or chilled. Fractures and head trauma can be associated with falls, especially when landing on hard surfaces. Cat attack is common, especially for freshly fledged juveniles. Some may arrive for care after striking windows or being hit by cars. Birds may arrive ill or debilitated for unknown reasons, necessitating a medical work up to determine a treatment plan. The specific protocols for medication in this chapter are those used by the author (GP) working largely from information that can be found in Hawkins et al. (2018), an excellent reference for drug doses in many species of birds.

## Record Keeping

See Chapter 1 for information regarding appropriate record keeping, and Appendix A for a sample bird record.

## Initial Care and Stabilization

See Chapter 1 for initial care information. As with all young birds presenting for care after trauma or misadventure, warm chicks to normal body temperature (103–106 °F/39.4–41.1 °C) prior to fluid administration. On presentation, icterids are commonly dehydrated, especially in the spring and summer months when the weather is hot. Once birds have warmed up and calmed down, give all new arrivals subcutaneous (SQ) fluids at 5% body weight of a balanced electrolyte, like lactated Ringer's solution warmed to 100–105 °F (38–41 °C). Deliver using a 25 gauge needle at the loose skin cranial to the knee while holding the syringe parallel to the thigh. Oral fluids delivered via syringe every 30 minutes is another option for rehydrating a dehydrated chick. Do not begin feeding birds until they begin passing droppings.

Some orphaned neonate grackles have an olive/yellow cast to their skin. These birds do fine when fed regularly and the odd coloring will eventually fade. Development may be slowed and adult size smaller than normal, but generally there will be no other problems if fed correctly.

## Common Medical Problems

Grackles and other icterids often nest near water. If a fallen neonate is found near water, listen for wheezes or clicks when breathing, which may indicate aspiration and possible pneumonia. Any such bird should be given a broad-spectrum antibiotic, such as amoxicillin with clavulanic acid, at 125 mg/kg orally twice daily for 7–14 days.

Birds with open wounds should always be similarly treated with antibiotics until the injury has resolved. If the cause of injury is cat attack, infection with *Pasteurella multocida* is an especial risk and the antibiotic chosen should cover this bacterium. Treatment should be started even if cat contact is only suspected. Cat claws are so sharp, that sometimes no wound is found, but pathogenic bacteria can nonetheless have been introduced. Infections due to cat contact can be severe and onset rapid. It is better to treat proactively than to wait for the bird to become sick.

Ideally, all open wounds should be closed or covered. Clean wounds with a gentle disinfectant (e.g. dilute povidone-iodine or chlorhexidine) and if a dressing is applied, change it every 2–3 days until healed. If possible, suture or apply surgical glue to the wound once it has been thoroughly cleaned. If this is not possible, one option is to cover the open lesion with a self-adhesive hydrocolloid dressing. This will keep the wound clean and protected, and will serve to prevent desiccation and speed healing. Air sacs can be damaged and pockets of air develop under the skin after cat attacks or severe trauma (e.g. falls or window strikes), a condition called subcutaneous emphysema. These birds should also be treated with antibiotics until the gas bubble is resolved, as in these species the problem is most commonly caused by cat attack. If the subcutaneous (SQ) air bubble is large enough to be causing the bird discomfort or impeding mobility, it can be drained with a sterile needle. These bubbles may re-inflate, requiring repeated punctures over several days to resolve (Figure 47.2). See Chapter 1 for more information on wound care.

If head trauma is known or suspected, or if the bird has a potentially painful injury or bone fracture, then begin a course of meloxicam at 0.5 mg/kg given orally twice daily. The first dose should be done as 1 mg/kg. The course can be as short as 3 days for mild injuries and 5–7 days for head trauma, however it can be extended if needed.

If possible, run fecal direct and float tests on all newly arriving birds. This becomes a necessity if birds are persistently emaciated or unthrifty and no other cause can be determined. Coccidia is common and can be treated with ponazuril at 20 mg/kg orally once daily for 5 days. Check the fecal

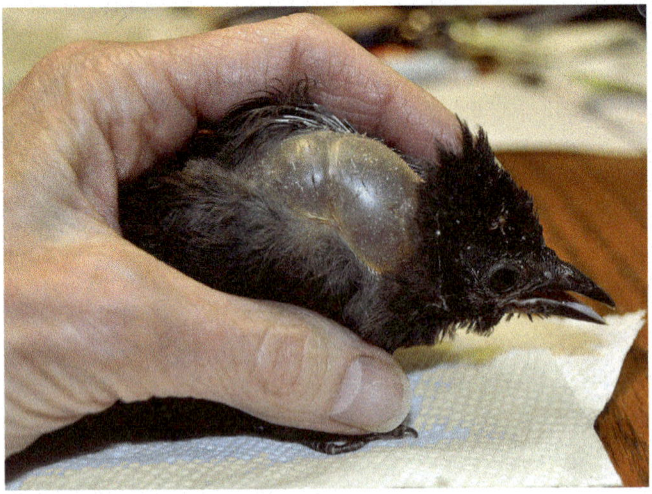

Figure 47.2 Common Grackle chick with a subcutaneous emphysema (air under the skin) due to attack by a cat resulting in the puncture of an internal air sac.

again on day 6. If the bird is still positive for coccidia, continue treatment for another 2–5 days. Coccidia is highly infectious and the oocysts found in the feces are environmentally stable. Isolate positive and exposed cagemates until fecals are negative, although each chick needs at least one companion to assist with social skill development. Change all caging, bedding, and feeding materials and disinfect soiled tools. Wear gloves and wash hands between cages.

Nematode eggs are occasionally seen in fecals. Treat with fenbendazole at 50 mg/kg orally once daily for 5 days. Treatment may need to be repeated after 14 days. Alternatively, nematode-positive birds can be given ivermectin 0.4 mg/kg once orally, then repeat on day 14.

Knemidocoptes, also called scaly-leg mites, appears as a thickening and crusty overgrowth of scales on the legs, most commonly seen on individuals such as Brewer's Blackbirds that live around shopping centers and fast food restaurants. Lesions can be mild to crippling, with the worst affected birds unable to stand. Neonates presenting with this may have subtle lesions. If suspected, look for mites by doing a skin scraping of the affected portions of the legs and examine under a microscope. The cornerstone of treatment is ivermectin, given as previously described. Wipe the legs with a cloth or gauze soaked in dilute chlorhexidine daily for 3 days then every third day until resolved. Some protocols recommend using ivermectin topically. If used in this way, be very careful to not overdose the bird, since this drug can be toxic. Systemic ivermectin is more likely to reach all mites on the bird. Quarantine affected birds and exposed cagemates.

Birds with feather lice or skin mites can be sprayed with a topical anti-arthropod spray like UltraCare Mite and Lice Bird Spray (8 in 1 Pet Products) or similar pyrethrin/piperonyl butoxide-based product; cover the bird's head when applying to avoid spraying in the eyes. Prevent inhalation of vapors by providing adequate ventilation during and after application.

Blackbirds and orioles may arrive with damaged or poorly developed flight feathers that are broken, have stress bars, or otherwise show abnormal growth. After the causal problem (e.g. malnutrition) has been addressed and corrected, the birds may still not be releasable due to poor feather quality. They can sometimes be kept in captivity until they molt, but this may be a prolonged period of many months or even a year or more. Alternatively, for smaller species, flight feathers can be plucked. Hold the affected feather at the base with a hemostat and pull quickly, straight out, while holding the wing firmly at the follicle base with your other hand. If targeting damaged feathers that are adjacent to one another, pull every third feather, then repeat a few days later and then again until all affected feathers have been removed. Give these birds meloxicam prior to plucking and once or twice daily until the process is completed. Plucking the feathers under anesthesia is also an option, but still it is best to avoid plucking adjacent feathers at the same time due to risks of damage. Be aware of housing needs: if a large enough number of feathers is removed, the bird will not be able to fly until regrowth has occurred. Provide a diversity of low perching so the patient can get up off the floor and make its way to higher perches. If the substrate is hard, like concrete, either have only low perches or move the bird into smaller housing until flight has returned. If the new feathers are also of poor quality, the chances of release are poor and euthanasia should be considered.

West Nile virus is spread by mosquitoes. Affected birds are often neurologically abnormal and may present with reduced mentation, nystagmus, incoordination, torticollis, trembling, and/or seizures. If WNV is suspected and clinical signs are not too severe, provide supportive care and place the bird on meloxicam for 7 days and monitor for improvement. If clinical signs worsen or remain static, then euthanasia is indicated. Birds presenting as severely affected on arrival should be euthanized since the prognosis is poor. Toxicities due to agricultural or pest-control chemicals may present similarly and it can be difficult to differentiate. When in doubt, supportive care with an assessment of improvement every few days is useful.

## Diet

A 100% insect diet is best for hatchlings and nestlings. See Chapters 43 and 44 for information on care and feeding of feeder insects and necessary supplementation for a 100% insect diet in Chapter 44, Box 44.1: "Supplements for Birds Hand-reared on an Insects-only Diet." Defrosted frozen or fresh cricket bodies (with the spiny legs removed) and gut-loaded mealworms are main foods. Drown gut-loaded whole small- or medium-size mealworms in water to kill them prior to feeding young chicks. Pull out a few at a time, dab them on a tissue or paper towel to reduce the amount of water, then feed with forceps. Weight gain may vary each day as they get older, but the bird should be gaining a minimum of 1–2 g every day. A few drops of water at the end of the day are well received.

When grackle fledglings begin to develop their primary wing feathers, add peanut suet balls, waxworms, some earthworms, fruit, and eggs scrambled in oil. Using yellow foods like fresh or defrosted frozen corn encourages them to learn how to self-feed. Another option is to use a mix of 50/50 powder-to-water (the consistency should look like thick sour cream) of Harrison's® Recovery Formula (Harrison's Bird Foods) or Emeraid® IC Carnivore (Lafeber Company) or Mazuri® Handfeeding Formula (PMI Nutrition International) as a supplement fed via syringe or as a dip for the insects, making sure the primary diet is insects. A 90% insect and 10% formula feeding ratio works well. Watch the bird's droppings to make sure it is properly digesting any of the pre-made formulas. Make sure mixed formulas are made fresh at least twice a day. Always smell the formula before feeding it to the birds. If it smells sour or "off," discard the whole batch.

Feeding insect-only diets to hatchlings, nestlings, and pre-weaned fledglings in a high-volume rehabilitation facility can be difficult due to expense, time constraints, and a rotating pool of sometimes inexperienced caregivers. One of the authors (GP) has had good outcomes raising Red-winged and Brewer's Blackbirds and Brown-headed Cowbirds using Basic Nestling Diet formula (see Table 41.3 for recipe). Once birds are out of the nest, a variety of solid foods should be offered even while the primary source of nutrition remains syringe-feeding. This is especially true as birds approach weaning age. Provide a low dish of chopped broccoli florets and cut-up grapes – these will often be the first things a growing bird will start to eat on its own. Cat or dog kibble can be offered either as a dry, ground crumble or soaked, whole kibble. A bowl of mealworms (deep enough for the worms to be unable to crawl out, but shallow enough for the birds to reach in) is a key motivation to self-feeding. Mealworms should be gut-loaded by housing in highly nutritious bedding for at least 24 hours prior to offering to birds. Game Bird Starter is a preferred substrate for mealworms. Provide moisture to the worms by placing thinly cut apple slices, broccoli stem slices, or other greens. Provide mixed cut fruit and a separate, shallow dish of finch seed. Change out these food items as they become depleted, soiled, or aged.

When birds start to have a long tail and are in playpens or their outdoor conditioning cages, add live crickets, summer suet, wild fruit on the stems, acorns, shell-free mix birdseed, millet, soaked raisins, a product like Nuts "n" Bugs (Wild Bird Store), and peanut butter suet balls. In the wild, these birds are "gapers," so to facilitate foraging practice, add a large dirt bowl filled with earthworms, beetles, and mealworms, especially if the flight cage flooring has no dirt/grassy spots. Use two water bowls since they sometimes like to dunk their food. Older fledglings and pre-release birds need to be acquainted with some of the adult diet items listed above. Oriole diets in the wild include various insects and invertebrates plus berries and a diversity of fruits and nectar. Older chicks should be offered these as well.

## Feeding Procedures

Grackles can be food flingers. Drown mealworms in water or pinch their heads before offering to the bird. Using hemostats, present the worm so that the bird has to lift its bill up. There is a sweet spot on top of their tongue in the back of the mouth and if food is placed there, no flinging occurs. For inexperienced birds and persistent food flingers, gently tip the bill from underneath with the hemostats as it swallows. Grackles are smart and usually figure out the process after a few feedings. It is okay to feed until the bird refuses food, they will not overeat. They are also very noisy birds if hungry or bored. Slightly altering the feeding schedule by a few minutes sooner or later (use a timer) will help cut down on the noise. They will figure out food is coming but not be conditioned to a set time. For smaller species being syringe-fed, see Table 47.1 for feeding frequencies and volumes.

### Foraging Enrichment

It may be necessary to house grackles away from more sensitive species if their calls are disruptive or stressful. They can be aggressive to conspecifics and other species of birds. Grackle fledges have been known to kill birds they are housed with. They are flock birds, so they should not be housed alone, but their attitude and behavior with other cagemates must be monitored carefully. Make sure they

Table 47.1 Protocol for syringe feeding Brewer's Blackbirds and Brown-headed Cowbirds.

| Age | Weight (g) | Amount (cc) | Minutes between feeds |
|---|---|---|---|
| Tiny hatchlings | 5–10 | 0.25–0.5 | 30 |
| Eyes open, mostly naked nestlings | 11–18 | 0.5–1 | 30 |
| Young nestlings | 18–28 | 1–1.5 | 30 |
| Older nestling-fledglings | 29+ | 1.5–2 | 45 |
| Ideal weaning weight 42+ g | | | |

Basic Nestling Diet. Use a 1 cc syringe, with a cannula tip for small chicks.

are in appropriately sized housing, have "something to do", and are not bored so they are more likely to get along with cagemates. Environmental enrichment is very important. Diversify the food items offered. Foods can be "hidden" in old paper towel tubes, buried in pans of dirt, or elsewhere in the enclosure. Natural tree branches with leaves and foraging opportunities should be available. Be creative and see what works best for the birds in care. Icterids have diverse diets in the wild and should be offered diverse opportunities to forage on different foods when learning to feed themselves.

## Weaning

Once blackbirds and cowbirds are nearing adult weight, are actively navigating their environment, and are nearly done growing feathers, they can be considered for weaning. Move the birds from the basket to a playpen well supplied with tasty food offerings. The motion of live insects like mealworms is an especially effective incentive. Offer a diverse diet to simulate wild conditions and provide ample nutritional opportunities. A mix of 60% mealworms, 30% crickets, and 10% waxworms has been effective and some facilities will add small dubia roaches. Orioles tend to be slower to total independence and will need more fruit offered, and some of this can be suspended to approximate natural food sources. Orioles enjoy orange slices hung on skewers and live fruit flies can also been offered. While in basket housing, formula feedings should be every 30–45 minutes as long as the lights are on (ideally for 16 hours a day and no less than 12). At the start of weaning in the playpen, offer formula every 1 hour for 2–3 days. If weights are stable or improved, change to offering formula every 2 hours for 2–3 days. If birds maintain their weight when being offered formula only once every 3 hours for 2 days, they can be considered self-feeding. If weights remain stable with no supplemental feeding for 2 days, move them to a pre-release flight aviary. Before the move, make sure they are fully independent of formula and in good body condition. Flocks can be rambunctious and the more timid birds, new to self-feeding, may be bullied away from food in large flight aviaries. Offer food in multiple dishes, so aggressive birds can't monopolize a single food source. If during the weaning process a bird loses 3 g, return to the previous feeding schedule for 2–3 days, then try again. Do not force-feed weaning birds. Weaning can be stressful for some birds with a subsequent drop in immune function. If birds have a continual weight loss or appear unthrifty, evaluate for illness.

## Expected Weight Gain

Common grackles are completely altricial at hatch but, like most passerines, grow rapidly. At about 2 days of age, weight ranges from 7 to 10 g. Fledging is around 14–17 days after hatching, when they are, on average, 65–70 g. Some birds may take a little longer depending on the weather and food availability.

## Housing

Icterid hatchlings should be kept in an incubator with the temperature maintained at 95–100 °F (35–38 °C) with 50–60% humidity, although bear in mind a whole nest full of large chicks will not need as much thermal support. Nests should be cup-shaped and easily cleaned. While still in the nestling stage, knitted nests work well, but the birds should rest on a bed of coiled or wadded up tissue paper which can be easily changed as it becomes soiled (Figure 47.3). Never house a hatchling or a nestling on a flat surface or the legs may become permanently splayed. Once fully feathered, chicks still in the nest can be moved into a 5-gal (18.9 l) plastic basket where the holes are covered with fiberglass window screening (attached with hot glue); the window screening serves to protect their feathers from abrasion against the plastic edges. The top of the basket can be covered with more screening held in place with clothes pins, metal office clamps, or tailored to fit with an elastic hem. Cover the front of the basket with light-colored cloth so that human activity is blocked, but leave the screen top uncovered to allow for light. Chicks need a normal day/night cycle throughout care, and adequate light is needed for birds to learn to eat on their own. The baskets can be on a heating pad on the "low" setting for the first 3 days after leaving the incubator, but this is usually not necessary as long as chicks are fully feathered and healthy. As soon as chicks start standing and moving about the basket, they should be offered food and water to explore. Water bowls should be stable; if tipping is a risk, add a rock for stability but not one so big that the bird cannot immerse its beak to drink.

Grackles can be housed with other species' nestlings while still in the nest, but must be watched carefully for aggressive behavior. As soon as they fledge, move them into larger housing and away from other species. Watch for aggression between individual conspecifics. Choose enclosures that allow the grackles to move about easily without damaging their excessively long tails.

Other icterids are typically very social birds and do not generally fight when housed in groups. Brewer's Blackbirds and similar sized species can be moved to a children's playpen when they reach weaning age at around 75% of adult weight. These rectangular folding playpens have mesh fabric walls and are about 40 × 29 × 29 in. (1 × 0.7 × 0.7 m). Clip opaque sheets to the walls as privacy screening, and fiberglass mesh screening makes an excellent ceiling. For ease in cleaning, cover the floor pad in a disposable plastic garbage bag (change between groups of birds) then cover with newspaper, which can be changed daily or when soiled. Suspend hanging perches from the upper edges – use natural branches with irregular surfaces. Do not use perches that are too big or too small. The bird's feet should wrap partially around the perch without the nails of the front and back digits touching. Provide food and water dishes. Water bowls can now be large enough to not

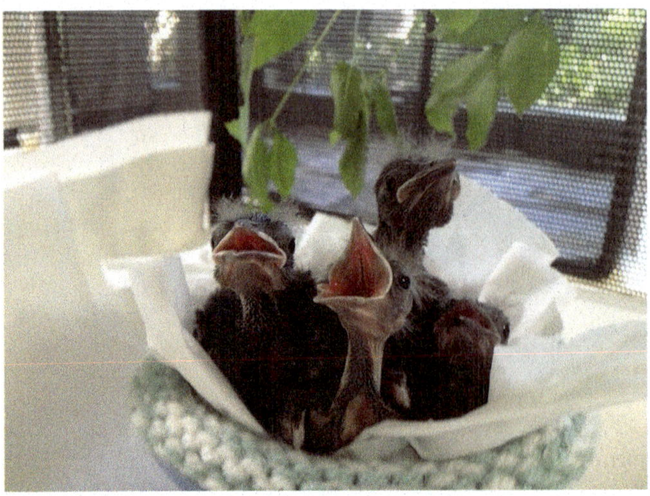

Figure 47.3 Brewer's Blackbird nestlings in a knit nest with tissue lining. *Source:* photo courtesy of Veronica Bowers.

tip and can allow birds to bathe. Adding a few rocks in the middle can be helpful. Disinfect between groups of birds.

Pre-release flight caging should be at least 4×8×8 ft. (1.2×2.4×2.4 m) for smaller icterids and 8×16×8 ft. (2.4×4.9×2.4 m) for larger species such as grackles (Miller 2012). Birds should be in these aviaries for 7–14 days before release. Do not keep smaller icterids longer than this without specific reasons (e.g. keeping for molt, recovery from injury). The longer birds are kept in care, especially when healthy and wild enough for release, the more likely they are to develop stress and captivity-related problems (e.g. injury in aviary, infectious disease).

Grackles are fed by their parents for several weeks after they fledge. Wait until almost all the feathers are in on the face and the bird becomes noticeably restless in the aviary before considering releasing (Figure 47.4). Usually at this point the eyes are starting to change color and are not as dark. They are short migrants in the wild, so flight and endurance must be strong.

## Release Criteria and Location

For all icterids, make sure the bird can forage and is eating a variety of natural foods on its own. Observe it surreptitiously in the aviary: can the bird perch, walk, and fly like a healthy wild bird? Are all birds normally averse to human presence? Condition of flight and contour feathers should be excellent. Do a physical exam on each bird before release: body weight must be good, mentation normal, with no signs of disease or injuries. If an individual has any abnormalities, consider holding it back until the next group is ready for release.

Icterids are diurnal birds and most are highly social. Choose a place for the release where conspecifics are commonly found. For example: look for flocks of Common Grackles feeding in backyards, open fields, or wetlands in the summer and fall. Release birds into a flock of the same species early in the day, which will allow them to begin the process of establishing themselves in the social structure, finding food and water, and learning where to roost for the night. Additional insight on potential release sites can be found by contacting local bird clubs or checking with eBird online (https://ebird.org). Time releases to coincide with 3 days of expected good weather and mild temperatures.

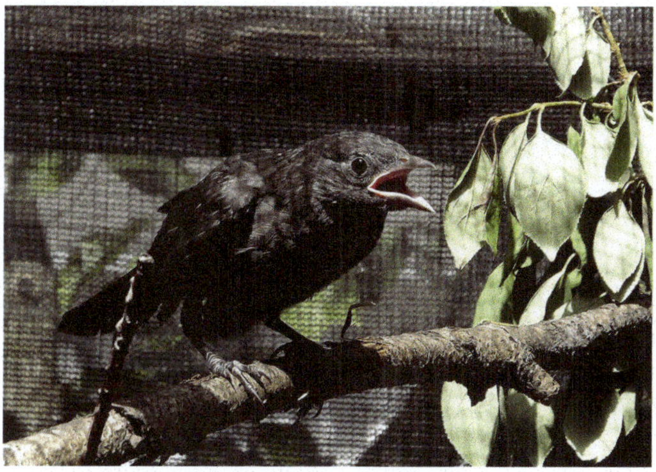

Figure 47.4 Common Grackle fledgling nearing release age.

## Acknowledgments

M. Eiger: Many thanks to Janine Perlman for always answering my nerdy questions about bird stuff, Jean Chamberlain for her unbiased input and for exchanging ideas, Jodi Swenson for her laughter and knowledge when I get stuck, and Suzie Gilbert for connecting me to other great rehabilitators on Facebook.

G. Purdin: Special thanks to Rebecca Duerr for all the work, dedication, and insight she's put into this book and so many other things. Thanks to Jason Williams for his friendship and good cheer through some tough nighttime crewshifts. Thanks also to the many rehabbers who have shared with me the adventure of wildlife rehabilitation.

## Sources for Products Mentioned

Emeraid IC Carnivore: Lafeber Company, 24981 N 1400 East Road, Cornell, IL 61319, (800) 842-6445, https://lafeber.com.

Harrison's Recovery Formula: Harrison's Bird Foods, 7108 Crossroads Blvd. Suite 325, Brentwood, TN 37027, (800) 346-0269, www.harrisonsbirdfoods.com.

Mazuri products: Mazuri, PMI Nutrition International, LLC, PO Box 66812, St. Louis, MO 63166, www.mazuri.com.

Nuts "n" Bugs: Wild Bird Store, 3160 East Fort Lowell Road, Tuscon, AZ, 520-322-9466, https://wildbirdsonline.com.

UltraCare Mite and Lice Bird Spray: 8 in 1 Pet Products, Hauppauge, NY, (800) 645-5154.

## References

Gill, F. and D. Donsker (eds). (2019). IOC World Bird List (v9.1). https://doi.org/10.14344/IOC.ML.9.1.

Hawkins, M.G., Barron, H.W., Speer, B.L. et al. (2018). Birds. In: *Exotic Animal Formulary*, 5e (eds. J.W. Carpenter and C.J. Marion), 167–375. St. Louis, MO: Elsevier.

Miller, E.A. (ed.) (2012). *Minimum Standards for Wildlife Rehabilitation*, 4e. St. Cloud, MN: National Wildlife Rehabilitation Association.

Peer, B.D. and Bollinger, E.K. (1997). Common grackle (*Quiscalus quiscula*), version 2.0. In: *The Birds of North America* (eds. A.F. Poole and F.B. Gill). Ithaca, NY, USA: Cornell Lab of Ornithology. https://doi.org/10.2173/bna.271.

# 48

# House Finches, Goldfinches, and House Sparrows

*Guthrum Purdin and Rebecca S. Duerr*

## Natural History

House Finches and goldfinches are classified in family Fringillidae, subfamily Carduelinae. Other members of family Fringillidae include chaffinches, bramblings, and Hawaiian honeycreepers. The cardueline finches also include some grosbeaks, siskins, canaries, crossbills, and redpolls, among others. The taxonomy of this group is somewhat controversial and may become revised with time. Adults of these species typically show pronounced sexual dimorphism, with males often possessed of striking plumage. There are approximately 150 species of fringillid finches worldwide, with 17 species occurring in North America (Elphick et al. 2001).

House Finches commonly nest near human habitation, including in hanging planters, under eaves, or on trellises. In temperate areas, pairs may produce up to three broods of four to five chicks per season. Unusual among North American passerines, they do not feed their young many (if any) insects; the chicks are fed regurgitated seeds (Badyaev et al. 2012). There are three species of goldfinches in North America: Lesser, American, and Lawrence's Goldfinches. These species lay four to six eggs per clutch and may have two broods per season. Young are fed largely regurgitated seeds (Watt et al. 2016; McGraw and Middleton 2017); Lesser Goldfinches also feed some regurgitated aphids (Watt and Willoughby 2014).

The European House Sparrow is an introduced and well-established species in North America and elsewhere, and is not especially closely related to native North American sparrows. There are also introduced Eurasian Tree Sparrows breeding in a small area of central North America, but this species is nowhere near as ubiquitous as the House Sparrow. These two species are classed in Family Passeridae, the Old World sparrows. House Sparrow populations have declined in some areas of their native range in recent years. House Sparrows often nest in urban areas: shopping malls, nest boxes intended for other species, eaves, drain spouts, Spanish tile roofs, and other enclosed spaces. As cavity-nesters, they may outcompete native species for nest sites, particularly Eastern Bluebirds and Cliff Swallows. House Sparrows have up to three broods of four to six chicks per season. Chicks are fed primarily insects (Lowther and Cink 2006); however, chicks hatched at shopping malls may be fed random human food debris, leading to developmental deficits.

### Finch versus Sparrow

House Finches and House Sparrows are among the most common chicks presented for rehabilitation in North America, with goldfinches presented less often. Chicks of these species are often confused with other species and with each other. All hatch small (<1–2 g) with distinctly

*Hand-Rearing Birds*, Second Edition. Edited by Rebecca S. Duerr and Laurie J. Gage.

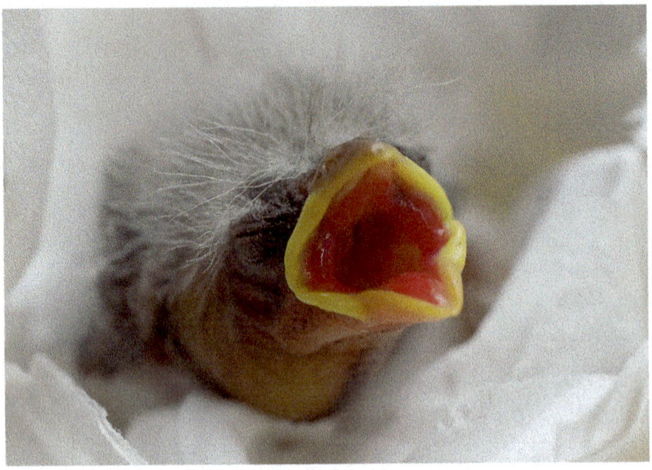

Figure 48.1 House Finch hatchlings have four rows of down on their heads. *Source:* photo courtesy of Jackie Wollner.

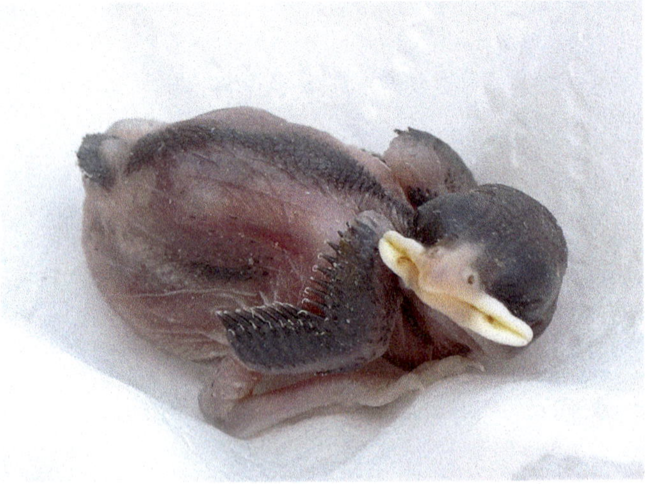

Figure 48.2 House Sparrow nestling with body and flight feathers just starting to come in. Note the complete lack of downy feathers. *Source:* photo courtesy of Jackie Wollner.

red-colored mouths and pink skin. These species all display the typical anisodactyl passerine toe arrangement with three toes forward and one back.

House Finch chicks have four rows of whitish down on their heads: two rows on the crown and a small row above each eye (Figure 48.1). Goldfinch chicks have one row of grayish down over each eye, and another row crossing the back of the head to form a triangle of down. The down on House Finches and goldfinches persists as the body feathers come in, and may give the chicks the appearance of having cobwebs on their heads. House Sparrow chicks do not have any down at all, but rather hatch completely naked. By the time their eyes begin to open at 3–5 days of age, they typically have feather tracts beginning to emerge with a "5 o'clock shadow" appearance (Figure 48.2). Well-nourished House Sparrow chicks may near adult weight before developing significant feathering. House Sparrows are the largest in this group, with House Finches slightly smaller. Goldfinches are approximately half the size and weight of the others at any given age as determined by feather development. Adult weights are as follows: House Sparrow 28 g, House

Finch 21 g, American Goldfinch 13 g, Lawrence's Goldfinch 11.5 g, Lesser Goldfinch 9.5 g (Sibley 2014). Young American Goldfinches can be differentiated from other goldfinches by the presence of distinctly black feathering on the wings with peach wing bars apparent as soon as feathers emerge. With experience, caregivers may also recognize each species' distinctive vocalizations.

## Criteria for Intervention

These species are common victims of cat attack. Any suspected direct cat contact is reason for intervention due to the likelihood of injury and risk of subsequent infection. Additionally, chicks may be found on the ground covered in mites. Chicks may be presented for care when drain spouts are cleaned, or when house painting or construction is occurring. Hot weather may make chicks restless in the nests, leading to falls. House Sparrow hatchlings frequently land on concrete when falling from urban nests and consequently may present with intraabdominal bleeding or leg fractures. House Finch fledglings are commonly "kidnapped" by well-meaning people who erroneously believe them to be abandoned.

## Record Keeping and Initial Care and Stabilization

Small plastic leg bands may be used to differentiate individuals from each other (Red Bird Products). Individual identity is important for regulatory agency reporting, monitoring progress, body weights, or tracking effectiveness of treatment. Records should be kept for each individual, not just for whole clutches. This will make weaning easier and help deal with health problems should they occur.

## Common Medical Problems and Solutions

Protocols for medication used in this chapter are those used by the authors working from information that can be found in Hawkins et al. 2018, an excellent reference for drug dosing in many species of birds.

### Wounds

All chicks with wounds, including subcutaneous emphysema, should be placed on a course of broad-spectrum antibiotics that is likely to cover *Pasteurella multocida,* such as amoxicillin with clavulanic acid, at 125 mg/kg orally twice daily until the problem resolves. Be sure antibiotics are not discontinued until the wound has completely healed. Some wildlife veterinarians continue antibiotics for several days after external wounds have healed to reduce the likelihood of complications, especially in cases of body cavity punctures. Those individuals with potentially painful injuries or head trauma should be given an NSAID like meloxicam at 0.5 mg/kg PO twice daily for 3–10 days once well hydrated.

Lacerations from predators should be cleaned, debrided, and have primary closure whenever possible, to speed healing and reduce development of stress bars on growing feathers. All debris should be removed from wounds, and the feathers carefully plucked within 3–5 mm of the margin, with the exception of flight feathers. Take care to avoid tearing skin by gently plucking in the direction of feather growth or toward the wound edge if close to margins. For very young chicks or for wounds that do not have much tension, surgical glue may provide adequate closure. Semipermeable self-adhesive dressings such as Tegaderm (3M®) or small pieces of self-adhesive hydrocolloid bandages may be used for wounds that cannot be sutured or glued. The authors' preference is to suture, glue, or dress all open wounds, especially in crowded wild bird nursery situations. Always work to facilitate the fastest possible wound healing in order to lead to rapid progress through rehabilitation and an expeditious release. The longer the bird must stay in captivity, the more likely it is to develop secondary problems.

Subcutaneous emphysema (air under the skin) is a common result of cat attack or severe impact, where one or more air sacs have been ruptured and leak air into subcutaneous spaces. This often resolves without any other treatment, but it may be helpful to remove the pressure if it is interfering with mobility or if it is causing the bird to become depressed. If necessary, puncture the bubble with a sterile needle, avoiding any visible skin blood vessels. Many cases will re-inflate quickly and may require repeat punctures several times over the course of a few days. This problem may manifest 24–48 hours after presentation.

### Fractures

Midshaft tibiotarsus fractures are quite common in these chicks and often heal well with little impact on time in captivity. The authors use a minimally restrictive splint reminiscent of a miniature hockey shin guard to splint these fractures. See Duerr et al. (2017) for information on management of fractures in small birds. Even tiny nestling goldfinches may be splinted with a neatly constructed lightweight splint. Splints for this fracture must hold the broken bone at the correct length to prevent the loose ends from overriding each other, and must provide rotational stability to keep the foot facing forward. As long as these requirements are met, it is not necessary to fully restrain the hock or knee joints, or bind the leg to the body. The goal should be for the bird to be able to use its leg as normally as possible while the fracture heals. Binding a rapidly growing leg to the body is not ideal. Splints that reduce mobility risk malunion, slow healing, may lead to dirty or damaged feathers, and can depress the patient thus reducing appetite, increasing time in care, and may compromise chance of recovery and release. Fractures heal extremely quickly in these chicks. Remove splints in 1 week. If any motion is detected at the fracture site, reapply the splint for 1 more week, with size adjusted for growth if necessary. The younger the chick and the smaller the species, the faster fractures heal. Wing fractures are much less common in this age group than in adults, but can be treated with a figure-8 wing wrap over a padded splint; be careful that any restrictive wraps do not interfere with growth of feathers or bones.

### Parasites

Intestinal parasites are uncommon in House Finches and goldfinches, but House Sparrows occasionally have coccidia. Diagnosis is by fecal float or smear. Treatment is with ponazuril at 20 mg/kg once daily for 5 days.

Trichomoniasis may be found in these chicks at admission, and is highly contagious. It may spread through a crowded facility. Many rehabilitation centers treat incoming animals for this disease prophylactically with carnidazole at 25 mg/kg orally once before birds are introduced into the nursery. House Finches typically display signs of vomiting, slow or absent crop emptying time, or nonspecific signs of illness. A House Finch with "trich" may appear completely normal one day, begin vomiting, and expire 24 hours later after infecting its basketmates. Close attention must be paid to disinfection of feeding implements and the hygiene of the caging. Each container of chicks should have its own food container to reduce potential spread of pathogenic organisms. Warmed formula containers should be discarded every 3–4 hours, and feeding implements replaced.

### Yeast Infections

Gastrointestinal yeast infections are not uncommon. Diagnosis is by fecal cytology or wet mount swabs of the crop. Treatment is with nystatin at 300 000 IU/kg twice daily for 7–14 days. These infections usually resolve in 7 days. Yeast is not a communicable disease, but may be secondary to another problem.

### Mycoplasma

*Mycoplasma gallisepticum* causes a highly infectious, often fatal disease manifesting in finches and goldfinches as mild to severe conjunctivitis. Treatment of infected birds is not recommended due to the speed with which outbreaks spread through a nursery and the risk of survivors developing a carrier state. All affected birds should be euthanized, all items they have been in contact with should be thoroughly disinfected, including baskets and shelving. Unaffected but directly exposed birds should be isolated and started on a course of tylosin at 50 mg/kg once daily for 14–21 days. A concurrent course of metronidazole (50 mg/kg orally once daily) is recommended for 7 days. If another bird in the group develops clinical signs, it should be euthanized and the tylosin extended. For fully self-feeding birds, the tylosin can be delivered in the drinking and bathing water at 1000 mg/l.

### Avian Pox

Avian pox most commonly first manifests in these birds as a smooth lump on the central ridge of upper bill between the eyes and the nares. This disease is also highly infectious and persistent in housing, as it may spread through exfoliated skin or scabs. Insect bites, or fomites such as caregivers, also can spread the disease. Affected birds should be euthanized and exposed cagemates isolated for 14 days.

### Poor Feather Condition in Sparrows

House Sparrows often require manual preening to remove the feather sheaths from their flight feathers. If this is not done, birds often develop stress marks at the spot where the sheath constricted the feather. To remove feather sheaths, gently scrape a thumbnail along the white, non-blood-feather portion of the feather to break the sheath. Do not attempt this higher on the growing feather or damage to the blood feather zone may result. House Finches and goldfinches do not generally require assistance preening.

Sparrows sometimes present as runts, with feather development suggesting an age far older than body size would indicate. These birds typically do not do well, and although they may be frisky on arrival, they often decline and die within a few days. Survivors remain unthrifty and do not develop normally. Feather condition is usually poor. Normal-size sparrows may present with abnormally white feathers, or feathers in terrible condition. These birds are often unable to grow normal feathers, neither with plucking nor with long-term care to wait for a normal molt. Birds with inadequate body feather coverage may do poorly once outside or even die abruptly in the aviary. Euthanasia should be considered for House Sparrows with extremely poor feather condition. Because possession of House Sparrows is not regulated in many areas of the United States, permanent captivity may be a viable option in some circumstances. Check with local wildlife agencies if uncertain of applicable regulations.

### Chronic Under- and Overfeeding

Many wildlife centers have problems raising House Finches and goldfinches. There is a tendency for caregivers to feed chicks meals that are too large at once, but to not feed them enough times per day or over enough hours. Consequently, chicks end up simultaneously over- and underfed, which leads to undernourished chicks that take extra-long to finish maturing and are at risk of becoming sickly (see below). Chronically undernourished chicks are highly stressed (caregivers too) and may do nothing but continue to beg all day, which can lead to more over- and underfeeding. Impatient caregivers also may be tempted to force the chicks to wean as soon as they start nibbling, long before they are ready. This prolongs their dependent period as they get physiologically stuck at the young fledgling developmental age. Counterintuitively, feeding these species intensively and attentively leads to a shorter period of dependence, because well-fed, confident chicks explore eating on their own sooner. Patient and attentive feeding also oddly leads to fewer mouths to feed simultaneously, because birds mature more promptly.

### Sickly House Finches

House Finches sometimes develop a disease syndrome colloquially known to rehabilitators as "Sudden Finch Death Syndrome," which may make them very frustrating birds to raise. It occurs as House Finches approach weaning age, when a significant portion of them may start to decline and eventually sicken and die. The authors' opinion on this issue is as follows:

- The onset of problems is not sudden if adequate attention is paid. Chicks that are in trouble have slowed crop clearance time, appear fluffed, may exhibit vomiting, or develop dirty feathers secondary to vomiting. These signs are seen 24–48 hours or more before deaths occur.
- Placing birds exhibiting signs of poor thrift on a cocktail of antibiotic, antiprotozoal, and antifungal medications turns many cases around quickly, which suggests an infectious organism may be the problem. Crop swabs of these birds often show high numbers of clostridial-type bacteria and/or budding yeast. Trichomonad trophozoites may also be present. Occasionally no pathogens are found in either crop swabs or fecals.
- Susceptibility to disease may be due to reduced immune function, which may be secondary to nutritional issues and stress. Premature weaning likely contributes to the decline. Overfeeding is also a common problem because finches will continue gaping when already overfull. Stretched-out crops have poor motility. A poorly motile, overly large crop provides an excellent site for growth of pathogenic organisms.
- For many wildlife veterinarians, including the authors, overgrowth of *Clostridium* spp. is the primary suspect agent. Problems appear reduced when at-risk House Finches are raised with a daily dose of metronidazole. This medication covers many anaerobic intestinal bacteria such as *Clostridium* and is effective against flagellates as well.

### Sick House Finch Recommendations

If a finch shows signs of illness, examine carefully and do a crop swab and fecal. If bacteria are seen, begin metronidazole 50 mg/kg once daily for all birds in the enclosure. This may need to continue until birds are fully weaned. If budding yeast is seen, begin Nystatin for 7 days – continue if crop swabs or fecals are still positive. If flagellates are seen during the crop swab, treat with carnidazole at 25 mg/kg once daily for 3 days before starting metronidazole. If chicks do not improve on metronidazole, add enrofloxacin at 30 mg/kg orally once daily. For those facilities without the ability to do crop swabs, treat empirically.

Increase biosecurity and separate sickly chicks from healthy chicks, and affected cages from healthy birds. Treat all affected and exposed chicks. Subcutaneous fluids may be needed for chicks with delayed crop emptying. Consult an avian veterinarian for diagnostic tests and further treatment.

## Diets

### Hand-feeding

Unusually among passerines, House Finch chicks are not fed a primarily insect diet during the early stages of life. The parents regurgitate a mixture of seeds, other plant material, and about 2% insect protein for the developing chicks. Thus, the most common passerine insect-based or insect-replacement diets are not ideal for these birds. Commercial diets for raising parrots are also problematic, yielding feathering of generally poor quality, likely due to parrot chicks' relatively low requirement for protein.

A mix of Kaytee exact® Hand Feeding Formula (Kaytee) and a high protein neonate formula such as Emeraid® IC Carnivore (Lafeber Company) will produce healthy House Finch fledglings with quality feathering, who reach maturity on roughly the same schedule as birds raised in the wild by their parents. Another benefit of the inclusion of Exact may be that it contains beneficial bacteria and digestive enzymes.

Mixing Kaytee exact and Emeraid Carnivore at a 50/50 ratio can be used for all ages, from hatchlings to weanlings. Mix the two diets as powder, then add water until a smooth, "cake-batter" consistency is achieved – this is usually at 2 : 1 ratio (water : powder). Some caregivers have started hatchlings on straight higher protein Emeraid IC Carnivore, then transitioned to straight Kaytee exact for weanlings with a gradation in between. However, this can prove difficult in high volume shelters and the end results – a healthy, independent, juvenile finch raised in a timely manner – is equally achievable with the 50/50 formulation. Goldfinches can also be raised on this formula, as the primary diet fed to chicks of these species is also regurgitated seeds.

House Sparrow chicks have a more normal passerine wild diet and can do well on any of the blended diets listed in Table 41.3, or when treated as insectivores (see Chapter 43). The author (GP) has had excellent results using Basic Nestling Diet (see Table 41.3) when rearing this species.

### Self-Feeding

Once birds are leaving the nest and starting to explore, a diverse mix of small seeds should be offered. "Canary Mix" or "Finch mix" or similar undyed mixes work well, especially if other seeds such as niger (thistle) are mixed in for variety. Goldfinches are particularly attracted to thistle seeds and millet spray. Fresh plant material such as broccoli florets, parsley sprigs, minced greens, and halved grapes are popular first foods. House Sparrows may also eat small insects and crumbled hard-boiled egg. Other possible foods include fennel, crushed nuts, currants, minced apple or cherries, and ground kitten kibble. Present food as an array of easily visible items. Shallow lids make excellent seed dishes, although scatter some seed on the floor as well. Broccoli florets and halved sideways grapes may be impaled on a bamboo skewer as "shish kabobs" and suspended within easy reach of perches. Another presentation option is to drill a hole in one side of the long arm of a wooden clothespin big enough to snugly fit a short bamboo skewer segment. Fill the skewer with fresh fruits and vegetable chunks, wedge one end in the clothespin, and then clamp the clothespin to the perch with the skewer sticking up. Broccoli and fruits can be chopped and offered in low dishes as well. Millet spray dangled next to perches may act as a needed enticement for reluctant eaters, but should not be the main food item. Shallow water dishes should also be offered as soon as the birds are out of the nest and exploring their environment. Keep food dishes low, large, and wide to maximize visual stimulus. Wall-mounted food dishes may be useful in some circumstances, but may end up serving as litter boxes instead when birds perch on them while facing toward the center of the basket. Water can be provided in very small, stable bowls – if the type of bowl may tip, or is large enough for birds to fall into, add small rocks for stability.

## Feeding Procedures

House Finches and goldfinches of all ages eat best when fed in small bites (0.05–0.2 ml per bite depending on age) delivered to the back of the mouth. Nestlings that are frightened may be stimulated to gape by gently tapping a clean syringe tip on the side of the beak. Next try gently tapping the edge of the nest to simulate the adult's arrival. It is helpful in encouraging gaping to imitate the species' begging noise in a soft whistle. Older chicks that are too frightened to gape may gape if beak tapping occurs while gently held in the feeder's hand, especially while the whistling begging sound is made. Be patient. Within a few feedings, healthy chicks will begin to understand that we are trying to feed them not eat them.

A 1 ml syringe with an attached cannula tip (Jorgensen) works well for all ages of House Finches and goldfinches, and hatchling House Sparrows. It provides a controlled amount of diet with less risk of dirtying the bird with spilled formula. Once House Sparrows have grown strong enough to pull on the cannula tip, at around 10 g, there is significant risk the bird will pull the cannula tip off the syringe and swallow it – never use cannula tips for sparrows after the hatchling stage; do use them for finches and goldfinches until they're weaned. Use a 1 ml syringe without the extra tip for older sparrows. Once a feeding syringe has been filled, all extraneous food should be wiped from the outside of the syringe and tip before feeding to reduce spillage.

When feeding a nest full of chicks, it is useful to give one bite to each bird and move around in a circle until all chicks have had enough. This allows each bird to fully swallow their last bite before receiving more. If a bird cannot clear its mouth of liquid quickly, it may aspirate. All these species, especially House Sparrows, are quite competitive for food. It is imperative to make sure each chick is receiving its share. The smallest, weakest chick in a clutch may end up on the bottom of the nest, necessitating the counting of heads when feeding (Figure 48.3).

Some rehabilitators use other feeding implements, including feeding picks and clean paintbrushes, to deliver food. In the authors' experience, the paintbrush technique tends to result in chicks that have been "painted" with food. In the hands of a dedicated caregiver, that is less likely the case, but this method can be problematic when feeding is being done by multiple volunteers. Feeding picks also may be problematic due to the propensity of finches for chaotic jumping around when begging, potentially brushing against a loaded pick and becoming dirty. Neither of these methods allows quantification of the amount fed.

### Hatchlings and Nestlings

Young chicks should be fed every 20–30 minutes for 14–16 hours a day. House Finch and goldfinch crops are easily visible on young chicks and should never be filled larger than 1/2 to 2/3 the

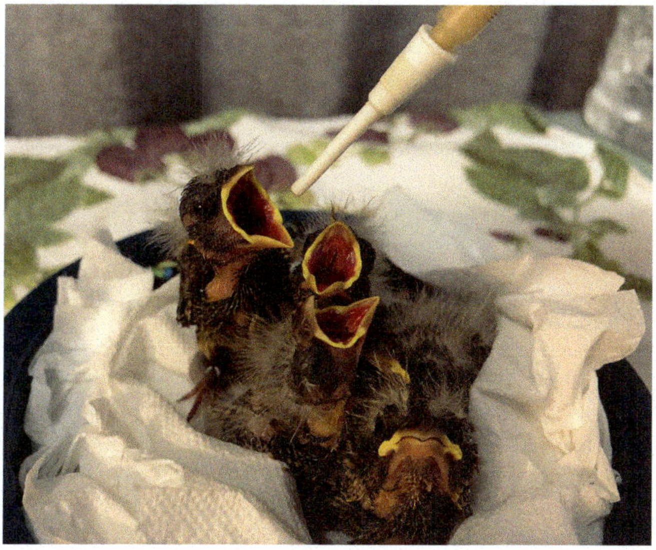

Figure 48.3 House Finch nestlings being fed with a cannula-tipped syringe.

size of the bird's head. This amount is approximately 5% of body weight (1 ml per 20 g body weight).

Crops should empty between feedings. If there is still a significant amount of diet in the crop by the next meal, skip the feeding. If the crop is still full at the next scheduled feeding time, carefully assess the bird. It may need to have formula gently drained from the crop (a "reverse feeding" with a soft catheter), may need fluids (either orally or subcutaneously), and there may be pathogenic organisms growing in the crop (best assessed by a crop swab). Additional heat may be necessary; chicks that are too cold do not digest well.

Hatchlings may weave their head while gaping. A cotton swab may be needed to steady the head during feedings, or gentle, steadying fingers. Sharp vision is required to feed tiny chicks, because it is easy to miss the mouth and get birds dirty. Hatchlings have a higher requirement for water than older chicks. Their diet should either be thinned to a runny but not watery consistency, or amounts of more solid formula should be kept small and a corresponding amount of water fed with the meal. Pay close attention to droppings. If droppings stop being produced with every meal or if the chick stops gaping, palpate the chick's abdomen; it should always feel soft. Hatchlings that are becoming dehydrated may lack enough fluid to move food through the gut and it may feel firm to the touch. Give these birds small amounts of oral fluids, or subcutaneous fluids if not swallowing well, until food currently in the body has passed. A very gentle massage of the abdomen may induce passing feces/urates. Once the abdomen is again soft and stools are being passed, start feeding the diet but with higher moisture content.

Keep birds in the incubator until fully feathered. As long as they're in the incubator, feed every 30 minutes. Once out of the incubator, feed every 45 minutes until weaning.

## Fledglings

Fledglings should be fed every 45 minutes for 14–16 hours a day. House Finches that stay in the nest until quite mature are the easiest to wean, and they tend to have relatively high body weights. Allow birds to stay in the nest as long as they want. As soon as birds are perching and moving about the cage, they should be offered solid foods. These species start nibbling on food items well in advance of being able to effectively crack open seeds, so caregivers may be prematurely fooled into thinking birds are self-feeding. Hand-feeding should continue until birds are no longer frantically begging. Continue using the 1 ml syringe with cannula tip for goldfinches and House Finches until weaning. Again, do not use cannula tips for House Sparrow fledglings. House Finches and House Sparrows at 15 g can be fed up to 0.75 ml of formula per feeding, while those 17 g and up can get as much as 1 ml as long as their crops are clearing between feeds.

## Expected Weight Gain

Weigh chicks daily until they are weaned; try to weigh birds at the same time each day so the evaluation of condition is consistent. All chicks should gain weight steadily until at or above adult weight at around 10 days of age. Plateaued weights below normal adult weights should trigger concern. A weight loss of more than 10% of this amount during weaning may indicate a chick is not ready to wean.

## Housing

Provide a calm, quiet environment. Do not keep House Finches or goldfinches next to noisy or predator species, such as starlings or corvids, or species that carry trichomonas, such as doves or pigeons. House Sparrows are susceptible to imprinting and habituation when raised alone. Singly raised House Sparrows may be aggressive if introduced to other birds at the aviary stage. Ensure that all birds have at least one conspecific companion in order to gain social skills. Never raise birds alone.

### Hatchlings

Hatchlings should be kept in appropriately-sized nest replacements inside an incubator such as an Animal Intensive Care Unit (Lyon Technologies). House Sparrows enjoy the security of having the nest covered with a tissue between feedings or using a cave-like structure as a nest (see Figure 44.2). Temperatures should be kept at 95–100 °F (35–38 °C) with 50–60% humidity.

Never keep chicks on flat surfaces because of the possible development of splayed legs. Nests must have texture on the inside and bottom that will allow growing feet and legs something to grip, such as coiled or crumpled tissue. Keep hatchlings scrupulously clean by removing fecal material or spilled food immediately, changing tissue as needed.

### Nestlings and Fledglings

When chicks are fully feathered nestlings, they may be moved out of the incubator. Place the nest in a large basket on a heating pad set on "low." Large laundry baskets with window screening covering all holes make excellent housing (Figure 48.4), as do reptariums (see Chapters 43 and 44). Use large pieces of window screening secured with clothespins as a ceiling on baskets, or sew elastic into screening to create fitted tops. Older House Sparrows are excellent escape artists and tend to hide under furniture once out and about, so be sure to adequately secure all caging lest caregivers have to waste time chasing birds around the facility.

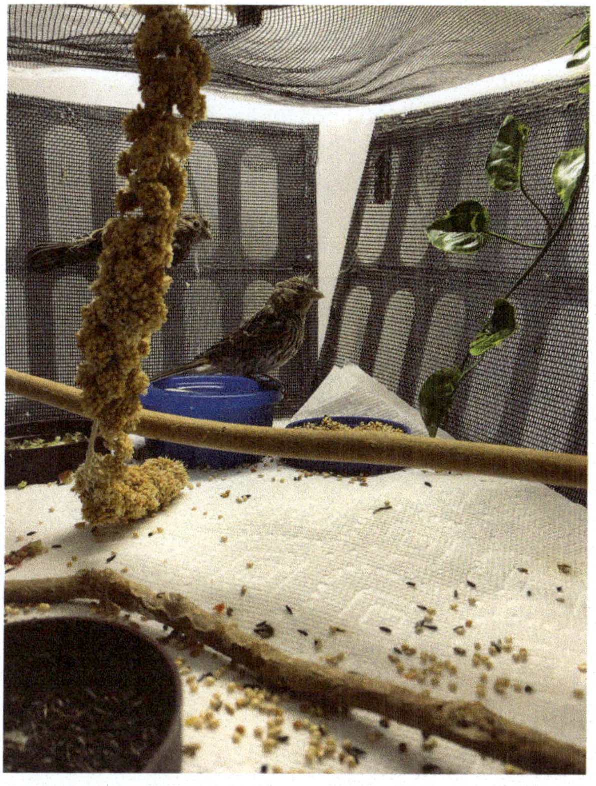

Figure 48.4 Laundry basket housing: screening over holes (attached with hot glue), perches, greenery, diverse food offerings. Full-spectrum lighting over the basket, and visual barriers to block views of people.

Baskets should have normal daylight-level illumination, preferably with a full-spectrum lighting fixture. Fledglings will be more difficult to wean if lighting levels are too dim. Block birds' view of human activities; cheesecloth or white sheet is a good choice for visual barrier. Birds require 8–10 hours of sleep nightly and will continue begging until the lights are turned out for the evening. Cleaning and other maintenance that requires light for human activity should take this need for darkness into account. If lights are left on while tasks are finished, birds will continue to be active and will go to bed hungry. Similarly, in the mornings, prepare food and keep the nursery area as dark as possible until ready to begin feedings.

As birds begin to leave the nest and explore their environment, add perching materials, such as wild collected sticks and trimmings cut to fit braced between opposite walls of the basket. A diversity of perch sizes with irregular surfaces helps prevent foot lesions. When perches become soiled, clean and soak in bleach (allow to dry before returning to bird enclosure) or discard and replace. Adding natural food items, including dandelion heads or green tips of small branches of unsprayed lilac, honeysuckle, or forsythia with buds, will help chicks learn to recognize the food they will encounter in the wild. Do not overfill baskets with natural vegetation, because birds will need easy access to food when weaning begins. Once birds no longer return to the nest, discontinue the supplemental heat. Keep perches placed close to the ground, because these species tend to perch on the highest spot available. Perches near the floor put fledglings in close proximity to food dishes.

House Sparrows may spend a lot of time hiding, as is to be expected from a cavity-nesting species. This can complicate ensuring that every chick gets enough to eat, because one chick may continually poke its head out to eat while others simply hide. It may occasionally be necessary to remove excessive hiding places and add them again when birds are well on their way to eating on their own. Count birds whenever feeding so none are missed.

Each morning, cage substrates for nursery birds should be cleaned and dry food refreshed. Old wet food as well as soiled dry food and cage furnishings should be changed each morning and during the day as needed. The flooring and sides of baskets can be wiped down with a mild disinfectant such as dilute chlorhexidine during morning substrate changes. Weigh birds during cleaning by putting them one-by-one into a small paper bag secured with a clothespin and recording weights; the bags can be disposed of when dirty. Alternatively, small plastic boxes are used for weights, but wipe them out with disinfectant between weighing each group. At all stages, maintain good hygiene standards – infectious disease outbreaks can spread through a nursery like wildfire.

## Weaning

### House Finches

It is critical to not try weaning small seed-eating birds too soon. It can be very tempting to reduce the number of daily feedings as soon as they are observed manipulating solid food, especially when raising large numbers of birds simultaneously. These birds are fed by their parents well after they have fledged from the nest. In the wild, chicks follow their parents from place to place learning how to forage. It is a common sight to see House Finch fledglings that appear very mature perching outdoors begging and being fed by an adult. This is a crucial period when fledglings experiment with finding food and perfecting their food-handling skills while their beaks continue to mature.

Weaning House Finches is a relatively easy procedure, but it involves scrupulous attention to detail to be successful. Once fledglings reach about 16g, they start becoming interested in solid foods. Many caregivers use this as a cue to cut back on formula feedings, thinking the birds are becoming self-sufficient; however, they are still too uncoordinated in handling seed and their beaks are too soft to properly shell a seed. Adults may pick up, shell, and swallow a seed in less than a second. Fledglings may carry the same seed around for 20 minutes, practicing manipulation. They may, in fact, simply lift and drop seed after seed. The amount of seed they consume is inadequate for health and the final stages of development. If formula feeding frequency for pre-weaning size finches is cut back, they are not stimulated to self-feed faster. Instead they will stop experimenting with forage, wasting the energy needed for growth on increasingly continuous, frantic begging.

Syringe-feeding must continue at 45-minute intervals. If a 16-g bird has copious seed in the crop, the ration size of 1 ml can be lowered, but with caution. Birds at this age that are not begging should be suspected of having a health problem and should be examined. Never try to wean a frantically begging bird or one that is weak, vomiting, depressed, or generally sickly.

Well-nourished fledglings will happily investigate offered food. To facilitate fledglings' experiments in self-feeding, provide fresh skewers of broccoli florets and halved grapes. It is also acceptable to offer broccoli florets and grapes in a small, low dish on the floor of the basket. These items are soft and highly palatable to finches. Cut strawberries are also a good first food. Use a separate dish or jar lid from the seed dish for easy disposal when wetter food items become chewed over. Make sure the produce is fresh and change often. House Finches eat green plant buds and green seeds in the wild; broccoli florets approximate these soft green buds. It will often be the first thing they eat on their own. They can become very excited when getting greens intermittently during the day. A small sprig of millet hung beside the perch is well received by young birds. It is best to use only a small sprig because millet is not especially nutritious. The key is to get them eating and to make it something pleasant for them to do.

The decision to start weaning House Finches is based on observation of the whole bird. Pre-weaning birds tend to perch with the body leaned forward, while weaning and adult finches have a more upright posture. The tail must be fully grown out and the notch in the distal tip noticeable. Birds unready for weaning will have a fluffy, immature appearance to the head feathers; body feathers often look ruffled. When old enough to wean, the head and body will look smooth and sleek. Be aware that when begging, they will erect those feathers and lean forward to look younger. Observe birds at rest when not being fed. The wispy, white natal down may be entirely absent by this point, but a few plumes can persist for quite a while. The beaks start to look somewhat heavier, with gape flanges nearly gone. If a bird bites the caregiver's finger, it may have noticeable pressure. Some birds in the basket may be showing less of the wild enthusiasm for the syringe seen in nestlings. Birds being weaned should be sleek and starting to have the silhouette of adults.

### Characteristics of House Finches Ready to Wean

- Sleek head feathers.
- Gape flanges regressed.
- Fully-grown tail (long, notched).
- Upright body posture.
- Vigorous, active demeanor, with no frantic begging.
- More than 18 g, plump breast muscles.

Weight is key at this point. House Finches can be best weaned at 18–21 g. On the morning of day 1, weigh all birds in the basket to be weaned. If all birds are at least 18 g, increase the feeding interval to every 1 hour. Provide a very large dish of seed and scatter seed on the floor. This should be a diverse mix of regular finch seed, thistle, and can include canary mix for diversity. Provide a skewer of fruits and vegetables. Continue hourly feedings the rest of the day. Weigh birds again the next morning. If all birds are behaving normally and accepting the syringe, there's no problem. If one or more birds are gaping frantically and look like they are starving, reevaluate those birds. If they are maintaining their weight at or above 18 g, leave them on the new schedule. If a bird's weight is below 18 g, consider moving that bird to a basket of younger birds. If several are losing weight, return to the previous 45-minute schedule. Do not force-feed healthy weanlings that are not taking food from the syringe unless they are losing weight.

The morning of day 3–4, weigh all birds. If weights are still 18 g or above, increase the feeding interval to once every 2 hours. Some birds may be fully self-feeding, but chances are that most are still begging. Give up to 1 ml of formula during feedings. Ample seed and water must always be available. Birds that act desperate for food at any point should be critically evaluated. It may be a signal of illness or a need for more time at more frequent feedings. Sometimes groups develop a personality and may appear especially dependent or independent. Some groups may all beg wildly. Others may refuse all syringe food on their first day. Look at the birds during each feeding and cleaning to get a sense for their condition. If there is any uncertainty, leave them at 1 hour intervals.

On day 5–6, check weights and follow the above observational recommendations. If all weights are still at or above 18 g, decrease formula feedings to every 3 hours. Many or all fledglings may be uninterested in the syringe. If birds can maintain weight for 1 day on this small amount of supplemental feeding, they must be eating significant amounts on their own because 1 ml every 3 hours is insufficient to maintain body weight. If any birds are still actively taking syringe food, it is fine to wait until day 7–8 to change the feeding schedule. Even if still begging, they can be safely cut off thereafter as long as they appear healthy and vigorous. Weigh them 24 hours after ending the last syringe feeding. If weight is maintained, they are self-feeders and can be considered for pre-release aviary time.

Record weights daily during weaning to monitor individual variation. Daily weighing is also a good idea before weaning if time permits and can be done while cleaning the basket. Some finches are small. The authors have found about 5% of House Finches mature at a smaller size, weaning at 17 g. If unable to weigh birds daily, monitor the keel musculature closely; birds should always have a rounded breast.

In summary, on day 1 increase the feeding interval from 45 minutes to 1 hour. On day 3, offer feedings every 2 hours. Baskets that are doing well can go to 3-hour feeds on day 5 and by day 7 are likely to be fully self-feeding. Advancement can be delayed at each step based on the needs of individual birds in each basket.

### House Sparrows

House Sparrows can be weaned on the same basic schedule with a few species-specific considerations. A sparrow of 20–27 g with tail feathers grown in to at least 1–1.5 in. (2–3 cm) long is likely ready for weaning. Sparrows ready to wean will have resorbed their bright yellow gape flanges. Their beaks will be turning gray-beige and hard. Their bites will become painful, and their bodies are fully feathered. They act restless in the basket and start to become an escape risk. Sparrows tend to progress very quickly to fully self-feeding once the daily number of syringe-feedings is reduced. Work from the basic weight check and increasing feed interval plan for finches; however, it may be found that all birds are refusing formula after a day or two. Do not force-feed, and just monitor weights. If they're staying over 20 g and appear bright and alert, they should be fine. After a few days, evaluate for transfer to the aviary.

### Goldfinches

Goldfinches notoriously gape long after their crops are full. Markers of maturity are similar to House Finches. Once they start eating on their own, monitor how full their crops are before syringe-feeding to avoid overfilling the crop. When offering solid food, mix in a liberal amount of thistle. Wean Lesser Goldfinches at 9–10 g, but, again, evaluate feathering and demeanor to determine maturity. Lesser Goldfinches are dangerously thin if they drop back down to 7 g. American Goldfinches generally run 2 g or so larger. Regional differences should be expected in any bird species. The weaning plan may need adapting to local variations in body size.

## Hints for Care in Large Facilities

If rotating volunteer caregivers are feeding chicks, training in feeding techniques is very important before allowing new persons to feed chicks. It only takes one feeder with poor technique to leave an entire room of chicks covered in food. See Appendix C for instructions on how to safely wash a songbird, should it become necessary.

These species do well in a shelter environment, but need consistent care and daily attention from management staff. Birds that become fluffed, stop producing droppings, or refuse food when not being weaned must be promptly evaluated. Hatchlings may require micromanagement-level attention several times daily, because troubleshooting problems in hatchling passerines is beyond the skill level of most general care volunteers. Having a highly trained individual or team specifically tasked with monitoring these species, and with the patience to mentor others, is ideal.

## Preparation for Wild Release

Aviaries for these species are recommended to be at least 4×8×8 ft. high (1.2×2.4×2.4 m) for four to six birds (Miller 2012). Aviaries should be constructed with 0.5×0.5 in. (1×1 cm) hardware cloth or wire mesh outer walls, and the interior should be fully lined with fiberglass window screen to prevent injury and damage to feathers. If flooring is dirt or pea gravel rather than concrete, provide protection from digging predators by having hardware cloth embedded below the substrate.

At least one-third of the ceiling, sides, and back of the aviary should be of solid material to provide shade and privacy. A variety of perching opportunities should be available, such as branches, shrubs, and sisal rope. The central area of the aviary should be left open to provide room for active flight exercise. As much natural food as possible should be provided, with seed mixes offered as well. Multiple elevated feeding dishes should be used to present food (Figure 48.5).

Birds should spend 7–10 days in the aviary before release. They must be strong flyers, waterproof, and able to forage on a wide variety of food items.

## Release

Goldfinches should be released into a flock if possible. Releasing House Finches back into the area each bird was found is an option, but since birds from different areas are often raised together, the authors prefer to release aviary birds as a group into good habitat with adults of the species nearby.

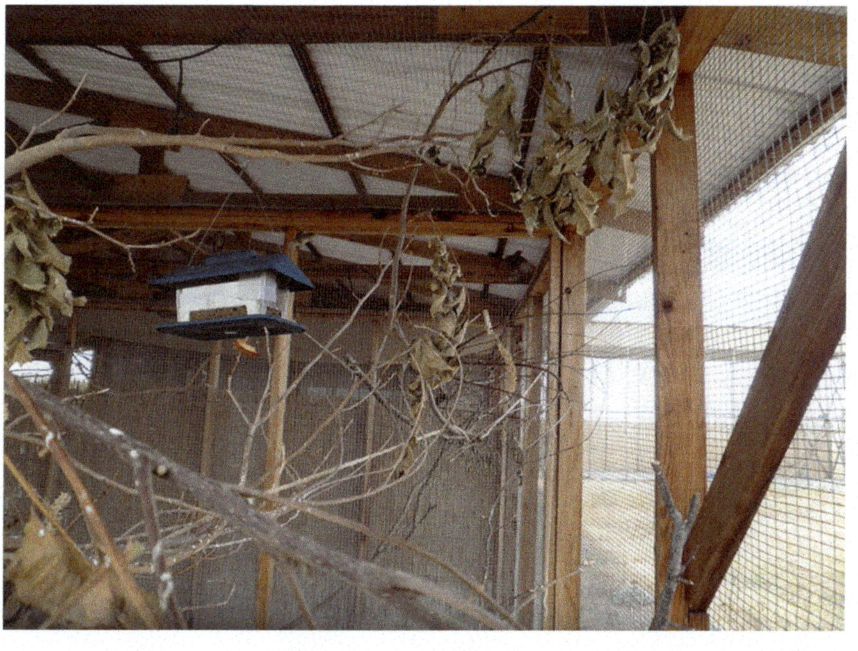

**Figure 48.5** Plentiful natural perches and elevated food offerings in a large outdoor aviary.

Release of nonnative House Sparrows is controversial. If birds are to be released, choose locations where there are already well-established populations. Do not release into naive habitat or into areas where they are known to be outcompeting native birds.

Because these species are diurnal, release in the morning, allowing birds to orient themselves before dark. Choose the release date with at least 3 days of nonextreme weather forecasted (no snow, rain, or excessive heat).

## Acknowledgments

Many thanks to the volunteers and staff at the wildlife shelters we've worked with over the years. Thanks to your enthusiasm and hard work, many thousands of animals who would otherwise have died, instead have gone on to live healthy lives in the wild. A special thank you to the thousands of finches and sparrows that have wound up in our hands, for teaching us about their needs, and enriching our lives.

## Sources for Products Mentioned

Animal Intensive Care Unit: Lyon Technologies, Inc., 1690 Brandywine Avenue, Chula Vista, CA. 91911, https://lyonvet.com.

Cannula tip for feeding (aka teat infusion cannula): Jorgensen Labs, 1450 Van Buren Ave, Loveland, Colorado 80538, (800) 525-5614, https://www.jorvet.com.

Emeraid IC Carnivore: Lafeber Company, 24981 N 1400 East Road, Cornell, IL 61319, https://lafeber.com.

Kaytee Exact Hand Feeding Formula: 521 Clay St, PO Box 230, Chilton, WI 53014, (800) KAYTEE-1, https://www.kaytee.com.

Leg Bands: Red Bird Products, P.O. Box 376, Mt. Aukum, CA 95656, (530) 620-7440, www.http://redbirdproducts.com.

Reptarium screen enclosures: LLLReptile and Supply Company Inc., 609 Mission Ave, Oceanside, CA 92054, (760) 439-8492, www.lllreptile.com.

Tegaderm: 3 M Corporate Headquarters, 3 M Center, St. Paul MN 55144-1000, (888) 364-3577.

## References

Badyaev, A.V., Belloni, V., and Hill, G.E. (2012). House Finch (*Haemorhous mexicanus*), version 2.0. In: *The Birds of North America* (ed. A.F. Poole). Ithaca, NY, USA: Cornell Lab of Ornithology. https://doi.org/10.2173/bna.46.

Duerr, R.S., Purdin, G.J., and Bowers, V. (2017). Small-bodied birds: passerines, doves, woodpeckers, others. In: *Topics in Wildlife Medicine, Vol. 4: Orthopedics* (eds. R.S. Duerr and G.J. Purdin), 53–74. St. Cloud, MN: National Wildlife Rehabilitators Association.

Elphick, C., Dunning, J.B. Jr., and Sibley, D.A. (2001). *The Sibley Guide to Bird Life and Behavior*, 588 pp. New York: Alfred A. Knopf Inc.

Hawkins, M.G., Barron, H.W., Speer, B.L. et al. (2018). Birds. In: *Exotic Animal Formulary*, 5e (eds. J.W. Carpenter and C.J. Marion), 167–375. St. Louis, MO: Elsevier.

Lowther, P.E. and Cink, C.L. (2006). House Sparrow (*Passer domesticus*), version 2.0. In: *The Birds of North America* (ed. A.F. Poole). Ithaca, NY, USA: Cornell Lab of Ornithology. https://doi.org/10.2173/bna.12.

McGraw, K.J. and Middleton, A.L. (2017). American Goldfinch (*Spinus tristis*), version 2.1. In: *The Birds of North America* (ed. P.G. Rodewald). Ithaca, NY, USA: Cornell Lab of Ornithology. https://doi.org/10.2173/bna.amegfi.02.1.

Miller, E.A. (ed.) (2012). *Minimum Standards for Wildlife Rehabilitation*, 4e. St. Cloud, MN: National Wildlife Rehabilitation Association.

Sibley, D.A. (2014). *The Sibley Guide to Birds*, 2e. New York: Alfred A. Knopf Inc.

Watt, D.J. and Willoughby, E.J. (2014). Lesser Goldfinch (*Spinus psaltria*), version 2.0. In: *The Birds of North America* (ed. A.F. Poole). Ithaca, NY, USA: Cornell Lab of Ornithology. https://doi.org/10.2173/bna.392.

Watt, D.J., Pyle, P., Patten, M.A., and Davis, J.N. (2016). Lawrence's Goldfinch (*Spinus lawrencei*), version 3.0. In: *The Birds of North America* (ed. P.G. Rodewald). Ithaca, NY, USA: Cornell Lab of Ornithology. https://doi.org/10.2173/bna.lawgol.03.

# 49

# Grosbeaks and Cardinals

*Veronica Bowers and Jessika Madison-Kennedy*

## Natural History

Black-headed Grosbeaks (*Pheucticus melanocephalus*), Rose-breasted Grosbeaks (*Pheucticus ludovicianus*), and Northern Cardinals (*Cardinalis cardinalis*) are North American passerines belonging to the family Cardinalidae. Other members of this family include Blue Grosbeaks, tanagers, buntings, Pyrrhuloxia, and Dickcissel. Pine, Kona, and Evening Grosbeaks are classified as Fringillid Finches. The Rose-breasted Grosbeak and Northern Cardinal nest east of the Rockies and the Black-headed Grosbeak nests west of the Rockies. Grosbeaks have earned their name due to their exceptionally large and powerful conical-shaped bill, or beak. Northern Cardinals have expanded their southeastern range to include the northern and eastern parts of the United States up toward the Canadian border. These species occupy diverse habitats within their breeding ranges, from mature pine forests and oak woodlands to urban developments, backyards, and orchards. Regardless of overall habitat, a well-developed understory combined with large trees appears to be a key habitat component for these species.

Although over 50% of the grosbeak diet consists of insects, they are considered omnivorous. The remainder of their diet includes seeds, nuts, wild and cultivated fruits, and other plant materials including buds and flowers from trees. Both species of grosbeak are migratory and depart from North America during late summer for the wintering grounds of Central America.

The diet of Northern Cardinals is also omnivorous and is made up of approximately 30% plant matter and 70% animal matter, depending on the time of year. They are known to consume at least 77 different types of plants but demonstrate a preference for oil-type and striped sunflower seeds, hulled sunflower seeds, buckwheat, cracked corn, safflower seeds, millet, and various fruits including wild grapes and berries. Cardinals also forage on dogwood and grasses such as smartweed and sedges. The insects that Northern Cardinals hunt include moths, butterflies, centipedes, flies, cicadas, crickets, beetles, leafhoppers, katydids, and spiders. Northern Cardinals do not migrate but congregate in large flocks during the nonbreeding season.

## Criteria for Intervention

Most grosbeaks received in rehabilitation facilities are cat-caught fledglings and juveniles that collided with a window. Accidental kidnapping is unusual due to the secretive nature of nesting

*Hand-Rearing Birds*, Second Edition. Edited by Rebecca S. Duerr and Laurie J. Gage.

grosbeaks and newly fledged young. Injured and orphaned Northern Cardinal chicks more easily find their way into rehabilitative care because of their tendency to nest in close proximity to human activity. Often opting to nest in backyards, any perceived reason to intervene is often noticed and acted upon by vigilant homeowners. Breeding pairs may have more than one brood per year and often have many failed nesting attempts due to nest predation. For this reason, rehabilitators may see a fair number of hatchling cardinals being admitted into their care very late in the breeding season.

## Record Keeping

As with all animals entering care, it is good practice to record the animal's origin and circumstances of rescue, plus prior care. Regulatory agencies in the United States have basic requirements for data that must be reported by holders of wildlife rehabilitation permits. Other countries likely have similar requirements for possession of wildlife.

## Initial Care and Stabilization

See Chapter 1.

## Common Medical Problems

The primary reason grosbeaks and cardinals enter care is known or suspected attacks by cats. Consequently, these chicks often have wing or leg fractures, abrasions, bruising, puncture wounds, or subcutaneous emphysema. Birds that have been attacked by cats often require wound care including dressings or suturing, plus splints and wraps to treat fractures. See Duerr et al. (2017) for information on treating orthopedic injuries of small birds. Cat-caught chicks should be placed on a course of broad-spectrum antibiotic, such as amoxicillin with clavulanic acid, at 125 mg/kg orally twice daily until after wounds have fully healed (Hawkins et al. 2018). Chicks with wounds that will make it impossible for the bird to lead a normal life after recovery should be humanely euthanized. Also see Chapter 1, and Chapter 48 for information about managing typical problems of small songbirds.

Generalized poor feather quality is a problem seen frequently in cardinal chicks (Figure 49.1). An assessment should be made to see if the sub-adult plumage will fill in and make the bird releasable (if the tail feathers are a little poor but the bird can fly perfectly and is adequately insulated, the bird may be releasable). If poor feather quality would render the bird nonreleasable in its current condition, the feather condition must be improved prior to release. Flight and tail feather issues that affect flight, or contour feathers that do not offer adequate insulation, are examples of this. Releasing first year Northern Cardinals with marginal plumage into wintery northern climates should be avoided as it puts large survival challenges on a first-year bird who is already at a disadvantage due to being raised in a captive setting. Strategic removal of damaged or poor flight or tail feathers should be considered (and performed by a veterinarian under light anesthesia) to speed up the rehabilitation and release time line. Contour feathers are not candidates for pulling and must fill in naturally. Overwintering birds is also an option, as is transferring a patient to a rehabilitation center in a warmer climate for release. If transferred, the transfer should be done

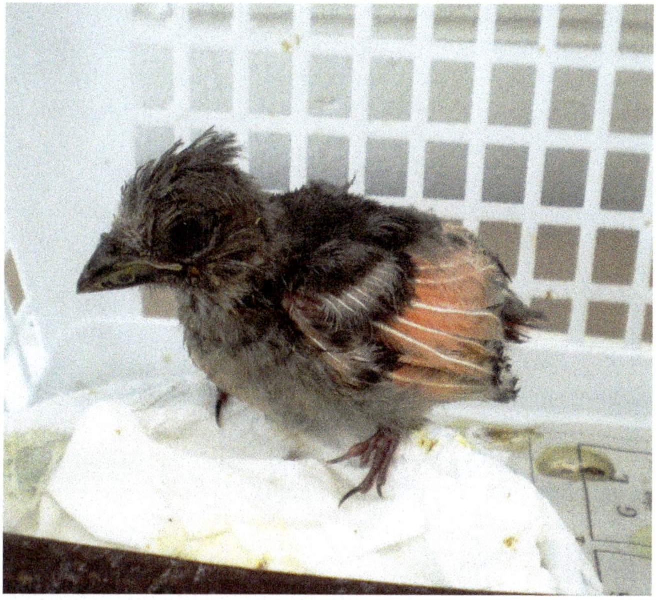

Figure 49.1 Poor quality plumage in a Northern Cardinal chick. *Source:* photo courtesy of Wildlife Rehabilitation Center of Minnesota.

according to state and federal laws and regulations and should be within the species' natural range. The specific patient's feather condition, general condition, location, time of year, and facilities should all be considered when determining a course of action. Each bird's plumage should be tested for waterproofing prior to release.

## Diets

Juvenile and adult diets consist mostly of insects. Depending on the season, fruit, seeds, and other vegetable matter can make up 30–50% of the diet. Parent birds feed their nestlings a diet that is comprised primarily of insects and approximately 20% fruit, pre-digested and regurgitated seed, and plant material.

### Hatchlings

Hatchling birds should be fed the Diet for Hatchling Passerines described in Chapter 43. Administer the diet using a 1 ml syringe. Hatchlings will expel a large fecal sac after every few feedings. If the young bird appears to be straining to produce a dropping, provide a small amount of oral fluids at the beginning of the next feeding or gently prod the cloaca area (as the parents do in the wild) using a warm, moistened swab. This action should prompt the chick to expel a dropping and keep the GI tract moving.

### Nestlings and Fledglings

Nestlings 4 days of age and older, and fledglings should be fed whole insects plus supplements shown in Box 44.1: "Supplements for Birds Hand-reared on an Insects-only Diet" in Chapter 44.

Pre-kill insects fed to younger nestlings. See Chapter 43, Box 43.1 for preparation of crickets and dubia roaches for handfeeding. Use curved or mosquito tipped hemostats to deliver the insects. Grosbeak and cardinal parents break apart insects in their beaks prior to feeding their chicks, so captive chicks should be fed insects that are soft-bodied and similarly prepared at this stage to avoid possible digestion issues.

Fruit such as blueberries can be hand-fed in small amounts (one blueberry every feeding). Grosbeaks and cardinals may continue gaping even after their crop is full. Use extreme caution when feeding a juicy berry as aspiration can occur if the crop is already full.

## Feeding Procedures

Respect and abide by the birds' natural schedule. Baby passerines require feeding from sunrise to sunset, 12–14 hours a day. A schedule of frequent and consistent feeding intervals will support a growing passerine's energetic demands for rapid growth and development.

- Feed hatchlings every 15–20 minutes.
- Feed very young nestlings every 20 minutes.
- Feed older nestlings every 20–30 minutes.
- Feed young fledglings every 30–45 minutes.
- Feed older fledglings every 45–60 minutes – at this point, their behavior and weight should be monitored. As the bird begins to transition to self-feeding, a slow gradual reduction in feeding frequency can be implemented.

### The "Weaning" Process: It Happens when it Happens

Baby passerines are at a developmental disadvantage as soon as they enter the doors of a rehabilitation facility. It is the role of the rehabilitator to support and care for them. Do not hurry them along before they are ready. Let the behavioral and physical development of the bird guide you and never impose the weaning process on a bird. Due to illness, injury, or delayed development for a variety of reasons, some individuals of the same species take longer than others to become self-sufficient.

At the fledgling stage, it is time to introduce whole foods for exploration and foraging. Research what types of food are appropriate for the species in care. Proper presentation of whole foods facilitates exploration, self-feeding, and enrichment. Consider the natural history of the bird and how it would explore and develop in the wild. And don't forget the basics: water for drinking and bathing, a dish of dirt and a dish of free-choice calcium (crushed cuttlebone or crushed sterilized eggshell).

Cardinals and grosbeaks will begin to make attempts at foraging for food around 10–12 days after fledging. They will continue to be fed regularly by their parents for 20–25 days after leaving the nest. Even though they are beginning to seek food on their own, young cardinals and grosbeaks will have ineffective foraging skills and many unsuccessful attempts at capturing prey. As mentioned before, weaning should not be rushed with these species and it is critical to keep a close eye on their weight. Caregivers should continue to hand-feed chicks until they are fully capable of catching live prey, cracking and eating shelled seeds, and no longer begging for food. In the wild, adult Northern Cardinal parents will continue to feed their young for at least 40 days after fledging, and have been observed feeding them for up to 56 days after fledging. Since these birds spend so much time following and learning from their parents, it is imperative to house fledglings with conspecifics. This provides opportunities for them to learn foraging from each other and prevents them from becoming too comfortable around their human caregivers. If young cardinals and grosbeaks become proficient at foraging during their first 2 to 3 weeks of independence, their chances of surviving their first year dramatically increase.

As cardinals and grosbeaks develop, their beak forms into a sturdy, cone-shaped structure that is well-equipped for cracking and grinding even the toughest seed husks. The upper part of the bill is supported and strengthened by bony struts called trabeculae. The trabeculae allow them to crack open thick shells without causing damage to their beak. The thick upper beak can make the safe administration of oral fluids via a 1 ml syringe somewhat difficult due to the position of the glottis and the angle that a syringe is guided into the mouth. Since it is not uncommon for a juvenile captive Northern Cardinal to beg at the sight of a syringe, caregivers should take care to avoid unintentional aspiration when offering oral fluids to a bird who no longer has a large mouth gape. It is safer to offer oral hydration with small pieces of chopped, watery fruit, or to administer fluids subcutaneously if the bird is particularly dehydrated.

Because effective foraging skills are critical for survival in the wild, food presentation should be varied and should mimic how it would be displayed in the natural environment. Be creative with food choices and presentation and consider the developmental stage the bird is at. Food as enrichment provides the opportunity to practice and develop essential foraging skills, such as the ability to capture, pluck, peck at, crack open, and consume foods. Newly-fledged birds may be enticed to pick at produce when it is chopped into small pieces and sample nuts and seeds that are out of the shell and chopped. However, as they grow older their food should be presented in in the way they might encounter it upon release. For example, a bunch of wild grapes, a spray of blackberries, or other wild fruits appropriate for the species can be collected and clipped to branches. "Berry branches" (Figure 49.2) can also be created by sticking small pieces of cut up fruit or berries onto the ends of leafless branches and clipped among the aviary's perches (Figure 49.3). Make sure to offer cut branches of food sources they will encounter in the wild such as Fir, Coffee Berry (*Rhamnus californica*), or Blue Elderberry (*Sambucus Mexicana*) for grosbeaks, and Dogwood

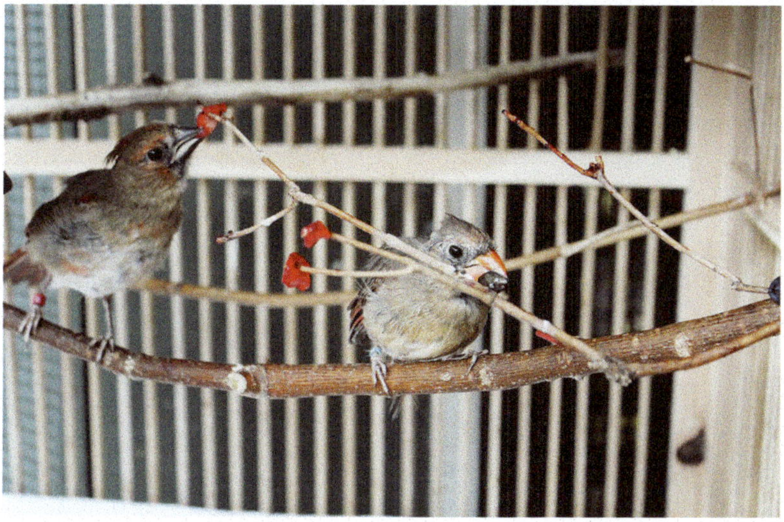

Figure 49.2 Northern Cardinal chicks foraging on fruit stuck onto twigs. *Source:* photo courtesy of Wildlife Rehabilitation Center of Minnesota.

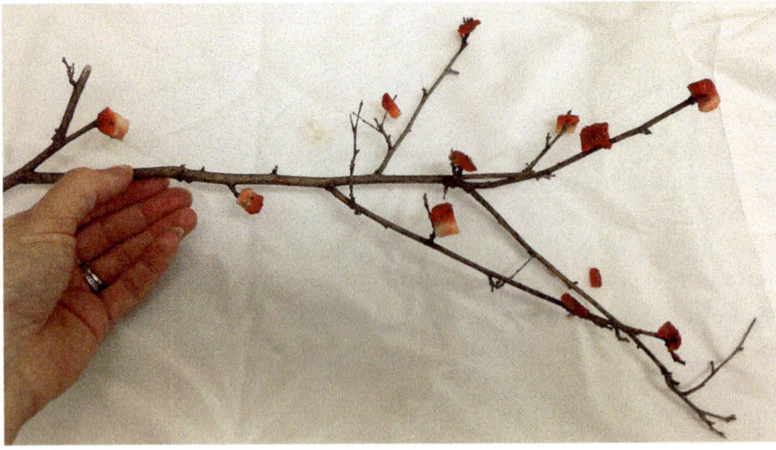

Figure 49.3 Strawberry pieces impaled on a branch make an excellent foraging opportunity for fledglings. *Source:* photo courtesy of Wildlife Rehabilitation Center of Minnesota.

(*Cornus florida*), Blackberries (*Rubus plicatus*), and Raspberries (*Rubus idaeus*) for Northern Cardinals. Northern Cardinals will often begin to eat from a dish that is at branch level before exploring the ground level of their enclosure. However, grosbeaks and cardinals will both opportunistically feed low and off the ground, so offer a variety of native grasses, weeds with seed heads, and scattered birdseed on a tray of soil. Place mealworms and other insects at various heights from "canopy" to ground level. Dishes filled with insects or seeds can be clipped into the enclosure's foliage using binder clips or hooks to guide young birds to forage in the trees and bushes as well as on the ground. Natural colored dishes, such as clay-colored, plastic plant pot saucers, brown peanut butter jar lids, clear plastic containers, and natural vessels such as small hollowed out rotten branches are excellent containers for seeds and insects. If the enclosure does not have wild vegetation growing in it, smartweed and similar wild grasses can be provided in pots. Provide a couple different styles of seed-filled bird feeders in the aviary to help them learn how to manage different perches and feeder ports.

Free-choice foods for fledglings includes the following: mealworms, crickets, moths, waxworms, fly larvae, dubia roaches, blackberries, blueberries, strawberries, soaked currants, grapes, cherries, walnuts, pine nuts, assorted seed and grains, black oil sunflower, peanut butter crumbles, suet cake, ripe fruits: pear, apricot, strawberry, plum, fig, wild fruits grape, coffeeberry, elderberry, blackberry. Offer new eaters large or difficult-to-open foods chopped into smaller pieces. Once birds are eating well, offer fruits and nuts whole or barely cracked open.

### Peanut Butter Crumble Recipe

- 1 cup (240 ml) creamy peanut butter (no salt added)
- 1½ cup (360 ml) cornmeal
- ½ cup (120 ml) freeze-dried mealworms
- ¼ cup (60 ml) dried currants

Mix together and store in fridge or freezer. Adapted from the Songbird Diet Index by Marcy Rule.

## Expected Weight Gain

Weight at time of hatching is approximately 3–3.5 g for Northern Cardinals and 4 g for grosbeaks. For both grosbeaks and cardinals, rapid growth occurs at 2 to 6 days of age at which time a nestling will gain approximately 3 g per day. Nestling grosbeaks and cardinals weigh 27–28 g just before fledging.

Cardinals and grosbeaks follow a similar developmental pattern. Young climb out of the nest at approximately 10–14 days of age and disperse among branches with thick cover near the nest. Fledglings are unable to fly until they are approximately 3 weeks old. Fledglings are relatively quiet during their flightless period but become very vocal once they are flighted. Young grosbeaks are independent approximately 3 weeks after fledging, whereas cardinals rely on their parents for approximately 6 weeks after fledging.

Sexes of Rose-breasted Grosbeaks can be distinguished at 5 days of age when the pink wing-linings of young males begin to show. Northern Cardinals will gradually reveal their sex as older juveniles when their feathers begin to fill in. Male plumage will slowly develop an overall red color, whereas females will develop plumage that is olive-green with only a trace of red.

## Developmental Needs

### Migratory Function

To complete their journeys north and south, grosbeaks and other migratory passerines use many cues for orientation and navigation, including geographical features, the stars, the sun, and the Earth's magnetic field. Some species may even use their olfactory and inertial (logging turns and acceleration of the route) senses. According to scientists and their research, most birds use a combination of these techniques.

Through numerous experiments, scientists have confirmed the use of a "star compass" in nocturnal migrant passerines. In the rehabilitation setting, nocturnal migrants such as grosbeaks should have exposure to a full view of the setting sun and night sky at approximately 3 weeks of age. This will help them learn to orient their direction by the stars.

### Song Development

Grosbeaks and cardinals belong to a suborder of Passeriformes known as Oscines, or "true songbirds." Most true songbirds must learn their songs. They learn their song from a model sound (usually their father) or a tutor (in rehab), memorize the model, and practice the sound until it matches their memory of the original sound. This period of learning is called the "sensitive period." The age at which the sensitive period begins and ends varies by species, but in general, lasts from days 8 to 60.

Some species will begin to practice singing as young as a few weeks old, although it is barely perceptible at that time. Other species will not begin practice singing until the following spring, but most songbirds begin to practice singing in late summer.

Vocal ability is socially important to passerines. Vocalizations help birds stay in contact with each other, warn each other of danger, or let flock members know where food is available. Song is an essential vocal skill that passerines, mostly males, use to attract a mate and claim territory.

In the rehabilitation setting, hand-raised songbirds (oscines) must have exposure to the songs of their species. It would be ideal if the nursery was surrounded by good habitat and singing conspecifics right outside the window. However, if the nursery is not surrounded by bird song or there is a bird in care that does not have a singing conspecific outside the window, you will need to provide a tutor for song.

Raw unprocessed geographically appropriate recordings of bird songs are available from Cornell's Lab of Ornithology Macaulay Library of sound (see resources). Research the available materials for the species in question. Download the sound file to a computer or smartphone and play the recording at dawn and dusk. It is also possible to make a recording of the song by visiting the location where the orphaned bird was found and recording the dawn song at that location. Birds in care should have access to their song from nestling through fledgling stage. Providing song at hatchling stage may be impractical as it is unlikely to be heard over the din of the incubator.

## Housing

Never raise a single baby bird. Single babies of any age should be with a conspecific or compatible species (Figure 49.4). You may need to call another center or rehabilitator in your area if you do not receive a conspecific or compatible species in a timely manner. Every effort should be made to raise young birds with others of their own species.

Food or feces stuck to any part of the baby must be gently removed immediately using a soft cotton swab moistened with warm water. Contaminants left on the skin can cause bacterial infection as well as feather development issues. Food covering an eye or the nares is an obvious problem and should be dealt with immediately.

Create a comfortable and stress-free environment. Never house corvids, starlings, or grackles with or near other passerine species; these birds are aggressive and/or predatory species that most passerines seek to avoid in the wild. Do not house passerines within sight or sound of other predatory species such as mammals, birds of prey, or domestic pets.

### Hatchlings

Hatchlings, days 0–3, are featherless, their eyes are closed, and they are unable to thermoregulate. They should be housed in an incubator set at 91–93 °F (32.8–33.9 °C). Incubators are ideal for

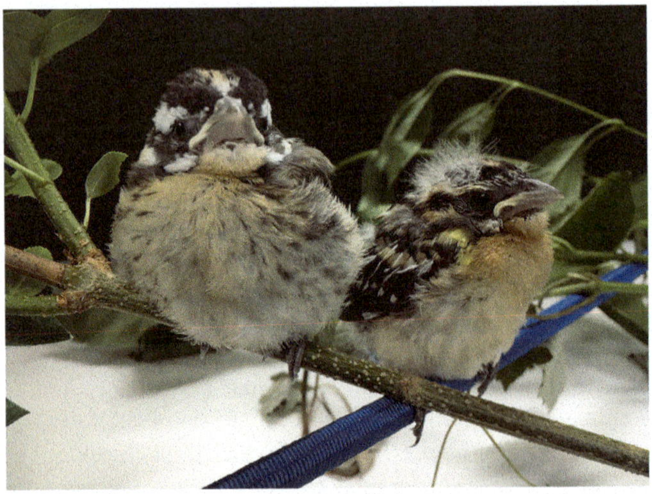

Figure 49.4 Black-headed Grosbeak fledglings. The one on the right is younger: note the downy tufts remaining on the head.

hatchlings as they provide much-needed humidity as well as the ability to maintain a consistent ambient temperature.

An artificial nest can be created using a small- to medium-sized round plastic container lined with a face cloth or similar fabric for insulation and softness. Fill the center of the nest with tightly crumpled tissue or an additional face cloth folded into a square and then folded to form the shape and cup of a natural nest. Ensuring the proper texture of the lining and shape of the nest interior is important to support the body of a developing young bird. Choose a size of container that will comfortably accommodate the number of birds to inhabit the nest. Simulate a brooding parent by placing a soft, lightweight cloth or tissue over hatchlings.

Keep baby birds and their nest clean. Use extreme care when handling hatchlings, as their skin is tender and sensitive. Well-formed fecal sacs can be carefully removed from the nest with tweezers or forceps. This will help reduce the handling of hatchlings and decrease the number of times nest substrate is changed throughout the day.

## Nestlings

Very young nestlings, days 4–5, will also benefit from the ambient heat (89–90 °F/31.7–32.2 °C) and humidity of an incubator. Healthy nestlings, 6 days and older, can be housed in their nest and placed in a reptarium (38-gal/144 l) or medium-sized mesh butterfly enclosure. Provide a supplemental heat source if necessary.

Lay a piece of soft felt or a folded tissue over hatchlings to simulate a brooding parent and provide warmth and security. The addition of a face cloth folded over the top of the nest to create a dome will help nestlings feel more secure and minimize stress (see Figure 44.2). Grosbeaks and cardinals are open-cup nesters, which means as soon as nestlings eyes are open, they have visual access to the world around them. Place greenery around the nest to naturalize their environment and provide a sense of security.

Ill and injured nestlings may require the ambient heat of an incubator or another heat source. Use the bird's health as your guide in determining the appropriate level of warmth and necessary support.

## Fledglings

A 175-gal reptarium (4 × 3 × 3 ft./1.2 × 0.9 × 0.9 m) or similar housing is suitable for two to three grosbeaks or cardinals who are recently fledged and not yet fully flighted. However, an enclosure of this size is less than ideal for flighted active fledglings. It is strongly recommended to move fledglings outdoors to an aviary to continue the hand-rearing process in a more natural environment. In an aviary, fledglings will have access to natural sunlight, exposure to the night sky, and more space to support physical and behavioral development.

Whether housed indoors or in an aviary, create a natural environment for fledglings by furnishing the enclosure with perches at different heights and a generous amount of fresh, leafy branches to provide cover and foraging opportunities. Not only will some natural wild insects be brought into the pre-release enclosure this way, but having lots of vegetation in the enclosure will nicely replicate the spaces where cardinals and grosbeaks will feed and roost once they are released into the wild.

Scatter leaf litter and grass on the bottom of the enclosure. Include a wide, shallow dish of water for drinking and bathing, a shallow dish of clean dirt, and a source of free-choice calcium, such as ground cuttlebone or crushed sterilized eggshell offered in a small dish. Provide dishes of mealworms, waxworms, and dubia roaches at varying heights in the enclosure. Provide and present other food choices as described in the section "Diets."

### Aviaries

The minimum aviary size recommended for these medium-sized songbirds is 4×8×4 ft. (1.2×2.4×1.2 m) for four to six birds (Miller 2012), but the authors recommend larger 6×10×8 ft. (1.8×3×2.1 m) for three to four birds or 8×16×8 ft. (2.4×4.8×2.4 m) for five to eight pre-release birds. Aviaries must be safe and predator-proof. Basic design includes 2×4 in. (5.1×10.2 cm) wood frame construction, with ½ in. (1.25 cm) hardware cloth on the outside, fiberglass screen on the inside, and solid plywood on the bottom 3 ft. of the walls. The wood frame will create a space between the exterior aviary wire and the interior fiberglass window screen. This important buffer prevents sneak attacks and strikes through the wire and screen from predators such as accipiters and free-roaming cats.

At least one-quarter of the structure should be fully enclosed with plywood on the roof, back, and sides (Figure 49.5). This provides shelter and a safe place to roost and escape from view of predators. Include a double-door entry, or interior screen door, to prevent accidental escapes upon entry into the enclosure.

Enclosure substrates can be gravel, sand, turf, dirt, or a combination. You must have the ability to clean and disinfect. A layer of hardware cloth (1/4 in./0.6 cm wire mesh) should be submerged under the dirt and gravel layer to prevent intrusions from rats, raccoons, and other predators. A well-placed, well-built structure provides access to sunlight, natural elements, good air circulation, room for full flight and normal flight patterns (banking, turning, sallying), and a view of the night sky.

## Pre-release Conditioning and Release Criteria

As prey species, passerines must have strength, stamina, and agile flight to evade predators and capture food. Pre-release conditioning in a secure, large outdoor aviary is the best way to support the development of these skills for a hand-raised passerine.

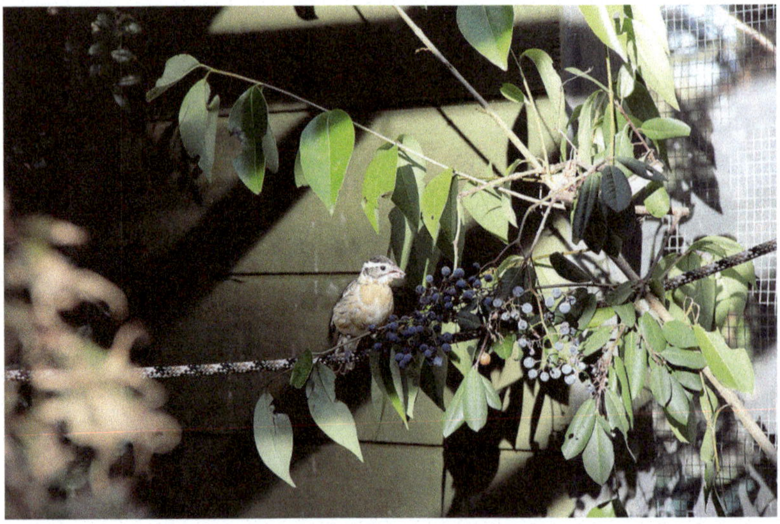

Figure 49.5 Black-headed Grosbeak in an aviary furnished with ample greenery, mixed solid and wire mesh walls, with natural foods offered for foraging practice.

If birds are not moved outside until they are self-feeding, they should be housed in an outdoor aviary for at least 14 days to build strength, stamina, and acclimate to the outdoors (weather, predators, observe natural behavior of wild conspecifics, etc.). A hand-raised passerine is not ready for release until it has met appropriate behavioral and physical criteria.

## Release

Birds should have excellent feather condition, be aerobically fit, at adult weight, waterproof, totally self-feeding, able to recognize their natural diet, able to forage for their natural diet successfully in the manner appropriate for the species, free of disease and parasites, fully recovered from injuries, and able to demonstrate a healthy fear of and respond appropriately to all predators, including humans.

Every effort should be made to release birds back to their natal territory. However, if that is not possible, select a location with appropriate habitat where the species is present. Releases should occur in the mid to late morning upon a forecast of 3 days of clear weather.

## Acknowledgments

Veronica Bowers offers sincere gratitude to the amazing passerines whose beauty and song grace this earth each day. Jessika Madison-Kennedy offers great thanks to those who have supported my avian rescue work over the years, to Janine Perlman Ph.D. for working so closely with me on solving nutritional issues for different species (as well as reviewing my work), and to the awe-inspiring birds, from the common to the rare, that we share this planet with.

## Sources for Products Mentioned

Freeze-dried insects: Arbico Organics, 10831 N. Mavinee Drive, Ste. 185, Oro Valley, AZ 85737-9531, (800) 847-2847, http://www.arbico-organics.com.

Mealworms, waxworms, dubia roaches, fly larvae, fruit flies and crickets: Rainbow Mealworms, 126 E. Spruce St, Compton, CA 90220, (800) 777-9676. https://www.rainbowmealworms.net.

Mesh butterfly enclosures: http://Amazon.com.

Mesh reptariums, logs, and bark: LLLReptile and Supply Company Inc., 609 Mission Ave, Oceanside, CA 92054, (760) 439-8492, www.http://lllreptile.com.

Recordings of song: Macaulay Library, Cornell Lab of Ornithology, 159 Sapsucker Woods Road, Ithaca, New York USA 14850 (607) 254-2404 www.macaulaylibrary.org.

Ultracare Mite and Lice Bird Spray: 8 in 1 Pet Products, Hauppauge, NY, (800) 645-5154.

## References

Duerr, R.S., Purdin, G.J., and Bowers, V. (2017). Small-bodied birds: passerines, doves, woodpeckers, others. In: *Topics in Wildlife Medicine, Vol. 4: Orthopedics* (eds. R.S. Duerr and G.J. Purdin), 53–74. St. Cloud, MN: National Wildlife Rehabilitators Association.

Hawkins, M.G., Barron, H.W., Speer, B.L. et al. (2018). Birds. In: *Exotic Animal Formulary*, 5e (eds. J.W. Carpenter and C.J. Marion), 167–375. St. Louis, MO: Elsevier.

Miller, E.A. (ed.) (2012). *Minimum Standards for Wildlife Rehabilitation*, 4e. St. Cloud, MN: National Wildlife Rehabilitation Association.

## Further Reading

Bowers, V. (2018). *Passerine Fundamentals*, 119 pp. Sebastopol, CA: Native Songbird Care and Conservation.

Elphick, C., Dunning, J.B., and Sibley, D.A. (eds.) (2001). *The Sibley Guide to Bird Life and Behavior*, 588 pp. New York: Alfred A. Knopf, Inc.

Halkin, S.L. and Linville, S.U. (1999). Northern cardinal (*Cardinalis cardinalis*), version 2.0. In: *The Birds of North America* (eds. A.F. Poole and F.B. Gill). Ithaca, NY, USA: Cornell Lab of Ornithology https://doi.org/10.2173/bna.440.

International Wildlife Rehabilitation Council (2003). *Wildlife Nutrition and Feeding*, 73 pp. Oakland, California: IWRC.

MacLeod, A. and Perlman, J. (2001). Adventures in avian nutrition: dietary considerations for the hatchling and nestling passerine. *Journal of Wildlife Rehabilitation* 24 (1): 10–15.

Ortega, C. and Hill, G.E. (2010). Black-headed grosbeak (*Pheucticus melanocephalus*), version 2.0. In: *The Birds of North America* (ed. A.F. Poole). Ithaca, NY, USA: Cornell Lab of Ornithology. https://doi.org/10.2173/bna.143.

# 50

# Java Sparrows

*Jo Gregson and Andrew Bowkett*

## Natural History

The Java Sparrow *Lonchura oryzivora* (Linneaus 1758), sometimes referred to as *Padda oryzivora*, is the largest species in the family Estrildidae, which also includes waxbills, grass finches, and munias. Java Sparrows are popular in aviculture due to their contrastingly patterned plumage, distinctive white cheeks, and large pinkish-red bills. Males and females are similar in appearance although males may have a more distinguishing eye-ring and deeper bill.

Java Sparrows feed predominantly on seeds, including rice, and inhabit a variety of lowland habitats including grassland, open woodland, cultivated land, and residential areas. They are a social species which feed in flocks, particularly during the nonbreeding season, and they generally breed communally. Breeding pairs build bulky nests made of grass which they strategically place in trees or cavities, including gaps in buildings and nest boxes (Kurniandaru 2008). Clutch size is generally three to seven eggs, which are incubated for up to 14 days and reach independence at 33–35 days in captivity (Payne 2016). Pairs lay up to three clutches per season (Yuda 2008).

Native to the Indonesian islands of Java, Bali, and probably Madura, Java Sparrows have been widely introduced to other Indonesian islands and around the world including various south-east Asian countries, China, Japan, Sri Lanka, Tanzania, Fiji, Mexico, and USA (Payne 2016). While formerly abundant enough to be considered a serious pest in rice paddies, the species has undergone a population collapse primarily driven by trapping for the cage-bird trade and is listed as Endangered by the World Conservation Union (Birdlife International 2018). Some introduced populations have also declined or gone extinct due to excessive trapping. Other potential threats in its native range include trapping for consumption, changes in farming practices, and competition with introduced species. Recommended conservation actions include enforcement of trade restrictions, protection of remaining wild populations, and captive-breeding to meet market demands in order to discourage trapping (Collar and Butchart 2014; Birdlife International 2017) (Figure 50.1).

## Criteria for Intervention

Java Sparrows generally breed readily in captivity and do not require intervention. The hand-rearing trials reported in this chapter were undertaken to gain experience in incubation and hand-feeding small seed-eating passerines and also to study the effects of hand-rearing on the

*Hand-Rearing Birds*, Second Edition. Edited by Rebecca S. Duerr and Laurie J. Gage.

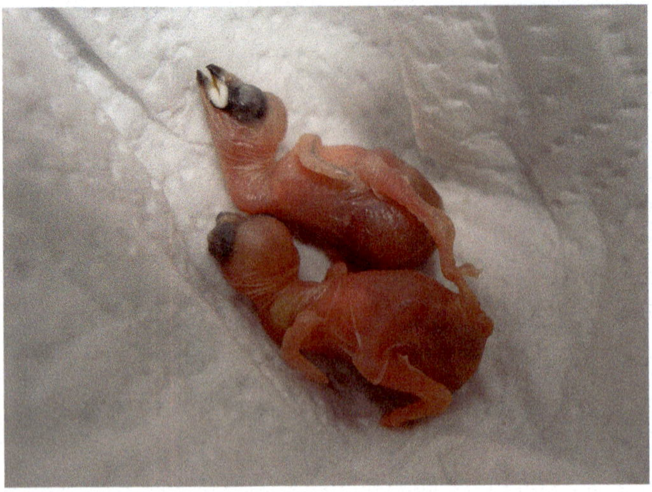

Figure 50.1 One day old Java Sparrow chicks in nesting bowl.

Table 50.1 Hand-rearing success with Java Sparrows collected as eggs or chicks over two breeding seasons at Paignton Zoo Environmental Park, UK.

| Breeding season | | Collected | Survived | % Survival |
|---|---|---|---|---|
| 2013/14 | Eggs | 11 | 4 | 36.4% |
| | Chicks | 7 | 5 | 71.4% |
| 2014/15 | Eggs | 9 | 5 | 55.6% |
| | Chicks | 3 | 3 | 100% |
| | **Total** | **30** | **17** | **56.7%** |

reproduction and behavior of hand-reared individuals. The aim was to develop a reliable protocol that would be a useful guideline for many other Estrildid finches. The trials included artificial incubation and rearing chicks from day 1. Several chicks were also harvested at the age of 6 days to compare growth and vigor with those harvested as an egg. Eggs and chicks were harvested from a captive flock kept at Paignton Zoo Environmental Park, UK, and fledglings released back into the same enclosure as used to house the adults. Survival was comparable to that in wild populations (Ricklefs 1969) and improved noticeably in the second year (Table 50.1). Similar methods were also employed to rear captive Cut-throat Finches *Amadina fasciata* (Gregson and Tooley 2016).

## General Husbandry

Java Sparrows at Paignton Zoo are housed in a large walkthrough glasshouse exhibit, measuring 40 × 15 × 7 m (131 × 49 × 23 ft.). The enclosure is maintained at an average temperature of 70.4 °F (23 °C) and contains tropical vegetation, a variety of substrates, and water sources. Fourteen other bird species are free-flying within the exhibit, which also contains separate units housing reptiles and amphibians. Java Sparrows are provided a seed mix consisting of millet seeds, millet sprays, and Vesele Laga NutriBird C15 pellets. Living in a mixed exhibit they also have access to the soft fruit, egg, and insectivore mix provided for softbill species. Feeding stations are cleaned and replenished each morning. The flock consisted of between 35 and 60 individuals over the course of the study (2013–2015) and breeds regularly without any intervention. Most pairs use nest boxes, although some choose to nest in dense foliage. Breeding typically begins in September and continues through to the end of March. Where possible, nests are visually inspected every week during the breeding season to record nest stage, clutch size, and chick survival.

## Incubation, Initial Care, and Stabilization

Eggs were incubated in an R.COM Digital Incubator at 99.5 °F (37.5 °C) for 15 days and were automatically turned every hour. The day after hatch they are moved to a brooder at 98.6 °F (37 °C). Once chicks are warm and settled, they are offered a few drops of water from a pipette. The first feed was offered from 3 to 12 hours after hatching.

Chicks were maintained in brooders at 98.6 °F (37 °C) until day 7 when the temperature was dropped to 96.8 °F (36 °C). The temperature was then decreased gradually to 86 °F (30 °C) by 20 days of age. Chicks cool down quickly when removed from the brooder and feeding should be carried out quickly, or with the chicks placed under a heat lamp to maintain body temperature (Figure 50.2).

The skin on newly hatched chicks is thin and therefore a very soft paper tissue should be used in the nesting bowl, avoiding harsher hand wipe rolls. Single chicks require support with tissue or, ideally, if there is another brood they can be nested together. As chicks grow stronger, they will need a nonslip substrate added to the nest. The liners used in hanging plant baskets can be cut to size and are an excellent replacement for sticks.

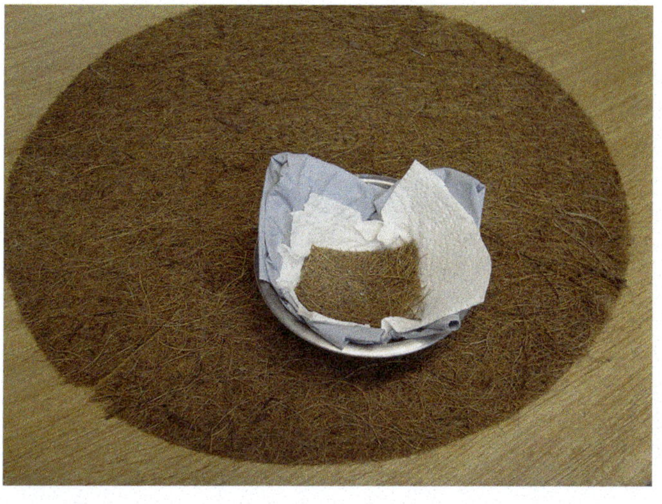

Figure 50.2 Prepared rearing bowl for chicks at 10 days.

## Hand-feeding Diets

Kaytee® exact® Hand-Feeding Formula was used successfully. This is a conventional hand-rearing formula more often used for parrots. Start with 1 part Kaytee Formula to 6 parts water and increase the strength of the formula to 4 parts water to 1 part Kaytee Formula on day 5 (Figure 50.3).

## Feeding Procedures

On day 1, feed the chicks every hour from 6:00 a.m. to 9:00 p.m. At day 18, reduce feeds to every 2 hours from 7:00 a.m. to 7:00 p.m. and at day 25 feed every 2 hours from 8:00 a.m. to 5:00 p.m. Java Sparrow chicks are blind until day 12. A soft whistle feeding signal was used to announce the approach of the caregivers. Alerting the birds in this way also helps to regulate defecation (Figure 50.4).

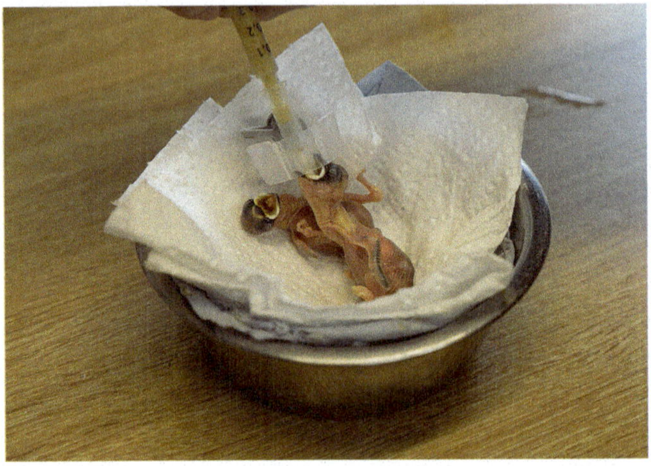

Figure 50.3 Pipette used to feed newly hatched chicks. *Source:* courtesy of Lesley O'Connor.

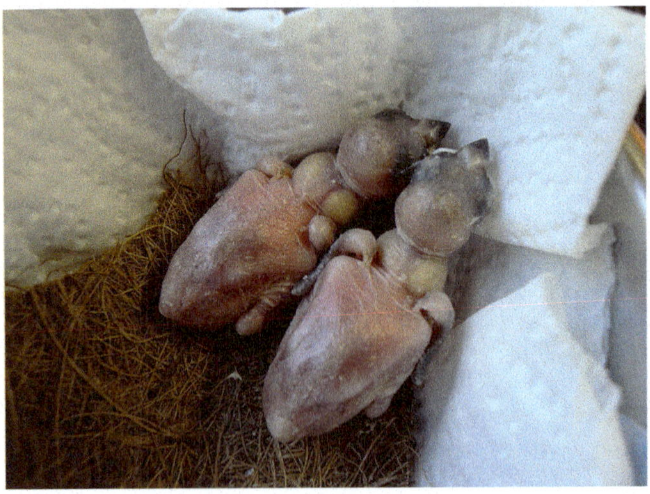

Figure 50.4 Java Sparrow chicks at 10 days of age.

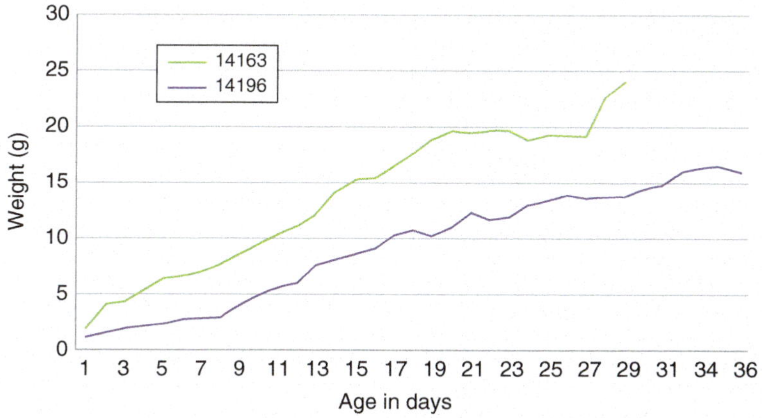


**Figure 50.5** Growth in body weight of two typical Java Sparrow chicks hand-reared from hatching.

The formula was offered in a small pipette. As the chicks grew, the formula was thickened and the chicks were fed from a 1 ml syringe. At day 10, ground flaked millet was introduced to the mix and increased to 25% of the mix over 4–5 days. No whole seed was offered until chicks began weaning and at that time soaked shelled millets were offered. Once the chicks were digesting seed they were introduced to millet sprays and the formula was gradually phased out by day 35.

Individual chicks were identified using metal rings and unique combinations of colored split rings (size K, Haith's). Color ring combinations were important to allow monitoring of birds after release into the large aviary, where reading of identification rings is not usually possible.

## Expected Weight Gain

See Figure 50.5 for a chart of typical growth of Java Sparrow chicks. Expected weight gains are 10–15% per day. Birds became difficult to weigh after fledging.

## Weaning

The chicks fledged from the nesting bowl at approximately 25 days. At this time, their weight leveled out for a few days and then began to increase again by day 28. Feeding times were reduced as the birds became less interested in food and more active. Once the chicks were mobile they were moved from the brooder to a canary breeding cage, 4.5 × 1 × 1.5 ft. (140 × 30 × 41 cm), where they could flex their wings and still feel secure. After a few days they were offered a small, shallow bowl of water for bathing. The finches began to self-wean at about 30 days of age. They were soon very mobile and would fly to the hand for seed and then return to the fledgling holding area. By day 36, they were less responsive to the keepers and appeared more nervous. They were moved to a small aviary before they were released into the exhibit at 45 days old. By then none of the birds were hand-tame. The perching branches used in both the small aviary and the canary cage were fine and flexible to encourage a wide range of foot movements (Figure 50.6).

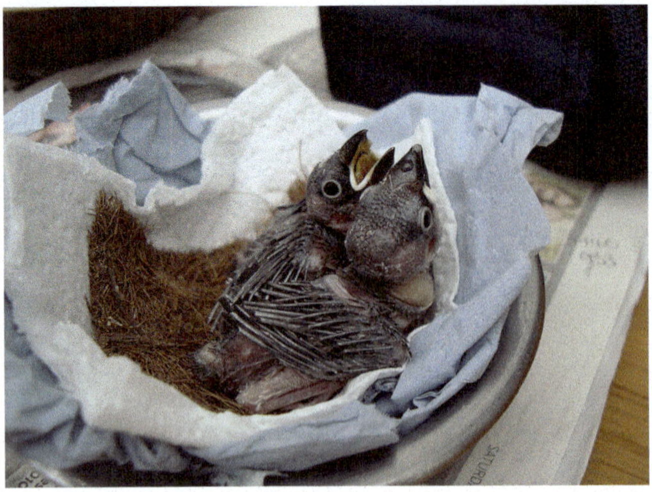

Figure 50.6 Java Sparrow chicks at 15 days of age. *Source:* courtesy of Lesley O'Connor.

## Preparation and Release into a Large Aviary

Hand-reared fledglings were transferred as a group to a release pen within the exhibit. After 1 week, when the door to the release pen was opened the birds were able to enter the main exhibit space and interact with adult Java Sparrows and other species. Most of the fledglings were reluctant to leave the release pen for the first 3 days and had to be encouraged to leave by placing food just beyond the door.

To monitor post-release behavior, the exhibit was divided into 10 zones, centered on feeding stations, each of which was observed for 20 minutes per day for two periods of 10 days each: 5 days and 4 weeks after release. These observations revealed that hand-reared sparrows did not associate preferentially with other hand-reared sparrows (hand-reared sparrows were in the same zone as parent-reared sparrows in more than 90% of observations) and were no more likely to be involved in aggressive interactions with other Java Sparrows or other bird species than parent-reared individuals. Hand-reared sparrows were displaced at feeding stations more frequently, on average, than parent-reared sparrows but this was probably due to their younger average age. No individuals were observed attempting to interact with people. Overall, the hand-reared sparrows appeared to integrate well into the flock and there was no evidence of negative behavioral effects.

## Reproductive Success of Hand-reared Individuals

The reproductive success of hand-reared Java Sparrows was monitored. Four of nine hand-reared sparrows established nest sites in their first breeding season (aged 9 to 12 months). There appeared to be no effect of rearing on mate preference. Hatching and fledging rates were similar for both hand-reared and parent-reared birds. Incidents of displacement and aggression were observed too infrequently to compare fledgling types, but the amount of time each spent with each other, with other fledgling types, and with adults was similar.

There was no obvious negative impact of hand-rearing on breeding success in the small number of hand-reared chicks in the study. Despite the negative effects of hand-rearing seen in some species (e.g. Myers et al. 1988) there are also potential positive effects linked to greater average body size in hand-reared individuals if the process reduces feeding competition within broods. Mate preference studies show that female Java Sparrows choose larger males (Hasegawa et al. 2011) and so there is a potential mechanism for hand-rearing to benefit reproductive success in this species, at least for males. The relative success of hand-rearing, in terms of survival, behavior, and reproduction, demonstrated here for captive Java Sparrows illustrates the potential for using this technique more widely in the conservation of threatened passerines.

## Acknowledgments

Thanks to Tom Tooley, Lesley O'Connor, and Peter Smallbones for hand-rearing the sparrows; Paul Jacques for caring for the birds in Reptile Tropics; and Bryony Baker and Charlotte Leaman for carrying out the behavioral observations and collating the growth weights and productivity data. Holly Farmer helped access zoo records and advised on behavioral observation methods.

## Sources for Products Mentioned

Haith's leg bands: John E Haith Ltd., The Bird Food Centre, Genesis Way, Europarc, Grimsby, NE Lincs, DN37 9TU, UK, www.haiths.com.

Kaytee products: 521 Clay St, PO Box 230, Chilton, WI USA 53014, (800) KAYTEE-1, https://www.kaytee.com.

Vesele Laga NutriBird C15 pellets: Versele-Laga, Kapellestraat 70, 9800 Deinze, Belgium, http://www.versele-laga.com.

## References

BirdLife International. (2017). Species factsheet: Lonchura oryzivora. www.birdlife.org (accessed 3 January 2017).

BirdLife International (2018). Lonchura oryzivora. The IUCN Red List of Threatened Species 2018. http://dx.doi.org/10.2305/IUCN.UK.2018-2.RLTS.T22719912A131809903.en (accessed 25 November 2019).

Collar, N.J. and Butchart, S.J.M. (2014). Conservation breeding and avian diversity: chances and challenges. *International Zoo Yearbook* 48: 7–28.

Gregson, J. and Tooley, T. (2016). Hand-rearing the cutthroat finch (Amadina fasciata) at Paignton zoo, UK. *Avicultural Magazine* 122: 27–28.

Hasegawa, A., Soma, M., and Hasegawa, T. (2011). Male traits and female choice in Java Sparrows: preference for large body size. *Ornithological Science* 10 (1): 73–80.

Kurniandaru, S. (2008). Providing nest boxes for Java Sparrows *Padda oryzivora* in response to nest site loss due to building restoration and an earthquake, Prambanan Temple, Java, Indonesia. *Conservation Evidence* 5: 62–68.

Myers, S.A., Millam, J.R., Roudybush, T.E., and Grau, C.R. (1988). Reproductive success of hand-reared vs parent-reared cockatiels (*Nymphicus hollandicus*). *Auk* 105 (3): 536–542.

Payne, R. (2016). Java Sparrow (*Lonchura oryzivora*). In: *Handbook of the Birds of the World Alive* (eds. J. del Hoyo, A. Elliot, J. Sargatel, et al.). Barcelona: Lynx Edicions. http://www.hbw.com/node/6184 (accessed 23 May 2016).

Ricklefs, R.E. (1969). An analysis of nesting mortality in birds. *Smithsonian Contributions to Zoology* 9: 1–48.

Yuda, P. (2008). Conservation genetics of the Java Sparrow (Padda oryzivora) and an analysis of its viability. Ph.D. thesis, James Cook University, Australia.

# Appendix A

## Record Sheet Example

An example of a rehabilitation animal record. The use of check-off boxes is handy for data entry into databases and when admitting large numbers of animals. Forms such as this can be laminated and reused after entering data into a database or used as a permanent paper medical record.

*Hand-Rearing Birds*, Second Edition. Edited by Rebecca S. Duerr and Laurie J. Gage.

Wildlife Care Association — Giving wildlife a second chance

**Species:** ______

**Date Admitted** ______ **Time** ______ am/pm

**Band #or mark:**

| Bird: | Mammal: | Other: | Sex: | Intaken at: |
|---|---|---|---|---|
| ☐ Hatchling | ☐ Newborn | ☐ Reptile | ☐ M | ☐ Nursery |
| ☐ Nestling | ☐ Infant | ☐ Amphibian | ☐ F | ☐ Rehabber |
| ☐ Fledgling | ☐ Juvenile | | ☐ U | |
| ☐ Adult | ☐ Adult | | | |

**DISPOSITION**

Date:

Released ☐

Transfer (to other org) ☐

DOA ☐

Expired ☐

EOA ☐

Euthanized ☐

Release site/zip code:

Group transferred to:

**Patient Record**

***Please promptly return completed forms to: WCA, POBox 60982, Sacramento, CA 95860***

**Initial Information:Examiner(s)** ______ **Date:**

| Mobility: | Respiration: | Stress/fear level: | Attitude: | Temp |
|---|---|---|---|---|
| ☐ Normal | ☐ Normal | ☐ Low/Calm | ☐ Bright/Alert | ☐ Hot |
| ☐ Favoring | ☐ limbFast/Panting | ☐ Moderate | ☐ Somewhat alert | ☐ Warm |
| ☐ Unbalanced | ☐ Slow | ☐ High | ☐ Depressed | ☐ Cool |
| ☐ Hock sitting | ☐ Gasping | **Dehydration status:** | ☐ Unresponsive | ☐ Cold |
| ☐ Head Tilt | ☐ Clicking/Crackling | ☐ None/Mild (0-5%) | **Color:** | |
| ☐ Prone | ☐ Open mouth breathing | ☐ Moderate (6-9%) | ☐ normal ☐ pale mouth | |
| | | ☐ Severe (>9%) | ☐ pale flesh | |

**Weight (g):** ______

**Physical exam:Examiner(s):** ______ **Date:** ______ ***Check areas with problems, detail below.***

| | | | |
|---|---|---|---|
| ☐ Head | ☐ EarsL / R | ☐ Grip | ☐ Stool |
| ☐ Tracking | ☐ Neck | ☐ Back | ☐ Fur/feathers: ☐ stress marks ☐ bald area(s) |
| ☐ Mouth | ☐ Throat | ☐ Chest | ☐ Fracture: |
| ☐ Bill/Teeth | ☐ Crop: ☐ full ☐ empty | ☐ Abdomen | ☐ Wounds: |
| ☐ Tongue | ☐ Wings/ForelegsL / R | ☐ Vent/Anus/Genitals | Nutritional State: ☐ Normal ☐ Thin ☐ Emaciated |
| ☐ EyesL / R | ☐ Legs/HindlegsL / R | ☐ Tail | |
| ☐ Nares/NostrilsL / R | ☐ FeetL / R | ☐ Ectoparasites: ☐ mites ☐ fleas ☐ lice ☐ fly-eggs ☐ flat flies | |

| Date | Exam/Progress notes | Initials |
|---|---|---|
| | Rehydration: ______ ml fluids given SQ or Orally at ______ am/pm | |
| | | |
| | | |
| | | |
| | | |
| | | |
| | Over ➡ | |

| Drug/Procedure/Treatment: | Dose: | Dates: | Procedure/Treatment: | Dose: | Dates: |
|---|---|---|---|---|---|
| ☐ Frontline | | | | | to |
| | | to | | | to |
| | | to | | | to |
| | | to | | | to |
| | | to | | | to |

| Date: | | | | | | | | | | | | | | | | | | |
|---|---|---|---|---|---|---|---|---|---|---|---|---|---|---|---|---|---|---|
| Wt (g): | | | | | | | | | | | | | | | | | | |

**Please fill out the box below with information about the animal.**

**Date found** ______ **Time found:** ______

**Reason rescued:** ☐ Cat contact ☐ Hit by car ☐ Hit window ☐ Fell from nest ☐ Orphaned ☐ Appears sick or injured:

Other:

**Describe any care given:** ______

**Street address or cross streets or city where found:** ______

**Area found (in road, lawn etc.):**

**Name** ______

**Address** ______

**Zip** ______

**Email** ______

**Phone (   )** ______

**Would you like to make a donation today? $** ______

***Your donation will help us continue to care for the animals.***

***All donations are tax deductible and much appreciated!***

# Appendix B

# Energy Requirements for Growing Birds

## B.1 General Information

See Tables B.1 and B.2 for energy requirements of growing birds. Sick and injured young birds have extremely high energy requirements but may have a reduced capacity to metabolize food. In such cases, growth may be delayed while healing occurs. Caregivers should provide the chick with as much high-quality diet as it is able to digest. Energy needs change daily in rapidly growing chicks.

## B.2 Calculations

- Passerine Bird Basal Metabolic Rate (BMR) = body weight in $\text{kgs}^{0.75} \times 129$
- Nonpasserine Bird Basal Metabolic Rate (BMR) = body weight in $\text{kgs}^{0.75} \times 78$
- Maintenance Energy Requirement (MER) in kcal/day = BMR × 1.5
- Adjustment for Growth = MER × 1.5–3.0
- Adjustment for Sepsis = MER × 1.2–1.5
- Adjustment for Mild Injury = MER × 1.0–1.2
- Adjustment for Severe Injury = MER × 1.1–2.0

*Source:* Carpenter, J.W. (ed.) (2005). *Exotic Animal Formulary*, 3e, 559 pp. St. Louis: Elsevier Saunders.

*Hand-Rearing Birds*, Second Edition. Edited by Rebecca S. Duerr and Laurie J. Gage.

Table B.1 Energy requirements of passerine chicks.

| Body Weight (grams) | Basal Metabolic Rate (BMR) | Maintenance Energy Requirement (MER) in kcal/Day | Kilocalories per Day for Growth when Healthy |
|---|---|---|---|
| 2 | 1.2 | 1.8 | 2.7–5.5 |
| 4 | 2.1 | 3.1 | 4.6–9.2 |
| 6 | 2.8 | 4.2 | 6.3–12.5 |
| 10 | 4.1 | 6.1 | 9.2–18.4 |
| 12 | 4.7 | 7.0 | 10.5–21.0 |
| 14 | 5.3 | 7.9 | 11.8–23.6 |
| 16 | 5.8 | 8.7 | 13.1–26.1 |
| 18 | 6.3 | 9.5 | 14.3–28.5 |
| 20 | 6.9 | 10.3 | 15.4–30.9 |
| 25 | 8.1 | 12.2 | 18.2–36.5 |
| 30 | 9.3 | 13.9 | 20.9–41.8 |
| 35 | 10.4 | 15.7 | 23.5–47.0 |
| 40 | 11.5 | 17.3 | 26.0–51.9 |
| 45 | 12.6 | 18.9 | 28.4–56.7 |
| 50 | 13.6 | 20.5 | 30.7–61.4 |
| 60 | 15.6 | 23.5 | 35.2–70.4 |
| 70 | 17.6 | 26.3 | 39.5–79.0 |
| 80 | 19.4 | 29.1 | 43.7–87.3 |
| 90 | 21.2 | 31.8 | 47.7–95.4 |
| 100 | 22.9 | 34.4 | 51.6–103.2 |
| 120 | 26.3 | 39.5 | 59.2–118.4 |
| 140 | 29.5 | 44.3 | 66.4–132.9 |
| 160 | 32.6 | 49.0 | 73.4–146.9 |

Table B.2 Energy requirements of nonpasserine chicks.

| Body Weight (grams) | Basal Metabolic Rate (BMR) | Maintenance Energy Requirement (MER) in kcal/Day | Kilocalories per Day for Growth when Healthy |
|---|---|---|---|
| 30 | 5.6 | 8.4 | 13–25 |
| 40 | 7.0 | 10.5 | 16–31 |
| 50 | 8.2 | 12.4 | 19–37 |
| 60 | 9.5 | 14.2 | 21–43 |
| 70 | 10.6 | 15.9 | 24–48 |
| 80 | 11.7 | 17.6 | 26–53 |
| 90 | 12.8 | 19.2 | 29–58 |
| 100 | 13.9 | 20.8 | 31–62 |
| 120 | 15.9 | 23.9 | 36–72 |
| 140 | 17.9 | 26.8 | 40–80 |
| 160 | 19.7 | 29.6 | 44–89 |
| 180 | 21.6 | 32.3 | 48–97 |
| 200 | 23.3 | 35.0 | 52–105 |
| 225 | 25.5 | 38.2 | 57–115 |
| 250 | 27.6 | 41.4 | 62–124 |
| 275 | 29.6 | 44.4 | 67–133 |
| 300 | 31.6 | 47.4 | 71–142 |
| 350 | 35.5 | 53.2 | 80–160 |
| 400 | 39.2 | 58.8 | 88–177 |
| 450 | 42.9 | 64.3 | 96–193 |
| 500 | 46.4 | 69.6 | 104–209 |
| 600 | 53.2 | 79.8 | 120–239 |
| 700 | 59.7 | 89.5 | 134–269 |
| 800 | 66.0 | 99.0 | 148–297 |
| 900 | 72.1 | 108.1 | 162–324 |
| 1000 | 78.0 | 117.0 | 176–351 |
| 1250 | 92.2 | 138.3 | 207–415 |
| 1500 | 105.7 | 158.6 | 238–476 |
| 1750 | 118.7 | 178.0 | 267–534 |
| 2000 | 131.2 | 196.8 | 295–590 |
| 2500 | 155.1 | 232.6 | 349–698 |
| 3000 | 177.8 | 266.7 | 400–800 |

# Appendix C

## Songbird Washing Instructions

*Veronica Bowers*

Use this procedure to wash songbirds with contaminated feathers.

**Rule #1:** NEVER wash a bird until it is stable. Make sure the bird has been properly warmed, rehydrated, and stabilized before washing.

**Rule #2:** If, at any time during the procedure, the bird becomes too stressed, STOP immediately and put the bird in an incubator to rest.

**Pre-treatment of sticky residues:** Sticky residue from rat traps, fly traps, and insect barriers can be pre-treated by using a syringe to apply small drops of heated methyl soyate or canola oil (102–104 °F/38.9–40 °C) to the affected areas – do not saturate the bird with oil. Allow the oil to sit for about 2 minutes before attempting to remove the residue. After the residue has softened, use the tips of your fingers and fingernails to gently roll the residue off toward the tip of the feather (go with the grain of the feather). Allow the bird to rest in a warm environment before proceeding with washing. See Rule #1.

**When a bird arrives still stuck in a sticky fly or rat trap (Figure C.1):** Sprinkle cornmeal on the exposed part of the trap to prevent further sticking (Figure C.2). Apply small drops of heated canola oil to the areas where the bird is stuck to the trap. Gently remove the bird from the trap as the oil softens the sticky adhesive. See Rule #1.

**Step one:** See Rule #1. Make sure the room is warm (75–78 °F/ 23.9–25.6 °C). Have the following supplies ready: small towels or wash cloths, two washing tubs or containers that will fit the entire bird, a soft child's toothbrush, a 10–20 cc syringe, 5 cc syringe of warm sterile saline, Seventh Generation or Dawn® dish soap, and a clean surface area adjacent to a sink with screened drain. Turn on the incubator to 95 °F/35 °C (or prepare an alternate warming unit that will provide sufficient heat for the bird to maintain body temperature while it preens and feathers dry).

**Step two:** See Rule #1. Prepare washing solution in the two containers. The solution should be 1 teaspoon (5 ml) of soap to 4 cups (946 ml) of water. Make sure water is 103–104 °F (39.4–40 °C). Make sure the water does not exceed that temperature range and that it remains at that temperature throughout the process. Placing a lid on the second tub until it is ready to be used will help maintain the temperature of the water.

**Step three:** Place the bird in the first container. Keep the head above the water. If a small area of the bird is contaminated, only submerge that part of the body. Agitate the washing solution through the feathers using your fingertips. Going with the grain of the feathers, brush the feathers with the soft toothbrush (Figure C.3). You can also draw up soapy water into a 10–20 cc syringe and gently squirt solution into feathers to help remove the contaminant. If you are removing a sticky

*Hand-Rearing Birds*, Second Edition. Edited by Rebecca S. Duerr and Laurie J. Gage.

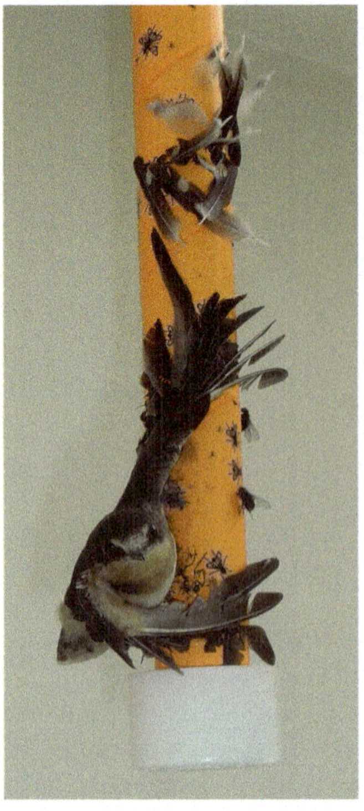

Figure C.1 Barn Swallow caught in a fly trap.

residue, such as insect barrier sticky resins or fly trap glue, feel the area with your fingers for remaining residue and roll the bits of glue off toward the tip of the feathers. Do not get soapy water in the bird's eyes. If this occurs, gently flush the eyes with saline as needed.

Place the bird in the second washing solution and repeat the process. Make sure the water temperature remains at 103–104 °F (39.4–40 °C). Flush the eyes with saline as needed.

**Step four:** Rinse the bird. This can be done by preparing a third container of clean water that is 103–104 °F (39.4–40 °C). Holding the bird over the sink, gently pour the water over the soapy areas until the bird is clean and residue free. Alternatively, if the sink is fitted with a spray nozzle (like a home kitchen sink), turn the water on and allow it to reach 103–104 °F (39.4–40 °C), then using low pressure, rinse the bird over the sink using the spray nozzle. This is the method the author uses and it works very well.

You will know when all of the soap and residue has been successfully rinsed from the feathers when the water beads off the surface of the feathers and down feathers will begin to fluff.

The entire process from wash to rinse should take no more than 10 minutes. If at any time during the process the bird becomes stressed, stop the process immediately. Songbirds are small, so this is usually a one-person job. However, a second person can be helpful to monitor consistent water temperature and observe the patient.

**Step five:** After the bird is rinsed, swaddle it in a towel and blot off excess water. Place the bird in the pre-heated incubator and allow it to rest and dry. This will take 15–20 minutes, depending on the size of the bird and how much of the bird needed to be washed.

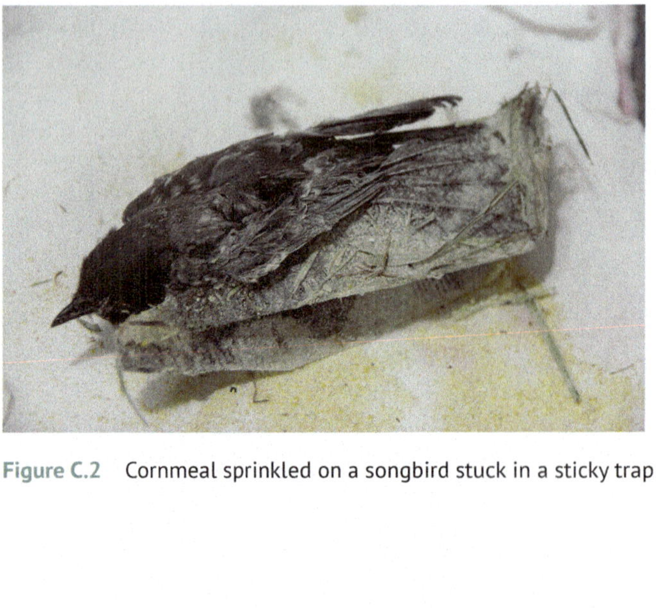

Figure C.2 Cornmeal sprinkled on a songbird stuck in a sticky trap to prevent further sticking.

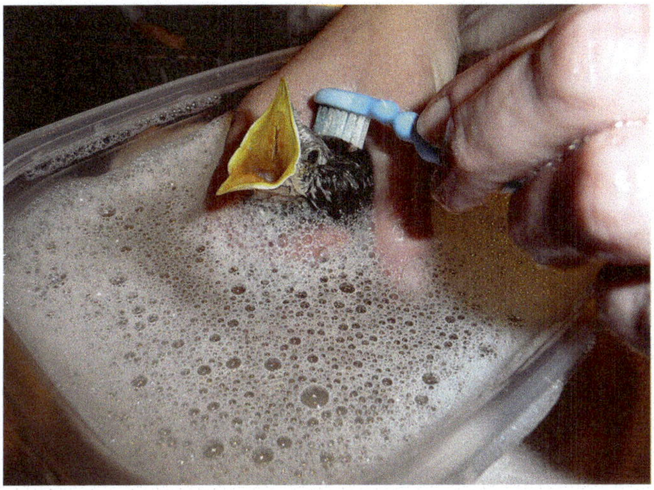

Figure C.3 Songbird chick being washed, note head being kept out of the water while feathers are gently washed with a soft toothbrush.

## Sources of Products Mentioned

Dawn Dish Soap: Procter & Gamble, (800) 725–3296, https://dawn-dish.com/en-us.

Dish Liquid – Free and Clear: Seventh Generation, 60 Lake Street, Burlington, VT 05401, (800) 211–4279, www.seventhgeneration.com.

# Index



*Hand-Rearing Birds*, Second Edition. Edited by Rebecca S. Duerr and Laurie J. Gage.